Contents

*New chapter.

PRINCIPLES & PRACTICE OF

Psychiatric Nursing

PRINCIPLES & PRACTICE OF
Psychiatric Nursing

GAIL WISCARZ STUART, PhD, RN, CS, FAAN

Administrator, Institute of Psychiatry
Professor, College of Nursing
Associate Professor, College of Medicine
Medical University of South Carolina
Charleston, South Carolina

SANDRA J. SUNDEEN, MS, RN, CNAA

Chief, Division of Human Resource Development
Mental Hygiene Administration
Maryland Department of Health and Mental Hygiene;
Adjunct Assistant Professor, School of Nursing
University of Maryland
Baltimore, Maryland

FIFTH EDITION

with 200 illustrations including 12 in color

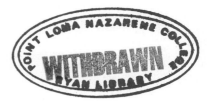

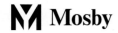 **Mosby**

St. Louis Baltimore Boston Carlsbad Chicago Naples New York Philadelphia Portland
London Madrid Mexico City Singapore Sydney Tokyo Toronto Wiesbaden

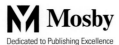

Mosby
Dedicated to Publishing Excellence

**A Times Mirror
Company**

Publisher: Alison Harrison
Managing Editor: Jeff Burnham
Associate Developmental Editor: Linda Caldwell
Project Manager: Patricia Tannian
Senior Production Editor: John P. Casey
Senior Book Designer: Gail Morey Hudson
Cover Designer: Teresa Breckwoldt
Manufacturing Supervisor: Karen Lewis
Cover Art: Photographs by CLG Photographics, Inc.
Illustration by Jeanne Robertson
PET scans from Dr. Lewis Baxter

FIFTH EDITION

Printed in the United States of America
Composition by Clarinda Company
Printing/binding by Von Hoffmann Press, Inc.

Mosby–Year Book, Inc.
11830 Westline Industrial Drive
St. Louis, Missouri 63146

Library of Congress Cataloging in Publication data
Principles and practice of psychiatric nursing / [edited by] Gail
    Wiscarz Stuart, Sandra J. Sundeen. —5th ed.
        p.   cm.
    Includes bibliographical references and index.
    ISBN 0-8016-7878-1
    1.   Psychiatric nursing.   I.   Stuart, Gail Wiscarz,   1949-
II. Sundeen, Sandra J.,   1940-
    [DNLM: 1. Psychiatric Nursing.   WY 160 P957 1995]
RC440.P69   1995
610.73'68—dc20
DNLM/DLC   94-36732
for Library of Congress   CIP

94 95 96 97 98 / 9 8 7 6 5 4 3 2 1

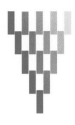

About the Authors

Dr. Gail Stuart is administrator of the Institute of Psychiatry at the Medical University of South Carolina, where she holds joint appointments as a professor in the College of Nursing and an associate professor in the Department of Psychiatry and Behavioral Sciences in the College of Medicine. She received her BSN from Georgetown University, her MS in psychiatric nursing from the University of Maryland, and her PhD in behavioral sciences from Johns Hopkins University, School of Hygiene and Public Health. She has been an American Nurses' Association Certified Specialist in psychiatric and mental health nursing since 1979 and is a Fellow in the American Academy of Nursing.

In her current position Dr. Stuart is responsible for the administration of all clinical services in psychiatry, focusing on interdisciplinary collaboration and new continuum of care initiatives. In addition to these administrative activities, she has over 20 years of experience as an educator and is active in clinical practice and research activities in the Department of Psychiatry. Dr. Stuart serves on national boards and represents nursing on a number of panels including those of the National Institute of Mental Health and the Agency for Health Care Policy and Research. She is frequently invited to speak and consult throughout the country and has written numerous articles that have been published in journals and textbooks. She has received many awards including the American Nurses' Association Distinguished Contribution to Psychiatric Nursing–Current Impact on Innovations in Health Care Delivery Systems and Health Policy Award. Dr. Stuart's clinical and research interests involve the study of depression, anxiety disorders, and mental health delivery systems.

Sandra J. Sundeen is chief of the Division of Human Resource Development and chief psychiatric nurse for the Maryland Mental Hygiene Administration. In this role she is involved in policy development that affects the practice of psychiatric nurses and other mental health professionals. She is also an adjunct assistant professor at the University of Maryland School of Nursing. She received her BSN from the University of Rochester and her MS in psychiatric nursing from the University of Maryland. She has served on advisory committees on nursing practice standards and mental health service delivery and is a member of the Mental Health Association and the National Alliance for the Mentally Ill. In 1993 she received the Psychosocial Nurse of the Year Award from the *Journal of Psychosocial Nursing and Mental Health Services*.

The focus of her practice is on continuing education for mental health service providers, policy development, services for elderly people who are mentally ill, and the rehabilitation of people who have serious and persistent mental illnesses. She is especially interested in becoming involved in partnerships with consumers of mental health services and their families. She speaks, writes, and consults about these areas of interest.

Gail Stuart and Sandra Sundeen have co-authored several nursing textbooks, including *Nurse-Client Interaction: Implementing the Nursing Process*, *The Pocket Nurse Guide to Psychiatric Nursing*, and *Principles and Practice of Psychiatric Nursing*, which has received the Book of the Year Award from the *American Journal of Nursing*.

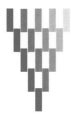

Contributors

BEVERLY A. BALDWIN, PhD, RN, FAAN

Sonya Ziporkin Gershowitz Professor of Gerontological
Nursing
School of Nursing
University of Maryland
Baltimore, Maryland

CAROLE F. BENNETT, MN, RN, CS

Family Outreach Program Chief
Institute of Psychiatry
Medical University of South Carolina
Charleston, South Carolina

SANDRA E. BENTER, DNSc, RN, CS

Psychotherapist and Consultant
Owing Mills, Maryland;
Visiting Assistant Professor
Department of Nursing
Towson State University
Towson, Maryland

CHRISTINE CAHILL HAMOLIA, MS, RN, CS

Adult Specialty Services Manager
Institute of Psychiatry
Medical University of South Carolina
Charleston, South Carolina

JACQUELINE C. CAMPBELL, PhD, RN, FAAN

The Anna D. Wolf Endowed Professor
School of Nursing
Johns Hopkins University
Baltimore, Maryland

CAROLYN E. COCHRANE, PhD, RN, CS

Associate Program Chief, Eating Disorders Program
Assistant Professor, College of Medicine
Department of Psychiatry and Behavioral Sciences
and College of Nursing
Medical University of South Carolina
Charleston, South Carolina

SUZANNE DOYLE FRIEDMAN, MS, RN, CS-P

Project Coordinator
Geriatric Mental Health Designated Bed Project
University of Maryland School of Nursing
Maryland Mental Health Hygiene Administration
Baltimore, Maryland

PATRICIA E. HELM, MSN, RN, CS

West Haven, Veterans Administration Medical Center
West Haven, Connecticut

LINDA V. JEFFERSON, PhD, RN, CS, CD

Research Manager
National Institute of Drug Abuse
Baltimore, Maryland

MICHELE T. LARAIA, MSN, RN

Assistant Professor, College of Medicine
Department of Psychiatry and Behavioral Sciences
and College of Nursing
Medical University of South Carolina
Charleston, South Carolina

ARTHUR J. LaSALLE, EdD, CCMHc

Psychotherapist, Consultant, Trainer
LaSalle Associates
Ellicott City, Maryland

PAULA CHELES LaSALLE, MS, RN, CS-P

Psychotherapist, Consultant, Trainer
LaSalle Associates
Ellicott City, Maryland

FRANCES G. LEHMANN, MSN, RN, CS

Group Manager, Field Operations
Joint Commission on Accreditation of Healthcare
Organizations
Oak Brook Terrace, Illinois

MARY D. MOLLER, MSN, ARNP, CS

Executive Director
The Center for Patient and Family
Mental Health Education
Nine Mile Falls, Washington

MILLENE FREEMAN MURPHY, PhD, APRN

Associate Professor
College of Nursing
Brigham Young University
Provo, Utah

LINDA D. OAKLEY, PhD, RN

Assistant Professor, School of Nursing
University of Wisconsin–Madison;
Clinical Specialist in Adult Psychiatric and Mental Health
Nursing
Madison, Wisconsin

BARBARA PARKER, PhD, RN, FAAN

Professor, School of Nursing
University of Virginia
Charlottesville, Virginia

CAROL K. PERLIN, MS, RN, CS-P

Associate Director of Nursing
Sheppard Pratt Health Systems
Towson, Maryland

SUSAN G. POORMAN, PhD, RN, CS

Associate Professor, School of Nursing
University of Pittsburgh
Psychotherapist and Consultant
Pittsburgh, Pennsylvania

VICTORIA A. QUEEN, MSN, RN, CNA

Administrative Nurse Manager
Institute of Psychiatry
Medical University of South Carolina
Charleston, South Carolina

AUDREY REDSTON-ISELIN, MA, RN, CS

Clinical Specialist, Children's Services
Soundview Throgs Neck Community Mental Health Center
Bronx, New York

GEORGIA L. STEVENS, PhD, RN, CS

Psychotherapist and Consultant
Adjunct Assistant Professor, School of Nursing
The Catholic University of America
Washington, DC

NANCY K. WORLEY, PhD, RN

Associate Professor, College of Nursing
Medical University of South Carolina
Charleston, South Carolina

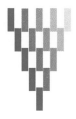

Reviewers

CAROLE-JEAN ADKISSON, MSN, RN

Assistant Professor, School of Nursing
Tennessee Technological University
Cookeville, Tennessee

JOYCE ADRIANCE, MSN, RN

Instructor, Department of Health Occupations
Napa Valley College
Napa, California

CLAUDETTE BACHAND, BSN, MSN, RN

Professor of Nursing
Bristol Community College
Fall River, Massachusetts

LINDA K. BLAZER, MEd, MS, RN

Instructor of Psychiatric/Mental Health Nursing
Lancaster General Hospital School of Nursing
Lancaster, Pennsylvania

MARJORIE CHILDERS, PhD, RN, C

Associate Professor of Nursing
College of Our Lady of the Elms
Chicopee, Massachusetts

VICTORIA CONN, MN, MA, RN

Chair, Curriculum and Training
National Alliance for the Mentally Ill
Newtown Square, Pennsylvania

PATRICIA DARDIS, MS, RN, CS, NP

Assistant Professor, School of Nursing
University of North Dakota
Jamestown, North Dakota

DONNA DARTY, BSN, MSN

Professor of Nursing
Jefferson State Community College
Birmingham, Alabama

MARY B. DAVIES, RN

Psychiatric Nurse/Case Manager
The Travelers
Waltham, Massachusetts

TOBIE DAY, BSN, MSN, RN

Instructor of Psychiatric Nursing
Department of Nursing
Bishop State Community College
Mobile, Alabama

PATRICIA DEAN, BSN, MSN, RN

Associate Professor, School of Nursing
Florida State University
Tallahassee, Florida

MARY ALICE DEDINSKY, MSN, PhD, RN, NCC

Nurse Educator
Milwaukee Area Technical College
Milwaukee, Wisconsin

JO ELBERG, RN, C, MAE

Nursing Instructor
Iowa Central Community College
Fort Dodge, Iowa

GINGER W. EVANS, MS, MSN, RN

Assistant Professor
University of Tennessee at Knoxville
Knoxville, Tennessee

ELLEN FISH-KINGSBURY, MS, RN

Associate Professor, Department of Nursing
Bunker Hill Community College
Charlestown, Massachusetts

ARLENE FREDERICK, BSN, MSN, EdD, MBA

President, Professional Health Education Consultants
Adjunct Faculty
Midlands Technical College
Columbia, South Carolina

ELAINE GALLIEN, MSN, RN, CS

Assistant Professor, Capstone College of Nursing
University of Alabama
Tuscaloosa, Alabama

RAUDA GELAZIS, RN, MNEd, PhDc

Associate Professor, Department of Nursing
Ursuline College
Pepper Pike, Ohio

JOYCE ROBERSON, PhD, RN

Level Coordinator, College of Nursing
University of Iowa
Iowa City, Iowa

MARY J. ROEHRIG, MSN, MA, LPC, RN

Associate Professor
Ferris State University
Private Practice
Big Rapids, Michigan

ELIZABETH ROMA, MS, RN

Professor of Nursing
North Shore Community College
Danvers, Massachusetts

BETTY ROSS, PhD, RN, CS

Assistant Professor, Department of Nursing
Fairleigh Dickinson University
Teaneck, New Jersey

CYNTHIA A. RUSSELL, DNSc, RN

Associate Professor, College of Nursing
Valparaiso University
Valparaiso, Indiana

PAMELA A. SCHROEDER, MEd, MS, RN

Former Associate Professor
South Dakota State University
Brookings, South Dakota

MARCY J.T. SMITH, MSN, RN

Professor, Department of Nursing
Cape Cod Community College
W. Barnstable, Massachusetts

SUSAN SPERAW, PhD, RN

Clinical Psychologist, Department of Behavioral Pediatrics
T.C. Thompson Children's Hospital;
Assistant Professor of Pediatrics, College of Medicine
University of Tennessee at Chattanooga
Chattanooga, Tennessee

STEPHANIE STOCKARD-SPELIC, MSN, CPC, RN, CS

Assistant Professor, Psychiatric–Mental Health Nursing
School of Nursing
Creighton University
Omaha, Nebraska

ELEANOR J. SULLIVAN, PhD, RN, FAAN

Dean and Professor, School of Nursing
University of Kansas
Kansas City, Kansas

ANITA THROWE, MS, RN, CS

Associate Professor, College of Nursing
Medical University of South Carolina
Florence, South Carolina

ANNA TICHY, PhD, RN

Professor, College of Nursing
University of Illinois–Chicago
Chicago, Illinois

MARGARET TRIMPEY, MSN, RN, C

Associate Professor, School of Nursing
University of Tennessee at Chattanooga
Chattanooga, Tennessee

JEAN WOLD, MSN, RN

Professor, Department of Nursing
California State University–Chico
Chico, California

LEE ANNE XIPPOLITOS, MS, CARN, RN, CS

Clinical Assistant Professor, School of Nursing
State University of New York at Stony Brook
Stony Brook, New York

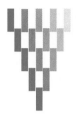

Preface

FOCUS AND APPROACH

It is with great excitement that we welcome you, both student and instructor, as our traveling partners to the fifth edition of this text. Since the first edition was published in 1979, enormous changes have occurred in mental health care and psychiatric treatment. These changes have been reflected in all aspects of psychiatric nursing practice and continue even as you read this preface. Health care is being propelled to assume the full spectrum of health promotion, illness management, and rehabilitative activities. Treatment settings have similarly become as diverse as the individuals who receive care. Perhaps most important, in the current era of health-care reform nurses are being asked to assume new and creative leadership roles that reflect their contributions to the care they provide individuals and families, as well as their skill in organizing and integrating health-care delivery systems. To face the challenges that lie ahead, psychiatric nurses need a text that will map out and guide the way in the uncharted territory of the art and science of contemporary psychiatric nursing. To that end we offer this fifth edition.

Innovative, progressive, evolving—these terms describe this new edition. To many of you, our colleagues and explorers in this brave new world, this will look like a completely new textbook. In some ways it is, since it has been totally reorganized and realigned with current and expanding knowledge in the field. For example, this edition contains eight entirely new chapters. Yet in other ways the text retains and builds on the strengths of earlier editions. Thus we continue the fundamental framework of psychiatric nursing principles and apply them in clinical practice. We have expanded and refined the original model of nursing practice to a stress adaptation model of human responses that now includes the full continuum of psychiatric nursing care. It remains the conceptual foundation of the book and reflects the theoretical basis for practice, treatment stages, and the evaluation component of nursing care.

We also recognize the growing importance of nursing practice based on sound and current research. Such practice must more fully reflect the holistic merging of the biopsychosocial aspects of care based on the most current findings in the field. This is reflected in the references and annotated suggested readings in each chapter of this edition. Nursing practice must also value the active participation of the patient and family, as evidenced by the special new feature of A Patient Speaks and A Family Speaks, which share treatment considerations from the consumer's point of view.

The 1990s have been called the "Decade of the Brain." In recognition of the importance of biology in psychiatric care, a new chapter is devoted solely to psychobiology with clinical implications identified for each disorder discussed. Included in this chapter is an eight-page full-color insert that visually depicts important psychobiological concepts. In addition, biology is integrated throughout each clinical disorder chapter, and the latest guidelines are presented for psychopharmacology.

Finally, the 1993 American Nurses' Association Standards of Psychiatric and Mental Health Clinical Nursing Practice are used throughout this edition, along with the 1994 DSM-IV medical diagnostic classifications and the most current NANDA nursing diagnoses. Thus the reader will truly be learning the dynamic future rather than the static past principles and practice of psychiatric nursing.

STRUCTURE AND ORGANIZATION

One of our primary goals for this new edition is to present the most up to date and comprehensive psychiatric nursing content in an open, accessible, clear, and concise way. It is our belief that people learn visually, and therefore we include over 200 illustrations and an eight-page full-color insert, which is the first of its kind in a psychiatric nursing text.

The book is divided into six units. Unit One presents psychiatric nursing principles that are fundamental to practice. First, the contemporary psychiatric nurse's roles and functions are addressed followed by a chapter on therapeutic relationship skills. A stress adaptation model of psychiatric nursing care is then presented along with separate chapters devoted to the biological, psychological, sociocultural, and legal contexts of practice. Finally, separate chapters in this unit focus on ANA professional practice and performance standards. The biological, psychological, and sociocultural contexts of psychiatric nursing and the ANA standards make up the five new chapters in this unit.

Unit Two addresses the continuum of care, including primary mental health prevention, crisis intervention, and psychiatric rehabilitation. These topics, unique in this textbook, are more important than ever, since health-care reform focuses on nontraditional settings and a wide range of treatment strategies.

Unit Three applies psychiatric nursing principles to specific clinical disorders, based on a continuum of adaptive-maladaptive coping responses, the six-step nursing process, and DSM-IV and NANDA diagnoses. There are separate chapters on anxiety, somatoform and sleep, dissociative, mood, psychotic, personality, substance use, eating, and sexual disorders, as well as suicidal behavior. The information in this unit has been reorganized to conform more closely to the DSM-IV classification. As a result there are now separate chapters on schizophrenia, eating disorders, and personality disorders. The substance-related disorders chapter has been extensively revised to reflect current thinking and practice in this important area.

Unit Four describes various modalities of psychiatric treatment, including a revision of the well-received chapter on psychopharmacology, and completely new chapters on somatic therapies, cognitive behavioral therapy, and managing aggressive behavior. Each of these areas is of emerging importance in the field, and together they join with chapters on therapeutic groups and family interventions to round out the repertoire of psychiatric nursing practice.

Unit Five begins with new chapters on inpatient and community-based psychiatric nursing care that reflect the most recent developments and current practice in these settings. Also included is a chapter on consultation liaison nursing, since health-care reform promises to emphasize the psychiatric nurse's abilities to collaborate, advise, and manage others in a rapidly changing health-care environment.

Unit Six concludes the text with a discussion of the unique issues and concerns in the psychiatric treatment of special populations including a completely rewritten chapter on children, revised chapters on adolescents, the elderly, and survivors of abuse and violence, and a new chapter about patients with HIV/AIDS.

SPECIAL FEATURES

We hope by now your appetite has been stimulated and you are ready to embark with us on this fascinating journey through the art and science of psychiatric nursing. On the way, look for other signposts and special features we have included in this edition to illuminate your journey. These include a dynamic, two-color design and considerably more boxes, tables, and figures than in previous editions. Many of the special features listed below have been highlighted by a special design or logo to enhance the teaching-learning process.

Clinical Examples, highlighted in second color, are taken from actual clinical situations. Many of them provide samples of nursing diagnoses related to the particular clinical situation.

Critical Thinking questions, interspersed throughout the narrative of each chapter, challenge students and promote independent clinical reasoning. At the same time they add interest to the textual information and encourage students to integrate the material with their own understanding of the world and nursing.

Case Studies are in-depth examples of clinical scenarios that discuss each step of the nursing process, providing students with realistic application of the nursing process in practice.

Competent Caring: A Clinical Exemplar of a Psychiatric Nurse is found at the end of the chapters in Units Two through Six. In this feature a practicing psychiatric nurse shares clinical experiences and insights related to the chapter topic.

Critical Thinking about Contemporary Issues. Every chapter presents a discussion of a current, controversial issue related to the chapter's topic and analyzed from current research findings in the field.

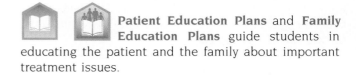 **A Patient Speaks** and **A Family Speaks** present relevant treatment issues from a patient's and family's point of view, giving students a better understanding of the patient's and family's perspective of the caregiving process.

Patient Education Plans and **Family Education Plans** guide students in educating the patient and the family about important treatment issues.

Nursing Care Plan Summaries present care plans based on the major disorders discussed in the book. The care plans include nursing diagnoses, expected outcomes, short-term goals, interventions, and rationales and serve as a guide for students in the nursing care related to the treatment of major disorders.

Medical and Nursing Diagnoses boxes present the DSM-IV and NANDA diagnoses applicable for a specific disorder to assist the student in understanding the relevance of complementary diagnoses in nursing care.

Detailed Diagnoses boxes present expanded examples of NANDA diagnoses applicable for a specific disorder and describe the essential features of related DSM-IV diagnoses.

The six steps of the **nursing process** are highlighted by individual symbols as they are discussed in the disorders chapters:

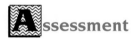 **A**ssessment

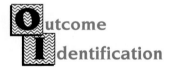 **N**ursing

Diagnosis

Outcome

Identification

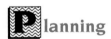 **P**lanning

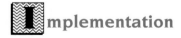 **I**mplementation

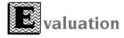 **E**valuation

Therapeutic Dialogues provide samples of appropriate verbal therapeutic interactions with patients to educate students about therapeutic communication skills.

Tables and boxes that discuss specific **pharmacology** information emphasize its importance in the treatment of psychiatric illnesses.

Perforated cards at the back of the book are useful learning tools and easy to use in the clinical setting. These cards detail nursing diagnoses and nursing interventions.

Learning objectives and a **topical outline** at the beginning of each chapter inform students of the basic concepts and organization of the chapter, and a chapter **summary** summarizes key points at the end of each chapter to help students grasp important concepts.

Annotated suggested readings at the end of each chapter refer students to other important and relevant sources of information for further in-depth study.

Key terms are highlighted in second color, and many are included in the **glossary** at the back of the book.

TEACHING AND LEARNING PACKAGE
Instructor's Resource Manual and Test Bank

The *Instructor's Resource Manual and Test Bank to Accompany Principles and Practice of Psychiatric Nursing* is designed to help you, the instructor, develop lectures, reinforce teaching through classroom and clinical activities, and evaluate student comprehension. This valuable resource manual follows the textbook chapter by chapter and includes learning objectives, critical thinking questions, future research boxes, learning resources, and a chapter glossary. Adapted outlines for courses of variable durations, student worksheets, and transparency masters are also featured. A *Test Bank* containing more than 800 test items in the NCLEX format has also been provided and includes an answer key with correlating page numbers as well as the applicable nursing process step and cognitive level of each question.

Transparencies

Mosby's Psychiatric Nursing Transparency Acetates provides 50 two-color transparencies that cover a variety of topics in psychiatric nursing, helping to increase understanding through visual learning aids.

Quick Psychopharmacology Reference

The second edition of this handy, pocket-sized reference accompanies every copy of the text. This guide focuses on key psychopharmacology information needed in the clinical area. Information is presented concisely in numerous boxes and tables, and a new drug index facilitates locating medication names. This reference will be very useful in clinical situations.

Computest 3

Available in IBM 3.5″ and Macintosh, Computest is the computerized version of the *Test Bank* from the *Instructor's Resource Manual*. Complete with an instruction guide, Computest allows users to edit, add, delete, or select questions on the computer.

Finally, we wish to communicate our respect for individuals and the roles they enact regardless of gender. To that end, we have attempted to avoid pronouns that express bias and to give recognition and support for the commitment of both men and women to the nursing profession. However, this sometimes creates difficult and tedious language for the reader. Therefore, for clarity and simplicity, the nurse is referred to in the third person, female gender, and the patient in the third person, masculine gender when necessary. It should also be noted that Ms. is used instead of Miss or Mrs. in examples in the text.

This completes your introduction to the journey before you. We invite you now to open the pages beneath your fingers and join us in a world of new ideas, challenging beliefs, and expanding competencies. We wish you well and look forward to meeting you in the empowering universe of psychiatric nursing practice.

Gail Wiscarz Stuart
Sandra J. Sundeen

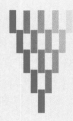

Contents in Brief

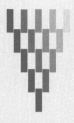

Contents

UNIT THREE

APPLYING PRINCIPLES IN NURSING PRACTICE

COLOR PLATES

PRINCIPLES & PRACTICE OF
Psychiatric Nursing

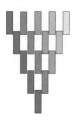

Principles of Psychiatric Nursing Care

Sit back and relax. You are about to begin a voyage to places and spaces you have never been before—the world of psychiatric and mental health nursing practice. In the olden days of nursing, students learned about pieces of people—an infected toe, a congested lung, a troubling twitch, or maybe even a broken heart— but pieces nonetheless. Today, students learn about the wholeness of people— a physically ill child struggling for safety in an abusive family, an adolescent coping with eating problems and self-concept issues, a young adult grieving over the diagnosis of HIV/AIDS, or an elder confused and disoriented at times of the day but frightened at the thought of going to a nursing home. This is the exciting world of contemporary psychiatric nursing. It is a world that integrates the biological, psychological, and sociocultural realities of life and weaves them together in a rich tapestry called psychiatric nursing practice.

This unit introduces you to parts of this world that may be new to you. It will help you explore how patients think, feel, and behave. It will assist you in learning how to talk with patients and families as partners and collaborators in the caregiving process. It will suggest that you think about people in terms of their overall functioning and adaptation rather than in relation to the symptoms of their specific illness. And, most important, it will define for you the responsibilities and obligations you have as a professional health-care provider who cares for and about the biological, psychological, and sociocultural problems of people. We hope you are ready to begin your journey, and we wish you curiosity about human nature, openness to new ways of thinking, and delight in the process of learning.

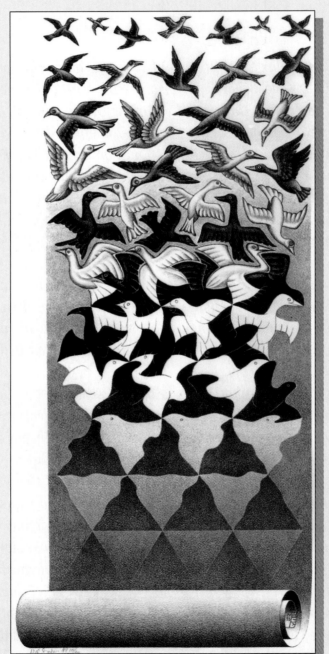

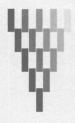

CHAPTER 1

Roles and Functions of Psychiatric Nurses: Competent Caring

GAIL W. STUART

And what they dare to dream of, dare to do.

James Russell Lowell

LEARNING OBJECTIVES

After studying this chapter the student should be able to:

▼ Describe the evolution of the psychiatric nursing role and functions

▼ Discuss the nature, scope, and setting of contemporary psychiatric nursing practice

▼ Analyze the factors that influence the psychiatric nurse's level of performance

▼ Critique areas of importance for psychiatric nursing's future agenda

The function of nursing or caring for the sick has existed since the beginning of civilization. Before 1860 the emphasis in psychiatric institutions was on custodial care, and attendants were prepared to maintain control of the patients. Frequently these attendants were little more than jailers or cellkeepers with very little training, and psychiatric care was poor. Nursing, as a profession, began to emerge in the late nineteenth century, and by the twentieth century it had evolved into a specialty with unique roles and functions.

HISTORICAL PERSPECTIVES

In 1873 Linda Richards graduated from the New England Hospital for Women and Children in Boston. She developed better nursing care in psychiatric hospitals and organized nursing services and educational programs in state mental hospitals in Illinois. For these activities she is called the first American psychiatric nurse. Basic to Richards' theory of care was her premise: "It stands to reason that the mentally sick should be at least as well cared for as the physically sick."[9]

The first school to prepare nurses to care for the mentally ill opened at McLean Hospital in Waverly, Massachusetts, in 1882. It was a 2-year program, but few psychological skills were addressed; the care was mainly custodial. Nurses took care of the patient's physical needs, such as medications, nutrition, hygiene, and ward activities. Until the end of the nineteenth century little changed in the role of psychiatric nurses. They had limited special training in psychiatry, and they primarily adapted the principles of medical-surgical nursing to the psychiatric setting. At that time psychological care consisted of kindness and tolerance toward the patients.

One of Linda Richards' more important contributions was her emphasis on assessing both the physical and emotional needs of the patients. In this early period of nursing history, nursing education separated these two needs; nurses were taught either in the general hospital or in the psychiatric hospital. In 1913 Johns Hopkins became the first school of nursing to include a fully developed course for psychiatric nursing in the curriculum. Other schools soon began to do likewise. It was not until the late 1930s that nursing education recognized the importance of psychiatric knowledge in general nursing care for all illnesses (Box 1-1).

An important factor in the development of psychiatric nursing was the emergence of various somatic therapies, including insulin shock therapy (1935), psychosurgery (1936), and electroconvulsive therapy (1937). These techniques all required the medical-surgical skills of nurses. Although these therapies did not foster the patient's insight, they did control behavior and make the patient more amenable to psychotherapy. Somatic therapies also increased the demand for improved psychological treatment for patients who did not respond.

As nurses became more involved with somatic therapies, they began the struggle to define their role as psychiatric nurses. An editorial in the *American Journal of Nursing*[10] in 1940 described the conflict between nurses and physicians as nurses tried to implement what they saw as appropriate care for psychiatric patients. This conflict continues to demand attention in current nursing practice (Box 1-2).

The period after World War II was one of major growth and change in psychiatric nursing. Because of the large number of service-related psychiatric problems and the increase in treatment programs offered by the Veterans Administration, psychiatric nurses with advanced preparation were in demand. The content of psychiatric nursing had now become an integral part of the generic nursing curriculum; its principles were applied to other areas of nursing practice, including general medical, pediatric, and public health nursing. By 1947 eight graduate programs in psychiatric nursing had been started.

Role Emergence

The role of psychiatric nursing began to emerge during this developmental period in the early 1950s. In 1947 Weiss[37] published an article in the *American Journal of Nursing* that reemphasized the shortage of psychiatric nurses and outlined the differences between psychiatric and general duty nurses. She described "attitude therapy" as the nurse's directed use of attitudes that contribute to the patient's recovery. In implementing this therapy the nurse observes the patient for small and fleeting changes, demonstrates acceptance, respect, and understanding of the patient, and promotes the patient's interest and participation in reality. More independent functions were described by Santos and Stainbrook[32] in 1949. They believed that nurses should perform "psychotherapeutic tasks" and should understand concepts related to therapy, such as transference.

An article by Bennett and Eaton[4] in the *American Journal of Psychiatry* in 1951 identified the following three problems affecting psychiatric nurses:

1. The scarcity of qualified psychiatric nurses
2. The underutilization of their abilities
3. The fact that "very little real psychiatric nursing is carried out in otherwise good psychiatric hospitals and units"

Box 1-1

A NURSE SPEAKS

We do not hesitate to emphasize the need of some psychiatric training in the life of every nurse who would represent her profession on the basis of modern standards. The psychiatrically trained nurse must remember, on the other hand, that all symptoms are not of mental origin. This fact has been long recognized, so nurses trained in mental hospitals have wisely requested affiliation in general hospitals, thus avoiding the danger of overspecialization. Does it not seem rational, therefore, that the general hospital shall guarantee its nurse an equivalent knowledge of the workings of the patient's mind as the psychiatric nurse has of the workings of his body? Modern psychology reveals the close interrelation of the two; it recognizes the ceaseless interaction of one on the other. Should we not then more consistently work toward the ideal that every hospital shall graduate nurses trained in preventive and curative methods of caring for the inevitably associated physically and mentally ill?

Annie L. Crawford, RN, BS
South Carolina Nurses' Association
Annual Convention Presentation
October 6, 1934

Box 1-2
A PHYSICIAN SPEAKS

I have spent all of my professional career in close association with, and close dependency on, nurses, and like many of my faculty colleagues, I've done a lot of worrying about the relationship between medicine and nursing.

The doctors worry that nurses are trying to move away from their historical responsibilities to medicine (meaning, really, to the doctors' orders). The nurses assert that they are their own profession, responsible for their own standards, coequal colleagues with physicians, and they do not wish to become mere ward administrators or technicians

My discovery as a patient is that the institution is held together, *glued* together, enabled to function as an organism, by the nurses and by nobody else.

The nurses make it their business to know everything that is going on. They spot errors before errors can be launched. They know everything written on the chart. Most important of all, they know their patients as unique human beings, and they soon get to know the close relatives and friends. Because of this knowledge, they are quick to sense apprehensions and act on them. The average sick person in a large hospital feels at risk of getting lost, with no identity left beyond a name and a string of numbers on a plastic wristband, in danger always of being whisked off on a litter to the wrong place to have the wrong procedure done, or worse still, *not* being whisked off at the right time. The attending physician or the house officer, on rounds and usually in a hurry, can murmur a few reassuring words on his way out the door, but it takes a confident, competent, and cheerful nurse, there all day long and in and out of the room on one chore or another through the night, to bolster one's confidence that the situation is indeed manageable and not about to get out of hand.

Knowing what I know, I am all for the nurses. If they are to continue their professional feud with the doctors, if they want their professional status enhanced and their pay increased, if they infuriate the doctors by their claims to be equal professionals, if they ask for the moon, I am on their side.

Lewis Thomas, MD
The Youngest Science
New York, 1983, Viking Press

---

role of the psychiatric nurse in psychotherapy, all nurses in psychiatric wards do psychotherapy of one kind or another by their contacts with patients."[5] Many of the issues raised in the article would be debated years later.

Do you think that the problems affecting psychiatric nurses described by Bennet and Eaton in 1951 continue to exist in the specialty today?

Also in 1951 Mellow[24] wrote of the work she did with schizophrenic patients. She called these activities "nursing therapy." A year later, Tudor[35] published a study in which she described the nurse-patient relationships she established, which were characterized by unconditional care, few demands, and the anticipation of her patients' needs. These articles by Mellow and Tudor were some of the earliest descriptions by psychiatric nurses of the nurse-patient relationship and the nature of its therapeutic process.

As nurses engaged in these kinds of activities, many questions arose. Are these activities therapeutic or are they therapy? What is a therapeutic relationship or a one-to-one nurse-patient relationship? How does it differ from psychotherapy? These questions were addressed by Dr. Hildegard Peplau, a dynamic nursing leader whose ideas and beliefs shaped psychiatric nursing.

In 1952 Peplau[28] published a book, *Interpersonal Relations in Nursing*, in which she described the skills, activities, and role of psychiatric nurses. It was the first systematic, theoretical framework developed for psychiatric nursing. Peplau defined nursing as a "significant, therapeutic process." She believed that the nurse-patient relationship was characterized by four overlapping and interlocking phases—orientation, identification, exploitation, and resolution. As she studied the nursing process in nurse-patient situations, she saw nurses emerge in various roles: as a resource person, teacher, leader in local, national, and international situations, surrogate parent, and counselor. She wrote, "Counseling in nursing has to do with helping the patient remember and to understand fully what is happening to him in the present situation, so that the experience can be integrated with rather than dissociated from other experiences in life."[28]

These psychiatrists believed that the psychiatric nurse should join mental health societies, consult with welfare agencies, work in outpatient clinics, practice preventive psychiatry, engage in research, and help educate the public. They supported the nurse's participation in individual and group psychotherapy and stated, "Despite the fact that most psychiatrists seem to ignore the

Compare the roles of psychiatric nurses identified by Hildegard Peplau in 1952 with your observations of contemporary psychiatric nursing practice.

Finally, two significant developments in psychiatry in the 1950s also affected nursing's role for years to come. The first was Jones' publication of *The Therapeutic Community: A New Treatment Method in Psychiatry*[15] in 1953. It encouraged using the patient's social environment to provide a therapeutic experience. The patient was to be an active participant in care and become involved in the daily problems of the community. All patients were to help solve problems, plan activities, and develop the necessary rules and regulations. Therapeutic communities became the preferred environment for psychiatric patients.

The second significant development in psychiatry in the early 1950s was the use of psychotropic drugs. With these drugs more patients became treatable, and fewer environmental constraints such as locked doors and straightjackets were required. Also more personnel were needed to provide therapy, and the roles of various psychiatric practitioners were expanded, including the nurse's role.

Evolving Functions

In 1958 the following functions of psychiatric nurses were described[12]:
▼ Dealing with patients' problems of attitude, mood, and interpretation of reality
▼ Exploring disturbing and conflicting thoughts and feelings
▼ Using the patient's positive feelings toward the therapist to bring about psychophysiological homeostasis
▼ Counseling patients in emergencies, including panic and fear
▼ Strengthening the well part of patients
The nurse-patient relationship was referred to by a variety of terms, including "therapeutic nurse-patient relationship," "psychiatric nursing therapy," "supportive psychotherapy," "rehabilitation therapies," and "nondirective counseling." The distinction between these terms and the exact nature of the nurse's role remained hazy.

Once again Peplau[29] clarified psychiatric nursing's position and directed its future growth. In "Interpersonal Techniques: The Crux of Psychiatric Nursing," published in 1962, she identified the heart of psychiatric nursing as the role of counselor or psychotherapist. Other functions such as mother surrogate, technician, manager, socializing agent, and health teacher were seen as subroles. In her article Peplau differentiated between (1) general practitioners who were staff nurses working on psychiatric units, and (2) psychiatric nurses who were specialists and expert clinical practitioners with graduate degrees in psychiatric nursing. Thus, from an undefined role involving primarily physical care, psychiatric

nursing was evolving into a role of clinical competence based on interpersonal techniques and use of the nursing process.

In the 1960s the focus of psychiatric nursing began to shift to primary prevention and implementing care and consultation in the community. Representative of these changes was the shift in the name of the field from "psychiatric" nursing to "psychiatric and mental health" nursing. This focus was stimulated by the Community Mental Health Centers Act of 1963, which made federal money available to states to plan, construct, and staff community mental health centers. This legislation was prompted by growing awareness of the value of treating people in the community and of preventing hospitalization whenever possible. It also encouraged the formation of multidisciplinary treatment teams by joining the skills and expertise of many professions to alleviate illness and promote mental health. This team approach continues to be negotiated. The issues of territoriality, professionalism, authority structure, consumer rights, and the use of paraprofessionals are still being debated.

The 1970s gave rise to the further development of the specialty. Psychiatric nurses became the pacesetters in specialty nursing practice. They were the first to:
▼ Develop a structure within the American Nurses' Association to focus on specialty practice
▼ Develop statements on scope of practice
▼ Establish generalist and specialist certification
The specialty was defined within a nursing framework of practice, and psychiatric nursing textbooks shifted away from the medical model and were organized around the nursing process, nursing diagnoses, and standards of psychiatric nursing practice.

At this same time, nursing, as a profession, was defining caring as a core element of all nursing practice, and the contributions of psychiatric nurses were embraced by nurses of all specialty groups. Partly as a result of this broader definition of psychiatric nursing practice and the perceived skills and competencies of psychiatric nurses, nursing education reorganized its approach to psychiatric nursing curriculum and began to integrate psychiatric nursing content into nonpsychiatric courses. This blending of content was evident in the second change in the name of the field in the 1970s from "psychiatric and mental health" nursing to "psychosocial" nursing. The integration of psychiatric nursing content into basic courses became so complete that faculty no longer viewed these areas as psychiatric nursing but saw them as an expanded, more holistic approach to nursing care. At the same time, clinical rotations focusing on the psychiatric illnesses of patients in psychiatric settings were often replaced by clinical rotations integrating psychosocial aspects of the care of physically ill patients on general medical-surgical units. Unfortunately, this trend often did not

EVOLUTIONARY TIMELINE IN PSYCHIATRIC NURSING

SOCIAL ENVIRONMENT

		PSYCHIATRIC NURSING
	1873	Linda Richards graduated from New England Hospital for Women and Children
	1882	First school to prepare nurses to care for the mentally ill opened at McLean Hospital in Massachusetts
American Journal of Nursing first published	1900	
Clifford Beer's book, A Mind That Found Itself, published	1908	
Florence Nightingale died	1910	
	1913	Johns Hopkins was first school of nursing to include a course on psychiatric nursing in its curriculum
Electroconvulsive therapy developed	1937	
National Mental Health Act passed by Congress, creating National Institute of Mental Health (NIMH) and providing training funds for psychiatric nursing education	1946	
	1950	National League for Nursing (NLN) required that to be accredited schools of nursing must provide an experience in psychiatric nursing
	1952	Hildegard Peplau published Interpersonal Relations in Nursing
Maxwell Jones published The Therapeutic Community	1953	
Development of major tranquilizers	1954	
Community Mental Health Centers Act passed	1963	Perspectives in Psychiatric Care published; Journal of Psychiatric Nursing and Mental Health Services published
	1973	Standards of Psychiatric–Mental Health Nursing Practice published; certification of psychiatric mental health nurse generalists established by the American Nurses' Association (ANA)
Report of the President's Commission on Mental Health	1978	
	1979	Issues in Mental Health Nursing published; certification of psychiatric mental health nurse specialists established by the ANA
Mental Health Systems Act passed	1980	Nursing: A Social Policy Statement published by the ANA
Mental Health Systems Act repealed	1981	
National Center for Nursing Research created in National Institute of Health (NIH)	1985	Standards of Child and Adolescent Psychiatric and Mental Health Nursing Practice published by the ANA
National Institute of Mental Health (NIMH) Task Force on Nursing created	1987	Archives of Psychiatric Nursing published; Journal of Child and Adolescent Psychiatric and Mental Health Nursing published
	1988	Coalition of Psychiatric Nursing Organizations (COPNO) established
	1990	Standards of Psychiatric Consultation Liaison Nursing Practice published by the ANA
Center for Mental Health Services created	1992	
	1994	Revised Standards of Psychiatric–Mental Health Clinical Nursing Practice published by the ANA
	1994	Psychopharmacology Guidelines for Psychiatric–Mental Health Nurses published by the ANA

provide students with an opportunity to also learn about new information that was emerging in the field of psychiatry and the broader behavioral sciences.

The 1980s were years of exciting scientific advances in the area of psychobiology. Advancements occurred in five basic areas:

▼ Brain imaging techniques
▼ Neurotransmitters and neuronal receptors
▼ Psychobiology of emotions
▼ Understanding the brain
▼ Molecular genetics related to psychobiology

While this information explosion advanced knowledge in the field, it lacked integration and was often of limited clinical usefulness. It has also been observed that psychiatric nurses in the 1980s were slow to make the paradigm shift away from primarily psychodynamic models of the mind to more balanced psychobiological models of psychiatric care.[1,3,17,21]

Psychiatric nurses thus entered the decade of the 1990s faced with the challenge of integrating the expanding bases of neuroscience into the holistic, biopsychosocial practice of psychiatric nursing. Advances in understanding the interrelationships of the brain, behavior, emotion, and cognition offered new opportunities for psychiatric nursing. Another issue that emerged in the 1990s was the importance of sociocultural factors in psychiatric care. Psychiatric nurses also saw the need to become realigned with care and caring, which represent the art of psychiatric nursing and give balance to the science and high technology of current health-care practices. These changes led to the revision of the *Standards of Psychiatric–Mental Health Clinical Nursing Practice* in 1994 and the publication of *Psychopharmacology Guidelines for Psychiatric–Mental Health Nurses* in the same year. Each of these exciting developments in the field is discussed in various chapters of this text.

The task for psychiatric nurses in the years ahead will be the need for greater differentiation and balance.[31] Psychiatric nursing practice needs to continue to differentiate between mental health and mental illness, medical and nursing models of care, adaptive and maladaptive responses, and psychiatric and psychosocial problems. For example, the anxiety felt by a patient before surgery is very different from the anxiety experienced by a patient with agoraphobia. So too, the care the nurse gives each patient varies based on whether the nurse is prepared to intervene from a psychosocial or psychiatric nursing perspective. As the specialty is able to better differentiate among these phenomena, a balance can be achieved in directing clinical practice, establishing research priorities, and preparing psychiatric nurses for the range of roles and functions they will be expected to assume in the next decade.

Compare the length of your clinical rotation in psychiatric nursing with your clinicals in medicine, surgery, and pediatrics. Given the prevalence of mental health problems such as depression and substance abuse, do you feel you have sufficient learning time in psychiatry?

CONTEMPORARY PRACTICE

Psychiatric nursing is an interpersonal process that promotes and maintains behavior that contributes to integrated functioning. The patient may be an individual, family, group, organization, or community. The American Nurses' Association *Statement on Psychiatric–Mental Health Clinical Nursing Practice* defines psychiatric nursing as "a specialized area of nursing practice employing theories of human behavior as its science and purposeful use of self as its art."[2] Psychiatric nurses deliver primary mental health care, which includes the continuous and comprehensive services necessary for the promotion of optimal mental health, prevention of mental illness, health maintenance, management of and referral of mental and physical health problems, the diagnosis and treatment of mental disorders and their sequelae, and rehabilitation.[11] The Center for Mental Health Services officially recognizes psychiatric nursing as one of the five core mental health disciplines. The other four disciplines are marriage and family therapy, psychiatry, psychology, and social work.

The current practice of psychiatric nursing is based on a number of underlying premises or beliefs. The philosophical beliefs of psychiatric nursing practice that this text is based on are described in Box 1-3. The psychiatric nurse uses knowledge from the psychosocial and biophysical sciences and theories of personality and human behavior. From these sources the nurse derives a theoretical framework on which to base nursing practice. The choice of a conceptual model or theoretical framework is an individual one. Various models of psychiatric treatment are described in Chapter 3. Chapter 4 presents a stress adaptation model of psychiatric nursing care developed by Gail Stuart that is used as the organizing framework for this text.

Finally, the contemporary practice of psychiatric nursing occurs within a social and environmental context (see Critical Thinking about Contemporary Issues). The professional psychiatric nursing role has grown in complexity from its original historical elements. It now includes the parameters of clinical competence, patient advocacy, fiscal responsibility, professional collaboration, social accountability, and legal and ethical obligations (Fig. 1-1). These factors influence the education,

---

Box 1-3

PHILOSOPHICAL BELIEFS OF PSYCHIATRIC NURSING PRACTICE

▼ The individual has intrinsic worth and dignity. Each person is worthy of respect solely because of each person's nature and presence.

▼ The goal of the individual is one of growth, health, autonomy, and self-actualization.

▼ Every individual has the potential to change and the desire to pursue personal goals.

▼ The person functions as a holistic being who acts on, interacts with, and reacts to the environment as a whole person. Each part affects the total response, which is greater than the sum of each separate component.

▼ All people have common, basic, and necessary human needs. These include physical needs, safety needs, love and belonging needs, esteem needs, and self-actualization needs.

▼ All behavior of the individual is meaningful. It arises from personal needs and goals and can be understood only from the person's internal frame of reference and within the context in which it occurs.

▼ Behavior consists of perceptions, thoughts, feelings, and actions. From one's perceptions thoughts arise, emotions are felt, and actions are conceived. Disruptions may occur in any of these areas.

▼ Individuals vary in their coping capacities, which depend on genetic endowment, environmental influences, nature and degree of stress, and available resources. All individuals have the potential for both health and illness.

▼ Illness can be a growth-producing experience for the individual. The goal of nursing care is to maximize positive interactions with the individual's environment, promote wellness, and enhance self-actualization.

▼ All people have a right to an equal opportunity for adequate health care regardless of gender, race, religion, ethics, sexual orientation, or cultural background. Nursing care is based on the needs of individuals, families, and communities and mutually defined goals and expectations.

▼ Mental health is a critical and necessary component of comprehensive health-care services.

▼ The individual has the right to participate in decision making regarding physical and mental health. The person has the right to self-determination. It is the decision of the individual to pursue health or illness.

▼ An interpersonal relationship has the potential for producing change and growth within the individual. It is the vehicle for the application of the nursing process and the attainment of the goal of nursing care.

---

research, and clinical components of contemporary psychiatric nursing practice.

Levels of Prevention

The concepts of primary, secondary, and tertiary prevention provide a framework for discussing contemporary psychiatric nursing activities.

Primary. **Primary prevention** involves lowering the incidence of illness in a community by changing causative factors before they can do harm. It is a concept that precedes disease and is applied to a generally healthy population. It includes health promotion, illness prevention, and protection against disease. Within this area lie many of nursing's independent functions, which have as their goal to decrease the vulnerability of individuals to illness and to strengthen their capacity to withstand stressors. Direct nursing care functions in this area include the following:

▼ Health teaching regarding principles of mental health

▼ Effecting changes in improved living conditions, freedom from poverty, and better education

▼ Consumer education in such areas as normal growth and development and sex education

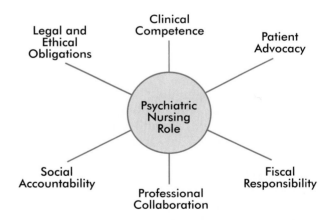

Fig. 1-1   Elements of the professional psychiatric nursing role.

▼ Making appropriate referrals before mental disorder occurs, based on assessment of potential stressors and life changes

▼ Assisting patients in a general hospital setting to avoid future psychiatric problems.

▼ Working with families to support family members and group functioning

▼ Becoming active in community and political activities related to mental health

CRITICAL THINKING ABOUT CONTEMPORARY ISSUES

Are Psychiatric Nurses Vulnerable or Valuable in an Era of Health-Care Reform?

One question that is often raised when nurses talk together about the health-care environment is whether psychiatric nurses will be vulnerable to being replaced as expensive and antiquated providers or be valued as competent clinicians who can function in a world of changing needs, processes, and structures. Potential areas of vulnerability have been identified and include the following:[34]

▼ Most psychiatric nurses work in inpatient units, yet health-care reform is stimulating the greater use of community-based settings.

▼ The skills of psychiatric nurses are often poorly utilized.

▼ Outcome studies that document the effectiveness of care delivered by psychiatric nurses are lacking.

▼ Psychiatric nurses continue to struggle to be perceived as revenue producers and to receive reimbursement for the services they provide.

▼ Role differentiation is lacking in the organizational structures and value systems of psychiatric nurses.

Each of these issues must be addressed if psychiatric nursing is to continue to develop as a specialty area. Nurses must move quickly into the continuum of care and be able to clearly articulate their skills, functions, and abilities. They must also demonstrate their cost effectiveness and differentiated levels of practice based on education, experience, and credentials. Other strategies that have been suggested are that psychiatric nurses assist in the development of national databases that list and define nursing phenomena of concern; continue to develop and use standards and guidelines for clinical practice; and participate in health-care payment reform that results in payment to the most cost-effective qualified provider.[6] Such strategies will position psychiatric nurses as visible, interdependent, central, and collaborating professionals who have much to offer a reformed health-care system. ▼

Secondary. **Secondary prevention** involves reducing actual illness by early detection and treatment of the problem. Direct nursing care functions in this area include the following:

▼ Intake screening and evaluation services
▼ Home visits for preadmission or treatment services
▼ Emergency treatment and psychiatric services in the general hospital
▼ Providing a therapeutic milieu
▼ Supervising patients receiving medication
▼ Suicide prevention services
▼ Counseling on a time-limited basis
▼ Crisis intervention
▼ Psychotherapy with individuals, families, and groups of various ages ranging from children to older adults
▼ Intervening with communities and organizations based on an identified problem

Tertiary. **Tertiary prevention** involves reducing the residual impairment or disability resulting from an illness. Direct nursing care functions in this area include the following:

▼ Promoting vocational training and rehabilitation
▼ Organizing aftercare programs for patients discharged from psychiatric facilities to ease their transition from the hospital to the community
▼ Providing partial hospitalization options for patients

In addition to direct nursing care functions, psychiatric nurses engage in indirect activities that affect all three levels of prevention. These activities include training nursing personnel in various educational programs; administrating in mental health settings to help provide optimal psychiatric care; supervising nursing personnel to improve the quality of nursing services; consulting with colleagues, other professionals, consumer groups, community care givers, and local and national agencies; and researching clinical nursing problems.

Continuum of Care

Traditional settings for psychiatric nurses include psychiatric facilities, community mental health centers, psychiatric units in the general hospital, residential facilities, and private practice. With health-care reform initiatives, however, alternative treatment settings throughout the continuum of care are emerging for psychiatric nurses. Such settings include home-based services, partial hospitalization programs, day treatment centers, foster care or group homes, hospices, visiting nurse associations, emergency departments, primary care clinics, schools, prisons, industry, managed care facilities, and health maintenance organizations.

The new opportunities for psychiatric nursing practice that are emerging throughout the continuum of mental health care are very exciting for the specialty. They require, however, that nurses be proactive in demonstrating their expertise in designing interventions, planning programs, implementing treatment strategies, and managing staff in a variety of traditional and non-traditional settings. Psychiatric nurses who have always worked in inpatient settings may feel a sense of bereavement when they leave the inpatient setting and move into the community.[19] They may also need to learn new skills and knowledge to make the transition to community-based psychiatric nursing practice.

Although these developments present challenges, psychiatric nurses must continue to demonstrate flexibility, accountability, and self-direction as they move forward into these expanding areas of practice. The continuum of care is not only providing new treatment options for patients, but also it is creating an opportunity for psychiatric nurses to evaluate the full range of their patients' coping responses. With this information, psychiatric nurses can then implement primary, secondary, and tertiary prevention functions from a holistic, biopsychosocial perspective.

Competent Caring

There are three domains of contemporary psychiatric nursing practice—direct care, communication, and management activities. Within these overlapping domains of practice, the teaching, coordinating, delegating, and collaborating functions of the role are expressed (Fig. 1-2). Often the communication and management domains of practice are overlooked when discussing the psychiatric nursing role. However, these integrating activities are critically important and very time-consuming aspects of a nurse's role. They are also likely to become more important in a reformed health-care system that places emphasis on efficient patient triage and management. Thus they should not be minimized or discounted when describing the contemporary psychiatric nursing role.

It is possible to further delineate the various activities engaged in by psychiatric nurses within each one of these three domains. Box 1-4 lists the range of specific nursing activities that could be enacted by a psychiatric nurse in each area. While not all nurses participate in all these activities, they do reflect the current nature and scope of competent caring by psychiatric nurses. In addition, psychiatric nurses are able to:

▼ Make biopsychosocial health assessments that are culturally sensitive

▼ Design and implement treatment plans for patients and families with complex health problems and comorbid conditions

▼ Engage in case management activities, such as organizing, accessing, negotiating, coordinating, and integrating services and benefits for individuals and families

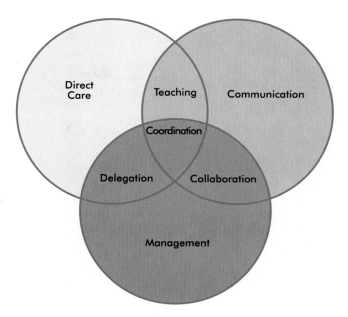

Fig. 1-2   Psychiatric nursing practice.

▼ Provide a "health-care map" for individuals, families, and groups to guide them to community resources for mental health—including the most appropriate providers, agencies, technologies, and social systems

▼ Promote and maintain mental health and manage the effects of mental illness through teaching and counseling

▼ Provide care for the physically ill with psychological problems and the psychiatrically ill with physical problems

▼ Manage and coordinate systems of care integrating the needs of patients, families, staff, and regulators

Psychiatric nurses need to be able to articulate both the general and the specific aspects of their practice as described in this chapter to patients, families, other professionals, administrators, and legislators. Only when such skills and competencies are identified will psychiatric nurses be able to ensure their appropriate role utilization, adequate compensation for the nursing care provided, and the most efficient use of scarce human resources in the delivery of mental health care.

LEVEL OF PERFORMANCE

The description of nursing roles and activities indicates a wide variation in levels of performance. Not all psychiatric nurses can perform each of these functions. Individual nurses have primary responsibility and accountability for their own practice; one aspect of accountability is that nurses define and adhere to the legitimate scope of their practice. Four major factors—laws, qualifications, setting, and personal initiative—

Box 1-4
PSYCHIATRIC NURSING ACTIVITIES

DIRECT CARE ACTIVITIES

Advocacy
Aftercare follow-up
Behavioral treatments
Case consultation
Case management
Cognitive treatments
Community education
Compliance counseling
Crisis intervention
Discharge planning
Family interventions
Group work
Health promotion
Health teaching
High-risk assessment
Home visits
Individual counseling
Intake screening and evaluation
Medication administration
Medication management
Mental health promotion
Milieu therapy
Nutritional counseling
Obtaining informed consent
Parent education
Patient triage
Physical assessment
Physiological treatments
Play therapy
Prescription of medications
Providing environmental safety
Psychosocial assessment
Psychotherapy
Relapse prevention
Research implementation
Self-care activities
Social skills training
Somatic treatments
Stress management

COMMUNICATION ACTIVITIES

Clinical case conferences
Developing treatment plans
Documentation of care
Forensic testimony
Interagency liaison
Peer review
Preparing reports
Professional nurse networking
Staff meetings
Transcribing orders
Treatment team meetings
Verbal reports of care

MANAGEMENT ACTIVITIES

Budgeting and resource allocation
Clinical supervision
Collaboration
Committee participation
Community action
Consultation/liaison
Contract negotiation
Coordination of services
Delegation of assignments
Grant writing
Marketing and public relations
Mediation and conflict resolution
Needs assessment and forecasting
Organizational governance
Outcomes management
Performance evaluations
Policy and procedure development
Professional presentations
Program evaluation
Program planning
Publications
Quality improvement activities
Recruitment and retention activities
Regulatory agency activities
Risk management
Software development
Staff scheduling
Staff and student education
Strategic planning
Unit governance
Utilization review

play a role in determining functions and the types of activities engaged in by each nurse.

Laws

Laws are the primary factor affecting the level of nursing practice. Each state has its own nurse practice act,

which regulates entry into the profession and defines the legal limits of nursing practice that must be adhered to by all nurses. Currently there are three general patterns of nurse practice acts: regulatory acts, expanded definition acts, and delegatory acts. Some acts recognize advanced practice of nurses; others do not.[27]

Nurses must be familiar with the nurse practice act of their state and define and limit their practice accordingly (see Chapter 8).

Qualifications

A nurse's qualifications include education, work experiences, and certification status (see Chapter 10). The American Nurses' Association[2] has identified two types of psychiatric nurse clinicians:

1. Nurses who are generalists, called *psychiatric–mental health nurses*
2. Nurses who are specialists, called *psychiatric–mental health nurse certified specialists*

The recommended educational preparation for the generalist role is a baccalaureate degree in nursing. The nurse also must demonstrate the profession's standards of knowledge, experience, and quality of care through formal review processes. The majority of nurses working in psychiatry are generalists.

In contrast, specialization involves adding to the generic base of nursing practice a systematized body of knowledge and competencies within a discrete area of nursing. The specialist in psychiatric and mental health nursing has a graduate education, supervised clinical experience, and depth of knowledge, competence, and skill in practice. The nurse specialist can apply this added knowledge to the solution of mental health problems. The minimal level of preparation for the specialist is a master's degree in psychiatric nursing, which requires academically supervised clinical practice and study in the theoretical bases for therapeutic intervention.

Another qualification is the nurse's relevant work experience. Although work experience does not replace education, it does provide an added and necessary dimension to the nurse's level of competence and ability to function therapeutically.

Practice Setting

The setting in which nurses practice also influences their level of performance. According to Peplau,[30] the role the nurse assumes in any psychiatric mental health setting depends on the following:

1. The competence brought to work as a consequence of basic or postbasic nursing education
2. The definition of mental illness that prevails in a given setting
3. The extent of consensus about whether each profession should have discrete and unique roles or whether there can be overlap
4. The cost of certain kinds of care, the difference in status and salary levels, and the number of persons needed and available to provide certain kinds of care

A basic consideration is the philosophy of the particular health care system—the way in which the setting defines mental illness. From this definition emerges the work of the patient and the role of the nurse. If the setting is that of an organization, additional constraints may be imposed on the nurse as a result of administrative policies, staff norms, or nursing service expectations.

Psychiatric nurses may practice in settings that vary widely in purpose, type, location, and administration. They may be employed by an organization or self-employed in private practice. Nurses employed by an organization are paid for their services on a salaried or fee-for-service basis. Most nurses work in such organized settings.[5,25] The administrative policies of these organizations can either foster or limit full use of the nurse's potential. Nurses who are self-employed are paid for their services through third-party payment and direct patient fees. Some self-employed certified specialists maintain staff privileges with institutional facilities.

 What qualities would you look for in an organization to see if it promoted professional nursing practice?

Personal Initiative

The personal competence and initiative of the individual nurse determine one's interpretation of the nursing role and the success of its implementation. The importance of this final factor should not be ignored; without a realization of clinical competence and the assumption of professional initiative, the nurse is significantly limited in performance.

Prolonged stress can cause depletion of a nurse's personal resources. Some common sources of stress for psychiatric nurses are:

▼ Conflict with supervisors, co-workers, or other team members
▼ Job dissatisfaction
▼ Heavy patient load
▼ High patient acuity
▼ Authority not equal to responsibility
▼ Lack of participation in decisions affecting work
▼ Inadequate staff support
▼ Lack of promotion potential
▼ Low salary
▼ Lack of autonomy

One study of stress among nurses in four specialty areas reported that psychiatric nurses experienced intense interpersonal involvement and frequent conflicts with patients, families, physicians, and colleagues.[7] They also experienced less social affirmation and recognition than intensive care nurses and less assistance than operating room nurses. These findings are noteworthy, especially in view of the fact that psychiatric nurses are expected to provide psychosocial assistance and support to their patients and, to some degree, to their peers.

Another study measured specific aspects of occupational stress as perceived by psychiatric nurses.[8] The study found that stressors related to the nursing role produced low levels of stress, but that stressors related to the organizational system produced high levels of stress. In fact, 50% of the high stressors and all the top 10 identified stressors were organizational in nature. The single most stressful experience involved not being notified of changes before they occurred.

Given the seriousness of the problem, it is important to plan and implement stress management strategies for psychiatric nurses. A supportive environment for psychiatric nurses should consider the importance of the following:

▼ The number and mix of staff
▼ Delegation of nonessential tasks
▼ Open communication
▼ Recognition of nurses' contributions
▼ Opportunity to influence the work context
▼ Involvement in clinical decision making
▼ Encouragement of professional activities
▼ Provision of new work roles or responsibilities
▼ Interdisciplinary respect

Another strategy for enhancing the personal growth and competence of the psychiatric nurse is the use of support groups. One model of a professional support group developed by Johnson and co-workers[14] has as its major purposes to provide practical help to one another, stimulate ideas, share professional experiences, and share relevant information. Possible group activities are described in Table 1-1.

Networking. Psychiatric nurses would also benefit from networking. Networks are groups of individuals drawn together by common concerns to support and help one another. Networks range from informal friendships to small groups providing contacts and advancement to large, open groups providing emotional support.

Forming networks can help nurses to unite and to value their profession. Meisenhelder[23] believes that nursing networking is needed on three levels. Networking at the grass roots or staff nurse level is crucial to the unity and survival of the profession. It would help nurses work toward caring for one another and having an influence on their work environment. A supportive staff network can extend beyond affirmation of the members and become an influential force in managing daily nursing care.

Table 1-1 Professional Support Group Activities

Purposes	Related activities
Practical help	Case presentations
	Evaluating record-keeping methods
	Interventions for staff performance problems
	Standardized nursing care plan development
	Position title changes
Stimulation of ideas	Educational meeting reports
	Individual role components discussion
Sharing of experiences	Discussion of difficult work experiences
	Description of successful interventions
Sharing information	Exchange of continuing education brochures
	Distribution of articles
	Update on new laws
	Sharing of institutional policies
	Suggestions of resources for additional information for problem solving

From Johnson R et al: J *Psychosoc Nurs Ment Health Serv* 20:9:1982.

The next level of networking is at the leadership level, where nursing leaders can unite for a common goal of increased power in the health-care system. Nurses at this level are in a position to make a significant contribution to the self-esteem of their fellow nurses through support and affirmation of their abilities and potential. The final level includes informational networks that are necessary for effective political action.

 What "networks" do you have in your life at this time and how do they help you? How might professional networks help you when you graduate?

PSYCHIATRIC NURSING AGENDA

Psychiatric nursing will continue to grow and evolve in the years ahead. Health-care reform, patient and family needs, scientific developments, economic realities, and societal expectations will each help to mold and shape the future roles and functions of psychiatric nurses. To best meet the challenges of the next decade, psychiatric nurses will need to focus their energies on three areas of importance—outcome evaluation, leadership skills, and political action.

Outcome Evaluation

Psychiatric nurses must be able to identify, describe, and measure the effect of the care they provide patients, families, and communities. Psychiatric nursing is noticeably absent from the numerous published reviews of the cost effectiveness of nursing, and the specialty has found it difficult to articulate the nature and outcomes of psychiatric nursing care. This has created problems in justifying the need for psychiatric nurses in various treatment settings and in giving psychiatric nurses the recognition they deserve based on their contributions to the mental health delivery system.

Outcomes are all those things that happen to the patient and family while they are involved in the healthcare system. They can include health status, functional status, quality of life, the presence or absence of illness, type of coping response, and satisfaction with treatment. Outcome evaluation can focus on a clinical condition, an intervention, or the caregiving process. The variety of outcomes that can be examined include clinical, functional, financial, and perceptual indicators related to the provision of psychiatric nursing (Box 1-5).

Outcome studies documenting the quality, cost, and effectiveness of psychiatric nursing practice must become an important part of the psychiatric nursing agenda. These studies should be able to stand up to the scientific review of the broader community of mental health professionals by being methodologically sound, empirically grounded, and replicated across the continuum of psychiatric care settings.[13,26] The results of these studies can then be used to provide a shared knowledge base, formulate practice guidelines, provide data on clinical course, and better manage mental health care outcomes.

The need to focus on ways to critically evaluate the outcomes of psychiatric nursing activities is a task for each and every psychiatric nurse regardless of role, qualifications, or practice setting. Psychiatric nurse clinicians, educators, administrators, and researchers all must assume responsibility for answering the question, What difference does psychiatric nurse caring make?

Leadership Skills

Psychiatric nurses, individually and collectively, need knowledge and strategies that enable them to exercise leadership and management in their work.[22] Such leadership has an effect on the care patients receive; it also strengthens and expands the contribution of psychiatric nursing to the larger health-care system.

Psychiatric nurses must use their leadership skills and work as change agents to a greater degree than they are doing at present. Mental health consumers need adequate, humane, and socially acceptable care. To this end nurses can initiate change; assist in change by supporting, participating, or implementing it; engage in joint ventures for planned change; and evaluate completed change. To do so, the psychiatric nurse needs the following key characteristics[20]:

1. The ability to take risks. The nurse must develop the ability to calculate potential risks surrounding the implementation of the change and then decide whether these risks are indeed worth taking.
2. A commitment to the efficacy of the change. The change agent must develop a commitment to investigating the worth, value, effectiveness, and necessity of the change before initiating it.
3. Three areas of competence: (1) a knowledge of nursing that combines research findings and basic scientific information, (2) clinical competence,

---

Box 1-5

CATEGORIES OF OUTCOME INDICATORS

CLINICAL OUTCOME INDICATORS

▼ High-risk behaviors
▼ Symptomatology
▼ Coping responses
▼ Relapse
▼ Recurrence
▼ Readmission
▼ Number of treatment episodes
▼ Medical complications
▼ Incidence reports
▼ Mortality

FUNCTIONAL OUTCOME INDICATORS

▼ Functional status
▼ Social interaction
▼ Activities of daily living
▼ Occupational abilities
▼ Quality of life
▼ Family relationships
▼ Housing arrangement

PERCEPTUAL OUTCOME INDICATORS
PATIENT-FAMILY SATISFACTION WITH

▼ Outcomes
▼ Providers
▼ Delivery system
▼ Caregiving process
▼ Organization

FINANCIAL OUTCOME INDICATORS

▼ Cost per treatment episode
▼ Revenue per treatment episode
▼ Length of inpatient stay
▼ Use of health-care resources
▼ Costs related to disability

Box 1-6

PSYCHIATRIC NURSING'S PRINCIPLES FOR HEALTH-CARE REFORM

▼ Equal availability and quality of treatment based on clinical needs for both mental and physical health conditions

▼ Policies of inclusion in insurance reform

▼ Access to appropriate mental health care at any point along the continuum of care in the least restrictive setting

▼ Flexibility and range of services that are tailored to the needs of consumers, community based, and readily accessible

▼ Nondiscriminatory access to social entitlement programs

▼ Multidisciplinary, cost-effective, culturally sensitive managed care services that address both cost and quality and emphasize coordination of care and provider choice

▼ Risk protection for out-of-pocket expenses associated with long-term catastrophic care

▼ Local authority for funding and delivery of mental health services

▼ Emphasis on consumer involvement in all aspects of service delivery

▼ Reimbursement for appropriate care and setting, based on service not provider, to all qualified providers

---

From Krauss J: *Health care reform: essential mental health services*, Washington, DC, 1993, American Nurses' Association.

and (3) skill in interpersonal relationships and communication.

Psychiatric nurses have the potential to be significant forces in the process of shaping the health care future of our society. To do so, they must learn to use their power and resources in the political arena—truly one of the most important targets for nursing action.

Political Action

Increasing psychiatric nurses' political awareness and skills is necessary to bring about needed changes in the mental health care delivery system. The political empowerment of nursing involves the development of three dimensions[18]:

1. Raising consciousness of sociocultural realities
2. Developing positive self-esteem
3. Acquiring political skills

These dimensions are overlapping and interactive and form the basis of political action by psychiatric nurses that is respectful of others, confirming of self, and directed toward the common good.

It is essential that psychiatric nurses recognize the value and legitimacy of their own voices. They then need to understand the many connections between their work and that of society and the world. This will allow nurses to mobilize their workplaces and effect community and legislative agendas that require political action. To do so effectively, nurses must become educated in legislative and regulatory processes.[36] They need to be involved in political campaigns and testify in legislative hearings.

Concerns about cost, access, and quality of health care in the United States have led to a variety of legislative proposals that would reform the health-care system and its financing. To date, health insurance benefits for mental illness, including substance abuse, have been treated differently from medical-surgical benefits, with stricter limits on outpatient visits and hospital days.[33] Nursing principles for a more equitable design of mental health reform are presented in Box 1-6.[16] In coalition with other mental health care providers and consumers, psychiatric nurses must lobby for government policies and legislation that provide adequate funding for mental health service delivery, parity in reimbursement for psychiatric illnesses, and support of psychiatric education and research.

Psychiatric nurses can then assert their right to an equitable share of the resources, given the value of the services they provide. Passive acceptance of decisions made by legislators, insurers, managed care companies, and other professionals should be replaced with proactive strategies. In this way the psychiatric nursing agenda of the next decade will advance nursing's commitment to caring in a mental health delivery system that is fair, sensitive, and responsible in meeting the biopsychosocial needs of patients, families, and communities.

SUMMARY

1. Psychiatric nursing began to emerge as a profession in the late nineteenth century, and by the twentieth century it had evolved into a specialty with unique roles and functions.
2. Psychiatric nursing is an interpersonal process that promotes and maintains behaviors that contribute to integrated functioning. The patient may be an individual, family, group, organization, or community.
3. Four factors that help to determine the level of a psychiatric nurse's performance are the law, the nurse's qualifications, the practice setting, and the nurse's personal initiative.
4. To best meet the challenges of the next decade, psychiatric nurses will need to focus their energies on three areas of importance—outcome evaluation, leadership skills, and political action.

REFERENCES

1. Abraham I, Fox J, Cohen B: Integrating the bio into the biopsychosocial: understanding and treating biological phenomena in psychiatric–mental health nursing, *Arch Psychiatr Nurs* 6:296, 1992.
2. American Nurses' Association: A *statement on psychiatric–mental health clinical nursing practice and standards of psychiatric–mental health clinical nursing practice, Washington*, DC, 1994, The Association.
3. Babich K, Tolbert R: What is biological psychiatry? How will the trend toward biological psychiatry affect the future of the psychiatric mental health nurse? *J Psychosoc Nurs Ment Health Serv* 30:33, 1992.
4. Bennett A, Eaton J: The role of the psychiatric nurse in the newer therapies, *Am J Psychiatry* 108:167, 1951.
5. Betrus P, Hoffman A: Psychiatric–mental health nursing: career characteristics, professional activities, and client attributes of members of the American Nurses' Association Council of Psychiatric Nurses, *Issues Ment Health Nurs* 13:39, 1992.
6. Billings C: Psychiatric–mental health nursing professional progress notes, *Arch Psychiatr Nurs* 7:174, 1993.
7. Cronin-Stubbs D, Brophy E: Burnout: can social support save the nurse? *J Psychosoc Nurs Ment Health Serv* 23:9, 1985.
8. Dawkins J, Depp F, Selzer N: Stress and the psychiatric nurse, *J Psychosoc Nurs Ment Health Serv* 23:9, 1985.
9. Doona M: At least as well cared for . . . Linda Richards and the mentally ill, *Image* 16:51, 1984.
10. Editorial, *Am J Nurs* 40:23, 1940.
11. Haber J, Billings C: Primary mental health care: a vision for the future of psychiatric–mental health nursing, *ANA Council Perspectives*, 2:1, 1993.
12. Hays D: Suggested clinical practice of psychiatric nurses recorded in the literature between 1946 and 1958. In *Psychiatric nursing 1946 to 1974: a report on the state of the art*, New York, 1975, American Journal of Nursing Co.
13. Jennings B: Patient outcomes research: seizing the opportunity, *Adv Nurs Sci* 14:59, 1991.
14. Johnson R et al: The professional support group: a model for psychiatric clinical nurse spcialists, *J Psychosoc Nurs Ment Health Serv* 20:9, 1982.
15. Jones M: *The therapeutic community: a new treatment method in psychiatry*, New York, 1953, Basic Books, Inc.
16. Krauss J: *Health care reform: essential mental health services*, Washington, DC, 1993, American Nurses' Association.
17. Lowry B: Psychiatric nursing in the 1990s and beyond, *J Psychosoc Nurs Ment Health Serv* 30:7, 1992.
18. Mason D, Backer B, Georges C: Toward a feminist model for the political empowerment of nurses, *Image* 23:72, 1991.
19. Massey P: Institutional loss: an examination of a bereavement reaction in 22 mental nurses losing their institution and moving into the community, *J Adv Nurs* 16:573, 1991.
20. Mauksch IG, Miller MH: *Implementing change in nursing*, St Louis, 1981, Mosby.
21. McEnany G: Psychobiology and psychiatric nursing: a philosophical matrix, *Arch Psychiatr Nurs* 5:255, 1991.

22. McNeese-Smith D: The impact of leadership on productivity, *Nurs Econ* 10:393, 1992.

23. Meisenhelder J: Networking and nursing, *Image* 14:77, 1982.

24. Mellow J: Nursing therapy, *Am J Nurs* 68:2365, 1968.

25. Merwin E, Fox J: Cost-effective integration of mental health professions, *Issues Ment Health Nursing* 13:139, 1992.

26. Mirin S, Namerow M: Why study treatment outcome? *Hosp Community Psychiatry* 42:1007, 1991.

27. Pearson L: Annual update of how each state stands on legislative issues affecting advanced nursing practice, *Nurse Pract* 19:11, 1994.

28. Peplau H: *Interpersonal relations in nursing,* New York, 1952, GP Putnam's Sons.

29. Peplau H: Interpersonal techniques: the crux of psychiatric nursing, *Am J Nurs* 62:53, 1962.

30. Peplau H: Psychiatric nursing: role of nurses and psychiatric nurses, *Int Nurs Rev* 25:41, 1978.

31. Pothier P, Stuart G, Puskar K, Babich K: Dilemmas and directions for psychiatric nursing in the 1990s, *Arch Psychiatr Nurs* 4:284, 1990.

32. Santos E, Stainbrook E: Nursing and modern psychiatry, *Am J Nurs* 49:107, 1949.

33. Sharfstein S, Stoline A, Goldman H: Psychiatric care and health insurance reform, *Am J Psychiatry* 150:7, 1993.

34. Stuart G: Vulnerable or valuable: psychiatric nursing's future in health care reform, *J Psychosoc Nurs* 32:7, 1994.

35. Tudor G: Sociopsychiatric nursing approach to intervention in a problem of mutual withdrawal on a mental hospital ward, *Psychiatry* 15:193, 1952.

36. Wakefield M: Influencing the legislative process, *Nurs Econ* 8:188, 1990.

37. Weiss MO: The skills of psychiatric nursing, *Am J Nurs* 47:174, 1947.

ANNOTATED SUGGESTED READINGS

*American Nurses' Association: A *statement on psychiatric–mental health clinical nursing practice and standards of psychiatric–mental health clinical nursing practice,* Washington, DC, 1994, The Association.

A *resource pamphlet that should be owned by all psychiatric nurses. It describes types of clinicians, settings, functions, and standards of practice.*

*Backer B: You can get there from here: guide to problem definition in policy development, *J Psychosoc Nurs Ment Health Serv* 29:24, 1991.

Discusses how nurses can formulate and implement health policy through assessment and clear problem definition.

*Billings C: Psychiatric–mental health nursing professional progress notes, *Arch Psychiatr Nurs* 7:174, 1993.

Reviews issues of importance to psychiatric nursing in the current political and professional environment. Enjoyable reading as well.

*Bushy A, Smith T: Lobbying: the hows and wherefores, *Nurs Manage* 21:39, 1990.

Details the steps involved in lobbying activities to help nurses become politically active. Practical, thorough, and needed information for all nurses.

*Church O: From custody to community in psychiatric nursing, *Nurs Res* 36:48, 1987.

Excellent review of the history of psychiatric nursing. Provides perspective and insight into current practice issues.

Health Affairs 11(3):1992.

The entire issue of this journal is devoted to mental health policy in America. Written by experts in the field, it is the best overview on the subject.

---

*Nursing reference.

*Jones J: Stress in psychiatric nursing. In Payne R, Firth-Cozens J, ed: *Stress in health professionals,* New York, 1987, John Wiley & Sons.

Literature is reviewed and summarized that addresses sources of stress for the psychiatric nurse.

*Krauss J: *Health care reform: essential mental health services,* Washington, DC, 1993, American Nurses' Assocation.

Presents nursing's position on the need for reform of America's essential mental health services and benefits.

*Lowry B: Psychiatric nursing in the 1990s and beyond, *J Psychosoc Nurs Ment Health Serv* 30:7, 1992.

Describes changes psychiatric nurses will face and ways in which the field will need to adapt to the larger social and economic environment.

*Mental health reform: New partnerships, new directions, *J Psychosoc Nurs Ment Health Serv* 31(8), 1993.

This issue is devoted to presentations from an invitational conference with leaders of psychiatric nursing who discuss the implications of healthcare reform for the field.

*Peplau H: *Interpersonal relations in nursing,* New York, 1952, GP Putnam's Sons.

Presents the first theoretical framework for the practice of psychiatric nursing. A "classic" in nursing literature.

*Smoyak S, Rouslin S, eds: *A collection of classics in psychiatric nursing literature,* Thorofare, NJ, 1982, Slack, Inc.

Collection of 37 articles written by luminaries in psychiatric nursing. Provides a clear sense of the field's early history.

Stein L, Watts D, Howell T: The doctor-nurse game revisited, *N Engl J Med* 322:546, 1990.

Addresses major changes in the doctor-nurse relationship over the past two decades. Highly recommended.

*Stuart G: An organizational strategy for empowering nursing, *Nurs Econ* 4:35, 1986.

Advocates nurses acting as a unified group and the impact they can have on the organizations in which they work.

*Nursing reference.

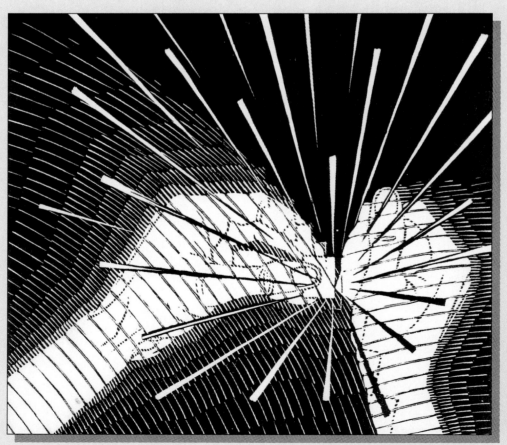

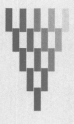

C H A P T E R 2

Therapeutic Nurse-Patient Relationship

GAIL W. STUART

When we treat man as he is, we make him worse than he is. When we treat him as if he already were what he potentially could be, we make him what he should be.

Johann Wolfgang von Goethe

The therapeutic nurse-patient relationship is a mutual learning experience and a corrective emotional experience for the patient. It is based on the underlying humanity of nurse and patient, with mutual respect and acceptance of ethnocultural differences. In this relationship the nurse uses personal attributes and clinical techniques in working with the patient to bring about insight and behavioral change.

CHARACTERISTICS OF THE RELATIONSHIP

The goals of a therapeutic relationship are directed toward the patient's growth and include the following:

1. Self-realization, self-acceptance, and an increased genuine self-respect
2. A clear sense of personal identity and an improved level of personal integration
3. An ability to form an intimate, interdependent, interpersonal relationship with a capacity to give and receive love
4. Improved functioning and increased ability to satisfy needs and achieve realistic personal goals

To achieve these goals, various aspects of the patient's life experiences are explored during the nurse-patient relationship. The nurse allows the patient to express thoughts and feelings and relates these to observed and reported actions, clarifying areas of conflict and anxiety. The nurse identifies and maximizes the patient's ego strengths and encourages socialization and family relatedness. Together the patient and nurse correct communication problems and modify maladaptive behavior patterns by testing new patterns of behavior and more adaptive coping mechanisms.

In the nurse-patient relationship differing values are respected. The two communicate through a dialogue, or discussion, not a monologue, affirming the patient's reality and worth and allowing the patient to more fully define ego identity. In Box 2-1 Rogers[40] summarizes the characteristics of a helping relationship that facilitate growth. All nurses working with patients may ask themselves these questions; their answers largely determine the progress of the relationship.

The therapeutic nurse-patient relationship is complex and merits further exploration. This chapter examines the nurse as helper, the phases of the relationship, facilitative communication, responsive and action dimensions, therapeutic impasses, and the therapeutic outcome (Fig. 2-1). Each of these factors influences the nurse's effectiveness.

THE NURSE AS HELPER

Nurses as helpers must be therapeutic, since their goal is to enable the patient to adapt as a unique individual to the stress being experienced. The self is the key help-

---

Box 2-1

CHARACTERISTICS THAT FACILITATE GROWTH IN HELPING RELATIONSHIPS

1. Can I be in some way that will be perceived by the other person as trustworthy, as dependable, or consistent in some deep sense?
2. Can I be expressive enough as a person that what I am will be communicated unambiguously?
3. Can I let myself experience positive attitudes toward this other person—attitudes of warmth, caring, liking, interest, and respect?
4. Can I be strong enough as a person to be separate from the other?
5. Am I secure enough within myself to permit him his separateness?
6. Can I let myself enter fully into the world of his feelings and personal meaning and see these as he does?
7. Can I be acceptant of each facet of the other person that he presents to me? Can I receive him as he is? Can I communicate this attitude? Or can I only receive him conditionally, acceptant of some aspects of his feelings and silently or openly disapproving of others?
8. Can I act with sufficient sensitivity in the relationship that my behavior will not be perceived as a threat?
9. Can I free him from the threat of external evaluation?
10. Can I meet this other individual as a person who is in the process of *becoming*, or will I be bound by his past and my past?

From Rogers C: On *becoming a person*, Boston, 1961, Houghton Mifflin.

---

ing tool the nurse can use in practice. Thus self-analysis is the first building block in providing quality nursing care.

Is it possible that nurses are alienated from their true selves and therefore do not allow patients to express all aspects of themselves? Jourard believes that the socialization process into nursing may destroy the nurse's spontaneity, and that the nurse may become detached from the real self:

Now, if a nurse is afraid or even ignorant of her own self, she is highly likely to be threatened by a patient's real-self expressions. . . . A nurse who is more aware of the breadth and depth of her own real self is in a much better position to empathize with her patients and to encourage (or at least not block) their self-disclosures.[21]

Research on counselor and teacher effectiveness suggests some essential qualities needed to help others. These qualities can be viewed as necessary characteristics for all nurses who wish to be therapeutic. These qualities help the nurse set goals for future growth.

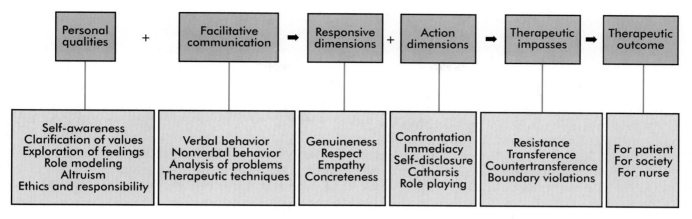

| Personal qualities | + | Facilitative communication | → | Responsive dimensions | + | Action dimensions | → | Therapeutic impasses | → | Therapeutic outcome |

Self-awareness
Clarification of values
Exploration of feelings
Role modeling
Altruism
Ethics and responsibility

Verbal behavior
Nonverbal behavior
Analysis of problems
Therapeutic techniques

Genuineness
Respect
Empathy
Concreteness

Confrontation
Immediacy
Self-disclosure
Catharsis
Role playing

Resistance
Transference
Countertransference
Boundary violations

For patient
For society
For nurse

Fig. 2-1   Elements affecting the nurse's ability to be therapeutic.

Awareness of Self

Theorists and practitioners agree that helpers must be able to answer the question, "Who am I?" Nurses who care for the biological, psychological, and sociocultural needs of patients see a broad range of human experiences; they must learn to deal with anxiety, anger, sadness, and joy in helping patients at all intervals of the health-illness continuum.

Self-awareness is a key component of the psychiatric nursing experience. The nurse's goal is to achieve authentic, open, and personal communication. The nurse must be able to examine personal feelings, actions, and reactions as a provider of care. A firm understanding and acceptance of self allows the nurse to acknowledge a patient's differences and uniqueness.

Campbell[7] has identified a holistic nursing model of self-awareness that consists of four interconnected components—psychological, physical, environmental, and philosophical.

1. The *psychological* component includes knowledge of emotions, motivations, self-concept, and personality. Being psychologically self-aware means being sensitive to feelings and to external elements that affect those feelings.

2. The *physical* component is the knowledge of personal and general physiology, as well as of bodily sensations, body image, and physical potential.

3. The *environmental* component consists of the sociocultural environment, relationships with others, and knowledge of the relationship between humans and nature.

4. The *philosophical* component refers to the sense of life having meaning. A personal philosophy of life and death may or may not include a superior being, but it does take into account responsibility to the world and the ethics of behavior.

Together these components provide a model that can be used to promote the self-awareness and self-growth of both nurses and the patients for whom they care.

| 1 Known to self and others | 2 Known only to others |
| 3 Known only to self | 4 Known neither to self nor to others |

Fig. 2-2   Johari Window. Each quadrant, or windowpane, describes one aspect of the self.

From Sundeen SJ et al: *Nurse-client interaction: implementing the nursing process,* ed 5, St Louis, 1994, Mosby.

Increasing Self-Awareness. No one ever completely knows the inner self as shown in the Johari Window (Fig. 2-2).[29] Quadrant 1 is the open quadrant; it includes the behaviors, feelings, and thoughts known to the individual and others. Quadrant 2 is called the blind quadrant because it includes all those things that others know but that the individual does not know. Quadrant 3 is the hidden quadrant; it includes those things about the self that only the individual knows. Quadrant 4 is the unknown quadrant, containing aspects of the self unknown to the individual and to others. Taken together, these quadrants represent the total self. The following three principles may help clarify how the self functions in this representation:

1. A change in any one quadrant affects all other quadrants.
2. The smaller the first quadrant, the poorer the communication.
3. Interpersonal learning means that a change has taken place, so quadrant 1 is larger and one or more of the other quadrants are smaller.

The goal of increasing self-awareness is to enlarge

the area of quadrant 1 while reducing the size of the other three quadrants. To increase self-knowledge, it is necessary to **listen to the self.** This means the individual allows genuine emotions to be experienced, identifies and accepts personal needs, and moves the body in free, joyful, and spontaneous ways. It includes exploring personal thoughts, feelings, memories, and impulses.

The next step in the process is to reduce the size of quadrant 2 by **listening to and learning from others.** Knowledge of self is not possible alone. As we relate to others, we broaden our perceptions of self, but such learning requires active listening and openness to the feedback others provide.

The final step involves reducing the size of quadrant 3 by **self-disclosing,** or revealing to others important aspects of the self. Self-disclosure is a symptom of personality health and a means of achieving healthy personality.

Compare A and B of Fig. 2-3. A represents a person with little self-awareness whose behaviors and feelings are limited in variety and scope. B, however, shows an individual with great openness to the world. Much of this person's potential is being developed and realized. B represents an individual who has an increased capacity for experiences of all kinds—joy, hate, work, and love.

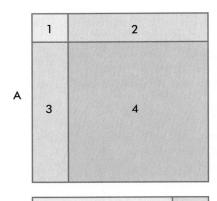

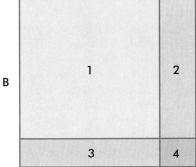

Fig. 2-3 Johari Windows showing varying degrees of self-awareness. **A,** Person with little self-understanding. **B,** Individual with great self-awareness.

From Sundeen SJ et al: *Nurse-client interaction: implementing the nursing process,* ed 5, St Louis, 1994, Mosby.

This person also has few defenses and can interact more spontaneously and honestly with others. This configuration represents a worthy goal for the nurse to attain.

 What does your Johari Window look like?

The Nurse and Self-Growth. People often assume that because a nursing education includes courses in the behavioral sciences, a nursing student is able to use self in a therapeutic manner in the clinical setting. However, although most nursing textbooks include a paragraph or two stressing the importance of self-awareness in quality nursing care, the process and components of the nurse's self-growth are seldom described. The patient's self-concept is also often treated in a cursory way. These omissions give an implicit message to the nursing student: Self-analysis is commendable, but a token assessment will do. This message is reinforced by the student's curriculum, which is burdened with tasks and reports that allow little time for quiet thought leading to self-growth.

Nurses need time to explore and define the many facets of their personalities. If nursing does involve perceiving, feeling, and thinking, nursing students should have the time and opportunity to study their own experiences. Authenticity in relationships must be learned and nurses must first experience openness and authenticity in relationships with instructors and supervisors. The student and instructor can participate in a relationship that accepts and respects their individual differences. Instructors can help students by (1) facilitating students' self-awareness, (2) increasing their level of functioning, (3) stimulating more self-direction, and (4) enabling students to cope more effectively with stressors.

Authenticity also involves being open to self-exploration of thoughts, needs, emotions, values, defenses, actions, communications, problems, and goals. Nursing students have many new experiences that provide opportunities for self-learning. Feelings related to these experiences should be focused on and discussed. Students might enter clinical settings with high ideals and unrealistic images. Perhaps they view nurses as all-knowing, all-caring "miracle workers." During initial encounters students may feel fearful, anxious, and inadequate, wondering how a nurse acquires the necessary knowledge. Nursing students might devalue their abilities and feel like an imposition on patients. At another time nurses may identify closely with patients and feel anger at the impersonal system and unresponsive personnel. The feelings involved in all of these situations should be identified, verbalized, and analyzed. Only then can nurses resolve them in a constructive manner.

A career in nursing is not easy if the nurse is still in adolescence. As a nurse the student will be faced with many adult responsibilities, such as disease, bizarre behavior, complex problems, and even death, when most of the student's friends are focusing on youth, enjoyment, and the future. This might alienate the nurse from some friends. Feelings of loneliness and sadness should be shared so that the nurse can work through personal needs.

Throughout the growing process the student needs the support and guidance of a noncritical but challenging instructor. Together they can analyze the student's behavior, and the student can then assess personal strengths and limitations. Also, it is often helpful to share these experiences with a peer group. Students can empathize, critique, and support each other as they learn more about themselves.

Finally, objective self-examination is not easy or pleasant particularly when findings conflict with self-ideal. However, like many painful experiences, discovering self-awareness presents a challenge: to accept self-limitations or to change the behaviors that support them.

Think back over the courses you have taken in your nursing program. How much time and importance in these courses were placed on developing your self-awareness as a person and a nurse?

Clarification of Values

Nurses should be able to answer the question, "What is important to me?" Awareness helps the nurse to be honest and to avoid the unethical use of patients to meet personal needs. Nurses should avoid the temptation to use patients for the pursuit of personal satisfaction or security. If nurses do not have sufficient personal fulfillment, they should realize it; their sources of dissatisfaction should then be clarified so that they do not interfere with the success of the nurse-patient relationship.

Value Systems. Values are concepts that are formed as a result of life experiences with family, friends, culture, education, work, and relaxation. The word *value* has positive connotations, since it denotes worth or significance. Yet values also imply negatives. If we value honesty, then it follows that we do not value dishonesty. People are likely to hold strong values in religious beliefs, family ties, sexual preferences, other ethnic groups, and sex role beliefs.

One of the many challenges facing psychiatric nurses today is the need to provide care for patients from many different ethnocultural backgrounds in both hospital and community settings. Because the goals of treatment are determined greatly by beliefs and values, establishing a therapeutic relationship with patients from different ethnocultural backgrounds requires particular skill and sensitivity (see Chapter 7).

Value systems also provide the framework for many daily decisions and actions. By being aware of their value systems, nurses can identify situations in which value systems are in conflict. Clarification of values also provides some insurance against the tendency to project values onto other people. Many therapeutic relationships test the nurse's values. A patient may describe a sexual behavior that the nurse finds unacceptable. The patient may talk about divorce, whereas the nurse may strongly believe that marriage contracts should not be broken. The patient may be a "born-again" Christian, but the nurse may have no belief in God or religion.

Can a nurse empathize with and help a patient solve a problem while maintaining personal values that are different from the values of the patient?

Value Clarification Process. Understanding personal values may be promoted by *value clarification*, which allows individuals to discover their values by assessing, exploring, and determining what those values are and what priority they hold in decision-making processes. Value clarification does not determine what the individual's values should be or what values should be followed. To prevent the imposition of values, value clarification focuses exclusively on the *process* of valuing, or on how people come to have the values they have.

Seven criteria are used to determine a value. These criteria should be considered in relation to a person's strongest value and tested against the person's own definition of a value. The seven criteria are broadly grouped into the three steps listed in Box 2-2.

The three criteria of **choosing** rely on the person's cognitive abilities; the two criteria of **prizing** emphasize the emotional or affective level; and the two criteria of **acting** have a behavioral focus.

A change takes place when certain contradictions are perceived in the person's value system. To eliminate the distress that follows such a realization, the person realigns values to coincide with the new view of self.

The Mature Valuing Process. Rogers[40] has described the valuing process in the mature person. The process is complex and the choices often perplexing and

---

Box 2-2

STEPS IN THE VALUE CLARIFICATION PROCESS

Choosing	1. Freely
	2. From alternatives
	3. After thoughtful consideration of the consequences of each alternative
Prizing	4. Cherishing, being happy with the choice
	5. Willing to affirm the choice publicly
Acting	6. Doing something with the choice
	7. Repeatedly, in some pattern of life

---

difficult. There is no guarantee that the choice made will prove to be self-actualizing. The valuing process in the mature person has the following characteristics[24]:

1. It is fluid and flexible, based on the particular moment and the degree to which the moment is enhancing, enriching, and actualizing. Values are continually changing.
2. The valuing experience is highly differentiated, that is, tied to a particular time and experience.
3. Personal experience provides the value information. Although the person is open to all evidence obtained from other sources, outside evidence is not considered as important as subjective responses. The psychologically mature adult trusts and uses personal wisdom.
4. In the valuing process the person is open to the immediacy of experience, trying to sense and clarify all its complex meanings. However, the immediate impact of the moment is colored by experiences from the past and conjecture about the future.

Exploration of Feelings

It is often assumed that helping others requires complete objectivity and detachment. This is definitely not true. Complete objectivity and detachment describe someone who is unresponsive, false, unapproachable, impersonal, and self-alienated—qualities that block the establishment of a therapeutic relationship. Rather, nurses should be open to, aware of, and in control of their feelings so that they can be used to help patients.

The feelings that nurses, as people, have serve an important purpose. They are barometers for feedback about themselves and their relationships with others. In helping others, nurses have many feelings—elation at seeing a patient improve, disappointment when a patient regresses, distress when a patient refuses help, and anger when a patient is demanding or manipulative.

Feelings of power can arise when patients express strong dependence on the nurse. When patients express profuse gratitude to the nurse, the nurse may wonder if the patients believe they helped themselves or whether the nurse did it for them.

Nurses who are open to their feelings understand how they are responding to patients and how they appear to patients. The nurse's feelings are valuable clues to the patient's problems. For example, despite the patient's statement that "things are going real well," the nurse might perceive a strong sense of despair or anger. So too, the nurse should be aware of the feelings conveyed to the patient. Is the nurse's mood one of hopelessness or frustration? If nurses view feelings as barometers and feedback instruments, their effectiveness as helpers will improve.

Serving as Role Model

Formal helping is a strong influence process, and nurses function as role models for their patients. Research has shown the power of role models for acquiring socially adaptive, as well as maladaptive, behavior. Thus a nurse has an obligation to model adaptive and growth-producing behavior. If a nurse has a chaotic personal life, it will show in the nurse's work with patients, decreasing the effectiveness of care. The nurse's credibility as a helper will also be questioned. The nurse may object, saying it is possible to separate personal life from the professional life, but in caring for patients this is not possible because psychiatric nursing *is* the therapeutic use of self.

This is not to imply, however, that the nurse must conform totally to local community norms or must live an idyllic, placid life. What is suggested is that the effective nurse has a fulfilling and satisfying personal life that is not dominated by conflict, distress, or denial, and that the nurse's approach to life conveys a sense of growing and adapting.

Altruism

It is vital for nurses to have an answer to the question, "Why do I want to help others?" Obviously, an effective helper is interested in people and tends to help out of a deep love for humanity. It is also true that everyone seeks a certain amount of personal satisfaction and fulfillment from work. The goal is to maintain a balance between these two needs. Helping motives can become destructive tools in the hands of naive or zealous users.

Another danger lies in subscribing to an extreme view of altruism. Altruism is concern for the welfare of others. It does not mean that an altruistic person should not expect adequate compensation and recognition or must practice denial or self-sacrifice. Only if personal needs have been appropriately met can the nurse expect to be maximally therapeutic.

Finally, a sense of altruism can also apply to more general social support and change motives. Activist helpers are needed who are primarily concerned with changing social conditions to meet human welfare needs. One goal of all helping professionals should be to create a people-serving and growth-facilitating society. As such, a legitimate and necessary role for the nurse is to work to change the larger structure and process of society in ways that will promote the individual's health and well-being.

Ethics and Responsibility

Personal beliefs about people and society can serve as conscious guidelines for action. The Code for Nurses (see Chapter 10) reflects common values regarding nurse-patient relationships and responsibilities and serves as a frame of reference for all nurses in their judgments about patient welfare and social responsibility. For psychiatric nurses, decisions are a part of daily functioning. Responsible ethical choice involves accountability, risk, commitment, and justice.

Related to the nurse's sense of ethics is the need to assume responsibility for behavior. This involves knowing limitations and strengths and being accountable for them. As a member of a health-care team, the nurse has the knowledge and expertise of other people readily available; these people should be used appropriately.

PHASES OF THE RELATIONSHIP

A vital characteristic of the nurse-patient relationship is the sharing of behaviors, thoughts, and feelings. Coad-Denton[11] describes this intimacy as the use of the nursing process to support patients as they explore areas of needs, solve problems, and acquire new coping skills. Table 2-1 identifies seven general components of relationships and contrasts social superficiality and therapeutic intimacy with these components. These elements evolve as the nurse moves through the various phases of the therapeutic relationship with the patient.

Four sequential phases of the relationship process have been identified: preinteraction phase; introductory, or orientation, phase; working phase; and termination phase. Each phase builds on the preceding one and is characterized by specific tasks. In one of the few studies in this area, Forchuk and Brown[15] developed an instrument with initial validity and reliability to measure the phases of the nurse-patient relationship based on observed behaviors. They believe that if nurses can accurately assess the phase of the relationship, appropriate interventions are more likely to be selected.

Preinteraction Phase

Concerns of New Nurses. The preinteraction phase begins before the nurse's first contact with the patient. The nurse's initial task is one of self-exploration. In the first experience working with psychiatric patients, the nurse brings the misconceptions and prejudices of the general public in addition to feelings and fears common to all novices (Box 2-3). An overriding one usually is anxiety or nervousness, which is provoked by new experiences of any kind. A related feeling is ambivalence or uncertainty; nurses may see the need for working with these patients but feel unclear about their ability.

There may also be a threat to the nurse's role identification, precipitated by the informal nature of psychiatric settings. Usually psychiatric patients do not wear hospital gowns or clothing, staff members do not wear uniforms, and the staff and patients mingle in a casual, relaxed, and apparently unstructured way. A common

Table 2-1 Contrast between Social Superficiality and Therapeutic Intimacy

Components of relationship	Social superficiality	Therapeutic intimacy
Mutual self-disclosure	Variable	Patient: self-disclosure; nurse: self-disclosure that promotes treatment goals
Focus of conversation	Unknown to participants	Known to nurse and patient
Pertinence of topic	Social, business, generalized, impersonal	Personal and relevant to nurse and patient
Relationship of experiences to topic	Sense of uninvolvement and use of indirect knowledge	Sense of involvement and use of direct knowledge
Time orientation	Past and future	Present
Use of feelings	Mutual sharing of feelings discouraged	Patient sharing of feelings encouraged by nurse
Recognition of individual worth	Not acknowledged	Fully acknowledged
Termination	Open-ended	Specified, agreed upon and honored

Modified from Coad-Denton A: Therapeutic superficiality and intimacy. In Longo D, Williams R, eds: *Psychosocial nursing: assessment and intervention,* New York, 1978, Appleton-Century-Crofts.

Box 2-3

COMMON CONCERNS OF PSYCHIATRIC NURSING STUDENTS

▼ Acutely self-conscious
▼ Afraid of being rejected by the patients
▼ Anxious because of the newness of the experience
▼ Concerned about personally overidentifying with psychiatric patients
▼ Doubtful of the effectiveness of skills or coping ability
▼ Fearful of physical danger or violence
▼ Inadequacy in therapeutic use of self
▼ Suspicious of psychiatric patients stereotyped as "different"
▼ Threatened in nursing role identity
▼ Uncertain about ability to make a unique contribution
▼ Uncomfortable about the lack of physical tasks and treatments
▼ Vulnerable to emotionally painful experiences
▼ Worried about hurting the patient psychologically

---

first reaction among students is a feeling of panic when they realize that they "can't tell the patients from the staff." The student's discomfort may be aggravated if a patient thinks the student is a newly admitted patient. Finally, it is unsettling for many students to give up their uniforms, stethoscopes, and scissors. Doing so dramatically emphasizes that, in this nursing setting, the most important tools are the ability to communicate, empathize, and solve problems. Without a tangible physical illness to care for, new students are likely to feel acutely self-conscious and hesitant about introducing themselves to a patient and initiating a conversation.

Many nurses express feelings of inadequacy and fears of hurting or exploiting the patient. They worry about saying the wrong thing, which might drive the patient "over the brink," or if, with their limited knowledge and experience, they will be of any value. They wonder how they can help or if they can really make a difference. Some nurses perceive the plight of psychiatric patients as hopeful; others perceive it as hopeless.

A common fear of nurses is related to the stereotype of psychiatric patients as abusive and violent. Because this is the picture portrayed by the media, many nurses are afraid of being physically hurt by a patient's outburst of aggressive behavior. Some nurses fear being psychologically hurt by a patient through rejection or silence. A final fear is related to nurses' questioning their mental health status. Nurses may fear mental illness and worry that exposure to psychiatric patients might cause them to lose their own grasp on reality. Nurses who are working on their own crises of identity and intimacy may

fear overidentifying with patients and using patients to meet their own needs. It has also been noted that students in their psychiatric nursing rotation may use humor as a cognitive coping strategy.[49]

The following clinical example contains many of the feelings and fears expressed by one nursing student in the preinteraction phase of self-analysis, as reported in the notes from her diary of her psychiatric rotation.

 CLINICAL EXAMPLE

When first told that I would have a clinical psychiatric nursing experience, I received this information with a blank mind. Mental overload, denial, repression, or whatever it was made me hear the words but put off dealing with it. Then, when given a chance to sort through my thoughts and feelings, I thought more about what this experience would entail. Having never been personally involved with any people who were psychiatrically ill before, I was unable to rely on past personal experiences. I did, however, have quite a "pseudoknowledge base" from my novels, television, and movie encounters. Do places like the hospitals in *One Flew Over the Cuckoo's Nest* or *Francis* really exist? Was the portrayal of *Sybil* accurate? How could I possibly help someone who has so many problems, like the boy in *Ordinary People*? After all, I have problems myself. I'm afraid these thoughts have raised more questions in me than they have answered.

Three things scare me the most about this experience. First, I feel that the behavior of a psychiatric patient is quite unpredictable. Would they get violent or aggressive without any warning? Would this aggression be directed toward me? If so, would I be hurt? Did I provoke them and was I wrong in my actions that caused this sudden shift?

The second, related to the first, is my feeling of inadequacy. I've been exposed to physically ill people and have learned how to respond to them. But, the psychologically ill are almost totally alien to me. How can I help? What if I do, or say, or infer something they could take offense to? Will I have the patience to persevere? I just don't know, and my not knowing makes me even more nervous.

My third fear is how seeing and being in contact with the psychiatrically ill will affect me. Although I know it's not contagious, the more exposure and knowledge I acquire in this area, the more I may begin to doubt my own stability and sanity. I mean, adolescence hasn't been easy for me, and I feel like I'm just now beginning to see things more clearly and feel better about myself. Will this experience stir up any past fears and doubts and, if so, how will I handle it? I am beginning to realize that there is a fine line between health and illness and that the psychiatric patients we'll meet have been unable to gather enough resources from within to cope with their problems. Help, reassurance, and understanding are their needs. I'm hoping I can help them . . . but I'm just not sure.

 What feelings, fears, and fantasies do you have about working with psychiatric patients?

Schoffstall[43] has described a method that can be used in the classroom to assess and reduce the anxiety of students who are about to begin their clinical experience in psychiatric nursing. In a group setting students were asked to anonymously write down a specific fantasy that they had about beginning their experience in psychiatric nursing. The fantasies were read aloud, and the group discussed the content and feelings in the responses. In a similar group discussion the students were then asked how they thought patients felt about being hospitalized. The exercise was found to be an effective way to handle the student's reluctance in expressing their concerns and to increase their empathy toward psychiatric patients.

Self-Assessment. Experienced nurses benefit by analyzing aspects of their practice. They may ask themselves the following questions:

1. Do I label patients with the stereotype of a group?
2. Is my need to be liked so great that I become angry or hurt when a patient is rude, hostile, or uncooperative?
3. Am I afraid of the responsibility I must assume for the relationship, and do I therefore limit my independent functions?
4. Do I cover feelings of inferiority with a front of superiority?
5. Do I require sympathy, warmth, and protection so much that I err by being too sympathetic or too protective toward patients?
6. Do I fear closeness so much that I am indifferent, rejecting, or cold?
7. Do I need to feel important and keep patients dependent on me?

The self-analysis that characterizes the preinteraction phase is a necessary task. To be effective, nurses should have a reasonably stable self-concept and an adequate amount of self-esteem. They should engage in constructive relationships with others and face reality to help patients do likewise. If they are aware of and in control of what they convey to their patients verbally and nonverbally, nurses can function as role models. To do this,

however, some nurses abandon their personal strengths and assume a facade of "professionalism" that alienates their authentic self. This facade immobilizes them and acts as a barrier to establishing mutuality with patients.

Additional tasks of this phase include gathering data about the patient if information is available and planning for the first interaction with the patient. The nursing assessment is begun, but most of the work related to it is accomplished with the patient in the second phase of the relationship. Finally, nurses review general goals of a therapeutic relationship and consider what they have to offer patients.

Introductory, or Orientation, Phase

It is during the introductory phase that the nurse and patient first meet. One of the nurse's primary concerns is to find out why the patient sought help and if this was voluntary (Table 2-2). Determining the patient's reason directly influences the establishment of mutuality between the nurse and the patient. The reason for seeking help forms the basis of the nursing assessment and helps the nurse to focus on the patient's problem and to determine patient motivation.

Formulating a Contract. The tasks in this phase of the relationship are to (1) establish a climate of trust, understanding, acceptance, and open communication and (2) formulate a contract with the patient. Box 2-4 lists the elements of a nurse-patient contract. The contract begins with the introduction of the nurse and patient, exchange of names, and explanation of roles. An explanation of roles includes the responsibilities and expectations of the patient and nurse, with a description of what the nurse can and cannot do. This is followed by a discussion of the purpose of the relationship, in which the nurse emphasizes that the focus of it will be the patient and the patient's life experiences and areas of conflict. Because establishing the contract is a mutual process, it is a good opportunity to clarify misperceptions held by either the nurse or patient.

With the "who" and the "why" determined, the "where, when, and how long" are discussed. Where will the meetings be held? When and how often will they occur? How long will each be and how long will the series of meetings be? The conditions for termination should be reviewed and may include a specified length of time, attainment of mutual goals, or the discharge of the patient if hospitalized. The issue of confidentiality is an important one to discuss with the patient at this time. Confidentiality involves the disclosure of certain information to another specifically authorized person (see Chapter 8). This means that information about the patient will be shared with people who are directly involved in the patient's care in the form of verbal reports

Table 2-2   Analysis of Why Patients Seek Psychiatric Help

Reasons for patients' seeking psychiatric care	Appropriate nursing approach	Sample response
Environmental change from home to treatment setting: They desire protection, comfort, rest, and freedom from demands of their usual home and work environments.	Emphasis should be placed on ability of environment to provide protection and comfort while healing process of mind occurs.	"Tell me what it was at home/on the job that made you feel so overwhelmed."
Nurturance: They wish for someone to care for them, cure their illnesses, and make them feel better.	Respond by acknowledging their nurturance needs and assuring them that help and caring are available to them.	"I'm here to help you feel better."
Control: They are aware of their destructive impulses to themselves or others but lack internal control.	Offer person sources of internal control such as medication, if prescribed, and reinforce external controls available through services of staff.	"We're not going to let you hurt yourself. Tell us when these thoughts come to mind and someone will stay with you."
Psychiatric symptoms: They describe symptoms of depression, nervousness, or crying spells. They know they need psychiatric help and actively want to help themselves.	Ask for clarification of symptom and strive to understand life experiences of patient.	"I can see that you're nervous and upset. Can you tell me about how things are at home/on the job so I can better understand?"
Problem solving: They identify a specific problem or area of conflict and express desire to reason it out and change.	Help patient look at problem objectively; utilize problem-solving process.	"How has drinking affected your life?"
Advised to seek help: Family member, friend, or health professional has convinced them to get treatment. They may feel angry, ambivalent, or indifferent.	Confirm facts surrounding seeking of help and set appropriate limits.	"I see that you're angry about being here. I hope that after we talk you might feel differently."

Modified from Burgess A, Burns J: *Am J Nurs* 73:314, 1973.

Box 2-4
ELEMENTS OF A NURSE-PATIENT CONTRACT

▼ Names of individuals
▼ Roles of nurse and patient
▼ Responsibilities of nurse and patient
▼ Expectations of nurse and patient
▼ Purpose of the relationship
▼ Meeting location
▼ Time of meetings
▼ Conditions for termination
▼ Confidentiality

---

and written notes. This is important in providing for the continuity and comprehensiveness of patient care and should be clearly explained to the patient.

Establishing a contract is a mutual process in which the patient participates as fully as possible. In some cases, such as with the psychotic or severely withdrawn patient, the patient may be unable to fully participate, and the nurse must take the initiative in establishing the contract. As the patient's contact with reality increases, the nurse should review the elements of the contract when appropriate and strive to attain mutuality.

It is also possible to use a written contracting model to work therapeutically with patients and groups. Loomis[28] describes a formal treatment contract as an openly negotiated, clearly stated set of mutual expectations that indicate what the nurse and patient expect of each other regarding the patient's health care. Such a contract establishes a set of shared objectives as well as an understanding of the structure and process of arriving at mutually determined outcomes. This model identifies four levels of change contracts (see Table 2-3). Each higher level implies the inclusion of all lower level contracts.

Level I, or care contracts, involves provision of physical and emotional safety. Level II, or social contracts, deals primarily with behaviors and situations that can be brought under the patient's conscious control. Level III, or relationship contracts, focuses on the repetitive or cyclical nature of patient problems as shown in their day-to-day relationships. Level IV contracts involve structural change and require intensive psychotherapy.

Table 2-3   Levels of Change Contracts

Level and type of contract	Focus of care	Nursing action
I Care contracts	Physical safety Emotional safety Avoid predictable negative outcomes	Provide physical care Protect from loss of functional abilities Provide safety
II Social control contracts	Self-care activities Problem-solving ability Alteration in time structuring Alteration in reinforcement patterns	Crisis intervention Brief therapy Support social systems Behavioral treatments
III Relationship contracts	Relationship patterns Life-script decisions Traumatic early scenes	Insight work Cognitive restructuring Marital, family, or relationship counseling
IV Structural change contracts	Parental modeling Persistent early injunctions	Script analysis Reparenting work Psychotherapy

Modified from Loomis M: J *Psychosoc Nurs Ment Health Serv* 23:10, 1985.

The emphasis here is on reworking the patient's ego structure, as well as the here-and-now relationship process. Nurse therapists entering into level IV contracts require master's degree preparation and specialized training in the theory and application of structural change treatment approaches. Since the level of contract can change over time, this contracting model allows the nurse and patient to evaluate their progress over time, renegotiate their work together, and determine the termination of a treatment relationship.

Exploring Feelings. Both the nurse and patient may experience some degree of discomfort and nervousness in the introduction phase of the relationship. The nurse may be well aware of personal anxieties and fears, but the patient's difficulty in receiving help may be overlooked:

1. It may be difficult to see or admit one's difficulties, first to oneself and then to another.
2. It is not easy to trust or be open with strangers.
3. Sometimes problems seem too large, too overwhelming, or too unique to share them easily.
4. Sharing personal problems with another person can pose a threat to one's sense of independence, autonomy, and self-esteem.
5. Solving a problem involves thinking about some things that may be unpleasant, viewing life realistically, deciding on a plan of action, and then, most important, carrying out whatever it takes to bring about a change. These activities place great demands on the patient's energy and commitment.

The nursing student's first psychiatric experience may be particularly stressful. Stacklum[45] identified a process that all new students go through in the beginning of their relationships. In the first stage, they experience a moderate to severe level of anxiety characterized by selective inattention to instructions, obsession with detail, dissociation of theory from practice, and avoidance behavior.

Stage two is characterized by the student's use of the defense mechanisms of denial of the patient's problems and strong identification with the patient. Social conversation with the patient predominates, and nursing actions tend to be concrete and simple. In stage three, students question their ability and experience feelings of anger and omnipotence. Hostility often is projected onto the staff.

From these early reactions students hopefully progress to a beginning adjustment stage, which marks the transition into the working phase of the relationship. Students now are truly able to hear what the patient is saying; their anxiety is decreased; their interactions show more depth and insight; and their nursing actions become more realistic. A therapeutic process has begun.

The tasks of the nurse in the orientation phase of the relationship include the following:

1. To explore the patient's perceptions, thoughts, feelings, and actions
2. To identify pertinent patient problems
3. To define mutual, specific goals with the patient

It is not uncommon for patients to display manipulative or testing behavior during this phase as they explore the nurse's consistency and intent. Patients may also show temporary regressions during the sessions as reactions to a large amount of self-disclosure in a previous meeting or to the anxiety created by a particular topic.

Finally, nurses need to be flexible in anticipating the length of time required for the orientation phase, particularly for patients who have a serious and persistent mental illness. Nurses might expect that more time will be required for patients who have had many or lengthy hospitalizations in the past.[14] Also, staff changes affect the patient's ability to progress in the therapeutic relationship and should be taken into account when planning nursing care.

 Talk with a friend or family member who has sought counseling. Why did they do so? What things made them uncomfortable about asking for help? What did the clinician do to put them at ease?

Working Phase

Most of the therapeutic work is carried out during the working phase. The nurse and the patient explore relevant stressors and promote the development of insight in the patient by linking perceptions, thoughts, feelings, and actions. These insights should be translated into action and integrated into the individual's life experiences. The nurse helps the patient to master anxieties, increase independence and self-responsibility, and develop constructive coping mechanisms. Actual behavioral change is the focus of this phase of the relationship.

Patients usually display resistance behaviors during this phase of the relationship because this phase encompasses the greater part of the problem-solving process. As the relationship develops, the patient begins to feel close to the nurse and responds by clinging to defensive structures and resisting the nurse's attempts to move forward. An impasse or plateau in the relationship results. Since overcoming resistance behaviors is crucial to the progress of the therapeutic relationship, these behaviors are discussed in greater detail later in this chapter.

Termination Phase

Termination is one of the most difficult but most important phases of the therapeutic nurse-patient relationship. During the termination phase learning is maximized for both the patient and the nurse. It is a time to exchange feelings and memories and to evaluate mutually the patient's progress and goal attainment. Levels of trust and intimacy are heightened, reflecting the quality of the relationship and the sense of loss experienced by both nurse and patient. Box 2-5 lists criteria identified by Campaniello[6] that can be used to determine whether the patient is ready to terminate.

Although agreement between the patient and the nurse is desirable in deciding when to terminate, this is

---

Box 2-5

CRITERIA FOR DETERMINING PATIENT READINESS FOR TERMINATION

1. The patient experiences relief from the presenting problem.
2. The patient's social function has improved, and isolation has decreased.
3. The patient has strengthened ego functions and attained a sense of identity.
4. The patient employs more effective and productive defense mechanisms.
5. The patient has achieved the planned treatment goals.
6. An impasse has been reached in the therapist-patient relationship because of resistance or countertransference that cannot be worked through.

---

not always possible. Nonetheless, the nurse's tasks during this phase revolve around establishing the reality of the separation. Together the nurse and the patient review the progress made in treatment and the attainment of specified goals. Feelings of rejection, loss, sadness, and anger are expressed and explored. It may be helpful to prepare the patient for termination by decreasing the number of visits, incorporating others into the meetings, or changing the location of the meetings. The reasons behind a change should be clarified so that the patient does not interpret it as rejection by the nurse. It may also be appropriate to make referrals at this time for continued care or treatment.

It is evident that successful termination requires that the patient work through feelings related to separation from emotionally significant people. The nurse can help by allowing the patient to experience and feel the effects of the anticipated loss, to express the feelings generated by the impending separation, and to relate those feelings to former symbolic or real losses.

Reactions to Termination. Patients may react to termination in a variety of ways. They may deny the separation or deny the significance of the relationship and impending separation, perhaps causing the inexperienced nurse to feel rejected by the patient. Patients may express anger and hostility, either overtly and verbally or covertly through lateness, missed meetings, or superficial talk. These patients may view the termination as personal rejection, which reinforces their negative self-concept. Patients who feel rejected by the nurse may terminate prematurely by rejecting the nurse before the nurse rejects them. It is also common to see the patient regress to an earlier behavior pattern, hoping to convince the nurse not to terminate because of the need for further help.

The nurse should be aware of these possible reactions and discuss them with the patient if they occur. For some patients termination is a critical therapeutic experience because many of their past relationships were terminated in a negative way that left them with unresolved feelings of abandonment, rejection, hurt, and anger. All these patient reactions have a similar goal—to cope with the anxiety about the separation and to delay the termination process. Levinson[27] has identified five factors that can influence the patient's reaction to termination (Box 2-6).

The patient's response will be significantly affected by the nurse's ability to remain open, sensitive, empathic, and responsive to the patient's changing needs. Helping the patient to work and grow through the termination process is an essential goal of each relationship. It is important that the nurse does not deny the reality of it or allow the patient to repeatedly delay the process. Particularly in this phase of the relationship, as in the orientation phase, the patient will be testing the nurse's judgment, and the issues of trust and acceptance will again predominate.

During the course of the relationship and with the attainment of nursing goals, the nurse and the patient come to realize a growing sense of equality. The impending termination therefore can be as difficult for the nurse as for the patient. Nurses who can begin reviewing their thoughts, feelings, and experiences will be more aware

of personal motivation and more responsive to patients' needs.

Learning to bear the sorrow of the loss while working positive aspects of the relationship into one's life is the goal of termination for both the nurse and the patient. The major tasks of the nurse during each phase of the nurse-patient relationship are summarized in Table 2-4.

 Watch the movies *The Dream Team* and *Awakenings* and discuss how staff-patient relationships are portrayed.

FACILITATIVE COMMUNICATION

Communication can either facilitate the development of a therapeutic relationship or serve as a barrier to its development. According to Carkhoff and Truax,[10] "The central ingredient of the psychotherapeutic process appears to be the therapist's ability to *perceive and communicate*, ac-

---

Box 2-6

FACTORS THAT INFLUENCE A PATIENT'S REACTION TO TERMINATION

1. The greater the degree of involvement the patient has had in the treatment and with the therapist, the more intense will be the nature of the reaction to termination.
2. Reaction to termination will vary with the degree of success and satisfaction the patient feels with the treatment.
3. The greater the degree of transference involvement and wished-for gratification or fulfillment of childlike wishes, the more intense will be the nature of the patient's reaction to termination.
4. Patients who have sustained earlier losses of significant persons in their lives will reexperience, as termination approaches, the arousal of affects and conflicts from those earlier periods.
5. Whether the patient has experienced key losses or not, the reaction to termination will be influenced by the level at which the patient has mastered the early separation-individuation crisis.

Table 2-4   Nurse's Tasks in Each Phase of the Relationship Process

Phase	Task
Preinteraction	Explore own feelings, fantasies, and fears
	Analyze own professional strengths and limitations
	Gather data about patient when possible
	Plan for first meeting with patient
Introductory, or orientation	Determine why patient sought help
	Establish trust, acceptance, and open communication
	Mutually formulate a contract
	Explore patient's thoughts, feelings, and actions
	Identify patient's problems
	Define goals with patient
Working	Explore relevant stressors
	Promote patient's development of insight and use of constructive coping mechanisms
	Overcome resistance behaviors
Termination	Establish reality of separation
	Review progress of therapy and attainment of goals
	Mutually explore feelings of rejection, loss, sadness, and anger and related behaviors

curately and with sensitivity, the feelings of the patient and the meaning of those feelings."

Every individual communicates constantly from birth until death.[64] All behavior is communication, and all communication affects behavior. This reciprocity is central to the communication process. The relevance of communication to nursing practice is threefold:

1. Communication is the vehicle for establishing a therapeutic relationship.
2. Communication is the means by which people influence the behavior of another and thus is critical to the successful outcome of nursing intervention.
3. Communication is the relationship itself, since without it, a therapeutic nurse-patient relationship is impossible.

Verbal Communication

Communication takes place on two levels, verbal and nonverbal. Verbal communication occurs through words, spoken or written. Taken alone, verbal communication can convey factual information accurately and efficiently. It is a less effective means of communicating feelings or nuances of meaning, and it represents only a small segment of total human communication.

Another limitation of verbal communication is that words can change meanings with different cultural groups or subgroups because words have both denotative and connotative meanings. The denotative meaning of a word is the concrete representation of it. For example, the denotative meaning of the word "bread" is "a food made of a flour or grain dough that is kneaded, shaped, allowed to rise, and baked." The connotative meaning of a word, in contrast, is its implied or suggested meaning. Thus the word "bread" can conjure up many different connotative or personalized meanings. Depending on a person's experiences, preferences, and present frame of reference, he may think of French bread, rye bread, a sesame seed roll, or perhaps pita bread. When used as slang, "give me some bread" may be understood to mean "give me some money." Thus the characteristics of the speaker and the context in which the phrase is used influence the specific meaning of verbal language.

When communicating verbally, many people assume that they are "on the same wavelength" as the listener. But since words are only symbols, they seldom mean precisely the same thing to two people. And if the word represents an abstract idea such as "depressed" or "hurt," the chance of misunderstanding or misinterpretation may be great. In addition, many feeling states or personal thoughts cannot be put into words easily. Nurses should strive to overcome these obstacles by checking their interpretation and incorporating information from the nonverbal level as well.

Finally, today more than ever before nurses need to be prepared to communicate effectively with people from a variety of ethnocultural backgrounds. Sensitivity to two language phenomena may help the psychiatric nurse to establish transcultural psychotherapeutic relationships based on mutual understanding. These are detachment effect and code switching.[12] The detachment effect refers to individuals who have a limited ability to express affect and to report early development events because they speak more than one language. Thus events that may have occurred before a person learned English or those that have a strong emotional component may not be easily communicated in English. In contrast, code switching refers to an individual who transfers values associated with one context to another situation. An example of this is inserting a cultural dialect into a conversation that may mark an affective change in the message.

The effective psychiatric nurse uses verbal communication sensitively as a tool to promote mutual respect based on understanding and acceptance of cultural differences. The nurse may also communicate respect for the patient's dialect by adapting slightly to the patient's linguistic style, such as by using fewer words, more gestures, or more expressive facial behaviors.

Nonverbal Communication

Nonverbal communication includes everything that does not involve the spoken or written word, including all of the five senses. It has been estimated that about 7% of meaning is transmitted by words, 38% is transmitted by paralinguistic cues such as voice, and 55% is transmitted by body cues.[32] Nonverbal communication is often unconsciously motivated and may more accurately indicate a person's meaning than the words being spoken. People tend to verbalize what they think the receiver wants to hear, whereas less acceptable or more honest messages may be communicated simultaneously by the nonverbal route.

Types of Nonverbal Behaviors. Various types of nonverbal behaviors have been identified. Each of these is greatly influenced by sociocultural background. Following are brief descriptions of five categories of nonverbal communication.

Vocal cues, or paralinguistic cues, include all the noises and sounds that are extraspeech sounds. Some examples include pitch, tone of voice, quality of voice, loudness or intensity, rate and rhythm of talking, and unrelated nonverbal sounds such as laughing, groaning, and nervous coughing and sounds of hesitation ("um," "uh"). These are particularly vital cues of emotion and can be powerful conveyors of information.

Action cues are body movements, sometimes referred to as kinetics. They include automatic reflexes, posture, facial expression, gestures, mannerisms, and actions of any kind. Facial movements and posture can be particularly significant in interpreting the speaker's mood.

Object cues are the speaker's intentional and non-intentional use of all objects. Dress, furnishings, and possessions all communicate something to the observer about the speaker's sense of self. These cues often are consciously selected by the individual, however, and therefore may be chosen to convey a certain "look" or message. Thus they can be less accurate than other types of nonverbal communication.

Space provides another clue to the nature of the relationship between two people. It must be examined based on sociocultural norms and customs. Hall[18] extensively researched the use of space between communicators, and identified the following four zones of space that are demonstrated interpersonally in North America:
1. Intimate space—up to 45.5 cm (18 inches). This allows for maximum interpersonal sensory stimulation.
2. Personal space—45.5 to 120 cm (18 inches to 4 feet). This is used for close relationships and touching distance. Visual sensation is improved over the intimate range.
3. Social-consultative space—270 to 360 cm (9 to 12 feet). This is less personal and less dependent. Speech must be louder.
4. Public space—360 cm (12 feet) and over. This is used in speech giving and other public occasions.

Observation of seating arrangements and use of space by patients can yield valuable information to the nurse, with implications for both the nurse's assessment of the patient and the way the nursing intervention should be implemented.

Touch involves both personal space and action. It is possibly the most personal of the nonverbal messages. A person's response to it is influenced by setting, cultural background, type of relationship, sex of communicators, ages, and expectations. Touch can express a striving to connect with another person as a way of meeting them or relating to them. It can be a way of expressing or conveying something to another, such as concern, empathy, or caring. Touch can also be used receptively as a way of sensing, perceiving, or allowing someone else to leave an imprint on another person. Finally, Krieger[25] has developed the concept of "therapeutic touch," or the nurse's laying hands on or close to the body of an ill person for the purpose of helping or healing. Krieger believes touch to be the imprimatur

of nursing and contends that the therapeutic, comforting effects of touch often have been overlooked.

Touch is a universal and basic aspect of all nurse-patient relationships. It is often described as the first and most fundamental means of communication. Nevertheless, relatively little is really known about touch as it relates to health.[50]

Interpreting Nonverbal Behavior. All types of nonverbal messages are important, but interpreting them correctly can present numerous problems for the nurse. It is impossible to examine nonverbal messages out of context, and sometimes the individual's body reveals a number of different and perhaps conflicting feelings at the same time.

Sociocultural background is also a major influence on the meaning of nonverbal behavior. In the United States, with its diverse ethnic communities, messages between people of different upbringing can easily be misinterpreted. For instance, Arabs tend to stand closer together when speaking, and Orientals tend to touch more; touching in the United States is often minimized because of perceived sexual overtones or because of Puritan heritage. Because the meaning attached to nonverbal behavior is so subjective, it is essential that the nurse check its meaning.

Nurses should respond to the variety of nonverbal behaviors displayed by the patient, particularly voice inflections, body movements, gestures, facial expression, posture, and physical energy levels. Incongruent behavior or contradictory messages are especially significant. The nurse should refer to the specific behavior observed and attempt to confirm its meaning and significance with the patient. If the nurse's words and tone of voice indicate a true attempt at clarification, suggestion, or validation, a defensive reaction usually is not evoked. The nurse may use three kinds of responses to the patient:
1. Questions or statements intended to increase the patient's awareness
2. Content reflections
3. Statements reflecting the nurse's responsiveness

These possible responses are illustrated in the following interaction.

PATIENT: (Shifting nervously in his chair, eyes scanning the room and avoiding the nurse) What . . . what do you want to talk about today?

NURSE RESPONSE #1: I sense that you are uncomfortable talking to me. Could you describe to me how you are feeling?

NURSE RESPONSE #2: You're not sure what we should be talking about, and you want me to start us off?

NURSE RESPONSE #3: You look very nervous, and I can feel those same feelings in me as I sit here with you.

The nurse's first possible response is a reflection and attempt to validate the patient's feelings. The purpose is to communicate to the patient the nurse's awareness of his feelings, to show acceptance of those feelings, and to request that he focus on them and elaborate on them. The nurse's second possible response deals with the content of the patient's message. The nurse is clarifying what the patient is trying to say. The third possible response shares both the nurse's perception of her patient's feelings and the personal disclosure that she has some of those same feelings. This type of response may help the patient feel that the nurse accepts and understands him.

Implications for Nursing Care. Besides responding to patients' nonverbal behavior, nurses should incorporate aspects of it into patient care. For example, patients who resist closeness will be disturbed by entry into their intimate space. The nurse can assess the patient's level of spatial tolerance by observing the distance the patient maintains with other people. The nurse can also be alert to the patient's response during their interaction. If the nurse sits next to the patient on the sofa, does the patient get up and move to a chair? If the nurse moves closer to the patient does the patient move away to reestablish the original space? Sometimes increasing the space between the nurse and an anxious patient can reduce the anxiety enough to allow the interaction to continue. A decrease in the distance the patient chooses to maintain from others may indicate a decrease in interpersonal anxiety.

Territoriality is a concept related to those of personal distance and personal space. Territoriality is the drive to acquire and defend territory to ensure species' survival. Whenever possible, the hospitalized patient should be allowed to control and enjoy personal possessions and private living space, no matter how small or seemingly insignificant. Specifically, patients should be allowed free access to their personal living quarters and, as soon as possible, free access out of doors or at least off the unit itself. Patients can also be encouraged to wear personal clothing and keep personal items.

Other spatial parameters are also interpersonally significant.[2] Height may communicate dominance and submission. Communication is made easier when both participants are at similar levels. Orientation of the participants' body positions is also significant. Face-to-face confrontation is more threatening than oblique (sideways) body positions. The physical setting also has spatial meaning. A patient may be more comfortable in his own room than in the therapist's office, unless the patient's room is also defined as bedroom. Control issues are minimized when communication takes place in a neutral area that belongs to neither participant. However, people quickly identify their own turf, even in unfamiliar settings, and then begin to exert ownership rights over this area. A common example of this can be observed in most college classes. At the beginning of the semester, people sit randomly, but the arrangement usually solidifies after a couple of classes. Students then feel vaguely annoyed if they arrive in class to find another person in "their seat." They are experiencing an invasion of personal space. Awareness of a patient's use of space can add a further dimension to the nurse's ability to understand the patient.

Touch also should be used judiciously. Patients who are sensitive to issues of closeness may experience a casual touch as an invasion or an invitation to intimacy, which may be even more frightening. Physical contact with a person of the same sex may be experienced by the patient as a homosexual advance and may precipitate a panic reaction. If procedures requiring physical contact must be carried out, careful explanations should be given both before and during the procedure. In addition, the nurse should always be aware of the potential for touch to be interpreted in a sexual way, thus creating problems related to the sexual conduct of the nurse within the nurse-patient relationship.

In spite of these issues, a study on the use of nonprocedural touch shows that it is a significant part of inpatient psychiatric nursing.[48] The researcher found that several elements went into the nurse's decision to touch a patient, such as the patient's age, gender, and needs and the nurse's knowledge of the patient. The nurse's feelings, beliefs, intuition, personal style, and expectations of the nursing role were also considered. Patient needs identified by the nurses included the following:
▼ Establishing contact with the patient
▼ Enhancing communication
▼ Communicating caring, interest, and recognition
▼ Providing reassurance and comfort

Results of this study indicate that touch is a part of psychiatric nursing practice and suggest the importance of studying patients' perceptions of its use and potential benefits and drawbacks.

Finally, nurses must be aware of not only patients' nonverbal cues but also of their own. The nurse's nonverbal cues can communicate interest, respect, and genuineness or disinterest, lack of respect, and an impersonal facade. La Crosse[26] did a study of nonverbal behaviors to determine which promoted relating to someone else and which prohibited it. He concluded that affiliative nonverbal behavior included smiles, positive head nods, gestures, 80% eye contact, and a 20% forward body lean. Unaffiliative nonverbal behavior included 40% eye contact, a 20% reclining body lean, and none of the other categories. Furthermore, affiliative counselors were perceived to be more attractive and persuasive than unaffiliative ones. Nurses, as therapeutic helpers, need to be aware of a spectrum of nonverbal behaviors in their patients and themselves and then incorporate them judiciously into their care.

Follow the treatment team making patient rounds and observe body positions. Are staff and patients at eye level? What personal space is maintained? Is touch used at all?

The Communication Process

Human communication is a dynamic process influenced by the psychological and physiological conditions of the participants. Ruesch[42] has identified three elements of the process: perception, evaluation, and transmission. *Perception* occurs by activation of the sensory end organs of the receiver. The impulse is then transmitted to the brain. Human beings are most reliant on visual and auditory stimuli for communications. Vision is the primary means of perceiving nonverbal communication, and hearing primarily responds to verbal stimuli. However, if one of the primary senses is dysfunctional, the other functional senses accommodate to improve the person's perception. For instance, the deaf person can learn sign language and lip-reading, which rely on vision, to compensate for not being able to hear the verbal component of communication.

When the sensory impulse reaches the brain, *evaluation* takes place. Personal experience is the matrix within which new experience is evaluated. If the person encounters a new experience for which there is no frame of reference, confusion results. Evaluation results in two responses: a cognitive response related to the informational aspect of the message, and an affective response related to the relationship aspect of the message. Most messages stimulate both types of responses.

When the evaluation of the message is complete, *transmission* takes place. This is perceived by the sender as feedback, thereby influencing the continued course of the communication cycle. It is impossible not to transmit some kind of feedback. Even lack of any visible response is feedback to the sender that the message did not get through, was considered unimportant, or was an undesirable interruption. Feedback stimulates perception, evaluation, and transmission by the original sender. The cycle continues until the participants agree to end it or one participant physically leaves the setting.

Theoretical models of the communication process show visual relationships more clearly and can aid in finding and correcting communication breakdowns or problems. Two models, the structural and transactional analysis models, are presented, since each gives a valuable but different perspective on the communication process.

Structural Model. The structural model has five functional components in communication: the sender, the message, the receiver, the feedback, and the context (Fig. 2-4). The **sender** is the originator of the message. The **message** is the information that is transmitted from the sender to the receiver. The **receiver** is the perceiver of the message. The verbal or behavioral response of the receiver is **feedback** to the sender. The fifth structural element of communication is the **context.** This is the setting in which the communication takes place. Knowledge of context is necessary to understand the meaning of the communication. For example, the phrase "I don't understand what you mean" may have different meanings in the context of a classroom or a courtroom. Context involves more than the physical setting for communication, however. It also includes the psychosocial setting, which includes the relationship between the sender and the receiver, their past experiences with each other, and past experiences with similar situations, and cultural values and norms. Consider again the meaning of "I don't understand what you mean" in the following contexts: two college students discussing a philosophy assignment, a wife responding to her husband's accusation of infidelity, and a Japanese tourist asking directions in San Francisco. Although the content of the message is the same, its meaning is different, depending on the context in which the communication takes place.

In the evaluation of the communication process with regard to the five structural elements, specific problems or potential errors become evident (Table 2-5). If the sender is communicating the same message on both the verbal and nonverbal levels, then the communication is termed **congruent.** If, however, the levels are not in agreement, the communication is termed **incongruent,** which can be problematic.

 CONGRUENT COMMUNICATION

VERBAL LEVEL: I'm pleased to see you.
NONVERBAL LEVEL: Voice sounds warm; continuous eye contact maintained; smile.

 INCONGRUENT COMMUNICATION

VERBAL LEVEL: I'm pleased to see you.
NONVERBAL LEVEL: Voice sounds cold and distant; eye contact avoided; neutral facial expression.

Incongruent, or double-level, messages produce a dilemma for the listener, who does not know to which level

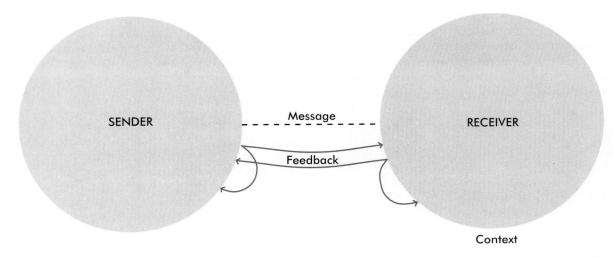

Fig. 2-4 Components of communication.

Table 2-5 Problems with the Structural Elements of the Communication Process

Structural element	Communication problem	Definition
Sender	Incongruent communication	Lack of agreement between the verbal and nonverbal levels of communication
	Inflexible communication	Exaggerated control or permissiveness by the sender
Message	Ineffective messages	Messages that are not goal directed or purposeful
	Inappropriate messages	Messages not relevant to the progress of the relationship
	Inadequate messages	Messages that lack a sufficient amount of information
	Inefficient messages	Messages that lack clarity, simplicity, and directness
Receiver	Errors of perception	Various forms of listening problems
	Errors of evaluation	Misinterpretation due to personal beliefs and values
Feedback	Misinformation	Communication of incorrect information
	Lack of validation	Failure to clarify and ratify understanding of the message
Context	Constraints of physical setting	Noise, temperature, or various distractions
	Constraints of psychosocial setting	Impaired previous relationship between the communicators

to respond, the verbal or nonverbal. Since both levels cannot be responded to, the listener is likely to feel frustrated, angry, or confused. Obviously, both patients and nurses can display incongruent communication if they are not aware of their internal feeling states and the nature of their communication.

Another problem initiated by the sender is inflexible communication that is either too rigid or too permissive. A rigid approach by the nurse does not allow for spontaneous expression by the patient, nor does it allow the patient to contribute to the flow or direction of the interaction. Exaggerated permissiveness, on the other hand, refers to the lack of a direction and mutuality in the interaction established by the nurse. The pa-

tient may interpret the nurse's behavior as lack of interest or incompetence.

The message of the communication process can also pose problems. Messages can be ineffective, inappropriate, inadequate, or inefficient. Ineffective messages serve at least to distract and at most to prevent the objectives of the nurse-patient relationship from being met. Inappropriate messages are not relevant to the progress of the relationship. They may include failures in timing, stereotyping the receiver, or overlooking important information. Inadequate messages lack sufficient information. In this case, senders assume that receivers know more than they actually do. Inefficient messages lack clarity, simplicity, and directness. Using more energy than is necessary, these messages confuse or complicate the information.

The third element, the receiver, may experience errors of perception. The receiver may miss nonverbal cues, respond only to content and ignore messages of affect, be selectively inattentive to the speaker's message because of physical or psychological discomfort, be preoccupied with other thoughts, or have a physiological hearing impairment. These errors are problems of listening. The receiver may also have problems in evaluating the message. The meaning of the message may be misinterpreted because the receiver views it in terms of the receiver's value system rather than that of the speaker.

Errors in the feedback element include all of those that apply to the message. Feedback can also convey to the sender incorrect information about the message. Another serious error exists when the receiver fails to use feedback to validate understanding of the message. Although feedback is the last step, it has the potential for correcting previous errors and clarifying the nature of the communication.

The fifth element of context can also contribute to communication problems. The setting may be physically noisy, cold, or distracting to one or both parties. So, too, the psychosocial context, or past relationship between the communicators, may be one of mistrust or harbored resentment. This analysis shows the complexity of the communication process. It may seem surprising that successful communication can occur, given all of these vulnerable areas. However, it can and does occur among people who understand the process and use appropriate techniques.

Transactional Analysis Model. Transactional analysis (TA) is the study of the communication or transactions that take place between people; it uncovers the sometimes unconscious and destructive ways ("games") in which people relate to each other. This approach to personality was developed by Berne, a psychiatrist who made transactional analysis a popular theory through his book, *Games People Play: The Psychology of Human Relationships.*[3] It is a method of therapy, as well as a model of communication.

The cornerstone of Berne's theory is that each person's personality is made up of three distinct components called **ego states.** An ego state is a consistent pattern of feeling, experiencing, and behaving. The three ego states that make up personality are the parent ego state (parent), adult ego state (adult), and child ego state (child) (Fig. 2-5). It is as though three "people" reside in each person; the "parent" incorporates all the attitudes and behaviors the individual was taught (directly or indirectly) by parents; the "child" contains all the feelings the individual had as a child; and the "adult" deals

with reality in a logical, rational, computer-like manner.

The parent and child ego states are made up of the feelings, attitudes, and behaviors that are remnants of the past but can be reexperienced under certain conditions. The parent ego state consists of all the nurturing, critical, and prejudicial attitudes, behaviors, and experiences learned from other people, especially parents and teachers. The adult ego state is the reality-oriented part of the personality. It gathers and processes information about the world and is objective, emotionless, and intelligent in its approach to problem solving. The child ego state is the feeling part of the personality. In it resides feelings of happiness, joy, sadness, depression, and anxiety.

Berne's model of communication makes it possible to diagram transactions using these ego states. A transaction or communication between two people can be complementary, crossed, or ulterior. In a **complementary transaction** (Fig. 2-6), the arrows in the ego state diagram are parallel, and the communication flows smoothly.

 COMPLEMENTARY TRANSACTION

PATIENT: I know that when I get mad at my boss, I take it out on my wife and kids.

NURSE: Are you ready to think about some other ways you can handle your anger?

If the arrows in the ego state diagram **cross,** however, communication breaks down (Fig. 2-7).

 CROSSED TRANSACTION

PATIENT: I know that when I get mad at my boss, I take it out on my wife and kids.

NURSE: Men always think that's okay, but the women have to suffer for it.

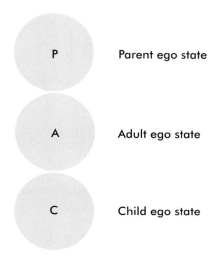

P — Parent ego state

A — Adult ego state

C — Child ego state

Fig. 2-5   Three ego states as described by Berne's theory of transactional analysis.

Patient   Nurse

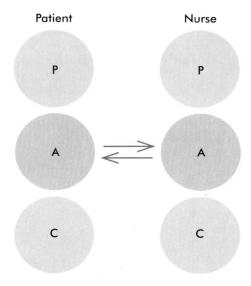

Fig. 2-6   Diagram of complementary transaction.

Patient   Nurse

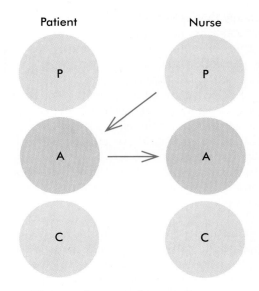

Fig. 2-7   Diagram of a crossed transaction.

The third type of transaction is **ulterior** transaction (Fig. 2-8). It takes place on two levels: the social, or overt, level and the psychological, or covert, level. These transactions tend to be destructive, because the communicators conceal their true motivations. One of the best known examples of this is the "Why Don't You . . . Yes But" (WDYYB) game. This game involves one person asking for a solution to a problem; however, every suggested solution is negated, until the helper is silenced. On the surface, the interaction is two adults problem solving; in reality, one person is using the child ego state to show what a bad parent the other person is.

 ULTERIOR TRANSACTION

PATIENT: I know that when I get mad at my boss, I take it out on my wife and kids, but I don't know what else to do.
NURSE: Do you think you could let your boss know how you're feeling?
PATIENT: He'll fire me for sure.
NURSE: Perhaps you could talk it over with someone you work with.
PATIENT: I don't have time to chat on the job like that. Besides, no one cares about someone else's beefs.
NURSE: Sometimes physical exercise helps people get rid of their anger. Have you ever tried it?
PATIENT: Sure. I work out a lot, but it doesn't help.
NURSE: Perhaps you can explain all this to your family.
PATIENT: My wife's tired of "all my talk" as she puts it. She says she wants some action.

The transactional analysis model of communication provides a framework for the nurse to use in

Patient   Nurse

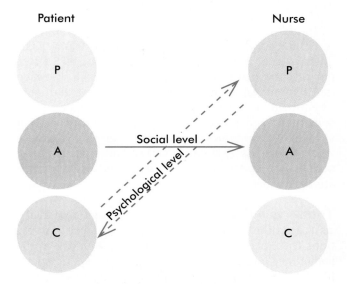

Fig. 2-8   Diagram of an ulterior transaction.

exploring the patient's recurrent behaviors, identifying patterns, postulating causes, and planning alternative ways to respond. Thus nonproductive communication patterns can be stopped and new, healthier, ones learned.

 Using the transactional analysis model, diagram a recent conversation you have had with a friend, your instructor, and a patient.

Therapeutic Communication Techniques

There are two basic requirements for effective communication:

1. All communication must be aimed at preserving the self-respect of both the helper and the helpee
2. The communication of understanding should precede any suggestions of information or advice giving

These requirements for therapeutic communication make the formation of the nurse-patient relationship and the implementation of the nursing process possible. The collection of data and the planning, implementation, and evaluation activities are carried out *with* the patient, not *for* the patient, when the nurse uses therapeutic communication skills.

Some nurses reject the notion of therapeutic communication techniques because they view them as unnatural, ineffective, or stereotypical. Although simple on the surface, these techniques are difficult and require practice and conscious thought to master. Because they are techniques, they are only as effective as the person using them. If they are worked into existing interpersonal skills, they can enhance the nurse's effectiveness. If they are used as automatic responses and are inappropriate to the nurse's manner of personal expression, they will negate both the nurse's and the patient's individuality and divest them of their dignity.

To ensure that the nurse is using these skills appropriately and effectively, the nurse needs to record interactions with the patient in some way and then analyze them. The nurse should also seek feedback from others. The nurse can benefit from maintaining a diary of thoughts, feelings, and impressions in relation to clinical work. This can prove valuable in working through difficult aspects of termination or counter-transference reactions.

The nurse may decide to tape record or videotape interactions with the patient. These are two of the most informative recording methods, and they also allow the nurse the freedom to concentrate on the patient. However, they do present problems. Sometimes another person is needed to operate the equipment; there is always the possibility of equipment failure; equipment can be expensive to obtain and operate and may be prohibited by the agency; and such equipment can raise questions about confidentiality.

Handwritten records are less expensive and do not require mechanical devices. They also allow the nurse to record thoughts and feelings along with the verbal and nonverbal behavior. However, they require more time and energy. If such records are written in the patient's presence, they can be very distracting. If they are written afterward, some aspects of the interaction

may be unconsciously forgotten or consciously ignored. Often these are significant omissions.

The advantages and disadvantages of the various methods of recording nurse-patient interactions must be considered, along with the nurse's and patient's preferences, before deciding on a particular method. Some form of recording that is as objective and comprehensive as possible is necessary. Only by analyzing the interaction can the nurse evaluate the degree of success in using therapeutic communication techniques.[47] Some of the more helpful techniques will now be described.

Listening. Listening is essential if the nurse is to reach any understanding of the patient. The only person who can tell the nurse about the patient's feelings, thoughts, and perception of the self in the world is the patient. Therefore the first rule of a therapeutic relationship is to listen to the patient. It is the foundation on which all other therapeutic skills are built.

Inexperienced nurses often find it difficult not to talk. This may be caused by their anxiety, the need to prove themselves, or their usual way of social interaction. It is helpful to remember that the patient should be talking more than the nurse during the interaction; the task of the nurse is to listen.

Real listening is difficult. It is an active, not a passive, process. The nurse should give complete attention to the patient and should not be preoccupied. The nurse should suspend thinking of personal experiences and problems and personal judgments of the patient. Listening is a sign of respect for the patient and is a powerful reinforcer. It reinforces verbalization by the patient, without which the relationship could not progress.[23]

Broad Openings. Broad openings such as "What are you thinking about?," "Can you tell me more about that?," and "What shall we discuss today?" confirm the presence of the patient and encourage the patient to select topics to discuss. They can also indicate that the nurse is there, listening to and following the patient. Also serving in this way are acceptance responses such as "I understand," "And then what happened?," "Uh huh," or "I follow you."

Restating. Restating is the nurse's repeating of the main thought the patient has expressed. It, too, indicates that the nurse is listening. Sometimes only a part of the patient's statement is repeated. This technique can serve as a reinforcer or bring attention to something important that might otherwise have been passed over.

Clarification. Clarification occurs when the nurse attempts to put into words vague ideas or thoughts that are implicit or explicit in the patient's talking. It is necessary because statements about emotions and behaviors are rarely straightforward. The patient's verbalizations, especially if the patient is upset or is overwhelmed with feelings, are not always clear and obvious. Nothing should be allowed to pass that the nurse does not hear or understand. Because of this uncertainty, clarification responses often are tentative or phrased as questions such as "I'm not sure what you mean. Are you saying that . . .?" or "Could you go over that again?" This technique is important because two functions of the nurse-patient relationship are to help clarify feelings, ideas, and perceptions and to provide an explicit correlation between them and the patient's actions.

Reflection. **Reflection of content** is also called validation; it lets the patient know that the nurse has heard what was said and understands the content. It consists of repeating in fewer and fresher words the essential ideas of the patient and is like paraphrasing. Sometimes it helps to repeat a patient's statement, emphasizing a key word.

PATIENT: When I walked into the room, I felt like I was going to faint. I knew I had tried to do too much too quickly, and I just wasn't ready for it.
NURSE: You thought you were ready to put yourself to the test, but when you got there, you realized it was too much too soon.

Reflection of feelings consists of responses to the patient's feelings about the content. These responses let the patient know that the nurse is aware of what the patient is feeling. Broad openings, restatements, clarifications, and reflections of content need not represent empathic understanding. But reflection of feeling signifies understanding, empathy, interest, and respect for the patient. It increases the level of involvement between the nurse and patient.

The purpose of reflecting feelings is to focus on feeling rather than content to bring the patient's vaguely expressed feelings into clear awareness; it helps the patient accept or "own" those feelings. The steps in reflection of feelings are to determine what feelings the patient is expressing, describe these feelings clearly, observe the effect, and judge by the patient's reaction whether the reflection was correct. Sometimes even inaccurate reflections can be useful because the patient may correct the nurse and state feelings more clearly.

Although reflecting techniques are some of the most useful, the nurse can also use them incorrectly. One common error is stereotyping of responses; that is, the nurse begins reflections in the same monotonous way,

such as "You think" or "You feel." A second error is in timing. Reflecting back almost everything the patient says provokes feelings of irritation, anger, and frustration in the patient because the nurse appears to be insincere and fails to be therapeutic. Other nurses may have trouble interrupting patients who continue talking in long monologues. Not only is it difficult to capture a feeling after it has passed, but also the nurse is failing to be a responsible, active partner in the relationship. Interruptions may at times be productive and necessary. Another error is inappropriate depth of feeling. The nurse fails by being either too superficial or too deep in assessing the patient's feelings. The final error is use of language that is inappropriate to the patient's sociocultural experience and educational level. Effective language is language that is natural to the nurse and readily understood by the patient.

Focusing. Focusing helps the patient expand on a topic of importance. Effectively used, it can help the patient become more specific, move from vagueness to clarity, and focus on reality.

By avoiding abstractions and generalizations, focusing helps the patient face problems and analyze them in detail. It helps a patient talk about life experiences or problem areas and accept the responsibility for improving them. If the goal is to change thoughts, feelings, or beliefs, the patient must first identify and own them.

PATIENT: Women always get put down. It's as if we don't count at all.
NURSE: Tell me how *you* feel as a woman.

Encouraging a description of the patient's perceptions, encouraging comparisons, and placing events in time sequence are focusing techniques that promote specificity and problem analysis.

Sharing Perceptions. Sharing perceptions involves asking the patient to verify the nurse's understanding of what the patient is thinking or feeling. The nurse can ask for feedback from the patient while possibly providing new information. Perception checking can consist of paraphrasing what the patient is saying or doing, asking the patient to confirm the nurse's understanding, and allowing the patient to correct that perception if necessary. "You seem to be very irritated with me. Am I right about that?" Perception checking can also note the implied feelings of nonverbal language. It is best to describe the observed behavior first and then reflect on its meaning. "You say you really care about her, but every time you talk about her, you clench your fists. I wonder if you don't feel betrayed by her?" Perception check-

ing is also a way to explore incongruent or double-blind communication. "You're smiling, but I sense that you're really angry with me." Perception checking conveys understanding to the patient and clears up confusing communication.

Theme Identification. Themes are underlying issues or problems experienced by the patient that emerge repeatedly during the course of the nurse-patient relationship. Once the nurse has identified the patient's basic themes, he or she can better decide which of the patient's many feelings, thoughts, and beliefs to respond to and pursue. Important themes tend to be repeated throughout the relationship. They can relate to feelings (depression or anxiety), behavior (rebelling against authority or withdrawal), experiences (being loved, hurt, or raped), or combinations of all three.

Silence. Silence on the part of the nurse has varying effects, depending on how the patient perceives it. To a vocal patient, silence on the part of the nurse may be welcome, as long as the patient knows the nurse is listening. When patients pause, they often expect and want the nurse to respond. If the nurse does not, patients may perceive this as rejection, hostility, or disinterest. With a depressed or withdrawn patient, the nurse's silence may convey support, understanding, and acceptance. In this case verbalization by the nurse may be perceived as pressure or frustration.

Silence can prompt the patient to talk. Some introverted people find out that they can be quiet but still be liked. Silence allows the patient time to think and to gain insights. Finally, silence can slow the pace of the interaction. In general, the nurse should allow the patient to break a silence, particularly when the patient has introduced it. Obviously, sensitivity is called for in this regard, and silence should not develop into a contest. However, if the nurse is unsure how to respond to a patient's comments, a safe approach is to maintain silence. If the nurse's nonverbal behavior communicates interest and involvement, the patient often will elaborate or discuss a related issue.

As a general technique, direct questioning has limited usefulness in the therapeutic relationship. Repetitive questioning takes on the tone of an interrogation and negates the element of mutuality. "Why" questions are particularly ineffective and are to be avoided, as are questions that can be answered yes or no. One consequence of it is that patients do not take the initiative and are discouraged or prevented from engaging in the process of exploration.

Humor. Humor is a basic part of the personality and has a place within the therapeutic relationship.[5,13,37,39]

As a part of interpersonal relationships, it is a constructive coping behavior. By learning to express humor, a patient may be able to learn to express other feelings. As a planned approach to nursing intervention, humor can promote insight by making conscious repressed material. A change in the expression of humor and the quality of interpersonal relationships may be indicators of significant change in the patient.

Humor can serve many functions within the nurse-patient relationship (Box 2-7). These can be either positive or negative. There are no rules for determining how, when, or where humor should be used in the therapeutic relationship. It depends on the nature and quality of the relationship, the patient's receptivity to such themes, and the relevance of the tale or witticism. Some occasions when the use of humor may be of therapeutic value include the following:

1. When the patient is experiencing mild to moderate levels of anxiety and humor serves as a tension reducer. It is inappropriate if a patient has severe or panic anxiety levels.
2. When it helps a patient cope more effectively, facilitates learning, puts life situations in perspective, decreases social distance, and is understood by the patient for its therapeutic value. It is inappropriate when it promotes maladaptive coping responses, masks feelings, increases social distance, and helps the individual avoid dealing with difficult situations.
3. When it is consistent with the social and cultural values of the patient and when it allows the patient to laugh at life, the human situation, or a particular set of stressors. It is inappropriate when it violates a patient's values, ridicules people, or belittles others.

The nurse must also be aware of the dangerous ways it can be used to hide conflicts, ward off anxiety, manipulate the patient, and serve the nurse's own need to be liked and admired. If it is used indiscriminately, humor meets only the nurse's needs and may be destructive to the relationship and frightening to the patient.

Box 2-7
FUNCTIONS OF HUMOR

Establishes relationships	Expresses emotion
Stress and tension reduction	Facilitates learning
Promotes social closeness	Reinforces self-concept
Provides social control	Voices social conflict
Cognitive reframing	Conflict avoidance
Reflects social change	Facilitates enculturation
Provides perspective	Instills hope

Box 2-8

THERAPEUTIC COMMUNICATION TECHNIQUES

Technique: LISTENING

Definition: An active process of receiving information and examining reaction to the messages received

Example: Maintaining eye contact and receptive nonverbal communication

Therapeutic value: Nonverbally communicates to the patient the nurse's interest and acceptance

Nontherapeutic threat: Failure to listen

Technique: BROAD OPENINGS

Definition: Encouraging the patient to select topics for discussion

Example: "What are you thinking about?"

Therapeutic value: Indicates acceptance by the nurse and the value of the patient's initiative

Nontherapeutic threat: Domination of the interaction by the nurse; rejecting responses

Technique: RESTATING

Definition: Repeating the main thought the patient expressed

Example: "You say that your mother left you when you were 5 years old."

Therapeutic value: Indicates that the nurse is listening and validates, reinforces, or calls attention to something important that has been said

Nontherapeutic threat: Lack of validation of the nurse's interpretation of the message; being judgmental; reassuring; defending

Technique: CLARIFICATION

Definition: Attempting to put into words vague ideas or unclear thoughts of the patient to enhance the nurse's understanding or asking the patient to explain what he means

Example: "I'm not sure what you mean. Could you tell me about that again?"

Therapeutic value: Helps to clarify feelings, ideas, and perceptions of the patient and provide an explicit correlation between them and the patient's actions

Nontherapeutic threat: Failure to probe; assumed understanding

Technique: REFLECTION

Definition: Directing back the patient's ideas, feelings, questions, and content

Example: "You're feeling tense and anxious and it's related to a conversation you had with your husband last night?"

Therapeutic value: Validates the nurse's understanding of what the patient is saying and signifies empathy, interest, and respect for the patient

Nontherapeutic threat: Stereotyping the patient's responses; inappropriate timing of reflections; inappropriate depth of feeling of the reflections; inappropriate to the cultural experience and educational level of the patient

Technique: HUMOR

Definition: The discharge of energy through the comic enjoyment of the imperfect

Example: "That gives a whole new meaning to the word *nervous*," said with shared kidding between the nurse and patient

Therapeutic value: Can promote insight by making conscious repressed material, resolving paradoxes, tempering aggression, and revealing new options, and is a socially acceptable form of sublimation

Nontherapeutic threat: Indiscriminate use; belittling patient; screen to avoid therapeutic intimacy

---

Informing. Informing, or information giving, is an essential nursing technique in which the nurse shares simple facts with the patient. It is a skill used by nurses in health teaching or patient education, such as in informing a patient when to take medication and about necessary precautions and side effects. Giving information, however, must be distinguished from giving suggestions or advice.

Suggesting. Suggesting is the presentation of alternative ideas relative to problem solving. As a therapeutic technique, it is a useful intervention in the working phase of the relationship when the patient has analyzed the problem area and is exploring alternative coping mechanisms. At that time, suggestions by the nurse will increase the patient's perceived options and choices.

Suggesting, or giving advice, can also be nontherapeutic. Some patients who seek help expect some pronouncement from the health-care professional on what to do. So, too, nursing students often perceive their function as giving "common sense" advice. In these instances giving advice shifts responsibility to the nurse and reinforces the patient's dependence.

Another limitation is that the patient may take the nurse's advice and still not have things work out. The patient then returns to blame the nurse for failure. Most commonly, though, patients do not follow the advice offered by others, as in the transactional analysis model. The request for advice is often a child's expression of dependency, and the patient really knows what to do. The nurse who falls into the trap and responds with advice receives the patient's anger and contempt. A more productive strategy is for the nurse to deal with the patient's feelings first—feelings of indecision, dependence, and perhaps fear. Then the request for advice can be looked at and responded to in its proper perspective.

Box 2-8—cont'd

THERAPEUTIC COMMUNICATION TECHNIQUES

Technique: INFORMING

Definition: The skill of information giving

Example: "I think you need to know more about how your medication works."

Therapeutic value: Helpful in health teaching or patient education about relevant aspects of patient's well-being and self-care

Nontherapeutic threat: Giving advice

Technique: FOCUSING

Definition: Questions or statements that help the patient expand on a topic of importance

Example: "I think that we should talk more about your relationship with your father."

Therapeutic value: Allows the patient to discuss central issues and keeps the communication process goal-directed

Nontherapeutic threat: Allowing abstractions and generalizations; changing topics

Technique: SHARING PERCEPTIONS

Definition: Asking the patient to verify the nurse's understanding of what the patient is thinking or feeling

Example: "You're smiling but I sense that you are really very angry with me."

Therapeutic value: Conveys the nurse's understanding to the patient and has the potential for clearing up confusing communication

Nontherapeutic threat: Challenging the patient; accepting literal responses; reassuring; testing; defending

Technique: THEME IDENTIFICATION

Definition: Underlying issues or problems experienced by the patient that emerge repeatedly during the course of the nurse-patient relationship

Example: "I've noticed that in all of the relationships that you have described, you've been hurt or rejected by the man. Do you think this is an underlying issue?"

Therapeutic value: Allows the nurse to best promote the patient's exploration and understanding of important problems

Nontherapeutic threat: Giving advice; reassuring; disapproving

Technique: SILENCE

Definition: Lack of verbal communication for a therapeutic reason

Example: Sitting with a patient and nonverbally communicating interest and involvement

Therapeutic value: Allows the patient time to think and gain insights, slows the pace of the interaction and encourages the patient to initiate conversation, while conveying the nurse's support, understanding, and acceptance

Therapeutic threat: Questioning the patient; asking for "why" responses; failure to break a nontherapeutic silence

Technique: SUGGESTING

Definition: Presentation of alternative ideas for the patient's consideration relative to problem solving

Example: "Have you thought about responding to your boss in a different way when he raises that issue with you? For example, you could ask him if a specific problem has occurred."

Therapeutic value: Increases the patient's perceived options or choices

Nontherapeutic threat: Giving advice; inappropriate timing; being judgmental

---

Suggesting is also nontherapeutic if it occurs early in the relationship before the patient has analyzed personal conflicts or if it is a technique the nurse uses frequently. Then it negates the possibility of mutuality and implies that the patient is incapable of assuming responsibility for thoughts and actions. This assumption is also present when suggestion by the nurse is really covert coercion, as the nurse tells patients how they *ought* to live their lives.

The nurse's intent in using the suggesting technique should be to provide feasible alternatives and allow the patient to explore their potential value for himself. The nurse can then focus on helping the patient explore the advantages and disadvantages and the meaning and implications of the alternatives. In this way suggestions can be offered in a nonauthoritarian manner with such phrases as "Some people have tried. . . . Do you think that would work for you?" When using the technique of suggesting, nurses must be careful about both the tim-

ing of their intervention and their underlying motivation.

The therapeutic communication techniques presented in this chapter are summarized in Box 2-8.

 Which therapeutic communication techniques listed in Box 2-8 are you skilled in using? Which techniques are more difficult for you?

RESPONSIVE DIMENSIONS

The nurse must achieve certain skills or qualities to initiate and continue a therapeutic relationship. These skills or qualities incorporate verbal and nonverbal behavior and the attitudes and feelings behind communication. Carkhoff, Berenson, and Truax[8-10] have identified specific core conditions for facilitative interpersonal relationships. They broadly divided these conditions into responsive dimensions and action dimensions.

The responsive dimensions include genuineness, respect, empathic understanding, and concreteness. A number of studies have reported that nurses are low in the qualities traditionally associated with therapeutic effectiveness in counseling—genuineness, nonpossessive warmth, and empathy.[38] One study is even more specific and suggests that nurses are most skilled in the authoritative interventions of prescribing, informing, and confronting patients and less skilled in the facilitative interventions of drawing out patient's emotions, encouraging their self-exploration, and confirming their self-worth.[34] Furthermore, the helping process can impede the patient's growth rather than enhance it, depending on the level of the nurse's responsive and facilitative skills.

The responsive dimensions are crucial in a relationship to establish trust and open communication between the nurse and the patient. The nurse's goal is to gain an understanding of the patient and to help the patient gain self-understanding and insight. These responsive conditions then continue to be useful throughout the working and termination phases.

Genuineness

Genuineness implies that the nurse is an open, honest, sincere person who is actively involved in the relationship. Genuineness is the opposite of self-alienation, which occurs when many of an individual's real, spontaneous reactions to life are repressed or suppressed. Genuineness means that the nurse's response is sincere rather than phony, that the nurse is not thinking and feeling one thing and saying something different. It is an essential quality because nurses cannot expect openness, self-acceptance, and personal freedom in patients if they lack these qualities themselves.

Genuineness does not mean that the nurse must make a complete self-disclosure, but whatever the nurse does show must be real and not merely a "professional" response that has been learned and repeated. Genuineness also does not imply that the nurse will behave in the same way as family, friends, or colleagues. In focusing on the patient, much of the nurse's personal need system is put aside, as well as some of the usual ways of relating to others. Carried to this extreme, genuineness can be destructive and work against the goals of a therapeutic relationship.

Following is an example of genuineness.

PATIENT: I'd like my parents to give me my freedom and let me do my own thing. If I need them or want

their advice, I'll ask them. Why don't they trust what they taught me? Why do parents have to make it so hard—like it's all or nothing?

NURSE: I know what you mean. My parents acted the same way. They offered advice, but what they expected was obedience. When they saw I could handle things on my own and used good judgment, they began to accept me as an individual. There are still times when they slip back into their old ways, but we understand each other better now. Do you think you and your parents need to share more openly and honestly your feelings and ideas?

Respect

Respect, also called *nonpossessive warmth* or *unconditional positive regard*, does not depend on the patient's behavior. *Caring, liking,* and *valuing* are other terms for respect. The patient is regarded as a person of worth and is respected. The nurse's attitude is nonjudgmental; it is without criticism, ridicule, or reservation. This does not mean that the nurse condones or accepts all aspects of the patient's behavior as desirable or likeable. Patients are accepted for who they are, as they are. The nurse does not demand that the patient change or be perfect to be accepted. Imperfections are accepted along with mistakes and weaknesses as part of the human condition. The inexperienced nurse may have difficulty accepting the patient without transferring feelings about the patient's thoughts or actions. However, acceptance means viewing the patient's actions as coping behaviors that will change as the patient becomes less threatened and learns more adaptive mechanisms. It involves viewing the patient's behavior as natural, normal, and expected, given the circumstances.

Although there should be a basic respect for the patient simply as a person, respect is increased with understanding of the patient's uniqueness. Respect can be communicated in many different ways: by sitting silently with a patient who is crying; by genuine laughter with the patient over a particular event; by accepting the patient's request not to share a certain experience; by apologizing for the hurt unintentionally caused by a particular phrase; by being open enough to communicate anger or hurt caused by the patient. Being genuine with and listening to the patient are also manifestations of respect.

When nurses communicate conditional warmth, they foster feelings of dependency in patients because nurses become the evaluator and superior in the relationship, making mutuality impossible. If dependency feelings should arise in patients, nurses can effectively deal with them by acknowledging and exploring these feelings with patients.

Empathic Understanding

Empathy has been defined by Kalisch[22] as "the ability to enter into the life of another person, to accurately perceive his current feelings and their meanings. It is an essential element of the interpersonal process. When communicated, it forms the basis for a helping relationship between nurse and patient." Rogers[41] described it as "to sense the client's private world as if it were your own, but without losing the 'as if' quality." Rogers believes that a high degree of empathy is one of the most potent factors in bringing about change and learning—"one of the most delicate and powerful ways we have of using ourselves."[40]

Accurate empathy involves more than knowing what the patient means. It also involves the nurse's sensitivity to the patient's current feelings and the verbal ability to communicate this understanding in a language attuned to the patient. It means frequently confirming with the patient the accuracy of personal perceptions and being guided by the patient's responses. It requires that the nurse lay aside personal views and values to enter another's world without prejudice.

Two types of empathy can be identified in the nursing literature.[1,51,52] The first type is basic empathy. It involves the natural, universal human capacity to feel for others. The second type is trained empathy, which is taught and learned in relation to helping others. Trained empathy is also called clinical empathy or professional empathy. Unfortunately, these two types of empathy are often confused when empathy is discussed in relation to the nurse-patient relationship. For example, it would be important to first assess a baseline of empathic ability in nursing students. After teaching this skill, nursing students can then be assessed for trained empathy and the impact it may have on the outcome of psychiatric nursing care.

Development of Empathy

Empathic understanding consists of a number of stages. If patients allow nurses to enter their private world and attempt to communicate their perceptions and feelings, nurses must be receptive to this communication. Next, nurses must understand the patient's communication by putting themselves in the patient's place. Nurses must then step back into their own role and communicate understanding to the patient. It is not necessary or desirable for nurses to feel the same emotion as the patient. Empathy should not be confused with sympathy. It is, instead, an appreciation and awareness of the patient's feelings. A good deal of research has been conducted on empathy. The discussion of the findings presented in Box 2-9 underscores its importance in counseling.

Rogers[41] expands on the profound consequences empathy can have in promoting constructive learning and change. In the first place, it dissolves the patient's sense of alienation by connecting the patient on some level to a part of the human race. The patient can perceive that "I make sense to another human being . . . so I must not be so strange or alien. . . . And if I am in touch with someone else, I am not so all alone." On the other hand, if not responded to empathically, the patient may believe, "If no one understands me, if no one can see what I'm experiencing, then I must be very bad off. . . . I'm sicker than even I thought." Another benefit of empathy, is that the patient can feel valued, cared for, and accepted as a person. Then perhaps come to think, "If this other person thinks I'm worthwhile, maybe I could value and care for myself. . . . Maybe I am worthwhile after all."

Empathic Responses. It is essential that the nurse first provide the contextual base for the relationship through genuineness and unconditional positive regard for the patient. Then, the understanding conveyed to the patient through empathy gives him his personhood or identity. The patient, incorporates these new aspects into a new, changing self-concept. And once self-concept changes, behavior also changes, thus producing the positive outcome of therapy.

Box 2-9

RESEARCH FINDINGS ABOUT EMPATHY

▼ Empathy is clearly related to positive outcome.

▼ Low empathy is related to a worsening in adjustment or pathological conditions.

▼ The ideal therapist is first of all empathic.

▼ Empathy is correlated with self-exploration and process movement.

▼ Empathy early in the relationship predicts later success.

▼ The patient comes to perceive more empathy in successful cases.

▼ Understanding is provided by, not drawn from, the therapist.

▼ The more experienced therapists are more likely to be empathic.

▼ Empathy is a special quality in a relationship, and therapists offer definitely more of it than even helpful friends.

▼ The better self-integrated the therapist, the higher the degree of empathy.

▼ Experienced therapists often fall far short of being empathic. Brilliance and diagnostic perceptiveness are unrelated to empathy.

▼ An empathic way of being can be learned from empathic persons.

Gazda and co-workers[16] have described the following guidelines for responding with empathy:

1. Verbal and nonverbal behavior should be focused on by the helper.
2. The helper should formulate responses of empathy in a language and a manner that are most easily understood by the patient.
3. The tone of the helper's response should be similar to that of the patient.
4. In addition to concentrating on what the patient is expressing, the helper should also be aware of what is not being expressed.
5. The helper must accurately interpret responses to the patient and use them as a guide in developing future responses.

A nursing study identified specific verbal and nonverbal behaviors that conveyed high levels of empathy to the patient[31]:

▼ Having nurses introduce themselves to patients
▼ Head and body positions turned toward the patient and occasionally leaning forward
▼ Verbal responses to the patient's previous comments, responses that focus on strengths and resources
▼ Consistent eye contact and response to the patient's nonverbal cues such as sighs, tone of voice, restlessness, and facial expressions
▼ Conveyance of interest, concern, and warmth by the nurse's own facial expressions
▼ A tone of voice consistent with facial expression and verbal response
▼ Mirror imaging of body position and gestures between the nurse and patient

Additional studies are needed in nursing to identify the behavioral indicators and outcomes of this important dimension of nursing care.[1,36]

Empathic Functioning Scale. Kalisch[22] devised the "Nurse-Patient Empathic Functioning Scale," which describes five categories of empathy (Table 2-6). High levels of empathy (categories 3 and 4) communicate "I am with you"; the nurse's responses fit perfectly with the patient's conspicuous current feelings and content. The nurse's responses also serve to expand the patient's awareness of hidden feelings through the use of clarification and reflection. Such empathy is communicated by the language used, voice qualities, and nonverbal behavior, all of which reflect the nurse's seriousness and depth of feeling.

At low levels of empathy (categories 0 and 1), the nurse ignores the patient's feelings, goes off on a tangent, or misinterprets what the patient is feeling. The nurse at this level may be uninterested in the patient or concentrating on the "facts" of what the patient says rather than on current feelings and experiences. The nurse is doing something other than listening, for example, evaluating the patient, giving advice, sermonizing, or thinking about personal problems or needs.

Empathic responses need to be properly timed within the nurse-patient relationship. Category 4 responses in the orientation phase may be viewed as too intense and intrusive. Usually a number of category 2 responses are required initially to build an atmosphere of trust and openness. In the later stages of the orientation phase and most particularly in the working phase, categories 3 and 4 responses are appropriate and most effective. Responses from categories 0 and 1 are nontherapeutic at all times and block the development of the relationship.

The various levels of empathy are evident in the following example:

PATIENT: I'm really jittery today, and I hope I can get things out right. It started when I saw Bob on Friday, and it's been building up since then.
NURSE: You're feeling tense and anxious, and it's related to a talk you had with Bob on Friday. (Category 2.)
PATIENT: Yes. He began putting pressure on me to have sex with him again.
NURSE: It sounds like you resent it when he pressures you for sex. (Category 3.)
PATIENT: I do. Why does he think things always have to be his way? I guess he knows I'm a pushover.
NURSE: It makes you angry when he wants his way even though he knows you feel differently. But you usually give in and then you wind up disappointed in yourself and feeling like a failure. (Category 4.)
PATIENT: It happens just like that over and over. It's as if I never learn.
NURSE: So when the incident's all over, you're left blaming yourself and wallowing in self-pity. (Category 4.)
PATIENT: I guess that's right.

Sociocultural differences between nurses and patients can be barriers to empathy if nurses are not sensitive to them. Differences in sex, age, religion, socioeconomic status, education, and culture can block the development of empathic understanding. However, the greater the nurse's cultural sensitivity and the greater the openness to the world view of others, the greater will be the potential for understanding people.

Identical or similar experiences are not essential for empathy. No man can really experience what it is like to be a woman; no white can experience what it is like to be black. It is not necessary to be exactly like another, but it is desirable for nurses to prepare themselves in any way they can to understand potential patients. It is

Table 2-6   Nurse-Patient Empathic Functioning Scale

Categories of nurse empathic functioning	Level of patient's feelings	
	Conspicuous current feelings	**Hidden current feelings**
0	Ignores	Ignores
1	Communicates awareness that is accurate at times and inaccurate at other times	Ignores
2	Communicates complete and accurate awareness of essence and strength of feelings	Communicates an awareness of presence of hidden feelings but is not accurate in defining their essence or strength; effort being made to understand
3	Same as category 2	Communicates an accurate awareness of hidden feelings slightly beyond what patient expresses
4	Same as category 2	Communicates without uncertainty an accurate awareness of deepest, most hidden feelings

From Kalisch B: Am J Nurs 73:1548, 1973. Copyright © 1973, American Journal of Nursing Company. Reproduced with permission from *American Journal of Nursing*, September, vol 73, no 9.

also important for nurses to realize that empathy can be learned and enhanced in a variety of ways, including staff development programs.

 Evaluate a recent interaction you had with a patient based on the empathy scale described in Table 2-6. Use it again at the end of your psychiatric nursing experience and note any differences.

Concreteness

Concreteness involves using specific terminology rather than abstractions when discussing the patient's feelings, experiences, and behavior. It avoids vagueness and ambiguity and is the opposite of generalizing, categorizing, classifying, and labeling the patient's experiences. It has three functions: (1) to keep the nurse's responses close to the patient's feelings and experiences, (2) to foster accuracy of understanding by the nurse, and (3) to encourage the patient to attend to specific problem areas.[9]

The level of concreteness should vary during the various phases of the nurse-patient relationship (Fig. 2-9). In the orientation phase, concreteness should be high; at this time it can contribute to empathic understanding. It is essential for the formulation of specific goals and plans. As patients explore various feelings and perceptions related to their problems in the working phase of the relationship, concreteness should be at a relatively low level to facilitate a thorough self-exploration. At the end of the working phase, when patients are engaging in action, and during the termination phase high levels of concreteness are again desirable.

Concreteness is evident in the following examples:

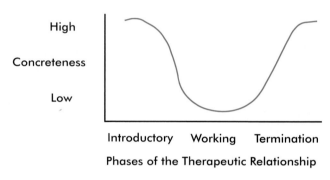

Fig. 2-9   Levels of concreteness in the therapeutic relationship.

 EXAMPLE 1

PATIENT: I wouldn't have any problems if people would quit bothering me. They like to upset me because they know I'm high strung.
NURSE: What people try to upset you?
PATIENT: My family. People think being from a large family is a blessing. I think it's a curse.
NURSE: Could you give me an example of something someone in your family did that upset you?

EXAMPLE 2

PATIENT: I don't know what the problem is between us. My wife and I just don't get along anymore. We seem to disagree about everything. I think I love her, but she isn't affectionate or caring—hasn't been for a long time.
NURSE: You say you're not sure what the problem is, and you think you love your wife. But the two of you argue often and she hasn't given you any sign of love or affection. Have you felt affectionate

toward her, and when was the last time you let her know how you felt?

These four responsive dimensions or conditions—genuineness, respect, empathic understanding, and concreteness—facilitate the formation of a therapeutic relationship. The therapeutic level at which nurses function is unknown at present. Additional research is greatly needed on nurse-patient interactions because there is little empirical evidence on which to base scientific practice in this area.

ACTION DIMENSIONS

Carkhoff[8] identified the action-oriented, or initiative, conditions for facilitative interpersonal relationships as confrontation, immediacy, and therapist self-disclosure. To these will be added the dimensions of catharsis and role playing. The separation of these therapeutic conditions into two groups—the understanding, or responsive, conditions and the initiating, or action, conditions—is not a distinct separation. To some extent all the dimensions are present throughout the therapeutic relationship. The action dimensions must have a context of warmth and understanding. This is important for inexperienced nurses to remember because they may be tempted to move into high levels of action dimensions without having established adequate understanding, empathy, warmth, or respect. The responsive dimensions allow the patient to achieve insight, but this is not enough. With the action dimensions, the nurse moves the therapeutic relationship upward and outward by identifying obstacles to the patient's progress and the need for both internal understanding and external action.

Confrontation

Confrontation usually implies venting anger and aggressive behavior. However, confrontation as a therapeutic action dimension is an assertive rather than aggressive action. Confrontation is an expression by the nurse of perceived discrepancies in the patient's behavior. Carkhoff[8] identifies three categories of confrontation:

1. Discrepancy between the patient's expression of what he is (self-concept) and what he wants to be (self-ideal)
2. Discrepancies between the patient's verbal self-expression and behavior
3. Discrepancies between the patient's expressed experience of himself and the nurse's experience of him

Confrontation is an attempt by the nurse to make the patient aware of incongruence in his feelings, attitudes, beliefs, and behaviors. It may also lead to the discovery of ambivalent feelings in the patient. Confrontation is not limited to negative aspects of the patient. It includes pointing out discrepancies involving resources and strengths that are unrecognized and unused. It requires that the nurse collect sufficient data about the patient's history and accumulate sufficient perceptions and observations of verbal and nonverbal communication so that validation of reality is possible.

The nurse must have developed an understanding of the patient to perceive discrepancies, inconsistencies in word and deed, distortions, defenses, and evasions. The nurse must be willing and capable of working through the crisis after confronting the patient. Without this commitment the confrontation lacks therapeutic potential and can be quite damaging to both nurse and patient. Without question the effects of confrontation are challenge, exposure, risk, and the possibility for growth. The nurse who uses confrontation is modeling an active role to the patient; the nurse is using insight and understanding to remove ambiguity and inconsistency and thus seek deeper understanding.

Timing in Relationships. Bromley[4] suggests that before confrontation, nurses should assess the following factors:
▼ The trust level in the relationship
▼ The timing
▼ The patient's stress level
▼ The strength of the patient's defense mechanisms
▼ The patient's perceived need for personal space or closeness
▼ The patient's level of rage and tolerance for hearing another perception

Patients have the capacity to deny or accept nurses' observations, and their response to the confrontation can serve as a measure of its success or failure. Acceptance indicates appropriate timing and patient readiness. Denial serves to allay any threat that the confrontation posed to the patient. It provides nurses with additional information; it tells them that patients are resisting change and are unwilling to enlarge their view of reality at this time.

Confrontation must be appropriately timed to be effective (Fig. 2-10). In the orientation phase of the relationship, the nurse should use confrontation infrequently and pose it as an observation of incongruent behavior. A simple "mirroring" of the discrepancy between a patient's actions and words is the most nonthreatening type of confrontation. The nurse might say, "You seem to be saying two different things." This type of confrontation closely resembles clarification at this time. Nurses might also identify discrepancies between how they and patients are experiencing their relationship, point out unnoticed patient strengths or untapped resources, or provide patients with objective but per-

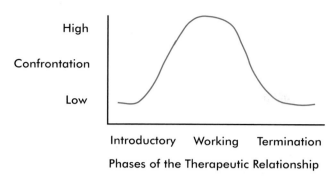

Fig. 2-10   Levels of confrontation in the therapeutic relationship.

haps different information about their world. According to Carkhoff,[8] "Premature direct confrontations may have a demoralizing and demobilizing effect upon an inadequately prepared helpee. To be effective, confrontation requires high levels of empathy and respect."

In the working phase of the relationship, more direct confrontations may focus on specific patient discrepancies. The nurse may confront the patient with areas of weakness or shortcomings or may focus on the discrepancy between the nurse's perception of the patient and the patient's self-perception. This expands the patient's awareness and helps the patient move to higher levels of functioning. Confrontation is especially important in pointing out when the patient has developed insight but has not changed behavior. This encourages the patient to act in a reasonable and constructive manner, rather than assuming a dependent and passive stance toward life.

Research indicates that effective counselors use confrontation frequently, confronting patients with their assets more often in earlier interviews and with their limitations in later interviews. Another study[33] found that therapists who rated significantly higher on empathy, genuineness, respect, and concreteness confronted their patients significantly more often than those therapists who were less facilitative. In the initial interview, these confrontations were based on attempts to clarify the relationship, eliminate misconceptions, give patients more objective information about themselves and their world, and emphasize patient strengths and resources.

Inexperienced nurses frequently avoid confrontation. It can be nontherapeutic when it is not associated with empathy or warmth or when it is used to vent the nurse's negative feelings of anger, frustration, and aggressiveness. However, carefully monitored confrontation can be viewed as an extension of genuineness and concreteness. It is a useful therapeutic intervention that can further the patient's growth and progress.

Following are seven examples of confrontation:

 EXAMPLE 1

NURSE: I see you as someone who has a lot of strength. You've been able to give a tremendous amount of emotional support to your children at a time when they needed it very much.

 EXAMPLE 2

NURSE: It was my understanding that we were meeting together to talk about the problems that brought you to the hospital. But every time I come, you ask me to play cards with you, share a game of table tennis, or toss around a basketball. It seems to me that we're not in agreement on what these meetings are all about.

 EXAMPLE 3

NURSE: The fact that Sue didn't accept your date for Friday night doesn't necessarily mean she never wants to go out with you. She could have had another date or other plans with her family or girlfriends. But if you don't ask her, you'll never find out why she refused you or if she'll accept in the future.

 EXAMPLE 4

NURSE: We've talked three different times now and you've told me that you don't really have a problem or that other people make trouble for you. But I've noticed that on the unit you seldom talk to the other patients and little accidents like the spilled coffee at lunch really seem to upset you.

 EXAMPLE 5

NURSE: You tell me that your parents don't trust you and never give you any responsibility, but each week you also tell me how you stayed out beyond your curfew or had friends over when your parents weren't home. Do you see a connection between the two?

 EXAMPLE 6

NURSE: You say you want to feel better and go back to work, but you're not taking your medicine, which will help you to do that.

 EXAMPLE 7

NURSE: We've been talking for 3 weeks now about your need to get out and try to meet some people. We even talked of different ways to do that. But so far you haven't made any effort to join aerobics, take a class, or do any of the other ideas we had.

Your friend tells you that she feels uncomfortable using confrontation with patients. Why do you think this might be and what advice would you give her?

Immediacy

Immediacy involves focusing on the current interaction of the nurse and the patient in the relationship. It is a significant dimension, because the patient's behavior and functioning in the relationship are indicative of functioning in other interpersonal relationships. Most patients experience difficulty in interpersonal relationships; thus the patient's functioning in the nurse-patient relationship must be evaluated. The nurse has the opportunity to intervene directly with the patient's problem behavior, and the patient has the opportunity to learn and change behavior.

Immediacy connotes sensitivity by the nurse to the patient's feelings and a willingness to deal with these feelings rather than ignore them. This is particularly difficult when the nurse must recognize and respond to negative feelings the patient expresses toward the nurse. The difficulty is compounded by the fact that patients often express these messages indirectly and conceal them in references to other people.

It is not possible or appropriate for the nurse to focus continually on the immediacy of the relationship. It is most appropriate to do so when the relationship seems to be stalled or is not progressing. It is also helpful to look at immediacy when the relationship is progressing particularly well. In both instances the patient is actively involved in describing what is helping or hindering the relationship.

As with the other dimensions, high-level immediacy responses should not be suddenly presented to the patient. The nurse must first know and understand the patient and have developed a good, open relationship. The nurse's initial expressions of immediacy should be tentatively phrased; for example, "Are you trying to tell me how you feel about our relationship?" As the relationship progresses, observations related to immediacy can be made more directly, and as communication improves, the need for immediacy responses may decrease.

Following are two examples of immediacy:

 EXAMPLE 1

PATIENT: I've been thinking about our meetings, and I'm really pretty busy now to keep coming. Besides, I don't see the point in them, and we don't seem to be getting anywhere.

NURSE: Are you trying to say you're feeling discouraged and you feel our meetings aren't helping you?

 EXAMPLE 2

PATIENT: The staff here couldn't care less about us patients. They treat us like children instead of adults.

NURSE: I'm wondering if you feel that I don't care about you or perhaps I don't value your opinion?

Nurse Self-Disclosure

Self-disclosures are (1) subjectively true, (2) personal statements about the self, and (3) intentionally revealed to another person. The nurse may share experiences or feelings that are similar to those of the patient and may emphasize both the similarities and differences. This kind of self-disclosure is an index of the closeness of the relationship and involves a particular kind of respect for the patient. It is an expression of genuineness and honesty by the nurse and is an aspect of empathy.

The rationale for nurse self-disclosure comes from the theoretical and research literature; it provides significant evidence that therapist self-disclosure increases the likelihood of patient self-disclosure.[54] Patient self-disclosure is necessary for a successful therapeutic outcome. However, the nurse must use self-disclosure judiciously, and this is determined by the quality, quantity, and appropriateness of the disclosures. Criteria for self-disclosure include[46]:

▼ To model and educate
▼ To foster the therapeutic alliance
▼ To validate reality
▼ To encourage the patient's autonomy

The number of self-disclosures appears to be crucial to the success of the therapy. Too few nurse self-disclosures may fail to produce patient self-disclosures, whereas too many may decrease the time available for patient disclosure or may alienate the patient. The problem for the nurse is knowing where the middle ground is. Clinical experience is necessary to determine the optimum therapeutic level.

The appropriateness or relevance of the nurse's self-disclosure is also important. The nurse should self-disclose in response to statements made by the patient. If the nurse's disclosure is far from what the patient is experiencing, it can serve to distract the patient from the problem or cause feelings of alienation. A patient who is experiencing severe or panic levels of anxiety may feel threatened or frightened by the nurse's self-disclosure. In these cases the nurse must be careful not to burden a patient with self-disclosures. Above all, disclosure by the nurse is always for the patient's benefit. The nurse does not disclose to meet personal needs or to feel better. When self-disclosing, the nurse should have a particular therapeutic goal in mind.

Guidelines that nurses can use to evaluate the potential usefulness of their self-disclosure are listed in Box 2-10. These guidelines govern the "dosage and timing" of self-disclosures and help the nurse assess the appropriateness, effectiveness, and anticipated response of the patient to the disclosure.

Self-disclosure by the nurse is evident in the following example:

PATIENT: When he told me he didn't want to see me again, I felt like slapping him and hugging him at the same time. But then I knew the problem was really me and no one could ever love me.

NURSE: When I broke off with a man I had been seeing, I felt the anger, hurt, and bitterness you just described. I remember thinking I would never date another man.

In this example the nurse self-disclosed to emphasize that the patient's feelings were natural. She also reinforced the external cause for the separation (boyfriend's decision to leave versus the patient's inadequacy) and implied that, with time, the patient will be able to resolve the loss.

Even though research has indicated the importance of this dimension for patient growth, it appears to be an area of some discomfort for nurses. Johnson[19,20] studied the level of reciprocal disclosure occurring between nurses and patients on four clinical units—medical, surgical, psychiatric, and critical care. She found that anxiety levels tended to decrease among nurses and patients as their levels of self-disclosure increased. In addition, she reported low reciprocal self-disclosure in the psychiatric unit despite the verbal nature of psy-

chiatric therapy and the lack of restrictions on talking about oneself. She concluded from her study that nurses and patients need to be assisted in learning to be therapeutically open and authentic in their interactions with each other.

Emotional Catharsis

Emotional catharsis occurs when the patient is encouraged to talk about things that are most bothersome. Catharsis brings fears, feelings, and experiences out into the open so that they can be examined and discussed with the nurse. The expression of feelings can be very therapeutic in itself, even if behavioral change does not result. The previously described responsive dimensions create an atmosphere within the nurse-patient relationship in which emotional catharsis is possible. The patient's responsiveness depends on the confidence and trust the patient has in the nurse.

The nurse must be able to recognize cues from the patient concerning readiness for discussion of problems. It is important that the nurse proceed at the rate chosen by the patient and provide support during discussion of difficult areas. Forcing emotional catharsis on the patient could precipitate a panic episode, since the patient's defenses are attacked without sufficient alternative coping mechanisms available.

Patients are often uncomfortable about expressing feelings. Nurses may be equally uncomfortable with expressing feelings, particularly sadness or anger. Frequently nurses assume they know the patient's feelings and do not attempt to specifically validate them. The dimensions of empathy and immediacy require the nurse to notice and express emotions. Unresolved feelings and feelings that are avoided can cause stalls or barriers in the nurse-patient relationship. Specific examples are transference and countertransference phenomena, which are discussed later in the chapter.

If patients have difficulty in expressing feelings, nurses may help by suggesting how they or others might feel in the patient's specific situation. Some patients respond directly to the question, "How did that make you feel?" Others intellectualize and avoid the emotional element in their answer. When patients realize they can express their feelings within an accepting relationship, they expand their awareness and potential acceptance of themselves.

The following example illustrates emotional catharsis:

NURSE: How did you feel when your boss corrected you in front of all those customers?

PATIENT: Well, I understood that he needed to set me

Box 2-10

GUIDELINES FOR SELF-DISCLOSURE

1. Cooperation—Will the disclosure enhance the patient's cooperation, which is necessary to the development of a therapeutic alliance?
2. Learning—Will the disclosure assist patients' ability to learn about themselves to set short- and long-term goals, and to deal more effectively with life's problems?
3. Catharsis—Will the disclosure assist the patient to express formerly held or suppressed feelings, important to the relief of emotional symptoms?
4. Support—Will the disclosure provide the patient with support or reinforcement for attaining specific goals?

straight, and he's the type that flies off the handle pretty easily anyhow.

NURSE: It sounds like you're defending his behavior. I was wondering how you felt at that moment.

PATIENT: Awkward . . . uh . . . upset, I guess (pause).

NURSE: That would have made me pretty angry if it had happened to me.

PATIENT: Well, I was. But you can't let it show, you know. You have to keep it all in because of the customers. But he can let it out. Oh *sure* (emphatically)! He can tell *me* anything he wants. Just *once* I'd like him to know how I feel.

Role Playing

Role playing involves acting out a particular situation. It increases the patient's insight into human relations and can deepen the ability to see the situation from another person's point of view. Sedgwick[44] identifies the intent of role playing as being to represent closely real life behavior that involves individuals holistically, to focus attention on a problem, and to permit individuals to see themselves in action in a neutral situation. It provides a bridge between thought and action in a "safe" environment in which the patient can feel free to experiment with new behavior. It is a method of learning that makes actual behavior the focus of study; it is action oriented and provides immediately available information. Role playing consists of the following steps:

1. Defining the problem
2. Creating a readiness for role playing
3. Establishing the situation
4. Casting the characters
5. Briefing and warming up
6. Acting
7. Stopping
8. Analyzing and discussing
9. Evaluation

When role playing is used for attitude change, it relies heavily on role reversal. The patient may be asked to play the role of a certain person in a specific situation or to play the role of someone with opposing beliefs. Role reversal can help a person reevaluate the other person's intentions and become more understanding of the other person's position. After role reversal, patients may be more receptive to modifying their own attitudes.

As a method of promoting self-awareness and conflict resolution, role playing may help the patient "experience" a situation rather than just "talk about it." Role playing can elicit feelings in the patient that are similar to those experienced in the actual situation. It provides an opportunity for insight and for the expression of affect. For these reasons it is a useful method for heightening a patient's awareness of feelings about a situation.

One of the specific ways in which role playing can be used to resolve conflicts and increase self-awareness is through a "dialogue" that requires the patient to take the part of each person or each side of an argument. If the conflict is internal, the dialogue occurs in the present tense between the patient's conflicting selves until one part of the conflict outweighs the other. If the conflict involves a second person, the patient is instructed to "imagine that the other person is sitting in the chair across from you." The patient is told to begin the dialogue by expressing wants and resentments about the other person. Then the patient changes chairs, assumes the role of the other person, and responds to what was just said. The patient assumes the first role again and responds to the other person. Using dialogue in this way not only serves as practice for the patient in expressing feelings and opinions but also gives a reality base for the probable response from the other party involved in the conflict. This can often remove the barrier that is keeping the patient from making a decision and acting on it.

Role playing is included as an action dimension because it can help the patient develop insight. Nurses need a variety of intervention skills. Role playing can be effective when an impasse has been reached in the patient's progress or when it is difficult for the patient to translate insight into action. In these instances it can reduce tension and allow the patient the opportunity to practice or test new behaviors for future use.

Table 2-7 summarizes the responsive and action dimensions for therapeutic nurse-patient relationships. In concluding this section on therapeutic dimensions, it must be emphasized that the nurse's effectiveness is based on openness to learning what works best with particular kinds of patients. Both the use of communication techniques and the therapeutic conditions must be individualized to the nurse's personality and the patient's needs. Rote application can be destructive. The nurse must be willing to try other approaches and techniques that seem potentially helpful when the current approach seems ineffective at a given time.

THERAPEUTIC IMPASSES

Therapeutic impasses are blocks in the progress of the nurse-patient relationship. They arise for a variety of reasons, but they all create stalls in the therapeutic relationship. Impasses provoke intense feelings in both the nurse and the patient that may range from anxiety and apprehension to frustration, love, or intense anger. Four specific therapeutic impasses and ways to overcome them are discussed here: resistance, transference, countertransference, and boundary violations.

Table 2-7   Responsive and Action Dimensions for Therapeutic Nurse-Patient Relationships

Dimension	Characteristics
RESPONSIVE DIMENSIONS	
Genuineness	Implies that the nurse is an open person who is self-congruent, authentic, and transparent
Respect	Suggests that the patient is regarded as a person of worth who is valued and accepted without qualification
Empathic understanding	Viewing the patient's world from the patient's internal frame of reference, with sensitivity to the patient's current feelings and the verbal ability to communicate this understanding in a language attuned to the patient
Concreteness	Involves the use of specific terminology rather than abstractions in the discussion of the patient's feelings, experiences, and behavior
ACTION DIMENSIONS	
Confrontation	The expression by the nurse of perceived discrepancies in the patient's behavior to expand self-awareness
Immediacy	Occurs when the current interaction of the nurse and patient is focused on and is used to learn about the patient's functioning in other interpersonal relationships
Nurse self-disclosure	Evident when the nurse reveals personal information, ideas, values, feelings, and attitudes to facilitate the patient's cooperation, learning, catharsis, or support
Emotional catharsis	Takes place when the patient is encouraged to talk about things that are most bothersome
Role playing	The acting-out of a particular situation to increase the patient's insight into human relations and deepen the ability to see a situation from another point of view. It also allows the patient to experiment with new behavior in a safe environment

Resistance

Resistance is the patient's attempt to remain unaware of anxiety-producing aspects. It is a natural reluctance or learned avoidance of verbalizing or even experiencing troubled aspects of self. The term *resistance* was initially introduced by Freud to mean the patient's unconscious opposition to exploring or recognizing unconscious or even preconscious material. Primary resistance is often caused by the patient's unwillingness to change when the need for change is recognized. Patients usually display resistance behaviors during the working phase of the relationship, because this phase encompasses the greater part of the problem-solving process.

Resistance may also be a reaction by the patient to the nurse who has moved too rapidly or too deeply into the patient's feelings or who has intentionally or unintentionally communicated a lack of respect. It may also simply be the result of a patient who is working with a nurse who is an inappropriate role model for therapeutic behavior.

Secondary gain is another cause of resistance. Favorable environmental, interpersonal, and situational changes occur, and material advantages may be secured as a result of the illness. Types of secondary gain include financial compensation, avoiding unpleasant situations, increased sympathy or attention, escape from responsibility, attempted control of people, and lessening of social pressures. Secondary gain can become a powerful force in the perpetuation and propagation of an illness, since it makes the environment more comfortable.

Resistance may take many forms. Box 2-11 lists some of the forms of resistance that patients display as identified by Wolberg.[53]

Transference

Transference is an unconscious response in which the patient experiences feelings and attitudes toward the nurse that were originally associated with significant figures earlier in life. They may be triggered by some superficial similarity, such as a facial feature or manner of speech, or by the patient's perceived similarity of the relationship. These reactions are an attempt to reduce or alleviate anxiety. The outstanding trait defining transference is the inappropriateness of the patient's response in terms of intensity.

Transference reduces self-awareness by helping the

Box 2-11
FORMS OF RESISTANCE DISPLAYED BY PATIENTS

▼ Suppression and repression of pertinent information
▼ Intensification of symptoms
▼ Self-devaluation and a hopeless outlook on the future
▼ Forced flight into health where there is a sudden, but short-lived recovery by the patient
▼ Intellectual inhibitions, which may be evident when the patient says he has "nothing on his mind" or that he is "unable to think about his problems" or when he breaks appointments, is late for sessions, or is forgetful, silent, or sleepy

▼ Acting out or irrational behavior
▼ Superficial talk
▼ Intellectual insight in which the patient verbalizes self-understanding with correct use of terminology yet continues destructive behavior, or use of the defense of intellectualization where there is no insight
▼ Contempt for normality, which is evident when the patient has developed insight but refuses to assume the responsibility for change on the grounds that normality "isn't so great"
▼ Transference reactions

---

patient maintain a generalized view of the world in which all people are seen in similar terms. Thus the nurse may be viewed as an authority figure from the past, such as a parent figure, or as a lost loved object, such as a former spouse. Transference reactions are harmful to the therapeutic process only if they remain ignored and unexamined.

Two types of transference present particular resistances in the nurse-patient relationship. The first is the **hostile transference.** If the patient internalizes anger and hostility, this resistance may be expressed as depression and discouragement. The patient may ask to terminate the relationship on the grounds that there is no chance of getting well. If the hostility is externalized, the patient may become critical, defiant, and irritable and may express doubts about the nurse's training, experience, or personal adjustment. The patient may attempt to compete with the nurse by reading books on psychology and challenging her.

Hostility may also be expressed by the patient in detachment, forgetfulness, irrelevant chatter, or preoccupation with childhood experiences. An extreme form of uncooperativeness and negativism is evident in prolonged silences. Some of the most frustrating moments for the nurse are those spent in total silence with a patient. This is not the therapeutic silence that communicates mutuality and understanding. Rather, it is the silence that seems to be hostile, oppressive, and eternal. It is particularly disturbing for the nurse in the orientation phase, before a relationship has been established. The nurse's task is to understand the meaning of the patient's silence and decide how to deal with it despite feeling somewhat awkward and useless.

A second difficult type of transference is the **dependent reaction transference.** This resistance is characterized by patients who are submissive, subordinate,

and ingratiating and who regard the nurse as a "godlike" figure. The patient overvalues the nurse's characteristics and qualities, and their relationship is in jeopardy because the patient views it as magical. In this reaction the nurse must live up to the patient's overwhelming expectations, which is impossible because these expectations are completely unrealistic. The patient continues to demand more of the nurse, and when these needs are not met, the patient is filled with hostility and contempt.

Overcoming Resistance and Transference

Resistances and transferences can pose difficult problems for the nurse. The psychiatric nurse must be prepared to be exposed to powerful negative and positive emotional feelings coming from the patient, often on a highly irrational basis. The relationship can become stalled and nonbeneficial if the nurse is not prepared to deal with the patient's feelings.

Sometimes resistances occur because the nurse and patient have not arrived at mutually acceptable goals or plans of action. This may occur if the contract was not clearly defined in the orientation stage of the relationship. The appropriate action here is to return to the goals, purpose, and roles of the nurse and patient in the relationship.

Whatever the patient's motivations, the analysis of the resistance or transference is geared toward the patient gaining awareness of these motivations and learning about being completely responsible for all actions and behavior. The first thing the nurse must do is listen. When the nurse recognizes the resistance, clarification and reflection of feeling can be used. Clarification gives the nurse a more focused idea of what is happening. Reflection of content may help patients become aware of what has been going on in their own minds.

Reflection of feeling acknowledges the resistance and mirrors it to the patient. The nurse may say, "I sense that you're struggling with yourself. Part of you wants to explore the issue of your marriage and another part says 'No—I'm not ready yet.' "

It is not sufficient, however, to merely identify that resistance is occurring. The behavior must be explored and possible reasons for its occurrence analyzed. The depth of exploration and analysis engaged in by nurse and patient is related to the nurse's experience and knowledge base.

Countertransference

Countertransference is a therapeutic impasse created by the nurse's specific emotional response generated by the qualities of the patient. This response is inappropriate to the content and context of the therapeutic relationship or inappropriate in the degree of intensity of emotion. It is transference applied to the nurse. Inappropriateness is the crucial element, as it is with transference, because it is natural that the nurse will have a warmth toward or liking for some patients more than others. The nurse will also be genuinely angry with the actions of certain patients. But in countertransference the nurse's responses are not justified by reality. In this case nurses identify the patient with individuals from their past, and personal needs will interfere with therapeutic effectiveness.

Countertransference reactions are usually of three types:

1. Reactions of intense love or caring
2. Reactions of intense disgust or hostility
3. Reactions of intense anxiety often in response to resistance by the patient

Through the use of immediacy the nurse can identify countertransference in one of its various forms (Box 2-12).

Forms of countertransference occur because the nurse is involved with the patient as a participant observer and is not a detached bystander. These reactions can be powerful tools in exploration and potent instruments for uncovering inner states. They are destructive only if they are brushed aside, ignored, or not taken seriously.

If studied objectively, these reactions can lead to further information about the patient. The ability to remain objective does not mean that the nurse may not at times dislike what the patient says or may not become irritated. The patient's resistance to acquiring insight and transforming it into action and the refusal to change maladaptive and destructive coping mechanisms can be frustrating. But the nurse's capacity to understand personal feelings helps to maintain a working relationship with the patient.

Countertransference may also be manifested as a group phenomenon. Psychiatric staff members can become involved in countertransference reactions when they overreact to a patient's aggressive behavior, ignore available patient data that would promote understanding, or become locked in a power struggle with a patient. Other types of countertransference might include ignoring patient behavior that does not fit the staff's diagnosis, minimizing a patient's behavior, joking about or criticizing a patient, or becoming caught up in intimidation. Although these have been reported as phenomena of group countertransference, they can also illustrate individual countertransference reactions.

The experienced nurse is constantly on the lookout for countertransference, becomes aware of it when it oc-

---

Box 2-12

FORMS OF COUNTERTRANSFERENCE DISPLAYED BY NURSES

▼ Inability to empathize with the patient in certain problem areas

▼ Depressed feelings during or after the session

▼ Carelessness about implementing the contract by being late, running overtime, etc.

▼ Drowsiness during the sessions

▼ Feelings of anger or impatience because of the patient's unwillingness to change

▼ Encouragement of the patient's dependency, praise, or affection

▼ Arguing with the patient or a tendency to push before the patient is ready

▼ Trying to help the patient in matters not related to the identified nursing goals

▼ Involvement with the patient on a personal or social level

▼ Dreaming about or preoccupation with the patient

▼ Sexual or aggressive fantasies toward the patient

▼ Recurrent anxiety, unease, or guilt feelings about the patient

▼ Tendency to focus repetitively on only one aspect or way of looking at the information presented by the patient

▼ Need to defend nursing interventions with the patient to others

curs, and holds it in abeyance or utilizes it to promote the therapeutic goals. In attempting to identify a countertransference, the nurse must apply the same standards of honest self-appraisal personally that is expected of the patient. The nurse should employ self-examination throughout the course of the relationship, particularly when the patient attacks or criticizes. The following questions may be helpful:

▼ How do I feel about the patient?
▼ Do I look forward to seeing the patient?
▼ Do I feel sorry for or sympathetic toward the patient?
▼ Am I bored with the patient and believe that we are not progressing?
▼ Am I afraid of the patient?
▼ Do I get extreme pleasure out of seeing the patient?
▼ Do I want to protect, reject, or punish the patient?
▼ Do I dread meeting the patient and feel nervous during the sessions?
▼ Am I impressed by or try to impress the patient?
▼ Does the patient make me very angry or frustrated?

If any of these questions suggests a problem, the nurse should pursue it. What is the patient doing to provoke these feelings? Who does the patient remind me of? The nurse must discover the source of the problem. Because countertransference can be detrimental to the relationship, it should be dealt with as soon as possible. When it is recognized, the nurse can exercise control over it. If the nurse needs help in dealing with countertransference, individual or group supervision can be most beneficial.

Problem Patients. Countertransference problems are most clearly evident when a patient is labeled a "problem patient." Usually such a patient elicits strong negative feelings such as anger, fear, and helplessness and is often described by nurses as "manipulative, dependent, inappropriate, and demanding." The label "problem patient" implies that the patient's behavior should change for the sake of the helper rather than for the patient's own benefit. This labeling often causes the patient and nurse to become adversaries, and the nurse avoids contact.

It is more productive for a nurse to view a "problem patient" as one who poses problems for the nurse. This turns the responsibility for action back onto the nurse. It forces the nurse to explore responses to the patient that reinforce the patient's unproductive behavior. In this way the nurse also makes patients responsible for their behavior. By stepping back and reviewing again the patient's needs and problems, the nurse becomes aware of failing to use the responsive dimensions of genuineness, respect, empathic understanding, and concrete-

ness. Without this therapeutic groundwork, a therapeutic outcome is impossible.

Boundary Violations

A final but very important therapeutic impasse is that of boundary violations. These occur when a nurse goes outside the boundaries of the therapeutic relationship and establishes a social, economic, or personal relationship with a patient. As a general rule, whenever the nurse is doing or thinking of doing something special, different, or unusual for a patient, often a boundary violation is involved. Examples of possible boundary violations are listed in Box 2-13.

Categorizing boundary violations may be helpful for the psychiatric nurse in examining this issue in greater detail. It is possible to categorize boundary violations under the following categories[47]:

1. **Role boundaries**—These are a core component of the psychiatric nurse's role. They are embodied in the question "Is this what a psychiatric nurse does"? Problems with role boundaries require the insight of the nurse and the setting of firm therapeutic limits with the patient.
2. **Time boundaries**—These address the conditions surrounding the time of day that the nurse implements treatment. Odd and unusual treatment hours that have no therapeutic necessity must be evaluated in light of boundary violations.

Box 2-13

POSSIBLE BOUNDARY VIOLATIONS RELATED TO PSYCHIATRIC NURSES

▼ The patient takes the nurse out to lunch or dinner
▼ The professional relationship turns into a social relationship
▼ The nurse attends a party at a patient's invitation
▼ The nurse regularly reveals personal information to the patient
▼ The patient introduces the nurse to family members, such as a son or daughter, for the purpose of a social relationship
▼ The nurse accepts free gifts from the patient's business
▼ The nurse agrees to meet the patient for treatment outside of the usual setting without therapeutic justification
▼ The nurse attends social functions of the patient
▼ The patient gives the nurse an expensive gift
▼ The nurse routinely hugs or holds the patient
▼ The nurse does business or purchases services from the patient

---

3. **Place and space boundaries**—This issue is related to where treatment actually takes place. An office or hospital unit is the usual locale for most treatment. Treatment out of the office usually merits special scrutiny. Most often treatment over lunch, in the car, or in the patient's home must have a good therapeutic rationale and explicit treatment goals. In an inpatient setting, any time spent by a nurse in a patient's room should be done so only if indicated and with appropriate action taken to respect boundary concerns, such as with the door open and in the presence of other staff.

4. **Money boundaries**—This issue relates to honoring the compensation for treatment established between the nurse and patient. Bartering or seeing an indigent patient for free should be carefully reviewed for potential boundary violations.

5. **Gifts and services boundaries**—Gift giving is a controversial issue in nursing (see Critical Thinking about Contemporary Issues). Gifts that are obvious boundary violations place undue obligations on the patient for the benefit of the nurse. Gifts can be divided into five types[35]:
   a. Gifts to reciprocate for care given
   b. Gifts intended to manipulate or change the quality of care given or the nature of the nurse-patient relationship
   c. Gifts given as perceived obligation by the patient
   d. Serendipitous gifts or gifts received by chance
   e. Gifts given to the organization to recognize excellence of care received
   The nurse must carefully consider how to respond to each of these categories based on the intention of the gift and the possibility of boundary violations.

6. **Clothing boundaries**—This pertains to the nurse's need to dress in an appropriate therapeutic manner. Suggestive or seductive clothing of the nurse is unacceptable and limits should be set on inappropriate dress by patients as well.

7. **Language boundaries**—This boundary raises questions of when patients should be addressed by their first or last names, the tone that the nurse uses when talking with the patient, and the nurse's choice of words in implementing care. Too familiar, sexual, or leading language clearly suggests boundary violations.

8. **Self-disclosure boundaries**—Inappropriately timed self-disclosure by the nurse or nurse self-disclosure that lacks therapeutic value are suspect for boundary violations as discussed previously in this chapter.

9. **Physical contact boundaries**—All physical contact with a patient must be evaluated for possible boundary violations. Sexual contact of any kind is never therapeutic within the nurse-patient relationship.

 ## CRITICAL THINKING ABOUT CONTEMPORARY ISSUES

Is Gift Giving Acceptable Behavior in the Therapeutic Nurse-Patient Relationship?

Gift giving is a controversial issue in nursing. There has been a long-accepted taboo in nursing on accepting gifts from patients. On the other hand, some have questioned the theoretical rationale for this position and suggest that gift giving can sometimes serve discrete therapeutic purposes.[35]

Gifts can take many forms. They can be tangible or intangible, lasting or temporary. Tangible gifts may include such items as a box of candy, a bouquet of flowers, a hand-knit scarf, or a hand-painted picture. Intangible gifts can be the expression of thanks to a nurse by a patient who is about to be discharged or a family member's sense of relief and gratitude at being able to share an emotional burden with another caring person. The underlying element of all of these gifts is that something of value is voluntarily offered to another person, usually to convey gratitude.

Because gifts can be so varied, it is inappropriate to lump them all together and uniformly arrive at an appropriate nursing action. Rather, the nurse's response to gift giving and the role it plays in the therapeutic relationship depends on the timing of the particular situation, the intent of the giver, and the contextual meaning of the giving of the gift. Occasionally it may be most appropriate and therapeutic for the nurse to accept a patient's gift; on other occasions it may be quite inappropriate and detrimental to the relationship.

The timing of the gift giving is an important consideration. In the introductory, or orientation, phase of the relationship, nurses may be asked, "Do you have a cigarette I can borrow?" or "Will you buy me a cup of coffee?" These seemingly minor requests may make the nurse feel uncomfortable refusing them. The nurse may rationalize compliance by thinking that it indicates interest in the patient and may help win his trust. But these responses indicate the nurse's failure to examine the patient's covert, or underlying, need and the nurse's own needs in complying with it. Also, in this early phase of the relationship, the nurse may

Continued.

be the one to initiate gift giving by giving the patient a book, plant, or some other item that expresses interest in the patient.

In the orientation phase of the relationship, gift giving can be detrimental because it often meets personal needs rather than therapeutic goals. The patient may be trying to manipulate the nurse as a way to control the relationship and set interpersonal limits on the level of intimacy that will be allowed. By giving gifts to the patient, the nurse is attempting to relate through objects instead of the therapeutic use of self and is avoiding exploring possible feelings of inadequacy or frustration.

As the relationship progresses, gift giving may take on a different significance. In the working phase, for example, the patient may one day offer to buy the nurse a cup of coffee. This can be an indication of the patient's respect for the nurse and of belief in the mutuality of their work together. As an isolated incident, the nurse's acceptance of it can enhance the patient's confidence, self-esteem, and sense of responsibility.

Gift giving most often arises in the termination phase of the relationship, and it is in this phase that the meaning behind it can be the most complex and difficult to determine. At this time gift giving can be tangible or intangible and can reflect a patient's need to make the nurse feel guilty, delay the termination process, compensate for feelings of inadequacy, or attempt to transform the therapeutic nurse-patient relationship into a social one that can possibly go on indefinitely. The nurse can initiate gift giving for similar reasons. The feelings evoked during the termination process can be very powerful, and they must be acknowledged and explored if termination is to be a learning experience for both participants. If feelings are identified and clarified, then a small gift that reflects gratitude and remembrance can be exchanged, accepted, and valued. ▼

EFFECTIVENESS OF THE NURSE

The nurse's effectiveness in working with psychiatric patients is related to knowledge base, clinical skills, and capacity for introspection and self-evaluation. The nurse and patient, as participants in an interpersonal relationship, are entwined in a pattern of reciprocal emotions that directly affect the therapeutic outcome. The nurse conveys feelings to the patient. Some of these are in response to the patient; others arise from the nurse's personal life and are not necessarily associated with the patient.

Many painful feelings arise within the nurse because of the nature of the therapeutic process, which can be stressful. These "normal" stresses are caused by a variety of factors. Although it is necessary to be a skilled listener, it is inappropriate for the nurse to discuss personal conflicts or responses, except when they may help the patient. This bottling up of emotions can be painful. The nurse is expected to empathize with the patient's emotions and feelings. At the same time, however, the nurse is expected to retain objectivity and not be caught up in a sympathetic response. This can create a kind of double bind.

Termination poses another stress when the nurse must separate from a patient she has come to know well and care for deeply. It is common to experience a grief reaction in response to the loss. Many nurses find it emotionally draining when a patient communicates a prolonged and intense expression of emotion, such as sadness, despair, or anger. Discomfort also arises when the nurse feels unable to help a patient who is in great distress. Suicide dramatizes this situation. Treating suicidal individuals can arouse intense and prolonged anxiety in the nurse.

The painful nature of these emotional responses makes the practice of psychiatric nursing challenging and stressful. The therapeutic use of self involves the nurse's total personality, and total involvement is not an easy task. It is essential that the nurse be aware of personal feelings and responses and receive guidance and support.

SUMMARY

1. The therapeutic nurse-patient relationship is a mutual learning experience and a corrective emotional experience for the patient. The nurse uses personal attributes and specified clinical techniques in working with the patient to bring about behavioral change.
2. The following qualities are needed by nurses to be effective helpers: awareness of self, clarification of values, exploration of feelings, ability to serve as a role model, altruism, and a sense of ethics and responsibility.
3. The structural and transactional analysis models were used to examine components of the communication process and to identify common problems. Helpful therapeutic communication techniques were also discussed.
4. The responsive dimensions of genuineness, respect, empathic understanding, and concreteness were presented.
5. The action dimensions of confrontation, immediacy, nurse self-disclosure, catharsis, and role playing stimulate and contribute to patient insight.
6. Therapeutic impasses such as resistance, transference, countertransference, and boundary violations are roadblocks in the progress of the nurse-patient relationship.
7. The nurse's effectiveness in working with psychiatric patients is related to knowledge base, clinical skills, and capacity for introspection and self-evaluation.

REFERENCES

1. Alligood M: Empathy: the importance of recognizing two types, J *Psychosoc Nurs* 30:14, 1992.
2. Argyle M: *Bodily communication*, ed 2, New York, 1988, Methuen.
3. Berne E: *Games people play: the psychology of human relationships*, New York, 1964, Grove Press.
4. Bromley G: Confrontation in individual psychotherapy, J *Psychiatr Nurs Ment Health Serv* 19:15, 1981.
5. Buxman K: Humor in therapy for the mentally ill, J *Psychosoc Nurs Ment Health Serv* 29:15, 1991.
6. Campaniello J: The process of termination, J *Psychiatr Nurs* 18:29, 1980.
7. Campbell J: The relationship of nursing and self-awareness, *Adv Nurs Sci* 2:15, 1980.
8. Carkhoff R: *Helping and human relations*, vols 1 and 2, New York, 1969, Holt, Rinehart & Winston.
9. Carkhoff R, Berenson B: *Beyond counseling and therapy*, New York, 1967, Holt, Rinehart & Winston.
10. Carkhoff R, Truax C: *Toward effective counseling and psychotherapy*, Chicago, 1967, Aldine Publishing.
11. Coad-Denton A: Therapeutic superficiality and intimacy. In Longo D, Williams R, eds: *Psychosocial nursing: assessment and intervention*, New York, 1978, Appleton-Century-Crofts.
12. Cravener P: Establishing therapeutic alliance across cultural barriers, J *Psychosoc Nurs Ment Health Serv* 30:11, 1992.
13. Davidhizar R, Bowen M: The dynamics of laughter, *Arch Psychiatr Nurs* 6:132, 1992.
14. Forchuk C: The orientation phase of the nurse-client relationship: how long does it take? *Perspect Psychiatr Care* 28:7, 1992.
15. Forchuk C, Brown B: Establishing a nurse-client relationship, J *Psychosoc Nurs Ment Health Serv* 27:30, 1989.
16. Gazda G et al: *Human relations development: a manual for educators*, Boston, 1971, Allyn & Bacon.
17. Guthiel T, Gabbard G: The concept of boundaries in clinical practice: theoretical and risk-management dimensions, *Am J Psychiatry* 150:188, 1993.
18. Hall E: *The silent language*, Garden City, NY, 1959, Doubleday & Co.
19. Johnson M: Self-disclosure and anxiety in nurses and patients, *Issues Ment Health Nurs* 2:41, 1979.
20. Johnson M: Self-disclosure: a variable in the nurse-client relationship, J *Psychiatr Nurs* 18:17, 1980.
21. Jourard S: *The transparent self*, New York, 1971, Litton Educational Publishing.
22. Kalisch B: What is empathy? *Am J Nurs* 73:1548, 1973.
23. Kemper B: Therapeutic listening, J *Psychosoc Nurs Ment Health Serv* 30:21, 1992.

24. Kirschenbaum H and Simon S, editors: *Readings in values clarification*, Minneapolis, 1973, Winston Press.

25. Krieger D: *The therapeutic touch: how to use your hands to help or to heal*, New York, 1979, Prentice Hall.

26. La Crosse M: Nonverbal behavior and perceived counselor attractiveness and persuasiveness, *J Counsel Psychol* 22:563, 1975.

27. Levinson H: Termination of psychotherapy: some salient issues. Paper presented at a meeting of the Illinois Society for Clinical Social Work, Chicago, Oct 1975.

28. Loomis M: Levels of contracting, *J Psychosoc Nurs Ment Health Serv* 23:9, 1985.

29. Luft J: *Of human interaction*, Palo Alto, Calif, 1969, National Press Books.

30. MacKay R, Hughes J, Carver E eds: *Empathy in the helping relationship*, New York, 1990, Springer.

31. Mansfield E: Empathy: concept and identified psychiatric nursing behavior, *Nurs Res* 22:525, 1973.

32. Mehrabian A: *Nonverbal communication*, Chicago, 1972, Aldine Publishing.

33. Mitchell K and Berenson B: Differential use of confrontation by high and low facilitative therapists, *J Nerv Ment Dis* 151:303, 1970.

34. Morrison P, Burnard P: Student's and trained nurse's perceptions of their own interpersonal skills: a report and comparison, *J Adv Nurs* 14:321, 1989.

35. Morse J: The structure and function of gift giving in the patient-nurse relationship, *West J Nurs Res* 13:597, 1991.

36. Morse J et al: Exploring empathy: a conceptual fit for nursing practice? *Image J Nurs Sch* 24:273, 1992.

37. Pasquali E: Learning to laugh: humor as therapy, *J Psychosoc Nurs Ment Health Serv* 28:31, 1990.

38. Peitchinis J: Therapeutic effectiveness of counseling by nursing personnel, *Nurs Res* 21:138, 1972.

39. Robinson V: *Humor and the health professions*, Thorofare, NJ, 1991, Slack.

40. Rogers C: *On becoming a person*, Boston, 1961, Houghton Mifflin.

41. Rogers C: Empathic: an unappreciated way of being, *J Counsel Psychol* 5:2, 1975.

42. Ruesch J: *Disturbed communication*, New York, 1972, WW Norton.

43. Schoffstall C: Concerns of student nurses prior to psychiatric nursing experience: an assessment and intervention technique, *J Psychosoc Nurs Ment Health Serv* 19:11, 1981.

44. Sedgwick R: Role playing: a bridge between talk and action, *J Psychiatr Nurs* 14:16, 1976.

45. Stacklum M: New student in psychology, *Am J Nurs* 81:762, 1981.

46. Stricker G, Fisher M: *Self-disclosure in the therapeutic relationship*, New York, 1990, Plenum Press.

47. Sundeen S et al: *Nurse-client interaction: implementing the nursing process*, ed 5, St Louis, 1994, Mosby.

48. Tommasini N: The use of touch with the hospitalized psychiatric patient, *Arch Psychiatr Nurs* 4:213, 1990.

49. Warner S: Humor: a coping response for student nurses, *Arch Psychiatr Nurs* 5:10, 1991.

50. Weiss S: Touch, *Annu Rev Nurs Res* 6:3, 1988.

51. Wheeler K: A nursing science approach to understanding empathy, *Arch Psychiatr Nurs* 2:96, 1988.

52. Williams C: Biopsychosocial elements of empathy: a multidimensional model, *Issues Ment Health Nurs* 11:155, 1990.

53. Wolberg L: *The technique of psychotherapy*, ed 4, Orlando, Fla, 1988, Grune & Stratton.

54. Young J: Rationale for clinician self-disclosure and research agenda, *Image J Nurs Sch* 20:196, 1988.

ANNOTATED SUGGESTED READINGS

Berne E: *Games people play*, New York, 1967, Grove Press.

The founder of transactional analysis uses that technique to explore a number of specific "games." A thought-provoking book that gives a different slant on relationships and challenges the reader to find ways to terminate destructive "games."

*Burnard P: *Learning human skills: an experiential guide for nurses*, Oxford, 1990, Heinemann Nursing.

Workbook style approach to help nurses learn interpersonal and therapeutic relationship skills.

Carkhoff R: *Helping and human relations*, vols 1 and 2, New York, 1969, Holt, Rinehart & Winston.

Explores elements of research and practice in helping relationships. Presents scales used to rate the "core therapeutic dimensions."

Cormier W, Cormier L: *Interviewing strategies for helpers*, Pacific Grove, Calif, 1990, Brooks/Cole Publishing.

Comprehensive coverage of skills and strategies associated with effective helping. Practical application with many examples and learning activities for the student.

Jourard S: *The transparent self*, New York, 1971, Litton Educational Publishing.

Proposes that a person can attain health only as he gains courage to be himself with others and finds goals that have meaning for him.

*La Monica E, Karshmer J: *Empathy: educating nurses in professional practice*, J Nurs Educ 17:3, 1978.

Describes a staff development program that was effective in raising nurses' abilities to perceive and respond with empathy.

*May C: *Research on nurse-patient relationships: problems of theory, problems of practice*, J Adv Nurs 15:307, 1990.

Challenges traditional notions and raises problems about nurse-patient relationships and interactions, particularly in nonpsychiatric settings. Interesting reading.

*Miles M: *The evolution of countertransference and its applicability to nursing*, Perspect Psychiatr Care 29:13, 1993.

Reviews the concept of countertransference and ways nurses can benefit from using it as a valuable therapeutic tool.

*Moller M, McBride A: *What clinical experiences are needed before entering psychiatric nursing?* J Psychosoc Nurs Ment Health Serv 30:41, 1992.

Two leaders in psychiatric nursing answer this often asked question. Both agree that a biopsychosocial approach is needed and that specific medical-surgical or other experiences are not necessary if the nurse is committed, has an inquiring mind, and practices in a supportive organization.

*Montgomery C: *Healing through communication: the practice of caring*, Newbury Park, Calif, 1993, Sage Publications.

Superb text that examines the concept of caring, the manifestations of caring, and the effects of caring. Important reading for every nurse.

*Sayre J: *Common errors in communication made by students in psychiatric nursing*, Perspect Psychiatr Care 16:175, 1978.

Should be required reading for all students in psychiatric nursing. Identifies many of the communication errors made in each phase of the nurse-patient relationship and gives a clinical example of each.

*Schoffstall C: *Concerns of student nurses prior to psychiatric nursing experience: an assessment and intervention technique*, J Psychosoc Nurs Ment Health Serv 19:11, 1981.

The authors describe a study they conducted to assess and reduce the anxiety of students about to begin their clinical experience in psychiatric nursing. Educators may find this useful.

*Scott A: *A beginning theory of personal space boundaries*, Perspect Psychiatr Care 29:12, 1993.

Thought-provoking article about the role of boundaries in protecting the person from environmental overload and possible disorganization with application to nursing practice.

*Sedgwick R: *Role playing: a bridge between talk and action*, J Psychiatr Nurs 14:16, 1976.

Describes the uses and steps of role playing. Techniques are included, with a brief description of how they are accomplished.

*Sundeen S et al: *Nurse-client interaction: implementing the nursing process*, ed 5, St Louis, 1994, Mosby.

Describes the nursing process, including concepts related to self, communication, phases of the nurse-client relationship, and stress and adaptation. A useful reference for developing relationship skills.

---

*Nursing reference.

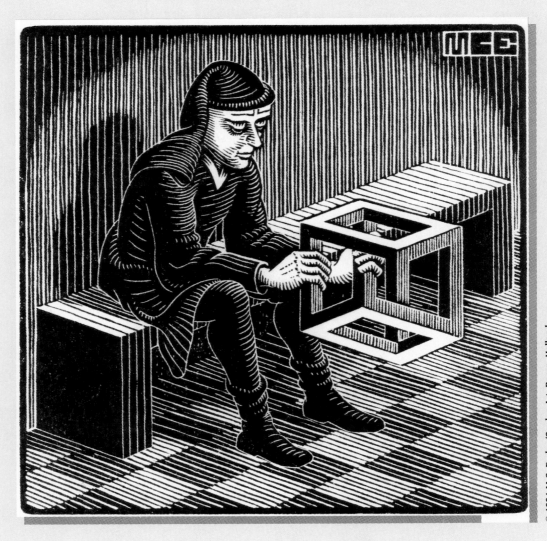

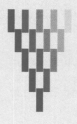

CHAPTER 3

Conceptual Models of Psychiatric Treatment

GAIL W. STUART

SANDRA J. SUNDEEN

Though this be madness, yet there is method in't.

William Shakespeare: *Hamlet*, Act II

LEARNING OBJECTIVES

After studying this chapter the student should be able to:

▼ Describe the psychoanalytical model including its view of behavioral deviations, therapeutic process, and roles of the patient and therapist

▼ Describe the interpersonal model including its view of behavioral deviations, therapeutic process, and roles of the patient and therapist

▼ Describe the social model including its view of behavioral deviations, therapeutic process, and roles of the patient and therapist

▼ Describe the existential model including its view of behavioral deviations, therapeutic process, and roles of the patient and therapist

▼ Describe the supportive therapy model including its view of behavioral deviations, therapeutic process, and roles of the patient and therapist

▼ Describe the medical model including its view of behavioral deviations, therapeutic process, and roles of the patient and therapist

TOPICAL OUTLINE

Psychoanalytical Model
   View of Behavioral Deviations
   Psychoanalytical Therapeutic Process
   Roles of Patient and Psychoanalyst
   Other Psychoanalytical Theorists
Interpersonal Model
   View of Behavioral Deviations
   Interpersonal Therapeutic Process
   Roles of Patient and Interpersonal Therapist
Social Model
   View of Behavioral Deviations
   Social Therapeutic Process
   Roles of Patient and Social Therapist
Existential Model
   View of Behavioral Deviations
   Existential Therapeutic Process
   Roles of Patient and Existential Therapist
Supportive Therapy Model
   View of Behavioral Deviations
   Supportive Therapeutic Process
   Roles of Patient and Supportive Therapist
Medical Model
   View of Behavioral Deviations
   Medical Therapeutic Process
   Roles of Patient and Medical Therapist

Most mental health professionals practice within the framework of a conceptual model of psychiatric treatment. A model is a way of organizing a complex body of knowledge, such as concepts related to human behavior. Models can help clinicians by suggesting:

▼ Reasons for observed behavior
▼ Therapeutic treatment strategies
▼ Appropriate role enactment for both patient and therapist

Models also provide for the organization of data. This allows the clinician to measure the effectiveness of the treatment process and facilitates research into human behavior.

This chapter presents an overview of some of the many conceptual models used by mental health professionals, including the psychoanalytical, interpersonal, social, existential, supportive, and medical models. Other models often used by nurses are discussed in other chapters of this text including cognitive behavioral (Chapter 28), group (Chapter 29), and family (Chapter 30). Finally, a stress adaptation model of psychiatric nursing is presented in detail in Chapter 4. This nursing model is the organizing conceptual framework for this text.

PSYCHOANALYTICAL MODEL

Psychoanalytical theory was developed by Sigmund Freud (Fig. 3-1) in the late nineteenth and early twentieth centuries.[8] It focused on the nature of deviant behavior and proposed a new perspective on human de-

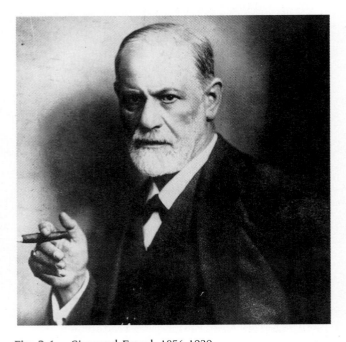

Fig. 3-1 Sigmund Freud, 1856-1939.
From The Bettman Archive.

velopment. Many of Freud's ideas were controversial, particularly in the Victorian society of that time. Objective observation of human behavior was a great contribution of the psychoanalysts, as was the identification of a mental structure. Such concepts as id, ego, superego, and ego defense mechanisms are still widely used. Most people also accept the existence of an unconscious level of mental functioning first introduced by Freud.

View of Behavioral Deviations

Psychoanalysts trace disrupted behavior in the adult to earlier developmental stages. Each stage of development has a task that must be accomplished. If too much emphasis is placed on any stage or if unusual difficulty arises in dealing with the associated conflicts, psychological energy (libido) becomes fixated in an attempt to deal with anxiety.

Psychoanalysts believe that neurotic symptoms arise when so much energy goes into controlling anxiety that it interferes with the individual's ability to function. They believe that everyone is neurotic to some extent. Everyone carries the burden of childhood conflicts and is influenced in adulthood by childhood experiences. Psychoanalysts in training must undergo personal analysis so that their own neurotic behavior does not hinder their objectivity as therapists.

According to psychoanalytic theory, symptoms are symbols of the original conflict. For instance, compulsive hand washing may represent the person's attempt to cleanse the self of impulses that a parent labeled unclean during the anal stage of development. However, the meaning of the behavior is hidden from the conscious awareness of the person, who usually is upset about these uncontrollable thoughts, actions, and feelings.

Freud developed most of his theories around neurotic symptoms. His theory is less well developed in the area of psychosis. However, other psychoanalytical theorists such as Frieda Fromm-Reichmann[9] have successfully worked with psychotic patients. They believe that the psychotic symptom occurs when the ego must invest most or all of the libido to defend against primitive id impulses. This leaves little, if any, energy to deal with external reality and leads to the lack of reality testing seen in psychosis.

Psychoanalytical Therapeutic Process

Psychoanalysis uses free association and dream analysis to reconstruct the personality. Free association is the verbalization of thoughts as they occur without any conscious screening or censorship. Of course, there is always unconscious censorship of thoughts and impulses that threaten the ego. The psychoanalyst searches for patterns in the areas that are unconsciously avoided. Conflictual areas that the patient does not discuss or recognize are identified as resistances. Analysis of the patient's dreams can provide additional insight into the nature of the resistances, since dreams symbolically communicate areas of intrapsychic conflict.

The therapist helps the patient recognize intrapsychic conflicts by using interpretation. Interpretation involves explaining to the patient the meaning of dream symbolism and the significance of the issues that are discussed or avoided. However, the process is complicated by transference, which occurs when the patient develops strong positive or negative feelings toward the analyst. These feelings are unrelated to the analyst's current behavior or characteristics; they represent the patient's past response to a significant other, usually a parent. Strong positive transference causes the patient to want to please the therapist and to accept the therapist's interpretations of the patient's behavior. Strong negative transference may impede the progress of therapy as the patient actively resists the therapist's interventions. Countertransference, or the therapist's response to the patient, can also interfere with therapy if the analyst is unaware of it or unable to deal with it.

Since the therapist can temporarily replace the significant other of the patient's early life experience, previously unresolved conflicts can be brought into the therapeutic situation. These conflicts can be worked through to a healthier resolution. This releases previously invested libido for mature adult functioning. Psychoanalytical therapy is usually long term. The patient is often seen five times a week for several years. This approach is therefore time consuming and expensive.

Roles of Patient and Psychoanalyst

The roles of the patient and the psychoanalyst were defined by Freud. The patient was to be an active participant, freely revealing all thoughts exactly as they occurred and describing all dreams. The patient often lies down during therapy to induce relaxation, which facilitates free association.

The psychoanalyst is a shadow person. The patient is expected to reveal all private thoughts and feelings, and the analyst reveals nothing personal. The analyst usually is out of the patient's sight to ensure that nonverbal responses do not influence the patient. Verbal responses are brief and noncommittal for the most part to prevent interference with the associative flow. For instance, the analyst might respond with "Uh huh," "Go on," or "Tell me more."

The therapist changes this communication style when interpreting behavior. Interpretations are presented for the patient to accept or reject, but rejections suggest resistance. Likewise, frustration that the patient expresses toward the analyst is interpreted as transference. By the end of therapy, the patient should be able to view the analyst realistically, having worked through conflicts and dependency needs.

 Do you think that the roles of the patient and psychoanalyst support patient empowerment or patient dependency?

Other Psychoanalytical Theorists

Much of Freud's theory is still used by psychotherapists. The theorists who followed him have modified and built on the original psychoanalytical theories.

Box 3-1 presents a list of several contemporary psychoanalytical theorists and a brief statement identifying their major contributions.

INTERPERSONAL MODEL

The theorist most representative of the interpersonal model is Harry Stack Sullivan, a twentieth-century American therapist.[23,24] In addition, attention is given to the interpersonal nursing theory of Hildegard Peplau[17] (Fig. 3-2). Her work represents a milestone in the conceptualization of the psychotherapeutic role of the nurse in the context of the interpersonal relationship.

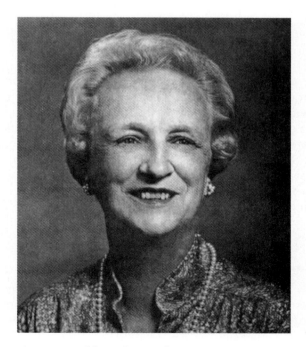

Fig. 3-2 Hildegard E. Peplau.
Courtesy Hildegard E. Peplau.

Box 3-1
CONTEMPORARY PSYCHOANALYTICAL THEORISTS

Erik Erikson[5]	Expanded Freud's theory of psychosocial development to encompass the entire life cycle
Anna Freud[7]	Expanded psychoanalytical theory in the area of child psychology
Melanie Klein[14]	Extended the use of psychoanalytical techniques to work with young children through development of play therapy
Karen Horney[13]	Focused on psychoanalytical theory relative to cultural and interpersonal factors; rejected Freud's view of feminine sexuality
Frieda Fromm-Reichmann[9]	Used psychoanalytical techniques with psychotic individuals
Karl Menninger[16]	Applied the concepts of dynamic equilibrium and coping to mental functioning

---

View of Behavioral Deviations

Interpersonal theorists believe that behavior evolves around interpersonal relationships. While Freudian theory emphasizes a person's intrapsychic experience, interpersonal theory emphasizes social or interpersonal experience. Sullivan, like Freud, traces a progression of psychological development. Sullivan's theory states that the person bases behavior on two drives: the drive for satisfaction and the drive for security. Satisfaction refers to the basic human drives, including hunger, sleep, lust, and loneliness. Security relates to culturally defined needs such as conformity to the social norms and value system of the individual's ethnic group. Sullivan states that when the nature of a person's self-system interferes with the ability to attend to the need for either satisfaction or security, the person will become mentally ill.

When Peplau defined nursing as an interpersonal process, she also discussed the importance of basic human needs. Needs must be met if a healthy state is to be achieved and maintained. For Peplau, the two interacting components of health are physiological demands and interpersonal conditions. These may be viewed as parallel to the drives of satisfaction and security identified by Sullivan, as evident in the following clinical example.

 ## CLINICAL EXAMPLE

Ms. Y an attractive 26-year-old woman, appeared at a psychiatric outpatient clinic requesting therapy. She described her problem as "I can't get close to people." She said that her childhood was happy and that she had loving parents and liked her sister. Her family were devout members of a fundamentalist Protestant church, so most of her activities were church related. She had many friends during childhood and then one close girl friend in early adolescence. She thought that her fear of closeness began when she slept over at her friend's house. During the night her friend began to fondle her in a way that she interpreted as sexual. She became very frightened and felt guilty about this. She did not tell her parents because of her guilt and, in fact, had told no one before entering therapy. Although she attended college, she never dated and would participate only in superficial social contacts. She realized that this was not healthy young adult behavior and, as the behavior continued into her twenties, Ms. Y decided that she needed to seek help.

From an interpersonal perspective, Ms. Y was unable to fulfill her needs for friendship and sexual love. Interpersonal theorists would view the unfulfilled sexual love dynamism as a lack of satisfaction, and her fear that she had deviated from the norm as a lack of security. Her anxiety stemmed from her conviction that her parents would disown her if they heard what had happened. This belief was based on their earlier responses to childhood sexual play. The therapist decided that Ms. Y first needed to experience intimacy on a nonsexual level. This was approached in therapy. When she began to feel comfortable sharing closeness with the therapist, Ms. Y. gradually explored friendships and later began dating.

Interpersonal Therapeutic Process

The interpersonal therapist, like the psychoanalyst, explores the patient's life history. The crux of the therapeutic process is the corrective interpersonal experience. The idea is that by experiencing a healthy relationship with the therapist, the patient can learn to have more satisfying interpersonal relationships. The therapist actively encourages the development of trust by relating authentically to the patient. The therapist must share feelings and reactions with the patient. The process of therapy is a process of reeducation.

The therapist helps the patient identify interpersonal problems and then encourages attempts at more successful styles of relating. For example, patients often have a fear of intimacy. The therapist allows the patient to become close while clearly showing that there is no threat of sexual involvement. It is believed that closeness within the therapeutic relationship builds trust, facilitates empathy, enhances self-esteem, and fosters growth toward healthy behavior. Peplau[17] describes this process as "psychological mothering," which includes the following steps:

1. The patient is accepted unconditionally as a participant in a relationship that satisfies needs.
2. There is recognition of and response to the patient's readiness for growth, as initiated by the patient.
3. Power in the relationship shifts to the patient, as the patient is able to delay gratification and to invest energy in goal achievement.

Therapy is completed when the patient can establish satisfying human relationships, thereby meeting basic needs. Termination is a significant part of the relationship that must be experienced and shared by both the therapist and the patient. The patient learns that leaving a significant other involves pain but can also be an opportunity for growth.

 Do you think that "psychological mothering" promotes maternalism or mutuality in the patient-therapist relationship?

Roles of Patient and Interpersonal Therapist

The patient-therapist dyad is viewed as a partnership in interpersonal therapy. Sullivan describes the therapist as a "participant observer" whose role is to engage the patient, establish trust, and empathize. There is an active effort to help the patient realize that other people have similar perceptions and concerns. An atmosphere of uncritical acceptance encourages the patient to speak openly. The therapist interacts as a real person who also has beliefs, values, thoughts, and feelings. The patient's role is to share concerns with the therapist and to participate as fully as possible in the relationship. The relationship itself is meant to serve as a model of adaptive interpersonal relationships. As the patient matures

in the ability to relate, life experiences with people outside the therapeutic situation can be enhanced.

Interpersonal nursing roles have been identified by Peplau[17] and are listed in Box 3-2. These roles may be assumed by the nurse or assigned to others. The therapist helps the patient meet the goals of therapy: need satisfaction and personal growth. In addition, through role performance the nurse also experiences growth and self-discovery. Self-awareness is essential to success as an interpersonal therapist.

SOCIAL MODEL

The two preceding models focused on the individual and intrapsychic processes and interpersonal experiences. The social model moves beyond the individual to consider the social environment as it affects the person and the person's life experience (see Chapter 7). Psychoanalytical theory has been criticized for not extending to other cultures and times. For example, Freud's view of women has been repeatedly challenged, particularly by feminists. Some theorists such as Thomas Szasz[25-27] and Gerald Caplan[3] believe that the culture itself is useful in defining mental illness, prescribing the nature of therapy, and determining the patient's future. In addition, the community mental health movement is an example of a governmental effort to respond to the philosophy of the social theorists (see Chapter 32).

View of Behavioral Deviations

According to the social theorists, social conditions are largely responsible for deviant behavior. Deviancy is cul-

---

Box 3-2

INTERPERSONAL NURSING ROLES IDENTIFIED BY PEPLAU

1. *Stranger*—the role assumed by both nurse and patient when they first meet
2. *Resource person*—provide health information to a patient who has assumed the consumer role
3. *Teacher*—assist the patient as learner to grow and learn from experience with the health-care system
4. *Leader*—assist the patient as follower to participate in a democratically implemented nursing process
5. *Surrogate*—assume roles that have been assigned by the patient, based on significant past relationships, similar to the psychoanalytical concept of transference
6. *Counselor*—help the patient integrate the facts and feelings associated with an episode of illness into the patient's total life experience

turally defined. Behavior considered normal in one cultural setting may be eccentric in another and psychotic in a third. An example is the African exchange student described in the following clinical example.

CLINICAL EXAMPLE

Early in the fall semester a black male exchange student from Africa was brought to the psychiatric emergency room. He had been walking around the campus carrying a spear and had been apprehended by the university security patrol. His speech was heavily accented and they could not understand his explanation of his behavior. Later evaluation revealed that in his culture one never went walking at night without a spear to defend against attack by wild beasts or hostile neighboring tribes. He was sent back to his dormitory after being convinced that his spear was not appropriate to the culture of the American college campus.

With this point of view, Szasz[25] writes of the "myth of mental illness." He believes that society must find a way of managing "undesirables," so it labels them as mentally ill. People who are so labeled usually are unable or refuse to conform to social norms, and this behavior usually leads to institutionalization. If these individuals then conform to social expectations, they are considered to be recovered and are allowed to return to the community. Institutionalization, then, performs the dual function of removing deviant members from the community and exerting social control over their behavior.

Szasz believes that people are responsible for their behavior. The person has control over whether to conform to social expectations. Those labeled as mentally ill may be scapegoats, but they participate in the scapegoating process by inviting it or by allowing it to occur. Szasz objects to describing deviant behavior as "illness." He believes that illness can occur in the body and that diseases of the body can influence behavior (e.g., brain tumors), but that no physiological disruption can be demonstrated to cause most deviancy. He distinguishes between the biological condition that is central to illness and the social role that is the focus of deviancy.

Caplan[3] also has studied deviant behavior from a social perspective. He has extended the public health model of primary, secondary, and tertiary prevention to the mental health field. He has focused particularly on primary prevention, since much attention has been given in the past to the secondary and tertiary levels. Lack of understanding of the cause of deviant behavior has hindered the development of primary prevention techniques.

Caplan believes that social situations can predispose a person to mental illness. Such situations include poverty, family instability, and inadequate education. Deprivation throughout the life cycle results in limited ability to cope with stress. The person has few available environmental supports. The result is a predisposition to maladaptive coping responses.

How do you distinguish between social deviancy and psychiatric illness? How do your friends and family?

Social Therapeutic Process

Szasz advocates freedom of choice for psychiatric patients. People should be allowed to select their own therapeutic modality and therapists. This also implies a well-informed consumer who can base this decision on knowledge of available modes of therapy (see Critical Thinking about Contemporary Issues). Szasz does not believe in involuntary hospitalization of the mentally ill. He questions whether any psychiatric hospitalization is truly voluntary. Szasz disapproves of the community mental health trend to place mental health care within the reach of every American. He questions government involvement in what he views as a private concern.

Caplan, on the other hand, supports community psychiatry. He sees the mental health professional as using consultation to combat societal problems. He believes that future psychiatric patients would benefit indirectly from positive social change.

Roles of Patient and Social Therapist

Szasz believes that a therapist can help the patient only if the patient requests help. The patient, then, initiates therapy and defines the problem to be solved. The patient also has the right to approve or reject the recommended therapeutic intervention. Therapy is successfully completed when the patient is satisfied with the changes made in lifestyle. The therapist collaborates with the patient to promote change. This includes making recommendations to the patient about possible means of effecting behavioral change, but it does not include any element of coercion, particularly the threat of hospitalization if the patient does not agree with the therapist's recommendations. The therapist's role also may involve protecting the patient from social demands for being treated unwillingly.

Caplan believes that society itself has a moral obligation to provide a wide range of therapeutic services covering all three levels of prevention. The patient has

CRITICAL THINKING ABOUT CONTEMPORARY ISSUES

What Kind of Psychotherapy Works Best, for Whom, under What Circumstances, and at What Cost?

Competition between the various models of psychiatric treatment has tended to distract attention from questions about what model of psychotherapy works best, for what type of patient, under what life conditions, and at what cost. Answering these questions has been difficult. For example, few studies focus on the cost effectiveness of psychotherapy.[15] Evaluating the outcomes of treatment is also difficult. At best, these have proven to be inexact and subjective processes that depend on one or more of the following factors:

▼ The therapist's evaluation of changes that have occurred
▼ The patient's report of changes
▼ Reports from the patient's family and friends
▼ Comparison of pretreatment and posttreatment behavioral rating scale scores
▼ Measures of changes in selected symptoms or behaviors

Unfortunately, each of these sources has serious limitations. In addition, these studies often fail to measure other critically important aspects of treatment, such as the nature of the therapeutic alliance, health belief systems of the patient and therapist, cost of treatment, and impact of treatment on the patient's overall biopsychosocial functioning and quality of life. What is needed is greater specificity about the people and problems for which psychotherapy can provide the greatest benefit, the methodology that would be most useful in providing these data, and comprehensive quantification of the indications for, cost of, and outcomes produced by psychotherapy. ▼

a consumer role and selects the appropriate level of help from a wide array of available services. Ideally, effective primary preventive services would decrease the need for secondary or tertiary care.

According to this model, therapists may be professionals or nonprofessionals with professional consultation. People such as clergy, police, bartenders, and beauticians can be trained to listen and to refer people who need professional help to appropriate resources. The therapist in the social context is not tied to the office but is involved in the community. Activities may include home visits, lectures to community groups, or consultation with other agencies. The rationale for this approach is that the more involved therapists are in the community, the greater the impact on the community's mental health. Community involvement also enhances the therapist's understanding of patients who live in that environment.

 Do you think bartenders and beauticians can be effective therapists? Why or why not?

EXISTENTIAL MODEL

The existential model focuses on the person's experience in the here and now, with much less attention to the person's past than in other theoretical models.

View of Behavioral Deviations

Existentialist theorists believe that behavioral deviations result when the individual is out of touch with the self or the environment. This alienation is caused by self-imposed restrictions. The individual is not free to choose from among all alternative behaviors. Deviant behavior frequently is a way of avoiding more socially acceptable or more responsible behavior.

The person who is self-alienated feels helpless, sad, and lonely. Self-criticism and lack of self-awareness prevent participation in authentic, rewarding relationships with others. Theoretically, the person has many choices in terms of behavior. However, existentialists believe that people tend to avoid being real and instead give in to the demands of others.

Existential Therapeutic Process

There are several existential therapies, all of which assume that the patient must be able to choose freely from what life has to offer. Although the approaches are somewhat different, the goal is to return the patient to an authentic awareness of being.

The existential therapeutic process focuses on the encounter. The encounter is not merely the meeting of two or more people; it also involves their appreciation of the total existence of each other. Through the encounter the patient is helped to accept and understand personal history, to live fully in the present, and to look forward to the future. Table 3-1 presents an overview of several existential therapies.

Roles of Patient and Existential Therapist

Existential theorists emphasize that the therapist and the patient are equal in their common humanity. The

Table 3-1   Overview of Existential Therapies

Therapy	Therapist	Process
Rational-emotive therapy (RET)	Albert Ellis[4]	An active-directive, cognitively oriented therapy. Confrontation is used to force patient to assume responsibility for behavior. Patients are encouraged to accept themselves as they are and are taught to take risks and to try out new behavior.
Logotherapy	Viktor E. Frankl[6]	A future-oriented therapy. The search for meaning (*logos*) is viewed as a primary life force. Without a sense of meaning, life becomes an "existential vacuum." The aim of therapy is to help patients assume personal responsibility.
Reality therapy	William Glasser[10]	Central theme is the need for identity, which is reached by loving, feeling worthwhile, and behaving responsibly. Patients are helped to recognize life goals and ways by which they keep themselves from accomplishing goals.
Gestalt therapy	Frederick S. Perls[18]	Emphasizes the here and now. The patient is encouraged to identify feelings. The increased awareness makes the patient more sensitive to other aspects of existence. Self-awareness is expected to lead to self-acceptance.
Encounter group therapy	Carl Rogers[21,22] (Fig. 3-3)	Focuses on the establishment of intimate interactions in a group setting. Therapy is oriented to the here and now. The patient is expected to assume responsibility for behavior. Feeling is stressed; intellectualization is discouraged.

therapist acts as a guide to the patient, who has gone astray in the search for authenticity. The therapist is direct in pointing out areas where the patient should consider changing. However, caring and warmth are also emphasized. The therapist and the patient are to be open and honest. The therapeutic experience is a model for the patient; new behaviors can be tested before risks are taken in daily life.

The patient is expected to assume and accept responsibility for behavior. Dependence on the therapist generally is not encouraged. The patient is treated as an adult. Frequently, illness is deemphasized. The patient is viewed as a person alienated from the self and others, but for whom there is hope if the therapist is trusted and directions are followed. The patient is always active in therapy, working to meet the challenge presented by the therapist.

SUPPORTIVE THERAPY MODEL

Supportive therapy is a relatively new mode of psychotherapy that is widely used in hospital and community-based psychiatric treatment settings. It differs from other models in that it is not dependent on any overriding concept or theory. Instead, it uses many psychodynamic theories to understand how people change. The aims of supportive psychotherapy include the following:

▼ Promote a supportive patient-therapist relationship
▼ Enhance patient's strengths, coping skills, and ability to use coping resources
▼ Reduce the patient's subjective distress and maladaptive coping responses
▼ Help the patient achieve the greatest independence possible based on the specific psychiatric or physical illness
▼ Foster the greatest amount of autonomy in treatment decisions with the patient

Controlled studies have shown it to be effective in treating schizophrenia, borderline conditions, affective and anxiety disorders, posttraumatic stress disorder, eating and substance abuse disorders, and the psychological component of a variety of physical illnesses.[20]

View of Behavioral Deviations

Supportive therapists are psychodynamically based, and they describe behavioral deviations as neurotic, borderline, or psychotic. They subscribe to the concepts of id, ego, and superego and emphasize the important role of psychological defenses in adaptive functioning.[19] Compared with other models of psychiatric treatment, however, their focus is more behavior oriented. They emphasize current biopsychosocial coping responses and the person's ability to use available coping resources.

Supportive Therapeutic Process

Supportive therapy is an eclectic form of psychotherapy; that is, it is not based on a particular theory of psychopathology. Rather, it can draw as needed from other models and may address different symptoms with different therapeutic methods. The methods and goals of supportive therapy are equally applicable to high-functioning patients in crisis and low-functioning patients suffering from psychosis or persistent mental illness. Its emphasis is on improving behavior and subjective feelings of distress, rather than on achieving insight or self-understanding.

Principles of supportive therapy include the following:

▼ Giving immediate help to the patient that may include a variety of treatment modalities
▼ Family and social support system involvement
▼ Focus on the present and not the past
▼ Anxiety reduction through supportive measures and medication if necessary
▼ Clarification of the patient's current problem using a variety of approaches including advice, supportive confrontation, limit setting, education, and environmental change
▼ Assisting the patient to avoid future crises and seek help early when under stress

Roles of Patient and Supportive Therapist

In supportive therapy the therapist plays an active and directive role in helping the patient improve social functioning and coping skills. The setting for supportive therapy should allow for a moderate to high level of activity in both the patient and therapist. Communication is viewed as an active two-way process, and the use of medications or other treatments and therapies is encouraged.

The therapist is involved and is willing to contribute to a true therapeutic alliance with the patient. Expressing empathy, concern, and nonjudgmental acceptance of the patient are important therapist qualities. The therapist supports the patient's healthy adaptive efforts, conveys a willingness to understand, respects the patient as a unique human being, and takes a genuine interest in the patient's life activities and well-being. Finally the therapist regards the patient as a partner in treatment and encourages the patient's autonomy to make treatment and life decisions. In turn, the patient is expected to demonstrate a willingness to talk about life events, to accept the therapist's supportive role, to participate

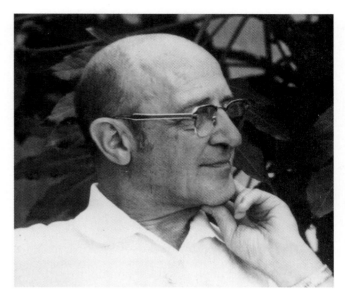

Fig. 3-3   Carl R. Rogers, 1902-1987.
From The Bettman Archive.

in the therapeutic program, and to adhere to the therapeutic structure.

What aspects of supportive therapy are similar to those of the therapeutic nurse-patient relationship? In what ways are they different?

MEDICAL MODEL

The medical model refers to psychiatric care that is based on the traditional physician-patient relationship. It focuses on the diagnosis of a mental illness, and subsequent treatment is based on this diagnosis. Somatic treatments, including pharmacotherapy and electroconvulsive therapy are important components of the treatment process. The interpersonal aspect of the medical model varies widely, from intensive insight-oriented intervention to brief sessions involving medical management of medications.

Much of modern psychiatric care is dominated by the medical model. Other health professionals may be involved in interagency referrals, family assessment, and health teaching, but physicians are viewed as the leaders of the team when this model is in effect. Elements of other models of care may be used in conjunction with the medical model. For instance, a patient may be diagnosed with schizophrenia and treated with phenothiazine medication. This patient may also be participating in a token economy program to encourage socially acceptable behavior.

A positive contribution of the medical model has been the continuous exploration for causes of mental illness using the scientific process. Recently, great strides have been taken in learning about the functioning of the brain and nervous system (see Chapter 5). This progress has led to a beginning understanding of the probable physiological components of many behavioral disorders and increasingly specific and sophisticated approaches to psychiatric care.

 What problems may the medical model pose for interdisciplinary collaboration in psychiatric treatment?

View of Behavioral Deviations

The medical model proposes that deviant behavior is a symptom of a central nervous system disorder.[12] As Andreasen writes, "Mental illness is truly a nervous breakdown—a breakdown that occurs when the nerves of the brain have an injury so severe that their own internal healing capacities cannot repair it."[2] She lists several types of brain disorders that could lead to mental illness: loss of nerve cells, excesses or deficits in chemical transmission, abnormal patterns of brain circuitry, problems in the command centers, and disruptions in the movement of messages along nerves.

Currently the exact nature of the physiological disruption is not well understood. It is thought that the psychotic disorders such as bipolar disorder, major depression, and schizophrenia involve an abnormality in the transmission of neural impulses. It is also thought that this difficulty occurs at the synaptic level and involves neurochemicals such as dopamine, serotonin, and norepinephrine (see Chapter 5).

Much research currently is taking place so that the brain's involvement in emotional response can be better understood. Another branch of research focuses on stressors and the human response to stress. Researchers are asking, "Why do some people seem to tolerate great stress and continue to function well, and others fall apart when a small problem arises?" These researchers suspect that humans may have a physiological stress threshold that may be genetically determined. These areas of research are intriguing but currently are not able to provide definitive guidelines for therapy.

Medical Therapeutic Process

The medical process of therapy is well defined and familiar to most patients. The physician's examination of the patient includes the history of the present illness, past history, social history, medical history, review of body systems, physical examination, and mental status examination. Additional data may be collected from significant others, and past medical records are reviewed if available. A preliminary diagnosis is then formulated, pending further diagnostic studies and observation of the patient's behavior. This process may take place on an ambulatory or an inpatient basis, depending on the patient's condition.

The diagnosis is stated and classified according to the *Diagnostic and Statistical Manual of Mental Disorders*, fourth edition, of the American Psychiatric Association. The names of the various illnesses are accompanied by a description of diagnostic criteria, associated general medical and psychiatric features, diagrams showing the longitudinal course of the disorder, and specific gender, age, and cross-cultural aspects of each illness. Changes in the manual reflect changes in the medical model of psychiatric care. DSM-I was first published in 1952,[11] and DSM-IV, published in 1994, is the most up-to-date edition.[1]

After the diagnosis is formulated, treatment is instituted. The physician-patient relationship is developed to foster trust in the physician and compliance with the treatment plan. If indicated, physicians help patients face stressful situations in their lives. Other health team members may contribute their expertise. Response to treatment is evaluated on the basis of the patient's subjective assessment and on the physician's objective observations of symptomatic behavior. Therapy is terminated when the patient's symptoms have remitted. For instance, some people who experience depression may be able to return to usual life-style after a course of medication and supportive therapy. Other patients may require long-term therapy, often including pharmacotherapy and periodic laboratory studies.

Roles of Patient and Medical Therapist

The roles of physician and patient have been well defined by tradition and apply in the psychiatric setting. The physician, as the healer, identifies the patient's illness and institutes a treatment plan. The patient may have some say about the plan, but the physician prescribes the therapy.

The role of the patient involves admitting being ill, which can be a problem in psychiatry. Patients sometimes are not aware of their disturbed behavior and may actively resist treatment. This is not congruent with the medical model. The patient is expected to comply with the treatment program and to try to get well. If observable improvement does not occur, caregivers and significant others often suspect that the patient is not trying hard enough. This can be frustrating to a patient who is trying to get well and is disappointed with the lack of progress. The patient also may have difficulty letting people extend care and at the same time be self-sufficient.

How would each conceptual model described in this chapter view the issue of patient non-adherence to the psychiatric treatment plan.

SUMMARY

Model (major theorists)	View of behavioral deviation	Therapeutic process	Roles of patient and therapist
Psychoanalytical (S. Freud, Erikson, A. Freud, Klein, Horney, Fromm-Reichmann, Menninger)	Based on inadequate resolution of developmental conflicts. Ego defenses inadequate to control anxiety. Symptoms result in effort to deal with anxiety and are related to unresolved conflicts.	Uses techniques of free association and dream analysis. Identifies problem areas through interpretation of patient's resistances and transferences.	Patient verbalizes all thoughts and dreams; considers therapist's interpretations. Therapist remains remote to encourage development of transference and interprets patient's thoughts and dreams.
Interpersonal (Sullivan, Peplau)	Anxiety arises and is experienced interpersonally. Basic fear is fear of rejection. Person needs security and satisfaction that result from positive interpersonal relationships.	Relationship between therapist and patient builds feeling of security. Therapist helps patient experience trusting relationship and gain interpersonal satisfaction.	Patient shares anxieties and feelings with therapist. Therapist uses empathy to perceive patient's feelings, and uses relationship as a corrective interpersonal experience.
Social (Szasz, Caplan)	Social and environmental factors create stress, which causes anxiety and symptoms. Unacceptable (deviant) behavior is socially defined.	Patient helped to deal with social system. May use crisis intervention, environmental manipulation, and social supports.	Patient presents problem to therapist, works with therapist, and uses community resources. Therapist explores patient's social system and resources available.
Existential (Perls, Glasser, Ellis, Rogers, Frankl)	Life is meaningful when the person can fully experience and accept the self. The self can be experienced through authentic relationships with other people.	Person aided to experience authenticity in relationships. Therapy frequently conducted in groups. Patient encouraged to accept self and to assume control of behavior.	Patient participates in meaningful experiences to learn about real self. Therapist helps patient recognize value of self, clarify realities of situation, and explore feelings.

SUMMARY—cont'd

Model (major theorists)	View of behavioral deviation	Therapeutic process	Roles of patient and therapist
Supportive therapy (Wermon, Rockland)	Problems are a result of bio-psychosocial factors. Emphasis on current maladaptive coping responses.	Reality testing and self-esteem enhancing measures. Social supports are enlisted, and adaptive coping responses are reinforced.	Patient actively involved in treatment. Therapist warm, empathic, and allies with patient.
Medical (Meyer, Kraeplin, Spitzer, Frances)	Behavioral disruptions result from a biological disease process. Symptoms result from a combination of physiological, genetic, environmental, and social factors.	Treatment is related to diagnosis and includes somatic therapies and various interpersonal techniques. Treatment approach adjusted depending on symptomatic response.	Patient complies with prescribed therapy and reports effects of therapy to physician. Therapist diagnoses illness and prescribes therapeutic approach.

REFERENCES

1. American Psychiatric Association: *Diagnostic and statistical manual of mental disorders*, ed 4, Washington, DC, 1994, The Association.
2. Andreasen NC: *The broken brain*, New York, 1984, Harper & Row.
3. Caplan G: *Principles of preventive psychiatry*, New York, 1964, Basic Books.
4. Ellis A: *Inside rational emotive therapy*, San Diego, 1989, Academic Press.
5. Erikson E: *Childhood and society*, ed 2, New York, 1963, WW Norton.
6. Frankl V: *Man's search for meaning*, New York, 1959, The Beacon Press.
7. Freud A: *The ego and the mechanisms of defense*, New York, 1966, International Universities Press.
8. Freud S: In Strachey J, ed: *The standard edition of the complete psychological works of Sigmund Freud*, London, 1953-1974, Hogarth Press.
9. Fromm-Reichmann F: *Principles of intensive psychotherapy*, Chicago, 1950, The University of Chicago Press.
10. Glasser W: *Reality therapy: a new approach to psychiatry*, New York, 1965, Harper & Row.
11. Grob G: Origins of DSM-I: a study in appearance and reality, *Am J Psychiatry* 148:421, 1991.
12. Guze S: Biological psychiatry: is there any other kind? *Psychol Med* 19:315, 1989.
13. Horney K: *The collected works of Karen Horney*, vols 1 and 2, New York, 1937-1950, WW Norton.
14. Klein M: *The psychoanalysis of children*, London, 1949, Hogarth Press.
15. Krupnick J, Pincus H: The cost-effectiveness of psychotherapy: a plan for research, *Am J Psychiatry* 149:1295, 1992.
16. Menninger KA: *The vital balance*, New York, 1963, Viking Press.
17. Peplau HE: *Interpersonal relations in nursing*, New York, 1952, GP Putnam's Sons.
18. Perls FS: *In and out of the garbage pail*, Lafayette, Calif, 1969, Real People Press.
19. Rockland L: *Supportive therapy: a psychodynamic approach*, New York, 1989, Basic Books.
20. Rockland L: A review of supportive psychotherapy, 1986-1992, *Hosp Community Psychiatry* 44:1053, 1993.
21. Rogers CR: *Client-centered therapy*, Boston, 1951, Houghton Mifflin.
22. Rogers CR: *Carl Rogers on encounter groups*, New York, 1970, Harper & Row.
23. Sullivan HS: *The interpersonal theory of psychiatry*, New York, 1953, WW Norton & Co.
24. Sullivan HS: *The psychiatric interview*, New York, 1954, WW Norton.
25. Szasz T: *The myth of mental illness*, New York, 1961, Hoeber-Harper.
26. Szasz T: *Insanity: the idea and its consequences*, New York, 1987, Wiley.
27. Szasz T: *A lexicon of lunacy*, New Brunswick, 1993, Transactional Publishers.

ANNOTATED SUGGESTED READINGS

*Burnard P: Existentialism as a theoretical basis for counselling in psychiatric nursing, Arch Psych Nurs 3:142, 1989.

Proposes an existential approach to counseling by nurses and contrasts it with Rogers' nondirective approach. The clearly presented contrast between the two models should stimulate thought and discussion.

Corsini R, Wedding D: Current psychotherapies, Itasca, Ill, 1989, FE Peacock.

Comprehensive introduction to the various models of psychotherapy. Uses an easy-to-follow format, clinical examples, and writings from leading figures in the field.

Frank J: Psychotherapy: the restoration of morale, Am J Psychiatry 131:271, 1974.

Classic article that shares a different view of psychotherapy by describing commonalities of psychotherapeutic rationales and rituals in combating demoralization.

Frank JD: Persuasion and healing, Baltimore, 1991, The Johns Hopkins University Press.

Thought-provoking comparison of psychotherapy to other forms of persuasion such as religious revivalism and thought reform; considers several models of psychiatric care in terms of this frame of reference.

Greenfield D, ed: Treating diverse disorders with psychotherapy, New Directions for Mental Health Services vol 55, 1992.

Entire volume of this journal addresses psychotherapy and related issues including the impact of culture on the psychotherapeutic process.

Kaplan H, Sadock B, eds: Synopsis of psychiatry, Baltimore, 1991, Williams & Wilkins.

Definitive source on the diagnosis and treatment of psychiatric illness based the medical model. Current and comprehensive.

Novalis P, Rojcewicz S, Peele R: Clinical manual of supportive psychotherapy, Washington, DC, 1993, American Psychiatric Press.

Excellent and easy-to-read overview of the principles, applications, and interactions of supportive psychotherapy. Useful for all psychiatric nurses.

*O'Toole A, Welt S: Interpersonal theory in nursing practice, New York, 1989, Springer.

Presents a selection of Peplau's best clinical and theoretical papers based on her theory of interpersonal relations. Excellent nursing reference.

Rosenhan DL: On being sane in insane places, Science 179:250, 1973.

Classic report of admission of several pseudopatients to psychiatric hospitals; raises interesting questions about the implications of labeling people as mentally ill. The experience of being a psychiatric patient is also recounted. Worthwhile reading for any nurse.

Wolberg LR: The techniques of psychotherapy, parts I and II, ed 4, New York, 1988, Grune & Stratton.

A thorough presentation of basic theories of psychotherapy, followed by a discussion of the practice of psychotherapy. An excellent resource for the experienced practitioner of psychiatric nursing.

---

*Nursing reference.

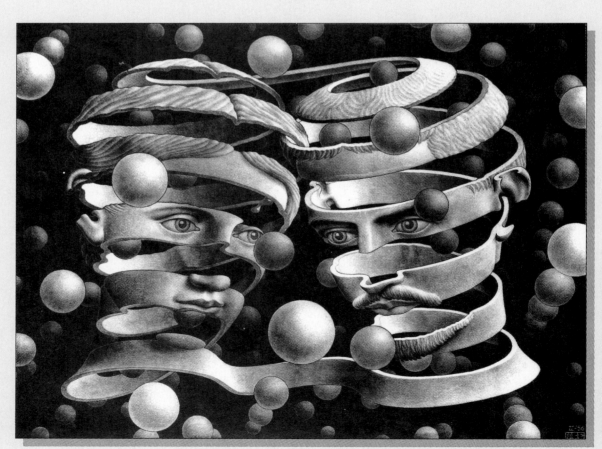

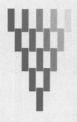

CHAPTER 4

A Stress Adaptation Model of Psychiatric Nursing Care

GAIL W. STUART

Much madness is Divinest Sense—To a discerning eye.
EMILY DICKINSON

LEARNING OBJECTIVES

After studying this chapter the student should be able to:

▼ Discuss the theoretical assumptions underlying the stress adaptation model of psychiatric nursing care
▼ Describe criteria of mental health and dimensions of mental illness in the United States
▼ Analyze the biopsychosocial components of the stress adaptation model of psychiatric nursing care
▼ Compare and contrast coping responses, nursing diagnoses, medical diagnoses, and health problems
▼ Evaluate nursing activities appropriate to the various stages of psychiatric treatment

TOPICAL OUTLINE

Theoretical Assumptions
Describing Mental Health and Illness
   Defining Mental Health
   Dimensions of Mental Illness
Biopsychosocial Components
   Predisposing Factors
   Precipitating Stressors
   Appraisal of Stressor
   Coping Resources
   Coping Mechanisms
Patterns of Response
   Nursing Diagnoses
   Relationship to Medical Diagnoses
   Classifying Mental Disorders
Treatment Activities
Appendix—DSM-IV classification

Models serve many purposes. They can help clarify relationships, generate hypotheses, and give perspective to an abstract idea or concept. They also can provide a structure for thinking, observing, and interpreting what is seen. Conceptual nursing models are particular frames of reference within which patients, their environments and health states, and nursing activities are described. They explain in general terms why individuals respond to stress in the way they do and help to provide an understanding of the process and desired outcomes of nursing interventions. Psychiatric nurses can enhance their practice if their actions are based on a model of psychiatric nursing care that is inclusive, ho-

listic, and relevant to the needs of patients, families, groups, and communities.[13]

This text is based on a stress adaptation model of psychiatric nursing care, originally developed by Gail Stuart in 1983 and further refined in this edition of the text. It integrates the biological, psychological, and sociocultural aspects of patient care into a unified framework for practice. It also recognizes that health-illness and adaptation-maladaptation are distinct concepts. Each exists on a separate continuum. Thus a person with a persistent illness, whether physical or psychiatric, can be adapting well to it. In contrast, a person without a diagnosed illness may have many maladaptive coping responses. These two continuums reflect the complementarity of nursing and medical models of practice. The stress adaptation model provides a framework for psychiatric nursing based on the continuum of coping responses and presents a holistic approach to psychiatric nursing practice in a variety of treatment settings.

THEORETICAL ASSUMPTIONS

A primary assumption of the stress adaptation model is that nature is ordered as a social hierarchy from the simplest unit to the most complex (Fig. 4-1). Each level within this hierarchy represents an organized whole with distinctive properties. Each level is also a component of the next higher level, so nothing exists in isolation. Thus the individual is a component of family, group, community, society, and the larger biosphere. Material and information flow across levels, and each level is influenced by all the others. For this reason, one level of organization, such as the individual, cannot be characterized as a dynamic system without incorporating the other levels of the social hierarchy. The most basic level of nursing intervention is the individual level. An exploration of this level must focus on its unique aspects without excluding its relationship to the whole, because "wholeness" is the essence of psychiatric nursing practice.

A second assumption of the model is that nursing care is provided within a biological, psychological, sociocultural, and legal context. Each of these aspects of care is described in detail in Chapter 5 to 8. They must be understood and integrated by the nurse to provide competent, holistic psychiatric nursing care. Thus the theoretical basis for psychiatric nursing practice is derived from nursing science as well as from the behavioral, social, and biological sciences. The range of theories used by psychiatric nurses includes nursing, developmental psychology, neurobiology, pharmacology, psychopathology, learning, sociocultural, cognitive, behavioral, legal-ethical, interpersonal, group, family, and milieu. Psychiatric nursing practice requires the use of many theories because of the variation in patients' responses, the philosophical backgrounds of psychiatric nurses, and the settings in which nurses work. No one theory is universally applicable to all patients. Rather the appropriate theory should be selected for its relevance to a particular patient, the presenting problem, and the environment of caregiving.

A third and final aspect of the stress adaptation model is that it is based on the use of the nursing process described in Chapter 9 and professional role behavior discussed in Chapter 10. Psychiatric nursing care is provided through assessment, diagnosis, outcome identification, planning, implementation, and evalua-

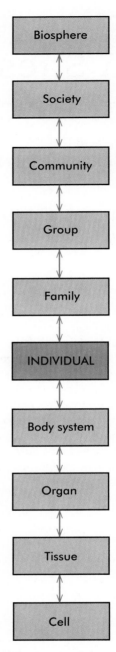

Fig. 4-1 Levels of organization that make up the social hierarchy.

tion (Fig. 4-2). Each step of the process is critically important, and the nurse assumes full responsibility for all nursing actions implemented and the enactment of a professional nursing role.

DESCRIBING MENTAL HEALTH AND ILLNESS

The mental health–mental illness continuum is asymmetrical. The standards of mental health are less clear

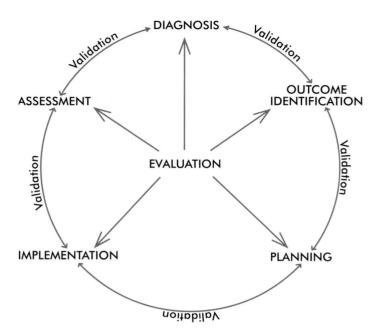

Fig. 4-2   The nursing process.

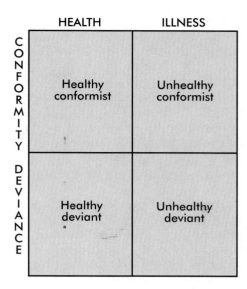

Fig. 4-3   Patterns of behavior.

and agreed upon than those of mental illness. Problems arise with viewing mental health as the average or mean of a group, since what is "average" may not necessarily be "healthy." It is similarly dangerous to equate social alternatives with illness, such as when an unusual lifestyle is regarded as sick or when aberrant behavior is taken to be a sign of personal abnormality. These problems can be avoided if it is recognized that health-illness and conformity-deviance are independent variables. Combining them generates four patterns: the healthy conformist, the healthy deviant, the unhealthy conformist, and the unhealthy deviant (Fig. 4-3). Psychiatric nurses must carefully consider the meaning of an individual's behavior and its context, since it may reflect an adaptation to realistic forces in the individual's life or conformity to group norms.

Defining Mental Health

Mental health is often spoken of as a state of well-being associated with happiness, contentment, satisfaction, achievement, optimism, or hope.[6] These are difficult terms to define, and their meanings change by person and life situation. Some have suggested that the idea of any single criterion of mental health should be abandoned because mental health cannot be confined to a simple concept or a single aspect of behavior.[12] Instead, mental health should be thought of as consisting of a number of criteria that exist on a continuum with gradients or degrees. These criteria should then be regarded as the optimum of mental health. They are not

absolute, however, and each person has limits. Although no one reaches the ideal in all the criteria, most people can approach the optimum.

 Do you think that a person with diabetes that is controlled with medication can still be regarded as healthy? How does this compare with a person who has schizophrenia that is controlled with medication?

Criteria of Mental Health. The following six criteria have been suggested as indicators of mental health[12]:
1. Positive attitudes toward self
2. Growth, development, and self-actualization
3. Integration
4. Autonomy
5. Reality perception
6. Environmental mastery

Positive attitudes toward self include an acceptance of self and self-awareness. A person must have some objectivity about the self and realistic aspirations that necessarily change with age. A healthy person must also have a sense of identity, wholeness, belongingness, security, and meaningfulness.

Growth, development, and **self-actualization** have been the objects of considerable research. Maslow and Rogers, for example, developed theories on the realization of the human potential. Maslow describes the concept of "self-actualization," and Rogers emphasizes the "fully functioning person." Both theories focus on the entire range of human adjustment. They describe a self engaged in a constant quest, always seeking new growth, development, and challenges. These theories focus on the total person and whether the person:

1. Is adequately in touch with the self to free the resources that are there
2. Has free access to personal feelings and can integrate them with intellectual and cognitive functioning
3. Is immobilized by inner conflicts and stresses or can interact freely and openly with the environment
4. Can share with other people and grow from such experiences

Maslow[17] identified 15 personality characteristics that distinguish "self-actualized" individuals—people moving in the direction of achieving their highest potential. Rogers[28] described seven essential personality traits of the "fully functioning person," who similarly is moving toward self-growth and fulfillment (Table 4-1).

Integration is a balance between what is expressed and what is repressed, between outer and inner conflicts and drives, and a regulation of moods and emotions. It

Table 4-1 Theories on the Realization of Human Potential

Maslow's "self-actualized" individual	Rogers' "fully functioning" person
Has accurate perception of reality	Moves away from facades that are not true to self
Has a high degree of acceptance of self, others, and human nature	Moves away from others' expectations
Exhibits spontaneity	Moves away from pleasing others who impose artificial goals
Is problem-centered as opposed to self-centered	
Has need for privacy	Moves toward becoming autonomous, self-directing, and self-responsible
Demonstrates high degree of autonomy and independence	
Has freshness of appreciation	Is open to change and exploring self-potential
Has frequent "mystic or peak" experiences	Is open to own self and the lives of others
Shows identification with mankind	As a self-trusting and self-valuing person, the individual dares to try new ways to be self-expressive
Shares intimate relationships with a few significant others	
Has democratic character structures	
Possesses strong ethical sense	
Demonstrates unhostile sense of humor	
Possesses creativeness	
Exhibits resistance to conformity	

includes emotional responsiveness and control and a unified philosophy of life. This consistent set of values provides a framework for continuity in all responses. This criterion can be measured at least in part by the person's ability to withstand stress and cope with anxiety. A strong but not rigid ego enables the person to handle change and grow from it.

Autonomy involves self-determination, a balance between dependence and independence, and acceptance of the consequences of one's actions. It implies that the person is self-responsible for decisions, actions, thoughts and feelings. Consequently the person can respect autonomy and freedom in others.

Reality perception is the individual's ability to test assumptions about the world by empirical thought. The mentally healthy person can change perceptions in the light of new information. This criterion includes empathy or social sensitivity, a respect for the feelings and attitudes of others.

Environmental mastery enables a mentally healthy person to feel success in an approved role in personal society or group. The person can deal effectively with the world, work out personal problems of living, and obtain satisfaction from life. This criterion incorporates the idea of social competence as well. The person should be able to cope with loneliness, aggression, and frustration without being overwhelmed. The mentally healthy person can respond to others, love and be loved, and cope with reciprocal relationships. This individual can build new friendships and have satisfactory social group involvement.

Finally, a person should not be assessed against some vague or ideal notion of health. Rather, each person should be seen in a group context and an individual context. The issue is not how well someone fits an arbitrary sociocultural standard, but rather what is reasonable for a particular person. Is there continuity or discontinuity with the past? Does the person adapt to changing needs throughout the life cycle? Such a view incorporates the concept of **psychobiological resilience,** which proposes that humans must weather periods of stress and change throughout life. Successfully weathering each period of disruption and reintegration leaves the person better able to deal with the next change.

Dimensions of Mental Illness

Mental disorders are a major contributor to the burden of illness in the United States. Both the seriousness and the persistence of some disorders cause great strain on affected individuals, their families and communities, and on the larger health-care system. Key facts about mental illness prepared by the National Institute of Mental Health[24] are presented in Box 4-1.

Box 4-1
KEY FACTS ABOUT MENTAL ILLNESS

EXTENT AND SEVERITY OF THE PROBLEM

▼ The full spectrum of mental disorders affects 22% of the adult population in a given year. This figure refers to *all* mental disorders and is comparable to rates for "physical disorders" when similarly broadly defined (e.g., respiratory disorders affect 50% of adults, and cardiovascular diseases, 20%).

▼ Severe mental disorders, i.e., schizophrenia, manic depressive illness and severe forms of depression, panic disorder, and obsessive compulsive disorder:

  Affect 2.8% of the adult population—approximately 5 million people

  Account for 25% of all Federal disability payments

▼ At least 7.5 million children in the United States under 18 years of age have a mental health problem severe enough to require treatment.

▼ Approximately 18 million persons in the United States 18 years of age and older have problems as a result of alcohol use. 10.6 million of these suffer from alcoholism.

▼ An estimated 23 million people in the United States currently use illicit drugs.

COST OF MENTAL DISORDERS

▼ In 1990 the Nation's health-care bill was $670 billion; direct cost of treating *all* mental disorders was 10%, or $67 billion.

  $148 billion: total costs (treatment plus indirect costs) of *mental disorders* in 1990

  $159 billion: total cost of *cardiovascular system* diseases in 1990

▼ Severe mental disorders: Total direct treatment costs are $20 billion per year plus $7 billion for long-term nursing home care.

  Indirect and related costs bring the total for severe mental disorders to $74 billion per year.

▼ It has been estimated that drug and alcohol abuse contribute to over $163.6 billion in health-care costs, lost productivity, and crime. Estimates of general hospital beds occupied by patients whose physical condition is complicated by alcohol and drug problems range from 25 to 50%.

▼ Alcohol or mental illness are involved in 94% of all suicides and suicide ranks as the second leading cause of death among persons aged 15-24.

▼ Alcoholism is the third leading cause of illness and disability in the U.S. and accounts for 10% of all deaths.

TREATMENT EFFICACY

▼ How *effective* are treatments for severe mental disorders as compared with treatments for physical illness?

Disorder	Treatment Success Rate (%)
Panic	80
Bipolar	80
Major depression	65
Schizophrenia	60
Obsessive compulsive	60
Cardiovascular treatments	
Atherectomy	52
Angioplasty	41

▼ The majority of alcoholics improve through treatment, and evidence suggests that alcoholism treatment is effective in containing costs throughout the health-care system and increasing worker productivity.

REIMBURSEMENT

▼ People who need help often cannot receive it. Approximately 30% of the 2.8 million people with severe mental illness receive active treatment in a given year; 70% to 80% of children needing mental health treatment do not receive appropriate services.

▼ 85% of all drug and alcohol abusers are not in treatment. Only 150,000 of an estimated 1.4 million intravenous drug abusers are currently in treatment.

▼ Under insurance plans offering full, comprehensive, and equitable coverage for mental disorders, the percent of cost represented by these disorders plateaus at about 10% to 11%.

  Inpatient care for treatment of severe psychiatric disorders has grown less rapidly than inpatient care for all health conditions.

▼ Under health-care reform, making mental health coverage for the severely mentally ill commensurate to other health-care coverage would:

  Add only $6.5 billion in new mental health care costs—10% more than is currently spent.

  Produce a 10% decrease in the cost and use of general medical services by people with severe mental disorders.

  Yield a $2.2 billion net saving for the United States.

From National Advisory Mental Health Council: *Am J Psychiatry* 150:1447, 1993.

Many myths and misunderstandings contribute to the stigmatization of persons with mental illness and to their often limited access to needed health-care services. For example, many Americans and policymakers are unaware of a solid body of research that documents the effectiveness of treatment for these illnesses. These studies demonstrate that mental disorders can be diagnosed and treated as effectively as physical illness. However, far too many Americans with severe mental illness and their families find that appropriate treatment is not available to them because they lack insurance coverage or the coverage they have is inequitable and inadequate. For example, private health insurance for mental disorders is often limited to 30 to 60 inpatient days per year, compared with 120 days or unlimited days for physical illnesses. Similarly, the Medicare program requires 50% copayment for outpatient care of mental disorders, compared with 20% copayment for outpatient treatment of physical illnesses.

Fair and equal coverage for Americans with mental illness will result in both human and economic benefits. Millions of Americans will be able to participate more productively at home, at work, and in the community. The enormous but often hidden costs of untreated or undertreated severe mental illness, which are now absorbed by the general health-care system and society at large, can be substantially reduced. Psychiatric nurses should work to make these benefits a reality by supporting national health-care reform initiatives and research funding that is equitable for the needs of the mentally ill.

Identify two key facts about mental illness from Box 4-1 that you didn't know. How will these facts change your views about needed health care reform in this country?

BIOPSYCHOSOCIAL COMPONENTS

The stress adaptation model of psychiatric nursing care developed by Stuart views human behavior from a holistic perspective that integrates biological, psychological, and sociocultural aspects of care. For instance, a man who has had a myocardial infarction may also be severely depressed because he fears he will lose his ability to work and to satisfy his wife sexually. He may also have a family history of depression. So too, a patient who seeks treatment for a major depression may also have gastric ulcers that are exacerbated as a result of the depressive state. The holistic nature of psychiatric nursing practice examines all aspects of the individual and the individual's social hierarchy. The specific biopsychosocial components of the stress adaptation

model are in shown in Fig. 4-4. Each component of the model will now be described.

Predisposing Factors

Predisposing factors are biological, psychological, and sociocultural in nature. They may be viewed as conditioning factors that influence both the type and amount of resources the person can elicit to handle stress. Genetic background, nutritional status, biological sensitivities, general health, and exposure to toxins are examples of **biological** predispositions. **Psychological** factors include but are not limited to intelligence, verbal skills, morale, personality, past experiences, self-concept, motivation, psychological defenses, and locus of control, or a sense of mastery over one's own fate.

Sociocultural characteristics include age, gender, education, income, occupation, social position, cultural background, religious upbringing and beliefs, political affiliation, socialization experiences, and level of social integration or relatedness. Together these factors provide a link with higher and lower levels of the social hierarchy and a backdrop against which all current experiences are given meaning and value.

 Explain why predisposing factors are also sometimes referred to as risk factors.

Precipitating Stressors

Precipitating stressors are stimuli that the individual perceives as challenging, threatening, or demanding. They require excess energy and produce a state of tension and stress within the individual. They may be biological, psychological, or sociocultural in *nature,* and they may *originate* from the person's internal or external environment. Besides describing the nature and origin of a stressor, it is important to assess the timing of the stressor. This *timing* has many dimensions, such as when the stressor occurred, the duration of exposure to the stressor, and the frequency with which it occurs. A final factor to be considered is the *number* of stressors an individual experiences within a certain period of time, because events may be more difficult to deal with when they occur close together.

Stressful Life Events. One group of stressors that has received much attention in the health-care literature are stressful life events. The relationship of stressful life events to the cause, onset, course, and outcomes of various psychiatric illnesses, such as schizophrenia, depression, and anxiety, has been the focus of much research.[20,21]

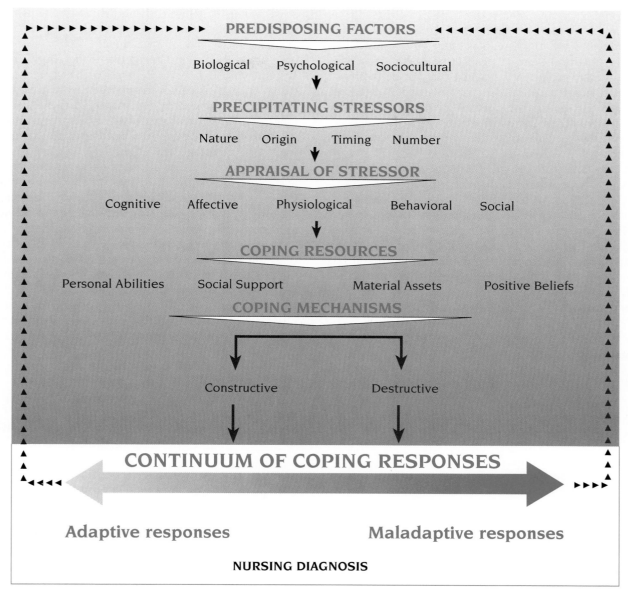

PREDISPOSING FACTORS

Biological   Psychological   Sociocultural

PRECIPITATING STRESSORS

Nature   Origin   Timing   Number

APPRAISAL OF STRESSOR

Cognitive   Affective   Physiological   Behavioral   Social

COPING RESOURCES

Personal Abilities   Social Support   Material Assets   Positive Beliefs

COPING MECHANISMS

Constructive   Destructive

CONTINUUM OF COPING RESPONSES

Adaptive responses   Maladaptive responses

NURSING DIAGNOSIS

Fig. 4-4   Biopsychosocial components of the stress adaptation model of psychiatric nursing care.

Holmes and Rahe[10] developed the "Social Readjust ment Rating Scale," which assigns a value to each life event on the basis of the coping behavior the event requires of the individual. As the score of the mean value increases, it is suggested that the likelihood of an illness increases. Rahe[27] has also developed a questionnaire called the *Schedule of Recent Experience*, which assesses life events for the individual during specific periods. The schedule determines the degree of change in a given period by totaling the mean values of reported life events. Rahe suggests that the schedule helps to identify the degree and type of life change experienced.

More recent issues related to life events as stressors focus on the nature of the event and the magnitude of change it represents. There appear to be three ways of categorizing events reported in the literature:

1. By social activity, which involves family, work, edu-

cational, interpersonal, health, financial, legal, or community crises

2. By the individual's social field. These events are defined as entrances and exists. An entrance is the introduction of a new person into the individual's social field; an exit is the departure of a significant other from the person's social field

3. By relating them to social desirability. In terms of the currently shared values of American society, one group of events can be considered generally desirable, such as promotion, engagement, and marriage. Another and proportionately larger group of events can be viewed unfavorably, such as death, financial problems, being fired, and divorce.

Unfortunately, conclusions about life events are far from definitive.[22] Although they have been correlated with the onset of anxiety and disease symptoms, the methodological and theoretical aspects of research in this area have been the subject of much criticism. Intervening or mediating variables often are not taken into account in the design and execution of studies. Also, the particular events in the scales may not be the most relevant to certain groups, such as students, working mothers, the elderly, the poor, or the persistently mentally ill. Finally, the life-events approach provides no clues to the specific processes by which the events affect health.

It may be more helpful, therefore, to suggest that stressful life events act along a continuum to influence the development of psychiatric illness. On one end of the continuum, they may act as "triggers" to precipitate an illness in predisposed individuals who would have developed the illness eventually for one reason or another. At the other end of the continuum, stressful life events may have a "vulnerability effect" in depleting an individual's resistance and coping resources and thus greatly advancing or bringing about psychiatric illness.

> What sociocultural norms and values need to be considered in evaluating the impact of potentially stressful life events?

Life Strains and Hassles. Life-events theory is built on the idea of change. However, much stress arises from chronic conditions such as boredom, continuing family tension, job dissatisfaction, and loneliness. This aspect is reflected in the work of Pearlin and Schooler,[26] who explored what people considered potential life strains. In their sample of 2300 people, 18 to 65 years of age, the following four areas were delineated:

1. Marital strains
2. Parental strains associated with teenage and young adult children
3. Strains associated with household economics
4. Overloads and dissatisfactions associated with the work role

These findings suggest more long-term life dissatisfactions than major episodic events.

Research indicates that small daily hassles or stresses may be more closely linked to and have a greater effect on a person's moods and health than do major misfortunes.[23] Hassles are irritating, frustrating, or distressing incidents that occur in everyday life. Such incidents may include disagreements, disappointments, and unpleasant surprises such as losing a wallet, getting stuck in a traffic jam, or arguing with a teenage son or daughter. Research suggests that hassles may be better predictors of psychological and

physical health than life events. The more frequent and intense the hassles people reported, the poorer their overall mental and physical health. Major events did have some long-term effects, but these effects may be accounted for by the daily hassles they precipitate. A study of the specific hassles and their frequency among persons with severe mental illness found that loneliness and boredom were serious concerns. Finances, crime, self-expression, and upward mobility were also important.[29]

A certain amount of stress is necessary for survival, and degrees of it can challenge the individual to grow in new ways. However, too much stress at inappropriate times can place excessive demands on the individual and interfere with integrated functioning. Stress does not reside within the particular life event itself or within the individual. Rather, it is in the interaction between the individual and situation. The questions that emerge therefore are "How much stress is too much?" and "What is a stressful life event?" These questions lead the nurse to explore the significance of the event for the individual's need-value system.

Appraisal of Stressor

Appraisal of a stressor refers to the processing and comprehension of the stressful situation that takes place on many levels for the individual. Specifically, it involves cognitive, affective, physiological, behavioral, and social responses. Appraisal is an evaluation of the significance of an event for a person's well-being. The stressor assumes its meaning, intensity, and importance by the unique interpretation and significance assigned to it by the person at risk.

Cognitive appraisal is a critical part of this health-illness model. Monat and Lazarus[23] believe that cognitive factors play a central role in adaptation, that they affect the impact of stressful events, the choice of coping patterns used, and the emotional, physiological, and behavioral reactions. Cognitive appraisal mediates psychologically between the person and the environment in any stressful encounter. That is, damage or potential damage is evaluated according to the person's understanding of the situation's power to produce harm and the resources the person has available to neutralize or tolerate the harm.

There are three types of primary cognitive appraisals to stress:

1. *Harm/loss,* referring to damage that has already occurred
2. *Threat,* referring to anticipated or future harm
3. *Challenge,* in which the focus is placed positively on potential gain, growth, or mastery rather than on the possible risks

The perception of challenge may play a crucial role

in psychological **hardiness** or resistance to stress. This theory proposes that psychologically hardy individuals are less likely than nonhardy people to fall ill as a result of stressful life events. Three parts of a hardy personality have been described and researched.[11,14,16] Hardy individuals are high in:

1. *Commitment*, the ability to involve oneself in whatever one is doing
2. *Challenge*, the belief that change rather than stability is to be expected in life, so events are seen as stimulating rather than threatening
3. *Control*, the tendency to feel and believe that they influence events, rather than feeling helpless in the face of life's problems

From this one might conclude that stress-resistant people have a specific set of attitudes toward life, an openness to change, a feeling of involvement in whatever they are doing, and a sense of control over events.[9] Such differences in cognitive appraisal affect the person's response to events. Those who view stress as a challenge are more likely to transform events to their advantage and thus reduce their level of stress. This is in contrast to more passive, hostile, avoidant, or self-defeating tactics, in which the source of stress does not go away. Additional research is needed in this important personality characteristic.[30,31]

Among the most important factors affecting a person's cognitive appraisal are commitments and beliefs.[15] *Commitments* express what is important to the individual, and they underlie the choices a person makes. Commitments can thus guide people into or away from situations that threaten, harm, or potentially benefit. *Beliefs* also determine how a person evaluates events. Personal control and beliefs are particularly relevant to stress reduction, since they influence the person's emotional response and potential coping ability.

An **affective** response is the arousal of a feeling state. In the appraisal of a stressor, the predominant affective response is a nonspecific or generalized anxiety reaction.

This generalized anxiety response becomes expressed as emotions. These may include joy, sadness, fear, anger, acceptance, distrust, anticipation, or surprise. Emotions may be further classified according to type, duration, and intensity—characteristics that change over time and events. For example, when an emotion is prolonged over time, it can be classified as a mood; when prolonged over a longer time, it can be considered an attitude.

Physiological responses reflect the interaction of several neuroendocrine axes involving growth hormone, prolactin, adrenocorticotropic hormone (ACTH), luteinizing and follicle-stimulating hormones, thyroid-stimulating hormone, vasopressin, oxytocin, epinephrine, norepinephrine, and insulin. The fight-or-flight physiological response stimulates the sympathetic division of the autonomic nervous system and increases activity of the pituitary-adrenal axis.

Behavioral responses reflect emotions and physiological changes as well as cognitive analysis of the stressful situation. Caplan[8] described four phases of an individual's responses to a stressful event.

▼ Phase 1 is behavior that changes the stressful environment or enables the individual to escape from it.
▼ Phase 2 is behavior to acquire new capabilities for action to change the external circumstances and their aftermath.
▼ Phase 3 is intrapsychic behavior to defend against unpleasant emotional arousal.
▼ Phase 4 is intrapsychic behavior to come to terms with the event and its sequelae by internal readjustment.

Finally, Mechanic[18] describes three aspects of a person's **social** response to stress and illness. The first aspect is the *search for meaning*, in which individuals seek information about their problem. This is a prerequisite for devising a coping strategy, because only through some formulation of what is occurring can reasonable response be devised.

The second aspect of social response is *social attribution*, in which the person tries to identify the unique factors that contributed to the situation. Patients who view their problem as resulting from their own negligence may be blocked from an active coping response. They may view their problems as a sign of their personal failure and engage in self-blame and passive, withdrawn behavior. Thus the way cause or etiology is viewed by both patients and health professionals can greatly affect successful coping.

The third aspect of social response is *social comparison*, in which individuals compare skills and capacities with those of others with similar problems. A person's self-assessment depends very much on those with whom comparisons are made. In many situations feelings and self-esteem may depend as much on this comparison process as on objective coping capacities. The outcome is an evaluation of the need for support from the person's social network or social support system. Both the person's predisposing factors such as age, developmental level, and cultural background, and the characteristics of the precipitating stressor determine the perceived need for social support.

In summary, the way a person appraises an event is the psychological key to understanding coping efforts and the nature and intensity of the stress response. Unfortunately, many nurses and other health professionals ignore this fact when they presume to know how certain stressors will affect an individual and thus provide "routine" care. Not only does this depersonalize the individual, but also it undermines the basis of nursing care. The patient's appraisal of life stressors with its cognitive, affective, physiological, behavioral, and social components must be an essential part of the psychiatric nurse's assessment.

 How might social attribution influence a nurse's response to a rape victim, a person with a substance abuse disorder, or a patient with HIV?

Coping Resources

Coping resources, options, or strategies help to determine what, if anything, can be done, as well as what is at stake. This component takes into account which coping options are available, the likelihood that a given option will accomplish what it is supposed to, and the likelihood that the person can apply a particular strategy effectively.

Mechanic[18] identifies five coping resources that help individuals adapt to the stress of illness. These coping resources are economic assets, individual abilities and skills, defensive techniques, social supports, and motivational impetus. They incorporate all levels of the social hierarchy represented in Fig. 4-1. Interrelationships between the individual, family, group, and society assume critical importance at this point of the model.

Lazarus and Folkman[15] add to these the resources of health and energy, positive beliefs, problem solving and social skills, and social and material resources. The role played by physical well-being is well documented in the literature. Similarly, viewing oneself positively can serve as a basis of hope and can sustain a person's coping efforts under the most adverse of circumstances. Problem-solving skills include the ability to search for information, identify the problem, weigh alternatives, and implement a plan of action. Social skills facilitate the solving of problems involving other people, increase the likelihood of enlisting cooperation and support from others, and in general give the individual greater social control. Finally, material assets refer to money and the foods and services that money can buy. Obviously, monetary resources greatly increase a person's coping options in almost any stressful situation.

Much research is being done on these coping resources. Antonovsky[4] is examining what he calls "generalized resistance resources"—characteristics of the person, group, or environment that can encourage more adaptive responses. He believes that knowledge and intelligence offer such a resource, since they allow people to see different ways of dealing with their stress. Other resources he identifies are a strong ego identity, commitment to a social network, cultural stability, a stable system of values and beliefs derived from one's philosophy or religion, a preventive health orientation, and genetic or constitutional strength. Thus research lends support to the relationship between predisposing factors and coping resources within a strong social community.

Coping Mechanisms

It is at this point in the model that coping mechanisms emerge. Thus this is an important time for nursing activities directed toward primary prevention. Coping mechanisms can be defined as any efforts directed at stress management. There are three main types of coping mechanisms:

1. **Problem-focused** coping mechanism; it involves tasks and direct efforts to cope with the threat itself. Examples of this type include negotiation, confrontation, and seeking advice.
2. **Cognitively focused** coping mechanism; the person attempts to control the meaning of the problem and thus neutralize it. Examples here include positive comparison, selective ignorance, substitution of rewards, and the devaluation of desired objects.
3. **Emotion-focused coping mechanism;** with this type the patient is oriented to moderating emotional distress. Examples include the use of ego defense mechanisms such as denial, suppression, or projection. A more detailed discussion of coping and defense mechanisms appears in Chapter 14.

Coping mechanisms may also be constructive or destructive. They can be considered **constructive** when anxiety is treated as a warning signal and the individual accepts it as a challenge to resolve the problem. In this respect anxiety can be compared to a fever—both serve as warnings that the system is under attack. Once employed successfully, constructive coping mechanisms modify the way past experiences are used to meet future threats. **Destructive** coping mechanisms ward off anxiety without resolving the conflict, using evasion instead of resolution.

PATTERNS OF RESPONSE

According to the stress adaptation model, an individual's coping response to stress is based on specific predisposing factors, the nature of the stressor, the perception of the situation, and an analysis of coping resources and mechanisms. Coping responses of the patient are then evaluated on a continuum of adaptation-

Box 4-2

NANDA-APPROVED NURSING DIAGNOSES
(Through the 10th Conference, 1992)

Activity intolerance
Activity intolerance, high risk for
Adjustment, impaired
Airway clearance, ineffective
Anxiety
Aspiration, high risk for
Body image disturbance
Body temperature, altered, high risk for
Breastfeeding, effective
Breastfeeding, ineffective
Breastfeeding, interrupted
Breathing pattern, ineffective
Cardiac output, decreased
Caregiver role strain
Caregiver role strain, high risk for
Communication, impaired verbal
Constipation
Constipation, colonic
Constipation, perceived
Coping, defensive
Coping, family: potential for growth
Coping, ineffective family: compromised
Coping, ineffective family: disabling
Coping, ineffective individual
Decisional conflict (specify)
Denial, ineffective
Diarrhea
Disuse syndrome, high risk for
Diversional activity deficit
Dysreflexia
Family processes, altered
Fatigue
Fear
Fluid volume deficit (1)
Fluid volume deficit (2)
Fluid volume deficit, high risk for
Fluid volume excess
Gas exchange, impaired
Grieving, anticipatory
Grieving, dysfunctional
Growth and development, altered
Health maintenance, altered
Health-seeking behaviors (specify)
Home maintenance management, impaired
Hopelessness
Hyperthermia
Hypothermia
Incontinence, bowel
Incontinence, functional
Incontinence, reflex
Incontinence, stress
Incontinence, total
Incontinence, urge
Infant feeding pattern, ineffective
Infection, high risk for
Injury, high risk for
Knowledge deficit (specify)
Mobility, impaired physical

Noncompliance (specify)
Nutrition, altered: less than body requirements
Nutrition, altered: more than body requirements
Nutrition, altered: high risk for more than body
   requirements
Oral mucous membrane, altered
Pain
Pain, chronic
Parental role conflict
Parenting, altered
Parenting, altered, high risk for
Peripheral neurovascular dysfunction, high risk for
Personal identity disturbance
Poisoning, high risk for
Post-trauma response
Powerlessness
Protection, altered
Rape-trauma syndrome
Rape-trauma syndrome, compound reaction
Rape-trauma syndrome, silent reaction
Role performance, altered
Self-care deficit, bathing/hygiene
Self-care deficit, dressing/grooming
Self-care deficit, feeding
Self-care deficit, toileting
Self-esteem disturbance
Self-esteem, chronic low
Self-esteem, situational low
Self-mutilation, high risk for
Sensory/perceptual alterations (specify) (visual,
   auditory, kinesthetic, gustatory, tactile, olfactory)
Sexual dysfunction
Sexuality patterns, altered
Skin integrity, impaired
Skin integrity, impaired, high risk for
Sleep pattern disturbance
Social interaction, impaired
Social isolation
Spiritual distress (distress of the human spirit)
Stress syndrome, relocation
Suffocation, high risk for
Swallowing, impaired
Therapeutic regimen (individual), ineffective
   management of
Thermoregulation, ineffective
Thought processes, altered
Tissue integrity, impaired
Tissue perfusion, altered (specify type) (renal, cere-
   bral, cardiopulmonary, gastrointestinal, peripheral)
Trauma, high risk for
Unilateral neglect
Urinary elimination, altered patterns
Urinary retention
Ventilation, inabilty to sustain spontaneous
Ventilatory weaning response, dysfunctional
   (DVWR)
Violence, high risk for: self-directed or directed at others

From North American Nursing Diagnosis Association: NANDA *nursing diagnosis: definitions and classifications*, 1992-1993, Philadelphia, 1992, The Association.

CRITICAL THINKING ABOUT CONTEMPORARY ISSUES

How Does Mind-Body Dualism Influence the Way Nurses Think about Patients and Their Illnesses?

In formulating nursing diagnoses, psychiatric nurses must be careful to avoid the mind-body dualism that characterizes the expression, diagnosis, and use of health-care services in the United States.[5,7] In most other cultures this division between mind and body does not exist. There is a wide range of behavior for expressing emotion and psychological disorders, and in America many people express their distress somatically and attribute their problems to physical illness rather than to psychological, social, or spiritual dilemmas. This can create a variety of problems.

One problem is that nurses can respond to patients' somatic complaints and treat them as problems of physical illness without questioning them about possible psychosocial causes. Many patients often want a somatic explanation and treatment and react with fear or anger to the suggestion that there may be a psychological component to their problem. These patients may receive treatment that results in harm or not receive treatment that is needed for their underlying psychological problem. Conversely, a physical illness with affective or cognitive symptoms might be misdiagnosed and inappropriately treated as a psychological problem. Another mistake is for nurses to believe that if a patient's problem is psychiatric then physical symptoms can be discounted or ignored.

As a consequence of mind-body dualism, therefore, patients are separated according to whether their illnesses are decided to be psychological or physical. They are then sent to different hospitals and are seen by different kinds of health-care providers. The practical consequence of this dualistic thinking is that it can interfere with a nurse's ability to understand people's reactions to events in their lives and the ways in which they cope and adapt. ▼

maladaption (see Fig. 4-4). Responses that support integrated functioning are viewed as adaptive. They lead to growth, learning, and goal achievement. Responses that block integrated functioning are viewed as maladaptive. They prevent growth, decrease autonomy, and interfere with mastery of the environment.

Nursing Diagnoses

Responses to stress, whether actual or potential, are the subject of nursing diagnoses. A **nursing diagnosis** is a clinical judgment about individual, family, or community responses to stress (see Critical Thinking about Contemporary Issues). It is a statement of the patient's nursing problem that includes both the adaptive and maladaptive health response and contributing stressors. These responses may be overt, covert, existing, or potential and may lie anywhere on the continuum of coping responses from adaptive to maladaptive. Formulating the diagnosis and implementing treatment are nursing functions for which the nurse is accountable. Box 4-2 lists the nursing diagnoses identified through the Tenth National Conference of the North American Nursing Diagnosis Association (NANDA). In addition, a task force of the Council on Psychiatric and Mental Health Nursing of the American Nurses' Association developed a classification system for human responses for psychiatric–mental health nursing practice.[25] They are now working with NANDA to create one classification system that all nurses can use.

Relationship to Medical Diagnoses

Medical diagnosis refers to the health problem or disease state of the patient. In the medical model of psychiatry these health problems are mental disorders or mental illnesses. It is important for psychiatric nurses to distinguish between nursing and medical models of care as shown in Fig. 4-5. In particular:

▼ Nursing diagnoses focus on the adaptive-maladaptive coping continuum of human responses
▼ Medical diagnoses focus on the health-illness continuum of health problems

A nurse may implement the nursing process for maladaptive responses based on the stress adaptation model whether or not a physician has diagnosed the presence of a psychiatric illness. So too, patients with a persistent psychiatric illness may be adapting well to it. Thus people can successfully adapt to an illness without necessarily recovering from it. This is an important aspect of the stress adaptation model because it suggests that psychiatric nurses can promote their patients' adaptive responses regardless of their health or illness state.

Classifying Mental Disorders

Mental illnesses can be broadly differentiated as neurotic or psychotic. **Neuroses** have the following characteristics[1]:

1. A symptom or group of symptoms is distressing and is recognized as unacceptable and alien to the individual.

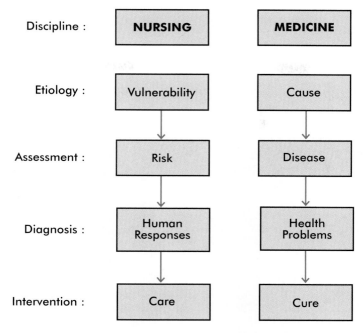

Discipline :	**NURSING**	**MEDICINE**
Etiology :	Vulnerability	Cause
Assessment :	Risk	Disease
Diagnosis :	Human Responses	Health Problems
Intervention :	Care	Cure

Fig. 4-5   Comparison of nursing and medical models of care.

2. Reality testing is grossly intact.
3. Behavior does not actively violate gross social norms (although functioning may be significantly impaired).
4. The disturbance is relatively enduring or recurrent without treatment and is not limited to a transitory reaction to stressors.
5. No demonstrable organic cause or factor is present.

In situations of severest conflict, however, the person may be powerless to cope with the threat by such patterns and may distort reality, as in **psychosis.** Psychosis consists of the following characteristics[1]:

1. A severe mood disorder
2. Regressive behavior
3. Personality disintegration
4. A significant reduction in level of awareness
5. Great difficulty in functioning adequately
6. Gross impairment in reality testing

This last characteristic is critical. When individuals demonstrate gross impairment in reality testing, they incorrectly evaluate the accuracy of their perceptions and draw incorrect inferences about external reality, even in the face of contrary evidence. Direct evidence of psychosis is the presence of either delusions or hallucinations without insight into their pathological nature. Psychotic health problems reflect the most severe level of illness.

Medical diagnoses are classified according to the *Diagnostic and Statistical Manual of Mental Disorders*, fourth edition (DSM-IV), of the American Psychiatric Association.[2] The various illnesses are accompanied by a description of diagnostic criteria, tested for reliability by psychiatric practitioners. DSM-IV uses a multiaxial system that gives attention to various mental disorders, general medical conditions, aspects of the environment, and areas of functioning that might be overlooked if the focus were exclusively on assessing a single presenting problem. The individual thus is evaluated on the following axes:

Axis I	Clinical syndromes
Axis II	Personality disorders
Axis III	General medical conditions
Axis IV	Psychosocial and environmental problems
Axis V	Global assessment of functioning

Axes I-V are presented in the Appendix at the end of this chapter. Axes I and II constitute the entire classification of mental disorders plus conditions that are not attributable to a mental disorder that are a focus of attention or treatment. Axis III allows the clinician to identify any physical disorder potentially relevant to the understanding or treatment of the individual. These three axes make up the diagnosis to be documented for any patient receiving psychiatric care. Axis IV is for reporting psychosocial and environmental problems that may affect the diagnosis, treatment, and prognosis of mental disorders. Axis V is for reporting the clinician's judgment of the individual's overall level of functioning. This information is useful in planning treatment and measuring its impact and in predicting outcomes. Psychiatric nurses use all five axes of the DSM-IV and integrate the axes with related nursing diagnoses.

A STRESS ADAPTATION MODEL OF PSYCHIATRIC NURSING CARE

THEORETICAL BASIS

- Nursing
- Psychopathology
- Neurobiology
- Developmental
- Learning
- Sociocultural
- Cognitive
- Behavioral
- Interpersonal
- Group
- Family
- Milieu
- Pharmacology
- Legal-Ethical

PREDISPOSING FACTORS
PRECIPITATING STRESSORS
APPRAISAL OF STRESSORS
COPING RESOURCES
COPING MECHANISMS

CONTINUUM OF COPING RESPONSES

Adaptive ←→ Maladaptive

NURSING DIAGNOSES

EVALUATION
ASSESSMENT
DIAGNOSIS
OUTCOME IDENTIFICATION
PLANNING
IMPLEMENTATION
EVALUATION

TREATMENT STAGE	HEALTH PROMOTION	MAINTENANCE	ACUTE	CRISIS
TREATMENT GOAL	Optimal Level of Wellness	Recovery	Remission	Stabilization
NURSING ASSESSMENT	Quality of Life and Well-Being	Functional Status	Symptoms and Coping Responses	Risk Factors
NURSING INTERVENTION	Inspire and Validate	Reinforcement Advocacy	Mutual Treatment Planning, Modeling, and Teaching	Manage Environment
EXPECTED OUTCOME	Attain Optimal Quality of Life	Improved Functioning	Symptom Relief	No Harm to Self or Others

Table 4-3   Summary of the Elements of the Stress Adaptation Model Developed by Stuart

Element	Definition	Examples
Predisposing factors	Risk factors that influence both the type and amount of resources the individual can elicit to cope with stress	Age, ethnicity, education, gender
Precipitating stressors	Stimuli that the individual perceives as challenging, threatening, or demanding and that require excess energy for coping	Life events, injury, hassles, strains
Appraisal of stressor	An evaluation of the significance of a stressor for a person's well-being, considering the stressor's meaning, intensity, and importance	Hardiness, perceived seriousness, anxiety, attribution
Coping resources	An evaluation of a person's coping options and strategies	Finances, social support, ego integrity
Coping mechanisms	Any effort directed at stress management	Problem-solving, compliance, defense mechanisms
Continuum of coping responses	A range of adaptive or maladaptive human responses	Social changes, physical symptoms, emotional well-being
Treatment stage activities	Range of nursing functions related to treatment goal, nursing assessment, nursing intervention, and expected outcome	Manage the environment, patient teaching, role model, advocacy

TREATMENT ACTIVITIES

The final aspect of the stress adaptation model is the integration of the theoretical basis, biopsychosocial components, patterns of response, and nursing activities based on the patient's treatment stage. The synthesis of all of the elements of the stress adaptation model of psychiatric nursing care developed by Stuart is depicted in Fig. 4-6. Once patterns of coping responses have been identified, the nurse determines which treatment stage the patient is in and implements the most appropriate nursing activities.

The model identifies four possible treatment stages: (1) health promotion, (2) maintenance, (3) acute, and (4) crisis. These stages reflect the range of the adaptive-maladaptive continuum and suggest a variety of nursing activities. For each stage the nurse identifies the treatment goal, focus of the nursing assessment, nature of the nursing intervention, and expected outcome of nursing care.

▼ In the **crisis stage of treatment** the nursing goal is the stabilization of the patient; the nursing assessment focuses on risk factors that threaten the patient's health and well-being; the nursing intervention is directed toward managing the environment to provide safety; and the expected outcome of nursing care is that no harm will come to the patient or others.

▼ In the **acute stage of treatment** the nursing goal is for the patient's illness to be placed in remission; the nursing assessment is focused on the patient's symptoms and maladaptive coping responses; the nursing intervention is directed toward treatment planning with the patient and the

modeling and teaching of adaptive responses; and the expected outcome of nursing care is symptom relief.

▼ In the **maintenance stage of treatment** the nursing goal is the complete recovery of the patient; the nursing assessment is focused on the patient's functional status; the nursing intervention is directed toward reinforcement of the patient's adaptive coping responses and patient advocacy; and the expected outcome of nursing care is improved patient functioning.

▼ In the **health promotion stage of treatment** the nursing goal is for the patient to achieve the optimal level of wellness; the nursing assessment is focused on the patient's quality of life and well-being; the nursing intervention is directed toward inspiring and validating the patient; and the expected outcome of nursing care is that the patient will attain the optimal quality of life.

This aspect of the model moves the field of psychiatric nursing beyond the usual activities associated with the stabilization of patients in crisis and the remission of the acutely ill patient's symptoms. It elaborates nursing responsibilities in the maintenance and health promotion treatment stages as improving patients' functional status and enhancing their quality of life.[3,19] These treatment stages have often been overlooked in traditional psychiatric nursing practice, yet they are essential aspects of the contemporary psychiatric nursing role.

The elements of the stress adaptation model are summarized in Table 4-3. Chapters 14 through 24 explore various maladaptive coping responses and related medical diagnoses. The phases of the nursing process are described for patients exhibiting maladaptive responses. Each chapter begins with a continuum of coping responses, followed by a discussion of behaviors, predisposing factors, precipitating stressors, coping resources, coping mechanisms, nursing diagnoses, and related interventions. Through consistent application of the stress adaptation model, the art and science of psychiatric nursing emerges.

SUGGESTED CROSS-REFERENCES

SUMMARY

1. The stress adaptation model assumes that nature is ordered as a social hierarchy and that psychiatric nursing care is provided through the use of the nursing process within a biological, psychological, sociocultural, and legal context.
2. The biopsychosocial components of the stress adaptation model include predisposing factors, precipitating stressors, appraisal of stressor, coping resources, and coping mechanisms.
3. Patterns of response include the individual's coping responses, which are the subject of nursing diagnoses, and health problems, which are the subject of medical diagnoses.
4. Psychiatric nursing activities were described for each of the four stages of treatment—crisis, acute, maintenance, and health promotion.

REFERENCES

1. American Psychiatric Association: *Diagnostic and statistical manual of mental disorders*, ed 3, revised, Washington, DC, 1987, The Association.
2. American Psychiatric Association: *Diagnostic and statistical manual of mental disorders*, ed 4, Washington, DC, 1994, The Association.
3. Anthony W: Recovery from mental illness: the guiding vision of the mental health service system in the 1990s, *Psychosoc Rehabil J* 16:11, 1993.
4. Antonovsky A: *Health, stress, and coping*, San Francisco, 1979, Jossey-Bass.
5. Boyle J, Andrews M: *Transcultural concepts in nursing care*, Glenview, Ill, 1989, Scott, Foresman/Little, Brown.
6. Bruckbauer E, Ward S: Positive mental attitude and health: what the public believes, *Image J Nurs Sch* 25:311, 1993.
7. Can your mind heal your body? *Consumer Reports* 58:107, 1993.
8. Caplan G: Mastery of stress: psychosocial aspects, *Am J Psychiatry* 138:41, 1981.
9. Friedman H, VandenBos G: Disease-prone and self-healing personalities, *Hosp Community Psychiatry* 43:1177, 1992.
10. Holmes T, Rahe R: The social readjustment rating scale, *J Psychosom Res* 11:213, 1967.
11. Hull J, Van Treuren R, Virnelli S: Hardiness and health: a critique and alternative approach, *J Pers Soc Psychol* 53:518, 1987.
12. Jahoda M: *Current concepts of positive mental health*, New York, 1958, Basic Books.
13. Johnston N, Baumann A: Selecting a nursing model for psychiatric nursing, *J Psychosoc Nurs Ment Health Serv* 30:7, 1992.
14. Kobasa S, Maddi S, Kan S: Hardiness and health: a prospective study, *J Pers Soc Psychol* 42:168, 1982.
15. Lazarus R, Falkman S: *Stress, appraisal, and coping*, New York, 1984, Springer.
16. Maddi S, Kobasa S: *Stress and coping: an anthology*, New York, 1991, Columbia University Press.
17. Maslow A: *Motivation and personality*, New York, 1958, Harper & Row.
18. Mechanic D: Illness behavior, social adaptation, and the management of illness, *J Nerve Ment Dis* 165:79, 1977.
19. Meyblooom-de Jong B, Smith R: How do we classify functional status? *Fam Med* 24:128, 1992.
20. Miller T: Advances in understanding the impact of stressful life events on health, *Hosp Community Psychiatry* 39:615, 1988.
21. Miller T: *Stressful life events*, Madison, Conn, 1989, International Universities Press.
22. Mirowsky J, Ross C: *Social causes of psychological distress*, New York, 1990, Aldine de Gruyter.
23. Monat A, Lazarus R: *Stress and coping*, New York, 1991, Columbia University Press.
24. National Advisory Mental Health Council: Health care reform for Americans with severe mental illnesses, *Am J Psychiatry* 150:1447, 1993.
25. O'Toole A, Loomis M: Revision of the phenomena of concern for psychiatric mental health nursing, *Arch Psychiatr Nurs* 3:288, 1989.
26. Pearlin LI, Schooler C: The structure of coping, *J Health Soc Behav* 19:2, 1978.
27. Rahe R: Life-change measurement as a predictor of illness, *Proc R Soc Med* 61:1124, 1968.
28. Rogers C: *On becoming a person*, Boston, 1961, Houghton Mifflin.
29. Segal S, VanderVoort D: Daily hassles of persons with severe mental illness, *Hosp Community Psychiatry* 44:276, 1993.

30. Tartasky D: Hardiness: conceptual and methodological issues, *Image J Nurs Sch* 25:225, 1993.
31. Wagnid G, Young H: Another look at hardiness, *Image J Nurs Sch* 23:257, 1991.

ANNOTATED SUGGESTED READINGS

Elizur J, Minuchin S: *Institutionalizing madness: families, therapy and society,* New York, 1989, Basic Books.

Using case studies, this book explores patients, families, and institutions and the culture-bound way the mental health field repsonds to people labeled patients.

Gordon J: Holistic medicine and mental health practice: toward a new synthesis, *Am J Orthopsychiatry* 60:357, 1990.

Outlines the holistic approach, which regards the spiritual dimension as a vital enlargement of the biopsychosocial model, and the way in which holism may shape the future of mental health practice.

*Gross D, Fogg L, Conrad B: Designing interventions in psychosocial research, *Arch Psychiatr Nurs* 7:259, 1993.

Excellent discussion on developing interventions that are based on a strong theoretical and empirical foundation, which is greatly needed in the field.

*Johnston N, Baumann A: Selecting a nursing model for psychiatric nursing, *J Psychosoc Nurs Ment Health Serv* 30:7, 1992.

Clearly describes the process that psychiatric nurses can use in selecting a nursing model for practice. Practical and relevant.

Kaysen S: *Girl, interrupted,* New York, 1993, Turtle Bay Books.

A first-person account about the author's psychiatric hospitalization as an adolescent. Sensitizing reading from a patient's perspective of mental illness.

*Molzahn A, Northcott, H: The social bases of discrepancies in health/illness perceptions, *J Adv Nurs* 14:132, 1989.

Thought-provoking article that summarizes the literature pertaining to discrepancies in health-illness perceptions between patients and health-care providers and social factors that may effect these perceptions.

Monat A, Lazarus R: *Stress and coping,* New York, 1991, Columbia University Press.

Compiles work on stress and coping into one readable text. Definitive text by experts in the field.

Mirowsky J, Ross C: *Social causes of psychological distress,* New York, 1990, Aldine de Gruyter.

Interesting discussion of social factors that explain why some people are more distressed than others. Thought provoking and socially relevant.

National Advisory Mental Health Council: Health care reform for Americans with severe mental illnesses, *Am J Psychiatry* 150:1447, 1993.

Summary of the latest findings, statistics, and progress in psychiatric illness with implications for health-care reform.

---

*Nursing reference.

A P P E N D I X
DSM-IV Classification*

AXIS I: CLINICAL SYNDROMES

Disorders Usually First Diagnosed in Infancy, Childhood, or Adolescence

Mental Retardation

317	Mild Mental Retardation
318.0	Moderate Retardation
318.1	Severe Mental Retardation
318.2	Profound Mental Retardation
319	Mental Retardation, Severity Unspecified

Learning Disorders (Academic Skills Disorder)

315.00	Reading Disorder (Developmental Reading Disorder)
315.1	Mathematics Disorder (Developmental Arithmetic Disorder)
315.2	Disorder of Written Expression (Developmental Expressive Writing Disorder)
315.9	Learning Disorder NOS

Motor Skills Disorder

315.4	Developmental Coordination Disorder

Pervasive Developmental Disorders

29.00	Autistic Disorder
299.80	Rett's Disorder
299.10	Childhood Disintegrative Disorder
	Asperger's Disorder (? placement)
299.80	Pervasive Developmental Disorder NOS (including Atypical Autism)

Disruptive Behavior and Attention-Deficit Disorders

Attention-Deficit/Hyperactivity Disorder

314.00	Predominantly inattentive type
314.01	Predominantly hyperactive-impulsive type
314.01	Combined type
314.9	Attention-Deficit/Hyperactivity Disorder NOS
313.81	Oppositional Defiant Disorder
312.8	Conduct Disorder
312.9	Disruptive Behavior Disorder NOS

Feeding and Eating Disorders of Infancy or Early Childhood

307.52	Pica
307.53	Rumination Disorder
307.59	Feeding Disorder of Infancy or Early Childhood

Tic Disorders

307.23	Tourette's Disorder
307.22	Chronic Motor or Vocal Tic Disorder
307.21	Transient Tic Disorder
307.20	Tic Disorder NOS

Communication Disorders

315.31	Expressive Language Disorder (Developmental Expressive Language Disorder)
315.31	Mixed Receptive/Expressive Language Disorder (Developmental Receptive Language Disorder)
315.39	Phonological Disorder (Developmental Articulation Disorder)
307.0	Stuttering
315.39	Communication Disorder NOS

---

*From American Psychiatric Association: *Diagnostic and statistical manual of mental disorders*, ed 4, Washington, DC, 1994, The Association.

Elimination Disorders

307.7	Encopresis
307.6	Enuresis

Other Disorders of Infancy, Childhood, or Adolescence

309.21	Separation Anxiety Disorder
313.23	Selective Mutism (Elective Mutism)
313.89	Reactive Attachment Disorder of Infancy or Early Childhood
307.3	Stereotypic Movement Disorder (Stereotypic/Habit Disorder)
313.9	Disorder of Infancy, Childhood, or Adolescence NOS

Delirium, Dementia, Amnestic and Other Cognitive Disorders

Deliria

293.0	Delirium Due to a General Medical Condition
---.	Substance-induced Delirium (refer to specific substance for code)
---.-	Delirium Due to Multiple Etiologies (use multiple codes based on specific etiologies)
293.89	Delirium NOS

Dementias

---.-	Dementia of the Alzheimer's Type
	With Early Onset: if onset at age 65 or below
	290.10 uncomplicated
	290.11 with delirium
	290.12 with delusions
	290.13 with depressed mood
	290.14 with hallucinations
	290.15 with perceptual disturbance
	290.16 with behavioral disturbance
	290.17 with communication disturbance
	With Late Onset: if onset after age 65
	290.00 uncomplicated
	290.30 with delirium
	290.20 with delusions
	290.21 with depressed mood
	290.22 with hallucinations
	290.23 with perceptual disturbance
	290.24 with behavioral disturbance
	290.25 with communication disturbance
---.-	Vascular Dementia (D:9)
	290.40 uncomplicated
	290.41 with delirium
	290.42 with delusions
	290.43 with depressed mood
	290.44 with hallucinations
	290.45 with perceptual disturbance
	290.46 with behavioral disturbance
	290.47 with communication disturbance

Dementias Due to Other General Medical Conditions

294.9	Dementia Due to HIV Disease (Code 043.1 on Axis III)
294.1	Dementia Due to Head Trauma (Code 905.0 on Axis III)
294.1	Dementia Due to Parkinson's Disease (Code 332.0 on Axis III)
294.1	Dementia Due to Huntington's Disease (Code 333.4 on Axis III)
290.10	Dementia Due to Pick's Disease (Code 331.1 on Axis III)

290.10	Dementia Due to Creutzfeldt-Jakob Disease (*Code* 046.1 *on Axis* III)
294.1	Dementia Due to Other General Medical Condition
---.-	Substance-Induced Persisting Dementia (Refer to specific substance for code)
---.-	Dementia Due to Multiple Etiologies (use multiple codes based on specific etiologies)
294.8	Dementia NOS

Amnestic Disorders

294.0	Amnestic Disorder Due to a General Medical Condition
---.-	Substance-Induced Persisting Amnestic Disorder (Refer to specific substance for code)
294.8	Amnestic Disorder NOS
294.9	Cognitive Disorder NOS

Mental Disorders Due to a General Medical Condition Not Elsewhere Classified

293.89	Catatonic Disorder Due to a General Medical Condition
310.1	Personality Change Due to a General Medical Condition
293.9	Mental Disorder NOS Due to a General Medical Condition

Substance Related Disorders

Alcohol Use Disorders

303.90	Alcohol Dependence
305.00	Alcohol Abuse
303.00	Alcohol Intoxication
291.8	Alcohol Withdrawal
291.0	Alcohol Delirium
291.2	Alcohol Persisting Dementia
291.1	Alcohol Persisting Amnestic Disorder
	Alcohol Psychotic Disorder
291.5	With delusions
291.3	With hallucinations
291.8	Alcohol Mood Disorder
291.8	Alcohol Anxiety Disorder
292.8	Alcohol Sexual Dysfunction
292.89	Alcohol Sleep Disorder
291.9	Alcohol Use Disorder NOS

Amphetamine (or Related Substance) Use Disorders

304.40	Amphetamine (or Related Substance) Dependence
305.70	Amphetamine (or Related Substance) Abuse
305.70	Amphetamine (or Related Substance) Intoxication
292.0	Amphetamine (or Related Substance) Withdrawal
292.81	Amphetamine (or Related Substance) Delirium
	Amphetamine (or Related Substance) Psychotic Disorder
291.11	With delusions
291.12	With hallucinations
292.84	Amphetamine (or Related Substance) Mood Disorder
292.89	Amphetamine (or Related Substance) Anxiety Disorder
292.89	Amphetamine (or Related Substance) Sexual Dysfunction
292.89	Amphetamine (or Related Substance) Sleep Disorder
292.9	Amphetamine (or Related Substance) Use Disorder NOS

Caffeine Use Disorders

305.90	Caffeine Intoxication
292.84	Caffeine Anxiety Disorder
292.89	Caffeine Sleep Disorder
292.9	Caffeine Use Disorder NOS

Cannabis Use Disorders

304.30	Cannabis Dependence
305.20	Cannabis Abuse
305.20	Cannabis Intoxication
292.81	Cannabis Delirium
	Cannabis Psychotic Disorder
291.11	With delusions
291.12	With hallucinations
292.89	Cannabis Anxiety Disorder
292.9	Cannabis Use Disorder NOS

Cocaine Use Disorders

304.20	Cocaine Dependence
305.60	Cocaine Abuse
305.60	Cocaine Intoxication
292.0	Cocaine Withdrawal
292.81	Cocaine Delirium
	Cocaine Psychotic Disorder
291.11	With delusions
291.12	With hallucinations
292.84	Cocaine Mood Disorder
292.89	Cocaine Anxiety Disorder
292.89	Cocaine Sexual Dysfunction
292.89	Cocaine Sleep Disorder
292.9	Cocaine Use Disorder NOS

Hallucinogen Use Disorders

304.50	Hallucinogen Dependence
305.30	Hallucinogen Abuse
305.30	Hallucinogen Intoxication
292.89	Hallucinogen Persisting Perception Disorder
291.11	Hallucinogen Delirium
	Hallucinogen Psychotic Disorder
291.11	With delusions
291.12	With hallucinations
292.84	Hallucinogen Mood Disorder
292.89	Hallucinogen Anxiety Disorder
292.9	Hallucinogen Use Disorder NOS

Inhalant Use Disorders

304.60	Inhalant Dependence
305.90	Inhalant Abuse
305.90	Inhalant Intoxication
292.81	Inhalant Delirium
292.82	Inhalant Persisting Dementia
	Inhalant Psychotic Disorder
291.11	With delusions
291.12	With hallucinations
292.84	Inhalant Mood Disorder
292.89	Inhalant Anxiety Disorder
292.9	Inhalant Use Disorder NOS

Nicotine Use Disorders

305.10	Nicotine Dependence
292.0	Nicotine Withdrawal
292.9	Nicotine Use Disorder NOS

Opioid Use Disorders

304.00	Opioid Dependence
305.50	Opioid Abuse
305.50	Opioid Intoxication
292.0	Opioid Withdrawal
292.81	Opioid Delirium
	Opioid Psychotic Disorder
291.11	With delusions

291.12	With hallucinations
292.84	Opioid Mood Disorder
292.89	Opioid Sleep Disorder
292.89	Opioid Sexual Dysfunction
292.9	Opioid Use Disorder NOS

Phencyclidine (or Related Substance) Use Disorders

304.90	Phencyclidine (or Related Substance) Dependence
305.90	Phencyclidine (or Related Substance) Abuse
305.90	Phencyclidine (or Related Substance) Intoxication
292.81	Phencyclidine (or Related Substance) Delirium
	Phencyclidine (or Related Substance) Psychotic Disorder
291.11	With delusions
291.12	With hallucinations
292.84	Phencyclidine (or Related Substance) Mood Disorder
292.89	Phencyclidine (or Related Substance) Anxiety Disorder
292.9	Phencyclidine (or Related Substance) Use Disorder NOS

Sedative, Hypnotic, or Anxiolytic Substance Use Disorders

304.10	Sedative, Hypnotic, or Anxiolytic Dependence
305.40	Sedative, Hypnotic, or Anxiolytic Abuse
305.40	Sedative, Hypnotic, or Anxiolytic Intoxication
292.0	Sedative, Hypnotic, or Anxiolytic Withdrawal
292.81	Sedative, Hypnotic, or Anxiolytic Delirium
292.82	Sedative, Hypnotic, or Anxiolytic Persisting Dementia
292.83	Sedative, Hypnotic, or Anxiolytic Persisting Amnestic Disorder
	Sedative, Hypnotic, or Anxiolytic Psychotic Disorder
291.11	With delusions
291.12	With hallucinations
292.84	Sedative, Hypnotic, or Anxiolytic Mood Disorder
292.89	Sedative, Hypnotic, or Anxiolytic Anxiety Disorder
292.89	Sedative, Hypnotic, or Anxiolytic Sleep Disorder
292.89	Sedative, Hypnotic, or Anxiolytic Sexual Dysfunction
292.9	Sedative, Hypnotic, or Anxiolytic Use Disorder NOS

Polysubstance Use Disorder

304.80	Polysubstance Dependence (E:27)

Other (or Unknown) Substance Use Disorders

304.90	Other (or Unknown) Substance Dependence
305.90	Other (or Unknown) Substance Abuse
305.90	Other (or Unknown) Substance Intoxication
292.0	Other (or Unknown) Substance Withdrawal
292.81	Other (or Unknown) Substance Persisting Dementia
292.83	Other (or Unknown) Substance Persisting Amnestic Disorder
	Other (or Unknown) Substance Psychotic Disorder
291.11	With delusions
291.12	With hallucinations
292.84	Other (or Unknown) Substance Mood Disorder
292.89	Other (or Unknown) Substance Anxiety Disorder
292.89	Other (or Unknown) Substance Sexual Dysfunction
292.89	Other (or Unknown) Substance Sleep Disorder
292.9	Other (or Unknown) Substance use Disorder NOS

Schizophrenia and Other Psychotic Disorders

	Schizophrenia
395.30	Paranoid type
295.10	Disorganized type
295.20	Catatonic type
295.90	Undifferentiated type
295.40	Residual type
295.40	Schizophreniform Disorder

295.70	Schizoaffective Disorder
297.1	Delusional Disorder
298.8	Brief Psychotic Disorder
297.3	Shared Psychotic Disorder (Folie a Deux)
	Psychotic Disorder Due to a General Medical Condition
293.81	With delusions
293.82	With hallucinations
---.--	Substance-Induced Psychotic Disorder (refer to specific substances for codes)
298.9	Psychotic Disorder NOS

Mood Disorders

Code current state of Major Depressive Disorder or Bipolar Disorder in fifth digit:

0 *unspecified*
1 *mild*
2 *moderate*
3 *severe, without psychotic features*
4 *severe, with psychotic features*
5 *in partial remission*
6 *in full remission*

Depressive Disorders

	Major Depressive Disorder
296.2x	Single episode
296.3x	Recurrent
300.4	Dysthymic Disorder
311	Depressive Disorder NOS

Bipolar Disorders

	Bipolar I Disorder
296.0x	Single manic episode
296.4	Most recent episode hypomanic
296.4x	Most recent episode manic
296.6x	Most recent episode mixed
296.5x	Most recent episode depressed
296.7	Most recent episode unspecified
296.89	Bipolar II Disorder (Recurrent major depressive episodes with hypomania)
301.13	Cyclothymic Disorder
296.80	Bipolar Disorder NOS
293.83	Mood Disorder Due to a General Medical Condition
--- --	Substance-Induced Mood Disorder (refer to specific substances for codes)
296.90	Mood Disorder NOS

Anxiety Disorders

	Panic Disorder
300.01	Without Agoraphobia
300.21	With Agoraphobia
300.22	Agoraphobia Without History of Panic Disorder
300.29	Specific Phobia (Simple Phobia)
300.23	Social Phobia (Social Anxiety Disorder
300.3	Obsessive-Compulsive Disorder
309.81	Posttraumatic Stress Disorder
300.3	Acute Stress Disorder
300.02	Generalized Anxiety Disorder (includes Overanxious Disorder of Childhood)
293.89	Anxiety Disorder Due to a General Medical Condition
--- --	Substance-Induced Anxiety Disorder (refer to specific substances for codes)
300.00	Anxiety Disorder NOS

Somatoform Disorders

300.81	Somatization Disorder
300.11	Conversion Disorder
300.7	Hypochondriasis
300.71	Body Dysmorphic Disorder
	Pain Disorder
307.80	Associated with Psychological Factors
307.89	Associated with Both Psychological Factors and a General Medical Condition
300.82	Undifferentiated Somatoform Disorder
300.89	Somatoform Disorder NOS

Factitious Disorders

	Factitious Disorder
300.16	With predominantly psychological signs and symptoms
300.17	With predominantly physical signs and symptoms
300.18	With combined psychological and physical signs and symptoms
300.19	Factitious Disorder NOS

Dissociative Disorders

300.12	Dissociative Amnesia
300.13	Dissociative Fugue
300.14	Dissociative Identity Disorder (Multiple Personality Disorder)
300.6	Depersonalization Disorder
300.15	Dissociative Disorder NOS

Sexual and Gender Identity Disorders

Sexual Dysfunctions

Sexual Desire Disorders

302.71	Hypoactive Sexual Desire Disorder
?302.79	Sexual Aversion Disorder

Sexual Arousal Disorders

302.72	Female Sexual Arousal Disorder
302.72	Male Erectile Disorder

Orgasm Disorders

302.73	Female Orgasmic Disorder (Inhibited Female Orgasm)
302.74	Male Orgasmic Disorder (Inhibited Male Orgasm)
302.75	Premature Ejaculation

Sexual Pain Disorders

302.76	Dyspareunia
306.51	Vaginismus

Sexual Dysfunctions Due to a General Medical Condition

607.84	Male Erectile Disorder Due to a General Medical Condition
608.89	Male Dyspareunia Due to a General Medical Condition
625.0	Female Dyspareunia Due to a General Medical Condition
608.89	Male Hypoactive Sexual Desire Disorder Due to a General Medical Condition.
625.8	Female Hypoactive Sexual Desire Disorder Due to a General Medical Condition
608.89	Other Male Sexual Dysfunction Due to a General Medical Condition
625.8	Other Female Sexual Dysfunction Due to a General Medical Condition
--- --	Substance-Induced Sexual Dysfunction (refer to specific substances for codes)
302.70	Sexual Dysfunction NOS

Paraphilias

302.4	Exhibitionism
302.81	Fetishism
?302.85	Frotteurism
302.2	Pedophilia
302.83	Sexual Masochism
302.84	Sexual Sadism
302.82	Voyeurism
302.3	Transvestic Fetishism
302.9	Paraphilia NOS
302.9	Sexual Disorder NOS

Gender Identity Disorders

	Gender Identity Disorder
302.6	In Children
302.85	In Adolescents and Adults
302.6	Gender Identity Disorder NOS

Eating Disorders

307.1	Anorexia Nervosa
307.51	Bulimia Nervosa
307.50	Eating Disorder NOS

Sleep Disorders

Primary Sleep Disorders

Dyssomnias

307.42	Primary Insomnia
307.44	Primary Hypersomnia
347	Narcolepsy
780.59	Breathing-Related Sleep Disorder
307.45	Circadian Rhythm Sleep Disorder (Sleep-Wake Schedule Disorder)
307.47	Dyssomnia NOS

Parasomnias

307.47	Nightmare Disorder (Dream Anxiety Disorder)
307.46	Sleep Terror Disorder
307.46	Sleepwalking Disorder
307.47	Parasomnia NOS

Sleep Disorders Related to Another Mental Disorder

307.42	Insomnia related to [Axis I or Axis II Disorder]
307.44	Hypersomnia related to [Axis I or Axis II Disorder]

Other Sleep Disorders

	Sleep Disorder Due to a General Medical Condition
780.52	Insomnia type
780.54	Hypersomnia type
780.59	Parasomnia type
780.59	Mixed type
--- --	Substance-Induced Sleep Disorder (refer to specific substances for codes)

Impulse Control Disorders Not Elsewhere Classified

312.34	Intermittent Explosive Disorder
312.32	Kleptomania
312.33	Pyromania
312.31	Pathological Gambling
312.39	Trichotilomania
312.30	Impulse Control NOS

Adjustment Disorders

	Adjustment Disorder
309.24	With Anxiety
309.0	With Depressed Mood
309.3	With Disturbance of Conduct
309.4	With Mixed Disturbance of Emotions and Conduct
309.28	With Mixed Anxiety and Depressed Mood
309.9	Unspecified

Other Conditions That May be a Focus of Clinical Attention

316 **(Psychological Factors) Affecting Medical Condition**

Choose name based on nature of factors:
Mental Disorder Affecting Medical Condition
Psychological Symptoms Affecting Medical Condition
Personality Traits or Coping Style Affecting Medical Condition
Maladaptive Health Behaviors Affecting Medical Condition
Unspecified Psychological Factors Affecting Medical Condition

Medication-Induced Movement Disorders

332.1	Neuroleptic-Induced Parkinsonism
333.92	Neuroleptic Malignant Syndrome
333.7	Neuroleptic-induced Acute Dystonia
333.99	Neuroleptic-induced Acute Akathisia
333.82	Neuroleptic-induced Tardive Dyskinesia
333.1	Medication-Induced Postural Tremor
333.90	Medication-Induced Movement Disorder NOS
995.2	Adverse Effects of Medication NOS

Relational Problems

V61.9	Relational Problem Related to A Mental Disorder or General Medical Condition
V61.20	Parent-Child Relational Problem
V61.12	Partner Relational Problem
V61.8	Sibling Relational Problem
V62.81	Relational Problem NOS

Problems Related to Abuse or Neglect

V61.21	Physical Abuse of Child
V61.22	Sexual Abuse of Child
V61.21	Neglect of Child
V61.10	Physical Abuse of Adult
V51.11	Sexual Abuse of Adult

Additional Conditions That May Be a Focus of Clinical Attention

V62.82	Bereavement
V40.0	Borderline Intellectual Functioning
V62.3	Academic Problem
V62.2	Occupational Problem
V71.02	Childhood or Adolescent Antisocial Behavior
V71.01	Adult Antisocial Behavior
V65.2	Malingering
62.89	Phase of Life Problem
V15.81	Noncompliance with treatment for a mental disorder
313.82	Identity Problem
V62.61	Religious or Spiritual Problem
V62.4	Acculturation Problem
780.9	Age-Associated Memory Decline

Additional Codes

300.9	Unspecified Mental Disorder
V71.09	No Diagnosis or Condition on Axis I
799.9	Diagnosis or Condition Deferred on Axis I
V71.09	No Diagnosis on Axis II
799.9	Diagnosis Deferred on Axis II

AXIS II: PERSONALITY DISORDERS

301.0	Paranoid Personality Disorder
301.20	Schizoid Personality Disorder
301.22	Schizotypal Personality Disorder
301.7	Antisocial Personality Disorder
301.83	Borderline Personality Disorder
301.50	Histrionic Personality Disorder
301.81	Narcissistic Personality Disorder
301.82	Avoidant Personality Disorder
301.6	Dependent Personality Disorder
301.4	Obsessive-Compulsive Personality Disorder
301.9	Personality Disorder NOS

AXIS III: ICD-9-CM GENERAL MEDICAL CONDITIONS

Infectious and Parasitic Diseases (001-139)

Neoplasms (140-239)

Endocrine, Nutritional, and Metabolic Diseases and Immunity Disorders (240-279)

Diseases of the Blood and Blood-Forming Organs (280-289)

Diseases of the Nervous and Sense Organs (320-389)

Diseases of the Circulatory System (390-459)

Diseases of the Respiratory System (460-519)

Diseases of the Digestive System (520-579)

Diseases of the Genitourinary System (580-629)

Complications of Pregnancy, Childbirth, and the Puerperium (630-676)

Diseases of the Skin and Subcutaneous Tissue (680-709)

Diseases of the Musculoskeletal System and Connective Tissue (710-739)

Congenital Anomalies (740-759)

Certain Conditions Originating in the Perinatal Period (760-779)

Symptoms, Signs, and Ill-Defined Conditions (780-799)

Injury and Poisoning (800-999)

AXIS IV: PSYCHOSOCIAL AND ENVIRONMENTAL PROBLEMS

Problems with Primary Support Group (Childhood [V61.9], Adult [V61.9], Parent-Child [V61.2]). These include: death of a family member; health problems in family; disruption of family by separation, divorce, or estrangement; removal from the home; remarriage of parent; sexual or physical abuse; parental overprotection; neglect of child; inadequate discipline; discord with siblings; birth of a sibling.

Problems Related to the Social Environment (V62.4). These include: death or loss of friend; social isolation; living alone; difficulty with acculturation; discrimination; adjustment to life cycle transition (e.g., retirement).

Educational Problems (V62.3). These include: illiteracy; academic problems; discord with teachers or classmates; inadequate school environment.

Occupational Problems (V62.2). These include: unemployment; threat of job loss; stressful work schedule; difficult work condition; job dissatisfaction; job change; discord with boss or coworkers.

Housing Problems (V60.9). These include: homelessness; inadequate housing; unsafe neighborhood; discord with neighbors or landlord.

Economic Problems (V60.9). These include: extreme poverty; inadequate finances; insufficient welfare support.

Problems with Access to Health Care Services (V63.9). These include: inadequate health care services; transportation to health care facilities unavailable; inadequate health insurance.

Problems Related to Interaction with the Legal System/Crime (V62.5). These include: arrest; incarceration; litigation; victim of crime.

Other Psychosocial Problems (V62.9). These include: exposure to disasters, war, other hostilities; discord with non-family caregivers (e.g., counselor, social worker, physician); unavailability of social service agencies.

AXIS V: GLOBAL ASSESSMENT OF FUNCTIONING (GAF) SCALE*

Consider psychological, social, and occupational functioning on a hypothetical continuum of mental health-illness. Do not include impairment in functioning due to physical (or environmental) limitations.

Code (Note: Use intermediate codes when appropriate, e.g., 45, 68, 72.)

100 Superior functioning in a wide range of activities, life's problems never seem to get out of hand, is sought out by others because of his many positive qualities. No symptoms.
91

90 Absent or minimal symptoms (e.g., mild anxiety before an exam), good functioning in all areas, interested and involved in a wide range of activities, socially effective, generally satisfied with life, no more than everyday problems or concerns (e.g., an occasional argument with family members).
81

80 If symptoms are present, they are transient and expectable reactions to psychosocial stressors (e.g., difficulty concentrating after family argument); no more than slight impairment in social, occupational or school functioning (e.g., temporarily falling behind in school work).
71

70 Some mild symptoms (e.g., depressed mood and mild insomnia) OR some difficulty in social, occupational, or school functioning (e.g., occasional truancy, or theft within the household), but generally functioning pretty well, has some meaningful interpersonal relationships.
61

60 Moderate symptoms (e.g., flat affect and circumstantial speech, occasional panic attacks) OR moderate difficulty in social, occupational, or school functioning (e.g., no friends, unable to keep a job).
51

50 Serious symptoms (e.g., suicidal ideation, severe obsessional rituals, frequent shoplifting) OR any serious impairment in social, occupational, or school functioning (e.g., no friends, unable to keep a job).
41

40 Some impairment in reality testing or communication (e.g., speech is at times illogical, obscure, or irrelevant) OR major impairment in several areas, such as work or school, family relations, judgment, thinking, or mood (e.g., depressed man avoids friends, neglects family, and is unable to work; child frequently beats up younger children, is defiant at home, and is failing at school).
31

30 Behavior is considerably influenced by delusions or hallucinations OR serious impairment in communication or judgment (e.g., sometimes incoherent, acts grossly inappropriately, suicidal preoccupation) OR inability to function in almost all areas (e.g., stays in bed all day; no job, home, or friends).
21

20 Some danger of hurting self or others (e.g., suicide attempts without clear expectation of death, frequently violent, manic excitement) OR occasionally fails to maintain minimal personal hygiene (e.g., smears feces) OR gross impairment in communication (e.g., largely incoherent or mute).
11

10 Persistent danger of severely hurting self or others (e.g., recurrent violence) OR persistent inability to maintain personal hygiene OR serious suicidal act with clear expectation of death.
1

0 Inadequate information.

---

*The GAF Scale is a revision of the GAS (Endicott J, Spitzer RL, Fleiss et al: The Global Assessment Scale: a procedure for measuring overall severity of psychiatric disturbance, *Arch Gen Psychiatry* 33:766, 1976) and the CGAS (Shaffer D, Gould MS, Brasic J et al: Children's Global Assessment Scale (CGAS), *Arch Gen Psychiatry* 40:1228, 1983). These are revisions of the Global Scale of the Health-Sickness Rating Scale (Luborsky L: Clinicians' judgments of mental health, *Arch Gen Psychiatry* 7:407, 1962).

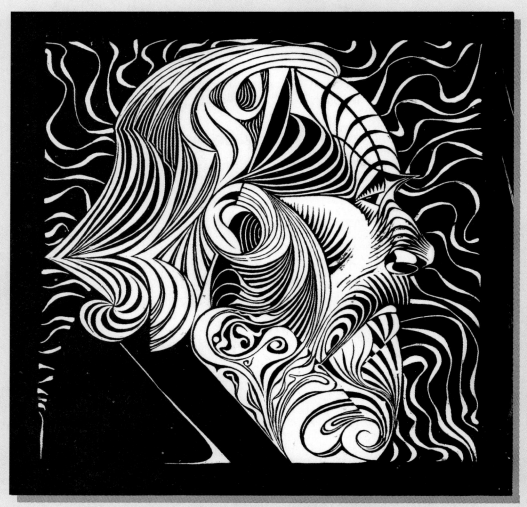

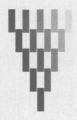

CHAPTER 5

Biological Context of Psychiatric Nursing Care

MICHELE T. LARAIA

We must recollect that all our provisional ideas in psychology will some day be based on an organic substructure. This makes it probable that special substances and special chemical processes control the operation.

Sigmund Freud

LEARNING OBJECTIVES

After studying this chapter the student should be able to:

▼ Relate the importance of understanding the structure and function of the brain for psychiatric nursing practice

▼ Describe neuroimaging techniques used in psychiatry

▼ Discuss the current status of genetic information related to psychiatric illness

▼ Identify the impact of circadian rhythms on a person's abilities and moods

▼ Describe the new field of psychoimmunology and its implications for psychiatry

▼ Demonstrate the ability to assess patients from a biological perspective

▼ Analyze the clinical implications of recent neuroscientific research related to schizophrenia, mood disorders, panic disorder, and Alzheimer's disease

TOPICAL OUTLINE

Structure and Function of the Brain
Neuroimaging Techniques
Genetics of Mental Illness
Circadian Rhythms
   Sleep
Psychoimmunology
Biological Assessment of the Patient
Biological Components of Mental Illness
   Schizophrenia
   Mood Disorders
   Panic Disorder
   Alzheimer's Disease
Decade of the Brain

Although interest in the brain and human behavior has a history as old as the human race, the twentieth century has witnessed a shift in how science views the brain and behavior, and thus human experience itself. The explosion in knowledge and technology in the neurosciences is unprecedented in the history of psychiatric care. This is evident in research that focuses on how the brain is structured, how the nervous system functions, how these systems affect health, and how they are af-fected by disease. Neuroscience research has begun to suggest causes of brain illnesses, interventions to treat these illnesses, and effective preventive measures. The field of neuroscience encompasses many disciplines including anatomy, physiology, biochemistry, genetics, neuroimaging, physics, pharmacology, neurology, neurosurgery, immunology, psychiatry, psychology, electronics, and computer science (Fig. 5-1).

New tools and techniques now help to explain the

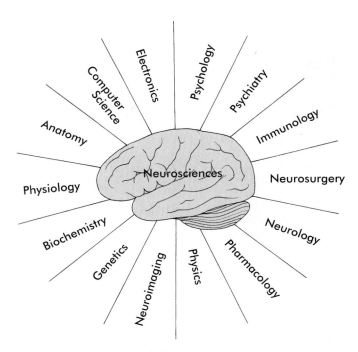

Fig. 5-1 The field of neurosciences.

way in which the brain works and how the brain, mind, and body interact. For example:

▼ Methods of staining nerve cells allow scientists to locate the precise position of these cells in the brain.

▼ Electrical activity of a single channel in a receptor cell membrane can be measured.

▼ Activities and functions of the living brain can be observed with computer, microscopy, and imaging technologies.

▼ Exogenous chemicals can be tagged, injected, and traced in the living brain.

▼ The search for specific genes that cause some brain dysfunctions has resulted in small scientific breakthroughs in the past few years.

These technologies, along with standardized behavioral tests, have allowed human behavior to be correlated with specific brain regions, functions, and dysfunctions. As a consequence, a revolution has begun in the study of how the human brain is understood and the way in which mental illness is conceptualized, recognized, and treated.

Psychiatric nursing has a key role to play in this endeavor. Nurses have always been in a pivotal position to integrate theories and technologies with therapeutic interventions and patient-centered approaches. They have demonstrated great ability to do this, for example, in the psychosocial areas of functioning. Now, psychiatric nurses must also integrate and use the biological context of psychiatric care to enhance nursing practice. Psychiatric nurses must also interpret this new biologi-

cal information and its potential for effective treatments to consumers of mental health services and other health-care providers, thus further reinforcing nurses' role as patient advocates. It is clear that the biological frontier presents great challenges, and if these challenges are accepted, psychiatric nursing can make a significant move forward in further defining the scope of its practice and the outcomes associated with psychiatric nursing care.

STRUCTURE AND FUNCTION OF THE BRAIN

The psychiatric nurse must have a working knowledge of the normal structure and function of the brain, particularly mental functions, just as the cardiac care nurse must know how the heart works. Much is known about various brain structures and how they are linked to some of the symptoms of mental illness. The reader is encouraged to review texts on basic anatomy and physiology or neurophysiology to learn more detailed information in these areas.[4,28] For the purposes of this chapter, a brief review of several key brain regions is presented in Color Plates 1 to 5 on pp. 129-132 and in Box 5-1 on pp. 126-128. This information can be used as a reference for topics discussed in this chapter.

The brain weighs about 3 pounds. It is composed of trillions of groups of cells that have formed structures that have changed over millions of years of evolution. These structures have complex functions and connections to each other that are not fully understood. There is some basic information, however, on how these structures function and communicate in health and illness. About 100 billion brain cells form groups of **neurons** that are arranged in networks. These neurons communicate with each other through **neurotransmission,** which gives rise to human activity, body functions, consciousness, intelligence, creativity, memory, and emotion. Neurotransmission is a key factor in understanding how various regions of the brain function and how biochemical interventions, such as medications, affect brain activity and behavior. There are also chemical messengers called **neurotransmitters.** These are manufactured in the neuron and released from the **axon,** or presynaptic cell membrane, into the **synapse,** which is the space between neurons. From there they are received by the **dendrite,** or postsynaptic membrane, of the next neuron. This neurotransmission process makes communication between brain cells possible (see Color Plate 6 on p. 132).

Like a key inserted into a lock, each of these chemicals fits into specific receptor cells, or proteins, embedded in the membrane of the dendrite, which recognize it. Then one of two things happens: the signal given by the neurotransmitter either (1) excites receiving cells, which causes them to fire and produce an action, or (2) inhibits cells from firing, which modifies the excitability of the receiving cell and stops an action. After release into the synapse and communication with receptor cells, these neurotransmitter chemicals are transported back from the synapse into the axon where they are stored for reuse or metabolized and inactivated by enzymes. The process of neurotransmitters returning to the presynaptic cell is known as **reuptake.**

A final structure is that of the **glial cells,** which are support cells that form the **myelin sheaths** providing insulation to the nervous system. They are thought to remove excess transmitters and ions from the extracellular spaces in the brain, provide glucose to some nerve cells, and direct the flow of blood and oxygen to various parts of the brain.

From this basic explanation it is evident that neurotransmitters perform vital functions in the normal working brain, and their absence or excess can play a major role in brain disease and behavioral disorders. It is also important to realize that a single neurotransmitter can activate several different subtypes of receptor cells, each located along tracks going to different regions of the brain. Thus one neurotransmitter can have different effects in different areas of the brain. Also, the number of receptors in the brain changes depending on the availability of the neurotransmitter. Nearly all of the known or suspected neurotransmitters fall into one of two categories: small amine molecules (monoamines, acetylcholine, and amino acids) and peptides. These are described in Table 5-1.

One clinical implication of this process is that abnormalities in the structure of the brain or in its activity in specific locations can cause or contribute to psychiatric disorders. For example, a communication problem in one small part of the brain can cause widespread dysfunction. It is also known that the following networks of nuclei that control cognitive, behavioral, and emotional functioning are particularly implicated in psychiatric disorders:

▼ The *cerebral cortex*, which is critical in decision making and higher order thinking, such as abstract reasoning
▼ The *limbic system*, which is involved in regulating emotional behavior, memory, and learning
▼ The *basal ganglia*, some of which coordinate movement
▼ The *hypothalamus*, which regulates hormones throughout the body and behaviors such as eating, drinking, and sex
▼ The *locus ceruleus*, which manufactures norepinephrine, involved in the body's response to stress
▼ The *raphe nuclei*, made up of serotonin neurons, which regulate sleep and are involved with behavior and mood

▼ The *substantia nigra*, dopamine-producing cells involved in the control of complex movements, thinking, and emotional responses

A second clinical implication is related to the use of psychotropic medications. These can work, for example, by blocking the reuptake of neurotransmitters or by decreasing the metabolism of the neurotransmitters, thus allowing more of the neurotransmitter to remain in the synapse. However, unless an intervention, such as a medication, is specific for the subtype of the receptor involved in the psychiatric symptomatology, it may activate many other receptor subtypes unnecessarily. This lack of specificity of many of today's drugs is one of the causes of drug side effects. By understanding the biological processes underlying psychiatric symptoms, the psychiatric nurse is able to select and measure the effects of appropriate interventions, maximize positive effects, minimize unwanted effects, and measure and predict outcomes of psychiatric nursing care.

How would you respond to a nursing colleague who says that psychiatric nurses do not need to know much about anatomy and physiology, since what they do primarily is talk to people?

NEUROIMAGING TECHNIQUES

Until recently the only way to study the brain itself was through surgery or autopsy. Brain imaging techniques that have evolved over the past 20 years allow for direct viewing of the structure and function of the intact, living brain. These techniques not only help in diagnosing some brain disorders but also are important because they are able to map the regions of the brain and correlate them with function. They are, in fact, pictures of the working brain. Table 5-2 describes some of the imaging techniques used in brain research, and Color Plates 7 (p. 133) and 10 (p. 135) show a positron emission tomography (PET) scan of the normal brain.

Computed tomography (CT) and magnetic resonance imaging (MRI) permit visualization of *brain structures*. They can detect structural abnormalities, changes in the volume of brain tissue, and enlargement of the cerebral ventricles. The function and activity of the brain can be studied using other techniques to determine damage or malfunctioning in specific regions. The techniques that show *brain activity* include brain electrical activity mapping (BEAM), which measures sensory input, PET, and single photon emission computed tomography (SPECT), which permits the study of brain metabolism and cerebral blood flow. PET, SPECT, and the newer MRI techniques can measure the use of glucose and the amount

Table 5-1   Neurotransmitters and Neuromodulators in the Brain

AMINES

Amines are neurotransmitters that are synthesized from amino molecules such as tyrosine, tryptophan, and histidine. Found in various regions of the brain, amines affect learning, emotions, motor control, and other activities.

Substance	Location	Effect	Function
Monoamines			
Norepinephrine (NE)	Derived from tyrosine, a dietary amino acid. Located in the brainstem (particularly the locus ceruleus).	Can be excitatory or inhibitory	Levels fluctuate with sleep and wakefulness. Plays a role in changes in levels of attention and vigilance. Involved in attributing a rewarding value to a stimulus and in the regulation of mood. Plays a role in affective and anxiety disorders. Antidepressants block the reuptake of NE into the presynaptic cell or inhibit monoamine oxidase from metabolizing it.
Dopamine (DA)	Derived from tyrosine, a dietary amino acid. Located mostly in the brainstem (particularly the substantia nigra).	Generally excitatory	Involved in the control of complex movements, motivation, cognition, and regulating emotional responses. Many drugs of abuse (such as cocaine and amphetamines) cause DA release, suggesting a role in whatever makes things pleasurable. Involved in the movement disorders seen in Parkinson's disease and in many of the deficits seen in schizophrenia and other forms of psychosis. Antipsychotic drugs block dopamine receptors in the postsynaptic cell.
Serotonin (5-HT)	Derived from tryptophan, a dietary amino acid. Located only in the brain (particularly in the raphe nuclei of the brainstem).	Mostly inhibitory	Levels fluctuate with sleep and wakefulness, suggesting a role in arousal and modulation of the general activity levels of the CNS, particularly the onset of sleep. Plays a role in mood and probably in the delusions, hallucinations, and withdrawal of schizophrenia. Involved in temperature regulation and the pain-control system of the body. LSD (the hallucinogenic drug) acts at 5-HT receptor sites. Plays a role in affective and anxiety disorders. Antidepressants block its reuptake into the presynaptic cell.

of blood flowing in a region of the brain (regional cerebral blood flow). These are the two basic indicators of brain activity. Thus the more active a region is, the more blood will flow through it and the more glucose it will use.

When these techniques are coupled with neuropsychological test results, deficits in a person's performance, such as language or cognitive and sensory information processing, can be linked to the activity of the region of the brain responsible for those functions. The remainder of this chapter describes new developments in the understanding of brain structure and function re-

Table 5-1   Neurotransmitters and Neuromodulators in the Brain—cont'd

Substance	Location	Effect	Function
Acetylcholine	Synthesized from choline. Located in the brain and spinal cord but is more widespread in the peripheral nervous system, particularly the neuromuscular junction of skeletal muscle.	Can have an excitatory or inhibitory effect	Plays a role in the sleep-wakefulness cycle. Signals muscles to become active. Alzheimer's disease is associated with a decrease in acetylcholine-secreting neurons. Myasthenia gravis (weakness of skeletal muscles) results from a reduction in acetylcholine receptors.
Amino acids			
Glutamate	Found in all cells of the body where they are used to synthesize structural and functional proteins. Also found in the CNS where they are stored in synaptic vesicles and used as a neurotransmitter.	Excitatory	Overexposure to glutamate can be toxic to neurons and may play a role in brain damage caused by stroke and in some degenerative diseases such as Huntington's disease. Drugs that block glutamate (which are under development) might prevent seizures and neural degeneration from overexcitation.
Gamma-aminobutyric acid (GABA)	A glutamate derivative, most neurons of the CNS have receptors.	Major transmitter for post-synaptic inhibition on the CNS	Drugs that increase GABA function, such as the benzodiazepines, are used to treat anxiety and to induce sleep.

PEPTIDES

Peptides are chains of amino acids found throughout the body. About 50 have been identified to date, but their role as neurotransmitters is not well understood. Although they appear in very low concentrations in the CNS, they are very potent. They also appear to play a "second messenger" role in neurotransmission; that is, they modulate the messages of the nonpeptide neurotransmitters.

Substance	Location	Effect	Function
Endorphins and enkephalins	Widely distributed in the CNS	Generally inhibitory	Can reduce pain. The opiates morphine and heroin bind to endorphin and enkephalin receptors on presynaptic neurons, blocking the release of neurotransmitters and thus reducing pain.
Substance P	Spinal cord, brain, and sensory neurons associated with pain	Generally excitatory	Found in pain transmission pathway. Blocking the release of substance P by morphine reduces pain.

lated to psychiatric illness that have been gained from some of these technologies.

GENETICS OF MENTAL ILLNESS

The search for the gene or genes that cause mental illness has been difficult and inconclusive but has stimulated significant scientific, political, and clinical debate (see Critical Thinking about Contemporary Issues). The Human Genome Project, funded by the National Institute of Mental Health, is the largest research project in the history of biology. The only gene that has been linked to any mental illness causes the development of Alzheimer's disease in about 10% of the people with the disorder. Nonetheless, the search for the identification of genes responsible for mental illness has captured the attention and potential funding of the political, scientific, and lay communities.

Success in the past decade in finding the genes responsible for a variety of physical illnesses such as

Table 5-2 Brain Imaging Techniques

Technique	How it works	What it images	Advantages/disadvantages
Computed tomography (CT)	Series of x rays that is computer-constructed into "slices" of the brain that can be stacked by the computer, giving a three-dimensional view	Brain structure	Provides clearer pictures of the brain than x rays alone
Magnetic resonance imaging (MRI)	A magnetic field surrounding the head induces brain tissues to emit radio waves that are computerized for clear and detailed construction of sectional images of the brain	Brain structure (newer MRI techniques show brain activity)	Avoids the use of harmful radiation, although MRI can be adapted to use radioactive materials also
Brain electrical activity mapping (BEAM)	Uses computed tomographic techniques to display data derived from electroencephalographic (EEG) recordings of brain electrical activity that can be sensory-evoked by specific stimuli, such as a flash of light or a sudden sound, or cognitive-evoked by specific mental tasks	Brain activity/function	Reflects the cumulative activity of broad areas of the brain, usually near the surface, making it difficult to locate areas of possible pathological states
Positron emission tomography (PET)	An injected radioactive substance travels to the brain and shows up as a bright spot on the scan; different substances are taken up by the brain in different amounts depending on the type of tissue and the level of activity	Brain activity/function	Allows the injection of labeled drugs for the study of neurotransmitter receptor activity or concentration in the brain
Single photon emission computed tomography (SPECT)	Similar to PET but uses more stable substances and different detectors to visualize blood flow patterns	Brain activity/function	Useful in diagnosing cerebrovascular accidents and brain tumors

Huntington's disease, cystic fibrosis, Duchenne's muscular dystrophy, and retinoblastoma has led to the use of similar techniques to search for genetic links to mental illness. However, unlike these physical illnesses, psychiatric illnesses do not appear to be simple Mendelian traits. Specifically, several problems involving human genetic research have confused the process of genetic discoveries for mental illness.

First, ethical problems are associated with human breeding experiments, so scientists must infer information from animal studies. It is then difficult to generalize the interpretation of genetic behavioral links from animals to humans, thus making the interpretation of cognitive and emotional elements relatively impossible. Other factors that also make research on the inheritance of mental illness difficult include the following:
▼ The changeable nature of the psychiatric diagnostic classification system

▼ The fact that a gene that sometimes produces a psychiatric disorder may not always do so
▼ The notion that several different genes may be necessary to produce a disorder
▼ The presence of nongenetic factors that may contribute to the development of a disorder

Although the search for the genes of mental illness continues to hold promise, current information regarding the transmission of mental illness is primarily based on investigations into human inheritance. There are three types of studies in this area:
1. **Adoption studies,** which compare a trait among biological versus adoptive family members or other control groups
2. **Twin studies,** which compare how often identical twins, who are genetically identical, and fraternal twins, who have the genetic similarity of nontwin siblings, are similar, or concordant, for a trait

CRITICAL THINKING ABOUT CONTEMPORARY ISSUES

Are the Mentally Ill Particularly Vulnerable to Attempts at Genetic Engineering?

In Nazi Germany and in the United States during the earlier part of this century, people with mental disorders were among the first targets of society's attempt to minimize the transmission of deleterious genes by reducing or preventing reproduction by individuals who might be carrying such genes. People with psychiatric illness were subject to immigration restrictions, involuntary sterilization, and extermination. More sophisticated technology and increased knowledge of genetics lead to speculation concerning the susceptibility of the mentally ill to future attempts to control people's choice to reproduce. For example, state sterilization laws still stand, as does the 1927 Supreme Court ruling that sterilization is constitutional.

However, most people believe that eugenics, the science of selective breeding, is not a major concern at this time.[9] Furthermore, current understanding of the cause of psychiatric disorders suggests that they do not have a simple genetic base and that nongenetic factors also play an important role. This country's emphasis on human rights also makes eugenics unlikely. However, it is not difficult to envision how indirect pressure not to have children may be placed on individuals who seem to have a greater risk for mental illness and how society may label them as irresponsible or immoral for transmitting illnesses to their children. Given the direct and indirect financial costs of mental illnesses to society and the public stigma surrounding these disorders, future scientific advances may introduce this problem in the days ahead. ▼

4. **Family studies,** which compare whether a trait is more common among first-degree relatives, such as parents, siblings, and offspring, than it is among more distant relatives or control groups
The limitation of all of these studies, however, is that they cannot identify a defect of a specific gene.

At this time the clinical implications of genetic information regarding mental illness are not well defined; thus only limited information can be provided to patients and their families. The nurse is often in the position to answer questions about the genetics of mental illness, and this information must be conveyed with the highest respect for the patient's and family's autonomy. The nurse can objectively share the results of studies to date while reminding people that this information is preliminary. Referral to a genetic counselor should also be considered when the questions are persistent and complex.

 Do you think there is a gene responsible for alcohol dependency, aggressive behavior, or sexual preference? How would your belief affect the nursing care you give patients?

CIRCADIAN RHYTHMS

The recognition that human activities and behaviors such as sleeping, eating, body temperature, menses, and, at times, mood are cyclical and tend to be correlated with certain external environmental stimuli is not new. Recently, biological research has hypothesized that these body rhythms are governed by internal circadian pacemakers located in specific areas of the brain and that they are subject to change by specific external cues.

Circadian rhythm is like a network of internal clocks that time and coordinate events within the body according to an approximate 24-hour cycle (Fig. 5-2). This cycle corresponds to the time it takes the earth to spin on its axis, exposing all of life to daily rhythms of light, darkness, and temperature. In turn, these rhythms affect every aspect of health and well-being including life-style, sleep, moods, eating, drinking, fertility, and illness.

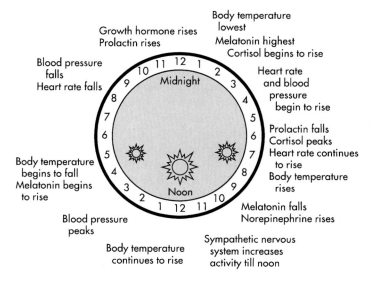

Fig. 5-2 The day within: a sample of the body's daily rhythms.

Because the body's fluids and tissues function according to circadian rhythms, physical and mental abilities and moods may vary widely from one time of day to another. To run according to the 24-hour clock, the circadian system must have a time cue from the external environment. That cue is usually sunlight, which sets the clock and synchronizes the body's complex set of rhythms.

Light enters the retina of the eye, which acts like an antenna of the brain. From the retina, electrical impulses in nerve cells transmit signals of light and dark through special pathways to the hypothalamus and to other regions of the brain (Fig. 5-3). Research suggests that one of the most important internal timekeepers is located in the hypothalamus. It consists of two clusters of nerve cells called the *suprachiasmatic nuclei* (SCN). A direct track leads from the retina to these two clusters of cells that in turn respond to the light signals from the retina.

The SCN is the pacemaker of circadian rhythm; it sends electrical and chemical messages to other tissues including the hypothalamus, the pituitary, pineal gland, and parts of the brainstem. These tissues send hormonal messages to other control systems in the body such as the heart, adrenal glands, liver, kidney, and intestines, keeping them regulated to the internal clock and modulating thoughts, moods, and activities.

Sleep

According to surveys, most people sleep 6 to 9 hours a night, with 8 to 9 hours reported most often. Few people sleep less than 5 or more than 10 hours. Usually people sleep in one nightly phase, although in some cultures and during some times of life a siesta, or afternoon nap, is common. Studies show that the sleep cycle is related to the timing of circadian rhythms, light and darkness, and temperature changes.

Generally, each night an individual's sleep passes through a repeated sequence of five stages. The first stage is that of "falling asleep," which is called *stage one sleep*. A person then progresses into sleep itself (stage two), followed by deep sleep, also called *delta sleep* (stages three and four). After a brief return to stage two sleep the person moves into stage five, or rapid eye movement (REM) sleep. Stages two through REM repeat themselves several times a night with deep sleep becoming briefer in the course of a night and REM sleep becoming progressively longer.

REM sleep occupies approximately 20% to 25% of the sleep time of adults; stage two about 50%; and stages three and four about 15%. Stages three and four occur primarily in the first half of the sleep period. The lighter stages of sleep and longer REM periods typically occur in the second half. Usually during REM sleep the indi-

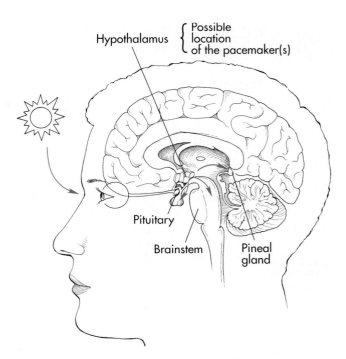

Fig. 5-3 From the sun to the brain.

vidual has vivid dreams, and the eyes show bursts of rapid movement beneath the closed lids. Studies show that REM sleep is excessive in depressed people and that dreams may be unusually intense.

PSYCHOIMMUNOLOGY

Evidence from a wide variety of sources in recent years suggests that psychosocial factors can have an important effect on a person's immune system at any point in time. In particular, psychosocial stressors and the mental state associated with them may depress immune function to the point of enhancing vulnerability to virtually any antigen to which an individual is exposed. It is also clear that the central nervous system would somehow be involved in mediating any such effects.

Psychoimmunology is a relatively new field that explores the psychological influences on the nervous system's control of immune responsiveness. Several diseases commonly encountered by neurologists are thought to have an autoimmune basis. This research has demonstrated the suppression of white blood cell reproduction following sleep deprivation, marathon running, space flight, death of a spouse, and during the course of depression. Another example is that of natural killer cells, which are believed to play a role in tumor surveillance and the control of viral infections.

Identifying a possible role for autoimmunity in the major psychiatric diseases has proven to be more problematic. Narcolepsy, a disease of the central nervous system characterized by excessive daytime drowsiness, appears to be closely linked to the immune system and may offer insights into mechanisms that could apply to some psychiatric disorders.

The evidence is compelling, however, that psychosocial stressors temporarily impair the immune response and thus contribute to the development of a variety of illnesses. Although efforts to relate specific stressors to specific diseases have not generally been successful, stress is recognized as a key to understanding the development and course of many illnesses. Presuming that all people have at least one vulnerable organ in their bodies, a high level of stress may eventually put an individual at risk for the breakdown of that organ and the development of clinical symptoms.

BIOLOGICAL ASSESSMENT OF THE PATIENT

Several steps are necessary in the assessment of psychiatric patients from a biological perspective. Brain disorders can be physical or psychiatric and can include many different diagnoses such as stroke, head and spinal cord injury, tumors, multiple sclerosis, alcoholism, and drug addiction. Schizophrenia, depression, anxiety disorders, and Alzheimer's disease are also considered brain disorders, although they are psychiatric in nature. As new understanding has been gained about mind-body connections, it has become clear that symptoms expressed by patients can more precisely be assigned to problems in specific organ systems, including the brain. Thus the ability to screen for undiagnosed physical disorders and distinguish them from psychiatric disorders has important implications for the psychiatric nurse in the approach to assessment of the presenting symptomatology, treatment selection, and the possible need for referral.

Undiagnosed physical illness, particularly organic brain disorders, can be costly and dangerous if treated incorrectly. For example, it has been estimated that 7% of patients seeking psychiatric help have a physical illness that directly causes psychiatric symptoms and that another 30% have a physical illness that contributes to psychiatric symptomatology.[13] Another study reported that more than 42% of the severely mentally ill have at least one chronic physical problem that limits their functioning.[18] In addition, patients who are psychiatrically ill often have limited access to general health-care services because of barriers of availability and associated stigmatization.

These facts make a compelling case for psychiatric nurses to include a thorough biological assessment in their evaluation of psychiatric patients. The psychiatric nurse is well suited to screen for the major signs of physical or organic disorders that may complicate a patient's psychiatric status, to identify physical illnesses that may have been overlooked, or to refer the patient for a thorough medical diagnostic work-up if indicated. In fact, this is one of the unique areas of expertise that the psychiatric nurse brings to the mental health treatment team, and it is essential that psychiatric nurses continue to demonstrate their competence in all aspects of their biopsychosocial assessment.

A complete health-care history of the patient, lifestyle review, physical examination, analysis of laboratory values, and discussion of presenting symptoms and coping responses are essential elements of a baseline biological assessment (Box 5-2). The nurse should be able to perform a basic physical examination to assess for gross abnormalities and be able to interpret the results of existing, more complex physical examinations. Appearance, gait, coordination, bilateral strength, tremors and tics, speech, and symptoms such as headaches, blurred vision, dizziness, vomiting, motor weakness, disorientation, confusion, and memory problems should be assessed in detail.

Obtaining permission from the patient to access other persons and documents that will help the nurse and health-care team gain a thorough view of the patient is an important step in the screening process. Particularly when brain disorders, whether physical or psychiatric, are suspected, the nurse should pay close attention to inconsistencies in the patient's account, between those of other persons, and in previous health care records. Throughout the course of the screening the nurse should be alert for any indications of head trauma at any time in the patient's life, such as through accidents, fevers, surgery, or seizures.

Only after a patient has been carefully screened can the nurse determine which of the patient's presenting problems are amenable to psychiatric intervention and which problems may need the attention of a consultant in another specialty. The identified problems that are appropriate for psychiatric intervention then become the target symptoms of specific interventions, and progress toward expected outcomes can be measured throughout the course of treatment.

Why is a history of psychiatric medications taken by a patient's first-degree relatives an important part of the psychiatric nurse's biological assessment?

BIOLOGICAL COMPONENTS OF MENTAL ILLNESS

The knowledge base related to the biology of mental illness is rapidly expanding. At this time, however, the

Box 5-2

BIOLOGICAL ASSESSMENT OF THE PSYCHIATRIC PATIENT

HEALTH CARE HISTORY

General health care
  Regular health-care provider
  Frequency of health-care visits
  Last medical examination and test results
  Any unusual circumstances of birth, including mother's
    preterm habits and condition

Hospitalizations and surgeries
  When
  Why indicated
  Treatments
  Outcome

Brain impairment
  Diagnosed brain problem
  Head trauma
  Details of any accidents or periods of unconsciousness
    for any reason—blows to the head, electrical shocks,
    high fevers, seizures, fainting, dizziness, headaches,
    falls

Cancer
  Full history, particularly consider metastases (lung,
    breast, melanoma, gastrointestinal tract, and kidney
    are most likely to metastasize)
  Results of treatments (chemotherapy and surgeries)

Lung problems
  Details of any condition or event that restricts the flow
    of air to the lungs for more than 2 minutes or ad-
    versely affects oxygen absorption (the brain uses
    20% of the oxygen in the body) such as with chronic
    obstructive pulmonary disease, near drowning, near
    strangulation, high altitude oxygen deprivation, re-
    suscitation events

Cardiac problems
  Childhood illnesses such as scarlet or rheumatic fever
  History of heart attacks, strokes, or hypertension

Blood diseases
  Anemia resulting in hypoxia
  Arteriosclerotic conditions
  HIV

Diabetes
  Stability of glucose levels

Endocrine disturbances
  Thyroid and adrenal function particularly

LIFE-STYLE

Eating
  Details of unusual or unsupervised diets, appetite,
    weight changes, cravings, and caffeine intake

Medications
  Full history of current and past psychiatric medications
    in self and first-degree relatives

Substance use
  Alcohol and drug use

Toxins
  Overcome by automobile exhaust or natural gas
  Exposure to lead, mercury, insecticides, herbicides, sol-
    vents, cleaning agents, lawn chemicals

Occupation (current and past)
  Chemicals in the workplace (farming, painting)
  Work-related accidents (construction, mining)
  Military experiences

Injury
  Safe sex practices
  Contact sports and sports-related injuries
  Exposure to violence or abuse

PHYSICAL EXAMINATION

Current health statistics
  Immunizations
  Allergies
  Last physical examination

Review of physiological systems
  Integumentary—skin, nails, hair, and scalp
  Head—eyes, ears, nose, mouth, throat, and neck
  Breast
  Respiratory
  Cardiovascular
  Hematolymphatic
  Gastrointestinal tract
  Urinary tract
  Genital
  Neurological
  Musculoskeletal
  Nutritive
  Restorative—sleep and rest
  Endocrine
  Allergic and immunological

LABORATORY VALUES

Blood, plasma, and serum
Urine
Steroid hormones
Polypeptide hormones
Thyroid hormones
Hematology
Cerebrospinal fluid

PRESENTING SYMPTOMS AND COPING RESPONSES

Description—nature, frequency, and intensity
Threats to safety of self or others
Functional status
Quality of life

amount of biological information about each psychiatric disorder varies considerably. In addition, what is known about the biology of the various mental illnesses is often incomplete, contradictory, and inconclusive. It is much like finding pieces of a jigsaw puzzle scattered throughout the house; while each piece by itself suggests a glimpse of the overall design, the full picture does not emerge until all the pieces are located and then put together to form an integrated whole.

In this section of the chapter four major psychiatric disorders are discussed in the context of neurobiological research. These illnesses were selected because of the amount of biological information available about them. Given the incomplete state of the science, the discussion will walk the reader through current areas of biological study related to these disorders and highlight their implications for clinical psychiatric nursing practice. The technologies described are also used in research of many other mental illnesses not focused on in this chapter.

The intention of this discussion is to expose the reader to emerging knowledge in the field and to provide a model that would allow the psychiatric nurse to keep abreast with the biological context of psychiatric nursing care. The psychiatric nurse should become familiar with these research findings and discuss these issues with patients, families, and colleagues. In addition, an overview of biological knowledge related to each of the various psychiatric disorders can be found in the chapters of Unit Three of this text (Chapters 14 to 24).

Schizophrenia

Neuroscientific research continues to make advances in the study of schizophrenia, although the complexity of this disorder and the range of symptoms have made progress slow and research directions unclear at times. The cause of schizophrenia is unknown, but it is widely believed that at least one biological cause exists. It also appears that schizophrenia is not one but several distinct disorders (see Chapter 19).

Genetics. There is a 1% lifetime risk of schizophrenia in the general population, unless an individual has a first- or second-degree relative with the disorder. It appears that schizophrenia is shaped by heredity (Table 5-3), although symptoms vary greatly within families. Although the gene for schizophrenia has not yet been identified, the biological transmission is established at approximately 80%. Thus schizophrenia is probably caused by or influenced by a genetic disorder, perhaps of brain development. Obviously, other unidentified factors are related to schizophrenia, since identical twins

Table 5-3 Genetic Risk of Schizophrenia

Monozygotic twin affected	50%
Dizygotic twin affected	15%
Sibling affected	10%
One parent affected	15%
Both parents affected	35%
Second-degree relative affected	2% to 3%
No affected relative	1%

with identical genes still only share a 50% concordance rate for the disease.

Biochemistry. Several brain chemicals have been implicated in schizophrenia, but research to date points most strongly to the following:

▼ An excess of the neurotransmitter, dopamine
▼ An imbalance between dopamine and other neurotransmitters
▼ Problems in the dopamine receptor systems

Several research strategies support the dopamine hypothesis.[14] For instance, drugs that increase levels of dopamine in the brain can produce psychosis.[21] These include the following:

▼ Amphetamines, which inhibit the reuptake of dopamine by the presynaptic membrane thereby increasing available dopamine in the synapse
▼ L-dopa, which increases the synthesis of dopamine thereby increasing the amount of dopamine produced
▼ Cocaine, which stimulates the release of dopamine at the presynaptic membrane thereby increasing dopamine in the synapse

Drugs that reduce dopamine function have antipsychotic effects as well. This is seen in the antipsychotic drugs that reduce the number of postsynaptic receptors that interact with dopamine.

Some studies have also shown an increase in the dopamine metabolites homovanillic acid (HVA) and vannilylmandelic acid (VMA) and the norepinephrine metabolite 3-methoxy-4-hydroxyphenylglycol (MHPG) in the plasma of untreated schizophrenic patients as compared with normal controls. This implies increased levels of these transmitters in the brain. When patients are treated with haloperidol, an antipsychotic drug, the levels of these transmitters decrease.[6] When patients are treated with clozapine, an atypical antipsychotic drug, an imbalance between the dopamine and serotonin systems occurs.[20] Although these strategies have not always yielded consistent results across studies, they do suggest that there is an increase of available dopamine in schizophrenics and that other neurotransmitter systems may be implicated, but the specific actions of these neurotransmitter balances remain unknown.

Brain Imaging. Various imaging techniques used in the study of schizophrenia focus on two specific areas of the brain:

1. The frontal cortex, which appears to be involved in the negative symptoms
2. The limbic system, which appears to be involved in the positive symptoms of schizophrenia

Although a consistent group of abnormalities seems evident in the brains of schizophrenics, exactly how these and other brain regions interact in the course of schizophrenia still is not understood. Imaging studies may continue to clarify this process and link abnormal brain structure and function with etiology, symptoms, and treatment of schizophrenia (see Color Plates 8 to 10 on pp. 134 and 135).

For instance, CT scans have demonstrated enlargement of the ventricles, particularly the lateral ventricle, of patients with chronic schizophrenia. This implies either a lack of brain development or a loss of brain tissue. MRI studies have replicated this finding and have also documented that several brain structures are smaller, such as the hippocampal region (which modulates emotional response and memory) in the limbic system in the temporal lobe of the cerebrum. Although a clear correlation with these findings and clinical symptoms has yet to emerge, there is a trend for large ventricles to be associated with two indicators of poor prognosis—early age of onset and poor premorbid functioning.

For the first time, PET studies have shown functional abnormalities in the brain by documenting activity in various regions of the brain of individuals who are given psychological tests. For example, the Wisconsin Card Sort Test (a test of working memory and abstract thinking) has been found to activate the cerebral blood flow in the prefrontal cortex in the brains of normal controls and in the nonaffected identical twins of schizophrenics.[30] Yet, this same region of the brain shows lower metabolism and reduced blood flow (hypofrontality) in schizophrenics who do worse on this test than normal controls regardless of the length of time they have been ill or whether or not they have been treated with antipsychotic drugs.

Viral Pandemics and Season of Birth. Although research in psychoimmunology related to schizophrenia has been difficult to conduct and interpret, some interesting data may be emerging. There is an excess of births of schizophrenics (approximately 5%) in Europe and the United States in the late winter and early spring months, and peaks of excess births can be correlated with pandemic viral outbreaks, particularly influenza, that occur during the third to sixth months of gestation. Although this information is inconclusive and is thought to account for a very small percentage of those with the disease, it is helpful in expanding information about the influences of biological and environmental factors on brain development and function.

Birth Events. Many attempts have been made to study the influences of maternal nutrition, infection, placental insufficiency, anoxia, hemorrhage, and trauma before or at birth as possible causes of schizophrenia. Much of this research is limited by its retrospective nature, since retrieving information about a complex event decades after its occurrence is very difficult. The best studies to date seem to indicate that it is unlikely that these events lead to any significant etiological basis of schizophrenia.

Clinical Implications: Biology of Schizophrenia. **Advances in molecular and cellular neurobiology have enabled science to capitalize on a variety of what were originally chance findings. In the early 1950s chlorpromazine was observed to have an antipsychotic effect. Today's technologies show that this effect is due to dopamine receptor blockade throughout the brain, accounting for the antipsychotic and side effect profiles of the typical antipsychotic drugs. These new technologies have also produced clozapine and risperidone, which specifically block the dopamine receptor implicated in schizophrenia (D2). They also act on other neurotransmitter systems. For these reasons, these two drugs avoid some of the usual antipsychotic side effects (see Chapter 25). This research direction holds the future promise of discovering drugs that are more and more specific in their actions, thus enhancing efficacy while eliminating troublesome and sometimes dangerous side effects.**

In the future, brain imaging technologies may direct the clinician to the most appropriate interventions (see Chapter 19), based on the area of the brain specifically involved in each patient's symptomatology. This approach could provide targeted treatment that eliminates the additional costs and adverse effects of strategies that may not be the first line of choice for a patient's particular symptom cluster.

What would you say to a man and woman who were debating about whether to have children because they both had relatives with schizophrenia?

Mood Disorders

Biological understanding of mood disorders has advanced in the past decade. Neuroscientific research has identified biological markers for mood disorders, and psychopharmacological interventions have yielded more specificity and fewer side effects and toxicities than the first-generation antidepressants of 40 years ago.

Genetics. As in schizophrenia, mood disorders run in families and tend to be inherited. The lifetime risk for mood disorders in the general population is 6%. Family, twin, and adoption studies have documented that the lifetime risk for relatives of people with depression is 20% and 24% for relatives of people with mania. A person with an identical twin with an affective disorder is at highest risk. No clear pattern of genetic mapping for these disorders has been found to date, but preliminary work points to a complex picture of genetic markers. Thus it is unlikely that a single gene causes mood disorders.

Biochemistry. Initially it was discovered that drugs like the tricyclics and monoamine oxidase inhibitors had antidepressant effects, stimulated a manic episode in individuals at risk, and prolonged the activity of norepinephrine (NE). NE is a member of the catecholamine family within the monoamine class of neurotransmitters. These findings led to the catecholamine hypothesis—that depression was caused by a shortage of NE, whereas mania was caused by an excess of NE.

Current theories of abnormal chemistry in unipolar and bipolar illness have moved beyond the original catecholamine hypothesis to more complex explanations of the biochemistry of mood disorders. More recently, biochemical studies of NE in mood disorders have shown conflicting results. Another factor that fails to support the catecholamine hypothesis is the lag time between the administration of antidepressants and their clinical effect. These drugs cause immediate increases in NE levels at the synapse, but patients must wait several weeks to obtain an antidepressant response. Thus the true mechanism of action of the antidepressants must involve additional actions not yet understood.

One current NE hypothesis focuses on a possible overactivity of the NE autoreceptor. Autoreceptors act as the neuron's own feedback system and inform the neuron when enough neurotransmitter has been released into the synapse. This theory proposes that instead of regulating the normal release of NE in the synapse, an overactive autoreceptor inhibits normal amounts of NE from entering the synapse. Since the antidepressant drugs also affect NE receptor cells after several weeks of ingestion, this might explain the lag time for clinical efficacy—it takes longer to change NE receptors than it does to increase NE in the synapse. An alternative explanation is that perhaps the antidepressant effect of these drugs is caused by an upregulation or increase of the NE receptor cells of the postsynaptic membrane, thus allowing more NE to be received.

Several findings support the hypothesis that other neurotransmitters are involved in mood disorders. For example, some studies have found that concentrations of serotonin are low in mood disorders, and low concentrations of serotonin have been found in people who commit suicide. In addition, the new class of antidepressants, the SSRIs (selective serotonin reuptake inhibitors), act almost exclusively on the serotonin system, supporting a role for serotonin in mood disorders. Acetylcholine has also been implicated in mood disorders. On the basis of drug effects, some investigators have proposed that too little acetylcholine can cause depression, and too much NE can cause mania, suggesting an imbalance between these two systems as the biological etiology of the mood disorders. Finally, gamma-aminobutyric acid (GABA), an inhibitory neurotransmitter, has a broad range of effects, and it has been proposed that it modulates the other neurotransmitter systems. This is supported by the paradoxical finding that increased GABA activity can have both an antidepressant and an antimanic effect. Thus GABA may play an important role in mood disorders as well.

Because of the inconsistent findings to date, one of the most popular current biological hypotheses for the development of mood disorders is the dysregulation hypothesis. This theory proposes a more generalized dysfunction in the overall mechanisms that regulate the activities of neurotransmission at the synapse and suggests that clinically effective drugs restore more efficient regulation. Additional support for this theory comes from the fact that the implicated neurotransmitter systems have been shown to interact with each other, and the activity of one affects and modulates the activities of the others. Based on available data it has been proposed that decreased activity within the NE-serotonin component of the system is associated with depression, and increased activity of the NE-dopamine component tends to cause mania.[11]

The evolution of biological hypotheses of mood disorders continues to stimulate much research, heated debate, and conflicting theories. This confusion seems particularly interesting, given that the pharmacological and somatic treatments of mood disorders have been some of the most effective in the mental health field to date.

If depression is partly due to disturbed biochemistry, does that mean that counseling and psychotherapy are inappropriate treatment strategies?

Brain Imaging. Imaging research into mood disorders has been largely inconclusive because various studies report contradictory results. This is primarily a result of a lack of standardization of research methodologies between investigators and difficulty in studying fluctuating illnesses. Generally, CT and MRI studies found larger ventricles in patients with affective disorders when compared with controls, particularly in the temporal horn in the right cerebral hemisphere, and reductions in cortical mass. However, the clinical significance of this remains obscure other than for screening for the presence of specific physical illnesses, such as tumors, manifesting as psychiatric illness.[25] One advantage to the use of MRI in affective disorders, however, is that MRI, unlike other scanning techniques, is without radiation risks, and thus multiple repeat scans of the same patient can be performed. This is of particular research importance as MRIs are repeated when the patient shifts mood, starts or stops treatment, or relapses.[12]

PET studies have demonstrated that depressive and manic patients show different metabolism rates and different patterns of cerebral activity as compared with normal controls. In depressed patients, investigators found hypometabolism in the prefrontal cortex of the frontal lobes in scans of glucose utilization that improved after treatment with antidepressant medication[2] (see Color Plate 11 on p. 135). Persons with bipolar disorder show a more general decrease in activity involving the whole cortex and the left frontal lobes, although the clinical significance of this finding is also uncertain.

In general, the studies to date suggest an association between mood disorders and abnormalities of large regions of the brain, especially the frontal and temporal lobes. An abnormal difference between the left (language and logical thinking) and right (spatial processing) hemispheres is also implied. Although these functions are different, they also overlap and exhibit different levels of activity that appear altered in mood disorders. Also, imaging studies have not been well correlated to date with neuropsychiatric testing, and results of the two techniques conflict, suggesting that diverse abnormalities are detected by different methodologies. Future methodologies promise to increase the use of imaging techniques as clinical and research tools for understanding affective disorders.

Seasonality and Circadian Rhythms. A variety of studies have linked seasonal variations, such as decreases in the length of daylight hours and wintertime decreases in available sunlight, to such human conditions as mood, sleeping, eating, and energy levels. Seasonal affective disorder (SAD) in particular has been shown to respond to geographical location closer to the equator or to phototherapy (light therapy), although rigorous placebo-controlled research documenting long-term efficacy has not been conducted at this time (see Chapter 26).[16]

The cause of SAD is not fully understood. It is proposed, however, that the neurotransmitter melatonin (a further synthesis of serotonin secreted by the pineal gland) is secreted with darkness and suppressed with bright light. It is further believed that melatonin regulates hypothalamic hormones involved in the generation of circadian rhythms and the synchronization of such rhythms to variations in environmental light in animals.[3] It is not yet clear, however, what role melatonin plays in humans or the effects of changes in melatonin levels on circadian rhythms.

What does appear to be clear is that the sleep cycle is linked to the timing of human circadian rhythms and to malfunctions in the brain's ability to follow environmental cues such as light and darkness, unusual environmental situations such as long, dark winters in northern latitudes, or disturbances in the intensity of the circadian rhythm such as those caused by sleep problems, body temperature changes, mood cycling, and cortisol and thyrotropin abnormalities. Thus the psychiatric nurse should be on the forefront of this research, since many patients with psychiatric symptoms suffer from disturbances of biological rhythms.[19]

Biological Markers. Perhaps more than in any other psychiatric diagnostic category, investigators have identified biological markers of clinical usefulness in the diagnosis and treatment of mood disorders. Research has identified certain biological markers in depression that are mediated by the hypothalamic-pituitary-adrenal (HPA) axis.[27] For example, in depressed patients sleep electroencephalographs (EEGs) are abnormal, with shortened REM latency experienced by 90% of depressed patients. Normally upon falling asleep the fifth stage of sleep—REM or dream sleep—occurs in 60 to 90 minutes. In depressed patients, it occurs in 5 to 30 minutes, thus indicating that there is sleep dysregulation in depression. As a consequence, depressed patients spend less time in the more refreshing slow wave stages of sleep, particularly stages three and four, and more time in REM sleep. This finding may explain why depressed patients complain of feeling tired and unrefreshed after a night's sleep.

Another biological marker is that plasma concentrations of the adrenal hormone, cortisol, are abnormally high in some depressed patients, and 60% of patients have abnormal results with the dexamethasone suppression test (DST). In normal controls cortisol levels are relatively flat from late afternoon until 3 or 4 AM, when they begin to increase and spike at regular intervals until about noon; then they gradually begin to level out again. In contrast, biologically depressed people have been shown to have erratic cortisol spikes over a 24-hour period.

The DST involves giving a small dose (1 mg) of the synthetic steroid dexamethasone. In normal people this is enough to turn down the pituitary production of adrenocorticotropic hormone (ACTH), thus blunting the adrenal production of cortisol for 24 hours. When plasma cortisol levels are drawn at intervals the next day (usually at 8 AM and 4 PM) in depressed people, they "escape" the cortisol suppression, and cortisol levels are high again, an indication of a dysregulation of the HPA axis in depression (see Fig. 5-4). The clinical implications of this marker for depression must be assessed cautiously, since this technology is not always accurate, but an abnormal DST appears to be a marker for biological depression. As such, positive DST results would support the use of antidepressant medications as a treatment strategy, although negative findings do not necessarily support withholding medication, especially in severe to moderate depression. Finally, a DST retest for a patient at a later time that indicates normal results might be a useful indicator that the biological depression has been corrected.

Finally, two other promising biological markers also deserve mention. The thyroid-stimulating hormone (TSH) response to a thyroid-releasing hormone (TRH) stimulation test is blunted in about 40% of patients with depression, and the growth hormone response to drugs that enhance the norepinephrine system, such as clonidine, is significantly blunted in depressed patients. These and other biological markers continue to stimulate interest from a research perspective and promise

to gain in their usefulness in clinical settings as the techniques are improved and their treatment implications are more fully understood.

> What are the implications of being able to identify biological markers for the diagnosis and treatment of depression?

Kindling. Animal studies of electrical or chemical kindling and behavioral sensitization may provide clues to the recurrence of mood disorders with increased frequency and intensity over time in some individuals. When an animal's brain is repeatedly stimulated by low-level electrical impulses or low-dose chemicals like cocaine, the result is an increased responsiveness to stable low doses of the stimulation over time, resulting eventually in seizures. Ultimately the animal becomes so sensitive that seizures occur spontaneously in the absence of the stimulation. This phenomenon is known as **kindling.** It is theorized that kindling underlies the addictive disorders and the cycling and recurrent psychiatric disorders, such as recurrent depression.

According to this theory, early episodes of an illness require precipitating events, but later episodes may occur spontaneously, and repeated exposure to precipitating events may lead to more frequent occurrence of episodes. This sequence is related to the idea that early episodes of mania and depression in humans may be precipitated by psychosocial stresses in vulnerable individuals, but later episodes can occur in the absence of any apparent external stimulus. Episodes may also occur with greater frequency and intensity over time.[22]

Additional evidence of a role for kindling in mood disorders is that the neurotransmitters most implicated in the mood disorders (NE, serotonin, and GABA) inhibit kindling. Also, lithium, an effective treatment for bipolar disorder, blocks behavioral sensitization, and carbamazepine, an anticonvulsant effective in the treatment of bipolar disorder, blocks kindling.[11] Thus the effect of the environment on a vulnerable brain is the focus of continued research interest.

Birth-Cohort Effects. Rates of depression, mania, and suicide over the past several generations have increased in the United States, Canada, and several European countries. These rates continue to rise as each new birth-cohort ages, even within the general population. Within the at-risk population, the relatives of depressed and manic patients from previous de-

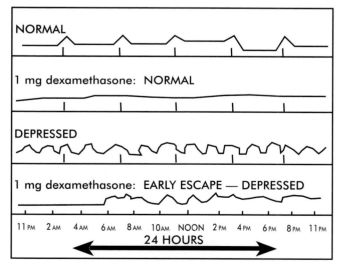

Fig. 5-4 Dexamethasone suppression test and cortisol levels.

cades are at even greater risk for these illnesses than were the siblings of their affected parents, showing a trend in increased genetic susceptibility in the at-risk population.

Another alarming trend noted in North America and Europe over the past 6 decades is the increase in birth-cohort suicide rates. Suicide rates among 15- to 19-year-olds were 10 times higher for those born in the 1950s than they were for those born in the 1930s. These epidemiological trends point to a yet unidentified interaction between genes and environment that continues to worsen over the decades.[10]

Birth-cohort studies such as these continue to generate much interest in psychiatric and epidemiological arenas and can have very important public health implications. They also serve to underscore the important point that the biological understanding of psychiatric illnesses cannot stand alone as the entire explanation of etiology. Rather, it underscores the need for integrated biopsychosocial models and multidimensional treatment strategies. Thus psychiatric nurses must continue to view the person in the context of the environment as well as biologically to understand and treat the individual holistically.

 What environmental factors might play a role along with genetics in the increased rate of suicide among adolescents in this country?

Clinical Implications: Biology of Depression.
There are many different pieces to the puzzle of the biology of mood disorders, and an all-inclusive hypothesis has not yet emerged. It is likely, however, that mood disorders occur because integrated control systems are disrupted, as evidenced by the suggestion of an overall dysregulation in neurotransmitter systems and by the fact that the brain mechanisms that control biological rhythms are implicated in mood disorders. What is clear is that the etiologies are diverse, and thus the treatments need to be both diverse and specific to the biopsychosocial context of the individual patient (see Chapter 17).

New information will provide clinicians with more specific drug treatments, again decreasing the cost, time, and adverse effects of treatments that may not be as effective as others for an individual patient. Markers such as the DST may also be able to tell the clinician and the patient when abnormal biology has normalized, thus providing more specific information about when treatments can be stopped. Phototherapy may hold promise for those with seasonal affective disorder, and sleep deprivation therapy may produce an antidepressant effect by

manipulating an individual's sleep cycle (see Chapter 26).

Panic Disorder

The biological study of anxiety has made significant advances in the past decade, resulting in many important findings that have helped in the understanding and treatment of this important and universal human experience. In panic disorder, in which the human alarm system seems to be triggered independently from appropriate appraisals of environmental cues, the results of neuroscientific exploration have been impressive. They are also a significant departure from earlier theories that have primarily emphasized psychodynamic causes for the anxiety disorders.

Genetics. Panic disorder, like schizophrenia and mood disorders, appears to have a genetic component, although there are less research data to support this.[24] While several family and twin studies have been conducted, adoption studies have yet to be completed. More studies are necessary to further document the genetic risk factors for anxiety disorders.

The few family studies conducted have found three to four times higher rates of panic disorder among first-degree relatives of people with these disorders as compared with control populations and to the relatives of people with other psychiatric disorders. In addition, these studies distinguish between panic disorder and the other anxiety disorders, suggesting separate mechanisms for the inheritance of each type of anxiety disorder. In families of individuals with both panic disorder and depression, first-degree relatives are at increased risk for panic disorder, depression, and other conditions. The few twin studies that have been conducted show that panic attacks, if not panic disorder, tend to have a genetic component. One early twin study remains the classic in this field and reports a significantly higher concordance for panic disorder in monozygotic versus dizygotic twins, although monozygotic twin concordance was only 31% as compared with 25% in first-degree relatives.[29] Thus genetic factors do not appear to be the only determinant of this disorder.

Biochemistry. Although it is unlikely that any one neurotransmitter system is solely responsible for panic anxiety, and research suggests a role for multiple brain neurochemical systems, the majority of studies to date strongly point to a dysfunction in norepinephrine regulation and transmission in the development of human anxiety disorders. Panic disorder is thought to be an overactivity of the noradrenergic system in the brain that mediates the fight-or-flight response, principally the locus ceruleus, which manufactures most of the brain norepinephrine and is thought to control an active response to anxiety-provoking stimuli. Neural tracks project from the locus ceruleus to other areas of the brain involved in anxiety, such as the amygdala and hippocampus in the limbic system and the cerebral cortex. The locus ceruleus may also play a critical role in responsiveness to changes in the internal and external environment. Also, various receptor systems within the noradrenergic system have been hypothesized to function abnormally.

Medications that decrease the activity of the locus ceruleus (noradrenergic antidepressant agents such as the tricyclics) effectively treat panic disorder. The hypothesis suggested by this is that panic attacks are caused by an inappropriate activation of the norepinephrine system in the locus ceruleus. Neuroanatomical, neurochemical, neurophysiological, and behavioral studies of the norepinephrine system provide a basis for relating increased activity of this system to the expression of anxiety and fear and to the somatic symptoms and cardiovascular changes that accompany severe anxiety states.[5]

There is sufficient research and treatment evidence to mention several other systems implicated in panic disorder. The GABA system is another area of research interest in panic disorder, since the benzodiazepines are some of the most effective antianxiety drugs and in high doses are effective in treating panic disorder. Benzodiazepines exert their antianxiety effects by increasing the action of the inhibitory neurotransmitter, GABA, thus turning off overly active brain cells. Although GABA receptors are located all over the brain, the areas of the brain where GABA receptors are coupled to benzodiazepine receptors include the hippocampus and the amygdala, both limbic system structures that function as the center of emotions such as rage, arousal, and fear. It is proposed that patients with panic disorder may have a decreased antianxiety ability of the benzodiazepine receptors in areas of the limbic system, making them more sensitive to anxiety-producing biological effects.

Serotonin and adenosine have also stimulated research interest in the past several years. For example, it has been proposed that transmission of serotonin in the midbrain may play a role in the etiology of panic attacks, and panic patients may have hypersensitive serotonin receptors. This etiology is supported by the fact that drugs that potentiate the regulation of serotonin (the SSRIs) suppress panic attacks. Clinically, it has also been documented that many people with panic disorder have noticed the panic effects of caffeine and have limited their ingestion of coffee and chocolate on their own. Although caffeine has some effects on a variety of neurotransmitter systems, its principal action in the brain is to block the receptors for the inhibitory neurotransmitter, adenosine. The role of this transmitter in panic disorder is unclear, however, and more research

is needed to define the interaction of all of these biochemical systems in panic disorder.

Brain Imaging. There have been several interesting findings using imaging technologies to study panic disorder (Fig. 5-5). CT and MRI scans consistently provide evidence of brain atrophy or underdevelopment, particularly in the frontal and temporal lobes of people with panic disorder, although the clinical significance of these findings is not yet clear.

Brain activity is also abnormal in panic patients. Under normal conditions, cerebral function leads to an increase in metabolic demand, resulting in an increase in cerebral blood flow. Cerebral blood flow studies using PET scans show that, at rest, panic disorder patients who have panic attacks during lactate infusions have increased cerebral blood flow to the parahippocampal gyrus, an area of the cerebral cortex that is associated with the limbic system. Normal controls and panic disorder patients who were not sensitive to lactate did not show this, suggesting a role for lactate sensitivity as a marker for certain types of panic disorder. Based on these preliminary data, it has been suggested that a parahippocampal abnormality is involved in a predisposition to panic disorder and that activation of a norepinephrine pathway to the parahippocampal gyrus initiates an attack.[23]

The brainstem reticular formation, with its widespread ascending and descending pathways and functionally specialized groups of neurons, is also associated with the mediation of arousal. Arousal refers to levels of generalized, diffuse activation of the brain and is associated with levels of consciousness and the sleep-wake cycle in humans. Correlations between blood flow to the brainstem and cerebellar regions and various states of arousal have been demonstrated. Reticular neurons effect activity in the regulation of norepinephrine and serotonin.[31] Thus while still preliminary this

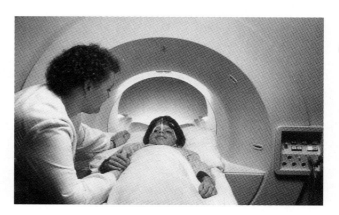

Fig. 5-5 Nurse preparing a patient for brain scanning.
Courtesy Division of Psychiatric Nursing, Medical University of South Carolina.

line of research promises to further explain the impact of levels of brain arousal on anxiety states.

The imaging research to date in panic disorder is preliminary and needs more standardized methodologies. Thus it is difficult to draw clinical implications from current findings. More studies are needed to understand structural and functional differences in patients with anxiety and panic disorders and how these changes may impact on behavior and ultimately on clinical interventions.

 How would you respond if a patient who is about to have an MRI scan asks you if the procedure is painful or harmful in any way and how exactly it will be helpful?

Challenge Tests and Basal Physiology Studies.

In the past 15 years two basic strategies have been devised to study the biology of panic disorder. The first, provocative challenge testing, is designed to cause panic attacks under controlled conditions so that the biology of the actual attack can be studied. The administration of chemicals like lactate or caffeine and inhalants like carbon dioxide cause panic attacks in vulnerable individuals. When people with panic disorder are given these challenges, they are more likely to have a panic attack than are normal controls and people with other psychiatric diagnoses. They are also less likely to have another attack when challenged again after adequate treatment with antipanic medications. This strategy may give clues to understanding the mechanism of panic attacks.

The second strategy involves studies of basal physiology, or the nonpanic state (between panic attacks), when the patient is still symptomatic with chronic high levels of anxiety and avoidance behavior. This strategy often leads to a better understanding of which parts of the brain may be important in triggering the panic state. For example, people with panic disorder have been shown to have blunted pituitary hormonal responses to several hypothalamic releasing hormones, suggesting either that the person cannot respond appropriately to stress, thus panic anxiety results, or the pituitary may adapt over time to repeated panic anxiety.

A final interesting physiological finding is that sleep-related panic attacks commonly occur in the transition from stage two to stage three sleep. Panic attacks occur in states of apparent deep relaxation and unconsciousness, rather than during dream (REM) sleep, when it could be suggested that the panic attack was in response to a disturbing dream. This further supports a biological component to panic.

Clinical Implications: Biology of Panic Disorder. **Although further research is needed to clarify the mechanisms for the cause of anxiety disorders, the clinical significance of the findings to date can be reassuring to patients. Patients can be told, for example, that panic anxiety is a dysregulation in the normal fight-or-flight response. The way in which it is manifested may be the combination of genetic vulnerability and an individual's reactions to life's experiences. Perhaps most important, patients should be told that panic disorder usually can be successfully treated by a variety of interventions. This information can give patients a sense of control over its seemingly uncontrollable and debilitating effects. They can then be taught to control their psychological, behavioral, and cognitive responses to anxiety and to actively participate in treatment in an informed partnership with health-care providers (see Chapter 14). Finally, in addition to the important role of patient educator, the psychiatric nurse can assess symptoms of anxiety disorders and select the most appropriate intervention based on the brain region implicated in the symptom and the treatment most likely to affect the function of that brain region (Table 5-4).**

Table 5-4 Biological Treatment Model of Panic Disorder

Symptom	Brain region	Function	Treatment
Phobic avoidance (a learned phenomenon)	Cerebral cortex (higher brain)	Learning and complex emotion	Desensitization and cognitive restructuring (see Chapter 28)
Anticipatory anxiety (possibly sensitized by hyperventilation)	Limbic lobe (midbrain: rich in benzodiazepine receptors)	Center for human emotions	Relaxation, breathing retraining, desensitization, antipanic medications
Panic attacks	Brainstem (lower brain: includes locus ceruleus and medulla)	Primitive emotion	Antipanic medication (see Chapter 25)

Modified from Gorman JM, Leibowitz MR, Fyer AJ, Stein J: *Am J Psychiatry* 146:2, 1989.

Alzheimer's Disease

The normal aging brain experiences a modest, gradual decline in enzyme activity and levels of selected proteins and neurons in certain brain regions. The aging individual may have decreased motor function and flexibility, slowness of movement, and a stooped, shuffling gait. However, changes in the brain appear to have little significant effect on mental functions such as thinking, except that these functions are slower.

Dementia, a decline of memory and other cognitive functions, is the most disabling psychiatric disorder of adulthood. It is not caused by the normal process of aging but rather appears to have many possible causes as identified in Box 5-3. About 45% of persons with dementia are diagnosed with Alzheimer's disease (AD), which

---

Box 5-3

POSSIBLE CAUSES OF DEMENTIA

HYPOXIA

Heart failure
Myocardial infarction
Postcardiac arrest
Respiratory disorders
Carbon monoxide poisoning

TRAUMA (2.5% to 15% of cases of dementia)
Head injury
Subdural hematoma

EPILEPSY

Psychomotor seizures
Postictal state
Nonconvulsive seizures

DEGENERATIVE DISORDERS

Presenile dementia including
    Alzheimer's disease (45% of cases of dementia)
    Pick's disease
    Prion disease
    Cortical lewy body disease (a 10% variant of AD cases)
    Huntington's chorea
    AIDS dementia ($<$ 1% of cases)
Senile dementia
Other disorders affecting the central nervous system including
    Multiple sclerosis
    Parkinson's disease (3% of cases)
    Normal-pressure hydrocephalus

DRUGS AND TOXIC DISORDERS

Alcohol
Barbiturates
Cocaine
Steroids
Digoxin
Antidepressants
L-dopa
Salicylates
Opiates
Cannabis
LSD
Industrial metals (lead, mercury, manganese)

VITAMIN DEFICIENCY

B_{12}
Thiamine
Nicotinic acid
Folic acid

SPACE-OCCUPYING LESIONS

Tumors
Subdural hematoma
Cerebral abscess

INFECTIONS

Meningitis
Encephalitis

CEREBRAL VASCULAR DISORDERS (15% of cases)
Transient ischemic attacks
Cerebral embolism
Subarachnoid hemorrhage

METABOLIC IMBALANCES

Electrolyte disturbance
Uremia
Hepatic encephalopathy
Hypoglycemia

ENDOCRINE DISEASES

Myxedema
Thyrotoxicosis
Diabetes mellitus
Cushing's disease
Addison's disease
Hypopituitarism

PSYCHIATRIC DISORDERS

Pseudodementias (sometimes seen in depression, schizophrenia, mania, and factitious disorder)
Chronic alcoholism

accounts for the fourth most common cause of death in the developed world after heart disease, cancer, and stroke. At a cost of $34 billion a year, AD afflicts 4 million people in the United States and results in 100,000 deaths annually. In light of today's aging population, AD has become a major health concern and the target of intensive research efforts nationwide. The causes of AD are not yet known, but a number of risk factors have been associated with it (Box 5-4).

Since head injury is a known risk factor for the dementing syndrome, what primary prevention strategies could society take to resolve this problem?

Genetics. It was not until 1991 that research in AD showed that genetic mutations cause some cases of AD. In early-onset AD (before age 65) these DNA mutations occur within chromosome 21, the same gene that forms beta-APP (amyloid precursor protein), the substance from which the protein beta-amyloid is made. The normal function of this protein is not fully understood, but its production is somehow accelerated in AD, and excessive deposits form both the senile plaques clustering outside each affected neuron and amyloid deposits in the walls of cerebral blood vessels. It is probably also related to the production of the neurofibrillary tangles seen within the neurons of AD patients. Approximately 50% of individuals in each generation of families with this genetic mutation develop AD. Interestingly, AD is also seen in the fourth and fifth decade of life in Down's syndrome patients, who have three rather than two copies of chromosome 21. Almost all of these patients develop senile plaques, neurofibrillary tangles, and clinical signs of dementia. In late-onset AD (after age 65) some cases have also been linked to chromosome 19 (probably a gene affecting beta-APP metabolism).

Another recent research finding is a link between combinations of a fairly common, cholesterol-trans-

---

Box 5-4

RISK FACTORS FOR ALZHEIMER'S DISEASE

AGE

▼ AD is a disease of old age.
▼ The population prevalence is less than 0.01% at age 45, 2% between age 65 and 70, 5% between 70 and 80, and over 20% at age 85.
▼ AD afflicts more women than men because women tend to live longer.
▼ An early age of onset (<65) is strongly associated with a positive family history.

FAMILY HISTORY

▼ A positive family history in first-degree relatives is the most persistent positive association for AD.
▼ Approximately 20% of AD cases are thought to be familial.

PARENTAL AGE

▼ Women who bear children before 20 and after 40 years of age have an increased incidence of AD in their offspring.
▼ This group of mothers also has increased risk of premature births, poor maternal fitness, and Down's syndrome babies.
▼ This suggests that children of older parents may have a chromosomal abnormality that makes them more susceptible to AD when they reach old age.

HEAD INJURY

▼ Descriptive reviews of case control studies often report the finding of a previous history of head injury in some AD patients.

▼ Support for head injury as a risk factor also comes from evidence that repetitive head trauma is known to cause a dementing syndrome in boxers (dementia pugilistica, or punchdrunk syndrome), which shows the same molecular pathology as AD.

POTASSIUM CHANNEL DYSFUNCTION

▼ One recent study[8] found that AD patients, when compared with both control groups and patients with other dementing illnesses, have a potassium (K+) channel dysfunction.
▼ K+ channels change during acquisition of memory in studies of mammals. Thus an abnormal K+ channel may serve as a marker for AD that would distinguish AD patients from age-matched controls and patients with non-AD neurological and psychiatric disorders.

ENVIRONMENTAL FACTORS

Although there have been anecdotal reports of other factors as risks for AD, systematic evidence is lacking. Some of these include:
▼ Aluminum—ingestion of foods stored in aluminum containers or use of deodorants and hairsprays with aluminum bases
▼ Bloodborne infections—blood transfusions if the blood donor has AD and it is transmitted by an infectious agent
▼ Chemicals—occupational exposure to chemicals

porting protein, Apo-E, and AD. Apparently many people with late-onset AD are born with a certain combination of Apo-E that attaches to beta-amyloid, perhaps then pulling bits of amyloid from the bloodstream and accumulating it in the brain. Thus developing AD may depend on which combination of Apo-E a person inherits. It remains to be seen if drugs can be developed that can prevent this form of Apo-E from doing its job.

Although at this time genetics accounts for only a small percentage of AD cases (perhaps 10%) and much of this work is still controversial, these discoveries are landmark scientific achievements. Genetic research in AD continues to be a high funding priority and promises to continue to unlock some of the mysteries of this devastating illness.

Biochemistry. Almost every neurotransmitter has been studied and implicated in AD, but the cholinergic hypothesis has commanded much of the attention as an explanation for AD. Disruption of the cholinergic system damages memory in animals and humans. Acetylcholine (ACh) is consistently reduced in AD. ACh is produced in a region of the basal nuclei selectively devastated in AD. It is thought that too little acetylcholine may allow a build-up of amyloid. Although over 10 experimental drugs are being tested for efficacy in AD, only a handful have shown promise. Tacrine (Cognex), which slows the natural breakdown of acetylcholine, has been approved for use in AD by the Food and Drug Administration, and it appears to be briefly effective in only a small group of AD patients.

In addition to cholinergic fibers, noncholinergic, serotonergic, and possibly dopaminergic fibers that innervate hippocampal and cortical areas are all severely affected by the disease. Glutamate and peptide transmitters are also affected in specific brain regions. Although correlations can be drawn between transmitter deficits and pathology and clinical symptoms of AD, they seem to reflect damage specific to affected regions of the brain rather than entire transmitter systems throughout the brain, providing little information about the underlying nature of the disease process itself. Another implication is that, unlike the neurochemistry of Parkinson's disease in which one transmitter deficit can be treated effectively by one drug intervention (L-dopa), it seems unlikely that AD can be effectively treated by neurotransmitter replacement therapy.

Brain Imaging. PET scans and performance tests indicate that the brains of healthy people in their eighties are almost as active and function nearly as well, although slower, on tests of memory, perception, and language as people in early adulthood.[26] Although diagnostic accuracy for AD requires neuropathological examination at autopsy, skillful neuropsychiatric examinations along with imaging techniques offer 80% to 90%

diagnostic accuracy. CT and MRI are useful to rule out space-occupying lesions, infarcts, or infection as causes of dementia but are not specific for the diagnosis of AD. Although early-onset AD patients may show cortical atrophy and ventricular enlargement with CT or MRI and a marked loss in brain weight, late-onset AD patients who develop the disease after age 75 usually show only age-related changes. PET scans show a typical pattern of frontal, parietal, and temporal hypometabolism (see Color Plate 12 on p. 136). These changes, however, are not specific to AD and thus cannot be used by themselves to make a definitive diagnosis. PET scans and SPECT studies have also shown results that appear to be specific to AD: a localized metabolic deficiency can be seen in the parietal, temporal, and eventually, the frontal lobes.[17]

Neuropathological Changes. It is not known how the excessive amyloid protein deposits lead to the plaques and tangles that cause extensive structural and biochemical changes in axons, dendrites, neuronal cell bodies, and glial cells. These changes reduce synaptic function by as much as 40% in affected regions and reduce protein synthesis and cellular processes. However, there is no doubt that this build-up of amyloid protein, combined with the formation of neurofibrillary tangles and other structural changes in neurons, contributes to a progressive breakdown of neuronal circuits necessary for communication in the brain. It is as if the limbic system, particularly the hippocampus and the association cortices, which are affected early in the AD process and are necessary to the organization of mental processes, becomes isolated and out of touch with other brain regions—thus the gradual impairment of memory, judgment, abstraction, and language. Eventually, motor and sensory regions are affected also, and the patient with AD becomes totally disabled.[7] Table 5-5 lists some of the affected brain regions and subsequent symptoms.

Clinical Implications: Biology of Alzheimer's Disease. Much research is being focused on understanding the molecular mechanisms underlying dementing diseases so that drugs can be designed to block these processes. In AD, future medications may be able to inhibit the enzymes that release excessive amounts of beta-amyloid protein from beta-APP, preventing it from entering cerebral tissue and causing the inflammatory and neurotoxic responses that result in CNS damage.

At present, although several drugs may lessen some of the disease processes for a time, there is no treatment for AD. Clinical intervention is targeted at differential diagnosis and managing the social and behavioral consequences of the progressive dementia of AD (see Chapters 21 and 36). The Advisory

Table 5-5 Some Brain Regions Affected by Alzheimer's Disease and Resulting Symptoms

Region affected	Function	Symptom
Limbic system: hippocampus	Memory, learning, and emotion	First, recent memories fade and then long-standing memories are affected. Symptoms of depression may occur, probably because of damage to the locus ceruleus.
Temporal-parietal-occipital association cortex	Visual impairment, aphasia, apraxia, and agnosia	Increasing difficulty recognizing even familiar faces, places, and objects. The ability to communicate, to use and understand language, to write, and to comprehend reading is lost. Hallucinations and delusions may occur. Seizures may occur.
Prefrontal cortex	Insight, planning, judgment, personality, behavior, and social propriety	Apathy, impaired insight, lack of judgment, concreteness, perseverance, and inefficient problem solving are seen.
Subcortical projections	Memory, learning, and behavior	More research is needed to correlate symptoms with changes seen in these areas, but it is clear that several important transmitter systems are affected: cholinergic basal forebrain, noradrenergic locus ceruleus, serotonergic raphe nuclei, and dopaminergic substantia nigra.
Motor cortex	Movement	Increasing difficulty walking, talking, and swallowing occur later in the disease process.

Panel on Alzheimer's Disease provides suggested minimum curricular requirements for nurses and other health-care providers for working with AD patients and their families.[1] These are outlined in Box 5-5. Another interesting line of nursing research shows that patients with AD who remain at home with a committed and loving caregiver live longer than patients with AD who live in nursing homes.[32] This may have interesting implications for society regarding the care and support of demented individuals and

their families, as well as the impact on the burden and cost of caregiving in this difficult population of extremely ill people.

One remedy to counter the effects of the aging process is for older individuals to stay physically fit. Older test subjects who regularly do aerobic exercises perform better on cognitive tests than do sedentary individuals in the same age group. Agents that interfere with the activity of the CNS should also be avoided by older persons. This includes alcohol and certain drugs, such as benzodiazepines and other depressants or stimulants of the CNS. People older than age 60 are particularly sensitive to these substances and perform poorly on cognitive tests compared with younger people taking these same drugs. It remains to be seen if early anecdotal reports of therapy with the antioxidant vitamin E or a lifetime of balanced, low caloric diets have positive effects on mental functions in elderly people.

DECADE OF THE BRAIN

The U.S. Congress has labeled the 1990s as the "Decade of the Brain" (Fig. 5-6), and there is a sense of excitement as each new discovery suggests new questions and new treatments that are explored in light of the latest brain research. Advances in the techniques used in the neurosciences, the scientific methodologies used in testing biological hypotheses, and the integration of nonbiological theories and findings in the clinical arena provide the biopsychosocial approach necessary for the study of psychiatric disorders in human beings.

Several well-researched lines of evidence support a

Box 5-5

MINIMUM CURRICULAR REQUIREMENTS FOR NURSES WORKING WITH ALZHEIMER'S DISEASE AND OTHER RELATED DEMENTIAS (ADRD)

▼ Introduction to aging focusing on both biological and psychological factors
▼ Cognitive functioning in the aged
▼ Behavior and nursing care problems
▼ Use of psychotropic medications
▼ Environmental restructuring, including the need for structure, consistency, and modified stimuli
▼ Social and emotional aspects of ADRD, including the role of the nurse in providing support for the family and the ADRD patient
▼ Methods for recognizing and preventing excess disability
▼ Methods for training, supervising, and evaluating nursing assistants in care of ADRD patients

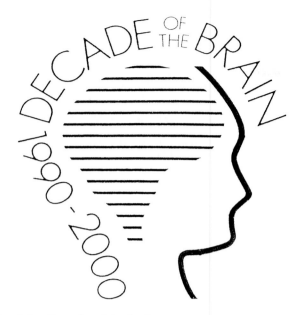

Fig. 5-6 Decade of the brain.
From The National Foundation for Brain Research, 1992.

biological link to mental illnesses, including the following:

1. Specific mental disorders can often be differentiated from each other by typical clinical features, epidemiological trends, and symptom presentations.
2. Exogenous chemicals can produce symptoms of mental illness or exacerbate existing symptoms, thus demonstrating that physical agents can be causative.
3. A biological cause of psychiatric illness is supported by in vitro simulations of some symptoms that can be replicated, such as the challenge studies in panic disorder.

4. Genetic studies show that psychiatric disorders are strongly influenced by inheritance: the closer the genetic structure, the more at risk the individual is for the disorder.
5. Many psychiatric disorders have associated "biological" symptoms or test results, such as altered sleep patterns and failure to suppress cortisol in the dexamethasone suppression test in depression.
6. Medications can suppress symptoms associated with psychiatric disorders, thus providing chemically mediated relief for many psychiatric illnesses.

As members of the mental health-care team, psychiatric nurses are faced with the challenge of integrating the new psychobiology with the long-standing biopsychosocial model of psychiatric nursing care. It is essential that psychiatric nurses make this paradigm shift and combine the enormous amount of information generated from the neurosciences with that of the other health sciences. They then need to apply this information and provide holistic, effective, and individualized psychiatric nursing care.

SUGGESTED CROSS-REFERENCES

Box 5-1

STRUCTURE AND FUNCTION OF THE BRAIN

CEREBRUM

Largest portion of the brain

Responsible for conscious perception, thought, and motor activity

Governs muscle coordination and the learning of rote movements

Can override most other systems

Divided into two hemispheres, each of which is divided into four lobes

Dominant hemisphere

Left side is dominant in most people (95% of right-handed and more than 50% of left-handed people)

Responsible for the production and comprehension of language, mathematical ability, and the ability to solve problems in a sequential, logical fashion

Nondominant hemisphere

Right side is nondominant in most people

Responsible for musical skills, recognition of faces, and tasks requiring comprehension of spatial relationships

Corpus callosum

Largest fiber bundle in the brain

Connects the two cerebral hemispheres and passes information from one to the other, welding the two hemispheres together into a unitary consciousness, allowing the "right hand to know what the left hand is doing"

Cerebral cortex

A few millimeters thick and about 2.5 sq. ft. in area

Sheet of gray matter containing 30 billion neurons interconnected by almost 70 miles of axons and dendrites

Forms the corrugated surface of the four lobes of the cerebral hemispheres

Connected to various structures of the brain and has a great deal to do with the abilities we think of as uniquely human, such as language and abstract thinking, as well as basic aspects of perception, movement, and adaptive response to the outside world

Functional areas have been "mapped," as can be seen in Fig. 5-3

Damage to certain cortical areas usually results in predictable deficits, depending on the area affected

Frontal lobes

Aid in planning for the future, motivation, control of voluntary motor function, and production of speech

Play an important part in emotional experience and expression of mood

Parietal lobes

Reception and evaluation of most sensory information (excluding smell, hearing, and vision)

Central sulcus

Groove or fissure on the surface of the brain that divides the frontal and parietal lobes

Temporal lobes

Receive and evaluate olfactory and auditory input and plays an important role in memory

Associated with brain functions such as abstract thought and judgment

Lateral fissure

Separates the temporal lobe from the rest of the cerebrum

Occipital lobes

Reception and integration of visual input

Clinical Example: Aphasia, absent or defective speech or comprehension, results from a lesion in the language areas of the cortex. The several types of aphasia depend on the site of the lesion. Damage to Broca's area, which contains the motor programs for the generation of language, results in expressive, or motor, aphasia, with difficulty producing either written or spoken words but no difficulty comprehending language. Damage to Wernicke's area, which contains the mechanisms for the formulation of language, results in receptive, or sensory, aphasia, where words are produced but their sequence is defective in linguistic content, resulting in paraphasia (word substitutions), neologisms (insertion of new and meaningless words), or jargon (fluent but unintelligible speech), and there is a general deficiency in the comprehension of language. If the lesion occurs in the connection between the two areas, conduction aphasia results, in which a person has poor repetition but relatively good comprehension.

DIENCEPHALON

Constitutes only 2% of the CNS by weight

Has extremely widespread and important connections, and the great majority of sensory, motor, and limbic pathways involve the diencephalon

Thalamus

Composes 80% of the diencephalon

All sensory pathways and many other anatomical loops relay in the thalamus

Takes sensory information and relays it to areas throughout the cortex

Influences prefrontal cortical functions such as affect and foresight

Influences mood and general body movements associated with strong emotions, such as fear or rage

Pineal gland

Endocrine gland involved in reproductive cycles

During darkness it secretes an antigonadotropic hormone called melatonin, which decreases during light, thus increasing gonadal function

Important in mammals with seasonal sexual cycles, its effects in humans are not yet clear, although tumors of the pineal gland affect human sexual development

May also be involved in the sleep-wake cycle

Box 5-1

STRUCTURE AND FUNCTION OF THE BRAIN—cont'd

Hypothalamus

Weighs only 4 g

Major control center for the pituitary gland, for maintaining homeostasis, and regulating autonomic, endocrine, emotional, and somatic functions

Controls various visceral functions and activities involved in basic drives and is very important in a number of functions that have emotional and mood relationships

Directly involved in stress-related and psychosomatic illnesses and with feelings of fear and rage

Regulates feeding and drinking behavior, temperature regulation, cardiac function, gut motility, and sexual activity

Coordinates responses for the sleep-wake cycle to other areas of the body

Contains the mamillary bodies, which are involved in olfactory reflexes and emotional responses to odors

BRAINSTEM

Connects the spinal cord to the brain

Location of cranial nerve nuclei

Controls automatic body functions like breathing and cardiovascular activity

Midbrain

Contains ascending and descending nerve tracks

Visual cortex center

Part of auditory pathway

Regulates the reflexive movement of the eyes and head

Aids in the unconscious regulation and coordination of motor activities

Contains the part of the basal ganglia, the substantia nigra, which manufactures dopamine

Pons

Contains ascending and descending nerve tracks

Relay between cerebrum and cerebellum

Reflex center

Contains the locus ceruleus, which manufactures most of the brain's norepinephrine

Medulla oblongata

Conduction pathway for ascending and descending nerve tracks

Conscious control of skeletal muscles

Involved in functions such as balance, coordination, and modulation of sound impulses from the inner ear

Center for several important reflexes: heart rate, breathing, swallowing, vomiting, coughing, sneezing

Reticular formation

Central core of the brainstem

Controls cyclic activities such as the sleep-wake cycle (called the reticular activating system, or RAS)

Plays an important role in arousing and maintaining consciousness, alertness, and attention

Contributes to the motor system, respiration, cardiac rhythms, and other vital body functions

Clinical Example: Damage to the RAS can result in coma. General anesthetics function by suppressing this system. It may also be the target of many tranquilizers. Ammonia (smelling salts) stimulate the RAS, resulting in arousal.

BASAL GANGLIA

Several deep gray matter structures that are related functionally and are located bilaterally in the cerebrum, diencephalon, and midbrain

Control muscle tone, activity, and posture

Coordinate large muscle movements

Major effect is to inhibit unwanted muscular activity

Cause extrapyramidal syndromes when dysfunctional

Clinical Example: Parkinson's disease, characterized by muscular rigidity, a slow, shuffling gait, and a general lack of movement, is associated with a dysfunction of the basal ganglia, probably a destruction of the dopamine-producing neurons of the substantia nigra (part of the basal ganglia but located in the midbrain).

LIMBIC SYSTEM

Forms the limbus, or border, of the temporal lobes and is intimately connected to many other structures of the brain

Concerned both with subjective emotional experiences and with changes in bodily functions associated with emotional states

Particularly involved in aggressive, submissive, and sexual behavior, and with pleasure, memory, and learning

Associated with mood, motivation, and sensations— all central to preservation

Clinical Example: Klüver-Bucy syndrome develops when the entire limbic system is removed or destroyed. Symptoms include fearlessness and placidity (absence of emotional reactions), an inordinate degree of attention to sensory stimuli (ceaseless and intrusive curiosity), and visual agnosia (the inability to recognize anything).

Hippocampus

Consolidates recently acquired information about facts and events, somehow turning short-term memory into long term

Contains large amounts of neurotransmitters

Continued.

Box 5-1
STRUCTURE AND FUNCTION OF THE BRAIN—cont'd

Clinical Example: Surgical removal of the hippocampus results in the inability to form new memories of facts and events (names of new acquaintances, day-to-day events, inability to remember why a task was begun), although long-term memory, intelligence, and the ability to learn new skills are unaffected. A similar memory problem is Korsakoff's syndrome in which patients have relatively intact intelligence but cannot form new memories. They typically confabulate (make up answers to questions), which occurs when the hippocampus and surrounding areas are damaged by chronic alcoholism. This is also seen in Alzheimer's disease in which the memory loss is profound, and there is extensive cellular degeneration in the hippocampus.

Amygdala

Generates emotions from perceptions and thoughts (presumably through its interactions with the hypothalamus and prefrontal cortex)
Contains many opiate receptors

Clinical Example: Electrical stimulation of the amygdala in animals causes responses of defense, raging aggression, or fleeing. In humans the most common response is fear and its related autonomic responses (dilation of the pupils, increased heart rate, and release of adrenalin). Conversely, bilateral destruction of the amygdala causes a great decrease in aggression, and animals become tame and placid. This is thought to be another kind of memory dysfunction that impairs the ability to learn or remember the appropriate emotional and autonomic responses to stimuli.

Fornix

Two-way fiber system that connects the hippocampus to the hypothalamus

CEREBELLUM

"Little brain"
Full range of sensory inputs finds its way here and in turn projects to various sites in the brainstem and thalamus
Although it is extensively involved with the processing of sensory information, it is also part of the motor system and is involved in equilibrium, muscle tone, postural control, and coordination of voluntary movements
More recently, it is thought that, because of connections to other brain regions, the cerebellum may be involved in cognitive, behavioral, and affective functions

Clinical Example: The malnutrition often accompanying chronic alcoholism causes a degeneration of the cerebellar cortex, resulting in the anterior lobe syndrome in which the legs are primarily affected, and the most prominent symptom is a broad-based, staggering gait and a general incoordination, or ataxia, of leg movements.

VENTRICLES

Each cerebral hemisphere contains a relatively large cavity, the lateral ventricle
A smaller midline cavity, the third ventricle, is located in the center of the diencephalon, between the two halves of the thalamus
The fourth ventricle is in the region of the pons and medulla oblongata and connects with the central canal of the spinal cord, which extends nearly the full length of the spinal cord

Clinical Example: Although the clinical significance of these findings is uncertain, imaging techniques have shown enlargement of the ventricles in many psychiatric disorders, suggesting an atrophy of the many critical structures in the brain with these illnesses

SPINAL FLUID

Cerebral spinal fluid (CSF) is procured from the blood choroid plexuses, located in the ventricles, and fills the ventricles, subarachnoid space (between the brain and the skull), and the spinal cord
CSF bathes the brain with nutrients, cushions the brain within the skull, and exits through the bloodstream
Approximately 140 ml of spinal fluid within the central nervous system travels from its point of origin to the bloodstream at approximately 0.4 ml per minute

Clinical Example: Neurotransmitters and their metabolites can be measured in the CSF, plasma, and urine and give an approximation of neurotransmitter production and metabolism in the brain. This provides clues to abnormal neurotransmission in some mental illnesses.

BLOOD-BRAIN AND BLOOD-CSF BARRIERS

Neuronal function requires a microenvironment that is protected from changes elsewhere in the body that may have an adverse effect
Blood-brain and blood-CSF barriers protect the CNS in several ways:
1. Large molecules, for example, plasma proteins, present in the blood are excluded from the CSF and nervous tissue
2. The brain and spinal cord are protected from neurotransmitters in the blood, for example, epinephrine produced by the adrenal gland
3. Neurotransmitters produced in the CNS are prevented from precipitously leaking into the general circulation
4. Toxins are excluded either because of their molecular size (too big) or because of their solubility (only substances soluble in water and cell-membrane lipids can pass these barriers)—thus many drugs are not able to enter the brain and spinal cord

COLOR ATLAS OF PSYCHOBIOLOGY

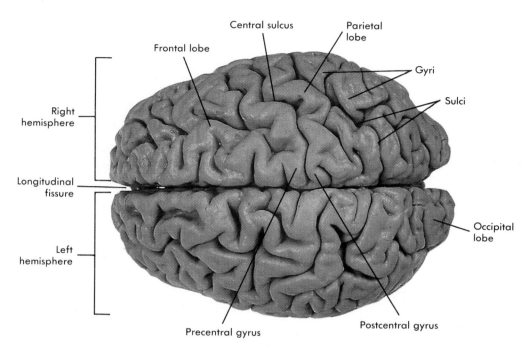

Color Plate 1   Superior view of the brain.
From Hutchings RT. In McMinn RMH, Hutchings RT: *Color atlas of human anatomy*, ed 2, Chicago, 1988, Year Book Medical Publishers.

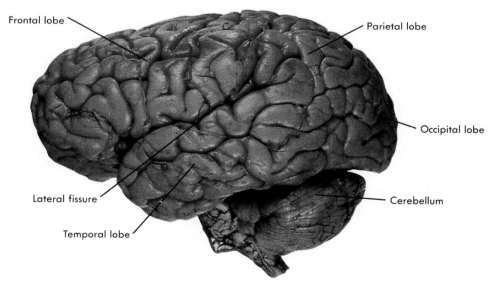

Color Plate 2   Lateral view of the left cerebral hemisphere of the brain.
From Hutchings RT. In McMinn RMH, Hutchings RT: *Color atlas of human anatomy*, ed 2, Chicago, 1988, Year Book Medical Publishers.

A

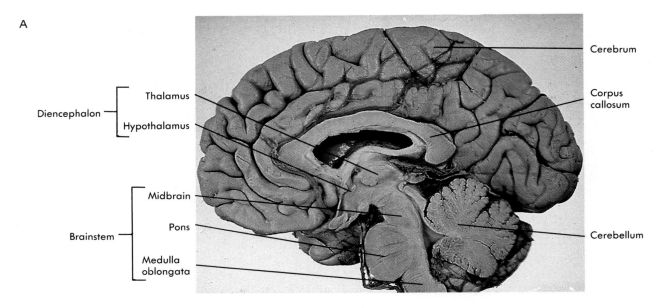

Diencephalon
— Thalamus
— Hypothalamus

Brainstem
— Midbrain
— Pons
— Medulla oblongata

Cerebrum

Corpus callosum

Cerebellum

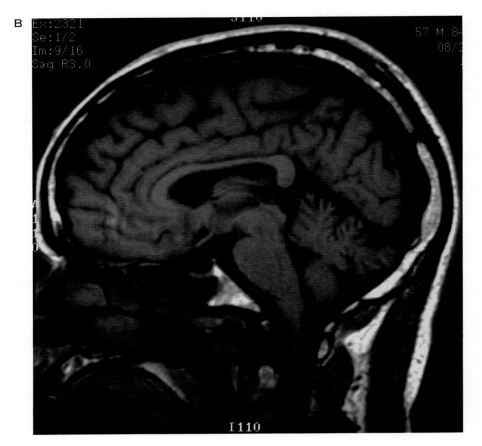

Color Plate 3   When the brain is cut between the two hemispheres down the middle (a midsagittal section) the main division can be clearly seen in an autopsy specimen **(A)**, a magnetic resonance imaging scan **(B)**, and a schematic representation **(C)**.

A from Hutchings RT. In McMinn RMH, Hutchings RT: *Color atlas of human anatomy*, ed 2, Chicago, 1988, Year Book Medical Publishers; **B** from Medical University of South Carolina.

C

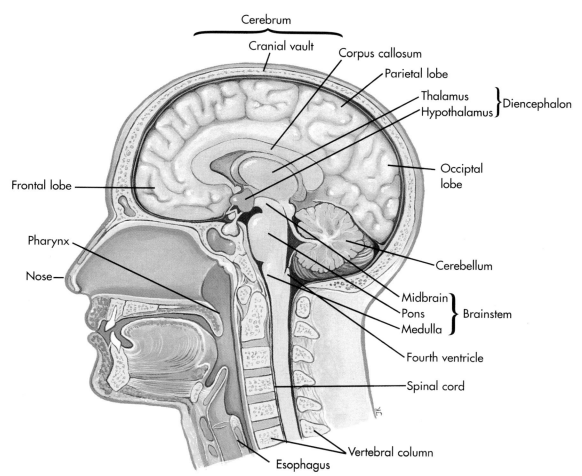

Cerebrum

Cranial vault

Corpus callosum

Parietal lobe

Thalamus
Hypothalamus } Diencephalon

Occiptal lobe

Frontal lobe

Pharynx

Nose

Cerebellum

Midbrain
Pons } Brainstem
Medulla

Fourth ventricle

Spinal cord

Vertebral column

Esophagus

Color Plate 3, cont'd
For legend see opposite page.

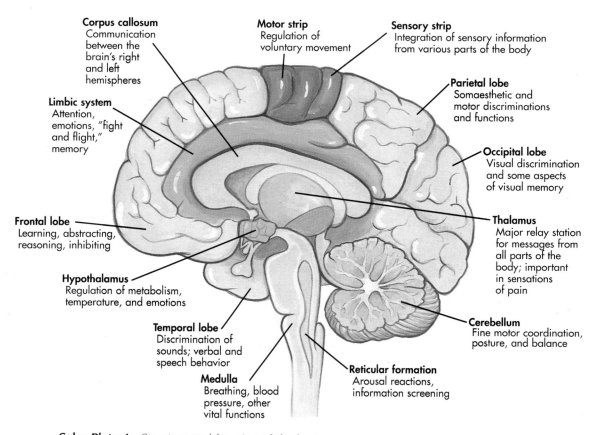

Corpus callosum
Communication between the brain's right and left hemispheres

Motor strip
Regulation of voluntary movement

Sensory strip
Integration of sensory information from various parts of the body

Parietal lobe
Somaesthetic and motor discriminations and functions

Limbic system
Attention, emotions, "fight and flight," memory

Occipital lobe
Visual discrimination and some aspects of visual memory

Frontal lobe
Learning, abstracting, reasoning, inhibiting

Thalamus
Major relay station for messages from all parts of the body; important in sensations of pain

Hypothalamus
Regulation of metabolism, temperature, and emotions

Temporal lobe
Discrimination of sounds; verbal and speech behavior

Cerebellum
Fine motor coordination, posture, and balance

Medulla
Breathing, blood pressure, other vital functions

Reticular formation
Arousal reactions, information screening

Color Plate 4   Structure and function of the brain.
From Carson RC, Butcher JN: *Abnormal psychology and modern life*, ed 9, New York, 1992, HarperCollins.

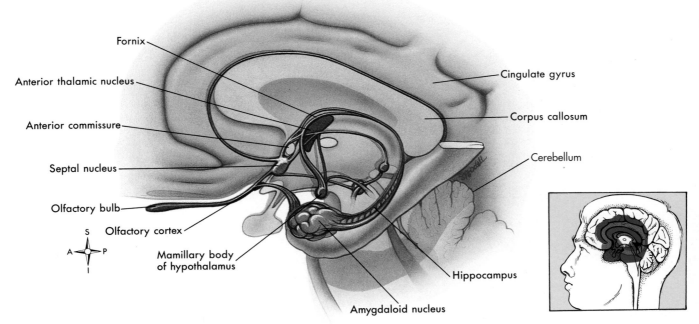

Color Plate 5   Structure of the limbic system.
Scott Bodell, illustrator.

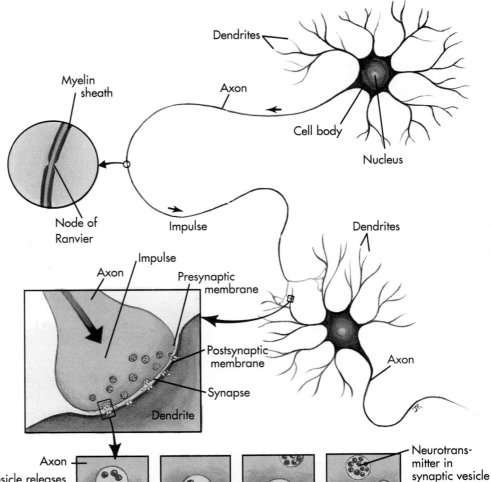

Color Plate 6   Neurotransmission. *Bottom*: 1, Neurotransmitter is released from presynaptic cell into synapse. 2, Neurotransmitter, reorganized by receptor cell, causes channel to open, and ions are exchanged. 3, Exchange of ions causes impulse, which causes reaction in receptor cell. 4, Neurotransmission has taken place; receptor channel closes, and neurotransmitter returns to presynaptic membrane (reuptake).

A

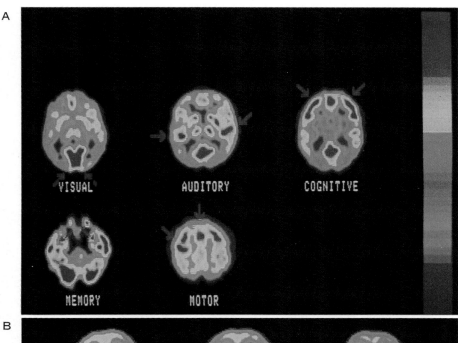

VISUAL　　AUDITORY　　COGNITIVE

MEMORY　　MOTOR

B

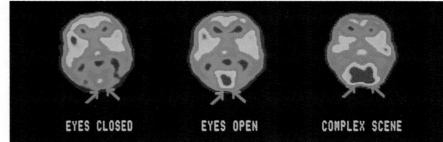

EYES CLOSED　　EYES OPEN　　COMPLEX SCENE

C

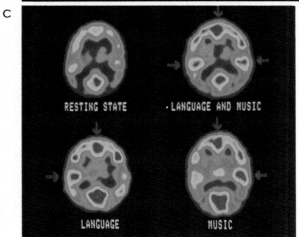

RESTING STATE　　·LANGUAGE AND MUSIC

LANGUAGE　　MUSIC

Color Plate 7 Positron emission tomography scan shows varying patterns of glucose consumption during different tasks. The color scale ranges from 2 (violet) to 45 (red). **A,** Different kinds of tasks cause increased glucose consumption in distinct areas of the brain. A checkerboard visual stimulus activates the occipital lobes. An auditory stimulus causes increased glucose consumption in the temporal lobes. When an individual is engaged in an active, cognitive task rather than passive perception of stimuli, glucose consumption increases in the frontal lobes. Subjects trying to remember information from a verbal stimulus (a story) show increased glucose consumption in the temporal lobes. Sequential movements of the fingers of the right hand activate the motor cortex on the left, as well as the supplementary motor arc (*vertical arrow*). **B,** Increasing complexity of a particular kind of task causes increased glucose consumption in progressively larger areas of the cortex. With the subject blindfolded ("eyes closed"), there is relatively little glucose consumption in the occipital lobes. With the eyes open, looking at a plain white light source activates the primary visual cortex of the occipital lobes. Looking at an outdoor scene ("complex scene") activates the visual association cortex in additional areas of the occipital lobes. **C,** The left hemisphere usually plays a dominant role in language functions, the right hemisphere in musical and certain other functions. When a subject listens simultaneously to a Sherlock Holmes story and a Brandenberg concerto, both superior temporal lobes and both frontal lobes are activated. Listening to just the story activates predominately the left hemisphere. Musical chords alone activate predominately the right hemisphere.

A and **B** from Phelps ME, Mazziotta JC: *Science* 228:799, 1985; **C** courtesy Dr. ME Phelps and Dr. JC Mazziotta, University of California School of Medicine.

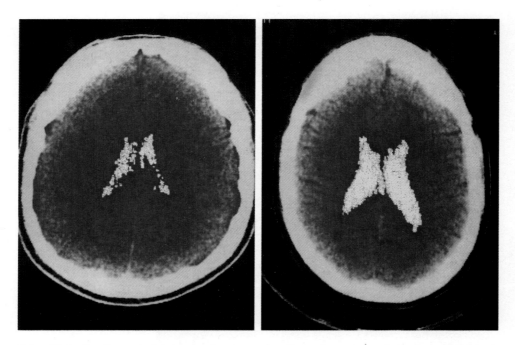

Color Plate 8 Computed tomography scans showing enlargement of the lateral cerebral ventricles in a chronic schizophrenic patient (*right*) as compared with a normal control (*left*). From Roberts GW, Leigh PN, Weinberger DR: *Neuropsychiatric disorders*, London, 1993, Wolfe.

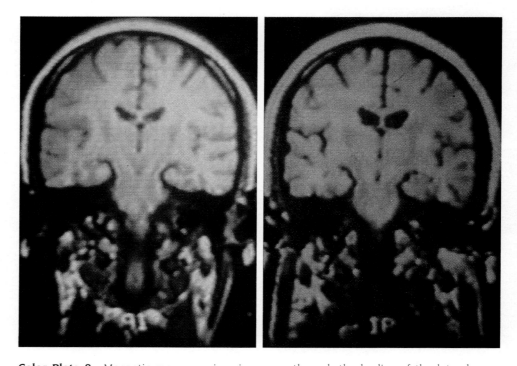

Color Plate 9 Magnetic resonance imaging scans through the bodies of the lateral ventricles in a pair of monozygotic twins who are discordant for schizophrenia. Note the increase in the cerebrospinal fluid spaces in the schizophrenic twin (*right*) as compared with the unaffected twin (*left*). From Roberts GW, Leigh PN, Weinberger DR: *Neuropsychiatric disorders*, London, 1993, Wolfe.

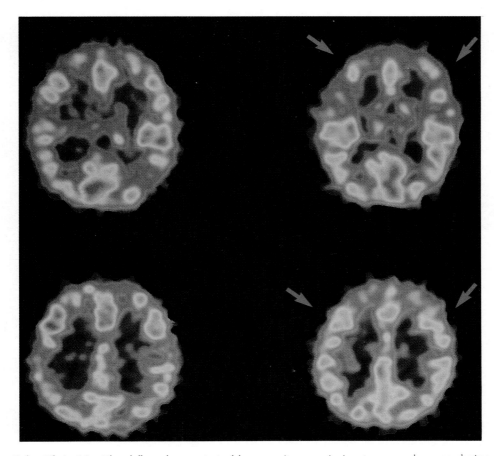

Color Plate 10 Blood flow demonstrated by a positron emission tomography scan during the performance of the Wisconsin Card Sort Task (a task that activates the prefrontal cortex in normal subjects) in a schizophrenic twin (*right column*) and an unaffected twin (*left column*). The arrows indicate the relatively focused failure of activation in the affected twin as compared with the unaffected twin.

From Roberts GW, Leigh PN, Weinberger DR: *Neuropsychiatric disorders*, London, 1993, Wolfe.

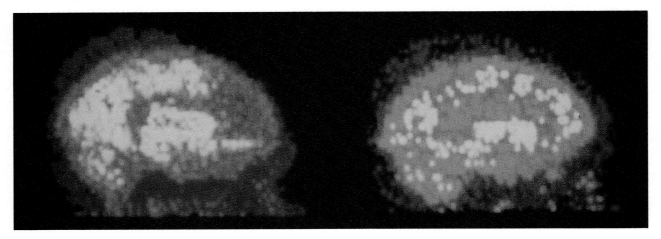

Color Plate 11 Positron emission tomography scans of glucose utilization in a depressed subject showing frontal hypometabolism (*left*), which improves after treatment with antidepressant medication (*right*).

Courtesy of Lewis Baxter, MD, UCLA School of Medicine, Los Angeles.

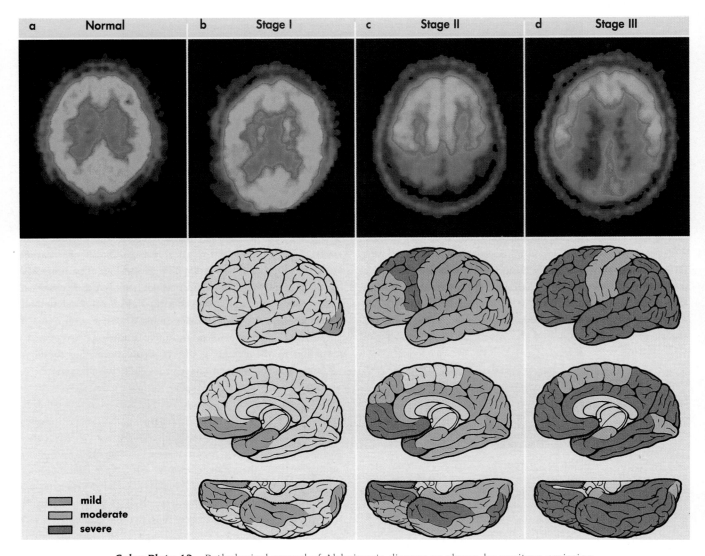

| a Normal | b Stage I | c Stage II | d Stage III |

mild
moderate
severe

Color Plate 12 Pathological spread of Alzheimer's disease as shown by positron emission tomography scans. **A,** Normal brain. **B,** Brain in stage I Alzheimer's disease. **C,** Brain in stage II Alzheimer's disease. **D,** Brain in stage III Alzheimer's disease. **E,** Diagrams show the spread of pathology in Alzheimer's disease.

From Roberts GW, Leigh PN, Weinberger DR: *Neuropsychiatric disorders,* London, 1993, Wolfe.

SUMMARY

1. It is essential that psychiatric nurses learn about the structure and function of the brain including the neurotransmission process to better understand the etiology, course, and most effective treatment strategies for psychiatric illnesses.

2. Brain imaging techniques such as CT, MRI, BEAM, PET, and SPECT allow for the direct viewing of the brain, which helps in diagnosing some brain disorders and correlating brain structure with function.

3. The search for the gene or genes that carry mental illness has been difficult and inconclusive to date but is a promising field for future research.

4. Circadian rhythm is like a network of internal clocks that time and coordinate events within the body including life-style, sleep, moods, eating, drinking, fertility, and illness according to an approximate 24-hour cycle.

5. Psychoimmunology is a new field that explores the influence of psychosocial factors on the nervous system's control of immune responses.

6. Psychiatric nurses need to be able to obtain a thorough history, perform a basic physical examination, and interpret the results of laboratory tests to screen for signs of physical or organic disorders and refer to specialists as indicated.

7. The clinical implications of neuroscientific research were discussed in relation to schizophrenia, mood disorders, panic disorder, and Alzheimer's disease.

8. The 1990s have been called the "Decade of the Brain," and psychiatric nurses are faced with the challenge of integrating the latest neuroscientific information into the biopsychosocial model of psychiatric nursing care.

REFERENCES

1. Advisory Panel on Alzheimer's Disease: *Second report of the Advisory Panel on Alzheimer's Disease*, DHHS Pub. No. (ADM) 91-1791, Washington, DC, 1991, US Government Printing Office.

2. Baxter L, Jeffrey M, Phelps M: Reduction of prefrontal cortex glucose metabolism common to three types of depression, *Arch Gen Psychiatry* 46:243, 1989.

3. Betrus P, Elmore S: Seasonal affective disorder: Part I. A review of the neural mechanisms for psychosocial nurses, *Arch Psychiatr Nurs* 5:357, 1991.

4. Bloom F, Lazerson A: *Brain, mind, and behavior*, New York, 1988, WH Freeman.

5. Charney D, Woods S, Nagy L, Southwick S, Krystal J, Heninger G: Noradrenergic function in panic disorder, *J Clin Psychiatry* 51:(suppl A):5, 1990.

6. Chen W, Chen T, Lin S, Hu W, Yeh E: Plasma catecholamine metabolites in schizophrenics: evidence for the two-subtype concept, *Biol Psychiatry* 27:510, 1990.

7. Chui H: Dementia: a review emphasizing clinicopathologic correlation and brain-behavior relationships, *Arch Neurol* 46:806, 1989.

8. Etcheberrigaray R, Ito E, Oka K, Tofel-Grehl B, Gigson E: Potassium channel dysfunction in fibroblasts identifies patients with Alzheimer's disease, *Proc Natl Acad Sci USA* 90:8209, 1993.

9. Garver K, Garver B: Eugenics: past, present, and future, *Am J Hum Genet* 49:1109, 1991.

10. Gershon ES, Rieder RO: Major disorders of mind and brain, *Sci Am* 267:133, 1992.

11. Goodwin W, Jamison K: *Manic depressive illness*, New York, 1990, Oxford University Press.

12. Hauser P: Magnetic resonance imaging in primary affective disorder. In Hauser P, ed: *Brain imaging in affective disorders*, Washington, DC, 1991, American Psychiatric Press.

13. Holmes C: *Recognizing brain dysfunction: a guide for mental health professionals*, Brandon, Ver, 1992, Clinical Psychology Publishing Company.

14. Joyce J: The dopamine hypothesis of schizophrenia: limbic interactions with serotonin and norepinephrine, *Psychopharmacology* 112:516, 1993.

15. Kety S: Paper presented at the IV World Congress of Biological Psychiatry, Philadelphia, September 12, 1985.

16. Lewy A, Sack R, Singer C, White D, Hoban T: Winter depression and the phase-shift hypothesis for bright light's therapeutic effects. In Rosenthal N, Blehar M, eds: *Seasonal affective disorder and phototherapy*, New York, 1989, The Guilford Press.

17. Margolin R: Neuroimaging. In Sadovoy J, Lazarus L, Jarvik L, eds: *Comprehensive review of geriatric psychiatry*, Washington, DC, 1993, American Psychiatric Press.

18. McCarrick A et al: Chronic medical problems in the chronically medically ill, *Hosp Community Psychiatry* 37:289, 1986.

19. McEnany G: Psychobiological indices of bipolar mood disorder: future trends in nursing care, *Arch Psychiatr Nurs* 4:29, 1990.

20. Meltzer H: Clozapine: mechanism of action in relation to its chemical advantages. In Kales A, Stefanis C, Talbott J, eds: *Recent advances in schizophrenia*, New York, 1990, Springer-Verlag.

21. Neylan J, van Kammen D: Biological mechanisms of schizophrenia: an update, *Psychiatr Med* 8:41, 1990.

22. Post R, Weiss S: Nonhomologous animal models of affective illness: clinical relevance of sensitization and kindling. In Koob G, Ehlers C, Kupfer D, eds: *Animal models of depression*, Boston, 1989, Birkhauser.

23. Reiman E: PET, panic disorder, and normal anticipatory anxiety. In Ballenger, ed: *Frontiers of clinical neuroscience*, vol 8, *Neurobiology of panic disorder*, New York, 1990, Alan R Liss.

24. Robins L, Regier D: *Psychiatric disorders in america: the epidemiologic catchment area study*, New York, 1991, Free Press.

25. Schlegel S: Computed tomography in affective disorders. In Hauser P, ed: *Brain imaging in affective disorders*, Washington, DC, 1991, American Psychiatric Press.

26. Selkoe D: Aging brain, aging mind, *Sci Am* 267:135, 1992.

27. Thase M, Frank E, Kupfer D: Biological processes in major depression. In Beckman E, Leber W, eds: *Handbook of depression*, ed 2, New York, 1993, The Guilford Press.

28. Thibodeau G, Patton K: *Anatomy and physiology*, ed 2, St Louis, 1993, Mosby.

29. Torgesen S: Twin studies in panic disorder. In Ballenger J, ed: *Neurobiology of panic disorder*, New York, 1990, Alan R Liss.

30. Weinberger D, Berman K, Zec R: Physiological dysfunction of dorsolateral prefrontal cortex in schizophrenia, *Arch Gen Psychiatry* 43:114, 1986.

31. Wilson W, Mathew R: Cerebral blood flow and metabolism in anxiety disorders. In Hoehn-Saric R, McLeod DR, eds: *Biology of anxiety disorders*, Progress in Psychiatry Series, no. 36, Washington, DC, 1993, American Psychiatric Press.

32. Wright L: *Alzheimer's disease and marriage: an intimate account*, Sage Series in Clinical Nursing Research, Newbury Park, Calif, 1993, Sage Publications.

ANNOTATED SUGGESTED READINGS

*Abraham IL, Fox JC, Cohen BT: Integrating the bio into the biopsychosocial: understanding and treating biological phenomena in psychiatric-mental health nursing, *Arch Psychiatr Nurs* 6:296, 1992.

The emergence of a new, holistic discipline of psychiatric nursing is described that integrates relationships between the brain, behavior, emotion, and cognition into nursing practice, research, and education.

*Abraham IL, Neundorfer MM: Alzheimer's: a decade of progress, a future of nursing challenges, *Geriatr Nurs* 5:116, 1990.

Describes the goal of comprehensive care for AD patients and their caregivers, nursing interventions shown to be effective, elements of a therapeutic milieu, and techniques for improving selected physical activities of daily living.

*Glod CA: Circadian dysregulation in abused individuals: a proposed theoretical model for practice and research, *Arch Psychiatr Nurs* 6:347, 1992.

Explores a possible model to link the sleep disruptions seen in abused children with circadian and rhythmic theories. Thought provoking with implications for nursing practice.

Gorman J, Kertzner R: *Psychoimmunology update*, Washington DC, 1991, American Psychiatric Press.

Examines current knowledge in the mind-body connection including findings related to schizophrenia, depression, and HIV infection.

*Harper-Jaques S, Reimer M: Aggressive behavior and the brain: a different perspective for the mental health nurse, *Arch Psychiatr Nurs* 6:312, 1992.

Presents a framework to understand the interrelationships among the limbic system and frontal and temporal lobes as they relate to the expression of aggressive behavior. Implications for psychiatric nurses include detecting contributing factors such as head injury, temporal epilepsy, alcoholism, and dietary imbalances and interpreting patient behaviors to colleagues.

Holmes C: *Recognizing brain dysfunction: a guide for mental health professionals*, Brandon, Ver, 1992, Clinical Psychology Publishing.

Provides an overview for mental health professionals on screening for brain dysfunctions based on history, physical, psychological, and cognitive signs and symptoms.

*Hundley J, Sullivan CH, Coburn KL: Computerized EEG: forming a mental picture. *J Psychosoc Nurs Ment Health Serv* 28:19, 1990.

Describes the expanding role of the nurse in relationship to the care of patients undergoing neuroimaging tests. Discusses the BEAM, what it does, its clinical implications, and its impact on the patient.

*Laraia MT: Biological correlates of panic disorder with agoraphobia: practice perspectives for nurses, *Arch Psychiatr Nurs* 5:373, 1991.

Reviews panic disorder with regard to epidemiological, environmental, cultural, psychological, family, and genetic factors. Neuroscience techniques, such as imaging and challenge tests, are discussed and treatment implications suggested.

*Nursing reference.

*McEnany GW: Psychobiology and psychiatric nursing: a philosophical matrix, *Arch Psychiatr Nurs* 5:255, 1991.

Articulates the challenge of integrating psychobiology with psychodynamics and suggests interesting and helpful ways psychiatric nurses can meet this challenge.

Melendez JC, McCrank E: Anxiety-related reactions associated with magnetic resonance imaging examinations, *JAMA* 270:745, 1993.

Reviews the epidemiology of anxiety-related reactions during MRI examinations, the feasibility of identifying patients at risk, and intervention strategies. Helpful for the nurse preparing a patient for imaging tests.

*Morin GD: Seasonal affective disorder, the depression of winter: a literature review and description from a nursing perspective, *Arch Psychiatr Nurs* 4:182, 1990.

Presents a literature review and description of seasonal affective disorder including theories indicating a chronobiological circadian etiology. Assessment, diagnoses, and interventions are discussed, as well as the implications for nurses who rotate shifts.

Seeley RR, Stephens TD, Tate P: *Anatomy and physiology,* ed 2, St Louis, 1992, Mosby.

Basic anatomy and physiology textbook that is well organized and easy to read. Up to date with many helpful pictures and tables. The presentation of the central nervous system is particularly well done, and brain structures and functions are described in detail.

*Simmons-Alling S: Genetic implications for major affective disorders, *Arch Psychiatr Nurs* 4:67, 1990.

Gives an overview of the methods and results of family, adoption, and twin studies for the affective disorders. The role of the psychiatric nurse, in collaboration with patients, families, and scientists, is discussed related to genetics.

*Thompson LW: The dopamine hypothesis of schizophrenia, *Perspect Psychiatr Care* 25:18, 1990.

Clear and up-to-date review of the neurobiology of the dopamine system and its implications in schizophrenia. Recent research is reviewed, and implications for psychiatric mental health nurses are discussed.

U.S. Congress, Office of Technology Assessment: *The biology of mental disorders,* OTA-BA-538, Washington DC, 1992, U.S. Government Printing Office.

Summarizes current research on biological factors associated with the major psychiatric disorders. Clear and easy to read.

Nursing reference.

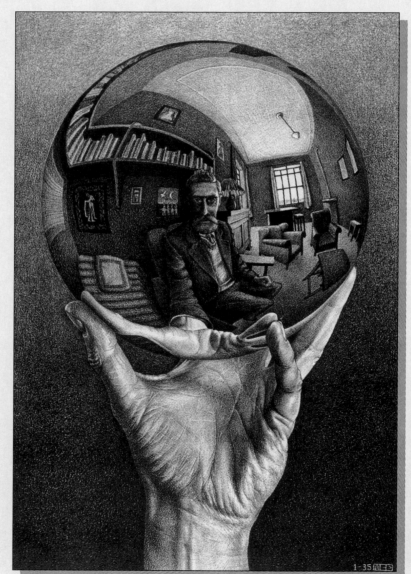

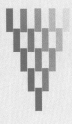

CHAPTER 6

Psychological Context of Psychiatric Nursing Care

GAIL W. STUART

Information is of no value for its own sake, but only because of its personal significance.

Eric Berne

LEARNING OBJECTIVES

After studying this chapter the student should be able to:

▼ Describe the nature, purpose, and process of the mental status examination

▼ Analyze the observations and clinical implications of each category of the mental status examination

▼ Identify commonly used psychological tests

▼ Discuss the value of behavioral rating scales in psychiatric nursing practice

TOPICAL OUTLINE

Mental Status Examination
    Eliciting Clinical Information
Content of the Examination
    Appearance
    Speech
    Motor Activity
    Interaction during the Interview
    Mood
    Affect
    Perceptions
    Thought Content
    Thought Process
    Level of Consciousness
    Memory
    Level of Concentration and Calculation
    Information and Intelligence
    Judgment
    Insight
    Documenting Clinical Information
    Mini-Mental State
Psychological Tests
Behavioral Rating Scales

Holistic psychiatric nursing care requires the nurse to complete an assessment of the patient's biological, psychological, and sociocultural health status. The part of the nursing assessment that focuses on the patient's psychological well-being should include the mental status examination. All nurses, regardless of the clinical setting, should be proficient in administering the mental status examination and be able to incorporate findings from it in the patient's plan of nursing care.

The mental status examination is a cornerstone in the evaluation of any patient with a medical, neurological, or psychiatric disorder that affects thought, emotion, or behavior. It is used to detect changes or abnormalities in a person's intellectual functioning, thought content, judgment, mood, and affect and can be used to suggest possible lesions in the brain.[2] The mental status examination is to psychiatric nursing what the physical examination is to general medical nursing.

MENTAL STATUS EXAMINATION

The mental status examination represents a cross-section of the patient's psychological life and the sum total of the nurse's observations and impressions at the moment. It also serves as a basis for future comparison to track the progress of the patient over time. The elements of the examination depend on the patient's clinical presentation, as well as the patient's educational and cultural background. It includes observing the patient's behavior and describing it in an objective, nonjudgmental manner.

The examination itself is usually divided into several parts. They can be arranged in different ways, as long as the nurse covers all the areas. Much of the information needed for the mental status examination can be gathered during the course of the routine nursing assessment. It should be integrated in the nurse's assessment in a smooth and flowing manner. Some parts of the mental status examination are completed through simple observation of the patient, such as by noting the patient's clothing or facial expressions. Other aspects require asking specific questions, such as those related to memory or attention span. Most of all, the nurse should remember that the mental status examination does not reflect how the patient was in the past or will be in the future; it is an evaluation of the patient's current state.

Information obtained during the mental status examination is used along with other objective and subjective data. These include findings from the physical examination, laboratory test results, patient history, description of the presenting problem, and information obtained from family, caregivers, and other health professionals. With these data the nurse is able to formulate nursing diagnoses and design the plan of care with the patient.

Do the nurses on the medical-surgical units routinely assess a patient's psychological status? Explain your findings given the fact that all nurses should be providing holistic, biopsychosocial nursing care.

Eliciting Clinical Information

The mental status examination requires a clinical rather than social approach to the patient. The nurse listens closely to what is said and reflects on what is not said, structuring the process in a way that allows for broad exploration of many areas for potential problems, as well as for more in-depth exploration of obvious symptoms or maladaptive coping responses. The patient is critically observed. Behaviors that the nurse might not normally attend to in more general situations must be carefully observed and described. Global and judgmental statements are not acceptable.

The skilled nurse attends to both the content and the process of the patient's communication (see Chapter 3). **Content** is the overtly communicated information. **Process** is how the communication occurs and includes feelings, intuition, and behaviors that accompany speech and thought. The content and process may not always be congruent. For example, a patient may deny feeling depressed and yet appear sad and cry. In this case, the stated message does not match the process, and the nurse should record this incongruity.

It is also important for nurses to monitor their feelings and reactions during the mental status examination. A nurse's gut reactions may signal subtle emotions being expressed by the patient. For example, a depressed patient may make the nurse feel sad, and a hostile patient may make the nurse feel threatened and angry. The nurse's feelings are useful information for the mental status assessment.

The nurse needs to be aware of these feelings and respond in a therapeutic manner toward the patient regardless of such feelings. The nurse should remain calm throughout the interview and simply reflect observations back to the patient. These observations should be related in an objective and nonthreatening manner, for example, "You are obviously quite upset about this," or "Do you feel safe here"? By conveying a sense of calm, the nurse will also demonstrate being in control, even if the patient is not.

The nurse should try to blend specific questions into the general flow of the interview. For example, questions about orientation, arithmetic problems, or proverbs may be introduced by soliciting patient comments about potential problems with concentration, memory, or understanding of written material. The nurse might then suggest that the patient try answering a few questions to determine if such problems are evident.

Finally, as with any other skill, nurses need to practice performing the mental status examination to gain proficiency and comfort. The nurse might start by observing a colleague conduct the examination. Videotapes of patient interviews are a particularly effective teaching-learning tool. The nurse should then be observed administering the mental status examination by a colleague or supervisor who can provide helpful feedback and identify ways to further enhance the nurse's competency.

CONTENT OF THE EXAMINATION

The mental status examination includes information pertaining to a number of categories (Box 6-1). It is one part of the complete psychiatric nursing assessment tool presented in Chapter 9. The content, observations, and clinical implications associated with each category are now described.[5,7] In completing this examination it is critically important that the nurse be aware that sociocultural factors can greatly influence the outcome of the examination (Box 6-2). In addition, biological expressions of psychiatric illness may also be evident in the interview process.

Box 6-1

CATEGORIES OF THE MENTAL STATUS EXAMINATION

GENERAL DESCRIPTION

Appearance
Speech
Motor activity
Interaction during interview

EMOTIONAL STATE

Mood
Affect

EXPERIENCES

Perceptions

THINKING

Thought content
Thought process

SENSORIUM AND COGNITION

Level of consciousness
Memory
Level of concentration and calculation
Information and intelligence
Judgment
Insight

Appearance

In the mental status examination the nurse takes note of the patient's general appearance. This part of the examination is intended to provide an accurate mental image of the patient as seen in the following clinical example.

 CLINICAL EXAMPLE

Mr. W is a middle-aged white man of average weight who appears older than his stated age. He was disheveled, dressed in a torn shirt and jeans, and was unshaven. He was slightly jaundiced, had a prominent red nose, and a scar on the left side of his cheek. He sat slumped in the chair and made little eye contact with the interviewer.

Observations. Areas that should be included are the following physical characteristics of the patient:
▼ Apparent age
▼ Manner of dress
▼ Cleanliness
▼ Posture
▼ Unusual gait
▼ Facial expressions
▼ Eye contact
▼ Pupil dilation or constriction
▼ General state of health and nutrition

Box 6-2

CLINICAL JUDGMENT OR SOCIOCULTURAL BIAS?

In completing the mental status examination clinicians need to be aware of the possibility of using subconscious and culturally determined criteria when judging a patient. Examples of potential sociocultural clinician bias include the following:

▼ How is the manner of dress judged? (i.e., what is unusual or expected dress?)
▼ Do all cultures accept the American norm of direct eye contact?
▼ What are the clinician's values about personal hygiene, and how do they influence assessment?
▼ Does a person's speech and use of language vary based on social class and life-style?
▼ How does body language and use of personal space vary by ethnicity and social group?
▼ Given the fact that over 20 to 30 million American adults lack basic educational skills, what is the expected "norm" regarding reading, writing, or problem-solving tasks?
▼ How "familiar" are common proverbs? Which interpretations of them are truly correct?

Clinical Implications. Dilated pupils are sometimes associated with drug intoxication, whereas pupil constriction may indicate narcotic addiction. Stooped posture is often seen in depression.

Speech

Speech is usually described in terms of rate, volume, and characteristics. Rate refers to the speed of the patient's speech, and volume refers to how loud a patient talks.

Observations. Speech can be described as follows:
▼ Rate—rapid or slow
▼ Volume—loud or soft
▼ Amount—paucity, mute, pressured
▼ Characteristics—stuttering, slurring of words, or unusual accents

Clinical Implications. Speech disturbances are often caused by specific brain disturbances. For example, mumbling may occur in patients with Huntington's chorea, and slurring of speech in intoxicated patients. Manic patients often show pressured speech, and people suffering from depression often have paucity of speech.

Motor Activity

Motor activity is concerned with the patient's physical movement.

Observations. The nurse should record the following:
▼ Level of activity—lethargic, tense, restless, or agitated
▼ Type of activity—tics, grimaces, or tremors
▼ Unusual gestures or mannerisms—compulsions

Clinical Implications. Excessive body movement may be associated with anxiety, mania, or stimulant abuse. Little body activity may suggest depression, organicity, catatonic schizophrenia, or drug-induced stupor. Tics and grimaces may suggest medication adverse effects (see Chapter 25). Repeated motor movements or compulsions may indicate obsessive-compulsive disorder. Repeated picking of lint or dirt off clothing is sometimes associated with delirium or toxic conditions.

Which category of psychotropic medications is most often associated with the adverse effects of tics and grimaces?

Interaction During the Interview

Interaction describes how the patient relates to the nurse during the interview as evident in this clinical example.

 CLINICAL EXAMPLE

The patient was interviewed in her room on the fourth day of hospitalization. She was a white woman slightly overweight, neatly dressed in jeans and a sweater, and appeared younger than her 36 years of age. Although she was cooperative, her guarded responses to all questions seemed excessively self-centered. She gave the interviewer the feeling that she didn't trust anyone and was preoccupied during the interview. When asked how other people treated her, she responded angrily, "I'd rather not say!"

Because this part of the examination relies heavily on nurses' emotional subjectivity, nurses must carefully examine their responses based on their personal and sociocultural biases. They must guard against overinterpreting or misinterpreting patients' behavior because of social or cultural differences (see Chapter 7).

Observations. Has the patient been hostile, uncooperative, irritable, guarded, apathetic, defensive, suspicious, or seductive? The nurse may explore this area by asking, "You seem irritated about something. Is that an accurate observation?"

Clinical Implications. Suspiciousness may be evident in paranoia. Irritability may suggest an anxiety disorder.

Mood

Mood is the patient's self-report of the prevailing emotional state and is a reflection of the patient's life situation.

Observations. Mood can be evaluated by asking a simple, nonleading question such as "How are you feeling today?" Does the patient report feeling sad, fearful, hopeless, euphoric, or anxious? Asking the patient to rate mood on a scale of 0 to 10 can help provide the nurse with an immediate reading of the patient's mood. It also can be valuable for comparison of changes that occur during treatment.

If the potential for suicide is suspected, the nurse should inquire regarding the patient's thoughts about self-destruction (see Chapter 18). Suicidal and homicidal thoughts must be addressed directly. Has the patient had the desire to inflict personal harm or injure someone else? Have any previous attempts been made, and if so, what events surrounded the attempts? To judge a patient's suicidal or homicidal risk, the nurse should assess the patient's plans, ability to carry out those plans (such as the availability of guns), the patient's attitude about death, and available support systems, as evident in the following clinical example.

 ## CLINICAL EXAMPLE

The patient responded to most of the questions in a flat, dull manner. Although he stated he felt sad about the recent changes in his life, his lifeless posture and tone of voice did not convey any emotional response. He denied any current suicidal or homicidal plans. He related having made two suicidal gestures in the past year by "taking pills."

Clinical Implications. Most people with depression describe feeling hopeless, and 25% of those with depression have suicidal ideation. Elation is most common in mania.

Affect

Affect is the patient's prevailing emotional tone observed by the nurse during the interview. The patient's statements of emotions and the nurse's empathic responses provide clues to the appropriateness of the affect.

Observations. Affect can be described in terms of the following:
- ▼ Range
- ▼ Duration
- ▼ Intensity
- ▼ Appropriateness

Does the patient report significant life events without any emotional response, indicating flat affect? Does the patient's response appear restricted or blunted in some way? Does the patient demonstrate great lability in expression by shifting from one affect to another quickly? Is the patient's response incongruent with speech content? For example, does the patient report being persecuted by the police and then laugh?

Clinical Implications. Labile affect is often seen in mania, and a flat, incongruent affect is often evident in schizophrenia.

Perceptions

There are two major types of perceptual problems: hallucinations and illusions. **Hallucinations** are defined as false sensory impressions or experiences. **Illusions** are false perceptions or false responses to a sensory stimulus.

Observations. Hallucinations may occur in any of the five major sensory modalities including:
- ▼ Auditory (sound)
- ▼ Visual (sight)
- ▼ Tactile (touch)
- ▼ Gustatory (taste)
- ▼ Olfactory (smell)

Command hallucinations are those that tell the patient to do something, such as to kill oneself, harm another, or join someone in afterlife. The nurse might inquire about the patient's perceptions by asking "Do you ever see or hear things"? or "Do you have strange experiences as you fall asleep or upon awakening"?

Clinical Implications. Auditory hallucinations are the most common and suggest schizophrenia. Visual hallucinations suggest organicity. Tactile hallucinations suggest organic mental disorder, cocaine abuse, and delirium tremors.

 You see in the chart that a nursing order has been written placing a patient with command hallucinations on one-to-one observation. What is the rationale for this nursing intervention?

Thought Content

Thought content refers to the specific meaning expressed in the patient's communication. It refers to the "what" of the patient's thinking.

Observations. Although the patient may talk about a variety of subjects during the interview, several content areas should be noted in the mental status examination (Box 6-3). They may be complicated and are often concealed by the patient as evident in this clinical example.

 ## CLINICAL EXAMPLE

The patient's speech was rapid, and he acknowledged feeling as if his thoughts were coming too fast, "My mind is racing ahead." The rapidity of his speech compounded the difficulty understanding him as he quickly moved

---

Box 6-3

THOUGHT CONTENT DESCRIPTORS

Delusion—false belief that is firmly maintained even though it is not shared by others and is contradicted by social reality

Religious delusion—belief that one is favored by a higher being or is an instrument of that being

Somatic delusion—belief that one's body or parts of one's body are diseased or distorted

Grandiose delusion—belief that one possesses greatness or special powers

Paranoid delusion—excessive or irrational suspiciousness and distrustfulness of others, characterized by systematized delusions that others are "out to get them" or spying on them

Thought broadcasting—delusion about thoughts being aired to the outside world

Thought insertion—delusion that thoughts are placed into the mind by outside people or influences

Depersonalization—the feeling of having lost self-identity and that things around the person are different, strange, or unreal

Hypochondriasis—somatic overconcern with and morbid attention to details of body functioning

Ideas of reference—incorrect interpretation of casual incidents and external events as having direct personal references

Magical thinking—belief that thinking equates with doing, characterized by lack of realistic relationship between cause and effect

Nihilistic ideas—thoughts of nonexistence and hopelessness

Obsession—an idea, emotion, or impulse that repetitively and insistently forces itself into consciousness, although it is unwelcome

Phobia—a morbid fear associated with extreme anxiety

---

from one topic to another in what appeared to be an unrelated manner. He denied any visual or auditory hallucinations; however, he believed that he could talk with God if he needed a consultant on his life situation. He felt this was a special blessing given to him over other men.

Tactful questioning by the nurse is needed to explore these areas. Does the patient have recurring, persistent thoughts? Is the patient afraid of certain objects or situations or worry excessively about body and health issues? Does the patient ever feel that things are strange or unreal? Has the patient ever experienced being outside of his or her body? Does the patient ever feel singled out or watched or talked about by others? Does the patient think that thoughts or actions are being controlled by an outside person or force? Does

the patient claim to have psychic or other special powers or believe that others can read the patient's mind? Throughout this part of the interview it is important that the nurse obtain information and not dispute the patient's beliefs.

Clinical Implications. Obsessions and phobias are symptoms associated with anxiety disorders. Delusions that are incongruent with mood suggest schizophrenia.

Thought Process

Thought process refers to the "how" of the patient's self-expression. A patient's thought process is observed through speech. The patterns or forms of verbalization rather than the content are assessed.

Observations. A number of problems can be assessed about a patient's thinking (Box 6-4). The nurse might ask a number of questions to evaluate the patient's thought process. Does the patient's thinking proceed in a systematic, organized, and logical manner? Is the patient's self-expression clear? Is it relatively easy for the patient to move from one topic to another?

Clinical Implications. Circumstantial thinking may be a sign of defensiveness or of paranoid thinking. Loose associations and neologisms suggest schizophrenia or other psychotic disorders. Flight of ideas indicates mania. Perseveration is often associated with brain damage and psychotic disorders. Word salad represents the highest level of thought disorganization.

Level of Consciousness

Mental status examinations routinely assess a patient's orientation to the current situation. Deciding whether or not a patient is oriented involves evaluating some basic cognitive functions.

Observations. A variety of terms can be used to describe a patient's level of consciousness, such as confused, sedated, or stuporous. In addition, the patient should be questioned regarding orientation to time, place, and person. Typically the nurse can determine this by the patient's answers to three simple questions:

1. What is your name?
2. Where are you today (such as in what city or in what particular building)?
3. What is today's date?

If the patient answers correctly the nurse can note "oriented times three." Level of orientation can be pursued in greater depth, but this area may be confounded by sociocultural factors.

Fully functioning patients may be offended by questions about orientation, so the skilled nurse should integrate questions pertaining to this area in the course of the interview and develop other ways of assessing this category. For example, the nurse could use some of the approaches listed in Box 6-5.

Clinical Implications. Patients with organic mental disorder may give grossly inaccurate answers, with orientation to person remaining intact longer than orientation to time or place. Patients with schizophrenic disorders may say that they are someone else or somewhere else or reveal a personalized orientation to the world.

Memory

A mental status examination can provide a quick screen of potential memory problems but not a definitive answer to whether a specific impairment exists. Neuropsychological assessment is required to specify the nature and extent of memory impairment. Memory is broadly defined as the ability to recall past experiences.

Observations. The following areas must be tested:
- ▼ Remote memory—recall of events, information, and people from the distant past
- ▼ Recent memory—recall of events, information, and people from the past week or so

- ▼ Immediate memory—recall of information or data to which a person was just exposed

Recall of remote events involves reviewing information from the patient's history. This part of the evaluation can be woven into the history-taking portion of the nursing assessment. This involves asking the patient questions about time and place of birth, names of schools attended, date of marriage, ages of family members, and so forth. The problem with an evaluation of the patient's remote memory is that the nurse is often unable to tell if the patient is reporting events accurately. This brings about the possibility of **confabulation,** which is when the patient makes up stories in response to situations or events that cannot be remembered. Thus the nurse may need to call on past records or the report of family or friends to confirm this historical information.

Recent memory can be tested by asking the patient to recall the events of the past 24 hours. A reliable informant may be needed to verify this information. Another test of recent memory is to ask the patient to remember three words (an object, a color, and an address) and then to repeat them 15 minutes later in the interview.

Immediate recall can be tested by asking the patient to repeat a series of numbers either forward or backward within a 10-second interval. The nurse should begin with a short series of numbers and proceed to longer lists.

Clinical Implications. Loss of memory occurs with organicity, dissociative disorder, and conversion disorder. Alzheimer's patients retain remote memory longer than recent memory. Anxiety and depression can impair immediate retention and recent memory.

Level of Concentration and Calculation

Concentration is the patient's ability to pay attention during the course of the interview. Calculation is the person's ability to do simple math. These and other areas of cognitive functioning may vary in expected and unexpected ways (Box 6-6).

Observations. The nurse should note the patient's level of distractibility. Calculation can be assessed by asking the patient to do the following:

1. Count from 1 to 20 rapidly
2. Do simple calculations, such as 2×3 or $21 + 7$
3. Serially subtract 7 from 100

If patients have difficulty subtracting 7 from 100, they can be asked to subtract 3 from 20 in the same way. Finally, more functional calculation skills can be assessed by asking practical questions such as "How many nickels are there in $1.35"?

Clinical Implications. The clinical implications of this part of the mental status examination must be carefully evaluated. Many psychiatric illnesses impair the ability to concentrate and complete simple calculations. It is particularly important to differentiate between organic mental disorder, anxiety, and depression.

Information and Intelligence

Information and intelligence are controversial areas of assessment, and the nurse should be cautious about judging intelligence after a brief and limited contact typical of the mental status examination (see Critical Thinking about Contemporary Issues). The nurse should also remember that information in this category is highly influenced by sociocultural factors of the nurse, the patient, and the treatment setting.

Observations. The nurse should assess the last grade of school completed, the patient's general fund of knowledge, and use of vocabulary. It is also critically important that the nurse assess the patient's level of literacy. The ability to conceptualize and abstract can be tested by having the patient explain a series of proverbs. The patient can be given an example of a proverb

CRITICAL THINKING ABOUT CONTEMPORARY ISSUES

Can a Person's Intellectual Functioning Be Validly Assessed in the Mental Status Examination?

The evaluation of an individual's intellectual functioning during the mental status examination has been subject to some controversy given both the brief nature of the interview and the sociocultural biases that may be brought to it. Nonetheless, knowing a patient's intellectual capacity is important to the nurse in evaluating the patient's coping resources and designing an effective treatment plan.

It has been suggested that there are three forms of intelligence[6]:

▼ Academic problem solving
▼ Practical intelligence
▼ Creative intelligence

For example, a patient may have excellent practical and creative intellectual skills as demonstrated by social competence, good street survival skills, and the ability to come up with solutions to many daily problems. However, this same patient may lack formal education and appear to have low intelligence if evaluated strictly from the perspective of academic problem-solving abilities. Thus nurses would benefit from a broader assessment of patients' intellectual functioning. This would allow them to identify the intellectual strengths, skills, and abilities of patients that may otherwise have been overlooked. ▼

with its interpretation and then asked to explain what several proverbs mean. Frequently used proverbs include the following:

▼ When it rains, it pours.
▼ A stitch in time saves nine.
▼ A rolling stone gathers no moss.
▼ The proof of the pudding is in the eating.
▼ People who live in glass houses shouldn't throw stones.
▼ A bird in the hand is worth two in the bush.

Most adults are able to interpret proverbs as symbolic of human behavior or events. However, sociocultural background should be considered when assessing a patient's information and intelligence.

If the patient's educational level is below the eighth grade, asking the patient to list similarities between a series of paired objects may better help the nurse assess the ability to abstract. The following paired objects are frequently used:

Box 6-6

SEX DIFFERENCES IN THE BRAIN

Women and men differ in physical attributes and in the way they think. It appears that the effect of sex hormones on brain organization occurs early in life, so the effects of the environment are secondary to the effects of biology. Behavioral, neurological, and endocrinologic studies help explain the processes giving rise to sex differences in the brain. Major sex differences in intellectual functioning seem to lie in patterns of ability rather than in overall level of intelligence. For example, the problem-solving tasks favored by women and men are shown below.*

PROBLEM-SOLVING TASKS FAVORING WOMEN

Women tend to perform better than men on tests of perceptual speed, in which subjects must rapidly identify matching items—for example, pairing the house on the far left with its twin:

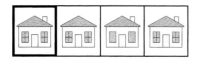

In addition, women remember whether an object, or a series of objects, has been displaced:

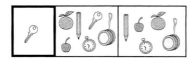

On some tests of ideational fluency, for example, those in which subjects must list objects that are the same color, and on tests of verbal fluency, in which participants must list words that begin with the same letter, women also outperform men:

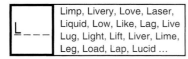

Women do better on precision manual tasks—that is, those involving fine-motor coordination—such as placing the pegs in holes on a board:

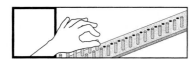

And women do better than men on mathematical calculation tests:

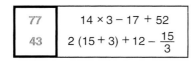

PROBLEM-SOLVING TASKS FAVORING MEN

Men tend to perform better than women on certain spatial tasks. They do well on tests that involve mentally rotating an object or manipulating it in some fashion, such as imagining turning this three-dimensional object

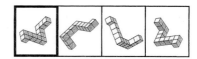

or determining where the holes punched in a folded piece of paper will fall when the paper is unfolded:

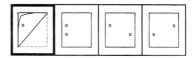

Men also are more accurate than women in target-directed motor skills, such as guiding or intercepting projectiles:

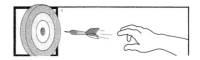

They do better on disembedding tests, in which they have to find a simple shape, such as the one on the left, once it is hidden within a more complex figure:

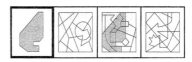

And men tend to do better than women on tests of mathematical reasoning:

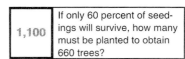

*From Kimura D: *Scientific American* 267:120, 1992 (Jared Schneidman, illustrator).

▼ Bicycle and bus
▼ Apple and pear
▼ Television and newspaper

A higher level reply would address function, while a description of structure would indicate more concrete thinking. To determine a patient's fund of general knowledge the nurse can ask the patient to name the last five presidents, the mayor, five large cities, or the occupation of a well-known person.

Clinical Implications. The patient's educational level and any learning disabilities should be carefully evaluated. Mental retardation should be ruled out whenever possible. Although the patient's level of literacy may be a general assessment, it will be an important factor in any health teaching or didactic information that is presented to the patient.

Judgment

Judgment involves making decisions that are constructive and adaptive. It involves the ability to understand facts and draw conclusions from relationships.

Observations. The patient's judgment can be evaluated by exploring a patient's involvement in activities, relationships, and vocational choices. For example, is the patient regularly involved in illegal or dangerous activities or frequently engage in destructive relationships with others? It is also useful to determine if the judgments are deliberate or impulsive. Finally, several hypothetical situations can be presented for the patient to evaluate:

1. What would you do if you found a stamped, addressed envelope lying on the ground?
2. How would you find your way out of a forest in the daytime?
3. What would you do if you entered your house and smelled gas?
4. If you won $10,000 what would you do with it?

Clinical Implications. Judgment is impaired in organic mental disorders, schizophrenia, intoxication, and borderline or below IQ.

What factors would you consider in evaluating the judgment of a man who engages in bungee jumping, rock climbing, and sky diving? How would this compare with a woman who has been in many relationships with abusive male partners?

Insight

Insight refers to the patient's understanding of the nature of the problem or illness.

Observations. It is important for the nurse to determine if the patient accepts or denies the presence of a problem or illness. In addition, the nurse should inquire whether the patient blames the problem on someone else or some external factors. Several questions may help to determine the patient's degree of insight. What does the patient think about the current situation? What does the patient want others, including the nurse, to do about it? The following clinical example illustrates a patient's level of insight.

 CLINICAL EXAMPLE

The patient described several problems he was having at work. He reluctantly stated that he might have to change, but really thought his difficulties were because of his wife's drinking. He believed he could do nothing until she changed.

Clinical Implications. Insight is impaired in organic mental disorder, psychosis, and borderline IQ and below. Whether or not a patient sees the need for treatment also critically affects the therapeutic alliance, setting of mutual goals, implementation of the treatment plan, and future adherence to it.

Documenting Clinical Information

Information from the mental status examination may be recorded in various ways. Some clinicians write a descriptive report such as the one presented in the case study on p. 154. Written reports should be brief, clear, and concise and address all categories of information. Others use an outline format that is completed with short answers. Still others use a format that is compatible with computerized information systems. Regardless of the format, important findings should be documented, and verbatim responses by the patient should be recorded whenever they add important information and support the nurse's assessment.

Mini-Mental State

There are times when it is not practical or desirable to complete a full mental status examination. On these occasions, nurses may find it helpful to use the mini-mental state examination.[3] It is a simplified scored form of the cognitive mental status examination. It consists of 11 questions, requires only 5 to 10 minutes to administer, and can therefore be used quickly and rou-

Box 6-7
MINI-MENTAL STATE

Maximum Score	Score	

ORIENTATION

5   ( )   What is the (year) (season) (date) (day) (month)?
5   ( )   Where are we (state) (county) (town) (hospital) (floor)?

REGISTRATION

3   ( )   Name three objects: Give 1 second to say each. Then ask the patient to repeat all three after you have said them.
Give 1 point for each correct answer. Then repeat them until the patient learns all three. Count trials and record.

ATTENTION AND CALCULATION

5   ( )   Serial sevens. Give 1 point for each correct. Stop after five answers. Alternatively, spell "world" backwards.

RECALL

3   ( )   Ask for three objects repeated above. Give 1 point for each correct.

LANGUAGE

9   ( )   Name a pencil and watch when pointed to (2 points)
Repeat the following, "No ifs, ands, or buts." (1 point)
Follow a three-stage command: "Take a paper in your right hand, fold it in half, and put it on the floor." (3 points)
Read and obey the following: "Close your eyes." (1 point)
Write a sentence. (1 point)
Copy design. (1 point)

Total Score _____

From Folstein M, Folstein S, McHugh P: J *Psychiatr Res* 12:189, 1975.

tinely. It is "mini" because it concentrates on only the cognitive aspects of mental functions and excludes questions concerning mood, abnormal psychological experiences, and the content or process of thinking. This examination is reproduced in Box 6-7.

PSYCHOLOGICAL TESTS

Psychological tests are of two types: those designed to evaluate intellectual and cognitive abilities and those designed to describe personality functioning. Some of these tests are described briefly in Table 6-1. Commonly used intelligence tests are the Wechsler Adult Intelligence Scale (WAIS) and the Wechsler Intelligence Scale for Children (WISC). Although intelligence tests often are criticized as culturally biased, their ability to determine an individual's strengths and weaknesses within the culture provides essential therapeutic information.

Material obtained from projective tests reflects aspects of an individual's personality function, including reality testing ability, impulse control, major defenses, interpersonal conflicts, and self-concept. A battery of tests is usually administered to provide comprehensive information. The Rorschach Test, Thematic Apperception Test (TAT), Bender Gestalt Test, and Minnesota Multiphasic Personality Inventory (MMPI) are commonly used by the clinical psychologist.

Table 6-1 Commonly Used Psychological Tests

Name	General classification	Description	Special features
Bellak Children's Apperception Test	Projective technique	Drawings of animals for children	Designed specifically for children
Bender (Visual-Motor) Gestalt Test	Graphomotor technique; may be used as projective technique	Geometric designs that the patient is asked to draw or copy, with design in view	Useful for detecting psychomotor difficulties correlated with brain damage
Draw-a-Person Test	Graphomotor projective technique	Patient asked to draw a person and then one of the sex opposite to the first drawing	Projects body image, how the body is conceived and perceived; sometimes useful for detecting brain damage; modifications include: draw an animal; draw a house, a tree, and a person (H-T-P); draw your family; draw the most unpleasant concept you can think of
Minnesota Multiphasic Personality Inventory (MMPI) (Forms: Individual, Group, and Shortened R)	Objective personality test	Questionnaire yielding scores for 9 clinical scales in addition to other scales	Includes scales related to test-taking attitudes; empirically constructed on basis of clinical criteria; computer interpretation services available
Rorschach Technique	Projective technique	Ten inkblots used as basis for eliciting associations	Especially revealing of personality structure; most widely used projective technique
Rosenzweig Picture Frustration Test	Projective technique	Cartoon situations, dialogue to be completed by subject	Designed specifically to assess patterns of reaction to typical stress situations; child, adolescent, and adult forms
Sentence Completion Test (SCT)	Varies from direct-response questionnaire to projective technique	Incomplete sentence stems that vary as to their ambiguity	Highly flexible; may be used to tap specific conflict areas; reveals generally more conscious, overt attitudes and feelings
Thematic Apperception Test (TAT)	Projective technique	Ambiguous pictures used as stimuli for making up a story	Especially useful for revealing personality dynamics; some pictures are designed specifically for women, men, adolescent girls, and adolescent boys
Wechsler Adult Intelligence Scale (WAIS)	Intelligence test	Eleven subtests: vocabulary, comprehension, information, similarities, digit span, arithmetic, picture arrangement, picture completion, object assembly, block design, and digit symbol	Most commonly used intelligence scale that yields a measure of intelligence expressed as IQ scores; differences in subtests can also be useful clinically
Wechsler Intelligence Scale for Children (WISC)	Intelligence test	Similar to the WAIS	Standardized for children ages 5 to 15
Wechsler Preschool and Primary Scale of Intelligence (WPPSI)	Intelligence test	Similar to the WAIS and WISC	Standardized for children ages 4 to 6½
Word-Association Technique	Projective technique	Stimulus words to which patient responds with first association that comes to mind	Flexible; may be used to tap associations to different conflict areas; generally not as revealing as SCT responses

Modified from Freedman AM, Kaplan HI, Sadock BJ, eds: *Comprehensive textbook of psychiatry*, ed 5, Baltimore, 1990, Williams & Wilkins.

Table 6-2 Behavioral Rating Scales

Content area	Scale	Content area	Scale
General psychiatric	Acculturation Scale Assessing Coping Strategies (COPE) Colorado Client Assessment Record (CCAR) Clinical Global Impression (CGI) Functional Status Questionnaire (FSQ) General Health Questionnaire (GHQ) Global Assessment Scale (GAS) Global Assessment of Functioning Scale (GAF) NIMH Global Consensus Rating Scales Nurse Observation Scale for Inpatient Evaluation (NOISE) Severity of Psychosocial Stressors Scale Symptoms Checklist-90 (SCL-90)	Eating disorders	Body Attitudes Test Diagnostic Survey for Eating Disorders (DSED) Eating Habits Checklist Eating Behaviors Diary Eating Disorders Inventory (EDI)
		Organic mental disorders	Alzheimer's Disease Rating Scale (ADAS) Cohen-Mansfield Agitation Inventory Blessed Dementia Scale Cornell Scale for Depression in Dementia Face-Hand Test Haycox Dementia Behavioral Scale Memory and Behavior Problem Checklist Neurobehavioral Rating Scale for Dementia (NRS)
Affective disorders	Assessment of Suicidal Potentiality Beck Depression Inventory (BDI) Carroll Self-Rating Scale Center for Epidemiologic Studies Depression Scale (CES-D) Geriatric Depression Scale (GDS) Hamilton Depression Scale (Ham-D) Inventory for Depressive Symptomatology (IDS) Manic-State Scale Montgomery-Asberg Depression Rating Scale (MADRS) Raskin Depression Scale Young Mania Scale Zung Self-Rating Depression Scale (ZSRDS)	Psychotic disorders	Andreasen Scale for Assessment of Negative Symptoms (SANS) Andreasen Scale for Assessment of Positive Symptoms (SAPS) Brief Psychiatric Rating Scale (BPRS) Life Skills Profile: Schizophrenia (LSP) University of Washington Paranoia Scale
		Substance use disorders	Addiction Severity Index (ASI) Brief Drug Abuse Screening Test (B-DAST) CAGE Clinical Institute Withdrawal Assessment-Alcohol (CIWA-AD) Michigan Alcoholism Screening Tool (MAST)
Anxiety disorders	Beck Anxiety Inventory Covi Anxiety Scale Dissociative Experience Scale Dissociative Disorders Interview Schedule (DDIS) Hamilton Rating Scale for Anxiety (Ham-A) Maudsley Obsessional Compulsive Inventory Spielberger Anxiety State-Trait Taylor Anxiety Scale Yale-Brown Obsessive Compulsive Scale (YBOC) Zung Anxiety Scale	Child/adolescent	Behavior Problems Checklist Brief Psychiatric Rating Scale for Children Child Behavior Checklist Children's Global Assessment Scale (CGAS) Competency Skills Questionnaire (CSQ) Conners Parent Rating Scale Home and School Questionnaire Self-Control Rating Scale Yale-Brown Obsessive Compulsive Scale (YBOCS) for Children
		Medication effects	Abnormal Involuntary Movement Scale (AIMS) Simpson-Angus Extrapyramidal Symptoms Scale

BEHAVIORAL RATING SCALES

The psychological context of psychiatric nursing care goes beyond the important assessment of a patient's mental status. Neither mental health nor mental illness can be measured directly. Rather, its measurement depends on gathering a number of behavioral indicators of adaptive or maladaptive responses, which together represent the overall concept.

Many behavioral rating scales and measurement tools have been designed to help clinicians do the following:

1. Measure the extent of the patient's problems
2. Make an accurate diagnosis
3. Track patient progress over time
4. Document the efficacy of treatment

Each one of these points is very important to the psychiatric nurse. The knowledge base for psychiatric care is expanding rapidly, and increased emphasis is being placed on clearly describing the nature of the patient's problems and the extent of the patient's progress toward obtaining the expected outcomes of treatment. Thus nurses must be able to demonstrate in a valid and reliable way what problems they are treating and what effect their nursing care is having on attaining the treatment goals.

Most psychiatric nurses have not routinely used behavioral rating scales in their practice, and there is little nursing literature on the subject.[1,4] Nonetheless, this is a critical area for contemporary psychiatric nursing practice. Nurses should become familiar with the many standardized rating scales that are available to enhance each stage of the nursing process. Some of the more commonly used behavioral rating scales are listed in Table 6-2. Any of these scales can be used by nurses with training. If the scales are to be used by a group of nurses, such as nurses working together in a specific treatment program or facility, interrater reliability among the nurses should be established.

These tools should not replace required nursing documentation. Rather, they can be used to complement nursing care and provide measurable indicators of treatment outcome. For example, if the nurse is caring for a patient with depression it would be useful to use one of the depression rating scales with the patient at the beginning of treatment. This would establish a baseline profile of the patient's symptoms and help confirm the diagnosis. The nurse might then administer the same scale at various times during the course of treatment to measure the patient's progress. Finally, completing the rating scale at the end of treatment would document the efficacy of the care provided.

The increasing focus in health care on high quality, cost containment, and documented effectiveness requires that psychiatric nurses be able to demonstrate the value of the services they provide. The psychological context of psychiatric nursing care suggests both the tools and the process nurses can use to meet this challenge.

 ## CASE STUDY

Ms. T was a stylishly dressed, neatly groomed, slender female in apparent good physical health who appeared her stated 22 years of age. She was cooperative during the interview but had difficulty expressing herself in specific terms. Her vague responses at times left the interviewer feeling perplexed about the difficulties she was describing.

The patient was alert and awake and oriented to person, place, and situation. Immediate recall and recent memory were intact, demonstrated in her ability to recall three unrelated objects immediately and again in 15 minutes. Some of the historical information given was inconsistent with historical facts reported by her father. Although the vocabulary used by Ms. T and her knowledge of general information was congruent with her twelfth-grade education and past employment, she had difficulty completing the serial sevens but performed serial threes with relative ease. She stated she was "nervous," which may be a factor related to performance. She was able to abstract two of three proverbs presented.

Proverb	Interpretation
Don't cry over spilled milk.	"If something happens, then forget about it. Maybe things will get better."

| A rolling stone gathers no moss. | "A good person gathers no enemies. If a person stays active, he won't get depressed." |
| People who live in glass houses shouldn't throw stones. | "The glass will break." |

Her responses to hypothetical situations were appropriate; however, the manner in which she coped with difficulties at work and home showed impaired judgment about personal issues.

Ms. T's speech was clear, coherent, and of normal rate and tone. Except for the vague tangential manner in which she discussed her concern for her aunt, her communication was goal directed. There were no apparent delusions, hallucinations, or illusions. She denied any obsessions, compulsions, or phobias.

The central theme during the interview was her fear of being irresponsible and hurting her aunt. Her sadness and concern about her behavior in relation to the aunt pervaded the interview. She appeared nervous (looking away, fidgeting) and cried whenever she talked about her aunt. She described her mood as "low" and rated it as a 4 on a scale of 1 to 10. She denied any suicidal or homicidal ideas or plan previously or at the present time.

Her insight was questionable, since she debated her need for treatment, although she agreed to return. She knew a problem existed but was unaware of the causative factors related to her behavior. ▼

SUMMARY

1. The mental status examination represents a cross-section of the patient's psychological life at that point in time. It requires that the nurse observe the patient's behavior and describe it in an objective, nonjudgmental manner.

2. The categories assessed in the mental status examination include the patient's appearance, speech, motor activity, mood, affect, interaction during the interview, perceptions, thought content, thought process, level of consciousness, memory, level of concentration and calculation, information and intelligence, judgment, and insight.

3. Psychological tests evaluate intellectual and cognitive abilities and describe personality functioning.

4. Behavioral rating scales help clinicians measure the extent of the patient's problem, make an accurate diagnosis, track patient progress over time, and document the efficacy of treatment. They should be used by psychiatric nurses to complement nursing care and provide measurable indicators of treatment outcome.

REFERENCES

1. Acron S: Use of the brief psychiatric rating scale by nurses, J *Psychosoc Nurs Ment Health Serv* 31:9, 1993.
2. Dilsaver S: The mental status examination, *Am Fam Physician* 41:1489, 1990.
3. Folstein M, Folstein S, McHugh P: Mini-mental state: a practical method for grading the cognitive state of patients for the clinician, J *Psychiatr Res* 12:189, 1975.
4. McGorry P, Goodwin R, Stuart G: The development, use, and reliability of the brief psychiatric rating scale (nursing modification)—an assessment procedure for the nursing team in clinical and research settings, *Compr Psychiatry* 29:575, 1988.
5. Sommers-Flanagan J, Sommers-Flanagan R: *Foundations of therapeutic interviewing*, Boston, 1992, Allyn & Bacon.
6. Sternberg R, Wagner R: *Practical intelligence: origins of competence in the everyday world*, New York, 1986, Cambridge University Press.
7. Trzepacz P, Baker R: *The psychiatric mental status examination*, New York, 1993, Oxford University Press.

ANNOTATED SUGGESTED READINGS

*Acron S: Use of the brief psychiatric rating scale by nurses, J *Psychosoc Nurs Ment Health Serv* 31:9, 1993.
 One of the few articles in the field to discuss the use of rating scales by nurses. Describes the BPRS and its use by psychiatric nurses.

Baker F: Screening tests for cognitive impairment, *Hosp Community Psychiatry* 40:339, 1989.
 Reviews five easily administered tests to screen for cognitive impairment.

*Bethot B, Lapierre E: What does it mean? A new scale for rating patients' behavior, J *Psychosoc Nurs Ment Health Serv* 27:25, 1989.
 Reports on the development and use of the Psychiatric Symptom Assessment Scale for assessing the symptomatology of patients with schizophrenia.

Dunner D: Diagnostic assessment, *Psychiatr Clin North Am* 16:431, 1993.
 Excellent overview of structured interviews and behavioral rating scales used in psychiatry.

Grotevant H, Carlson C: *Family assessment: a guide to methods and measures*, New York, 1989, The Guilford Press.
 Comprehensive presentation with detailed descriptions and critiques of current measurement tools in the field of family studies.

McDowell I, Ottawa C: *Measuring health: a guide to rating scales and questionnaires*, New York, 1987, Oxford University Press.
 Reviews the current status of health measurements and describes leading scales and questionnaires related to general well-being, symptoms of illness, and functional abilities.

*McGorry P, Goodwin R, Stuart G: The development, use, and reliability of the brief psychiatric rating scale (nursing modification)—an assessment procedure for the nursing team in clinical and research settings, *Compre Psychiatry* 29:575, 1988.
 Reports on training nurses to use the BPRS based on the belief that nurses should engage in systematic ratings of patient psychopathology.

Morrison J: *The first interview: a guide for clinicians*, New York, 1993, The Guilford Press.
 Good, clear discussion of interviewing with psychiatric patients.

Sommes-Flanagan J, Sommers-Flanagan R: *Foundations of therapeutic interviewing*, Boston, 1992, Allyn & Bacon.
 Excellent overview of points to consider in interviewing patients, including the mental status examination.

*Nursing reference.

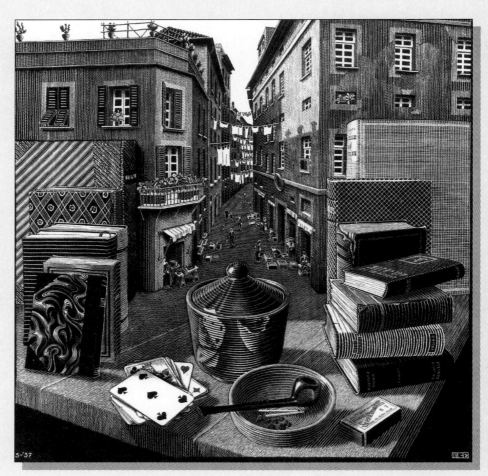

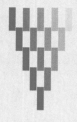

CHAPTER 7

Sociocultural Context of Psychiatric Nursing Care

LINDA D. OAKLEY

We know what we belong to, where we come from, and where we are going.
We may not know it with our brains, but we know it with our roots.

Noel Coward: This Happy Breed

LEARNING OBJECTIVES

After studying this chapter the student should be able to:

▼ Describe the qualities of a culturally sensitive psychiatric nurse

▼ Discuss the importance of the sociocultural risk factors of age, ethnicity, gender, education, income, and belief system in developing, experiencing, and recovering from psychiatric disorders

▼ Identify sociocultural stressors that hinder the delivery of quality psychiatric care

▼ Analyze the impact of sociocultural factors on coping responses

▼ Apply knowledge of sociocultural risk factors to the process of nursing assessment and diagnosis

▼ Discuss the treatment implications of culturally sensitive psychiatric care

TOPICAL OUTLINE

Cultural Sensitivity
Sociocultural Risk Factors
  Age
  Ethnicity
  Gender
  Education
  Income
  Belief System
Sociocultural Stressors
Impact on Coping Responses
Nursing Assessment and Diagnosis
Treatment Implications
  Counseling
  Family Systems
  Religion
  Psychobiology

Holistic psychiatric nursing care embraces all aspects of the individual in the assessment, diagnosis, and treatment process. An important element of this holistic perspective is the nurse's sensitivity to the sociocultural context of care. In each interaction with the patient the nurse is aware of the broader world in which the patient lives and knows that the perception of health and illness, help-seeking behavior, and treatment adherence depend on the individual's unique beliefs, social norms, and cultural values. Consequently, quality psychiatric nursing care must incorporate the unique aspects of the individual into every element of practice.

Knowledge of culture and its impact on mental health is gradually unfolding, and nurses need to keep abreast of new information and the implications it may have in psychiatric nursing practice.

CULTURAL SENSITIVITY

In recent years greater attention has focused on culturally relevant mental health care.[8,11,21] Nursing expectations are also evolving from a superficial knowledge of differences in age, sex, and ethnic groups to the implementation of culturally sensitive nursing care.[28,38]

Culturally sensitive nurses have the awareness, knowledge, and skills to intervene successfully in the lives of patients from culturally diverse backgrounds. They are able to view each patient as a unique individual while also considering the common developmental challenges faced by all people along with the specific experiences of the patient's particular cultural background. The nurse then applies this information in nursing interventions that are consistent with the life experiences and cultural values of patients.

Finally, culturally sensitive nurses are in touch with their own personal and cultural experiences as unique human beings who happen to be caring professionals. These nurses provide individualized patient care and are aware of actions that may potentially offend a patient who is not a member of the nurses' ethnic, social, or cultural group.[37] The culturally sensitive nurse understands the importance of social and cultural forces on the individual, realizes the uniqueness of these aspects, respects nurse-patient differences, and incorporates sociocultural information into psychiatric nursing care. Understanding cultural diversity, therefore, encompasses many skills that are a part of the repertoire of good psychiatric nurses—empathizing with the patient, questioning the validity of personal perceptions and assumptions, attaining mutuality, and continually evaluating and reassessing their analysis and treatment plan.

SOCIOCULTURAL RISK FACTORS

The concept of risk factors is important to understanding how people acquire, experience, and recover from illness. Risk factors are the same as the predisposing factors that nurses assess in the stress adaptation model of psychiatric nursing (see Chapter 4). They include specific traits, variables, and qualities of a person that both define who a person is and help to explain responses to external events. Understanding the risk factors involved in health and illness has helped in the prevention, early detection, and effective treatment of people with a variety of physiological illnesses such as cardiac, pulmonary, and hepatic diseases.

Identifying risk factors also is valuable when providing psychiatric care. Risk factors for psychiatric disorders refer to those characteristics of an individual that can significantly increase the potential for developing a psychiatric disorder, significantly decrease the potential for recovery, or both. Perhaps the most important outcome associated with the inclusion of risk or predisposing factors in the nurse's practice is the development of individualized, culturally sensitive, and socially relevant mental health care.

A variety of demographic, biological, psychological, social, and cultural factors have been associated with psychiatric disorders among various population groups.

The sociocultural perspective of risk factors described in this chapter focuses on age, ethnicity, gender, education, income, and belief system. No one or two of these factors alone adequately describes the sociocultural context of nursing care; however, together they provide a sociocultural profile of the patient that is essential to quality psychiatric nursing practice. These risk factors determine social norms, cultural beliefs, and personal values, as well as influence the patient's exposure to stressors, appraisal of stressors, coping resources, and coping responses as described in the stress adaptation model (Fig. 7-1).

The sociocultural risk factors of age, ethnicity, gender, education, income, and belief system are predisposing, or conditioning, factors that influence the amount and type of coping resources available to an individual. These risk factors do not cause future events. For example, being female may be a predisposing factor for the development of depression, but it does not *cause* depression. In fact, some of these factors may be a consequence of the illness. For example, being poor may be the result of a substance abuse disorder rather than the cause of it. These risk factors are important because they influence the individual's vulnerability to, development of, and recovery from a variety of psychiatric disorders. Finally, it is important to realize that these sociocultural risk factors can interact so that different factors become important at different times for the individual.

This sociocultural view does not assume that individual members of groups based on age, ethnicity, gender, education, income, or belief systems will all have

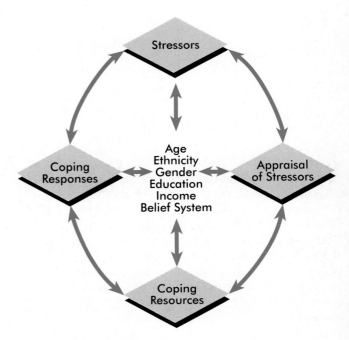

Fig. 7-1 Sociocultural context of psychiatric care.

the same risk of developing a psychiatric disorder. Neither does it assume that an individual's risk for developing a psychiatric disorder is constant. Rather, individual differences between the members of a group and contextual variations in individual risk are key principles of this perspective. Most important, this view does not draw generalizations about groups based on age, ethnicity, gender, education, income, or belief system. Literature that describes and summarizes the values or beliefs of specific populations such as blacks, Hispanics, and Asians often creates new stereotypes, and these generalizations can further depersonalize nursing care. In contrast, the sociocultural view of psychiatric disorder risk factors is based on the assessment and reassessment of risk factors for each person over time as change occurs within the individual and within the social environment.

Important health-related differences do exist between various groups in society. Group differences have been reported and examined in relation to a number of physical and psychiatric illnesses.[30] For example, researchers have noted that more females than males are diagnosed and treated for depression regardless of age, ethnicity, education, or income.[7,18] Findings such as this have led to the development of epidemiological and social models of psychiatric disorders that focus on group differences rather than on individual risk. Yet some researchers have questioned the usefulness of this approach because it is not known whether the different prevalence of a psychiatric disorder between groups is an indicator of clinical differences, cultural differences, or both.[31]

Specifically, it is not known whether the prevalence of depression among females is greater than that among males because the two groups are clinically different or because females are exposed to more social or cultural stressors that precipitate depression. If the latter were true, it would suggest that if males were exposed to the same stressors and were taught the same coping style as females, the rate of depression for the two groups would, theoretically, be equal.

This example also highlights other limitations of epidemiological and social models of psychiatric illness including the incorrect assumption that all members of a group behave, think, and feel similarly. Finally, this approach can discount the importance of biological, psychological, and cultural contributions and the need to integrate all these areas to understand more fully the dimensions of mental health and psychiatric illness.

Much research on sociocultural risk factors for psychiatric disorders is relevant to psychiatric nursing practice. However, the scope of the field is beyond that of this chapter, so the nurse is referred to other sources for more detailed information.[8,11,19] Some findings related to each risk factor, as well as their possible effects on holistic psychiatric nursing care, are described in the following sections. Box 7-1 provides some sociocultural trends and their influences on the health-care system.

> Think of a group you belong to based on one of your sociocultural characteristics. What stereotypes exist about this group, and do you, as an individual, fit these stereotypes?

Box 7-1

SOCIOCULTURAL DIVERSITY AND THE HEALTH-CARE SYSTEM

Current U.S. data suggest the following sociocultural trends will influence the health-care system and the way health care is provided:

1. The population will increase by 60% to almost 400 million by the year 2050.
2. Growth will be concentrated at the two ends of the age spectrum. By 2050 the population aged 65 and over will more than double, and the population 85 years and older will be the fastest-growing age group.
3. The U.S. population is becoming more diverse by race and ethnicity. Hispanics will be the largest ethnic group, making up one quarter of the population.
4. The United States has become a predominantly urban nation with the population occupying only 2.5% of the land mass.

These trends will have a profound impact on the health-care system for the following reasons:

1. As the aging population grows, there will be an increase in chronic conditions and chronic diseases related to behavior that will exact a greater toll on the health-care system.
2. A rise in the number of young people will bring new waves of problems typically committed by the young, such as murder, rape, robbery, and assault. Almost half of all violent crimes are committed by people under age 24, with those 15 to 19 years of age responsible for most. The overall crime rate has increased 500% since 1960.
3. Minority populations are currently underserved, a problem that may only intensify. In addition, there is an expected increase in low–birth weight babies among the minority populations.
4. Minority populations are underrepresented in all health-care professions, causing concern about whether health-care providers will understand health problems within a cultural context and be able to provide culturally sensitive care.

From *Advances*, Newsletter of the Robert Wood Johnson Foundation, Fall 1993.

Age

It has been reported that the frequency of seeking mental health treatment decreases with age and that help-seeking behavior peaks between 25 and 44 years of age and then declines.[23] It has also been observed that persons over 65 are more likely to seek help for psychiatric symptoms from nonpsychiatrists.[14]

A recent review examining the major factors related to depression in the elderly revealed the importance of a variety of social factors.[20] Among the elderly the prevalence of depression in women is higher than in men, and elders with high socioeconomic status and levels of education were less likely to be depressed than those with low socioeconomic status and less education. Thus female sex, low income, and less education were identified as risk factors for depression in the elderly.

Although the relationship between ethnicity and depression in the elderly was not clear, the relationship between age and depression was; as age increased, the prevalence of depression decreased. Even when compared with younger age groups, elders tended to recover from depression more quickly and were less likely to have a recurrence. Thus younger age emerged as a risk factor for depressive illness, possibly because elders who are socioeconomically stable may also be more resilient to depression, since they may have developed effective coping strategies and have less demanding or less stressful social roles than younger adults.[16]

Ethnicity

The term *ethnicity* as used in this chapter includes an individual's racial, national, tribal, linguistic, or cultural origin or background. Ethnicity has been shown to influence the development of and recovery from psychiatric disorders. Specifically, significant differences exist in the prevalence of certain disorders among various ethnic groups and in their use of mental health services. For example, the most severe labels of psychopathology tend to be diagnosed in black patients, with blacks being underrepresented in affective disorders and overdiagnosed as schizophrenic.[25] In addition, blacks and Native Americans have much higher admission rates to state and county mental hospitals than other ethnic groups. Hispanics have the next highest rate, and Asians have rates lower than all other groups.[33]

Regarding the use of mental health services, one study sampled almost 27,000 adults and found that Asians, Hispanics, and whites tended to use outpatient mental health services, whereas blacks tended to use emergency mental health services.[15] Significant differences were found in use based on sex and education. Asian, Hispanic, and white females used more services than their male counterparts, thereby improving their probability of recovery. However, the reverse was true for blacks; black males used more mental health services than black females. In terms of education, utilization rates were highest for Asians and Hispanics with less than 8 years of education. The reverse was true for blacks and whites. The highest utilization rate of mental health services was among blacks with 12 years of education and whites with more than 12 years of education. In terms of age, adults between the ages of 25 and 44 had the highest utilization rates for all ethnic groups.

The authors concluded that because blacks relied on emergency services that are often very brief, they tended to receive less treatment than those in other ethnic groups. In a similar study that included a measure of improvement in patient functioning after treatment, blacks showed the lowest rate of positive treatment outcome despite a high utilization rate and the fact that the patients and providers were members of the same ethnic group.

 How might ethnicity influence a patient's maladaptive responses and the specific symptoms expressed?

Gender

As a predisposing risk factor, gender is similar to ethnicity in that at first glance there appear to be distinctive male and female patterns of risk. However, when all psychiatric disorders are included, the prevalence of mental illness among males and females is relatively equal.[3] The actual difference between the two groups is in the type of disorder that is most commonly diagnosed. Substance abuse and antisocial personality disorder are the most prevalent psychiatric disorders among males, whereas mood disorders and somatization disorders are most prevalent among females. In contrast, the prevalence of schizophrenia and manic episodes for males and females is about equal.

These findings support the idea that male and female role socialization in contemporary American society is a significant determinant of the perception of health and illness and that the risk for psychiatric disorder may be sex typed by sociocultural factors. Specifically, it has been proposed that males are taught to aggressively externalize their psychological experiences, whereas females are taught to passively internalize their social experiences.

In a study aimed at measuring gender differences in schizophrenia, the authors found that males and females had the same psychiatric disorder but that for females, femininity may have delayed the onset of severe symptoms.[6] Specifically the mean age of disorder onset was 41 years for females and 31 years for males. This is an important difference because the age of onset is a critical factor in the prognosis for schizophrenia, in that early onset is associated with a longer course of illness and poorer treatment outcome. Thus men have a poorer prognosis for schizophrenia than do women in terms of both symptoms and course of illness. There is also evidence that men face a less tolerant social reaction to functional impairment and may experience greater pressure to assume social responsibilities.[13]

This study also illustrates the interactions of risk factors; gender appears to be significant in the development of schizophrenia, but age seems to be more important than gender in recovery from the illness. A similar relationship between early onset and more difficult course of illness has been reported for male and female depression. Specifically, as compared with males, females develop depression at an earlier age and have longer episodes of depression once diagnosed with the disorder.[34]

The following clinical example demonstrates the interaction of ethnicity and gender and the way in which they can affect a person's response to stress.

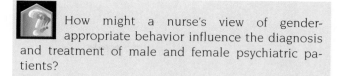

How might a nurse's view of gender-appropriate behavior influence the diagnosis and treatment of male and female psychiatric patients?

Education

Mental status examinations are often used to determine diagnosis and treatment for various psychiatric disorders. A study was conducted to compare the scores of black and white patients on the mini-mental state examination in an effort to determine if education level influenced scores on a measure of dementia.[27] For both blacks and whites, individuals with less than an eighth grade education had higher scores for dementia than subjects with ninth grade or higher education. Studies have also reported that education is more important than income in determining use of mental health services. Those with the highest educational level used mental health services most often.[14]

The clinical example that follows illustrates the effect ethnicity, gender, and education can have on an individual's ability to interact with others effectively.

CLINICAL EXAMPLE

Jose Rodriguez is a 36-year-old Hispanic man. Jose planned to graduate from a MBA program in May and marry his fiancee, Lisa, in June. The couple met in class 2 years ago and have dated for 1 year. Jose visited Lisa's family for the first time during spring break. Lisa's parents are of German descent, and they were shocked when Lisa told them she planned to marry Jose in 3 months. Lisa's father informed her that if she goes through with her wedding plans he will disown her. He said that her mother and brothers agreed with him and that she had to choose between Jose and her family. When she told Jose about her father's reaction he felt they should leave immediately, but Lisa said she could not go with him if it meant going against her family.

Jose drove back to school and on the way was cited twice for speeding. When he returned to his room he spent 2 days alone drinking beer. He did not shave, shower, or change his clothes. On the third day he went out for more beer and while walking past a group of men, one of them called him a "dirty wetback." When Jose got home he destroyed his room and everything in it, including his completed master's thesis, which he needed to hand in the next day in order to graduate in May.

CLINICAL EXAMPLE

Ms. Wong is a 22-year-old Chinese-American woman. She is employed at a university computer center and is a part-time law student. Her roommate is a second-year English major and has an active social life. Because her courses are demanding and her family expects her to be successful, Ms. Wong spends all of her free time studying. While studying one Friday afternoon, her roommate came home with several friends, including a young man from Ms. Wong's law class that she thought was very attractive. She was excited about seeing him and acted extremely friendly toward him until she realized that he was her roommate's date for the evening. Ms. Wong felt humiliated by her behavior and abruptly left the apartment. As she was leaving, she heard her roommate say, "Now that Miss Perfect is gone, we can party."

Ms. Wong did not know what to do or in whom to confide. She walked around town for hours. Although she was becoming exhausted, she did not stop to rest, eat, or drink. She continued to walk and smiled at the romantic couples she passed, but became sad again when they did not smile back at her. Ms. Wong noticed a wig store across the street from where she stood and went in and bought a curly blonde wig that she immediately put on. She wore this wig everyday since then and insisted that from now on everyone call her Patty, her new American name.

Income

The negative effects of poverty on mental health are severe regardless of age, ethnicity, or gender, as evidenced by many community surveys that report a relationship between lower economic status and higher level of psychiatric symptoms.[5] However, the prevalence of poverty among women, elders, and ethnic minorities is significant. Some researchers believe that the difference in risk for psychiatric disorders between groups is primarily a measure of social stratification and poverty, with those at the bottom facing more daily problems than those at the top.[32] Others suggest that the combination of poverty with other risk factors such as gender and ethnicity predicts both the onset of stress-related psychiatric disorders and the use of mental health services.[4]

The following clinical example describes the effect of ethnicity and income on self-esteem.

 ## CLINICAL EXAMPLE

John Willis is a 20-year-old black man. He has been looking for work since he graduated from high school 2 years ago and has had several job interviews with local employers. Over the phone, all of these employers seemed very interested in hiring John, but he never received a job offer. Each time he called back after an interview, he was told that the position had been filled and that his application would be kept on file. Last fall, John obtained an interview for an entry position at a local bank. He felt that his luck had changed and this would be the perfect job for him.

He arrived early for his interview, and after waiting an hour to meet with the interviewer, John was told that the position had been filled. John was very surprised to hear this. He felt that he had not been treated fairly and that the interviewer just wanted to look him over and decided that he did not like what he saw. John asked the interviewer, "Did the position get filled before or after I got here, or don't you know that either?" The interviewer alerted security and asked John to leave. John was angry and embarrassed and asked the interviewer why he was being treated like a criminal when he came here to apply for a job. Before the interviewer could answer, John left the building. Since then, John has refused to look for work or go to another interview. He has been unemployed for 2 years and continues to live with his parents, sleeping until noon everyday and spending all of his time "hanging out" with his male friends.

 Most single-parent households in this country are headed by women, and many of them are below the poverty level. What implications might this have for the mental health of the children living in these situations?

Belief System

A person's belief system, worldview, religion, or spirituality can also have a positive or negative impact on mental health. Human beings in general have a need to make sense out of and explain their life experiences. This is especially true when suffering or in distress. In the process of this quest for meaning, culturally determined belief systems play a vital role in determining whether a particular explanation and associated treatment plan will have meaning to the patient and others in the patient's social network. Incompatibility between the patient's and provider's belief systems often determines the patient's satisfaction with treatment, medication compliance, and treatment outcome.[12]

Adaptive belief system responses can enhance well-being, improve the quality of life, and speed recovery from illness. Maladaptive belief system responses may lead to poor adjustment to changing health status, refusal of necessary treatment, or even self-injury. For example, a strong relationship exists between certain religious beliefs and the avoidance of alcohol, illicit drugs, and cigarette smoking. Spiritually based intervention programs, such as 12-step programs, which encourage the individual to surrender control to an external supreme being, are commonly used treatments for addictive disorders.

Another indicator of the importance of a belief system emerges from a study of suicide and religious beliefs in which it was found that suicide was inversely related to religious commitment for women but not for men. Still other research reports that being Catholic does not reduce suicide rates except when Catholics live in a Catholic culture. These studies suggest that integration into a larger shared social belief system may be an important factor in mental health and well-being.[19]

In summary, age, ethnicity, gender, education, income, and belief system are psychiatric disorder risk factors that can increase the onset of psychiatric illness and decrease the likelihood of a positive treatment outcome. In particular, age, ethnicity, and gender become powerful risk factors for psychiatric illness when combined with poverty and low education.

> Think about two patients you took care of last week. Did you discuss with them their belief systems about their health and current illnesses? How might this information have influenced your nursing interventions with them?

SOCIOCULTURAL STRESSORS

Some of the sociocultural stressors that hinder the delivery of quality psychiatric care are listed in Table 7-1. Disadvantagement creates profound problems in the prevention, diagnosis, and treatment of psychiatric disorders. In addition to lacking basic resources, individuals who are poor and poorly educated are often stereotyped in society as freeloaders or lazy. Such individuals are often the focus of other negative attitudes and behaviors such as intolerance, stigma, prejudice, discrimination, and racism.

For example, consider a woman who is obese. In American society thinness is highly valued and obesity is stigmatized regardless of the person's ethnicity or age. However, obese males are stigmatized less than obese females. Despite the fact that the fashion industry now markets to the "big woman," "big" has yet to be-

Table 7-1 Sociocultural Stressors

Stressor	Definition
Disadvantagement	The lack of socioeconomic resources that are basic to biopsychosocial adaptation
Stereotype	A depersonalized conception of individuals within a group
Intolerance	Unwillingness to accept different opinions or beliefs from people of different backgrounds
Stigma	An attribute or trait deemed by the individual's social environment as different and diminishing
Prejudice	A preconceived, unfavorable belief about individuals or groups that disregards knowledge, thought, or reason
Discrimination	Differential treatment of individuals or groups not based on actual merit
Racism	The belief that inherent differences among the races determine individual achievement and that one race is superior.

come an acceptable standard of femininity in contemporary society. In addition, while obese women and men may encounter the same amount of employment discrimination, obese women are often also viewed as asexual because of their failure to follow the social rule of thinness as a norm of female sexuality. As a result, in comparison to the overweight or obese male, obese females are more likely to be single. Since married and partnered adults consistently report less stress than adults who are single or divorced, it is evident that sociocultural attitudes and values serve as stressors and increase the risk of psychiatric disorders for some individuals in society.

Racism is another sociocultural impediment in which, by virtue of ethnicity alone, an individual can be exposed to significant stress.[29] For example, consider the impact of racism on individuals with hypertension, which affects 25% of blacks in this country. A study aimed at measuring the association between anger and blood pressure reactivity found that anger related to racism increased the systolic and diastolic blood pressures of black students more than anger that was not related to racism.[1] The relationship between racism and psychiatric disorders has not yet been tested, but the relationship between stress and psychiatric disorders has been demonstrated, and for ethnic minorities, racism is a significant sociocultural stressor.

IMPACT ON COPING RESPONSES

The coping responses used by individuals and the ways in which symptoms of mental illness are expressed also vary according to culture. Coping responses and the meaning assigned to them are greatly influenced by sociocultural norms, values, beliefs, and expectations. Symptoms that indicate a problem in the context of one group may be tolerated or even ignored by another group for two reasons.[9] First, if a behavior or symptom is widespread, it may be considered normal. Second, if the behavior fits in with social values it may similarly be accepted. For example, hallucinations in Western society are considered a sign of serious illness because the social values emphasize rationality and control. In contrast, visions, hexes, and hearing voices are not necessarily considered signs of psychosis among other cultures, nor is communicating with the dead. In addition, some cultural groups would view symptoms typically associated with mental illness as signs of normality, meanness, laziness, sin, or spiritual distress.

Finally, there are many culture-specific ways of expressing distress. For example, black schizophrenic patients have been observed to show more anger and suspicion toward others than white schizophrenic patients. For some black patients, anger and suspicion are coping responses to chronic sociocultural stress. This coping response may be ineffective, however, in that anger and suspicion do not necessarily decrease feelings of distress, nor signal to others the need for support.

Still other questions are raised by observed cross-cultural differences in the ratio of cases of major depression to bipolar disorders, with Western nations showing a 4:1 ratio compared with a 1:1 ratio in more traditional, alcohol-free cultures. These differences raise diagnostic questions and concerns about cultural factors that may mask or accentuate symptoms.

NURSING ASSESSMENT AND DIAGNOSIS

Cultural self-awareness is an essential first step for the psychiatric nurse in the delivery of culturally sensitive nursing care.[17] To prepare to be culturally responsive to a patient, the nurse should answer the following questions:

   ▼ What about the patient's appearance or behavior makes me think that what I am seeing or hearing is pathological?
   ▼ What label am I subconsciously applying to this patient and where did it come from?
   ▼ What social class am I assuming this patient comes from and what are my prejudices about that group?
   ▼ What other explanations might account for this patient's unusual behavior?
   ▼ What personal characteristics of the patient have I noted and what are my positive and negative reactions to those characteristics?

In effect, psychiatric nurses need to qualify their clinical assessments by offering cultural explanations for their patients' problems.

Assessment of the patient's sociocultural risk factors and stressors greatly enhances the nurse's ability to establish a therapeutic alliance, identify the patient's problems, and develop a psychiatric nursing treatment plan that is accurate, appropriate, and culturally relevant. Box 7-2 presents questions the nurse might ask related to each of the risk factors described in this chapter.

A culturally sensitive psychiatric nursing diagnosis takes into account sociocultural risk factors and stressors that affect the patient's coping responses. Often, nurses exclude sociocultural information in their analysis because they want to avoid stereotyping the patient, feel that the patient's health-care problems are not related to the patient's age, ethnicity, gender, income, education, or belief system, or incorrectly assume that the patient shares their worldview. However, sociocultural information must be included in each and every phase of the nursing process because it has a significant influence on the patient's adaptive or maladaptive coping responses. Talking to patients about their sociocultural attitudes, feelings, beliefs, and experiences will not stereotype individuals, but not talking to patients about these important areas of their lives will.

> Do you think it is possible that two patients displaying the same symptoms could receive two different diagnoses based on the sociocultural factors of age, ethnicity, and gender of either the patient or the clinician?

TREATMENT IMPLICATIONS

There is growing awareness that the psychotherapeutic treatment process is influenced by the cultural and ethnic context of both the patient and the health-care provider (see Critical Thinking about Contemporary Issues). In terms of treatment planning, it is clear that the psychiatric nurse needs to be sensitive to sociocultural issues but also must transcend them. Together, the nurse and patient need to agree on the nature of the patient's coping responses, the means for solving problems, and the expected outcomes of treatment. A central responsibility of the nurse is to understand what the illness means to the patient and the way in which the patient's belief system can help to mediate the stressful events or make them easier to bear by redefining them as opportunities for personal growth.

Counseling

Culturally responsive counseling strategies should consider ethnic identity and acculturation, family influences, sex-role socialization, religious and spiritual influences, and immigration experiences.[21] In addition, sociocultural differences between the nurse and patient can be a source of misunderstanding by the nurse and resistance by the patient. Alternatively, these differences can serve as a vehicle for discussing important issues in counseling, thereby enriching the experience for both members of the therapeutic relationship.[2]

Family Systems

Family systems can be major sources of strength for persons with mental illness, and nurses should view them as allies and integral components of the treatment process. Families can provide an important economic and emotional buffer against the burden imposed by the patient's illness and allow the patient a supportive environment for recovery.

Box 7-2

QUESTIONS RELATED TO SOCIOCULTURAL RISK FACTORS

AGE

Questions

What is the patient's current stage of development?

What are the developmental tasks of the patient?

Are those tasks age-appropriate for the patient?

What are the patient's attitudes and beliefs regarding the patient's specific age group?

With what age-related stressors is the patient currently coping?

What impact does the patient's age have on mental and physical health?

Example

Assessment. Jim is 38 years old and trying to come to terms with balancing his need for intimacy with that of finding his own identity and sense of purpose in life. He describes feelings of anxiety along with waves of hopelessness. He states, "At my age I should stop acting like I'm twenty-something and accept myself, but I just can't seem to do that."

Analysis. Jim is worried that he will never settle down into an adult life-style, but he is more afraid of the high stress and loss of social attractiveness that he associates with being middle-aged.

ETHNICITY

Questions

What is the patient's ethnic background?

What is the patient's ethnic identity?

Is the patient traditional, bicultural, multicultural, or culturally alienated?

What are the patient's attitudes, beliefs, and values regarding the patient's specific ethnic group?

With what ethnic-related stressors is the patient currently coping?

What impact does the person's ethnicity have on mental and physical health?

Example

Assessment. Landa is a black woman. She strongly endorses African-American values and considers herself to be culturally traditional. Landa believes that African-American values are superior to Western values and that there would be less poverty and crime in black communities if all black people shared her beliefs. She spends much of her time reading about traditional African ways and has become isolated from her friends and family.

Analysis. Landa lacks the social support she needs to feel good about her ethnicity without having to idealize or reject members of her own or other ethnic groups. She is experiencing difficulty integrating her values with those of her family and friends.

GENDER

Questions

What is the patient's sex?

What is the patient's gender identity?

How does the patient define gender-specific roles?

What are the patient's attitudes and beliefs regarding males and females and masculinity and femininity?

With what gender-related stressors is the patient currently coping?

What impact does the person's gender have on mental and physical health?

Example

Assessment. Kelly is male, and enacting the male role is very important to him. As a man, he feels he must provide for his family by working hard, making money, and being smart. Kelly feels that his wife should respect how hard he works and support his plans for providing for her. Recently, he and his wife have had increasing marital conflict. He states "I am doing what is right for both of us. All my wife has to do is help me." Yet Kelly states that his wife does not want him to work 7 days a week and that she does not want to wait until he builds their house before she can go to college. He reports drinking more in the past couple of months and admits that it is difficult for him to express his emotional needs or to respond to those of his wife.

Analysis. Kelly defines masculinity as authority, and it is extremely important to his self image. He is unable to express feelings and is struggling to maintain a self-ideal that is in conflict with his wife's needs for her own growth as an individual as well as a spouse.

EDUCATION

Questions

What is the patient's education level?

What were the patient's educational experiences like?

What are the patient's attitudes and beliefs regarding education in general and the patient's own education in particular?

With what education-related stressors is the patient currently coping?

What impact does the patient's education have on mental and physical health?

Example

Assessment. Ron completed the eighth grade and then dropped out of school. He learned to be a plumber by working with a family friend that owned a plumbing business. Recently the friend retired and sold the business to Ron. Ron wants his son to work with him and learn the business, but his son wants to go to college. Ron and his son have been having violent fights about this issue, and Ron has told him, "College is what you do when you don't know anything. Do you think that by going to college you'll be better than me?"

Continued.

Box 7-2

QUESTIONS RELATED TO SOCIOCULTURAL RISK FACTORS—cont'd

Analysis. Ron feels bad about his lack of formal education and the negative stereotypes people hold about plumbers. His insecurity makes him unable to support his son's desire to attend college because he fears that his relationship with his son will suffer and that his son will think less of him in the future.

INCOME
Questions

What is the patient's income?

What is the source of the patient's income?

How does the patient describe one's specific income group?

What are the patient's attitudes and beliefs regarding personal socioeconomic status?

With what economic-related stressors is the patient currently coping?

What impact does the patient's income have on mental and physical health?

Example

Assessment. Amanda is unemployed. She has always believed that if a person is in good health they should work; however, Amanda has never been employed. She married a wealthy, older man when she was 19 years old, and for 10 years he supported her. Then with no warning, her husband left the country with a younger woman and filed for divorce. Amanda states, "He left me. I'm penniless. I'm homeless. I'm nothing." Her family is middle-income and is willing to help her if she gets a job, but she is unwilling to interview for a job because the concept of paid employment conflicts with her self-concept as a wealthy wife.

Analysis. Amanda's self-concept and self-esteem were based on her marriage and financial status. She never imagined being without these things, and she feels unprepared and resentful of the changes she needs to make to live on her own.

BELIEF SYSTEM
Questions

What are the patient's beliefs about health and illness?

What was the patient's religious or spiritual upbringing?

What are the patient's current religious or spiritual beliefs?

Who is the patient's regular health-care provider?

With what belief system–related stressors is the patient currently coping?

What impact does the patient's belief system have on mental and physical health?

Example

Assessment. Xiao believes that illness of the mind is correct punishment. Since her mother's death 2 months ago, she has experienced insomnia, fatigue, and weight loss. She and her mother argued frequently, including the morning her mother had a fatal car accident on her way to work. Xiao now avoids her family and for the last week has been unable to go to work. Xiao states, "I did not love my mother and now I am being punished. No one can help me."

Analysis. Xiao is unable to resolve her feelings about her mother and to grieve her loss adaptively. She feels guilt about her arguments with her mother and welcomes depression as a correct punishment. Because of this belief, seeking help is unacceptable.

Involving the family, however, does not mean imposing family therapy models based on unwarranted presumptions of family pathology, which families claim do little to help them or the patient.[10] Rather, psychoeducational, behavioral, supportive, and family-consultation models are preferable[26] (see Chapter 30). These models are directly responsive to families' requests for information, support, and techniques for managing their relatives' illnesses.

Religion

Religion can also be a core social and spiritual resource.[36] Among blacks, for example, the church often provides collective support, opportunities for self-expression, and the sense of helping others, which can

give meaning to life. Supernatural belief systems may also provide a natural support system for mentally ill persons, as well as a culturally understandable model for the illness.

Psychobiology

Sociocultural factors also influence various aspects of psychopharmacology and psychobiology[24] (see Chapters 5 and 25). For example, ethnicity represents one of the most important variables that contribute to variations in patients' responses to medications. Racial and ethnic differences in response to psychotropic drugs include the following:

▼ Extrapyramidal effects at lower dosage levels for Asians

CRITICAL THINKING ABOUT CONTEMPORARY ISSUES

Should Ethnic Minority Patients Be Treated by White Therapists?

Controversy exists over the effectiveness of psychotherapy for ethnic minority patients, especially when treated by white therapists. Some researchers and practitioners believe that ethnic patients are less likely to benefit from treatment. Others maintain that ethnic patients are just as likely as whites to show favorable outcomes from treatment and that ethnic or racial matching of patients studies have failed to show different outcomes on the basis of the race or the ethnicity of the patients and clinicians.

It has been proposed that ethnicity or race by itself tells very little about the values, attitudes, and experiences of individuals, whether patient or clinician, who engage in the treatment process.[35] Thus ethnic matches can result in cultural mismatches, as patients and clinicians from the same ethnic group may show markedly different values. Conversely, ethnic mismatches may be cultural matches because patients and clinicians from different ethnic groups may share similar values, lifestyles, and expectations. Thus sociocultural sensitivity refers to respect for individual differences regardless of one's age, ethnicity, gender, education, income, or belief system. The consideration of all of these characteristics and the ability to individualize patient care appear to be the best predictors of treatment outcome. ▼

▼ Lower effective dosage levels and a lower threshold for side effects for antidepressants among Hispanics

▼ Better response by black patients to phenothiazine and tricyclic antidepressants

▼ Higher red blood cell plasma/lithium ratio in blacks

In addition, sociocultural characteristics, including belief systems, appear to have a significant impact on treatment compliance, and there may also be normative cultural preferences for the different ways in which medication can be taken.[22] These findings have implications for treatment outcome and reinforce the need for sociocultural sensitivity when planning nursing care.

Equally important is the fact that numerous studies have documented that "indigenous" systems of health beliefs and practices persist in all societies including those exposed to modern Western medicine. The nurse should keep in mind that, despite the availability of Western medicine, traditional herbal medicines continue to be used extensively by many different cultural groups living in the United States. Some of these drugs have active pharmacologic properties that may interfere with psychotropic drugs. Clearly the use of alternative healing methods warrants additional research.

SUGGESTED CROSS-REFERENCES

SUMMARY

1. The culturally sensitive nurse is one who has the awareness, knowledge, and skills to intervene successfully in the lives of patients from culturally diverse backgrounds.

2. Sociocultural risk factors for psychiatric disorders refer to predisposing factors of the individual that can significantly increase a person's potential for developing a psychiatric disorder, significantly decrease a person's potential for recovery, or both. They include age, ethnicity, gender, education, income, and belief system.

3. A variety of sociocultural stressors hinder the delivery of quality psychiatric care including disadvantagement, stereotyping, intolerance, stigma, prejudice, discrimination, and racism.

4. Coping responses used by individuals and the ways in which symptoms of mental illness are expressed also vary by culture.

5. Assessment of the patient's presdisposing sociocultural risk factors and precipitating stressors greatly enhances the nurse's ability to identify the patient's problems and develop a psychiatric nursing treatment plan that is accurate, appropriate, and culturally sensitive.

6. Together, the nurse and patient need to agree on the nature of the patient's coping responses, the means for solving problems, and the expected outcomes of treatment within a sociocultural context.

REFERENCES

1. Amstead C et al: Relationship of racial stressors to blood pressure responses and anger expression in black college students, *Health Psychol* 8:541, 1989.
2. Blue H, Gonzalez C: The meaning of ethnocultural differ-

ence: its impact on and use in the psychotherapeutic process, *New Dir Ment Health Serv* 55:73, 1992.

3. Bourdon K et al: Estimating the prevalence of mental disorders in US adults from the epidemiologic catchment area survey, *Public Health Rep* 107:663, 1992.

4. Briones D et al: Socioeconomic status, ethnicity, psychological distress, and readiness to utilize a mental health facility, *Am J Psychiatry* 147:1333, 1990.

5. Bruce M, Takeuchi D, Leaf P: Poverty and psychiatric status: longitudinal evidence from the New Haven Epidemiologic Catchment Area study, *Arch Gen Psychiatry* 48:470, 1991.

6. Castle D, Wessely S, Murray R: Sex and schizophrenia: effects of diagnostic stringency and associations with pre-morbid variables, *Br J Psychiatry* 162:658, 1993.

7. Closser M, Blow F: Special populations: women, ethnic minorities, and the elderly, *Psychiatr Clin North Am* 16:199, 1993.

8. Comas-Diaz L, Griffith E: *Clinical guidelines in cross-cultural mental health*, New York, 1988, John Wiley & Sons.

9. Flaskerud J; Transcultural concepts in mental health nursing. In Boyle J, Andrews M, eds: *Transcultural concepts in nursing care*, Glenview, Ill, 1989, Scott, Foresman.

10. Francell C, Conn V, Gray D: Families' perceptions of burden of care for chronic mentally ill relatives, *Hosp Community Psychiatry* 39:1296, 1988.

11. Gaw A: *Culture, ethnicity, and mental illness*, Washington, DC, 1993, American Psychiatric Press.

12. Giglio J: The impact of patients' and therapists' religious values on psychotherapy, *Hosp Community Psychiatry* 44:768, 1993.

13. Goldstein M, Kreisman D: Gender, family environment, and schizophrenia, *Psychol Med* 18:861, 1988.

14. Horwitz A: Help-seeking processes and mental health services, *New Dir Ment Health Serv* 36:33, 1987.

15. Hu T et al: Ethnic populations in public mental health: services choice and level of use, *Am J Public Health* 81:1429, 1991.

16. Huges D, DeMallie D, Blazer D: Does age make a difference in the effect of physical health and social support on the outcome of a major depressive episode? *Am J Psychiatry* 150:728, 1993.

17. Hughes C: Culture in clinical psychiatry. In Gaw A, ed: *Culture, ethnicity, and mental illness*, Washington, DC, 1993, American Psychiatric Press.

18. Jones-Webb R, Snowden L: Symptoms of depression among blacks and whites, *Am J Public Health* 83:240, 1993.

19. Killian T, Killian L: Sociological investigations of mental illness: a review, *Hosp Community Psychiatry* 41:902, 1990.

20. Kurlowicz L: Social factors and depression in late life, *Arch Psychiatr Nurs* 7:30, 1993.

21. Lee C, Richardson B: *Multicultural issues in counseling: new approaches to diversity*, Alexandria, Va, 1991, American Association of Counseling and Development.

22. Lefley H: Culture and chronic mental illness, *Hosp Community Psychiatry* 41:277, 1990.

23. Lewinsohn P et al: Age cohort changes in the lifetime occurrence of depression and other mental disorders, *J Abnorm Psychol* 102:110, 1993.

24. Lin K, Poland R, Nakasaki G: *Psychopharmacology and psycho-*

biology of ethnicity, Washington, DC, 1993, American Psychiatric Press.

25. Loring M, Powell B: Gender, race, and DSM-III: a study of objectivity of psychiatric diagnostic behavior, *J Health Soc Behav* 29:1, 1988.

26. Marsh D: *Families and mental illness*, New York, 1992, Praeger.

27. Murden R et al: Mini-mental state exam scores vary with education in blacks and whites, *J Am Geriatr Soc* 39:149, 1991.

28. Murphy K, Clark J: Nurses' experiences of caring for ethnic minority clients, *J Adv Nurs* 18:442, 1993.

29. Outlaw F: Stress and coping: the influence of racism on the cognitive appraisal processing of African-Americans, *Issues Ment Health Nurs* 14:399, 1993.

30. Regier D et al: The de facto US mental and addictive disorders service system, *Arch Gen Psychiatry* 50:85, 1993.

31. Robins L: Cross-cultural differences in psychiatric disorder, *Am J Public Health* 79:1479, 1989.

32. Rogler L, Cortes D: Help-seeking pathways: a unifying concept in mental health care, *Am J Psychiatry* 150:554, 1993.

33. Rosenstein M, Milazzo-Sayre L, MacAskil R: Use of inpatient psychiatric services by special population. In Manderscheid R, ed: *Chronic mental disorder in the United States*, Rockville, Md, 1987, National Institute of Mental Health.

34. Sorenson S, Ritter C, Aneshensel C: Depression in the community: an investigation into age of onset, *J Consult Clin Psychol* 59:541, 1991.

35. Sue S: Psychotherapeutic services for ethnic minorities: two decades of research findings, *Am Psychol* 43:301, 1988.

36. Sue S et al: Community mental health services for ethnic minority groups: a test of the cultural responsive hypothesis, *J Consult Clin Psychol* 59:533, 1991.

37. Waldfogel S, Wolpe P: Using awareness of religious factors to enhance interventions in consultation-liaison psychiatry, *Hosp Community Psychiatry* 44:473, 1993.

38. Wilkins H: Transcultural nursing: a selective review of the literature, 1985-1991, *J Adv Nurs* 18:602, 1993.

ANNOTATED SUGGESTED READINGS

*American Academy of Nursing: Culturally competent health care, *Nurs Outlook*, 40:277, 1992.

Describes the 10 recommendations of the AAN's expert panel designed to stimulate the development and implementation of knowledge related to culturally competent nursing care.

Comas-Diaz L, Griffith E: *Clinical guidelines in cross-cultural mental health*, New York, 1988, John Wiley & Sons.

Excellent text reviewing essential aspects of culturally relevant mental health assessment and treatment with separate chapters devoted to the various ethnic groups.

*Connors D: Women's "sickness": a case of secondary gains or primary losses, *Adv Nurs Sci* 7:1, 1985.

Extensive discussion of the historical and sociopolitical context of sickness and the overlap between the medical control of sickness and male control over females lives.

Devine P et al: Prejudice with and without compunction, *J Pers Soc Psychol* 60:817, 1991.

---

*Nursing reference.

Interesting study on the difference between how people respond and how they feel they should respond to contact with black people and with homosexual men.

*Facione NC: The triandis model for the study of health and illness behavior: a social behavior theory with sensitivity to diversity, Adv Nurs Sci 15:49, 1993.

Describes a model that can be used to achieve cultural sensitivity in the design of nursing research based on gender, ethnicity, social class, and sexual orientation.

Flaskerud J, Hu L: Racial/ethnic identify and amount and type of psychiatric treatment, Am J Psychiatry 149:379, 1992.

Describes a large study of the number of treatment sessions, treatment modality, treatment setting, and therapist discipline for patients from different ethnic groups with different socioeconomic status.

*Foster S: The pragmatics of culture: the rhetoric of difference in psychiatric nursing, Arch Psychiatr Nurs 4:292, 1990.

Critical examination of the rhetoric versus the reality of the implementation of culturally sensitive psychiatric nursing care.

Gaw A: Culture, ethnicity, and mental illness, Washington, DC, 1993, American Psychiatric Press.

Perhaps the best text available to describe the expression and treatment of mental illness in the context of culture. Should be on the bookshelf of all psychiatric nurses.

Killian T, Killian L: Sociological investigations of mental illness: a review, Hosp Community Psychiatry 41:902, 1990.

Review of sociological research dealing with the effects of social class, race, gender, marital status, and age on the development, diagnosis, and treatment of mental illness.

Lee C, Richardson B: Multicultural issues in counseling: new approaches to diversity, Alexandria, Va, 1991, American Association of Counseling and Development.

Brings together new directions for multicultural counseling practice with culturally diverse groups. Easy to read and practical in focus.

Lefley H: Culture and chronic mental illness, Hosp Community Psychiatry 41:277, 1990.

Relationship of culture to chronic mental illness is reviewed in a cross-national and cross-ethnic perspective. Key questions are explored.

*Outlaw F: Stress and coping: the influence of racism on the cognitive appraisal processing of African-Americans, Issues Ment Health Nurs 14:399, 1993.

Describes a model to guide nursing practice, research, and education about the influence of racism on the cognitive appraisal, stress, and coping of African-Americans.

Rogler L: The meaning of culturally sensitive research in mental health, Am J Psychiatry 146:296, 1989.

Focuses on the entire process of research in analyzing ways to make it culturally sensitive. An important area for nursing research initiatives.

---

*Nursing reference.

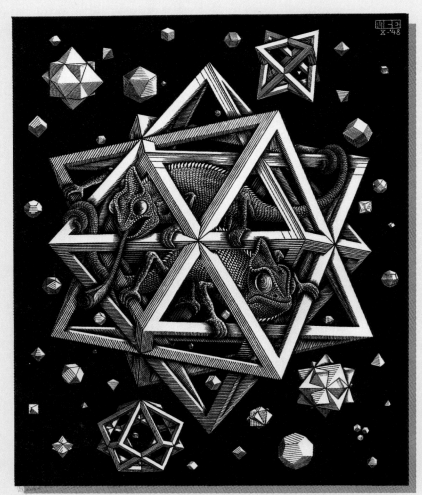

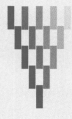

CHAPTER 8

Legal Context of Psychiatric Nursing Care

GAIL W. STUART

Pinel immediately led Couthon to the section for the deranged, where the sight of the cells made a painful impression on him. Couthon asked to interrogate all the patients. From most, he received only insults and obscene apostrophes. It was useless to prolong the interview. Turning to Pinel, Couthan said: "Now, citizen, are you mad yourself to seek to unchain such beasts?" Pinel replied calmly: "Citizen, I am convinced that these madmen are so intractable only because they have been deprived of air and liberty."

Philippe Pinel: Traite Complet du Regime Sanitaire des Alienes 56 (1836)

LEARNING OBJECTIVES

After studying this chapter the student should be able to:

▼ Compare and contrast the three types of admission to a psychiatric hospital and the issues raised by commitment
▼ Describe the various ways patients can be discharged from a psychiatric hospital
▼ Discuss outpatient commitment and its implications for improving the care received by psychiatric patients
▼ Analyze the common personal and civil rights retained by psychiatric patients and controversies related to them
▼ Identify current legislative initiatives that affect the psychiatric care provided in the United States
▼ Discuss the insanity defense and the criteria used in the United States to determine a mentally ill person's criminal responsibility
▼ Evaluate the rights, responsibilities, and potential conflict of interest that arise from the three legal roles of the psychiatric nurse

TOPICAL OUTLINE

Hospitalizing the Patient
   Informal Admission
   Voluntary Admission
   Involuntary Admission (Commitment)
   Commitment Dilemma
Discharge
   Conditional Discharge
   Absolute Discharge
   Judicial Discharge
Outpatient Commitment
Patients' Rights
Legislative Initiatives
   Omnibus Budget Reconciliation Act
   Protection and Advocacy Act
   Americans with Disabilities Act
   Advanced Directives
Psychiatry and Criminal Responsibility
   M'Naghten Test
   Irresistible Impulse Test
   American Law Institute's Test
   Disposition of Mentally Ill Offenders
Legal Role of the Nurse
Nurse as Provider
Nurse as Employee
Nurse as Citizen

The relationship between psychiatry and the law reflects the tension between individual rights and social needs. They are alike in that both psychiatry and the law deal with human behavior and the relationships and responsibilities that exist among people. Both also play a role in controlling socially undesirable behavior, and together they analyze whether the care psychiatric patients receive is therapeutic, custodial, repressive, or punitive.

Differences also exist between psychiatry and the law. For example, psychiatry is concerned with the meaning of behavior and the life satisfaction of the individual. In contrast, the law addresses the outcome of behavior and the enforcement of a system of rules to encourage orderly functioning among groups of people.

The legal context of care is important for all psychiatric nurses because it focuses concern on the rights of patients and the quality of care they receive. In the past two decades civil, criminal, and consumer rights of patients have been established and expanded through the legal system. The mentally ill and their families are now using the law to express legitimate grievances and to fight for needed changes in the way psychiatric care is provided in the United States. Many of the laws vary from state to state, and psychiatric nurses must become familiar with the legal provisions of the state in which they practice. This knowledge enhances the freedom of both the nurse and the patient and ultimately results in better care for psychiatric patients.

HOSPITALIZING THE PATIENT

Hospitalization can be either traumatic or supportive for the individual depending on the institution, attitude of family and friends, response of the staff, and type of admission. There are three major types of admission: informal, voluntary, and involuntary. Table 8-1 summarizes their distinguishing characteristics.

What were your first impressions as you walked through the doors of a psychiatric hospital for the first time? How might you use your perceptions and responses to provide better nursing care for patients being admitted for inpatient treatment?

Informal Admission

Informal admission to a psychiatric hospital is like admission to any general hospital. Entry into and release from the hospital may be requested orally. The individual is free to leave at any time. If patients leave before treatment is completed, they are often asked to sign themselves out "against medical advice" (AMA) but are not required to do so.

Voluntary Admission

Under voluntary admission any citizen of lawful age may apply in writing (usually on a standard admission form) for admission to a public or private psychiatric hospital. The individual agrees to receive treatment and abide by hospital rules. Individuals may seek help based on their personal decision or the advice of family or a health professional. If someone is too ill to apply but voluntarily seeks help, a parent or legal guardian may request admission. In most states children under the age of 16 years may be admitted if their parents sign the required application form.

Voluntary admission is preferred because it is similar to a medical hospitalization. It indicates that the individual acknowledges problems in living, seeks help in coping with them, and will probably actively participate

Table 8-1 Characteristics of the Three Types of Admission to Psychiatric Hospitals

	Informal admission	Voluntary admission	Involuntary admission
Admission	Orally requested by patient	Written application by patient	Application did not originate with patient
Discharge	Initiated by patient	Initiated by patient	Initiated by hospital or court but not by patient
Status of civil rights	Retained in full by patient	Retained in full by patient	Patient may retain none, some, or all, depending on state law
Justification	Voluntarily seeks help	Voluntarily seeks help	Mentally ill and one or more of the following: 1. Dangerous to self or others 2. Need for treatment 3. Unable to meet own basic needs

in finding solutions. Most patients who enter private psychiatric units of general hospitals do so voluntarily.

When admitted in this way, the patient retains all civil rights, including the right to vote, possess a driver's license, buy and sell property, manage personal affairs, hold office, practice a profession, and engage in a business. It is a common misconception that all admissions to a mental hospital involve the loss of civil rights.

Although voluntary admission is the most desirable, it is not always possible.[6] Sometimes a patient may be acutely disturbed, suicidal, or dangerous to self or others, yet rejects any therapeutic intervention. In these cases involuntary commitments are necessary.

> Should a psychotic person be allowed to sign forms for voluntary admittance to the hospital? If not, should all voluntary patients be screened for competence before hospitalization?

Involuntary Admission (Commitment)

In the late 1940s the World Health Organization reported that almost 90% of admissions to state mental hospitals in the United States were involuntary and approximately 10% were voluntary. The trend has shifted to more voluntary admissions. In 1963, 30% were voluntary, by 1980 nearly half of all admissions to psychiatric hospitals were voluntary, and currently about 73% of the 1.6 million yearly admissions to psychiatric hospitals are voluntary.[35] This trend has resulted from the greater variety of admission statuses and stricter rules regarding involuntary commitment.

Although involuntary commitment has come under intense scrutiny, the United States Supreme Court continues to recognize it based on two legal theories. First, under its police power, the state has the authority to protect the community from the dangerous acts of the mentally ill; and second, under its *parens patriae* powers, the state can provide care for citizens who cannot care for themselves, such as some mentally ill persons. In the past 20 years the police power rationale for civil commitment has been emphasized over the *parens patriae* doctrine, using dangerousness as the standard for commitment. There has also been a trend toward increasing the requirements for procedural due process for such commitments and the need for proof of mental illness and dangerousness by clear and convincing evidence.

Involuntary commitment means that the patient did not request hospitalization and may have opposed it or was indecisive and did not resist it. The standards for commitment vary among states and reflect the confu-

sion in the medical, social, and legal systems of society. Most laws permit commitment of the mentally ill on the following three grounds:

1. Dangerous to self or others
2. Mentally ill and in need of treatment
3. Unable to provide for own basic needs

Generally, each state identifies which criteria are required and what each criterion means. In addition to individuals with mental illness, certain states have laws that allow for the involuntary hospitalization of three other groups:

1. Developmentally disabled (mentally retarded) individuals
2. Substance abusers
3. Mentally disabled minors

The Commitment Process. State laws vary, but they try to protect the individual who is not mentally ill from being detained in a psychiatric hospital against the individual's will for political, economic, family, or other nonmedical reasons. Certain procedures are standard. The process begins with a sworn petition by a relative, friend, public official, physician, or any interested citizen stating the person is mentally ill and needs treatment. Some states allow only specific individuals to file such a petition. One or two physicians must then examine the patient's mental status; some states require that at least one of the physicians be a psychiatrist.

The decision whether to hospitalize the patient is made next. Precisely who makes this decision determines the nature of the commitment. **Medical** certification means a specified number of appointed physicians and sometimes psychologists make the decision. This power to certify is given to all physicians, not just psychiatrists. A judge or jury decides on **court** or **judicial** commitment in a formal hearing. In this case the court is required to notify patients so that they can retain a lawyer if they want to contest commitment. A jury trial is not mandatory in most states but can be requested by patients. Most states recognize patients' right to legal counsel, but only about half actually appoint a lawyer for patients if they do not have one. **Administrative** commitment is determined by a special tribunal of hearing officers. The Fourteenth Amendment to the U.S. Constitution protects citizens against infringements on liberty without "due process of the law." Because of this, medical certification is used rarely, primarily in emergencies, and administrative commitment is subject to judicial review.

If treatment is deemed necessary, the individual is hospitalized. The length of hospital stay varies, depending on the patient's needs. Fig. 8-1 diagrams the involuntary commitment process. It identifies three types of hospitalization: emergency, temporary, and indefinite.

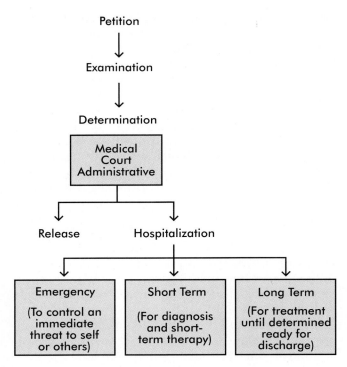

Petition
↓
Examination
↓
Determination

Medical
Court
Administrative

Release   Hospitalization

Emergency
(To control an immediate threat to self or others)

Short Term
(For diagnosis and short-term therapy)

Long Term
(For treatment until determined ready for discharge)

Fig. 8-1   Diagram of the involuntary commitment process.

Most states specify that any physician, not necessarily a psychiatrist, can certify a person for involuntary commitment to a psychiatric hospital? Do you agree with this? What is required by law in your state?

Emergency Hospitalization. Almost all states permit emergency commitment for patients who are acutely ill. The goals are short term and are primarily intended to control an immediate threat to self or others. In those states lacking such a law, police often jail the acutely ill individual on a disorderly conduct charge, which is a criminal charge. Such a practice is inappropriate and often harmful to the patient's mental status.

To obtain an emergency commitment, the patient's family, a physician, or someone designated by the state must file a petition that includes a supporting report by a psychiatrist. It is reviewed by a judge or hospital official, and hospitalization is provided. Most state laws limit the length of emergency commitment to 48 to 72 hours. Emergency hospitalization allows detainment in a psychiatric hospital only until proper legal steps are taken to provide for additional hospitalization.

Short-Term or Observational Hospitalization. This type of commitment is primarily used for diagno-

sis and short-term therapy and does not require an emergency situation. Again, the commitment is for a specified time that varies greatly from state to state. The commitment process is similar to that for emergency hospitalization. Some states require a court order for all temporary commitments, whereas others require one only if the person protests. If at the end of the period the patient is still not ready for discharge, a petition can be filed for a long-term commitment.

Long-Term Hospitalization (Formal Commitment). A long-term commitment provides for hospitalization for an indefinite time or until the patient is ready for discharge. The process is usually a court commitment. Patients in public or state hospitals more frequently have indefinite commitments than patients in private hospitals. Even when committed, these patients maintain their right to consult a lawyer at any time and to request a court hearing to determine if additional hospitalization is necessary. The hospital ultimately discharges the patient, however, and a court order is not necessary to do this. Periodic reviews for long-term hospitalization may be made every 3, 6, or 12 months.

 Do you agree with the criteria for committing patients to psychiatric hospitals? How would you assess whether or not a person met these criteria?

Commitment Dilemma

In a few states involuntary commitment assumes incompetency and patients lose their civil rights. In those states patients may not be able to make contracts, vote, drive, obtain a professional license, serve on a jury, marry, or enter into civil litigation. In addition, the patient must suffer the stigma attached to the label "committed" in all future activities. Because of the many people affected by involuntary commitment and the loss of personal rights that it can entail, it becomes a matter of great legal, moral, social, and psychiatric significance. In general medicine there is no equivalent loss of individual rights, except for rare cases requiring quarantine for carriers of potentially epidemic diseases.

The question may be asked, "How ill does a person need to be to merit commitment?" It is not necessary to be psychotic, as shown by the number of elderly, addicted, and neurotic patients hospitalized, as well as by the many psychotic individuals who remain free. Perhaps a person's dangerousness to self or others is a more pertinent consideration. Certainly psychiatric professionals consider hospitalization in this instance as a humanitarian gesture that protects both the individual and society. "Dangerousness," however, is a vague term.

Dangerousness. Interestingly, courts guard the freedom of people who are mentally healthy but dangerous. For example, after a prison sentence is served, the individual is automatically released and can no longer be retained. However, someone who is mentally ill and dangerous can be confined indefinitely.

Most mentally ill persons are not dangerous to themselves or others. Studies show that the incidence of violence among psychiatric patients is the same as that among the general population. Only with certain mental disorders and under certain conditions does mental illness result in violence. For example, Teplin[39] observed over 1000 police-citizen contacts in an urban area. She found that police contact with people who had signs of serious mental disorder was relatively rare. In addition, no differences were found between mentally disordered and nonmentally disordered suspects regarding the type of crimes committed. Research studies such as this one help to dispel the myth that the mentally ill are more dangerous and more prone to violent crime. Yet the idea of preventive detention does not exist in most areas of the law, since the ability to predict an action does not confer the right to control it in advance. Only illegal acts result in prolonged confinement for most citizens—except the mentally ill.

Another issue is that there are no reliable indicators of dangerousness. Even if some mentally ill individuals are potentially dangerous, psychiatrists cannot necessarily predict future violence. Frequently psychiatrists overpredict patients' potential for dangerous acts and the extent of their illness.

This may result from psychiatrists' medical training, which cautions that underdiagnosis is more harmful than overdiagnosis. It is complicated by their conflicting roles as an agent of both the patient and the community, which require them to be therapist, warden, and judge. If psychiatrists underpredict a psychiatric illness and the patient later causes harm, the community holds them responsible. If they overpredict illness, however, a patient is subjected to treatment unwillingly. Thus multidisciplinary teams rather than psychiatrists alone should be involved in determining dangerousness. Input from those familiar with the patient's home setting and sociocultural background might also improve evaluations.

Five components of dangerousness have been defined by legal scholars. These may be useful as a decision-making guide for judges, jurors, probation officers, and mental health professionals. They are[7]:

1. *Nature of harm or conduct.* Does the person threaten bodily harm, harm to property, or psychological harm?

2. *Magnitude of the harm.* Does the person threaten murder, assault, or verbal abuse?
3. *Probability.* How likely is it that the harmful act will occur?
4. *Imminence.* When will the threatened action take place?
5. *Frequency.* How often will the threatened action take place? Will it be repeated, or will it be a single act of violence?

The answers to these questions can be very subjective, which suggests that the underlying issue is noncomformity in ways that offend others. In this context, social role becomes important. For example, before the law all men and women are equal, but it is also true that most committed patients are members of the lower classes. This raises questions regarding the sociocultural context of psychiatric care (see Chapter 7) and the role of mental health professionals as the enforcer of social rules and norms.

Thus the behavioral standard of dangerousness has the potential of changing the function of the psychiatric hospital from a place of therapy for mental illness to a place of confinement for offensive behavior. This suggests that the psychiatric hospital's covert function can be social control. This idea is supported by the various behavioral disorders that result in commitment, including drug addiction, alcoholism, and sexual offenses.

How do you explain the fact that society condones certain kinds of dangerous behavior, such as race car driving, but objects to other kinds?

Freedom of Choice. The legal and psychiatric question thus raised is freedom of choice. Some professionals believe that at certain times the individual cannot be self-responsible. To protect both the patient and society, it is necessary to confine him and make decisions for him. An example is the suicidal patient. In most states suicide is against the law, so law and psychiatry join to protect the person and help individuals resolve personal conflicts.

How does this compare with cancer or cardiac patients who may reject medical advice and the prescribed treatment? Should society, through law and medicine, attempt to cure these patients against their will? Some physicians view civil commitment as basically a benevolent system that makes treatment available. They disagree with the assumption that mentally ill persons are competent to exercise free will and make decisions in their own best interest, such as whether to take medications or remain outside a hospital. They contend that there are mentally ill people who may not be physically dangerous but still endanger their own prospects for a normal life. Since institutions can at least protect them and in many cases help them, they think it would be immoral to abolish involuntary civil commitment.[13]

Other people, such as Szasz, oppose intervention. Szasz favors responsibility for self and the right to choose or reject treatment. If an individual's actions violate criminal law, he suggests the individual be punished through the penal system.[37]

Currently there appears to be a growing movement among state legislatures to revise commitment laws to respond better to the needs of the seriously mentally ill before they become a danger to themselves or others. An increasing effort by patient advocates, families, mental health professionals, and state lawmakers is being made to move away from the narrowly defined dangerousness standard as the primary criterion for commitment. A middle ground is being sought between meeting the needs of the severely mentally ill and preserving their legal rights and freedom of choice.[7]

> Who should decide what is in the patient's best interest if a patient is involuntarily committed? Should it be the patient, a family member, a health-care professional or the judicial system?

Ethical Considerations. All nurses must analyze their beliefs regarding commitment. What should be done if the nonconformist does not wish to change behavior? Do the nonconformists maintain freedom to choose even if their thinking appears to be irrational or abnormal? Is coercion fair? Can social interests be served by less restrictive methods such as outpatient therapy? All nurses are responsible for reviewing commitment procedures in their state and working for necessary clinical, ethical, and legal reforms.

The commitment dilemma exposes current practices and opens areas of controversy for the future. The present psychiatric hospital has been described as a jail, hospital, poorhouse, and home for the elderly. It protects, treats, feeds, maintains, and houses socially incompetent individuals who are often feared by society. When discharged, they often lack alternatives and come to the attention of law enforcement agencies or welfare offices.

Studies conducted during the 1980s showed that more than half of the homeless population have psychiatric or substance abuse disorders.[40] Homeless mentally ill persons have a wider array of service needs than homeless persons who use only social services. Many seriously mentally ill persons cannot obtain or maintain access to community resources such as housing, a stable source of income, or treatment and rehabilitative services.[36] Homeless individuals lack supportive social networks and underutilize psychiatric, medical, and welfare programs. Many avoid the mental health system entirely, often because they are too disorganized to respond to offers of help. As a consequence, they are often admitted into acute psychiatric hospitals or jailed because of their lack of shelter and other resources, even though such restrictive environments may not best address their psychiatric needs.[41]

Unfortunately, local communities often deny the problem by resisting the establishment of halfway houses or sheltered homes in their neighborhoods. Third-party insurance seldom covers extended outpatient psychiatric care. In today's mobile society, family and friends are often unable to care for the newly released patient, who may end up in a boarding house with little to do but watch television.

These issues must be addressed by psychiatric nurses, patients, and citizens across the United States. The value of commitment, goals of hospitalization, quality of life, and rights of patients must be preserved through the judicial, legislative, and health care systems.

DISCHARGE

The patient who is informally admitted to the hospital can leave at any time, limited only to reasonable hours, such as daytime hours or weekdays. The voluntarily admitted patient can be discharged by the staff when "maximum benefit" has been received from the treatment. Voluntary patients may also request discharge. Most states require written notice of patients' desire to leave and also that patients sign a form that states they are leaving "against medical advice" (AMA). This form then becomes part of patients' permanent record.

In some states voluntarily admitted patients can be released immediately; in others they can be detained 24 to 72 hours after submitting a discharge request. This allows hospital staff time to confer with the patient and family members and decide if additional inpatient treatment is indicated. If it is and the patient will not withdraw the request for discharge, the family may begin involuntary commitment proceedings, thereby changing the patient's status. Voluntarily admitted patients who elope from the hospital can be brought back only if they agree. Staff frequently attempt to contact such patients and discuss alternatives. If they refuse to return, either they must be discharged or involuntary commitment procedures must begin.

An involuntarily committed patient has lost the right to leave the hospital when he wishes. Temporary and emergency commitments specify the maximum length of detainment. Indefinite commitments do not, although the patient's status should be reviewed periodically. The patient may also apply for another commitment hearing. If a committed patient leaves secretly, the staff has the legal obligation to notify the police and committing courts. Frequently these patients return home or visit family or friends and can be easily located. The legal authorities then return the patient to the hospital. Additional steps are not necessary, since the original commitment is still effective.

There are three kinds of discharges: conditional, absolute, and judicial.

Conditional Discharge

Specified leaves of absence or liberties help many committed patients make the transition from hospital to community. These are known as conditional discharges because certain things are expected of patients. Most frequently they are required to attend outpatient therapy through the hospital or community mental health center. During this time the commitment order is still in effect, and, should patients relapse while in the community, they can be brought back to the hospital.

This type of discharge planning allows the patient a gradual integration into the community, and many patients have benefited from it. Other advantages include the greater ease of readmitting patients should it be necessary; the sense of support conveyed to patients, who know that at this difficult time they have not been abandoned by the hospital; and the ability to continue to provide needed services to patients such as the provision of free medication to a financially indigent patient or continued access to occupational or other therapy programs. If at the end of the conditional period the patient has adjusted well, the hospital can issue an absolute discharge.

Absolute Discharge

As the name implies, an absolute discharge terminates the patient's relationship with the hospital. It is a final discharge, and if the patient needs to return to the hospital at some future time, new admission proceedings must begin. Usually the hospital is required to notify the court when a committed patient receives an absolute discharge.

This type of discharge occurs most often when the patient has made substantial progress and can function well in the community. However, there are also cases when patients who have not improved and are unlikely to do so in the future are granted absolute discharges.

In these instances, families or guardians are contacted to arrange satisfactory care for the patient. In addition, some laws require that the hospital notify other state officials.

Judicial Discharge

Nearly 40 states have laws allowing patients or their families the right to appeal for a discharge even though the hospital does not agree with the discharge request. The process and requirements for such cases vary from state to state, but they give patients another option if they believe hospitalization is no longer appropriate. Such laws may be important for further defining patients' rights in future years.

OUTPATIENT COMMITMENT

Outpatient commitment is the process by which the courts can order patients "committed" to a course of outpatient treatment specified by their clinicians. It is one alternative for the pressing problem of the homeless but nondangerous mentally ill individual who is in need of psychiatric treatment and stabilization in the community. It may be most beneficial for revolving-door patients—those who stop taking their medication shortly after discharge, rapidly deteriorate, and soon require rehospitalization.[34]

Almost every state has provisions for outpatient commitment, but relatively few use them regularly because of the following reasons[45]:

▼ Lack of clinical and administrative structures needed to carry out court-ordered outpatient treatment
▼ Judicial unfamiliarity with the concept
▼ Absence of good criteria for outpatient commitment and enforcement mechanisms

North Carolina, Hawaii, Arizona, and Tennessee have implemented outpatient commitment. They have created different criteria for outpatient than for inpatient commitment. The criteria focus on the likelihood of relapse that would result in future dangerousness, and sometimes require evidence of a pattern of dangerous behavior when the patient is unmedicated.

In addition, Geller[19] has proposed 10 guidelines to determine a patient's appropriateness for involuntary outpatient treatment (Box 8-1). They are sequential in that a patient is not evaluated for appropriateness under a guideline unless the criteria for all preceding guidelines have been met. The guidelines also assume that the patient has a serious and persistent mental illness and a history of dangerousness to self or others. The few studies that have been conducted in this area show varying results of outpatient commitment.[45] It is

Box 8-1
GUIDELINES FOR THE USE OF OUTPATIENT COMMITMENT

1. The patient must express an interest in living in the community.
2. The patient must have previously failed in the community.
3. The patient must have that degree of competency necessary to understand the stipulations of his or her involuntary community treatment.
4. The patient must have the capacity to comply with the involuntary community treatment plan.
5. The treatment or treatments being ordered need to have demonstrated efficacy when used properly by the patient in question.
6. The ordered treatment or treatments must be such that they can be delivered by the outpatient system, are sufficient for the patient's needs, and are necessary to sustain community tenure.
7. The ordered treatment must be such that it can be monitored by outpatient treatment agencies.
8. The outpatient treatment system must be willing to deliver the ordered treatments to the patient and must be willing to participate in enforcing compliance with those treatments.
9. The public-sector inpatient support system must support the outpatient system's participation in the provision of involuntary community treatment.
10. The outpatient must not be dangerous when complying with the ordered treatment.

From Geller J: *Innovations & Research* 2:23, 1993.

an interesting approach that merits careful study as different models of care are implemented.

 How might sociocultural factors influence a nurse's interpretation of the guidelines listed in Box 8-1? How might nurses guard against potential bias based on their personal worldview?

PATIENTS' RIGHTS

In 1973 the American Hospital Association issued a Patient's Bill of Rights that many hospitals and community-based settings throughout the United States have adopted.[1] These were reaffirmed in 1990. Frequently, these rights are posted for reading in a location that is easily accessible to patients. In some hospitals they may be given to patients on admission and read or explained to them.

This process, however, does not ensure that psychiatric patients have knowledge of their civil rights. For example, one study reported that reading patients their rights on admission and giving them a copy did not necessarily result in understanding or retaining the information. Two important rights—the right to withdraw from treatment and the right to participate in the development of the treatment plan—were not understood by more than a fourth of the patients in the study.[46] This suggests that a change may be needed in how psychiatric patients are informed about their rights and empowered to participate in the treatment process.

 In your experience, are patients in general hospital settings granted their patient rights? How about patients in psychiatric inpatient units? What specific actions could nurses implement to see that these rights are honored in all hospitals?

Allowing for great variation among states, psychiatric patients currently have the following rights:
▼ Right to communicate with people outside the hospital through correspondence, telephone, and personal visits
▼ Right to keep clothing and personal effects with them in the hospital
▼ Right to religious freedom
▼ Right to be employed if possible
▼ Right to manage and dispose of property
▼ Right to execute wills
▼ Right to enter into contractual relationships
▼ Right to make purchases
▼ Right to education
▼ Right to habeas corpus
▼ Right to independent psychiatric examination
▼ Right to civil service status
▼ Right to retain licenses, privileges, or permits established by law, such as a driver's or professional license
▼ Right to sue or be sued
▼ Right to marry and divorce
▼ Right not to be subject to unnecessary mechanical restraints
▼ Right to periodic review of status
▼ Right to legal representation
▼ Right to privacy
▼ Right to informed consent
▼ Right to treatment
▼ Right to refuse treatment
▼ Right to treatment in the least restrictive setting
Some of these deserve more discussion.

Right to Communicate with People Outside the Hospital

This right allows patients to visit and hold telephone conversations in privacy and send unopened letters to anyone of their choice, including judges, lawyers, families, and staff. Although the patient has the right to communicate in an uncensored manner, the staff may limit access to the telephone or visitors when it could harm the patient or be a source of harassment for the staff. The hospital can also limit the times when telephone calls are made and received and when visitors can enter the facility. On occasions hospital staff have intercepted and destroyed letters presumed to be threatening or abusive. In states where this is not illegal, such activity raises the ethical question of individual freedom vs. the good of the community.

Right To Keep Personal Effects

The patient may bring clothing and personal items to the hospital, taking into consideration the amount of storage space available. The hospital is not responsible for their safety, and valuable items should be left at home. If the patient brings something of value to the hospital, the staff should place it in the hospital safe or otherwise provide for safekeeping. The hospital staff is also responsible for maintaining a safe environment and should take dangerous objects away from the patient if necessary.

How are patients informed of their rights on your psychiatric unit? Talk to some of the patients and see if they can recall any of the rights that were explained to them.

Right To Execute Wills

A person's competency to make a will is known as **testamentary capacity.** Patients can make a valid will if the following conditions are met:

1. They know they are making a will
2. They know the nature and extent of their property
3. They know who their friends and relatives are and what the relationships mean

Each of these criteria must be documented for the will to be considered valid. This means patients must not be mentally confused at the time they sign their will. It does not imply that they must know exact details of their property holdings or specific bank account figures, but they cannot attempt to give away more than they possess. Furthermore, the law requires that patients know who their relatives are but does not require them to bequeath anything to them.

A patient's commitment or a diagnosis of psychosis does not immediately invalidate the will. It is still valid if it was made during a lucid period and the patient met the three criteria. The problem most debated in determining testamentary capacity involves the delusional patient. The important question is whether the false belief or delusion caused the person to dispose of property differently than would have been done otherwise.

Two or three people must witness the will by watching the patient sign it and watching each other as they sign it. Later a nurse may be summoned to testify to the patient's condition at the time of writing the will. The nurse's testimony should relate to the three criteria just listed. It is important for the nurse to report pertinent observations, recall information as accurately as possible, and express thoughts concisely and objectively. Hospital charts and the nurse's notes may also be used in the court proceedings.

Right To Enter into Contractual Relationships

The court considers contracts valid if the person understands the circumstances of the contract and its consequences. Once again, a psychiatric illness does not invalidate a contract, although the nature of the contract and degree of judgment needed to understand it would be influencing factors.

Incompetency. Related to this right is the issue of mental incompetency. Every adult is assumed to be mentally competent, mentally able to carry out personal affairs. To prove otherwise requires a special court hearing to declare an individual "**incompetent.**" This is a legal term without a precise medical meaning. To prove incompetence, it must be shown that the individual:

1. Has a mental disorder
2. This disorder causes a defect in judgment
3. This defect makes the individual incapable of handling personal affairs

All three elements must be present, and the exact diagnostic label is not as important in this case. If a person is declared incompetent, the court will appoint a legal guardian to manage the individual's affairs. This frequently is a family member, friend, or bank executive. Incompetency rulings are most often filed for persons with senile dementia, cerebral arteriosclerosis, chronic schizophrenia, and mental retardation.

The legislative trend is to separate the concepts of incompetency and involuntary commitment, since the reasons for each are essentially different. Incompetency arises from society's desire to guard its citizens' assets from their inability to understand and transact business. Involuntary commitments are intended to protect patients from themselves (in the case of suicide), protect others from dangerous patients (as in homicide), and administer treatment. However, many states still consider the two equivalent.

If ruled incompetent, a person cannot vote, marry, drive, or make contracts. A release from the hospital does not necessarily restore competency. Another court hearing is required to reverse the previous ruling before the individual can once again manage private affairs.

> How is education provided for emotionally ill children living in the community? Should they be mainstreamed in the school system, given special educational resources, or both?

Right to Education

Many parents exercise this right on behalf of their emotionally ill or mentally retarded children. The U.S. Constitution guarantees this right to everyone, although many states have not provided adequate education to all citizens and are now required to do so.

> How is the right to education honored in a children's psychiatric inpatient setting? How does this compare with the education provided children in a pediatric hospital?

Right to Habeas Corpus

Habeas corpus is an important constitutional right patients retain in all states even if they have been involuntarily hospitalized. Its goal is the speedy release of any individual who claims being detained illegally. A committed patient may file a writ at any time on the grounds of being sane and eligible for release. The hearing takes place in court, where those who wish to restrain the patient must defend their actions. A jury is sometimes impaneled to determine the patient's sanity. Patients are discharged if they are judged as sane.

Right to Independent Psychiatric Examination

Under the Emergency Admission Statute, the patient has the right to demand a psychiatric examination by a physician of choice. If this physician determines that the patient is not mentally ill, the patient must be released.

Right to Privacy

The right to privacy implies the individual's right to keep some personal information completely secret. **Confidentiality** involves the disclosure of certain information to another person, but this is limited to authorized individuals. Every psychiatric professional is responsible for protecting a patient's right to confidentiality, including even the knowledge that an individual is in therapy or in a hospital. Revealing such information might damage the patient's reputation or hamper the ability to obtain a job. The protection of the law applies to all patients. This can create ethical and professional dilemmas, such as the one experienced by the nurse described in this clinical example.

 ## CLINICAL EXAMPLE

On a Wednesday morning in 1981 in Springfield, Illinois, a man walked into Lauterbach's Cottage Hardware Store, grabbed an ax, and began swinging. When he left, one person was dead and two others were critically injured. Ten days later, police received a call from Mr. K, who was a patient in the 49-bed psychiatric unit at St. John's Hospital. Mr. K told the police that his roommate at the hospital confessed the crime. However, he didn't know his roommate's name. He asked Nurse M to identify him but she refused to do so, since she believed his name was shielded by a state law guaranteeing the privacy of mental health records. Hospital administrators supported her decision even after she was fined $250 by a county judge for refusing to give the man's name to a grand jury. Nurse M did tell the police that the suspect was not a patient in St. John's at the time of the murder and that he resembled their composite sketch.

The issue of confidentiality is becoming increasingly important. Various agencies demand information about a patient's history, diagnosis, treatment, and prognosis, and sophisticated methods for obtaining information (e.g., wiretapping and computer banks) have developed. These threaten the individual's right to privacy. Clinicians are free from legal responsibility if they release information with the patient's written and signed request. Written consent is desirable for two reasons: (1) it makes clear to both parties that consent has been given; (2) if questions should arise about the consent, a documentary record of it exists. Therefore it should be made a part of the patient's permanent chart. As a rule, it is best to reveal as little information as possible and discuss with the patient what will be released.

Little research has been done on how patients feel about this important issue. One study found that psychiatric inpatients valued confidentiality highly and worried about the possibility of unauthorized disclosures, particularly to employers.[31] They were unfamiliar, however, with their legal rights or options should breaches in confidentiality occur. This study emphasizes the importance of confidentiality and the need for additional research and patient education in this area.

Confidentiality builds on the element of trust necessary in a patient-therapist relationship. Patients place themselves in the care of others and reveal vulnerable aspects of their personal life. In return they expect high-quality care and the protection of their interests. Thus the patient-therapist relationship is an intimate one that demands trust, loyalty, and privacy.

One of the adolescent girls on your unit elopes on the way to the cafeteria. When you speak to the girl's mother to let her know what has happened, the mother asks you to please call the radio and television stations and have them announce it so that she can be discovered. How would you respond to this request?

Privileged Communication. The legal phrase **privilege**, or more accurately, **testimonial privilege,** applies only in court-related proceedings. It includes communications between husband and wife, attorney and client, and clergy and church member. The right to reveal information belongs to the person who spoke, and the listener cannot disclose the information unless the speaker gives permission. This protects the patient, who could sue the listener for disclosing privileged information. It also gives the patient the confidence necessary to make a full account of symptoms and conditions so that treatment can be administered.

Testimonial privilege between health professionals and patients exists only if established by law. Because of the variety of state laws, the bases of privilege may vary greatly among professions even within the same state. A minority of the states provide for privilege between nurses and patients. Nurses may also be covered in states that have adopted privileges between psychotherapists and patients. The psychotherapist-patient privilege is usually limited. It applies only when a therapist-patient relationship exists, and only communications of a professional nature are protected. Third persons present during the communication between the

therapist and the patient may be required to testify and are not included in privilege.

What is the law in your state regarding testimonial privilege between nurses and patients? How would you go about changing the law if it does not include nurses?

This discussion is summarized by the circle of confidentiality presented in Fig. 8-2. Within the circle, patient information may be shared. Those outside the circle require the patient's permission to receive information. Within the circle are treatment team members, staff supervisors, health-care students and their faculty working with the specific patient and those consultants who actually see the patient. All of these individuals must be informed about the patient's clinical condition to be able to help. The patient is also inside the circle—an obvious point but one that is often overlooked. Patients can reveal any and all aspects of their life, problems, treatments, and experiences to anyone at all. This is an important point for the nurse to remember in those ambiguous situations where the requirements of confidentiality are uncertain.

A number of individuals are outside the circle. Family members and legal representatives are not automatically entitled to clinical information. Neither are outside or previous therapists, health-care professionals who are not directly involved with the patient, nor the police. However, in some situations breaching confidentiality and testimonial privilege is both ethical and legal. These exceptions are listed in Box 8-2.

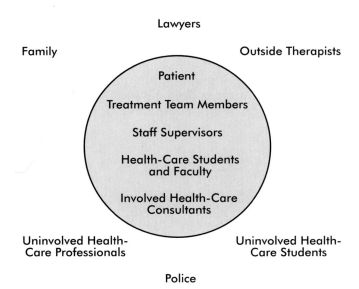

Fig. 8-2   The circle of confidentiality.

Box 8-2

EXCEPTIONS ALLOWING THE RELEASE OF INFORMATION WITHOUT THE PATIENT'S CONSENT

Emergency situations when acting in the patient's best interests
Court-ordered evaluations
If the patient is incompetent and consent is obtained from a guardian or is not available
Commitment proceedings
Criminal proceedings
Acting to protect third parties
Child custody disputes
Court-ordered reports
Reports required by state law—contagious diseases, gunshot wounds, child abuse
Patient-litigant exceptions
Child abuse proceedings

Patient Records. Most hospitals keep psychiatric records separately so that they are less accessible than medical records. The law and psychiatric profession view them as more sensitive than medical records. Many states allow or require that patients have access to their records. If a patient makes such a request, the clinician should explore the reasons for the request, determine the laws that apply in the particular state, prepare the patient for the review, and be present with the patient to discuss any questions the patient might have. The clinician must not release material from any other sources and must not alter or destroy any part of the record before the patient sees it.

Finally, it is important for the nurse to realize that the physical record itself is the property of the hospital or therapist; however, the information contained in the record belongs to the patient. Thus the original record should never be given to the patient; only a copy of it should be provided. A hospital chart can be brought into court and its contents used in a lawsuit, since privilege does not apply to hospital charts.

The parents of one of your patients arrive on the unit asking for information about their adult son. The patient has been very verbal about not wanting to see his family and not wanting them to know anything about his treatment. How would you respond?

Protecting a Third Party. Another dimension to the concepts of confidentiality and privilege stems from the case of *Tarasoff v. Regents of the University of California et al.*[38]

In this case the psychotherapist did not warn Tatiana Tarasoff or her parents that his client had stated he intended to kill her when she returned from summer vacation. In the lawsuit that followed Tatiana's death, California's Supreme Court decided that the treating therapist has a duty to warn the intended victim of a patient's violence. When a therapist is reasonably certain that a patient is going to harm someone, the therapist has the responsibility to breach the confidentiality of the relationship and warn or protect the potential victim.

Most states now recognize some variation of the duty to warn. This duty obliges the clinician to:

1. Assess the threat of violence to another
2. Identify the person being threatened
3. Implement some affirmative, preventive act

Since *Tarasoff*, over 70 legal cases have been published in which psychiatrists, psychotherapists, hospitals, and other health-care facilities have been sued for allegedly breaching the duty to protect a third party.[9]

Among the most problematic areas in which the duty to protect may apply is the protection of sexual partners of persons infected with the human immunodeficiency virus (HIV). Laws in some states forbid disclosure of patients' HIV status to sexual partners, whereas others allow it. No statutes yet mandate disclosure, but they appear to be gaining public support and may be on the horizon.

Right to Informed Consent

Informed consent means a physician must give the patient a certain amount of information about the proposed treatment and must attain the patient's consent, which must be competent, understanding, and voluntary. The physician should explain the special treatment and possible complications and risks. The reasonable information to be disclosed in obtaining informed consent is listed in Box 8-3.

The patient must be able to consent and not be a minor or judged legally incompetent. Even though a patient is psychotic, the physician is not relieved from attempting to obtain informed consent for treatment. Psychosis does not necessarily mean that an individual is unable to consent to treatment, and many psychotic patients are capable of giving informed consent. To help clinicians decide if a patient is competent to give consent, a number of techniques have been suggested.[18,21] For patients who are not able to consent and for minors informed consent should be obtained from a substitute decision maker.

The doctrine of informed consent is consistent with the provision of good clinical care. It allows patients and clinicians to become partners in the treatment process and respects patients' autonomy, needs, and values. Furthermore, informed consent should be viewed as a

---

Box 8-3

OBTAINING INFORMED CONSENT

INFORMATION TO DISCLOSE

▼ *Diagnosis*: description of the patient's problem
▼ *Treatment*: nature and purpose of the proposed treatment
▼ *Consequences*: risks and benefits of the proposed treatment including physical and psychological effects, costs, and potential resulting problems
▼ *Alternatives*: viable alternatives to the proposed treatment and their risks and benefits
▼ *Prognosis*: expected outcome with treatment, with alternative treatments, and without treatment

PRINCIPLES OF INFORMING

▼ Assess patients' ability to give informed consent
▼ Simplify the language so that laypersons can understand
▼ Offer opportunities for the patient and family to ask questions
▼ Test the patient's understanding after the explanation
▼ Reeducate as often as needed
▼ Document all relevant factors including what was disclosed, the patient's understanding, competency, voluntary agreement to treatment, and the actual consent

---

continuing educational process rather than a procedure performed merely to comply with the law. In obtaining informed consent the clinician should adhere to the principles listed in Box 8-3.

Consent forms usually require the signature of the patient, a family member, and two witnesses. Nurses are often called on to be a witness. The form then becomes part of the patient's permanent record.

In accordance with this doctrine, informed consent should be obtained for all psychiatric treatments including medication, particularly neuroleptics because of the risk of tardive dyskinesia; somatic therapies, such as electroconvulsive therapy (ECT); and experimental treatments. Whether consent should be obtained for psychotherapy is unclear at present, and other aspects related to obtaining informed consent remain controversial in many states.[42,44]

How is informed consent obtained in your psychiatric treatment setting? Ask if you can observe this process and evaluate it based on the criteria listed in Box 8-3.

Right to Treatment

The concept of the right to treatment originated in 1960 when Birnbaum,[10] a graduate student in both medicine and law, wrote, "there does not appear to have been any significant and realistic consideration given, from a legal viewpoint, to the problem of whether or not the institutionalized mentally ill person receives adequate medical treatment so that he may regain his health, and therefore his liberty, as soon as possible." In a 1966 case in the District of Columbia (*Rouse v. Cameron*), the court held that mental patients committed by criminal courts had the right to adequate treatment. Furthermore, confinement without treatment was imprisonment and transformed the hospital into a penitentiary. The case affirmed that the purpose of involuntary hospitalization was treatment, not punishment. If treatment was not provided, the patient could be transferred, released, or even awarded damages. The hospital did not need to show that the treatment would improve or cure the patient, only that there was a true attempt to do so.

A 1972 case (*Wyatt v. Stickney*) in Alabama extended the right to treatment to all mentally ill and mentally retarded persons who were involuntarily hospitalized.[47] The court defined three criteria for adequate treatment:

1. A humane psychological and physical environment
2. A qualified staff with a sufficient number of members to administer adequate treatment
3. Individualized treatment plans

The keystone of the *Wyatt* decision is the requirement for an individualized treatment plan. Failure to provide it means patients must be discharged unless they agree to remain voluntarily. This decision was upheld in a recent ruling that revised the standards related to the development of treatment plans, placed more stringent restrictions on the use of seclusion and restraint and electroconvulsive therapy, and expanded the definition of a qualified mental health professional.[26]

There were two cases that reached the nation's highest court as well. The Supreme Court made a landmark decision in 1975 in the case of *Donaldson v. O'Connor*, which freed a Florida State psychiatric patient after 15 years of involuntary confinement. The court ruled that he was not dangerous and was not receiving treatment. Therefore continuing to confine him would violate his right to liberty. Then again in 1982, in *Youngberg v. Romeo*, the court ruled that involuntary patients were entitled only to that treatment required to ensure freedom from unnecessary restraint and preventable assault.

The right to treatment is not a guarantee of treatment for all patients. It applies only to involuntary or committed patients. In addition, the right to treatment identifies minimal treatment standards, not optimal treatment; it does not guarantee that adequate treatment occurs; and it does not require that a range of treatments be available—one treatment choice is adequate. Thus, while much has been gained through this legislation, much remains to be done.

This right also poses several questions. One involves the appropriateness of treatment and whether confinement itself can be therapeutic. A second question deals with the untreatable patient. Should such a patient be released after a certain time? Another problem is the unwilling patient. Might a person refuse treatment and then seek release, claiming that the right to adequate treatment was denied? A more pressing question is whether the public is willing to pay the costs required to provide adequate treatment to the mentally ill in public institutions. In current times of reduced government funds, programs often struggle to survive at existing funding levels, let alone expansion. Thus budget constraints may play an even greater role than judicial decisions in affecting the care of the mentally ill.

Right to Refuse Treatment

The relationship between the right to treatment and the right to refuse treatment is complex (see Critical Thinking about Contemporary Issues). The right to refuse treatment includes the right to refuse involuntary hospitalization. It has been called the "right to be left alone." Some people believe therapy can control a person's mind, regulate thoughts, and change personality, and the right to refuse treatment protects the patient against this. This argument states that involuntary therapy conflicts with two basic legal rights: freedom of thought and the right to control one's life and actions as long as they do not interfere with the rights of others.

In recent years, there has been an increase in the number of lawsuits concerning the right to refuse treatment, especially treatment involving psychotropic drugs. Many states have guidelines for the administration of electroconvulsive therapy and psychosurgery; however, the controversy over refusal of medication is a more recent one. Related to this is the right to refuse experimentation. Any experimental treatment requires the written consent of the patient.

The 1979 landmark case that established this right for psychiatric patients was *Rogers v. Okin*.[30] This upheld the rights of hospitalized psychiatric patients to refuse medication. It emphasized that restraint may be used only in cases of emergency, such as the occurrence or serious threat of extreme violence, personal injury, or attempted suicide. The court's decision meant that committed psychiatric patients were presumed competent to make decisions regarding treatment in nonemergencies.

On the other hand, the 1982 Supreme Court decision in *Youngberg v. Romeo*[48] noted that patients' rights could

CRITICAL THINKING ABOUT CONTEMPORARY ISSUES

Is the Value of Treatment More Important Than a Person's Right to Liberty?

This question has been debated over the years and is still not resolved for psychiatric patients. The most publicized case examining this issue was that of Billie Boggs, a 40-year-old black woman who lived on the street for a year near a warm-air grate on New York's fashionable Upper East Side and who panhandled money for food. She attracted the attention of a mental health team who decided to hospitalize her believing she was mentally ill and not able to care for herself.[11]

The legal questions raised in this case were whether Billie Boggs was mentally ill and whether she was dangerous. At trial, psychiatrists from one side testified that she was both mentally ill and dangerous. However, psychiatrists who interviewed Billie after she was hospitalized and had received medication, been bathed, rested, dressed adequately, and fed testified that she was not mentally ill. The questions that emerged were:

▼ What behavior is socially acceptable?
▼ How is mental illness determined?
▼ How is dangerousness defined?

Although the legal actions proceeded, the hospital discharged Billie because she refused to accept further antipsychotic medication.

The Billie Boggs case has raised more unanswered questions and dramatized the problem of mentally ill street people. What it has not done is address the compelling needs of the chronically mentally ill in this country. ▼

be limited in the interest of treatment as long as professional judgment was made by qualified personnel.

The right-to-refuse-treatment concept raises many questions. Does the right apply to all treatments, including medications, or only to those that are hazardous, intrusive, or severe, such as psychosurgery? How can staff meet their obligation for the right to treatment when a patient refuses to be treated? How can refusal, resisting treatment, and noncompliance be differentiated, and does each of these require a different response? No solutions exist to these complex issues, but they concern nurses, who are frequently responsible for delivering prescribed treatments such as medications.

A recent review of the literature on the refusal of medication shows that, although short-term refusal is common, continuing long-term refusal is rare.[24] Symptomatology such as delusions and denial may cause the refusal, and patients who refuse medication are generally sicker than those who comply.[33] A study of patient's attitudes after involuntary medication suggests that for most patients the decision to refuse medication is a sign of the patient's illness and does not reflect autonomous functioning or consistent beliefs about mental illness or its treatment.[32]

 Is the refusal of treatment the same as noncompliance? If not, how would you distinguish between them and what nursing intervention would be most appropriate for each?

Rhoden[29] provides an additional perspective. She suggests that staff members who overrule a patient because they believe they are doing "what is best for the patient" may sacrifice increased patient-staff communication and cooperation. Although drug treatment may help patients, taking their views seriously by not forcing the medication shows respect for them and may, in itself, be therapeutic.

Staff members faced with the patient who is refusing medication have several options. First, they can offer the patient a lower dosage—or no medication at all. A second option would be to discharge the patient against medical advice if no other staff action can relieve the patient's symptoms and the patient does not meet the criteria for commitment. Another approach would be to have the patient declared incompetent and seek a court order permitting the medication. Similarly, a guardian can consent to medication when the patient's refusal can be shown to result from incompetence and resultant inability to make a rational decision.

Nurses should judge each situation on a case-by-case basis. The Task Force on Behavior Therapy has examined the issue of coerced treatment and suggested three criteria that may justify it[8]:

1. The patient must be judged to be dangerous to self or others.
2. It must be believed by those administering treatment that it has a reasonable chance to benefit the patient and those who are related.
3. The patient must be judged to be incompetent to evaluate the necessity of the treatment.

Even if these three conditions are met, the patient should not be deceived but should be informed regarding what will be done, the reasons for it, and its probable effects.

Nurses are frequently on the front line in dealing with patients who refuse treatments and medications. It is clear that voluntary patients have the right to refuse any and all treatments and should not be forcibly medicated except in exceptional situations when the patient is actively violent to self and others and when all less restrictive means have been unsuccessful. The behavior of the patient should be clearly documented and all interventions recorded.

Nurses must know the guidelines identified by the courts and the legislature in the state in which they practice in order to administer medication properly to involuntarily committed patients. Some questions that can help guide the nurse's decision are[27]:

1. Has the patient been given a psychiatric diagnosis?
2. Is the treatment consistent with the diagnosis?
3. Is there a set of defined "target symptoms?"
4. Has the patient been informed about the treatment outcome and side effects?
5. Have medical and nursing assessments been completed before introducing drug therapy?
6. Are the therapeutic effects of treatment being monitored?
7. Are side effects being monitored?
8. Is the patient over or under medicated?
9. Is drug therapy being changed too quickly?
10. Are PRNs and stat doses being used too often?
11. Is drug therapy being prescribed for an indefinite period of time?

Finally it is important for the nurse to remember that a therapeutic nurse-patient relationship is critical in working with a patient who refuses to take medication. A positive, caring relationship between the nurse and patient can play a vital role in reversing treatment refusal.

Imagine that your mother was admitted to a psychiatric hospital in need of treatment. Once there, however, she refused to take any medication. How would you feel if the staff forced medication on her? How would you feel if they honored her right to refuse treatment? What could you, as a family member, do to help your mother get the treatment she needed?

Right to Treatment in the Least Restrictive Setting

The right to treatment in the least restrictive setting is closely related to the right to adequate treatment. Its goal is evaluating the specific needs of each patient and maintaining the greatest amount of personal freedom, autonomy, dignity, and integrity in determining treatment. Table 8-2 presents six clinical dimensions of the concept of restrictiveness in psychiatric

Table 8-2   Six Dimensions of the Concept of Restrictiveness

Dimension	Component
Structural	Type of treatment setting and objective means of physical restraint or limitations on physical freedoms
Institutional policy	Rules, procedures, routines, and regulations for operating the institution and degree of patient involvement in planning
Enforcement	Staff-determined consequences of rule breaking or inability of the patient to leave the setting
Treatment	Use and level of antipsychotic medications and the use of other somatic treatments such as electroconvulsive therapy or psychosurgery
Psychosocial atmosphere	Status difference between patients and staff and degrees of staff authoritarianism
Patient characteristics	Patients' ability to manage their care and level of functioning as influenced by the severity of their disorder

From Garritson S: J *Psychosoc Nurs Ment Health Serv* 21:9, 1983.

nursing. This right applies to both community- and noncommunity-based programs. Greater consideration of this right might limit some of the controversy surrounding commitment and the right to refuse treatment.

The cases behind this right assert that if patients can function in some setting other than a mental hospital, the court has the responsibility of placing them in that setting. In the 1973 case *Dixon v. Weinberger*, the judge ruled that patients in Washington, D.C., have a statutory right to confinement in the least restrictive facility.[14] Washington, D.C., and the federal government were responsible for developing a plan to identify those who should be transferred to community-based facilities and the means for achieving this transfer, including creating new facilities if necessary. Although progress has been made, the court is still supervising the D.C. mental health system.

The right to the least restrictive alternative tends to support patients' needs for normalization more effectively than right-to-treatment cases. However, this is complicated by the need for new models, more facilities, and larger budgets for aftercare so that discharged and chronically ill patients can be supported and treated in the community.

Which do you think is more restrictive—to be living in the community while actively psychotic or to be involuntarily committed to a psychiatric hospital for treatment?

This right to treatment in the least restrictive setting raises a number of difficult questions. How do mental health professionals balance human rights with the human needs of patients? Will sufficient funds be available to provide adequate supportive care in the community? What will happen to the chronically ill patients who are not discharged into less restrictive settings? Will the community centers be able to provide better care than institutions? How can one counter community resistance to local placement of mentally ill patients? And most important, given economic constraints, how can limited resources be used wisely to provide a full range of mental health services? For further discussion of these issues see Chapter 13.

A final consideration in the right to the least restrictive alternative is that it applies not only to when a person should be hospitalized but also to how a person is cared for within the hospital setting. It requires that a patient's progress be carefully monitored so that treatment plans can be changed based on the patient's current condition.

Issues related to the use of seclusion and restraints are of particular concern. There must be adequate rationale for the use of these practices. Documentation should include a description of the precipitating event that led to seclusion or restraint, alternatives attempted or considered, the patient's behavior while secluded or restrained, nursing interventions, and ongoing evaluation of the patient. It is important to remember that seclusion and restraint must be therapeutically indicated and justified (see Chapter 26). Nurses may find it helpful to refer to the guidelines developed on them by a task force of the American Psychiatric Association.[4]

Nursing's Role in Patients' Rights

The National League for Nursing in 1977 issued a statement on the nurse's role in patients' rights.[25] It identified respect and concern for patients and assurance of competent care as basic rights, along with patients receiving the necessary information to understand their illness and make decisions about their care. The League urged nurses to get involved in assuring patients' human and legal rights.

The League identified many of the previously mentioned rights, plus the following[4]:

▼ Right to health care that is accessible and that

meets professional standards, regardless of the setting

▼ Right to courteous and individualized health care that is equitable, humane, and given without discrimination as to race, color, creed, sex, national origin, source of payment, or ethical or political beliefs

▼ Right to information about their diagnosis, prognosis, and treatment, including alternatives to care and risks involved

▼ Right to information about the qualifications, names, and titles of health-care personnel

▼ Right to refuse observation by those not directly involved in their care

▼ Right to coordination and continuity of health care

▼ Right to information on the charges for services, including the right to challenge these

▼ Above all, the right to be fully informed about all their rights in all health-care settings

Perhaps the single most important factor is the attitude of mental health professionals. Sensitivity to patients' rights cannot be imposed by the court, the legislature, administrative agencies, or professional groups. If nurses ignore them, implement them casually, or are outwardly hostile about honoring them, patients' rights remain an empty legal concept. But if professionals are sensitive to patients' needs in all aspects of their relationships with them, they will secure these human and legal rights.

LEGISLATIVE INITIATIVES

The interface between psychiatry and the law is becoming increasingly complex. Historically the mental health delivery system had only two components—mental health professionals and patients. Now, however, the system has grown to include six forces, each of which must be taken into account when dealing with any mental health problem. These are patients, families, providers of services, government regulators and lawmakers, the judiciary, and third-party insurers (Fig. 8-3). These groups have related, but slightly different, interests. The patient is concerned that services be available when and where he wishes them, that they are appropriate, and that he is involved in establishing their priorities. The family desires what is best for their family member and is concerned about issues related to quality of life, support, education, and empowerment. The provider has clinical and professional biases. If outside controls must exist, the provider wants them applied fairly, with responsibilities and liabilities clearly defined. The government wants citizens to have quality care at the lowest cost and wants providers to be accountable for their care. The courts, after years of neglect, are focusing on patients' constitutional rights and have begun to scru-

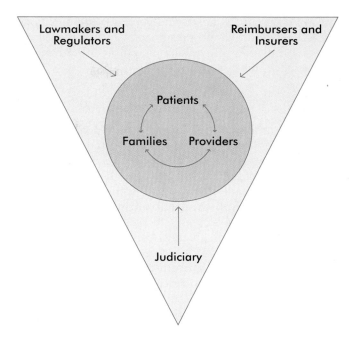

Fig. 8-3   Forces affecting psychiatric care.

tinize patient care and treatment. Finally, insurance companies are concerned with making a profit and paying for covered services by appropriately licensed and credentialed professionals. The changing priorities and interactions of these six forces affect the quality, availability, and responsiveness of mental health services in the United States. At present there are simultaneous trends toward adequate treatment of the psychiatrically ill and protection of their constitutional rights. Both trends are occurring at a time of fiscal restraint.

Mental health professionals are concerned about the quantity and quality of psychiatric care. Legal reformers are indignant about perceived violations of patients' rights. Judges are angry that in the day-to-day implementation of the commitment law, their only option is to prosecute the mentally ill defendant. Psychiatric hospitals are understaffed, underfunded, and attacked on all sides for their inability to "care for" and "cure" psychiatric patients. Community programs are few and poorly supported, often resulting in deinstitutionalized patients living without treatment in urban ghettos or being treated as criminals. The public is frightened at the thought of psychiatric patients in their neighborhoods. Concerned citizens demand that mental health programs exercise greater control over this population, whom they perceive as dangerous.

Clearly, mechanisms are needed by which patients, families, mental health professionals, attorneys, and concerned citizens can work together to advance mental health care and the rights of all patients. The mentally ill need protection not only of their legal rights but also of their clinical needs and general welfare. No one profession can fulfill all these needs, but increased cooperation among the various mental health advocates can achieve this goal.

Omnibus Budget Reconciliation Act

Other legislation has also changed the nature of psychiatric care and service delivery in the United States. One major event was the Omnibus Budget Reconciliation Act (OBRA) first passed in 1981. It placed the mental health services programs formerly administered by the federal government through the National Institute of Mental Health (NIMH) into alcohol and drug abuse and mental health services block grant to be administered by the states. The intent of OBRA was to reduce federal spending on health care and give states more flexibility in decision making about the allocation of funds for mental health. It also decreased the federal role in the coordination of these activities. Overall, this had a negative impact on the quality of mental health services provided throughout the country, since each state now was able to allocate resources to mental health based on its own priorities and political climate. Although some states made significant progress in developing community-based systems, in most state governments mental health funding was not given high priority.

Since that time, other changes have been mandated through this same annual legislative process. For example, in 1985 the Consolidated OBRA (COBRA) prohibited indigent patients with acute medical conditions from being transferred from general medical hospitals or emergency departments to public psychiatric hospitals that are ill equipped to provide medical care.[16] This helped the mentally ill. However, the OBRA passed in 1987 established criteria for Medicaid- or Medicare-certified nursing homes to use in admitting or retaining mentally ill patients. The effect of this law was to continue the trend of shifting costs from federal programs to the states, and it has the potential of increasing homelessness and continuing a pattern of failure to adequately serve patients with severe mental illness.[15]

Protection and Advocacy Act

Under the Protection and Advocacy for Mentally Ill Individuals Act of 1986, all states must designate an agency that is responsible for protecting the rights of the mentally ill. The following three areas of advocacy would help to maximize the fulfillment of patients' rights:

1. To educate the mental health staff and to implement policies and procedures that recognize and protect patients' rights
2. To establish an additional procedure to permit the speedy resolution of problems, questions, or disagreements that occur based on legal rights
3. To provide access to legal services when patients' rights have been denied

A model patients' rights advocacy program in Maryland includes a four-level appeal process that tries to resolve problems through mediation between patients, state hospital staff, and legal representatives.[22] In this program the majority of complaints were resolved without legal intervention at the first stage of the appeal process, usually in a meeting between a rights advisor, the patient, and the patient's primary clinician.

Although the advocacy movement has helped to bring about many positive changes in the health-care system, it has also been criticized for inadequate definition of terms and irresponsibility. "Advocate," "legal representative," and "ombudsman" are often defined differently in different programs. "Legal advocacy" and "legal services" are also confused, and "information" and "advice" are often equated with "advocacy." It has also been noted that the patients' rights activist has power without clinical responsibility, and major problems can result when power is wielded by people who do not understand the complex clinical needs of the severely mentally ill. Mental health professionals, therefore, must distinguish responsible advocacy from irresponsible lobbying. One suggestion is that advocates be required to have in-depth experience with severely disturbed patients for 6 months to a year and that advocates be rigorously screened.

Americans with Disabilities Act

The Americans with Disabilities Act, passed in 1990, protects over 43 million Americans with one or more physical or mental disabilities from discrimination in jobs, public services, and accommodations.[3,43] It prohibits discrimination against people with physical and mental disabilities in hiring, firing, training, compensation, and advancement in employment. Employers are prohibited from asking job applicants whether they have a disability, and medical examinations and questions about disability may be required only if the concerns are job related and necessary.[28]

This act promises to have a substantial impact on those with physical disabilities, but its impact on those with mental illness may not be as great.[20] It does, however, constitute a cultural as well as legal mandate to include people with disabilities in the social and economic mainstream. It is not likely to totally eliminate the myths, fears, and discrimination faced by people with disabilities, but it does contribute to the educational effort needed to combat widespread misinformation, biases, and misperceptions about people with disabilities, including mental illness.

Advanced Directives

Advanced directives came about as a result of the Patient Self-Determination Act (PSDA) of 1990. They are documents, written while a person is competent, that specify how decisions about treatment should be made if the person were to become incompetent. Use of advanced directives seems particularly appropriate for persons with mental illness who may alternate between periods of competence and incompetence. They could, for example, formalize a patient's wishes about forced medication or treatment setting.

Some states are already encouraging patients to fill out advanced directive forms. In addition, federal regulations that took effect in 1991 require all facilities that receive Medicare or Medicaid to inform patients, including psychiatric patients, at admission about their rights under state law to sign advanced directives. To date, advanced directives have not had a major impact on psychiatric treatment but that may change in the near future.[5]

Does your psychiatric setting comply with federal law that requires having patients sign advanced directives? If so, talk with some patients and ask them what this document means to them.

PSYCHIATRY AND CRIMINAL RESPONSIBILITY

The determination of criminal responsibility concerns the accused person's condition when the crime was committed. It has received much public attention as the "insanity defense." This proposes that a person who has committed an act usually considered criminal is not guilty by reason of "insanity." This is a difficult decision to make. Usually defense attorneys and prosecutors offer many arguments pro and con and frequently call on psychiatrists to testify. Nurses are seldom directly involved, but they should understand the law in this area as both citizens and psychiatric professionals.

This defense is based on the humanitarian rationale that individuals should not be blamed for crimes if they "did not know what they were doing" or "could not help themselves." With the complexity of today's society and judicial system, however, many believe this defense is being abused, and it is highly controversial. Some of this controversy stems from John Hinckley's shooting of President Reagan in 1981, from which he was acquitted by the verdict of "not guilty by reason of insanity" (Fig. 8-4). One recent change is the movement away from using the defense "not guilty by

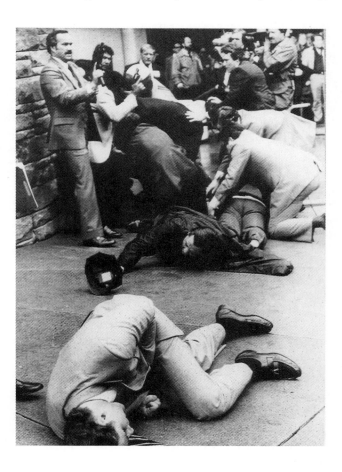

Fig. 8-4 John Hinckley's shooting of President Reagan and two other men in 1981 resulted in acquittal on grounds of insanity.
AP/Wide World Photos.

reason of insanity" (NGBI) to the more recent "guilty but mentally ill" (GBMI).

At present three sets of criteria are used in the United States to determine the criminal responsibility of an offender who is mentally ill: the M'Naghten Test, the Irresistible Impulse Test, and the American Law Institute's Test, the one most frequently used (Table 8-3).

M'Naghten Test

This law originated with the 1832 London trial of Daniel M'Naghten, who was tried for the murder of Edward Drummond. M'Naghten had suffered from delusions of persecution and had complained to public authorities many times. Receiving no help, however, he decided to resolve the situation himself. He began watching the house of Sir Robert Peele and one evening, under the belief he was shooting Peele, shot Edward Drummond as he left the house. His attorney entered an appeal of "partial insanity." M'Naghten was declared of unsound mind and committed to an institution for the criminally

Table 8-3 Three Sets of Criteria Used To Determine the Criminal Responsibility of a Mentally Ill Offender

Name of test	Criteria
M'Naghten Test	1. The individual did not know the nature and quality of the act. 2. The individual did not know that the act was wrong.
Irresistible Impulse Test	An individual is impulsively driven to commit the criminal act with lack of premeditation and a strong urge to do so. This test is usually used with the M'Naghten Test.
American Law Institute's Test	An individual lacks the capacity to "appreciate" the wrongfulness of an act or to "conform" conduct to the requirements of the law. It excludes the sociopath and is a popular criterion for determining criminal responsibility.

insane. In deciding the case the judges identified two rules to determine the criminal responsibility of a person who pleads insanity. The first rule states that the individual at the time of the crime did not "know the nature and quality of the act." The second states that if he did know what he was doing, he did not know that it "was wrong." These two rules are called the "nature and quality" rule and "right from wrong" test. This case was the first major test of criminal responsibility, and it is still used in most states and criminal courts.

Irresistible Impulse Test

A number of states have adopted the Irresistible Impulse Test along with the M'Naghten Test. It is never used in isolation. According to this test, a person may know the difference between right and wrong but feels impulsively driven to commit the criminal act. It is usually necessary to show a lack of premeditation and that the urge was so strong that it would have been followed regardless of the circumstances.

This test is a frequent defense for sudden, violent behavior displayed under stress. For example, it was the test used by the defense in the 1994 case of Lorena Bobbitt, who was found not guilty by reason of insanity. The jury concluded that she could not resist the impulse to sever her husband's penis. Mrs. Bobbitt was committed to a psychiatric hospital for observation and was released when she was found not to be psychiatrically ill.

American Law Institute's Test

The American Law Institute's Test is similar to the combination of the M'Naghten Test and Irresistible Impulse Test. It states that individuals are not responsible for criminal acts if they lack the capacity to "appreciate" that it is wrong or to "conform" their conduct to the law. It also excludes "an abnormality manifested only by repeated criminal or otherwise antisocial conduct," which excludes the sociopath who has repeated criminal conduct. This popular test is now used by all the federal circuit courts and a number of states' courts.

Disposition of Mentally Ill Offenders

Those found not guilty by reason of insanity (NGBI) are rarely set free. In some states they may be committed at the court's discretion, and in almost a third of the states they are automatically hospitalized. Some offenders are treated in special hospitals, others are sent to state mental hospitals, and still others go to prison treatment facilities. Those found guilty but mentally ill (GBMI) are never freed. Since the insanity defense is used most frequently in capital offenses, it is usually better to have good security, and penal institutions or maximum security forensic psychiatric hospitals are the best option.

After hospitalization and recovery, the patient may be discharged by the court that ordered the commitment. In other states the governor may discharge the patient. Still others allow the mental institution to make that decision. The major criteria for discharge are that the patient is not likely to repeat the offense and that it is relatively safe to release the patient to the community.

 Do you believe in both legal defenses—NGBI and GBMI? What are the pros and cons of each insanity defense?

LEGAL ROLE OF THE NURSE

Professional nursing practice is not determined by simply following patients' rights. Rather, it is an interplay between the rights of patients, the legal role of the nurse, and concern for quality psychiatric care (Fig. 8-5). There are three roles that the psychiatric nurse moves in and out of while completing professional and personal responsibilities: provider of services, employee or contractor of services, and private citizen. These roles are simultaneous, and each carries certain rights and responsibilities.

Nurse as Provider

Malpractice. All psychiatric professionals have legally defined duties of care and are responsible for their own

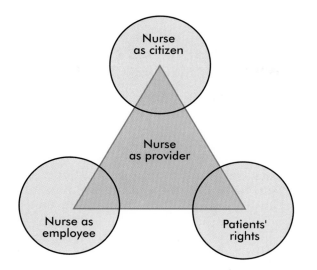

Fig. 8-5   Legal influences on psychiatric nursing practice.

work. If these duties are violated, malpractice exists. Malpractice involves the failure of professionals to provide the proper and competent care that is given by members of their profession, resulting in harm to the patient. Nurses are held to national and not local standards of care.

Most malpractice claims are filed under the law of negligent tort. A **tort** is a civil wrong for which the injured party is entitled to compensation. Because, under the law, individuals are responsible for their own torts, each nurse can be held responsible in malpractice claims. Under the law of negligent tort the plaintiff must prove the following:

1. A legal duty of care existed.
2. The nurse performed the duty negligently.
3. Damages were suffered by the plaintiff as a result.
4. The damages were substantial.

When patients are admitted to a psychiatric hospital, the problems of litigation in connection with their care are many and varied. The Bill of Rights in the Mental Health Systems Act, which was repealed, nevertheless helps clarify the sometimes conflicting roles of mental health professionals. It asserts that a health professional is not obligated to: administer treatment contrary to clinical judgment, prevent the discharge of any person for whom appropriate treatment is impossible as a result of the person's refusal to consent, admit any person who has repeatedly frustrated treatments in the past by withholding consent, or provide treatment to anyone admitted solely for diagnostic or evaluative purposes.[23] Such legislation helps to shed some light on the role of health providers in such issues as right to treatment and right to refuse treatment.

Litigation. Lawsuits alleging malpractice in psychiatric diagnosis or treatment, once rare, are now increas-

ing. Some of the most frequent sources of malpractice suits against psychiatrists between 1980 and 1985 include the following[7]:

▼ Incarceration and suicide attempts
▼ Drug overdose and addiction
▼ Failure to diagnose physical condition
▼ Breach of contract
▼ Psychotherapy/depression
▼ Failure to treat psychosis
▼ Complications of restraints—paralysis or fracture
▼ Sexual misconduct

Similarly, lawsuits against nurses were relatively uncommon. However, they can occur when the nurse errs while acting either dependently or independently.[17] Box 8-4 describes three recent cases involving psychiatric nurses. A study of nursing malpractice litigation between 1967 and 1977 indicated that approximately 14 cases occurred in psychiatric hospitals.[12] Most incidents involved administration of treatments or medications, communications, and supervision of patients.

The most common causes of malpractice suits against psychiatric nurses are negligence in suicide precautions and while assisting in ECT. When a patient is believed to be suicidal, the psychiatrist writes an order for suicide precautions. The nurse then has the responsibility to follow that order in a way that ensures the patient's safety. The exact procedure varies from hospital to hospital, but it should include close observation, limiting the patient's activity to the ward only, and removing any potentially harmful objects (see Chapter 18). Another potential problem area concerns the patient receiving ECT. The nurse must take proper precautions to prepare patients before the treatment and to monitor their status afterward until they are fully conscious and alert (see Chapter 26).

Legal Responsibilities. The nurse is responsible for reporting pertinent information to co-workers involved in the patient's care. The degree of nursing care depends on the patient's condition, with the seriously ill demanding a higher degree of care to protect them from injury and self-destruction.

Reporting information includes written as well as oral communication, and accurate records are crucial. Box 8-5 lists characteristics of good nursing records. For example, notes that record specific suicidal precautions clarify the nurse's actions. The nurse should also record all patient and family education such as explaining the food precautions needed when taking monoamine oxidase (MAO) inhibitor medication. Such a note would provide a good defense against a possible lawsuit should the patient violate dietary restrictions and become ill. Accurate reporting is an element of good nursing care that should be completed promptly and thoroughly.

Box 8-4
SELECTED LITIGATION INVOLVING PSYCHIATRIC NURSES

Case 1: Valentine v. Strange (597 F. Supp. 1316 Va)

Problem: Nurses were sued when psychiatric patient set self on fire

Facts: Despite two previous attempts to burn herself, the health-care providers permitted the patient to keep her cigarettes and lighter. Patient subsequently set fire to her clothing and suffered third-degree burns.

Legal Lesson: The failure of health-care professionals to take precaution in the face of imminent danger to the life of an involuntarily committed patient constitutes a violation of liberty interests protected by the due process clause of the Fourteenth Amendment.

Case 2: Vattimo v. Lower Bucks Hospital (428 A. 2nd 765—Pa.)

Problem: Need for restraint and supervision of patients by psychiatric nurses

Facts: A patient with a psychotic fascination with fire set fire to his hospital room, resulting in the death of the other occupant. The patient had been diagnosed as a paranoid schizophrenic, and staff had been warned of his preoccupation with fire.

Legal Lesson: The hospital was required to exercise reasonable care under the circumstances to restrain, supervise, and protect mentally deficient patients.

Case 3: Delicata v. Bourlesses (404 N.E. 2nd 667—Mass.)

Problem: Nursing psychiatric assessment vs. the psychologist's

Facts: A nursing assessment indicated that a depressed patient should be closely supervised as potentially suicidal. An evaluation by the staff psychologist advised that suicidal precautions were *not* necessary. The patient subsequently killed herself in a locked bathroom.

Legal Lesson: Medical orders by a staff psychiatrist or an evaluation by a staff psychologist must be questioned when there is a change or deterioration in a patient's condition. Nursing assessments should include the evaluation of such changes in the patient's apparent physical and psychological condition. The responsibility of assessment includes the necessity for making appropriate nursing judgments and implementing nursing actions based on these assessments.

Box 8-5
CHARACTERISTICS OF GOOD NURSING RECORDS

Clear	Concise	Legible
Factual	Accurate	Objective
Complete	Timely	

Unlike patients' charts, some hospital records, such as incident reports, are not admissible in court to prove facts but they can cast doubt on the credibility of the involved parties. Currently, more insurance companies are requiring hospitals to keep incident reports, and more state and federal agencies are demanding the right to review them. Because they can be seen and used by so many people, what a nurse writes on an incident report should be carefully considered, and unfounded statements, opinions, interpretations, and vague descriptions should be avoided.

The legal responsibilities of nonphysician therapists have not yet been well defined. The nurse can follow these preventive measures to avoid possible lawsuits:

1. Implement nursing care that meets the *Standards of Psychiatric–Mental Health Clinical Nursing Practice* as described by the American Nurses' Association.[2]
2. Know the laws of the specific state, including the rights and duties of the nurse as well as the rights of the patients.
3. Keep accurate and concise nursing records.
4. Maintain the confidentiality of patient information.
5. Maintain current malpractice liability insurance coverage.
6. Consult a lawyer should any questions arise.

Nurse As Employee

The role of employee, or contractor of service, is less frequently studied but also very important. It involves the practitioner's rights and responsibilities in relation to employers, partners, consultants, and other professional colleagues. Professionals often do not know the rights and responsibilities of employees and contractors of service. However, these are the basis of the practitioner's economic security, professional future, and peer relationships.

As employees, nurses have the responsibility to supervise and evaluate those under their authority for the quality of care given. They must also observe their employer's rights and responsibilities to clients and other employees, fulfill the obligations of the contracted service adequately, inform the employer of circumstances and conditions that impair the quality of care, and report negligent care by others when and where appropriate. This includes the legal duty to communicate any concerns about other mental health professionals.

 You have observed a colleague sexually touching a patient on the unit. What should you do based on your legal and professional obligations?

In return, nurses can expect certain rights from their employer. These include consideration for service, adequate working conditions, adequate and qualified assistance where necessary, and the right to respect all of their other rights and responsibilities.

 You arrive for work one morning and are told that you and an aide are the only staff assigned to work the day shift on a 25-bed closed psychiatric unit. Based on your legal roles, rights, and responsibilities how should you respond?

Nurse As Citizen

The third role that the nurse plays is that of citizen. This is particularly significant because all other roles, rights, responsibilities, and privileges are awarded because of the inherent rights of citizenship. The U.S. government grants these as inherent: civil rights, property rights, right to protection from harm, right to a good name, and right to due process. These form the foundation for the nurse's other legal relationships.

Conflict of Interest. Unfortunately the best interests of the patient, nurse, and employer do not always coincide. Conflict can occur when, for example, the nurse's right to live and work without threat to personal security is violated by a patient who harms the nurse. Take the case of a psychotic patient who has hallucinations that are adequately controlled with psychotropic medications but who refuses to take them. Intervention with this patient must consider the following possibilities:

▼ Failing to medicate may deny the patient's right to treatment.
▼ Failing to medicate the patient could have harmful side effects, such as the unnecessary and possibly irreversible continuation of illness.
▼ Failing to medicate the patient may lead to a psychotic episode and result in injury to self, other patients, or the staff.
▼ Failing to medicate the patient may lead to a psychotic episode but no violence.

▼ Medicating the patient in the absence of an emergency situation and without a clear threat of violence violates the patient's right to refuse treatment.

In the following case the staff decided not to medicate the patient. When the night nurse checked on the patient in his room that evening, he struck the nurse in the face, resulting in severe bruises and the loss of several teeth. This development leads to new questions:

▼ Was the patient competent and legally liable for his actions?
▼ What were the circumstances of the incident?
▼ Was the nurse sufficiently aware of the potential hazard and, if so, was she responsible for assuming the risk?
▼ Was staffing adequate to discourage, respond to, and control a potentially violent situation?
▼ Was there a provision in the unit for potentially violent patients and, if so, why wasn't it used for this patient?

Obviously, there are no simple or perhaps even equitable solutions to such dilemmas; yet they are real and ever present. All mental health professionals must focus on prevention. This requires a knowledge of legislation, rights, responsibilities, and potential conflicts.

Nurses in Maryland have developed a bill of rights for registered nurses (Box 8-6). This commendable document educates nurses and the public and also clarifies rights and responsibilities. In addition, professional nursing judgment requires examining the context of nursing care, the possible consequences of nurses' actions, and practical alternatives. Only then do rights and responsibilities become meaningful.

SUMMARY

1. There are three types of admission to a psychiatric hospital: informal, voluntary, and involuntary commitment. Involuntary commitment poses many legal and ethical issues for patients, the law, and psychiatric professionals.

Box 8-6

MARYLAND NURSES' ASSOCIATION: THE BILL OF RIGHTS FOR REGISTERED NURSES

We, the Council on Human Rights of the Maryland Nurses' Association, in order to promote increased knowledge and understanding of the rights and responsibilities of all registered nurses, have developed the Bill of Rights for Registered Nurses. We propose that this Bill will aid in educating consumers and health care professionals about the rights of registered nurses, as well as their corresponding responsibilities. Therefore we submit the Bill of Rights for Registered Nurses as a position statement of the Maryland Nurses' Association.

The nurse has a right:	**The nurse has a responsibility:**

The nurse has a right:

INDIVIDUAL

To practice according to the Maryland Nurse Practice Act.
To make independent nursing judgments.
To question any delegated medical order or any plan of care that may cause possible harm to the patient/client or others.
To refuse to carry out any delegated medical order or any plan of care that may cause possible harm to the patient/client or others.
To pursue quality continuing education.
To teach individuals and groups health care practices that facilitate treatment, prevent illness, and provide optimal wellness.

EMPLOYMENT

To competitive hiring and promotion which is based on knowledge and experience and which is unrestricted by consideration of sex, race, age, creed, or national origin.
To realistic assignments that can assure the patient/client quality care that includes safety, dignity, and comfort.
To negotiate salary and individual conditions of employment.
To work in a safe and adequately equipped environment.
To work with qualified, competent nursing personnel.
To periodic, fair, objective evaluations by peers.
To pay increases based on demonstrated performance.
To due process whenever accused of unethical, incompetent, illegal, or unqualified practice or of prejudicial or inappropriate conduct.
To be an advocate for the patient/client and the public when health care and safety may be affected by incompetent, unethical, or illegal practices.
To representation by a negotiator in labor matters.

The nurse has a responsibility:

To assume personal accountability for individual nursing judgments and actions which consider the individual value systems and the uniqueness of each patient/client.
To implement the nursing process in providing individualized nursing care.
To safeguard the patient/client and the public from incompetent, unethical, or illegal health care practices.
To refuse to perform any nursing action which will jeopardize the patient/client or the public, and the obligation to communicate the rationale to the proper authority.
To avail one's self of opportunities which will broaden knowledge and refine and increase skills.
To educate the patient/client and the public.

To maintain competence and prepare one's self adequately for promotion.
To evaluate one's own work environment and to communicate and document unrealistic work loads through appropriate channels.
To make known individual convictions and preferences prior to hiring.
To assess, evaluate, document, and correct unsafe conditions and to communicate such information to the appropriate authority promptly.
To objectively document and report to appropriate authority evidence of competent, as well as incompetent performance and to evaluate, inform, counsel, and teach nursing personnel when indicated.
To participate in the development of reliable and valid evaluation criteria for peer review.
To maintain competence, incorporate new techniques and knowledge, and continuously upgrade the quality of health care.
To participate in the planning, establishment, and implementation of procedures to ensure due process.
To be alert to any instances of incompetent, unethical, or illegal practices by any member of the health care system and to take appropriate action regarding these practices.
To select and utilize a knowledgeable and impartial negotiator.

Box 8-6
MARYLAND NURSES' ASSOCIATION; THE BILL OF RIGHTS FOR REGISTERED NURSES—cont'd

The nurse has a right:	The nurse has a responsibility:
PROFESSIONAL	
To receive support from the nursing profession at all levels.	To participate in activities that contribute to the ongoing development of the profession's body of knowledge.
To belong to an autonomous nursing organization.	To be an active member and to participate in the nursing organization's effort to implement and improve standards of nursing.
To have expert testimony supplied by the nursing organization for both legal and legislative issues.	
To full and equal representation on all decision-making bodies concerned with health care.	To provide knowledgeable, objective, articulate expert testimony.
To be involved actively in the political decision-making process at all levels of the government.	To provide knowledgeable, active, and effective collaborating with members of the health professions.
	To be knowledgeable, active, and effective in the legislative process by direct involvement, effective education and selection of representative legislators, lobbying, and creating citizen awareness in promoting local, state, and national efforts to meet the health needs of the public.

---

2. There are three types of discharge from a psychiatric hospital for committed patients: conditional, absolute, and judicial.

3. Outpatient commitment mandates patients to a course of outpatient treatment specified by their clinicians.

4. Psychiatric patients have a wide variety of personal and civil rights. They should be informed of these rights, and hospitals must honor them. Some of these rights are controversial and create dilemmas for psychiatric professionals.

5. Current legislative initiatives that affect psychiatric care provided in the United States include OBRA, the Protection and Advocacy Act, the Americans with Disabilities Act, and Advanced Directives.

REFERENCES

1. American Hospital Association: A *patient's bill of rights*, Chicago, 1990, The Association.
2. American Nurses' Association: *Statement on psychiatric–mental health clinical nursing practice and standards of psychiatric–mental health nursing practice*, Washington, DC, 1994, The Association.
3. Anfield R: Americans with disabilities act of 1990, *J Occup Med* 34:503, 1992.
4. APA task force issues guidelines for use of seclusion and restraint in inpatient settings, *Hosp Community Psychiatry* 36:677, 1985.
5. Appelbaum P: Advance directives for psychiatric treatment, *Hosp Community Psychiatry* 42:983, 1991.
6. Appelbaum P: Voluntary hospitalization and due process: the dilemma of *Zinermon v. Burch*, *Hosp Community Psychiatry* 41:1059, 1990.
7. Appelbaum P, Gutheil T: *Clinical handbook of psychiatry and the law*, ed 2, Baltimore, 1991, Williams & Wilkins.
8. Arkin A et al: Behavior modification, *NY State J Med* 76:190, 1976.
9. Beck J: Current status of the duty to protect. In Beck J, ed: *Confidentiality versus the duty to protect: foreseeable harm in the practice of psychiatry*, Washington, DC, 1990, American Psychiatric Press.
10. Birnbaum M: The right to treatment, *Am Bar Assoc J*, p 499, 1960.
11. Brooks A: Law and ideology in the case of Billie Boggs, *J Psychosoc Nurs Ment Health Serv* 26:22, 1988.
12. Campazzi B: Nurses, nursing, and malpractice litigation: 1967-1977, *Adv Nurs Sci* 4:1, 1980.
13. Chodoff P: The case for involuntary hospitalization of the mentally ill, *Am J Psychiatry* 133:496, 1976.
14. *Dixon v Weinberger*, No 74285 (CDDC Feb 14, 1974).
15. Eichmann M et al: An estimation of the impact of OBRA-87 on nursing home care in the United States, *Hosp Community Psychiatry* 43:781, 1992.
16. Elliott R: Patient dumping, COBRA, and the public psychiatric hospital, *Hosp Community Psychiatry* 44:155, 1993.
17. Fiesta J: Liability issues: patients with psychiatric problems, *Nurs Management* 22:14, 1991.
18. Galen K: Assessing psychiatric patients' competency to agree to treatment plans, *Hosp Community Psychiatry* 44:361, 1993.
19. Geller J: On being "committed" to treatment in the community, *Innovations & Research* 2:23, 1993.
20. Haimowitz S: Americans with disabilities act of 1990: its significance for persons with mental illness, *Hosp Community Psychiatry* 42:23, 1991.
21. Janofsky J, McCarthy R, Folstein M: The Hopkins competency assessment test: a brief method for evaluating

patients' capacity to give informed consent, *Hosp Community Psychiatry* 43:132, 1992.

22. Krajewski T, Bell C: A system for patients' rights advocacy in state psychiatric inpatient facilities in Maryland, *Hosp Community Psychiatry* 43:127, 1992.

23. Mental Health Systems Act, Report No 96-980, Amendment to Senate Bill 1177, Sept 23, 1980.

24. Miller R: *Involuntary civil commitment of the mentally ill in the post-reform era*, Springfield, Ill, 1987, Charles C Thomas.

25. National League for Nursing: *Nursing's role in patient's rights*, Pub No 11-1671, New York, 1977, The League.

26. News & Notes: Recent court ruling in Alabama's Wyatt case modifies 20-year-old patient care standards, *Hosp Community Psychiatry*, 43:851, 1992.

27. Rapoport D, Parry J, eds: *The right to refuse antipsychotic medication*, Washington, DC, 1986, The American Bar Association's Commission on the Mentally Disabled.

28. Ravid R, Menon S: Guidelines for disclosure of patient information under the Americans with disabilities act, *Hosp Community Psychiatry* 44:280, 1993.

29. Rhoden N: The presumption for treatment: has it been justified? *Law Med Health Care* 13:65, 1985.

30. *Rogers v Okin*, 478, Fed Supp 1342, 1979.

31. Schmid D, Applebaum P, Roth L, Lidz C: Confidentiality in psychiatry: a study of the patient's view, *Hosp Community Psychiatry* 34:353, 1983.

32. Schwartz H, Vingiano W, Perez C: Autonomy and the right to refuse treatment: patient's attitudes after involuntary medication, *Hosp Community Psychiatry* 39:1049, 1988.

33. Sheline Y, Beattie M: Effects of the right to refuse medication in an emergency psychiatric service, *Hosp Community Psychiatry* 43:640, 1992.

34. Simon R: *Clinical psychiatry and the law*, ed 2, Washington, DC, 1992, American Psychiatric Press.

35. Simon R: *Psychiatry and law for clinicians*, Washington, DC, 1992, American Psychiatric Association Press.

36. Smith P: *Moving forward: a national agenda to address homelessness in 1990 and beyond and a status report of homelessness in America*, New York, 1989, Partnership for the Homeless.

37. Szasz T: *Ideology and insanity*, New York, 1970, Doubleday.

38. *Tarasoff v Regents of the University of California et al*, 529 p 2d 553.

39. Teplin L: The criminality for the mentally ill: a dangerous misconception, *Am J Psychiatry* 142:593, 1985.

40. Tessler R, Dennis D: *A synthesis of NIMH-funded research concerning persons who are homeless and mentally ill*, Rockville, Md, 1989, National Institute of Mental Health.

41. Torrey E et al: Criminalizing the seriously mentally ill: the abuse of jails as mental hospitals, *Innovations & Research* 2:11, 1993.

42. Trudeau M: Informed consent: the patient's right to decide, *J Psychosoc Nurs Ment Health Serv* 31:9, 1993.

43. Walk E et al: Americans with disabilities act: *J Burn Care Rehabil* 14:92, 1993.

44. Weiss F: The right to refuse: informed consent and the psychosocial nurse, *J Psychosco Nurs Ment Health Serv* 28:25, 1990.

45. Wilk R: Implications of involuntary outpatient commitment for community mental health agencies, *Am J Orthopsychiatry* 58:580, 1988.

46. Wolpe P, Schwartz S, Sanford B: Psychiatric inpatients' knowledge of their rights, *Hosp Community Psychiatry* 42:1168, 1991.

47. *Wyatt v Stickney*, 344, Fed Supp 373, 375, 1972.

48. *Youngberg v Romeo*, 102 Supreme Ct 2452, 1982.

ANNOTATED SUGGESTED READINGS

Appelbaum P, Gutheil T: *Clinical handbook of psychiatry and the law*, ed 2, Baltimore, 1991, Williams & Wilkins.

Excellent text on legal issues in psychiatry written by experts in the field.

*Bergerson S: More about charting with a jury in mind, *Nursing* 88:51, 1988.

Written by an attorney, this practical article advises nurses how to chart to avoid legal difficulties. Highly recommended for all nurses.

*Brooks A: Law and ideology in the case of Billie Boggs, *J Psychosoc Nurs Ment Health Serv* 26:22, 1988.

Describes the highly publicized case of a homeless woman who was hospitalized and contested her involuntary commitment.

*Colorado Society of Clinical Specialists in Psychiatric Nursing: Ethical guidelines for confidentiality, *J Psychosoc Nurs Ment Health Serv* 28:43, 1990.

Presents guidelines for confidentiality in psychiatric nursing practice in a clear, concise way.

*Garritson S, Davis A: Least restrictive alternative: ethical considerations, *J Psychosoc Nurs Ment Health Serv* 21:17, 1983.

Critically evaluates how the principles and assumptions underlying the least restrictive alternative concept relate to the human rights versus human needs dilemma that confronts practitioners. Addresses rights, paternalism, autonomy, and needs.

Innovations & Research 2(1):1993.

The volume of this new journal addresses the issue of involuntary treatment from the perspective of the patient, family, and society. Excellent, sensitizing reading.

*Journal of Psychosocial Nursing and Mental Health Services 31:1993.

This volume is devoted entirely to forensic nursing. Articles discuss death investigations, false allegations, responsibilities of the legal nurse consultant, working with perpetrators and hostage negotiation teams, nurses' role with battered women, and a survey report on nurses who work in psychiatric forensic facilities.

*Laben J, MacLean C: Legal issues and guidelines for nurses who care for the mentally ill, ed 2, Thorofare, NJ, 1989, Charles B Slack.

Explores basic legal concepts in clear, concise language. Well-researched, reference discusses both issues and case decisions with application to nurses.

Munetz M, Geller J: The least restrictive alternative in the postinstitutional era, *Hosp Community Psychiatry* 44:967, 1993.

Challenges the view that the least restrictive alternative means anything but treatment in a state hospital. Suggests that this right includes consideration of the patient's needs and all alternatives be explored.

*Rabinow J: Where you stand in the eyes of the law, *Nursing* 15:34, 1989.

Brief overview of important nursing and legal issues. Clearly presented.

*Saunders J, Du Plessis D: An historical view of right to treatment, *J Psychosoc Nurs Ment Health Serv* 23:12, 1985.

---

*Nursing refernce.

Analyzes the professional nurse's responsibilities in the right-to-treatment issue. Describes providing active, individualized psychiatric treatment and monitoring the patients' environment, thus safeguarding the legal rights of the mentally ill.

Simon R: *Psychiatry and law for clinicians*, Washington, DC, 1992, American Psychiatric Association Press.

Best paperback handbook on the legal context of psychiatric care. Should be in the library of every psychiatric nurse.

*Stern S: Privileged communication: an ethical and legal right of psychiatric patients, *Perspect Psychiatr Care* 26:22, 1990.

Reviews the legal and ethical issues posed by testimonial privilege. Addresses implications for psychiatric nursing research, education, and clinical practice.

*Weiss F: The right to refuse: informed consent and the psychosocial nurse, *J Psychosoc Nurs Ment Health Serv* 28:25, 1990.

Excellent discussion of the role of the nurse in informed consent, advocacy, and accountability in psychiatric treatment.

*Zakarias L, Robinson D: Mental health review board: a new concept, *J Psychosoc Nurs Ment Health Serv* 30:6, 1992.

Describes a new approach for working with difficult patients involving the formulation of a nonnegotiable treatment contract. Thought provoking and innovative.

---

*Nursing reference.

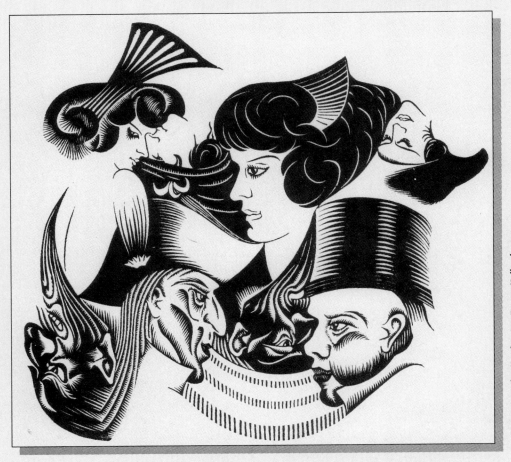

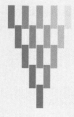

C H A P T E R 9

Implementing the Nursing Process: Standards of Care

GAIL W. STUART

To be what we are, and to become what we are capable of becoming, is the only end of life.

Robert L. Stevenson: *Familiar Studies of Men and Books*

The nurse-patient relationship is the vehicle for applying the nursing process. The goal of nursing care is to maximize the patient's positive interactions with the environment, promote a level of wellness, and enhance self-actualization. By establishing a therapeutic nurse-patient relationship and using the nursing process, the nurse strives to promote and maintain patient behavior that contributes to integrated functioning. This is the essence of the nursing therapeutic process and the framework on which this text is based.

The American Nurses' Association defines nursing as "the diagnosis and treatment of human responses to actual or potential health problems."[1] This definition suggests four defining characteristics of nursing*:

1. *Phenomena.* Nursing addresses a wide range of

---

*From American Nurses' Association: *Nursing: a social policy statement*, Kansas City, Mo, 1980, The Association.

health-related responses seen in both sick and well people.

2. *Theory.* Nurses use concepts, principles, and processes to guide their observations, understand the phenomena of human responses, and determine nursing actions to be taken.

3. *Actions.* Nursing actions attempt to prevent illness and promote health. They are related by theory to the phenomena of human responses and expected outcomes of care.

4. *Effects.* By evaluating the results of nursing actions, nurses determine whether their activities have enhanced adaptive responses and integrated functioning.

These characteristics describe nursing as an applied science with a focus of care, theoretical basis, documented interventions, and specified outcomes of care. They also reflect the integration of education, practice, and research activities (Fig. 9-1).

For psychiatric nurses, the characteristic of **phenomena** suggests the need to understand the range of actual and potential biopsychosocial health problems of patients and their possible responses to them. **Theory** maintains that nurses need a theoretical basis and conceptual model for psychiatric–mental health nursing practice. **Action** requires that the nursing process be a problem-solving process. **Effects** identifies the need for standards of psychiatric nursing practice to evaluate the quality of nursing care provided.

This chapter discusses each component of the therapeutic nursing process in relation to the new 1994 American Nurses' Association (ANA) *Standards of Psychiatric–Mental Health Clinical Nursing Practice.** The standards of professional performance are described in Chapter 10.

THE NURSING PROCESS

The nursing process is an interactive, problem-solving process. It is a systematic and individualized way to achieve the outcomes of nursing care. Since it is a deliberate and organized approach, it requires knowledge, judgment, and experience. The nursing process respects the individual's autonomy and freedom to make decisions and be involved in nursing care. Thus the nurse and patient emerge as partners in a relationship built on trust and directed toward maximizing the patient's strengths, maintaining integrity, and promoting adaptive response to stress.

In dealing with psychiatric patients, the nursing process can present unique challenges. Emotional problems may be vague and elusive, not tangible or visible like many physiological disruptions. Emotional problems also can show different symptoms and arise from a number of causes. Similar past events may lead to very different forms of present behavior. Many psychiatric patients are initially unable to describe their problems. They may be withdrawn, highly anxious, or out of touch with reality. Their ability to participate in the problem-solving process may also be limited if they see themselves as powerless victims or if their illness impairs them from fully engaging in the treatment process.

Geach[9] has identified three aspects of problem solving with psychiatric patients:

1. The nurse involves the patient in the process.
2. The problem that the nurse and patient address has immediate relevance to what is happening between them, at least initially.
3. The nurse and patient form some sort of relationship so that they can solve problems within a relationship rather than in isolation.

It is essential that the nurse and the patient become partners in the problem-solving process. Nurses may be tempted to exclude patients, particularly if they avoid or resist becoming involved, but this should be avoided for two reasons. First, learning is most effective when patients participate in the learning experience. Second, by including patients as active participants in the nursing process, the nurse helps restore their sense of control over life and their responsibility for action. It reinforces the message that patients, whether they have an acute crisis or a serious and persistent mental illness, can choose either adaptive or maladaptive coping responses.

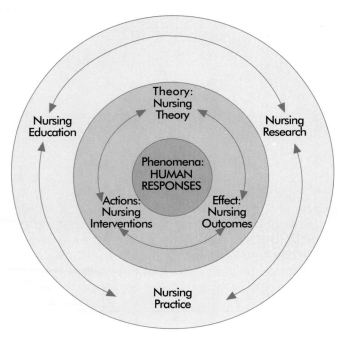

Fig. 9-1   Elements of nursing as an applied science.

*From American Nurses' Association: *A statement on psychiatric–mental health clinical nursing practice and standards of psychiatric–mental health clinical nursing practice,* Washington, DC, 1994, The Association.

The phases of the nursing process as described by the *Standards of Psychiatric–Mental Health Clinical Nursing Practice* are assessment, diagnosis, outcome identification, planning, implementation, and evaluation. Validation is part of each step, and all phases may overlap or occur simultaneously. The nursing conditions and nursing behaviors related to each one of these phases is shown in Fig. 9-2. Each of these phases as it applies to psychiatric nursing practice is now described.

 Some psychotic patients are discouraged and dispirited by their illness. As a result, they may be difficult to engage in the treatment process. What strategies might you use to connect with these patients and develop a therapeutic alliance with them?

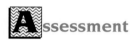ssessment

STANDARD I—ASSESSMENT

The psychiatric–mental health nurse collects client health data.

▼ *Rationale*

The assessment interview—which requires linguistically and culturally effective communication skills, interviewing, behavioral observation, database record review, and comprehensive assessment of the client and relevant systems—enables the psychiatric–mental health nurse to make sound clinical judgments and plan appropriate interventions with the client.

▼ *Nursing conditions*

Self-awareness
Accurate observations
Therapeutic communication
Responsive dimensions of care

▼ *Nursing behaviors*

Establish nursing contract
Obtain information from patient and family
Validate data with patient
Organize data

▼ *Key elements*

Identify the patient's reason for currently seeking help
Assess for risk factors related to the patient's safety including potential for:
    Suicide or self-harm
    Assault or violence
    Substance abuse withdrawal
    Allergic reaction or adverse drug reaction
    Seizure
    Falls or accidents
    Elopement (if hospitalized)
    Physiological instability

Complete a biopsychosocial assessment of patient needs related to this treatment encounter including:
    Patient and family appraisal of health and illness
    Previous episodes of psychiatric care in self and family
    Current medications
    Physiological coping responses
    Mental status coping responses
    Coping resources including motivation for treatment and functional supportive relationships
    Adaptive and maladaptive coping mechanisms
    Psychosocial and environmental problems
    Global assessment of functioning
    Knowledge strengths and deficits

In the assessment phase, information is obtained from the patient in a direct and structured manner through observations, interviews, and examinations. An assessment tool or nursing history form can provide a systematic format that becomes part of the patient's written record. This format provides the facts on which the nurse can assess the patient's level of functioning and serves as a basis for diagnosis, outcome identification, planning, implementation, and evaluation of nursing care. Using a specified data collection format helps ensure that the necessary information is obtained. It also reduces repetition of the patient's medical history and provides a source of information available to all health-team members. The assessment tool the nurse uses to collect data ideally should be derived from a conceptual model of psychiatric nursing.

The nurse may also use a variety of psychological assessment tools and behavioral rating scales (see Chapter 6). These can help define current pretreatment aspects of the patient's problems, document both the patient's progress over time and the efficacy of the treatment plan, and compare a patient's responses to groups of people with the same illness. This information can help formulate diagnoses and treatment goals and plans.

The patient data identified in the key elements of Standard I relate to all of the components of the stress adaptation model (Fig. 9-3) developed by Gail Stuart and used in this text—predisposing factors, precipitating stressors, appraisal of stressor, coping resources, coping mechanisms, and coping responses as described in Chapter 4. Appendices A and B at the end of this chapter present two psychiatric nursing assessment tools developed by nurses in the Division of Psychiatric Nursing at the Medical University of South Carolina. These forms were designed based on the stress adaptation model in a format that is consistent with the computerization of psychiatric nursing documentation.

Appendix A contains a risk factor assessment tool that addresses the Standard I elements related to ensuring the safety of the patient and others. The tool itself and directions for its use are described in Appen-

DATA COLLECTION

NURSING CONDITIONS

    Self-awareness
    Accurate observations
    Therapeutic communication
    Responsive dimensions of care

NURSING BEHAVIORS

    Establish nursing contract
    Obtain information from patient and family
    Validate data with patient
    Organize data

NURSING DIAGNOSIS

NURSING CONDITIONS

    Logical decision making
    Knowledge of normal parameters
    Inductive and deductive reasoning
    Sociocultural sensitivity

NURSING BEHAVIORS

    Identify patterns in data
    Compare data with norms
    Analyze and synthesize data
    Problems/strengths identified
    Validate problems with patient
    Formulate nursing diagnosis
    Set priorities of problems

OUTCOME IDENTIFICATION

NURSING CONDITIONS

    Critical thinking skills
    Partnership with patient
    and family

NURSING BEHAVIORS

    Hypothesizing
    Specify expected outcomes
    Validate goals with patient

PLANNING

NURSING CONDITIONS

    Application of theory
    Respect for patient and family

NURSING BEHAVIORS

    Prioritize goals
    Identify nursing activities
    Validate plan with patient

IMPLEMENTATION

NURSING CONDITIONS

    Past clinical experiences
    Knowledge of research
    Responsive and action
    dimensions of care

NURSING BEHAVIORS

    Consider available resources
    Implement nursing activities
    Generate alternatives
    Coordinate with other team members

EVALUATION

NURSING CONDITIONS

    Supervision
    Self-analysis
    Peer review
    Patient and family participation

NURSING BEHAVIORS

    Compare patient's responses and expected
    outcome
    Review nursing process
    Modify nursing process as needed
    Participate in quality improvement activities

Fig. 9-2   Nursing conditions and behaviors related to the standards of care.

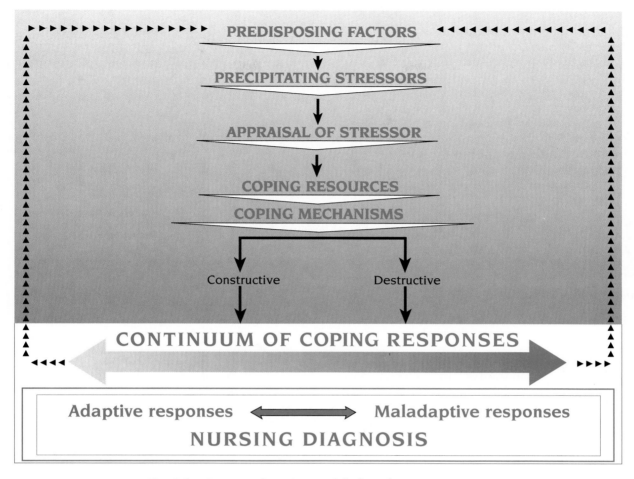

PREDISPOSING FACTORS

PRECIPITATING STRESSORS

APPRAISAL OF STRESSOR

COPING RESOURCES

COPING MECHANISMS

Constructive   Destructive

CONTINUUM OF COPING RESPONSES

Adaptive responses ⟷ **Maladaptive responses**

NURSING DIAGNOSIS

Fig. 9-3   A stress adaptation model of psychiatric nursing care

dix A. It is to be completed during the first contact with the patient, since safety is always the highest psychiatric nursing priority. If there is a positive response to any of the eight potential risk factors, a more complete assessment of the patient related to that specific risk factor is completed (see Chapters 18 and 27 for examples of these specific risk factor assessment tools.) Clinical nursing protocols are then initiated as indicated.

Appendix B contains a psychiatric nursing assessment tool that can be used by psychiatric nurses in any setting in the continuum of care. As such, it allows the nurse to collect patient data that can be evaluated over time, as the patient progresses in treatment and moves among various treatment settings. If used in an inpatient setting, however, some items must be completed by a psychiatric nurse within 8 hours and all items within 24 hours of the patient's admission. It incorporates data related to the biological, psychological, sociocultural, and legal contexts of psychiatric nursing care (see Chapters 5 to 8) and was designed to provide an integrated nursing assessment interview. It includes patient behaviors, perceptions, and some standardized

rating scales. The tool itself and directions for its use are described in detail in Appendix B.

The baseline data should reflect both content and process, and the patient is the ideal source of validation. The nurse should select a private place, free from noise and distraction, in which to interview the patient. Interviewing is a goal-directed method of communication that is required in a formal admission procedure. It should be focused but as open ended as possible, progressing from general to specific and allowing spontaneous patient self-expression. The nurse's role is to maintain the flow of the interview and to listen to the verbal and nonverbal messages being conveyed by the patient. Nurses must also be aware of their responses to the patient.

Although the patient should be regarded as a source of validation, the nurse should also be prepared to consult with family members or other persons knowledgeable about the patient. This will be particularly important when the patient is unable to provide reliable information because of the symptoms of the psychiatric illness. The nurse might also consider using a variety of other information sources, including the patient's health-care record, nursing rounds, change-of-shift reports, nursing care plan, and the evaluation of other health professionals such as psychologists, social workers, or psychiatrists. In using secondary sources, nurses should not simply accept the assessment of another health team member. Rather, they should apply the information they obtain to their nursing framework for data collection and formulate their own impressions and diagnoses. This brings another perspective to the work of the health-care team and an unbiased receptivity to patients and their problems.

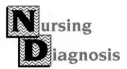

Nursing Diagnosis

STANDARD II—DIAGNOSIS

The psychiatric–mental health nurse analyzes the assessment data in determining diagnoses.

▼ *Rationale*

The basis for providing psychiatric–mental health nursing care is the recognition and identification of patterns of response to actual or potential psychiatric illnesses and mental health problems.

▼ *Nursing conditions*

Logical decision making

Knowledge of normal parameters

Inductive and deductive reasoning

Sociocultural sensitivity

▼ *Nursing behaviors*

Identify patterns in data

Compare data with norms

Analyze and synthesize data

Problems and strengths identified

Validate problems with patient

Formulate nursing diagnoses

Set priorities of problems

▼ *Key elements*

Diagnoses should reflect adaptive and maladaptive coping responses based on nursing frameworks such as those of the North American Nursing Diagnosis Association (NANDA)

Diagnoses should incorporate health problems or disease states such as those identified in the Diagnostic and Statistical Manual of Mental Disorders (DSM-IV)

Diagnoses should focus on the phenomena of concern to psychiatric–mental health nurses as described in Box 9-1.

After collecting all data, the nurse compares the information to documented norms of health and adaptation. Since standards of behavior are culturally determined, the nurse should allow for both the patient's in-

---

Box 9-1

PSYCHIATRIC–MENTAL HEALTH NURSING'S PHENOMENA OF CONCERN

ACTUAL OR POTENTIAL MENTAL HEALTH PROBLEMS OF CLIENTS PERTAINING TO:

▼ The maintenance of optimal health and well-being and the prevention of psychobiological illness

▼ Self-care limitations or impaired functioning related to mental and emotional distress

▼ Deficits in the functioning of significant biological, emotional, and cognitive systems

▼ Emotional stress or crisis components of illness, pain, and disability

▼ Self-concept changes, developmental issues, and life process changes

▼ Problems related to emotions such as anxiety, anger, sadness, loneliness, and grief

▼ Physical symptoms that occur along with altered psychological functioning

▼ Alterations in thinking, perceiving, symbolizing, communicating, and decision making

▼ Difficulties in relating to others

▼ Behaviors and mental states that indicate the patient is a danger to self or others or has a severe disability

▼ Interpersonal, systemic, sociocultural, spiritual, or environmental circumstances or events that affect the mental and emotional well-being of the individual, family, or community

▼ Symptom management, side effects/toxicities associated with psychopharmacological intervention and other aspects of the treatment regimen

From American Nurses' Association: A *statement on psychiatric-mental health clinical nursing practice and standards of psychiatric mental health clinical nursing practice,* Washington, DC, 1994, The Association.

---

dividual characteristics and the larger social group to which the patient belongs.

The nurse then analyzes the data and derives a nursing diagnosis. **A nursing diagnosis is a statement of the patient's nursing problem that includes both the adaptive or maladaptive health response and contributing stressors.** These nursing problems concern aspects of the patient's health that may need to be promoted or with which the patient needs help in adapting to stress. The subject of nursing diagnoses therefore is the patient's behavioral response to stress. This response, as represented in Fig. 9-3, may lie anywhere on the coping continuum from adaptive, to maladaptive. Nursing diagnoses identify problems that may be overt, covert, existing, or potential. The professional nurse assumes the responsibility for therapeutic decisions regarding these patients' health responses.

According to the North American Nursing Diagnosis Association (NANDA),[14] a nursing diagnostic statement ideally consists of three parts:

1. Health problem
2. Etiological or contributing factors
3. Defining characteristics

The first part, the *health problem*, identifies the behavioral disruption or threatened disruption that can be improved through nursing intervention. The second part, the *etiological factors*, identifies stressors that contribute to the problem. The third part, the *defining characteristics*, describes the signs and symptoms that relate to the identified health problem. All three components are important in formulating a nursing diagnosis. The defining characteristics are particularly helpful because they reflect the objective and subjective behaviors that are the target of nursing intervention. They also provide specific indicators for evaluating the outcomes of nursing interventions and for determining whether the expected goals of the nursing care were met. Some examples of possible nursing diagnoses include the following:

▼ Body image disturbance related to cerebrovascular accident, evidenced by lack of acceptance of body limitations
▼ Altered thought processes related to Alzheimer's disease, evidenced by inaccurate interpretation of environment, deficit in recent memory, and impaired ability to reason
▼ Altered sexuality patterns related to embarrassment about the body after a mastectomy, evidenced by lack of desire for sex

Psychiatric nurses must continue to define and describe what they do in the psychiatric setting, and this requires the use of nursing diagnoses. Nursing diagnoses pinpoint what exactly it is that nurses treat. Only if psychiatric nurses can name the health responses they treat will they be able to talk with legislators, reimbursers, administrators, other health-care professionals, patients, families, and even other nurses about the contribution nursing makes to health care.

NANDA has been working on identifying, defining, and describing a classification system of nursing diagnoses. Additional work is needed both in defining the phenomena of concern to psychiatric nurses and in testing the identified diagnoses. If nurses diagnose problems, record their observations and conclusions, and describe the health responses they treat, the body of nursing knowledge will increase, as will the credibility of and value placed on nursing care.

Relationship to Medical Diagnosis

Nursing does not exist in a vacuum. Although nurses are the largest group of health-care professionals, they must work with other groups, such as physicians. Each group of health-care providers serves as a resource to the others as they cooperate to improve the patient's health.

The interrelationship between medicine and nursing includes sharing information, ideas, and analyses and developing appropriate care plans for the patient. Interventions are based on the nursing assessment as well as the medical evaluation and ensure a thorough and coordinated plan of treatment for the psychiatric patient. Therefore, while formulating nursing diagnoses and using the nursing process, nurses should also be familiar with medical diagnoses and treatment plans.

Medical diagnosis refers to the health problem or disease states of the patient. In the medical model of psychiatry, the health problems are mental disorders or mental illnesses. These are classified in the DSM-IV,[3] which comprehensively describes the symptoms of various mental disorders but does not attempt to discuss cause or how the disturbances come about. However, specific diagnostic criteria are provided for each mental disorder. Chapters 3 and 4 of this text discuss the medical model and the DSM-IV in greater detail.

Nursing and medical diagnoses may complement each other, but one is not a component of another. A patient with one specific medical diagnosis may have a number of complementary nursing diagnoses related to the patient's range of health responses. On the other hand, a patient may have a specific nursing diagnosis without any identified medical diagnosis.

It is interesting to note that the DSM was first published in 1952, whereas the first NANDA diagnoses were put forth in 1973. Given the use of multidisciplinary teams in psychiatry and the relative infancy of nursing diagnoses, some psychiatric nurses prefer using the DSM-IV or do not see the relevance of NANDA diagnoses in their practice. Malone[11] notes, however, that those nurses who opt to use only the DSM-IV do not contribute to understanding the phenomena relevant to psychiatric nursing practice, perpetuate the invisibility of nursing to patient care, and invite turf battles with other professions. What is needed is for psychiatric nurses to be familiar with both DSM-IV and NANDA diagnoses and to use both to conceptualize patient problems, needs, and treatment strategies.

Some psychiatric nurses have proposed that nursing diagnoses be added as another axis to the DSM-IV. What problems would this create for psychiatric nurses' autonomy, reimbursement for psychiatric nursing services, and interdisciplinary collaboration?

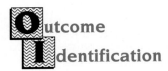

Outcome Identification

STANDARD III—OUTCOME IDENTIFICATION

The psychiatric–mental health nurse identifies expected outcomes individualized to the client.

▼ *Rationale*

Within the context of providing nursing care, the ultimate goal is to influence health outcomes and improve the client's health status.

▼ *Nursing conditions*

Critical thinking skills

Partnership with patient and family

▼ *Nursing behaviors*

Hypothesizing

Specify expected outcomes

Validate goals with patient

▼ *Key elements*

Outcomes should be mutually identified with the patient

Outcomes should be identified as clearly and objectively as possible

Well-written outcomes help nurses determine the effectiveness and efficiency of their interventions

Before defining expected outcomes, the nurse must realize that patients frequently seek treatment with goals of their own. These goals may be expressed as relieving symptoms or improving functional ability. Sometimes a patient cannot identify specific goals or may describe them in general terms. Translating nonspecific concerns into specific goal statements is not easy. The nurse must understand the patient's coping responses and the factors that influence them. Krumboltz and Thorensen[10] describe some of the difficulties in defining goals as follows:

1. The patient may view a personal problem as someone else's behavior. This may be the case of a parent who brings his adolescent son in for counseling. The parent may view the son as the problem, whereas the adolescent may feel his only problem is his father. One approach to this situation is to help the person who brings the problem into treatment, since he "owns" the problem at that moment. The nurse might suggest, "Let's talk about how I could help you deal with your son. A change in your response might lead to a change in his behavior also."

2. The patient may express a problem as a feeling, such as, "I'm lonely," or "I'm so unhappy." Besides trying to help the patient clarify the feeling, the nurse might ask, "What could you do to make yourself feel less alone and more loved by others?" This helps patients see the connection between actions and feelings and increase their sense of responsibility for themselves.

3. The patient's problem may be one of lacking a goal or an idea of exactly what is desired out of life. In this case it might be helpful for the nurse to point out that values and goals are not magically discovered but must be created by people for themselves. The patient can then actively explore ways to construct goals or adopt the objectives of a social, service, religious, or political group with whom the patient identifies.

4. The patient's goals may be inappropriate, undesirable, or unclear. However, the solution here is not for the nurse to impose goals on the patient. Even if the patient's desires seem to be against self-interests, the most the nurse can do is reflect the patient's behavior and its consequences. If the patient then asks for help in setting new goals, the nurse can help.

5. The patient's problem may be a choice conflict. This is especially common if all the choices are unpleasant, unacceptable, or unrealistic. An example is a couple who wishes to divorce but do not want to see their child hurt or suffer the financial hardship that would result. Although undesirable choices cannot be made desirable, the nurse can help patients use the problem-solving process to identify the full range of alternatives available to them.

6. The patient may have no real problem but may just want to talk. Nurses must then decide what role to play and carefully distinguish between a social and a therapeutic relationship.

Clarifying goals is an essential step in the therapeutic process. Out of this clarification emerges the mutually agreed on goals on which the patient-nurse relationship is based. A well-intentioned nurse sometimes overlooks the patient's goals and devises a care plan leading to an outcome that the nurse believes is better. However, this approach may be one of the conflict-producing situations that the patient has previously experienced. Therefore the experience of working cooperatively with the nurse to evolve mutually acceptable goals is extremely valuable. If the patient does not share one of the nurse's goals, it may be best to defer it until the patient agrees on its importance.

Specifying Goals

Once goals are agreed on, the nurse must state them explicitly. Box 9-2 lists qualities of well-written outcome criteria. The more specifically the goals of treatment can be stated, the more likely these goals can be achieved. These goals also serve to guide later nursing actions and enhance the evaluation of care. Goals should be written in behavioral terms. This means that the verb used to state the objective should represent a behavior that may be observed and should have as few interpretations

Box 9-2
QUALITIES OF WELL-WRITTEN OUTCOME CRITERIA

▼ Specific rather than general
▼ Measurable rather than subjective
▼ Attainable rather than unrealistic
▼ Current rather than outdated
▼ Adequate in number rather than too few or too many
▼ Mutual rather than one sided

as possible. Goals should realistically describe what the nurse wishes to accomplish within a specific time span. Often nurses err by using general statements that apply to all patients, such as the goals of forming a relationship or relieving depression. Although valid in general terms, they are not adequate in and of themselves.

 Review some of the nursing care plans on your unit. Are the expected outcomes and short-term goals well written given the qualities listed in Box 9-2?

Expected outcomes and short-term goals should be developed, with short-term objectives contributing to the longer-term expected outcomes. Following are sample expected outcomes and short-term goals:

Expected outcome:
The patient will travel about the community independently within 2 months.

Short-term goals:
1. At the end of 1 week the patient will sit on the front steps at home.
2. At the end of 2 weeks the patient will walk to the corner and back home.
3. At the end of 3 weeks the patient, accompanied by the nurse, will walk around the block.
4. At the end of 4 weeks the patient will walk around the block alone.

The hierarchy would continue until the desired expected outcome is achieved. Each goal is stated in terms of observable behavior and includes a period of time in which it is to be accomplished. It also includes any other relevant conditions, such as whether the patient is to be alone or accompanied by the nurse.

Finally it is important for psychiatric nurses to realize that expected outcomes can be classified into three domains: cognitive, affective, and psychomotor.[16] These are described in Table 9-1, which presents the content, an example, and verbs representative of each domain. Correctly identifying the domain of the expected outcome is very important in planning nursing interventions. Some psychiatric nurses assume that the only outcomes that are necessary are those related to learning new information. They forget about the equally important needs of patients to acquire new values or master new psychomotor skills.

For example, it would be of limited help to teach a patient about medication if the patient did not value taking medications based on a personal belief system or previous life experiences. It would be equally unsuccessful to engage in medication education if the patient did not know how to take public transportation to fill the prescription.

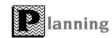

Planning

STANDARD IV—PLANNING

The psychiatric–mental health nurse develops a plan of care that prescribes interventions to attain expected outcomes.

▼ *Rationale*
A plan of care is used to guide therapeutic intervention systematically and achieve the expected client outcomes.

▼ *Nursing conditions*
Application of theory
Respect for patient and family

▼ *Nursing behaviors*
Prioritize goals
Identify nursing activities
Validate plan with patient

▼ *Key elements*
The plan of nursing care must always be individualized for the patient
Planned interventions should be based on current knowledge in the field and contemporary clinical psychiatric–mental health nursing practice
Planning is done in collaboration with the patient, the family, and the health-care team
Documentation of the plan of care is an essential nursing activity

One of the most important tasks facing the nurse and patient is to assign priorities to goals. Frequently, several goals can be pursued simultaneously. Those related to protecting the patient from self-destructive impulses always receive top priority. When identifying both expected outcomes and short-term goals, the nurse must keep the proposed time sequence firmly in mind.

Since the nursing care plan is dynamic and should adapt to the patient's coping responses throughout contact with the health care system, priorities are constantly changing. If the focus is always on the patient's behavioral responses, priorities can be set and modified as the patient changes. This personalizes nursing

Table 9-1   Domains of Expected Outcomes

Domain	Example	Representative verbs
Cognitive		
Outcomes associated with acquired knowledge or intellectual abilities	Learning the signs and symptoms of major depression	Define, list, relate, describe, discuss, explain, identify, apply, interpret, analyze, compare, contrast, examine, construct, create, design, organize, plan, assess, critique, evaluate, revise
Affective		
Outcomes associated with changes in attitude, values, or beliefs	Deciding that previous eating habits needed to be changed	Accept, realize, recognize, comply, observe, accept, believe, defend, prefer, seek, value, display, judge, weigh, express, share, internalize
Psychomotor		
Outcomes associated with developing motor skills	Completing self-care activities	Place, position, prepare, imitate, inject, repeat, build, set up, coordinate, operate, change, develop, supply, construct, design, produce, demonstrate, practice, perform, administer, give

care, and the patient participates in its planning and implementation.

Once the goals are decided, the next task is to outline the plan for achieving them. The nursing care plan applies theory from nursing and related biological and behavioral sciences to the unique responses of the individual patient. This assumes that as the nurse identifies patient needs, appropriate resources will be consulted. Failure to approach nursing care in this scientific manner can result in illogical decisions and a plan based on tradition, intuition, or trial and error. Although these decision-making methods may result in a valid plan, consistency of depth and accuracy over time will suffer, as will the overall care of the patient. Skilled psychiatric nursing requires a commitment to the ongoing pursuit of knowledge that will enhance professional growth.

The patient's active involvement leads to more successful care plans. If nurses collect data, return to their work station, consult textbooks, and then write up a plan of care, an important step has been missed. After writing a tentative care plan, nurses must validate this plan with the patient. This saves time and effort for them both as they continue to work together. It also communicates to the patient a sense of self-responsibility in getting well. The patient can tell the nurse that a proposed plan is unrealistic regarding financial status, lifestyle, value system, or, perhaps, personal preference. Usually there are several possible approaches to a patient's problem. Choosing the one most acceptable to the patient improves the chances for success.

If a goal answers the question of "what," the plan of care answers the questions "how" and "why." The plan chosen obviously depends on the nursing diagnosis, the nurse's theoretical orientation, and the nature of the goals pursued. In general, the goals influence the selection of therapeutic techniques. Failure to reach a goal

through one plan can lead to the decision to adopt a new approach or reevaluate the goal. These activities commonly occur in the working phase of the relationship.

Documentation

In 1991 the Joint Commission on Accreditation of Healthcare Organizations (JCAHO)[4] applied a new set of nursing standards across the country related to patient documentation. The revised standards specify that the nursing plan of care must contain the six elements listed in Box 9-3 and that the primary place to document the nursing process is in the patient's health-care record. The new standards also include the following changes:

▼ Recognition of nursing diagnoses for the first time
▼ Permission to use collaborative patient problems
▼ Acceptance of new documentation formats such as clinical protocols, critical pathways, clinical practice guidelines, and computerized care plans that can be individualized

---

Box 9-3

ESSENTIAL ELEMENTS OF THE NURSING PLAN OF CARE

▼ Initial assessment and reassessment
▼ Nursing diagnoses or patient care needs
▼ Interventions identified to meet the patient's nursing care needs
▼ Nursing care provided
▼ Patient's response to and the outcomes of the nursing care provided
▼ Ability of the patient or significant other to manage continuing care needs after discharge

---

▼ Allowance of charting by exception
▼ Mandate for the nursing plan of care to be permanently integrated into the clinical information system

Since these new standards were released, many changes have been made regarding the documentation of the nursing plan of care. Psychiatric nurses are beginning to use a variety of formats that often differ from the traditional nursing care plan. Many of these changes have been prompted by patients' shortened length of stay in inpatient settings, as well as by the advanced computer technology that is currently available (Fig. 9-4).

For example, computerized programs have been developed that can provide rapid entry of patient data, retrieve psychiatric treatment plans, and produce a finished document that is clinically useful and highly readable.[15,19] Another advantage of a computerized information system is its ability to store clinical data that can also be used for outcome research, quality improvement activities, and resource management.[21] In addition to computerized plans of care, psychiatric nurses are beginning to use clinical practice guidelines, clinical protocols, teaching protocols, flow sheets, and clinical pathways in their practice settings.[12]

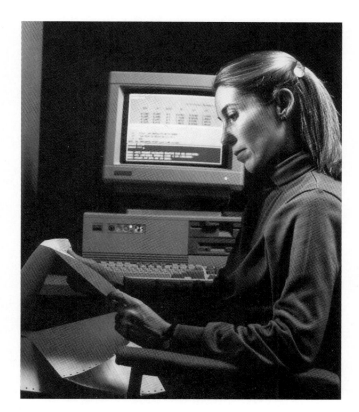

Fig. 9-4 Nurse reviewing patient data from a computerized information system.
Courtesy Division of Psychiatric Nursing, Medical University of South Carolina.

Clinical Pathways

A **critical**, or **clinical**, **pathway** (also known as care paths and Care Maps) is a shortened version of the plan of care for a particular individual. It lists key nursing and medical processes and corresponding time lines to which the patient must adhere to achieve standard outcomes within a specified period. The development of a clinical pathway includes reviewing for efficiency and necessity the events that occur the minute the patient enters the health-care facility and through discharge and aftercare. This includes preadmission work-ups, tests, consultations, treatments, activities, diet, and health teaching. A clinical pathway is a written plan that serves as a map and timetable for the efficient and effective delivery of health care.

An example of the format of a general clinical pathway for psychiatric treatment through the four stages of the continuum of care is presented in Fig. 9-5. Any one stage of psychiatric treatment (crisis, acute, maintenance, or health promotion) identified in this clinical pathway can be singled out and developed with a specific time frame for a single nursing diagnosis, medical diagnosis, or patient problem. In general, tools such as a clinical pathway are valuable because they:

▼ Help to target the focus of treatment
▼ Specify expected outcomes with time lines
▼ Identify individualized treatment strategies
▼ Minimize unnecessary documentation
▼ Allow for the evaluation of patient care activities and goal achievement

These formats continue to be developed and refined for use by nurses with psychiatric patients.

 Many health-care providers believe that clinical pathways are more difficult to develop in psychiatry than in other specialty areas. What problems would be particularly challenging in designing critical or clinical pathways for psychiatric treatment?

Implementation

STANDARD V—IMPLEMENTATION

The psychiatric–mental health nurse implements the interventions identified in the plan of care.

▼ *Rationale*

In implementing the plan of care, psychiatric–mental health nurses use a wide range of interventions designed to prevent mental and physical illness and promote, maintain, and restore mental and physical health. Psychiatric–mental health nurses select interventions according to their level of practice. At the basic level,

STAGE OF TREATMENT	CRISIS ←→	ACUTE ←--→	MAINTENANCE ←→	HEALTH PROMOTION
GOAL	**STABILIZATION**	**REMISSION**	**RECOVERY**	**OPTIMAL LEVEL OF WELLNESS**
TREATMENT FOCUS	High-risk behaviors	Symptoms and coping responses	Functional status	Quality of life
ASSESSMENTS	Risk factor assessment Nursing assessment	Nursing assessment Medical assessment Supplemental scales	Functional status scale	Well-being scale
EXPECTED OUTCOME	NO HARM TO SELF OR OTHERS	SYMPTOM RELIEF	IMPROVED FUNCTIONING	OPTIMAL QUALITY OF LIFE
Consults				
Tests/labs				
Symptom management				
Medications				
Treatments				
Activity				
Safety				
Teaching				
Nutrition				
Discharge planning				

Fig. 9-5   General clinical pathway for psychiatric care

the nurse may select counseling, milieu therapy, self-care activities, psychobiological interventions, health teaching, case management, health promotion and health maintenance, and a variety of other approaches to meet the mental health needs of clients. In addition to the intervention options available to the basic-level psychiatric–mental health nurse, at the advanced level the certified specialist may provide consultation, engage in psychotherapy, and prescribe pharmacological agents where permitted by state statutes or regulations.

▼ *Nursing conditions*
Past clinical experiences
Knowledge of research
Responsive and action dimensions of care

▼ *Nursing behaviors*
Consider available resources
Implement nursing activities
Generate alternatives
Coordinate with other team members

▼ *Key elements*
Nursing interventions should reflect a holistic, biopsychosocial approach to patient care
Nursing interventions are implemented in a safe, efficient, and caring manner

The level at which a nurse functions and the interventions implemented are based on the:
Nurse practice acts in one's state
One's qualifications including education, experience, and certification
Caregiving setting
Nurse's own personal initiative

STANDARD Va—COUNSELING

The psychiatric–mental health nurse uses counseling interventions to assist clients in improving or regaining their previous coping abilities, fostering mental health, and preventing mental illness and disability.

STANDARD Vb—MILIEU THERAPY

The psychiatric–mental health nurse provides, structures, and maintains a therapeutic environment in collaboration with the client and other health-care providers.

STANDARD Vc—SELF-CARE ACTIVITIES

The psychiatric–mental health nurse structures interventions around the client's activities of daily living

to foster self-care and mental and physical well-being.

STANDARD Vd—PSYCHOBIOLOGICAL INTERVENTIONS

The psychiatric–mental health nurse uses knowledge of psychobiological interventions and applies clinical skills to restore the client's health and prevent further disability.

STANDARD Ve—HEALTH TEACHING

The psychiatric–mental health nurse, through health teaching, assists clients in achieving satisfying, productive, and healthy patterns of living.

STANDARD Vf—CASE MANAGEMENT

The psychiatric–mental health nurse provides case management to coordinate comprehensive health services and ensure continuity of care.

STANDARD Vg—HEALTH PROMOTION AND HEALTH MAINTENANCE

The psychiatric–mental health nurse employs strategies and interventions to promote and maintain mental health and prevent mental illness.

ADVANCED PRACTICE INTERVENTIONS Vh-Vj

The following interventions (Vh-Vj) may be performed only by the certified specialist in psychiatric–mental health nursing.

STANDARD Vh—PSYCHOTHERAPY

The certified specialist in psychiatric–mental health nursing uses individual, group, and family psychotherapy, child psychotherapy, and other therapeutic treatments to assist clients in fostering mental health, preventing mental illness and disability, and improving or regaining previous health status and functional abilities.

STANDARD Vi—PRESCRIPTION OF PHARMACOLOGICAL AGENTS

The certified specialist uses prescription of pharmacological agents in accordance with the state nursing practice act to treat symptoms of psylchiatric illness and improve functional health status.

STANDARD Vj—CONSULTATION

The certified specialist provides consultation to health-care providers and others to influence the plans of care for clients and to enhance the abilities of others to provide psychiatric and mental health care and effect change in systems.

Implementation refers to the actual delivery of nursing care to the patient and the response to that care. Good planning increases the chances of successful implementation. Such factors as available people, equipment, resources, time, and money must be considered as nursing actions are planned. Well-planned nursing care also takes into account the personalities and experiences of the nurse and the patient and their interaction.

The most valid basis for nursing action applies the scientific method to nursing practice. It is also acceptable to use theory selectively from the biological and behavioral sciences. In most situations there is more than one way to accomplish the stated goals. It is helpful when planning care to identify alternative nursing actions that are also appropriate to the goal. If this is done, the nurse is not left floundering should the first approach fail. Considering several alternatives makes the implementation phase of the nursing process highly flexible.

In implementing psychotherapeutic interventions, the nurse helps the psychiatric patient do two things: (1) develop insight and (2) carry out a plan of positive action. These two areas for nursing intervention correspond with the responsive and action dimensions of the nurse-patient relationship described in Chapter 2. Insight refers to the patient's development of new emotional and cognitive organizations. Often the patient becomes more anxious as defense mechanisms are broken down. This is the time when resistance commonly occurs. But knowing something on an intellectual level does **not** inevitably lead to a change in behavior. Nurses who terminate their interventions at this point are not fully carrying out the therapeutic process to the patient's benefit. An additional step is needed. Patients must decide if they will revert to maladaptive coping mechanisms, remain in a resisting, immobilized state, or adopt new, adaptive, and constructive approaches to life.

The first step in helping a patient translate insight into action is to build adequate incentives to abandoning old patterns of behavior. The nurse should help the patient see the consequences of actions and that old patterns do more harm than good and inflict much suffering and pain. The patient will not learn new patterns until the motivation to acquire them is greater than the motivation to retain old ones. The nurse should encourage the patient's desires for mental health, emotional growth, and freedom from suffering. The nurse also should continue to motivate and support patients as they test new behaviors and coping mechanisms. The individual's social support system is vital in this regard. This is relevant to all levels of nursing intervention—primary, secondary, and tertiary—and all patient populations.

Within the nurse-patient relationship the patient can

actively work toward adaptive goals. It is important to allow sufficient time for change. Many of the patient's maladaptive patterns have been building up over years; the nurse cannot expect the patient to change them in a matter of days or weeks. Finally, the nurse must help the patient evaluate these new patterns, integrate them into life experiences, and practice problem solving to prepare for future experiences. In this way secondary prevention nursing interventions also fulfill primary and tertiary prevention goals.

The standards of care and related measurement criteria for implementation are detailed and explicit. The standards identify the range of activities psychiatric nurses use at both the basic and advanced levels. The measurement criteria detail the many specific activities involved. Information related to each of these implementation standards appear in various chapters throughout this text.

It is evident from reviewing this standard that psychi-atric nurses need to be skilled in biological, psychological, and sociocultural skills to implement these nursing interventions. The current psychiatric population has a higher level of acuity and greater complexity of problems than in the past. Specifically, a large number of people seeking psychiatric treatment have concurrent and often undiagnosed physical illnesses. Thus it is essential that psychiatric nurses stay current with their biomedical as well as their psychosocial skill development.[5]

Ten years ago, graduating nursing students were advised to work in a medical-surgical setting before going into psychiatry so that they could learn "basic nursing skills." Discuss why this suggestion is no longer valid given contemporary psychiatric patients and treatment settings.

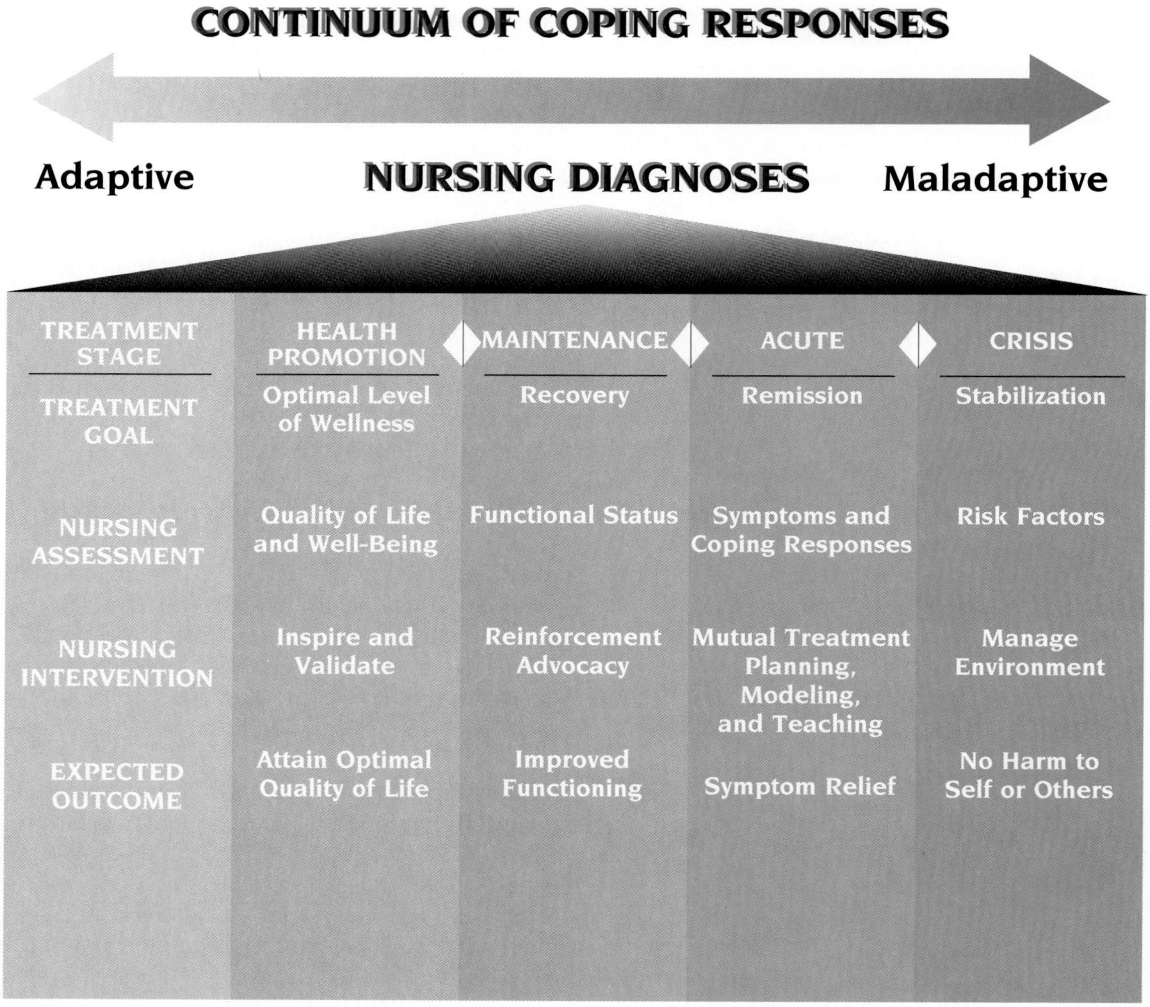

CONTINUUM OF COPING RESPONSES

Adaptive   **NURSING DIAGNOSES**   **Maladaptive**

TREATMENT STAGE	HEALTH PROMOTION	MAINTENANCE	ACUTE	CRISIS
TREATMENT GOAL	Optimal Level of Wellness	Recovery	Remission	Stabilization
NURSING ASSESSMENT	Quality of Life and Well-Being	Functional Status	Symptoms and Coping Responses	Risk Factors
NURSING INTERVENTION	Inspire and Validate	Reinforcement Advocacy	Mutual Treatment Planning, Modeling, and Teaching	Manage Environment
EXPECTED OUTCOME	Attain Optimal Quality of Life	Improved Functioning	Symptom Relief	No Harm to Self or Others

Fig. 9-6   Treatment stages related to implementation of nursing care.

Treatment Stages

A final issue for the psychiatric nurse to consider in the implementation process is that there are four possible treatment stages:

1. Health promotion
2. Maintenance
3. Acute
4. Crisis

These stages reflect the range of adaptive-maladaptive coping responses, and patients can move between these stages at any time. The goal, assessment, intervention, and expected outcome varies with each stage, as seen in Fig. 9-6. It is critically important for psychiatric nurses to appropriately determine the patient's stage of treatment and then implement nursing activities that target the agreed upon treatment goal in the most cost-effective and efficient manner.

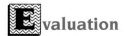 **valuation**

STANDARD VI—EVALUATION

The psychiatric–mental health nurse evaluates the client's progress in attaining expected outcomes.

▼ *Rationale*

Nursing care is a dynamic process involving change in the client's health status over time, giving rise to the need for new data, different diagnoses, and modifications in the plan of care. Therefore evaluation is a continuous process of appraising the effect of nursing interventions and the treatment regimen on the client's health status and expected health outcomes.

▼ *Nursing conditions*

Supervision
Self-analysis
Peer review
Patient and family participation

▼ *Nursing behaviors*

Compare patient's responses and expected outcome
Review nursing process
Modify nursing process as needed
Participate in quality improvement activities

▼ *Key elements*

Evaluation is an ongoing process
Patient and family participation in evaluation is essential
Goal achievement should be documented, and revisions in the plan of care should be implemented as appropriate
When evaluating care the nurse should review all previous phases of the nursing process and determine whether the expected outcomes for the patient have been met. Key words for the evaluation phase of the

nursing process are *mutual, continuous, adequate, effective, appropriate, efficient,* and *flexible.* Fig. 9-7 shows the overall flow of the nursing process. The nurse must make many decisions throughout the process including:

1. Was my conceptual model appropriate to this particular patient situation?
2. Was my data collection adequate, and were all relevant coping responses, objective signs, and subjective symptoms identified?
3. Were my nursing diagnoses accurate and based on the analysis and synthesis of relevant data, the application of theory, and the appropriateness of nursing treatment?
4. Were the expected outcomes and plan of care relevant and mutual, showing appropriate priorities and the consideration of all realistic alternatives?
5. Were my nursing interventions effective and efficient in time and energy?

 ## CRITICAL THINKING ABOUT CONTEMPORARY ISSUES

Does Psychiatric Nursing Care Really Make a Difference?

Most nurses reading this question would automatically and emphatically say, "Yes, of course it does!" But does it really? More specifically, what evidence exists that the care provided by psychiatric nurses actually results in a decrease in patients' symptoms, improvement in patients' functional status, or increased quality of life? What evidence would you provide a hospital administrator who was proposing that all but one of the psychiatric nursing positions on the units be replaced with counselors? How would you convince the director of a community mental health program for the seriously mentally ill that, as a nurse, you should be hired to work with this population rather than the social worker that is also being interviewed?

In fact, very few well-designed psychiatric nursing studies have demonstrated the effectiveness of psychiatric nursing care. Five major reports have reviewed the nursing literature with a focus on the cost effectiveness and the impact of nurses on health outcomes.[6-8,13,17] Of the hundreds of articles cited in these reviews, only three psychiatric nursing studies are mentioned, and one of these was conducted in England. It is clear that at this time psychiatric nurses believe they make a valuable contribution to the health care of patients. However, providing the evidence to support this is long overdue. ▼

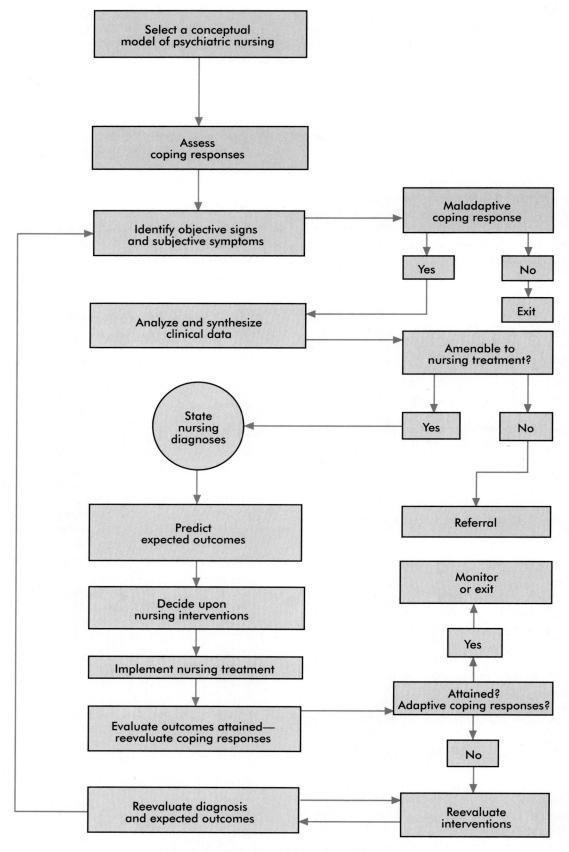

Fig. 9-7   Flowchart of the nursing process.

6. Were the expected outcomes achieved and, if not, did I reevaluate previous steps in the nursing process?

Often, progress with psychiatric patients is slow and occurs in small steps rather than dramatic leaps. Realizing that progress has been made can produce growth and inspire new enthusiasm in both the patient and the nurse.

The nurse also needs to remain flexible to modify interventions according to the patient's changing needs and the nurse's ongoing evaluation. Modifying a plan of care does not mean nursing care has failed. Failure occurs if the plan is not relevant to the patient's needs or is not revised as needs change. Thus reassessment, reordering priorities, setting new goals, and revising the nursing plan of care are all essential evaluation activities.

Above all, evaluation is a mutual process based on the patient's and family's previously identified goals and level of satisfaction. Patients, families, and psychiatric nurses often have different views of treatment and the effectiveness of the care they have received.[18,20] It is therefore critical that psychiatric nurses have a systematic and objective way to learn from patients and families which aspects of the nursing care provided were helpful, and what additional nursing actions may have further enhanced their well-being.

Finally, evaluation is a continuous, active process that begins early in the relationship and continues throughout. It is an activity that needs greater documentation by psychiatric nurses so that they can demonstrate the value of psychiatric nursing services to consumers, administrators, reimbursers, and other healthcare providers (see Critical Thinking about Contemporary Issues). Perhaps more than any other phase of the nursing process, evaluation and outcome measurement will be the key aspects of psychiatric nursing activities in the decade to come.

 # CASE STUDY

This case study describes the use of the nursing process with a psychiatric patient. It illustrates the interrelationship of the phases of the nurse-patient relationship, the therapeutic dimensions, and the various activities as the nurse works with the patient to foster adaptive coping behavior and more integrated functioning.

▼ ASSESSMENT

Ms. G came to the psychiatric outpatient department of the local hospital requesting treatment with a female therapist. The psychiatric nurse specialist agreed to perform the initial screening and evaluation and consider serving as her primary therapist.

To collect the initial data, the nurse followed the admission format required by the department. A description of the presenting problem revealed that Ms. G was a 29-year-old single woman who was neat in appearance and markedly overweight. She reported feelings of "confusion and depression" and said that superficially she appeared "outgoing and friendly and played the role of a clown." In reality, however, she said she had few close friends, felt insecure about herself, felt unsuccessful in her job, and believed she "overanalyzed her problems." She said she had feelings of worthlessness and loss of pleasure in her daily activities on and off for the past 2 years.

Additional information was obtained in other significant areas of her life. Her psychosocial history revealed a disrupted family situation. Her mother died of tuberculosis when she was 11 years of age. Her father, age 73, was alive but had been an alcoholic "for as long as Ms. G could remember." She had one sister, age 20, who married at age 16 and was now divorced. She also had one stepsister, age 45, who was married, had two adopted sons, and lived out of state. In exploring this family information, Ms. G revealed that her stepsister was her natural mother, but she had continued to call her father's wife "mother." After her "mother" died, her stepsister took over the house. Two years later, however, this stepsister married and moved out of state. Ms. G reported feeling closest to this stepsister and felt abandoned when she left. Ms. G then took charge of the house until age 14, when her father placed her and her sister in a group home where she had difficulty making friends.

She completed high school and college. In college she had four good friends who were all married now. Her only close heterosexual relationship was in high school, and this boyfriend eventually married her best friend. Since that time she had never dated and stated she had no desire to marry.

After college she obtained a job as a "girl Friday" for a law firm and expressed much pleasure with it. She then saw the opportunity to make more money as a waitress and switched jobs. She currently worked at a restaurant, and her schedule involved day and night rotations as well as weekend shifts. She expressed dissatisfaction with many aspects of her job but was unable to identify alternatives. Her goal in life was to have a fulfilling career.

She lived alone. Her best friend was her immediate

supervisor at work. She currently had no male friends and only two other female acquaintances.

Pertinent medical history revealed a major weight problem. She was 36 kg (80 pounds) overweight and extremely conscious of it. She viewed her body negatively and believed others were also "repulsed" by her weight. She also recently recovered from infectious hepatitis. She drank an occasional beer when out with friends (once or twice a month), denied any drug use, and smoked three fourths of a pack of cigarettes a day.

▼ DIAGNOSIS

After consultation the psychiatric nurse agreed to work with Ms. G as primary therapist. In the following session they established a contract for working together, and a fee was set by the agency's financial secretary. At this time they explored her expressed guilt over seeking help, the reason for her request for a female therapist, their mutual roles, and the confidential nature of the relationship. The nurse also shared with Ms. G the maladaptive coping responses she had noted and the inferences she had made. They discussed these areas, and the following nursing diagnoses were identified:

1. Self-esteem disturbance related to childhood rejection and unrealistic self-ideals as evidenced by feelings of worthlessness
2. Social isolation related to ambivalence regarding male-female relationships and lack of socialization skills as evidenced by lack of close friends
3. Altered role performance related to job dissatisfaction with working hours and nature of the work as evidenced by feeling unsuccessful in her job
4. Body image disturbance related to weight control problem as evidenced by negative feelings

Ms. G's DSM-IV diagnosis was identified as dysthymia, one of the mood disorders.

▼ OUTCOME IDENTIFICATION

They mutually agreed to work on her problem areas in weekly therapy sessions. After 3 months they would evaluate the achievement of the following expected outcomes:

1. Ms. G will describe her expectations of the therapeutic process and her commitment to it.
2. Aspects of Ms. G's self-ideal will be identified.
3. Factors influencing her self-concept and negative, stereotyped self-perceptions will be evaluated.
4. Interpersonal relationships will be analyzed to include her patterns of relating, her expectations of others, and specific areas of difficulty.
5. Alternative employment opportunities will be identified.
6. The advantages and disadvantages of a job change will be compared.

▼ PLANNING

In discussing these areas they agreed that nursing diagnosis 1 was a central one and problems 3 and 4 directly contributed to it. Her coping mechanisms included intellectualization and denial, and she compensated for her self-doubts by an outward appearance that was social, joking, and friendly, yet superficial. Nursing diagnosis 5 presented an immediate demand on the therapeutic relationship. The strengths Ms. G brought to the therapy process included her introspective nature and ability to analyze events, her openness to new ideas, the resource people available to her in her immediate environment, and a genuine sense of humor.

▼ IMPLEMENTATION

Since they were in the introductory phase of the relationship, many of the goals involved areas needing further assessment. During this phase of treatment Ms. G displayed much anxiety, testing behavior, and ambivalence, and the nursing actions were focused on promoting respect, openness, and acceptance and minimizing her anxiety. Through the nurse's use of empathic understanding, Ms. G became less jovial and superficial and began to attain some intellectual insight into her behavior. With guidance she began to appraise her own abilities and became more open in expressing feelings.

She feared intimate personal involvement and could not tolerate physical closeness. The nurse incorporated this into nursing actions by initially minimizing confrontation, setting limits on anxiety-producing topics, and arranging the office seating to allow the patient to select her proximity to the nurse.

As they discussed the patient's relationships, the nurse confronted her with the dependent role Ms. G played and the unrealistic expectations she placed on others in the exclusiveness and amount of time she demanded from them. Her pattern of relating was also manipulative in that she elicited a sympathetic response and then used it to meet her own needs. She had great difficulty with mutuality and autonomy in relating to others. She was inexperienced in heterosexual relationships and missed many of the normal adolescent growth experiences in this area. Finally, she had much emotion and fear vested in her family of origin. The only trusting relationship Ms. G could recall was with her stepsister-mother. When this stepsister abruptly left home to marry, Ms. G perceived this as a personal rejection. She had since isolated herself from her family and continued to blame herself for her rejection by others, thus lowering her self-esteem and ability to trust others.

At the end of 2 months Ms. G was being considered for a promotion at work to hostess but on the basis of an evaluation by her best friend and supervisor was rejected for it. This precipitated a suicide attempt, which

Ms. G revealed at her next regular session. At this point the issue of trust within the relationship became critical, as well as her inability to express anger because she feared rejection. The nurse now began more actively confronting Ms. G in her areas of ambivalence and inconsistency, setting limits on her self-destructive behavior, and suggesting alternatives. Ms. G then revealed that her relationship with her friend-supervisor was also a sexual one, and she expressed fears of homosexuality and loss of identity.

In later sessions Ms. G's relationship with this friend would become a critical therapeutic issue because it reflected many of her conflicts. The therapy process presented a threat to the unhealthy parts of this relationship, and during the course of therapy Ms. G decided she needed to choose between maladaptive behaviors and more growth-producing options.

The relationship had now moved into the working phase where focus was placed on specifics, and problem-solving activities began. After 3 months the nursing diagnoses were reevaluated to include the following:

1. Potential for self-directed violence related to perceived rejection by friend as evidenced by suicide attempt
2. Personal identity disturbance related to childhood rejection and unrealistic self-ideals as evidenced by self statements
3. Social isolation related to inability to trust, lack of socialization skills, and feelings of inadequacy as evidenced by relationship patterns
4. Powerlessness related to fear of rejection by others as evidenced by perceived lack of control over life events
5. Altered role performance related to job dissatisfaction with working hours and nature of the work as evidenced by feeling unsuccesssful in her job

At this time the nurse sought consultation as she further evolved her plan of care. Neither medication nor hospitalization were indicated. These formulations were shared with Ms. G, and together they collaborated about her future progress. They agreed to focus on changing Ms. G's maladaptive behavior by exploring past events and conflicts and helping her learn more productive patterns of living. Ms. G was now ready to commit herself to the work of therapy and interpersonal change, and she began to assume increased responsibility for this therapeutic work.

Because her self-ideal was unrealistically high, specific short-term goals became essential. The nurse's theoretical orientation incorporated the dynamics of Sullivan's and Peplau's interpersonal theories, Beck's cognitive framework, and Glasser's reality therapy. The relationship was focused on frequently through the use of immediacy and became a model for examining many of her conflicts. This proved to be an excellent learning opportunity as Ms. G and the nurse dealt with resistance, transference, and countertransference reactions. During the next year Ms. G made much progress, including the following changes:

1. She moved into an apartment with another girlfriend.
2. She left her previous job and resumed working in an office where she received more personal satisfaction and a work schedule that would allow her to increase her social activities.
3. She began a diet regimen.
4. She participated in additional activities, such as a dancing class and a health spa.
5. She learned to verbalize her anger more freely with the nurse, friends, and others at work. This included discussing the many relationships in her past that were terminated without her agreement and in which she had internalized her anger.
6. She contacted her stepsister-mother and visited her. This was an important therapeutic goal because it allowed her to review her early experiences and provided her with actual feedback from those involved. Consequently, many of her misperceptions became evident and open to exploration in therapy.
7. She was able to admit her ambivalent feeling about her friend-supervisor and discuss the negative aspects of the relationship. She stopped further sexual contact with her because she felt exploited. Over time, the nature of this relationship changed, and it eventually became a casual acquaintance.
8. She learned about the variety of sexual feelings and responses and saw her needs in this area as appropriate developmental tasks. She became open to evaluating both heterosexual and homosexual expressions of her own sexual feelings.
9. Her perception of personal space changed, and her tolerance for physical closeness increased.
10. She developed new male and female friends and socialized frequently with them.

▼ EVALUATION

The terminating phase of the relationship began after about 8 months. At this time Ms. G was independently solving problems and, in therapy, the nurse primarily validated and supported her thinking. She was now receiving and accepting much positive feedback from others, had lost 15 kg (40 pounds), was continuing to diet, was planning future career goals, and had achieved more satisfactory interpersonal relationships with both men and women. The mutual goals for therapy had been met.

Terminating was difficult because of the close, trusting bond that had developed between them. The nurse had feelings of pleasure in Ms. G's growth, as well as personal satisfaction in her effectiveness as therapist. Ms. G openly described her feelings about terminating and raised the question of a possible social relationship between them. Over the course of the sessions she came to realize that the premise of the relationship was therapy and changing individual perceptions or patterns of relating would not be feasible or desirable. Most important, she had control for terminating this relationship and the opportunity to work it through in a positive way. The sessions were spaced to monthly intervals and considerable time was spent reviewing initial problem areas and the progress she had made in them. After 10 months the nurse and patient mutually agreed to terminate regular sessions. ▼

SUMMARY

1. The nursing process is an interactive, problem-solving process used by the nurse as a systematic and individualized way to fulfill the goal of nursing care.
2. Assessment should reflect both content and process and information relative to the patient's biopsychosocial world. Data collection is facilitated by a systematic assessment tool that ideally is based on a conceptual model of psychiatric nursing.
3. The nursing diagnosis should include the patient's adaptive or maladaptive health response, defining characteristics of that response, and contributing stressors. Knowledge of both NANDA and DSM diagnoses is needed by psychiatric nurses.
4. Outcome identification involves setting goals that are mutual, congruent, realistic, and appropriately timed.
5. The plan of care should include prioritized nursing diagnoses and expected outcomes, as well as prescribed nursing strategies to achieve those outcomes.
6. Nursing interventions should be directed toward helping the patient develop insight and resolve problems through carrying out a positive plan of action. Psychiatric nursing practice includes both basic and advanced activities.
7. Evaluation involves reviewing all previous phases of the nursing process and determining the degree to which expected outcomes were attained.

REFERENCES

1. American Nurses' Association: *Nursing: a social policy statement*, Kansas City, Mo, 1980, The Association.
2. American Nurses' Association: A *statement on psychiatric–mental health clinical nursing practice and standards of psychiatric–mental health clinical nursing practice*, Washington, DC, 1994, The Association.
3. American Psychiatric Association: *Diagnostic and statistical manual of mental disorders*, ed 4, Washington, DC, 1994, The Association.
4. Brider P: Who killed the nursing care plan? Am J Nurs 1991:35, 1991.
5. Dunn J: Medical skills and knowledge: how necessary are they for psychiatric nurses? J *Psychosoc Nurs Ment Health Serv* 31:25, 1993.
6. Fagin C: The economic value of nursing research, Am J Nurs 1982:1844, 1982.
7. Fagin C: Nursing as an alternative to high-cost care, Am J Nurs 1982:56, 1982.
8. Fagin C: Nursing's value proves itself, Am J Nurs 1990:17, 1990.
9. Geach B: The problem-solving technique as taught to psychiatric students, *Perspect Psychiatr Care* 12:9, 1974.
10. Krumboltz J, Thorensen C: *Behavioral counseling: cases and techniques*, New York, 1969, Holt, Rinehart & Winston.
11. Malone J: The DSM-III-R versus nursing diagnosis: a dilemma in interdisciplinary practice, *Issues Ment Health Nurs* 12:219, 1991.
12. National Quality of Care Forum: Bridging the gap between theory and practice: exploring clinical practice guidelines, J *Qual Improv* 19:384, 1993.
13. Naylor M, Brooten D: The roles and functions of clinical nurse specialists, *Image* 25:73, 1993.
14. North American Nursing Diagnosis Association: NANDA *nursing diagnoses: definitions and classification* 1993-1994, Philadelphia, 1994, The Association.
15. Ormiston S, Barrett N, Binder R, Molyneux V: A partially computerized treatment plan, *Hosp Community Psychiatry* 40:531, 1989.
16. Redman B: *The process of patient teaching*, St Louis, 1993, Mosby.
17. Safriet B: Health care dollars and regulatory sense: the role of advanced practice nurses, *Yale J Regulat* 9:419, 1992.
18. Sullivan C, Yudelowitz I: Staff and patients: divergent views of treatment, *Perspect Psychiatr Care* 27:1991.
19. Teague D, Laraia M: Success factors for automated systems in the clinical environment: the MUSC experience, *Top Health Inform Manage* 14:21, 1994.
20. Yoder S, Rode M: How are you doing? Patient evaluations

of nursing actions, *J Psychosoc Nurs Ment Health Serv* 28:26, 1990.

21. Zielstorff R, Jette A, Barnett G: Issues in designing an automated record system for clinical care and research, *Adv Nurs Sci* 13:75, 1990.

ANNOTATED SUGGESTED READINGS

*Bond S, Thomas L: Issues in measuring outcomes of nursing, *J Adv Nurs* 16:1492, 1991.

Excellent overview outlining problems in outcome measurement and ways of moving forward in this much needed area of nursing research.

*Burdick M, Stuart G, Lewis L: Measuring nursing outcomes in a psychiatric setting, *Issues Ment Health Nurs* 15:137, 1994.

Reports the result of a study examining whether the use of nursing documentation based on NANDA human response patterns would positively affect the quality of nursing diagnoses, patient outcome criteria, and perceived patient improvement.

Hoffman P: Critical path method: an important tool for coordinating clinical care, *J Qual Improv* 19:235, 1993.

Clearly describes one hospital's experience of the developmental process and lessons learned in developing critical paths. Very helpful to anyone undertaking this task.

*Karshmer J: Expert nursing diagnoses: the link between nursing care plans and patient classification systems, *J Nurs Adm* 21:31, 1991.

Describes the process and outcome of developing a comprehensive system that merged two major clinical management problems in a psychiatric setting. Interesting and useful reading.

*Malone J: The DSM-III-R versus nursing diagnosis: a dilemma in interdisciplinary practice, *Issues Ment Health Nurs* 12:219, 1991.

Excellent comparison of the DSM and nursing diagnostic systems and discussion of the dynamics of interdisciplinary practice.

Mirin S, Gossett J, Grob M: *Psychiatric treatment: advances in outcome research*, Washington, DC, 1991, American Psychiatric Press.

Summarizes much of the work to date in the area of psychiatric treatment outcome research. Only one chapter is contributed by a nurse, and it focuses on quality assurance.

Modai I, Rabinowitz J: Why and how to establish a computerized system for psychiatric case records, *Hosp Community Psychiatry* 44:1091, 1993.

Answers practical questions about why and how to computerize and describes the many advantages of computerized psychiatric records.

*Nathenson P, Johnson C: The psychiatric treatment plan, *Perspect Psychiatr Care* 28:32, 1992.

Describes the conceptual framework for the treatment planning process at one institution using current HCFA and JCAHO standards.

*Pesut D: Aim versus blame: using an outcome specification model, *J Psychosoc Nurs Ment Health Serv* 27:26, 1989.

Excellent discussion of using outcome specification as a major therapeutic technique of neurolinguistic programming (NPL) with psychiatric patients.

*Sullivan C, Yudelowitz I: Staff and patients: divergent views of treatment, *Perspect Psychiatr Care* 27:1991.

Describes a patient-staff survey focusing on the efficacy of treatment and aftercare that showed inconsistencies in the way staff perceived treatment given patients. Thought-provoking reading.

Weiss K, Chapman H: A computer-assisted inpatient psychiatric assessment and treatment planning system, *Hosp Community Psychiatry* 44:1097, 1993.

Gives an example of one computerized treatment planning system developed for a psychiatric unit. Clear and practical.

*Wheeland R: Focus charting in a psychiatric facility, *J Psychosoc Nurs Ment Health Serv* 31:15, 1993.

Presents a structured method of documentation that allows psychiatric nurses to consider interventions and patient responses, as well as observations of the patient.

*Yoder S, Rode M: How are you doing? Patient evaluations of nursing actions, *J Psychosoc Nurs Ment Health Serv* 28:26, 1990.

Interesting report of a study on nursing actions perceived as helpful by psychiatric patients.

---

*Nursing reference.

A P P E N D I X   A
Risk Factor Assessment

RISK FACTOR ASSESSMENT DIRECTIONS

The purpose of this assessment is to formulate a nursing diagnosis based on the identification of risk factors that potentially present an immediate threat to the patient. A registered nurse must complete this assessment within the **FIRST HOUR** of the patient's encounter with the health-care system.

The space labeled "Informants" should identify by name any source of information used to assess the patient. Examples are the patient, family member, an accompanying individual, or the referral source. The "Reason for This Encounter" should quote the patient when possible.

The tool comprises eight (8) areas of potential risk. Positive findings in any area directs the nurse to initiate a more specific assessment or to initiate appropriate precautions. At the end of the risk factor assessment, the nurse must list the nursing diagnoses and total number of risk factors identified. A nursing care plan must be initiated immediately to address any nursing diagnosis that reflects an identified risk factor.

RISK FACTOR ASSESSMENT TOOL

INFORMANTS: _____   DATE:_____

_____

REASON FOR THIS ENCOUNTER:_____

_____

_____

RISK FACTORS:

1. Potential for Suicide/Self-Harm:

☐ yes ☐ no   Is there evidence of active or recent suicidal or self-harm ideation or attempt?
☐ yes ☐ no   Is there a history of suicidal or self-harm ideation or attempt?

*If yes to either question, initiate a Suicide/Self-Harm Assessment.

2. Potential for Assault/Violence:

☐ yes ☐ no   Is there a history of assaultive, destructive, or violent behavior?
☐ yes ☐ no   Does the patient express feelings of anger or aggression?

*If yes to either question, initiate an Assault/Violence Assessment.

3. Potential for Substance Abuse Withdrawal (alcohol, illicit drugs, prescription drugs, or inhalants):

☐ yes ☐ no   Have you ever felt the need to cut down on your drinking or drug use?
☐ yes ☐ no   Have people annoyed you by criticizing your drinking or drug use?
☐ yes ☐ no   Have you ever felt badly or guilty about your drinking or drug use?
☐ yes ☐ no   Have you ever had a drink first thing in the morning (eye opener)?

*If yes to any question, initiate a Substance Withdrawal Assessment.

4. Potential for Allergic Reaction/Adverse Drug Reaction

☐ yes ☐ no   Food
☐ yes ☐ no   Medication
☐ yes ☐ no   Other

*If yes to any item, initiate an Allergy Assessment.

5. Potential for Seizure:

☐ yes ☐ no   Is there a history of seizures?

*If yes to this question, initiate a Seizure Assessment.

6. Potential for Falls/Accidents:

☐ yes ☐ no   Ages 70 or older/5 or under
☐ yes ☐ no   History of confusion
☐ yes ☐ no   History of falls/accidents
☐ yes ☐ no   Sensory deficits
☐ yes ☐ no   Impaired mobility/balance
☐ yes ☐ no   Medications (check as many as apply)
      ☐ yes ☐ no   Sedatives/tranquilizers/narcotics
      ☐ yes ☐ no   Anesthetics
      ☐ yes ☐ no   Diuretics/antihypertensives
      ☐ yes ☐ no   Laxatives
      ☐ yes ☐ no   Substance Abuse
      ☐ yes ☐ no   Psychotropics

*If yes to two or more items, initiate Fall Precautions.

7. Potential for Elopement:

☐ yes ☐ no   Does the patient wish or intend to leave?
☐ yes ☐ no   Does the patient have a history of elopement?

*If yes to either question, initiate Elopement Precautions.

8. Potential for Physiologic Instability:

☐ yes ☐ no   Existing unstable physical problem?

Vital signs: T_____   P_____   R_____

BP stand_____   BP Sit_____   Weight_____   Height_____

*If yes to unstable problem or data out of normal range, initiate Physical Assessment.

Total number of risk factors identified (1-8)_____

IDENTIFIED NURSING DIAGNOSES:

☐ yes ☐ no   Potential for violence (self-directed)
☐ yes ☐ no   Potential for violence (other-directed)
☐ yes ☐ no   High Risk for self-mutilation
☐ yes ☐ no   Potential for injury, related to_____

RN Signature: _____ Date: _____ Time: _____

APPENDIX B

Psychiatric Nursing Assessment

PSYCHIATRIC NURSING ASSESSMENT DIRECTIONS

This assessment is intended to assist the nurse in identifying patient needs that should be addressed during the current treatment episode. It can be used in any psychiatric setting throughout the continuum of care. The tool has shaded and unshaded areas. In an inpatient setting, items in the shaded areas must be completed by a registered nurse within eight (8) hours of the patient's admission. All other items, including those in the unshaded areas, must be completed by a registered nurse within twenty-four (24) hours of the patient's admission.

The NURSING ASSESSMENT has ten (10) main areas:

1. Patient/Family Appraisal of Health and Illness
2. Predisposing Factors
3. Coping Responses—Physical
4. Coping Responses—Mental Status
5. Coping Resources and Discharge Planning Needs
6. Coping Mechanisms
7. Psychosocial and Environmental Problems
8. Global Assessment of Functioning
9. Knowledge Deficits
10. Nursing Diagnosis

Section I   Patient/Family appraisal of Health and Illness

This section of the tool is intended to assist the nursing staff in understanding the patient's and family's beliefs, values, and perceptions regarding the current problem, goals for treatment, and health care in general. Often, patients, families, and clinical staff have different perceptions of these issues based on their different sociocultural backgrounds and experiences. Yet it is critically important for these issues to be assessed so that the nursing staff can provide culturally sensitive and mutually planned care.

Section II   Predisposing Factors— Psychiatric Treatment

This section is designed to collect historical information about the patient and family that may affect the formulation of the treatment plan and the patient's receptivity to treatment.

Section III   Coping Responses—Physical

The nursing assessment of the patient's physical coping responses is intended to complement the thorough medical examination received by all patients. This section of the database assesses each of the patient's major physiological categories and identifies any dysfunctional coping responses or unhealthy patterns.

This section has twelve (12) categories to be assessed. The categories of physical coping responses are as follows:

Category	Assess
EENT	Eyes, ears, nose, throat—anatomy and associated functions
RESP	Respiratory anatomy and associated functions
CV	Cardiovascular anatomy and associated functions
GI	Gastrointestinal anatomy and associated functions
GU and REPRO	Genitourinary and reproductive anatomy and associated functions
NEURO	Neurological anatomy and associated functions
MS and SKIN	Musculoskeletal and integumental anatomy and associated functions
NUTRITION	Nutritional health status and eating behaviors
SLEEP	Sleep/wake behaviors and patterns
ENDO	Endocrinological functioning
TOXINS	Actual and potential exposure to environmental and occupational toxins
SELF-CARE	Degree to which functional assistance is required in activities of daily living

It is important to understand that **all dysfunctional patterns may not be addressed during this encounter.** Rather, the nurse will IDENTIFY all problems, and then make a determination as to whether or not the problem is a PRIORITY FOR THIS HEALTH-CARE CONTACT.

Courtesy of Division of Psychiatric Nursing, Medical University of South Carolina.

Section IV Coping Responses— Mental Status

This section of the nursing assessment relates to the patient's current mental status. It has fifteen (15) categories to be assessed:

Appearance
Speech
Motor activity
Mood
Affect
Interaction during interview
Perceptions
Thought content
Thought process
Level of consciousness
Memory
Level of concentration and calculation
Information and intelligence
Judgment
Insight

It is important to understand that **all dysfunctional patterns may not be addressed during this encounter.** Rather, the nurse will IDENTIFY all problems and then make a determination as to whether or not the problem is a PRIORITY FOR THIS HEALTH-CARE CONTACT.

Section V Coping Resources and Discharge Planning Needs

This section of the tool is designed to document the nurse's assessment of the patient's strengths, resources, and needs that can be addressed in the nursing care of plan. It also allows the nurse to better prepare the patient for discharge. If the patient is a minor, is mentally retarded, or has an organic mental disorder, the nurse should complete the assessment with the patient's primary caregiver.

Section VI Coping Mechanisms

This section of the tool documents the types and numbers of adaptive and maladaptive coping mechanisms that the patient utilizes. The nurse may have gathered sufficient data previously in the assessment process to categorize this information, or the nurse may need to ask pertinent questions to elicit additional information.

Section VII Psychosocial and Environmental Problems (Based on Axis IV: Severity of Psychosocial Stressors, DSM-IV)

This section of the tool provides the nurse with Axis IV of the DSM-IV, which is used to report psychosocial and environmental problems that may affect the diagnosis,

treatment, and prognosis of mental disorders. In general, the nurse should note only those psychosocial and environmental problems that have been present during the past year. However, the nurse may choose to note problems occurring before the past year if these contribute to a psychiatric problem or have become a focus of treatment. For convenience, the problems are grouped together in the following categories:

▼ **Problems with primary support group**—e.g., death of a family member; health problems in family; disruption of family by separation, divorce, or estrangement; removal from the home; remarriage of parent; sexual or physical abuse; parental overprotection; neglect of child; inadequate discipline; discord with siblings; birth of a sibling

▼ **Problems related to the social environment**—e.g., death or loss of friend; inadequate social support; living alone; difficulty with acculturation; discrimination; adjustment to life-cycle transition (such as retirement)

▼ **Educational problems**—e.g., illiteracy; academic problems; discord with teachers or classmates; inadequate school environment

▼ **Occupational problems**—e.g., unemployment; threat of job loss; stressful work schedule; difficult work conditions; job dissatisfaction; job change; discord with boss or co-workers

▼ **Housing problems**—e.g., homelessness; inadequate housing; unsafe neighborhood; discord with neighbors or landlord

▼ **Economic problems**—e.g., extreme poverty; inadequate finances; insufficient welfare support

▼ **Problems with access to health-care services**—e.g., inadequate health care services; transportation to health care facilities unavailable; inadequate health insurance

▼ **Problems related to interaction with the legal system/crime**—e.g., arrest; incarceration; litigation; victim of crime

▼ **Other psychosocial and environmental problems**—e.g., exposure to disasters, war, other hostilities; discord with nonfamily caregivers such as counselor, social worker, or physician; unavailability of social service agencies

Section VIII Global Assessment of Functioning—(Based on Axis V, DSM-IV)

This section of the tool provides the nurse with a standardized rating scale, the Global Assessment of Functioning (GAF), Axis V of DSM-IV. It assesses a person's functioning relative to one's mental health or illness. This tool allows the nurse to make an overall judgment about a patient's psychological, social, and occupational functioning at the time of the interview. It may be useful to track the clinical progress of an individual in global terms over time. It is rated as follows: Consider psychological, social, and occupational functioning on a hypothetical continuum of mental health–illness. Do not include impairment in functioning due to physical (or environmental) limitations.

Code (*Note*: Use intermediate codes when appropriate, e.g. 45, 68, 72.)

100 **Superior functioning in a wide range of activities, life's problems never seem to get out of hand, is sought out by others because of his or her many
91 positive qualities. No symptoms.**
90 **Absent or minimal symptoms** (e.g., mild anxiety before an exam), **good functioning in all areas, interested and involved in a wide range of activities, socially effective, generally satisfied with life, no more than everyday problems or concerns** (e.g.,
81 an occasional argument with family member).
80 **If symptoms are present, they are transient and expectable reactions to psychosocial stressors** (e.g., difficulty concentrating after family argument); **no more than slight impairment in social, occupational, or school functioning** (e.g., temporarily fall-
71 ing behind in schoolwork).
70 **Some mild symptoms** (e.g., depressed mood and mild insomnia) **OR some difficulty in social, occupational, or school functioning** (e.g., occasional truancy, or theft within the household), **but generally functioning pretty well, has some meaningful
61 interpersonal relationships.**
60 **Moderate symptoms** (e.g., flat affect and circumstantial speech, occasional panic attacks) **OR moderate difficulty in social, occupational, or school functioning** (e.g., few friends, conflicts with peers or
51 co-workers).
50 **Serious symptoms** (e.g., suicidal ideation, severe obsessional rituals, frequent shoplifting) **OR any serious impairment in social, occupational, or school
41 functioning** (e.g., no friends, unable to keep a job).
40 **Some impairment in reality testing or communication** (e.g., speech is at times illogical, obscure, or irrelevant) **OR major impairment in several areas, such as work or school, family relations, judgement, thinking, or mood** (e.g., depressed man avoids friends, neglects family, and is unable to work; child frequently beats up younger children, is
31 defiant at home, and is failing at school).
30 **Behavior is considerably influenced by delusions or hallucinations OR serious impairment in communication or judgement** (e.g., sometimes incoherent, acts grossly inappropriately, suicidal preoccupation) **OR inability to function in almost all areas** (e.g.,
21 stays in bed all day; no job, home, or friends).
20 **Some danger of hurting self or others** (e.g., suicide attempts without clear expectation of death; frequently violent; manic excitement) **OR occasionally

fails to maintain minimal personal hygiene (e.g., smears feces) **OR gross impairment in communi-
11 cation** (e.g., largely incoherent or mute).
10 **Persistent danger of severely hurting self or others** (e.g., recurrent violence) **OR persistent inability to maintain minimal personal hygiene OR serious
1 suicidal act with clear expectation of death.**
0 Inadequate information.

Section IX   Knowledge Deficits

This section of the tool allows the nurse to identify areas in which the patient is in need of health teaching including the following the areas:

Understanding of psychiatric illness	Assess patient's understanding of illness including diagnosis, etiology, signs and symptoms, course of illness, prognosis, and treatment.
Precipitating stressors	Assess patient's understanding of those stressors that result in a recurrence or exacerbation of symptoms.
Coping skills	Assess whether patient can successfully utilize effective coping skills to manage symptoms.
Access to resources	Assess patient's ability to purchase and obtain medications. Assess patient's ability to obtain emergency medical or psychiatric help.
Medications	Assess whether patient understands the medications prescribed, including their purpose, dosage, side effects, potential adverse effects, and symptoms or toxicity.
Understanding of physical illness	Assess patient's understanding of illness including diagnosis, course of illness, prognosis, treatment, and impact on psychiatric illness.

Section X   Nursing Diagnosis

This checklist of possible NANDA nursing diagnoses is included to provide the nurse with a brief, time-efficient mechanism to document the initial synthesis of the data that have been collected in the assessment process. To complete this section, the nurse should first blacken the square in front of each diagnosis that corresponds to problems identified as a priority for this health-care contact.

Once the targeted diagnoses have been highlighted, they should then be prioritized by rank ordering them in the spaces provided in front of each diagnosis (e.g., I indicates the diagnosis with the highest priority, 2 indicates the diagnosis with the next highest priority, and so on).

PSYCHIATRIC NURSING ASSESSMENT TOOL

Age: _____   Sex: ☐ male ☐ female   Race: ☐ White ☐ Black ☐ Native American ☐ Hispanic ☐ Asian ☐ Other

I. PATIENT/FAMILY APPRAISAL OF HEALTH AND ILLNESS

1. What problem led you to seek help at this time?   ☐ Unable or unwilling to answer

_____

2. What situations, events or stressors led to this problem?   ☐ Unable or unwilling to answer

_____

3. What is your goal while here and how can we help you?   ☐ Unable or unwilling to answer

_____

4. Whom do you see for your regular health care (physician, nurse, root doctor, healer, chiropractor, minister, priest, etc)?

_____

5. Have you been satisfied with your previous health care?   ☐ yes ☐ no
    If no, why not?

_____

II. PREDISPOSING FACTORS—PSYCHIATRIC TREATMENT

1. Have you been treated for a psychiatric illness in the past? ☐ yes ☐ no
    If yes: diagnosis _____
            treatment ☐ inpatient ☐ outpatient ☐ medication ☐ ECT ☐ other
    If inpatient: when _____ how long _____
    If outpatient: when _____ how long _____
    Was medication prescribed: ☐ Yes ☐ No   If yes, list: _____
    If other treatment: what _____ where _____ when _____

2. Past adherence to prescribed treatment   ☐ good   ☐ fair   ☐ poor

3.
	Victim	Witness	Age			Victim	Witness	Age
Physical Abuse	☐	☐	___	Domestic Violence		☐	☐	___
Sexual Abuse	☐	☐	___	Violent Crime		☐	☐	___
Neglect	☐	☐	___					

    Describe: _____

_____

4. Is there a psychiatric history in family: ☐ Yes   ☐ No
    Relative   Diagnosis   Medication/Treatment History

    _____   _____   _____

    _____   _____   _____

5. ALL CURRENT MEDICATIONS	Is the patient currently taking medication? ☐ Yes ☐ No			
Name	Dose	Frequency	Time of last dose	Side Effects

III. COPING RESPONSES—PHYSICAL

	Place an (X) in area of abnormality then describe. If unable to assess, indicate reason.
E E N T	**ASSESS EYES, EARS, NOSE, THROAT FOR CURRENT OR PAST PROBLEM** Yes No Yes No Eyes ☐ ☐ Nose ☐ ☐ Ears ☐ ☐ Throat ☐ ☐ Describe: _____	Priority for this encounter ☐ yes ☐ no
R E S P	**ASSESS CHEST, AND RESPIRATORY RATE, DEPTH, PATTERN FOR CURRENT OR PAST PROBLEM** Yes No Upper respiratory ☐ ☐ Lower respiratory ☐ ☐ Describe: _____	Priority for this encounter ☐ yes ☐ no
C V	**ASSESS HEART RATE, RHYTHM, PULSE, CIRCULATION, FLUID RETENTION FOR CURRENT OR PAST PROBLEM** Yes No Central cardiac ☐ ☐ Peripheral vascular ☐ ☐ Describe: _____	Priority for this encounter ☐ yes ☐ no
G I	**ASSESS ABDOMEN, BOWEL HABITS, SWALLOWING FOR CURRENT OR PAST PROBLEM** Yes No Ingestion ☐ ☐ Digestion ☐ ☐ Elimination ☐ ☐ Describe: _____	Priority for this encounter ☐ yes ☐ no

ASSESS GENITOURINARY FREQUENCY, CONTROL, COLOR, ODOR, BLEEDING, DISCHARGE COMFORT AND REPRODUCTIVE SYSTEM FOR CURRENT OR PAST PROBLEM	

<table>
<tr>
<td rowspan="2" align="center">G
U

AND

R
E
P
R
O</td>
<td>
Birth control method _____ Last menstrual period _____.___
                                  Last pap _____
Practices safe sex ☐ yes ☐ no   Urine Pregnancy Test ☐ + ☐ − ☐ na

	Yes	No		Yes	No
Urinary-renal	☐	☐	Reproductive	☐	☐
Genital	☐	☐	Sexual	☐	☐

Describe: _____
</td>
<td>Priority for this encounter
☐ yes ☐ no</td>
</tr>
</table>

ASSESS SENSATION, MOTOR FUNCTION FOR CURRENT OR PAST PROBLEM	

<table>
<tr>
<td rowspan="2" align="center">N
E
U
R
O</td>
<td>

	Yes	No
Cranial	☐	☐
Spinal	☐	☐
Peripheral	☐	☐

Describe: _____
</td>
<td>Priority for this encounter
☐ yes ☐ no</td>
</tr>
</table>

ASSESS MOBILITY, JOINTS, SKIN COLOR, TURGOR, INTEGRITY FOR CURRENT OR PAST PROBLEM	

<table>
<tr>
<td rowspan="2" align="center">M
S

AND

S
K
I
N</td>
<td>

	Yes	No		Yes	No
Muscular	☐	☐	Joint	☐	☐
Skeletal	☐	☐	Skin	☐	☐
			Pediculosis	☐	☐

Describe: _____
</td>
<td>Priority for this encounter
☐ yes ☐ no</td>
</tr>
</table>

ASSESS EATING, DIET HISTORY FOR CURRENT OR PAST PROBLEM	

<table>
<tr>
<td align="center">N
U
T
R
I
T
I
O
N</td>
<td>
Are you satisfied with your eating patterns? ☐ yes ☐ no
If no, why not? _____
Do you eat in secret? ☐ yes ☐ no Describe: _____
Number of meals per day _____ Number of snacks per day _____
appetite ☐ increased ☐ decreased   ☐ binging   ☐ purging
weight   ☐ increased ☐ decreased   highest weight _____
                                   lowest weight _____
☐ Special diet _____
</td>
<td>Priority for this encounter
☐ yes ☐ no</td>
</tr>
</table>

ASSESS SLEEP, REST FOR CURRENT OR PAST PROBLEM

S L E E P	Do you have problems with your sleep habits? ☐ yes ☐ no Normal HS time _____ Normal awakening time _____ Total hours _____ Do you feel rested after a night's sleep? ☐ yes ☐ no What helps you sleep? _____ Check all that apply: ☐ difficulty falling asleep How long does it take? _____ ☐ middle of night awakening Number of times? _____ ☐ early morning awakening What time? _____ ☐ restless sleep ☐ nightmares ☐ night terrors ☐ snoring ☐ somnambulism ☐ talking in sleep ☐ sleep apnea ☐ fatigue Do you normally nap? ☐ yes ☐ no How often _____ How long _____ Describe: _____	Priority for this encounter ☐ yes ☐ no

ASSESS ENDOCRINE AND METABOLIC SYSTEMS FOR CURRENT OR PAST PROBLEM

E N D O	Yes No Diabetes ☐ ☐ Thyroid ☐ ☐ Describe: _____	Priority for this encounter ☐ yes ☐ no

ASSESS EXPOSURE TO TOXIC SUBSTANCES

T O X I N S	Yes No Yes No Pesticide ☐ ☐ Asbestos ☐ ☐ Fertilizer ☐ ☐ Lead paint/pipes ☐ ☐ Poison ☐ ☐ Moonshine ☐ ☐ Describe: _____	Priority for this encounter ☐ yes ☐ no

ASSESS ACTIVITIES OF DAILY LIVING

S E L F C A R E	Is the patient independent in activities of daily living? ☐ yes ☐ no Needs Assistance Needs Total Care Bathing ☐ ☐ Hygiene ☐ ☐ Feeding ☐ ☐ Toileting ☐ ☐ Dressing ☐ ☐ Describe: _____	Priority for this encounter ☐ yes ☐ no

Significant Patient/Family History: _____

_____

Total number priorities for this encounter (0–12): _____

IV. COPING RESPONSES—MENTAL STATUS

Place an (X) in <u>ALL</u> items that apply

ASSESS APPEARANCE

| ☐ unkempt ☐ inappropriate dress | ☐ unusual gait ☐ minimal eye contact | ☐ appears older than stated age ☐ appears younger than stated age | Problem identified ☐ yes ☐ no Priority for encounter ☐ yes ☐ no |

Describe: _____

ASSESS SPEECH

| ☐ Rapid ☐ Slow ☐ Incoherent | ☐ Loud ☐ Soft ☐ Paucity | ☐ Pressured ☐ Mute | ☐ Stuttering ☐ Slurring | Problem identified ☐ yes ☐ no Priority for encounter ☐ yes ☐ no |

ASSESS MOTOR ACTIVITY

| ☐ lethargic ☐ tics | ☐ tense ☐ grimaces | ☐ restless ☐ tremors | ☐ agitated ☐ compulsions | Problem identified ☐ yes ☐ no Priority for encounter ☐ yes ☐ no |

ASSESS MOOD

| ☐ sad ☐ anxious | ☐ fearful | ☐ hopeless | ☐ euphoric | Problem identified ☐ yes ☐ no Priority for encounter ☐ yes ☐ no |

ASSESS AFFECT

| ☐ flat | ☐ blunted | ☐ labile | ☐ incongruent | Problem identified ☐ yes ☐ no Priority for encounter ☐ yes ☐ no |

ASSESS INTERACTION DURING INTERVIEW

| ☐ hostile ☐ apathetic | ☐ uncooperative ☐ defensive | ☐ irritable ☐ suspicious | ☐ guarded ☐ seductive | Problem identified ☐ yes ☐ no Priority for encounter ☐ yes ☐ no |

ASSESS PERCEPTIONS

| Hallucinations: ☐ auditory ☐ olfactory | ☐ visual ☐ command | ☐ tactile | ☐ gustatory | Problem identified ☐ yes ☐ no Priority for encounter ☐ yes ☐ no |

Describe: _____

ASSESS THOUGHT CONTENT

☐ obsessions   ☐ phobias   ☐ hypochondriasis
☐ depersonalization ☐ ideas of reference ☐ magial thinking

Delusions: ☐ religious   ☐ somatic   ☐ grandiose
☐ paranoia   ☐ thought broadcasting ☐ thought insertions ☐ nihilistic

Describe: _____

Problem identified
☐ yes ☐ no
Priority for encounter
☐ yes ☐ no

ASSESS THOUGHT PROCESS

☐ circumstantial ☐ tangential   ☐ loose associations
☐ flight of ideas ☐ thought blocking ☐ perseveration

Problem identified
☐ yes ☐ no
Priority for encounter
☐ yes ☐ no

ASSESS LEVEL OF CONSCIOUSNESS

☐ confused   ☐ sedated   ☐ stuporous

Not oriented to: ☐ time   ☐ place   ☐ person

Problem identified
☐ yes ☐ no
Priority for encounter
☐ yes ☐ no

ASSESS MEMORY

☐ poor remote   ☐ poor recent   ☐ poor immediate   ☐ confabulation

Problem identified
☐ yes ☐ no
Priority for encounter
☐ yes ☐ no

ASSESS LEVEL OF CONCENTRATION & CALCULATION

☐ distractible   ☐ unable to pay attention   ☐ unable to do simple math

Problem identified
☐ yes ☐ no
Priority for encounter
☐ yes ☐ no

ASSESS INFORMATION AND INTELLIGENCE

Last grade completed _____   Illiterate ☐
Learning disability type: _____
Intelligence (estimated _____ or diagnosed _____)
☐ average or above   ☐ moderate retardation   ☐ profound retardation
☐ mild retardation   ☐ severe retardation   IQ if known _____

Problem identified
☐ yes ☐ no
Priority for encounter
☐ yes ☐ no

ASSESS JUDGMENT

☐ mildly impaired   ☐ significantly impaired

Problem identified
☐ yes ☐ no
Priority for encounter
☐ yes ☐ no

ASSESS INSIGHT

☐ denial of illness   ☐ blames outside factors

Problem identified
☐ yes ☐ no
Priority for encounter
☐ yes ☐ no

Total number mental status problems identified (0–16): _____

Total number priorities for this encounter (0–16): _____

V. Coping Resources and Discharge Planning Needs*

		Number resources
1.	The patient is able to provide for: Yes No — ☐ ☐ food — Yes No — ☐ ☐ clothing — Yes No — ☐ ☐ shelter ☐ ☐ safety — ☐ ☐ transportation — ☐ ☐ money ☐ ☐ healthcare	Number resources (0–7): _____
2.	The patient is able to: — Yes No anticipate own needs — ☐ ☐ make decisions in own best interest — ☐ ☐ manage own treatment regime — ☐ ☐	Number resources (0–3): _____
3.	Motivated for treatment: — Yes No — ☐ ☐	Number resources (0–1): _____
4.	The patient has functional supportive relationships: Yes No — ☐ ☐ family — Yes No — ☐ ☐ friends/peers ☐ ☐ professional/therapeutic — ☐ ☐ social/clubs/church	Number resources (0–4): _____
5.	The adult patient enjoys fulfilling work, industrious activity — Yes No or hobbies: — ☐ ☐ If no, has the patient done so in the past?	Number resources (0–1): _____
*If the patient is a minor, mentally retarded or has an organic mental disorder assess caregiver instead of patient.		**Total Number Resources (0–16):** _____

VI. Coping Mechanisms

How does the patient cope with stress and conflict? Adaptive ☐ talks things out ☐ effective problem solving ☐ relaxation techniques ☐ balanced exercise ☐ constructive activity ☐ other: _____	Maladaptive ☐ excessive alcohol/drugs ☐ overeating or undereating ☐ overworking ☐ avoidance ☐ self-injury ☐ aggression ☐ other: _____	**Number adaptive (0–5):** _____ **Number maladaptive (0–6):** _____

VII. Psychosocial and Environmental Problems

☐ Problems with primary support group *Specify*: _____ ☐ Problems related to the social environment *Specify*: _____ ☐ Educational problems *Specify*: _____ ☐ Occupational problems *Specify*: _____ ☐ Housing problems *Specify*: _____ ☐ Economic problems *Specify*: _____ ☐ Problems with access to health care services *Specify*: _____ ☐ Problems related to interaction with the legal system/crime *Specify*: _____ ☐ Other psychosocial and environmental problems *Specify*: _____	**Number of problems (0-9):** _____

VIII. Global Assessment of Functioning

_____ 91–100 Superior	_____ 51–60 Moderate symptoms	_____ 11–20 Some danger
_____ 81–90 Minimal symptoms	_____ 41–50 Serious symptoms	_____ 1–10 Persistent danger
_____ 71–80 Transient symptoms	_____ 31–40 Difficulty functioning	_____ 0 Inadequate information
_____ 61–70 Mild symptoms	_____ 21–30 Inability to function	

IX. Knowledge Deficits

☐ understanding of psychiatric illness
☐ precipitating stressors
☐ coping skills
☐ accessing resources
☐ medications
☐ understanding of physical illness
☐ other: _____

Number deficits
(0–7): _____

X. Nursing Diagnoses

PATTERN 1: EXCHANGING
_____ ☐ Altered Nutrition: More than body requirements
_____ ☐ Altered Nutrition: Less than body requirements
_____ ☐ High Risk for Infection
_____ ☐ Hypothermia
_____ ☐ Hyperthermia
_____ ☐ Constipation
_____ ☐ Diarrhea
_____ ☐ Bowel Incontinence
_____ ☐ Altered Urinary Elimination
_____ ☐ Altered Tissue Perfusion (renal, cerebral, cardiopulmonary, gastrointestinal, peripheral)
_____ ☐ Fluid Volume Excess
_____ ☐ Fluid Volume Deficit
_____ ☐ Impaired Gas Exchange
_____ ☐ Ineffective Breathing Pattern
_____ ☐ High Risk for Injury
_____ ☐ High Risk for Disuse Syndrome
_____ ☐ Impaired Tissue Integrity
_____ ☐ Altered Oral Mucous Membrane
_____ ☐ Impaired Skin Integrity

PATTERN 2: COMMUNICATING
_____ ☐ Impaired Verbal Communication

PATTERN 3: RELATING
_____ ☐ Impaired Social Interaction
_____ ☐ Social Isolation
_____ ☐ Altered Role Performance
_____ ☐ Altered Parenting
_____ ☐ High Risk for Altered Parenting
_____ ☐ Sexual Dysfunction
_____ ☐ Altered Family Process
_____ ☐ Caregiver Role Strain
_____ ☐ High Risk for Caregiver Role Strain
_____ ☐ Parental Role Conflict
_____ ☐ Altered Sexuality Patterns

PATTERN 4: VALUING
_____ ☐ Spiritual Distress (distress of the human spirit)

PATTERN 5: CHOOSING
_____ ☐ Ineffective Individual Coping
_____ ☐ Impaired Adjustment
_____ ☐ Defensive Coping
_____ ☐ Ineffective Denial
_____ ☐ Ineffective Family Coping: Disabling
_____ ☐ Ineffective Family Coping: Compromised

_____ ☐ Family Coping: Potential for Growth
_____ ☐ Ineffective Management of Therapeutic Regimen
_____ ☐ Noncompliance (Specify)
_____ ☐ Decisional Conflict (Specify)
_____ ☐ Health Seeking Behaviors (Specify)

PATTERN 6: MOVING
_____ ☐ Impaired Physical Mobility
_____ ☐ Activity Intolerance
_____ ☐ Fatigue
_____ ☐ High Risk for Activity Intolerance
_____ ☐ Sleep Pattern Disturbance
_____ ☐ Diversional Activity Deficit
_____ ☐ Impaired Home Maintenance Management
_____ ☐ Altered Health Maintenance
_____ ☐ Feeding Self-Care Deficit
_____ ☐ Impaired Swallowing
_____ ☐ Bathing/Hygiene Self-Care Deficit
_____ ☐ Dressing/Grooming Self-Care Deficit
_____ ☐ Toileting Self-Care Deficit
_____ ☐ Altered Growth and Development
_____ ☐ Relocation Stress Syndrome
_____ ☐ Body Image Disturbance

PATTERN 7: PERCEIVING
_____ ☐ Self Esteem Disturbance
_____ ☐ Personal Identity Disturbance
_____ ☐ Sensory/Perceptual Alterations (Specify) (visual, auditory, kinesthetic, gustatory, tactile, olfactory)
_____ ☐ Hopelessness
_____ ☐ Powerlessness

PATTERN 8: KNOWING
_____ ☐ Knowledge Deficit (Specify)
_____ ☐ Altered Thought Processes

PATTERN 9: FEELING
_____ ☐ Pain
_____ ☐ Dysfunctional Grieving
_____ ☐ Anticipatory Grieving
_____ ☐ High Risk for Violence: Self-directed
_____ ☐ High Risk for Violence: Directed at others
_____ ☐ High Risk for Self-Mutilation
_____ ☐ Post-Trauma Response
_____ ☐ Rape-Trauma Syndrome
_____ ☐ Anxiety
_____ ☐ Fear

RN signature _____   Date _____

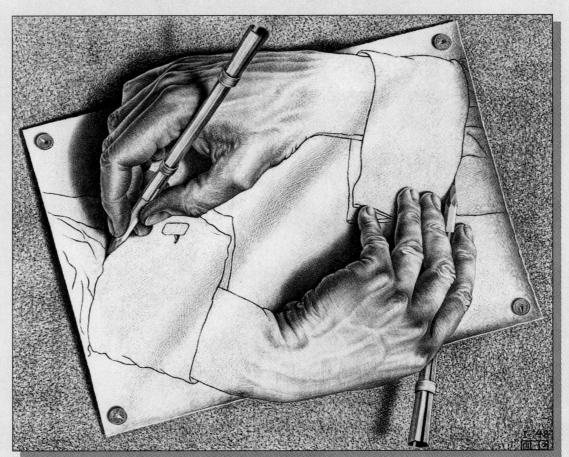

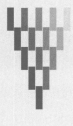

CHAPTER 10

Actualizing the Psychiatric Nursing Role: Professional Performance Standards

GAIL W. STUART

The professional motive is the desire and perpetual effort to do the thing as well as it can be done, which exists just as much in the Nurse, as in the Astronomer in search of a new star, or in the Artist completing a picture.

Florence Nightingale

LEARNING OBJECTIVES

After studying this chapter the student should be able to:

▼ Describe how accountability and autonomy relate to the psychiatric nurse's professional role responsibilities

▼ Analyze the conditions and behaviors of the psychiatric nurse related to quality of care activities

▼ Analyze the conditions and behaviors of the psychiatric nurse related to performance appraisal

▼ Analyze the conditions and behaviors of the psychiatric nurse related to education

▼ Analyze the conditions and behaviors of the psychiatric nurse related to collegiality

▼ Analyze the conditions and behaviors of the psychiatric nurse related to ethics

▼ Analyze the conditions and behaviors of the psychiatric nurse related to collaboration

▼ Analyze the conditions and behaviors of the psychiatric nurse related to research

▼ Analyze the conditions and behaviors of the psychiatric nurse related to resource utilization

TOPICAL OUTLINE

Accountability and Autonomy
Standard I—Quality of Care
  Systems Evaluation
  Consumer Evaluation
  Clinical Evaluation
Standard II—Performance Appraisal
  Differentiated Practice
  Clinical Supervision
Standard III—Education
  Certification
Standard IV—Collegiality
Standard V—Ethics
  Ethical Standards
  Power and Paternalism
  Ethical Dilemmas
  Ethical Decision Making
  Model for Ethical Decision Making
Standard VI—Collaboration
  Interdisciplinary Mental Health Teams
Standard VII—Research
Standard VIII—Resource Utilization

The standards of care from the American Nurses' Association (ANA) *Standards of Psychiatric–Mental Health Clinical Nursing Practice* as presented in Chapter 9 describe what the psychiatric nurse does; the standards of professional performance from the same document presented in this chapter describe the context in which the psychiatric nurse performs these activities.* Neither set of standards can be taken in isolation; rather, together they complete the picture of contemporary psychiatric nursing practice. They also clarify the many elements that influence enactment of the psychiatric nursing role.

ACCOUNTABILITY AND AUTONOMY

Psychiatric nursing is characterized by rules of competency and service. The standards of professional performance apply specifically to self-regulation and accountability for practice that must be shown by psychiatric nurses, both individually and as a group. They also address issues of professional autonomy and self-definition. As such, the standards of performance are critically important.

Accountability means to be answerable to someone for something. It focuses responsibility on the individual nurse for personal actions, or perhaps, lack of actions. The preconditions of accountability include ability, responsibility, and authority. Accountability also includes formal review processes and an attitude of integrity and vigilance.

Autonomy implies self-determination, independence, and shared power. It is the condition that allows for definition of and control over a work domain. For psychiatric nursing, attaining autonomy means being able to define the domain of nursing and being able to exercise control over psychiatric nursing practice. This idea of shaping destiny, rather than letting outside forces be in control, views power as a positive force that allows nurses to attain goals. It involves a conscious decision to identify objectives, plan strategy, assume responsibility, exercise authority, and be held accountable.

Autonomy has two major and interrelated components. The first is **control over nursing tasks,** which means:

1. Having the opportunity for independent thought and action
2. Having use of time, skills, and ability by being able to eliminate, refuse, and delegate nonnursing tasks
3. Having the authority and responsibility for implementing goals related to quality nursing care

4. Being able to initiate changes and innovations in practice

The second component of autonomy is **participation in decision making.** It requires the nurse's participation in the following:

1. Determining and implementing standards of quality nursing care
2. Making decisions affecting each nurse's job context, including salary, staffing, and professional growth
3. Setting institutional policies, procedures, and goals

This second component of participation in decision making is particularly problematic for nursing. Most nurses are employed in health-care organizations in which authority rests primarily with administrators, physicians, and board members. Furthermore, nurses often are expected to do tasks they are overqualified for, such as housekeeping, dietary, and clerical duties. This results in underutilization of their many important skills.

Nurses are thus caught in the crosswind. They staff clinical areas around the clock, make important decisions, and shoulder major responsibility for coordinating and managing patient care, but they often lack legitimate decision-making authority as to the allocation of resources. Because nurses are usually not compensated on a fee-for-service basis, they are often not viewed as a source of revenue by administrators and therefore lack a critical base for power. It is not surprising that if nurses do not have a role in organizational decision making, they will have only a limited ability to exercise control of their practice.

The 1991 Joint Commission on Accreditation of Healthcare Organizations (JCAHO) nursing standards help to address this problem. Specifically, they address collaborative and decision-making functions required of hospital-employed registered nurses and the chief nurse executive. They state that "The nurse executive and other nursing leaders participate with leaders from the governing body, management, medical staff, and clinical areas in the hospital's decision-making structure and processes."[15] Thus collaboration is promoted by requiring the leadership group to work together to foster continuous improvement in the hospital's patient care structures and processes.

This is an important change that helps to support nursing's accountability and autonomy, but full realization of nursing's potential will be obtained only through a negotiated process with other health professionals, consumers, and society at large. It requires increased access to resources, demonstration of expertise, and acknowledgment by other professionals, as shown in interdependent collaboration. Nurses are sometimes not fully accepted as professionals by other disciplines and

---

*From American Nurses' Association: A *statement on psychiatric–mental health clinical nursing practice and standards of psychiatric–mental health clinical nursing practice*, Washington, DC, 1994, The Association.

often are not allowed to function at their full potential. Yet psychiatric nursing is practiced largely in collaboration, coordination, and cooperation with a variety of other professionals working with and on behalf of the patient. Nurses will progress in this area as they are able to communicate with other professionals and as their clinical skills demand recognition and respect. As nurses view themselves in a positive way, they will increase their ability to assert themselves and function effectively. The nursing conditions and nursing behaviors related to each standard of professional performance are shown in Fig. 10-1. Each of these standards is now discussed.

Quality of Care

STANDARD I—QUALITY OF CARE

The psychiatric–mental health nurse systematically evaluates the quality of care and effectiveness of psychiatric–mental health nursing practice.

▼ *Rationale*

The dynamic nature of the mental health care environment and the growing body of psychiatric nursing knowledge and research provide both the impetus and the means for the psychiatric–mental health nurse to be competent in clinical practice, to continue to develop professionally, and to improve the quality of client care.

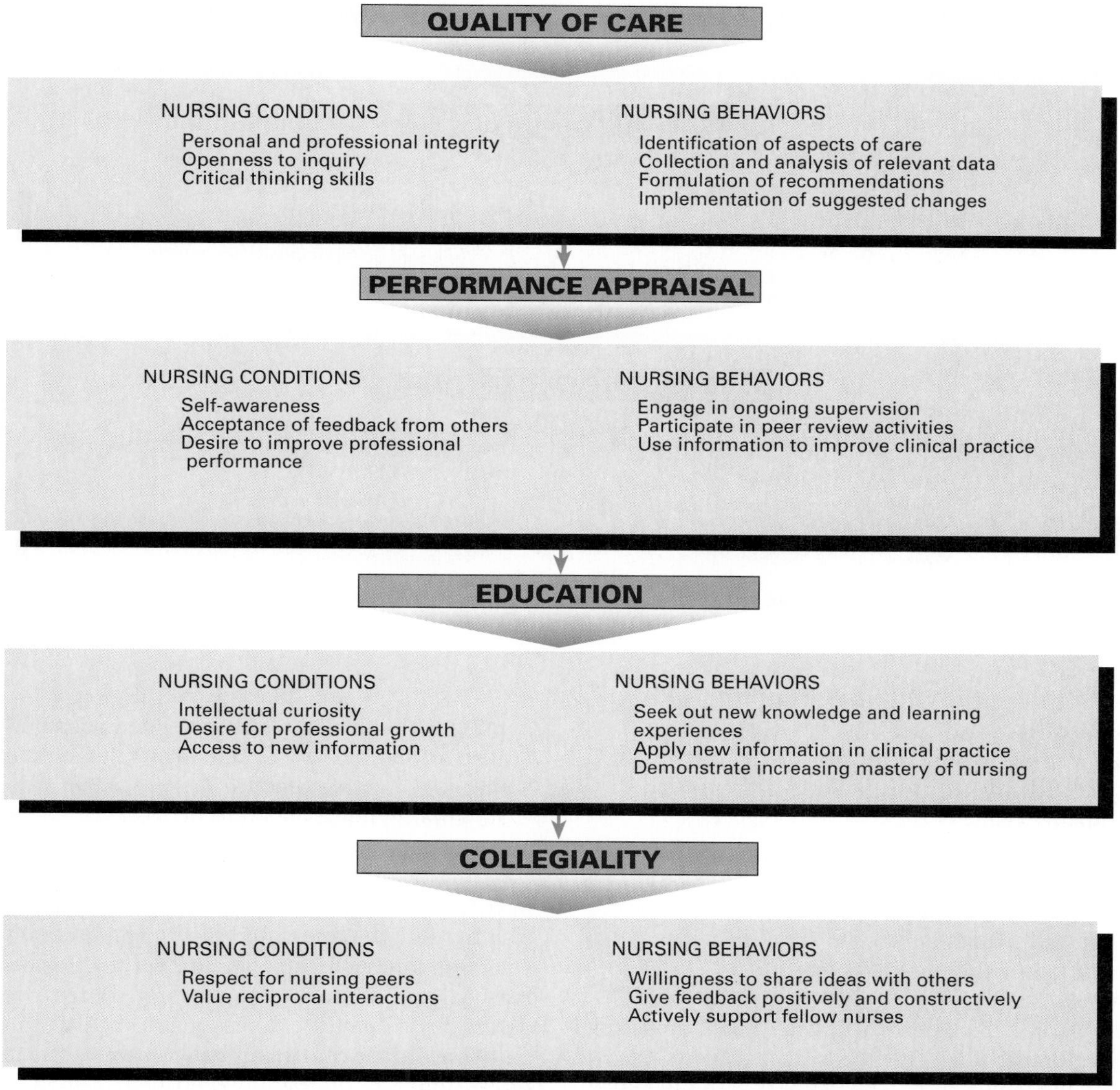

QUALITY OF CARE

NURSING CONDITIONS
- Personal and professional integrity
- Openness to inquiry
- Critical thinking skills

NURSING BEHAVIORS
- Identification of aspects of care
- Collection and analysis of relevant data
- Formulation of recommendations
- Implementation of suggested changes

PERFORMANCE APPRAISAL

NURSING CONDITIONS
- Self-awareness
- Acceptance of feedback from others
- Desire to improve professional performance

NURSING BEHAVIORS
- Engage in ongoing supervision
- Participate in peer review activities
- Use information to improve clinical practice

EDUCATION

NURSING CONDITIONS
- Intellectual curiosity
- Desire for professional growth
- Access to new information

NURSING BEHAVIORS
- Seek out new knowledge and learning experiences
- Apply new information in clinical practice
- Demonstrate increasing mastery of nursing

COLLEGIALITY

NURSING CONDITIONS
- Respect for nursing peers
- Value reciprocal interactions

NURSING BEHAVIORS
- Willingness to share ideas with others
- Give feedback positively and constructively
- Actively support fellow nurses

Fig. 10-1   Nursing conditions and behaviors related to the standards of professional performance.

Continued.

ETHICS

NURSING CONDITIONS	NURSING BEHAVIORS
Ability to engage in introspection	Guide practice by the Code for Nurses
Sensitivity to social and moral issues	Practice with legal and ethical responsibility
Commitment to the value clarification process	Act as patient and family advocate

COLLABORATION

NURSING CONDITIONS	NURSING BEHAVIORS
Positive self-concept	Assertively contribute one's professional expertise
Clear professional identity and accountability	Share planning and decision making with others
Ability to work with others in a cooperative manner	Make referrals when appropriate

RESEARCH

NURSING CONDITIONS	NURSING BEHAVIORS
Quest for new knowledge or answers to questions	Review reports of nursing research
Acute observational and analytical skills	Generate questions and identify clinical problems
Persistence and attention to detail	Implement research findings in practice

RESOURCE UTILIZATION

NURSING CONDITIONS	NURSING BEHAVIORS
Knowledge of the political and economic environment	Fact-based decision making
Ability to evaluate costs versus benefits of treatment	Cost-effective allocation of resources
Skill in negotiating and accessing resources	Patient advocacy on an individual and collective basis

Fig. 10-1 cont.

▼ *Nursing conditions*
Personal and professional integrity
Openness to inquiry
Critical thinking skills
▼ *Nursing behaviors*
Identification of aspects of care
Collection and analysis of relevant data
Formulation of recommendations
Implementation of suggested changes
▼ *Key elements*
The nurse should be open to critically analyzing the caregiving process
The patient and family should be partners with the nurse in the evaluation of care activities

Improving the quality of care provided goes beyond discussion and analysis to actually implementing actions that will improve practice

Psychiatric nurses need to actively participate in the formal organizational evaluation of overall patterns of care through a variety of quality improvement activities. In these activities the focus is not on the nurse clinician but on the patient and the overall program of care. The current growth and commitment to critically reviewing health care stems from several sources: consumer demand for quality but reasonable health care; third-party payors for controlled health-care costs; increased professional accountability; and regulatory and federal groups that monitor the quality of care. A comprehensive quality-of-care evaluation should include the following:

▼ Systems evaluation of treatment and allocation of resources
▼ Consumer evaluation of patient needs and satisfaction
▼ Clinical evaluation of treatment outcome and process

Systems Evaluation

Systems evaluation assesses the organization of the delivery system, including patient flow, paperwork, procedures for scheduling patients, staff-patient ratio, disciplinary mix, and use of resources. It supplements clinical evaluation and has three components:

▼ Systems analysis
▼ Economic analysis
▼ Operations research

Systems analysis attempts to simplify and improve the organization. Economic analysis emphasizes money spent and what, in turn, it produces. Operations research helps management allocate available resources most effectively. Together these analyses, by evaluating the actual organization of treatment, have the potential to improve the performance of the clinical operation.

Consumer Evaluation

Consumer evaluation has not received as much attention in the psychiatric literature as it has in other areas of health care. Assessing consumer satisfaction with nursing care is difficult because the health-care team works together and numerous variables can explain the findings. Nevertheless, additional studies are needed to both evaluate nursing services and document their cost effectiveness from the perspective of patients and families.

Clinical Evaluation

Clinical evaluation of ongoing programs takes place through various quality improvement activities that include both evaluation and corrective action. These programs are often called *quality monitoring programs*.

A quality monitoring program begins with selection of a specific issue, problem, or activity, which is called an *aspect of care*. Three basic types of aspects of care can be monitored:

▼ Clinical
▼ Professional
▼ Administrative

They can be further categorized as:

▼ High volume
▼ High risk
▼ Problem prone

Once the aspect of care to monitor has been determined, specific indicators of quality and acceptable thresholds need to be identified. In the quality monitoring forms shown in Fig. 10-2 one aspect of care is *clinical, high volume* (patient medication-taking behaviors), and the other is *administrative, high volume and problem prone* (nursing process documentation).

The next step involves data collection for each identified indicator. Often the method of collection is specific to the type of information desired. Most methods are either qualitative or quantitative. Qualitative data collection methods include interviews and surveys, which can be helpful in understanding patients' or families' perceptions and experiences of the care they received. In contrast, quantitative methods usually include counting the times something occurred, such as health teaching about a patient's illness or documentation of nursing care during the seclusion of a patient.

It is particularly important for the nurse to remember that all perspectives should be considered in determining the quality of care provided. This includes those of patients, families, staff, administration, and regulatory agencies.

Collected data are then analyzed for the presence or absence of the selected indicators. The degree to which these indicators are present or absent suggest opportunities for changes in practice. Nurses are professionally obligated to seek out these opportunities and identify and implement specific improvement strategies. Validation of excellence in practice occurs through quality monitoring and through the recognition of change opportunities.

The last step is the action that is taken to address the opportunities identified for improvement. This concept of corrective action, or actually making improvements, differentiates quality improvement from program evaluation and evaluation research. Sometimes administrative changes in policies or procedures are required. Often a staff education program directed toward the area of need can produce the recommended changes. Regardless, it is the responsibility of the nurse to see that the required changes are made, since evaluating and monitoring the quality of care are important aspects of the professional accountability of psychiatric nursing practice.

DIVISION OF PSYCHIATRIC NURSING
NURSING QUALITY COUNCIL
Monitoring and Evaluation Form

Unit: _____   Date: _____

Monitor: **PATIENT MEDICATION-TAKING BEHAVIORS**

__X__ clinical   _____ professional   _____ administrative

__X__ high volume   _____ high risk   _____ problem prone

Standard: The nurse evaluates patient responses to nursing interventions in order to review the database, nursing diagnoses and the NCP.

Expected
Outcome: When used to refine the nurse's approach with a patient, knowledge of that patient's behaviors improves the nurses ability to effect more productive health behaviors in the patient.

Special
Instruction: Select three patients on long-term medication regimens for their psychiatric dysfunction. While still in inpatient care, survey RN staff and the selected patients for the indicators enumerated below. Within 6 weeks after discharge, contact the patient's follow-up provider to obtain remaining information.

Threshold: 100%   **A** = always, **S** = sometimes, **SE** = seldom, **N** = never

INPATIENT INDICATORS	A	S	S E	N	N/A or COMMENTS
1. The patient shows up to take his or her medications at the prescribed time without prompting.					
2. The patient verbalizes agreement as to the need for the medications prescribed.					
3. The patient states willingness to take his or her medications as prescribed after discharge.					
4. The patient can identify any barriers that may interfere with him or her maintaining the prescribed medication regimen.					
5. If the patient has identified barriers in #4 above, s/he lists realistic strategies for dealing with them before a lapse in medication taking occurs.					

POST-DISCHARGE INDICATORS	YES	NO	CAN'T CONFIRM	COMMENTS
1. Patient is taking his or her medications as prescribed (as confirmed by the patient's follow-up provider or responsible and knowledgeable other).				

Fig. 10-2   A, Quality monitoring form for patient medication-taking behaviors (clinical and high volume).

Courtesy Division of Psychiatric Nursing, Medical University of South Carolina.

DIVISION OF PSYCHIATRIC NURSING
NURSING QUALITY COMMITTEE
Monitoring and Evaluation Form

Unit: _____ Date: _____

Monitor: **NURSING PROCESS DOCUMENTATION**

_____ clinical _____ professional __X__ administrative

__X__ high volume _____ high risk __X__ problem prone

Standard: The nurse collects and analyzes patient health data. The nurse determines appropriate diagnoses, identifies expected outcomes and develops a plan of care to meet those outcomes. The nurse implements those interventions and evaluates the patient's progress toward stated outcomes.

Expected
Outcome: This process is accurately and thoroughly documented in the patient's record.

Special
Instruction: Review five hospital records of patients with a significant risk factor (e.g., suicidality, violence, falls, withdrawal, elopement or seizure) for the indicators enumerated below.

Threshold: 100%

INDICATORS	MET	NOT MET	N/A or COMMENTS
1. The significant risk factor is identified upon admission on the nursing assessment forms.			
2. The appropriate nursing diagnosis for the risk factor is listed on the patient's nursing care plan (NCP).			
3. The necessary interventions (standards of care) for that nursing diagnosis are listed on the patient's NCP.			
4. The daily nursing documentation (as appropriate) shows those interventions were implemented as prescribed on the patient's NCP.			
5. The nursing weekly summary documents the patient's progress (or regress) relative to that nursing diagnosis.			
6. The patient's NCP was changed as needed to reflect any progression or regression for that nursing diagnosis that was mentioned in the nursing weekly summary note.			

Fig. 10-2, cont'd. **B,** Quality monitoring form for nursing process documentation (administrative, high volume, and problem prone).
Courtesy Division of Psychiatric Nursing, Medical University of South Carolina.

Performance Appraisal

STANDARD II—PERFORMANCE APPRAISAL

The psychiatric–mental health nurse evaluates own psychiatric–mental health nursing practice in relation to professional practice standards and relevant statutes and regulations.

▼ *Rationale*
The psychiatric–mental health nurse is accountable to the public for providing competent clinical care and has an inherent responsibility as a professional to evaluate the role and performance of psychiatric–mental health nursing practice according to standards established by the profession and regulatory bodies.

▼ *Nursing conditions*
Self-awareness
Acceptance of feedback from others
Desire to improve professional performance
▼ *Nursing behaviors*
Engage in ongoing supervision
Participate in peer review activities
Use information to improve clinical practice
▼ *Key elements*
Supervision should be viewed as an essential and on-
going aspect of one's professional life
The nurse should strive to grow and develop in one's
professional knowledge, skills, and expertise

Performance appraisal for the psychiatric nurse is generally provided in two forms: (1) administrative and (2) clinical. Administrative performance appraisal involves the review, management, and regulation of competent psychiatric nursing practice. It involves a supervisory relationship in which a nurse's work performance is compared with role expectations in a formal way, such as in a nurse's annual performance evaluation. Administrative performance evaluations should identify areas of competency and areas in need of improvement. There should also be a method for recognizing quality performance (see Critical Thinking about Contemporary Issues).

Many nursing departments have adopted clinical advancement programs or other formal mechanisms to recognize nursing excellence. Clinical advancement programs have been established to formally validate nurses for increasing mastery in practice. They allow the nurse to be promoted and economically rewarded for providing direct patient care.[9] Such programs identify levels of professional development in nursing based on increased critical thinking and advanced application of nursing skills (Fig. 10-3). These characteristics result in greater quality of care provided by psychiatric nurses throughout their professional career.

Differentiated Practice

Although controversial, the American Organization of Nurse Executives and the American Hospital Association have endorsed the concept of differentiation of nursing practice according to demonstrated competence, experience, and education.[6] A study of Chief Nurse Executives found they predicted that there would be an increase in the differentiation of nursing practice by education in the years to come.[23]

Future expectations of psychiatric nursing roles within the mental health care delivery system must take into account the diverse education and experiences represented by psychiatric nurses.[11] Thus role descriptions and functional assignments need to better differentiate among psychiatric nurses based on education, experience, and competency.[12] In addition, responsibilities of

CRITICAL THINKING ABOUT CONTEMPORARY ISSUES

What Kind of Recognition Do Staff Nurses Value?

It is well known that recognition is central to nurses' morale. However, it is less clear what type of recognition is valued and why it is given. A recent survey asked 239 staff nurses about this issue.[13] They found that verbal feedback was identified as the most meaningful type of recognition. This was followed by letters of praise for performance or achievement, organizational awards, honors or public announcements of outstanding performance, promotion or a prestigious assignment with increased responsibility, being personally thanked and praised during an evaluation, and finally monetary bonuses, salary increases, or gifts.

The main reasons given for receiving recognition included outstanding performance in patient care and positive attitude, followed by demonstrated expertise, assuming extra work, involvement in professional activities, receiving certification or a degree, and years of service in an organization. Finally, recognition came most often from the head nurse, followed by the nurse administrator, patients and families, coworkers, physicians, and hospital administrators. Studies such as this help to clarify meaningful aspects of administrative performance appraisals and ways to best commend nurses for a job well done. ▼

psychiatric nurses should clearly reflect their unique nursing knowledge base and biopsychosocial competencies that directly contribute to quality patient care.

One of your nursing colleagues tells you that she thinks nurses' pay should be based on their experience and not their education. After all, she argues, if two nurses do the same job, what does it matter if they have different educational degrees. How would you respond?

Clinical Supervision

Clinical performance appraisal is guidance provided through a mentoring relationship with a more experienced, skilled, and educated nurse. The professional psychiatric nurse is aware of the need for ongoing mentorship to achieve increasing levels of mastery of psychiatric nursing practice. Clinical supervision not only reviews one's clinical care but also functions as a sup-

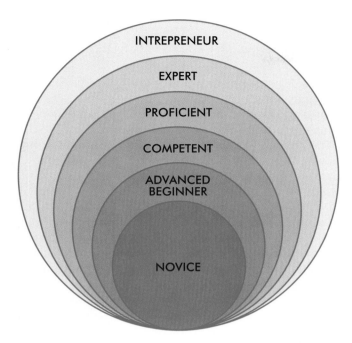

Fig. 10-3 Levels of differentiated nursing practice.

port system for the nurse providing care, since nurses must care about themselves before being able to care for others.

In many ways the process of supervision parallels the nurse-patient relationship. Both involve a learning process that takes place in the context of a deep and meaningful relationship that facilitates positive change. Self-exploration is a critical element of both. The supervisor should provide the same responsive and action dimensions present in the nurse-patient relationship to help the supervised nurse become a person who can live effectively with self and others.

There are four common forms of supervision:
1. The dyadic, or one-on-one, relationship, in which the supervisor meets the supervisee in a face-to-face encounter
2. The triadic relationship, in which a supervisor and two nurses of similar experience and training meet for supervision
3. Group supervision, in which several supervised nurses meet for a shared session with the supervisory nurse
4. Peer review, in which nurses meet together without a supervisor to evaluate their clinical practice

All four forms have a similar purpose—exploring the problem areas and maximizing the strengths of the supervisees.

Process of Supervision. The process of supervision requires the nurse to record the interactions with the patient. Both written processed recordings and audio recordings have been used for this purpose, but neither yields as accurate and complete information as that provided by videotape recordings. Videotaped sessions minimize distortion of data. The supervised nurse then analyzes the data, extracts themes, and identifies problems relevant to nursing care. The nurse reviews the literature, draws inferences, evaluates effectiveness, and formulates plans for the next session. In the supervision conference the nurse shares this analysis and receives feedback from the supervisor or peers, if it is a group or peer conference.

Supervision can be viewed as a didactic process, in which the theory and concepts related to nursing practice are reviewed, or it can be a quasitherapeutic process that explores countertransference problems, attitudes, values, and the nurse's emotional needs and personal biases. The latter is the more widely accepted view.

Three methods of supervision have been described:
1. **Patient centered,** in which the clinician brings technical problems with the patient to the supervisor and is given advice.
2. **Clinician centered,** in which the focus is on the clinician's blind spots and countertransference reactions. This helps clinicians see their influence on the therapeutic process. The danger with this method is that in its extreme, the patient is lost from sight and the supervision evolves into personal therapy for the supervisee.
3. **Process centered,** in which the emphasis is on what is happening between the clinician, patient, and supervisor. The supervisor makes use of the analogy between the nurse-patient relationship and the nurse-supervisor relationship to help the supervisee use personal experience of emotional difficulties in receiving help from the supervisor to facilitate understanding of the patient's situation.

Ekstein and Wallerstein[7] have developed a process-centered model of supervision that is neither personal therapy nor simply a didactic process of conveying information on theory and technique. In their model the supervisor is an active participant in an affectively charged learning process, the focus of which is learning and personal growth rather than psychotherapy for the supervisee. The authors describe how problems between the clinician and the supervisor can shed light on problems that exist between the clinician and patient. The very problems experienced in the one relationship affect and are reflected in the other relationship.

The goal of supervision, however, is not to eliminate these problems; it is to use them to achieve greater understanding of the ongoing dynamic processes at work in therapy. The problems become the vehicles through which therapeutic progress may be made. Thus the most effective supervision depends on active insight into the many forces in the parallel processes of therapy and supervision. Finally, it is important to remember that tension in the supervisory relationship is inevitable, but when understood and handled skillfully, it can be very helpful to the clinician's growth.

Purpose and Goals. Despite its intensity, supervision is not therapy. The essential difference between the two is a difference of purpose. The aim of supervision is to teach psychotherapeutic skills, whereas the goal of therapy is to alter a person's characteristic patterns of coping to function more effectively in all areas of life. In contrast, the supervisee's problems in the supervisory and therapeutic relationships are dealt with only to the extent that they affect the nurse's ability to learn from the supervisor and be effective with patients. Therefore the problems are limited in scope and depth; they do not include all other aspects of the supervisee's life situation. With the resolution of the particular problem, the focus of supervision returns to the teaching of psychotherapeutic skills and their implementation by the nurse. The therapeutic implications for the supervisee are therefore related to the primary goal of supervision—the teaching of psychotherapeutic skills.

Supervision or consultation is necessary for the practicing psychiatric nurse. Although it is crucial for novices, it is equally as important for experienced practitioners.[21] Personal limitations create a need for assistance in remaining objective throughout the therapeutic process and the "normal" stresses it presents. Obviously supervision is only as helpful as the skill of the supervisor, the openness of the supervised nurse, and the motivation of both to learn and grow.

Education

STANDARD III—EDUCATION

The psychiatric–mental health nurse acquires and maintains current knowledge in nursing practice.

▼ *Rationale*
The rapid expansion of knowledge pertaining to basic and behavioral sciences, technology, information systems, and research requires a commitment to learning throughout the psychiatric–mental health nurse's professional career. Formal education, continuing education, certification, and experiential learning are some of the means the psychiatric–mental health nurse uses to enhance nursing expertise and advance the profession.

▼ *Nursing conditions*
Intellectual curiosity
Desire for professional growth
Access to new information

▼ *Nursing behaviors*
Seek out new knowledge and learning experiences
Apply new information in clinical practice

Demonstrate increasing mastery of nursing
▼ *Key elements*
Professional learning should be regarded as a lifelong process
The nurse should pursue a variety of educational opportunities
New knowledge should be translated into professional nursing practice

The nature of psychiatry, the mental health delivery system, and the boundaries of nursing are changing rapidly. Two of the most recent developments include the revised American Nurses' Association (ANA) *Statement and Standards of Psychiatric–Mental Health Clinical Nursing Practice*, and the ANA's newly released *Psychopharmacology Guidelines for Psychiatric–Mental Health Nurses*. In addition, the scientific basis for practice is expanding at a rapid pace, and psychiatric nurses need to keep up with this knowledge explosion.

Psychiatric nurses are expected to engage in a continual learning process to maintain currency with the latest information in the field. They may do this in the following ways:
  ▼ Formal educational programs
  ▼ Continuing education programs
  ▼ Lectures, conferences, and workshops
  ▼ Credentialing
  ▼ Certification
Reading journals and textbooks and collaborating with colleagues are other important ways to remain current with expanding areas of knowledge. Fig. 10-4 lists journals that relate to psychiatric nursing practice and provide a good source of new knowledge and information.

Do you believe that continuing education should be mandated for all nurses by state law? Defend your position and describe its implications for the role of professional performance standards in nursing.

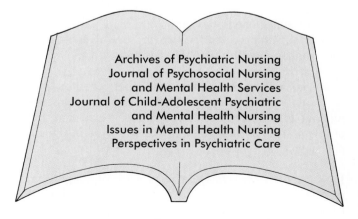

Archives of Psychiatric Nursing
Journal of Psychosocial Nursing
and Mental Health Services
Journal of Child-Adolescent Psychiatric
and Mental Health Nursing
Issues in Mental Health Nursing
Perspectives in Psychiatric Care

Fig. 10-4 Psychiatric nursing journals.

Certification

The certification process is a formal review of the clinical practice of nurses that has evolved within the American Nurses' Association. The objectives of certification are to:

1. Assure the public of quality care
2. Provide credentials to expedite employment and third-party reimbursement for services rendered
3. Expand opportunities for vertical and horizontal mobility and career advancement
4. Attain greater prestige and peer recognition for achieving clinical expertise
5. Improve clinical practice

Psychiatric nursing has two levels of certification: the **generalist,** who may be a staff nurse, and the **specialist,** who specializes in either adult or child and adolescent psychiatric nursing. As of 1993 there were 18,231 certified nurse generalists, 5306 certified nurse specialists in adult psychiatric mental health nursing, and 619 certified nurse specialists in child and adolescent psychiatric mental health nursing.

To become a **certified generalist** the psychiatric nurse must demonstrate expertise in practice, knowledge of theories concerning personality development and behavior patterns in treating mental illness, and the relationship of such treatments to nursing care. Special requirements include:

1. Practice as a psychiatric and mental health nurse for a minimum of 1600 hours within 2 of the last 4 years
2. Current work in psychiatric and mental health nursing for a minimum of 8 hours per week

To become a **certified specialist** the nurse must show a high degree of proficiency in interpersonal skills, in the use of the nursing process, and in psychological and milieu therapies. Following are five requirements for certification as a specialist in psychiatric and mental health nursing:

1. Current involvement in psychiatric and mental health nursing practice at least 4 hours per week
2. A master's or higher degree in nursing, with a specialization in psychiatric and mental health nursing OR a nurse may apply for individual consideration if he or she has a master's or higher degree in nursing or a mental health field with a minimum of 24 graduate academic credits in psychiatric and mental health theory and supervised training in two psychotherapeutic treatment modalities
3. Experience in at least two different treatment modalities
4. Have at least 800 hours of direct patient/client contact in advanced clinical practice of psychiatric and mental health nursing; up to 400 of these hours may be earned through the clinical practicum in a master's program of study
5. Document 100 hours of individual or group clinical consultation/supervision and submit endorsement(s) from the consultant/supervisor(s)

On successful completion of the certification examination and written documentation, the nurse is identified as certified (C.) if a generalist or as a certified specialist (C.S.) in psychiatric mental health nursing. Although any specialist nurse may be certified, it is expected that nurses who are self-employed in the practice of psychotherapy will obtain certification to assure the public of their ability to perform as competent nurse psychotherapists.

Collegiality

STANDARD IV—COLLEGIALITY

The psychiatric–mental health nurse contributes to the professional development of peers, colleagues, and others.

▼ *Rationale*

The psychiatric–mental health nurse is responsible for sharing knowledge, research, and clinical information with colleagues through formal and informal teaching methods to enhance professional growth.

▼ *Nursing conditions*

Respect for nursing peers

Value reciprocal interactions

▼ *Nursing behaviors*

Willingness to share ideas with others

Give feedback positively and constructively

Actively support fellow nurses

▼ *Key elements*

The nurse should regard other nurses as colleagues and trusted partners in care-giving

Mentorship within nursing is important both to nurses as individuals and to the nursing profession as a whole

Collegiality is an essential aspect of professional practice. It requires that nurses view their nurse peers as collaborators in the caregiving process who are valued and respected for their unique contributions, regardless of educational, experiential, or specialty background. It suggests that nurses must view themselves as members of an organized professional group or unit and that nurses trust, remain loyal, and demonstrate commitment to other nurses.

Many have observed that nursing, as a profession, has sometimes struggled with this concept. For example, complaints about "ivory-tower" nurse educators, "nonsupportive" nurse administrators, "nonintellectual" nurse clinicians, and "irrelevant" nurse researchers have been voiced by nurses about each other in the past. So, too, psychiatric nurses in various institutions or organizations have had difficulty joining forces and working together on a common psychiatric nursing agenda. However, this intradisciplinary interaction is not consistent with professional performance standards. It has also prevented the profession from acting as a united group in pursuing health-care initiatives at local, regional, and national levels.

Rather, nurses need to work together as colleagues to blend their various skills and abilities in creating a better health-care system and enhancing the quality and quantity of psychiatric nursing services provided to patients, families, and communities. One positive move toward such collegiality was the establishment of the Coalition of Psychiatric Nursing Organizations (COPNO) in 1988. This coalition brings together four major nursing organizations:

1. American Nurses' Association
2. American Psychiatric Nursing Association
3. Association of Child and Adolescent Psychiatric Nurses
4. Society for Education and Research in Psychiatric–Mental Health Nursing

With the formation of COPNO, psychiatric nurses across the country have begun working together in partnership to influence health-care reform and the mental health needs of the population.

What do you know about the four psychiatric nursing organizations? Find out about the purpose, membership, and activities of each one. Then consider joining one or more and become involved in their efforts at a local, regional, or national level.

Ethics

STANDARD V—ETHICS

The psychiatric–mental health nurse's decisions and actions on behalf of clients are determined in an ethical manner.

▼ *Rationale*

The public's trust and its right to humane psychiatric–mental health care are upheld by professional nursing practice. The foundation of psychiatric–mental health nursing practice is the development of a therapeutic relationship with the client. The psychiatric–mental health nurse engages in therapeutic interactions and relationships that promote and support the healing process. Boundaries need to be established to safeguard the client's well-being and to prevent the development of intimate or sexual relationships.

▼ **Nursing conditions**
Ability to engage in introspection
Sensitivity to social and moral issues
Commitment to the value clarification process
▼ **Nursing behaviors**
Guide practice by the Code for Nurses
Practice with legal and ethical responsibility
Act as patient and family advocate
▼ **Key elements**
Nurses should be sensitive to the social, moral, and ethical environment in which they practice
Patient and family advocacy is a core aspect of nursing practice
Ethical conduct is foundational to the nurse-patient relationship
Ethical considerations combine with legal and therapeutic issues to affect all aspects of psychiatric nursing practice. The legal context of psychiatric nursing care is discussed in Chapter 8. Boundary violations related to the nurse-patient relationship are described in Chapter 2.

Ethical Standards

An **ethic** is a standard of behavior or a belief valued by an individual or group. It describes what ought to be, rather than what is—a goal to which an individual aspires. These standards are learned through socialization, growth, and experience. As such, they are not static but evolve to reflect social change.

Groups, such as professions, can also hold a code of ethics. Such a code guides the profession in serving and protecting consumers. It also provides a framework for decision making for members of the profession. Two major purposes for a code of ethics are "structuring" and "sensitizing."[19] Structuring is preventive and aims to restrain impulsive and unethical behavior. The second purpose, sensitizing, is educative, with the goal of raising members' ethical consciousness.

The American Nurses' Association[1] published a code of ethics for nurses (Box 10-1). It emphasizes the nurses' accountability for the quality of care and their duty to act as patient advocates in ensuring the quality of care given by others.

Psychiatric nurses should follow these professional standards as they deliver health care. If nurses know their values and implement them within the framework of the code, they can increase both the quality of the care they give and the satisfaction they receive from practice.

Power and Paternalism

A discussion of ethics and psychiatric nursing must also consider the crucial element of power. In the psychiat-

---

Box 10-1

AMERICAN NURSES' ASSOCIATION CODE FOR NURSES

1. The nurse provides services with respect for human dignity and the uniqueness of the client unrestricted by considerations of social or economic status, personal attributes, or the nature of health problems.
2. The nurse safeguards the client's right to privacy by judiciously protecting information of a confidential nature.
3. The nurse acts to safeguard the client and the public when health care and safety are affected by the incompetent, unethical, or illegal practice of any person.
4. The nurse assumes responsibility and accountability for individual nursing judgments and actions.
5. The nurse maintains competence in nursing.

6. The nurse exercises informed judgment and uses individual competence and qualification as criteria in seeking consultation, accepting responsibilities, and delegating nursing activities to others.
7. The nurse participates in activities that contribute to the ongoing development of the profession's body of knowledge.
8. The nurse participates in the profession's efforts to implement and improve standards of nursing.
9. The nurse participates in the profession's efforts to establish and maintain conditions of employment conducive to high-quality nursing care.
10. The nurse participates in the profession's effort to protect the public from misinformation and misrepresentation and to maintain the integrity of nursing.
11. The nurse collaborates with members of the health professions and other citizens in promoting community and national efforts to meet public health needs.

From American Nurses' Association: *Code for nurses with interpretive statements*, Kansas City, Mo, 1985, The Association.

---

ric setting the nurse can function in many roles, from a custodial keeper of the keys to a skilled therapist. Each of these roles includes a certain amount of power, since all nurses have the ability to influence the patient's treatment and serve as the major source of information regarding a patient's behavior. This is particularly true in inpatient settings, in which a nurse and patient spend more time together and the nursing staff is the only group to work a 24-hour day. Nurses also participate in team meetings, individual and group psychotherapy, and behavior modification programs. Finally, nurses can greatly influence decisions about patient medications, such as type, dosage, and frequency.

The literature describes the ethical dilemmas that arise from health-care professionals' "paternalistic" attitude toward their patients. Paternalism can be defined as deciding what is best for another person without consideration of the person's thoughts or feelings. It occurs when something is done "for the patient's own good" even though the patient would likely disagree with the action. This attitude reduces adult patients to the status of children and interferes with their freedom of action.

To avoid this potential danger, nurses should realize that ethical obligations span a wide range of individuals, including the patient, the patient's family or support system, themselves, their own family, other health-care professionals, the health-care institution or organization in which they work, and the larger social community. Furthermore, their ethical obligations arise within a context of laws and government regulations that may, at times, create dilemmas. By remaining aware of these laws, nurses can examine these problems from both clinical and ethical perspectives.

Ethical Dilemmas

An ethical dilemma exists when moral claims conflict with one another. It can be defined as:

1. A difficult problem that seems to have no satisfactory solution
2. A choice between equally unsatisfactory alternatives

Ethical dilemmas pose such questions as "What should I do?" and "What is the right thing to do?" They can occur both at the nurse-patient-family level of daily nursing care and at the policy-making level of institutions and communities. Although ethical dilemmas arise in all areas of nursing practice, some are unique to psychiatric and mental health nursing.[8] Many of these dilemmas fall under the umbrella issue of behavior control.

At first glance, behavior control may seem a simple issue—behavior is a personal choice, and any behavior that does not impose on the rights of others is acceptable. Unfortunately, this does not help to address complex situations. For example, a severely depressed person may choose suicide as an alternative to an intolerable existence. This is, on one level, an individual choice not directly harming others, yet suicide is strongly forbidden in American society. In many states it is a crime that can be prosecuted. As another example, in some states it is illegal for consenting adults of the same sex to have sexual relations, although it is not illegal for a man to rape his wife. These examples raise difficult questions: When is it appropriate for society to regulate personal behavior? Who will make this decision? Is its goal personal adjustment, personal growth, or adaptation to social norms? And finally, how do we measure the costs and benefits of attempting to control personal freedom in a free society?

One of the most fundamental problems is that psychiatry lacks definitions for mental health, normalcy, mental illness, and insanity. These terms have been debated for centuries, yet there are no universally accepted definitions. This demonstrates the blurry line between science and ethics in the field of psychiatry.[4] Theoretically, science and ethics are separate entities. Science is descriptive, deals with "what is," and rests on validation; ethics is predictive, deals with "what ought to be," and relies on judgment. However, psychiatry is neither purely scientific nor value free.

Despite these ambiguities, mental health professionals must identify their professional commitment. Are they committed to the happiness of the individual or the smooth functioning of society? Ideally, these values should not conflict, but in reality they sometimes do. The patient's rights to treatment, to refuse treatment, and to informed consent highlight this conflict-of-interest question. Nurses must consider if they are forcing patients to be socially or politically acceptable at the expense of patients' personal happiness. Nurses may not be working for either the patient's best interests or their own; they may be acting as agents of society and not be aware of it.

All nurses participate in some therapeutic psychiatric regimens whose scientific and ethical bases are ambiguous. The American health-care system continues to apply a medical model of wellness and illness to human behavior. Wellness is socially acceptable behavior, and illness is socially unacceptable. It becomes critically important for each nurse to analyze such ethical dilemmas as freedom of choice versus coercion, helping versus imposing values, and focusing on cure versus prevention. The nurse must also become active in defining adequate treatment and deciding resource allocations.

Ethical Decision Making

Ethical decision making involves trying to determine right from wrong in situations without clear guidelines. There are three dimensions to ethical decision making, each of which influences analysis of the dilemma and related decisions:

1. The existence and awareness of a code of value judgments or ethics
2. The awareness of personal moral beliefs and values
3. A complex social and legal context

Nurses should relate the code of nursing ethics to

their own personal value system and identify areas of similarity and difference. This will allow nurses to base ethical decisions on behavior that involves responsibility, accountability, risk, and commitment. Responsibility requires the capacity for rational, moral decision making. Accountability signifies action. Risk involves taking the chance of peril, jeopardy, or loss, and commitment implies loyalty, trust, and a pledge of self. In addition, the nurse's ethical choice must consider the circumstances, social customs, and any legal ramifications.

Model for Ethical Decision Making

A decision-making model can help identify factors and principles that affect a decision. Curtin[5] proposed a model for critical ethical analysis (Fig. 10-5) that describes steps or factors that the nurse should consider in resolving an ethical dilemma. The first step is **gathering background information** to obtain a clear picture of the problem. This includes finding available information to clarify the underlying issues. The next factor is **identifying the ethical components** or the nature of the dilemma, such as freedom versus coercion or treating versus accepting the right to refuse treatment. The next step is the **clarification of the rights and responsibili-**

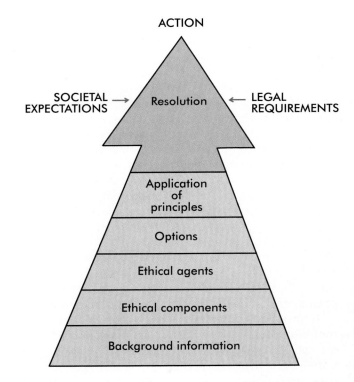

Fig. 10-5 Model for ethical decision making. Societal expectations and legal requirements may sway the resolution of the conflict one way or another. However, the notions of what is legal (or expected) with what is good, right, or proper—they may or may not coincide.

From Curtin L: *Nurs Forum* 17:12, 1978.

ties of all ethical agents, or those involved in the decision making. This can include the patient, the nurse, and possibly many others, including the patient's family, physician, health-care institution, clergy, social worker, and perhaps even the courts. Those involved may not agree on how to handle the situation, but their rights and duties can be clarified. All possible options must then be explored in light of everyone's responsibilities, as well as the purpose and potential result of each option. This step eliminates those alternatives that violate rights or seem harmful. The nurse then engages in the application of principles, which stem from the nurse's philosophy of life and nursing, scientific knowledge, and ethical theory. Ethical theories suggest ways to structure ethical dilemmas and judge potential solutions. Here are four possible approaches:

1. **Utilitarianism** focuses on the consequences of actions. It seeks the greatest amount of happiness or the least amount of harm for the greatest number: "the greatest good for the greatest number."
2. **Egoism** is a position in which the individual seeks the solution that is best personally. The self is most important, and others are secondary.
3. **Formalism** considers the nature of the act itself and the principles involved. It involves the universal application of a basic rule, such as "do unto others as you would have them do unto you."
4. **Fairness** is based on the concept of justice, and benefit to the least advantaged in society becomes the norm for decision making.

The final step is resolution into action. Within the context of social expectations and legal requirements, the nurse decides on the goals and methods of implementation. Table 10-1 summarizes these steps and suggests questions nurses can ask themselves in making complex ethical choices in psychiatric nursing practice.

 Think of an ethical problem you have encountered in caring for a psychiatric patient and family. Use the model for ethical decision making to decide on the best course of action.

Table 10-1   Steps and Questions in Ethical Decision Making

Steps	Relevant questions
Gathering background information	Does an ethical dilemma exist? What information is known? What information is needed? What is the context of the dilemma?
Identifying ethical components	What is the underlying issue? Who is affected by this dilemma?
Clarification of agents	What are the rights of each involved party? What are the obligations of each involved party? Who should be involved in the decision making? For whom is the decision being made? What degree of consent is needed by the patient?
Exploration of options	What alternatives exist? What is the purpose or intent of each alternative? What are the potential consequences of each alternative?
Application of principles	What criteria should be used? What ethical theories are subscribed to? What scientific facts are relevant? What is the nurse's philosophy of life and nursing?
Resolution into action	What are the social and legal constraints and ramifications? What is the goal of the nurse's decision? How can the resulting ethical choice be implemented? How can the resulting ethical choice be evaluated?

Collaboration

STANDARD VI—COLLABORATION

The psychiatric–mental health nurse collaborates with the client, significant others, and health-care providers in providing care.

▼ *Rationale*

Psychiatric–mental health nursing practice requires a coordinated, ongoing interaction between consumers

and providers to deliver comprehensive services to the client and the community. Through the collaborative process, different abilities of health-care providers are used to solve problems, communicate, plan, implement, and evaluate mental health services.

▼ *Nursing conditions*

Positive self-concept

Clear sense of professional identity and accountability

Ability to work with others in a cooperative manner

▼ *Nursing behaviors*
Assertively contribute one's professional expertise
Share planning and decision making with others
Make referrals when appropriate
▼ *Key elements*
Respect for others grows out of respect for self
The nurse should be able to clearly articulate one's professional abilities and areas of expertise to others
Collaboration involves the ability to negotiate and formulate new solutions with others

Collaboration is the shared planning, decision making, problem solving, goal setting, and assumption of responsibilities by individuals who work together cooperatively and with open communication. Three key ingredients are needed for collaboration:

1. Active and assertive contributions from each person
2. Receptivity and respect for each person's contribution
3. Negotiations that build on the contributions of each person to form a new way of conceptualizing the problem

It is important for psychiatric nurses to realize that they have many potential collaborators, including patients and families, interdisciplinary colleagues, and nursing peers (Fig. 10-6). Each of these groups allows the psychiatric nurse an opportunity to problem solve in new ways and thus better plan and implement nursing care.

Interdisciplinary Mental Health Teams

An essential part of contemporary practice is to work with other health-care providers. Nurses may be members of three different types of teams: **unidisciplinary,**

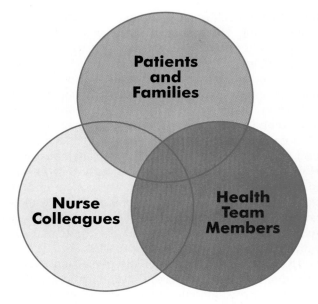

Fig. 10-6 Collaborative relationships for psychiatric nurses.

having all team members of the same discipline; **multidisciplinary,** having members of different disciplines who each provide specific services to the patient; and **interdisciplinary,** having members of different disciplines involved in a formal arrangement to provide patient services while maximizing educational interchange. Most organized mental health settings employ an interdisciplinary team approach, which requires highly coordinated and frequently interdependent planning based on the separate and distinct roles of each team member (Table 10-2).

However, interdisciplinary collaboration does not al-

Table 10-2   Mental Health Personnel, Training, and Roles

Personnel	Training	Role
Psychiatric nurse	Registered nurse (RN) with specialized training in the care and treatment of psychiatric patients. May have an AD, BS, MS, or PhD degree	Accountable for the biopsychosocial nursing care of patients and their milieu
Psychiatrist	Medical doctor with internship and residency training in psychiatry	Accountable for the medical diagnosis and treatment of patients
Social worker	BS, MSW, or PhD degree with specialized training in mental health settings	Accountable for family casework and community placement of patients
Psychologist	PhD or PsyD degree with research and clinical training in mental health	Accountable for psychological assessments and testing
Activity therapist	May have a BS degree with training in mental health settings	Accountable for recreational, occupational, and activity programs
Case worker	Varying degrees of training and usually works under supervision	Accountable for assisting patients to be maintained in the community and receive needed services
Substance abuse counselor	Varying degrees of training in alcohol and substance use disorders	Accountable for evaluating and managing patients with substance use problems

ways proceed smoothly. There are many barriers to interdisciplinary collaboration including inappropriate education and training of mental health team members, traditional organizational structures, goal and role conflict, competitive and accommodating interpersonal interactions, power and status inequities, and personal qualities of individuals that do not promote shared problem solving. If roles, functions, and channels of communication among the various team members are not clarified and agreed on, confusion, resentment, crossing of boundaries, and inappropriate use of psychiatric team members are likely to result. In addition to discrete and agreed on role descriptions, certain personal qualities and activities are necessary for collaborative practice (Table 10-3).

Finally, psychiatric nurses must assess if they as a group are ready to engage in collaborative practice. Questions that should be considered include the following:

1. Can psychiatric nurses define, describe, and appropriately defend psychiatric nursing roles and functions?
2. Is the nursing leadership ready for collegial practice?
3. Are psychiatric nursing roles and functions appropriate for nurses' education, experience, and expertise?
4. Is nurse staffing appropriate in numbers, patterns, and ratios?
5. Are inservices, education, credentialing, and certification valued and rewarded?

6. Are there necessary structural and human support systems?
7. Are the other disciplines prepared for and supportive of collaboration?
8. Is the organizational climate conducive to collaboration?

With positive answers to these questions, psychiatric nurses should be able to move forward in implementing collaborative practice. Steps that can be taken to facilitate the formation of interdisciplinary teams are listed in Box 10-2.

> Most people think that there are more collaborative interdisciplinary relationships in psychiatry than in other specialty areas because of the nature of the work. Others believe, however, that there is more interdisciplinary conflict in psychiatry because roles overlap and boundaries are often unclear. What position would you take on this issue based on your observation of the mental health care team?

Research

STANDARD VII—RESEARCH

The psychiatric–mental health nurse contributes to nursing and mental health through the use of research.

▼ *Rationale*

Nurses in psychiatric–mental health nursing are responsible for contributing to the further development of the field of mental health by participating in research. At the basic level of practice, the psychiatric–mental health nurse uses research findings to improve clinical care and identifies clinical problems for research study. At the advanced level, the psychiatric–mental health nurse engages and/or collaborates with others in the research process to discover, examine, and test knowledge, theories, and creative approaches to practice.

▼ *Nursing conditions*

Quest for new knowledge or answers to questions
Acute observational and analytical skills
Persistence and attention to detail

▼ *Nursing behaviors*

Review reports of nursing research
Generate questions and identify clinical problems
Implement research findings in practice

▼ *Key elements*

Research links nursing theory and practice and is essential to the development of a profession

Table 10-3 Analysis of Interdisciplinary Teams

Personal qualities vital to interdisciplinary team function	Activities necessary for interdisciplinary team function
Accept differences/ perspectives of others	Establish new professional interaction patterns
Function interdependently	Accept changes in authority and status
Negotiate role with other team members	Develop modes of conflict resolution and decision making
Form new values, attitudes, and perceptions	Accept shared authority and responsibility
Tolerate constant review and challenge of ideas	Tolerate risk-taking behavior
Possess personal identity and integrity	
Accept team philosophy of care	

From Given B, Simmons S: *Nurs Forum* 16:165, 1977.

Box 10-2
STEPS FOR INTERDISCIPLINARY TEAM BUILDING

▼ Define roles and responsibilities
▼ Understand and respect other disciplines
▼ Develop and agree on a treatment philosophy
▼ Specify lines of authority and decision-making procedures
▼ Communicate regularly, openly, and clearly
▼ Utilize multidisciplinary treatment plans
▼ Encourage the use of support systems
▼ Strive for consistent leadership and low staff turnover

Outcome research with help establish the value of nursing in an era of health care reform

The relationship between theory, practice, and research is interactive and reciprocal. For theory to be useful, it must have implications for practice, and for practice to be tested and validated, it must be based in theory. Theory that arises out of practice is validated by research, which returns to direct practice and has implications for clinical care.

This cyclical relationship, as diagrammed by O'Toole,[20] is represented in Fig. 10-7. It shows how the casual, nonsystematic observation of a problem in practice leads to a more systematic observation and definition of terms, including the nature of the problem and influencing factors. Descriptive, observational, and exploratory research can further define a problem. Hypotheses may be developed concerning relationships between identified variables, which may be tested in correlational or survey research designs. Cause-and-effect relationships between the variables might then be tested in various experiments with natural or controlled settings. Only after establishing cause-and-effect can specific interventions aimed at changing the clinical problem be prescribed and tested. In this way prescriptive studies feed knowledge back into practice to improve health care.

This progression of observing from practice, theorizing, testing in research, and subsequently modifying practice must become an essential part of psychiatric nursing. The gap between research and practice must be bridged. One solution is to encourage closer collaboration between nurse researchers and nurse clinicians to ensure that the right questions are asked and the right variables are tested. Another solution is to more clearly define how nurses with different educational backgrounds can participate in research. Table 10-4 summarizes the research expectations for nurses based on educational preparation. Finally, one research study on psychiatric nurses' attitudes toward involvement in nursing research found that the three major blocks to clinical nursing research were lack of time, lack of knowledge, and lack of administrative support.[22] They found that positive attitudes toward nursing research were re-

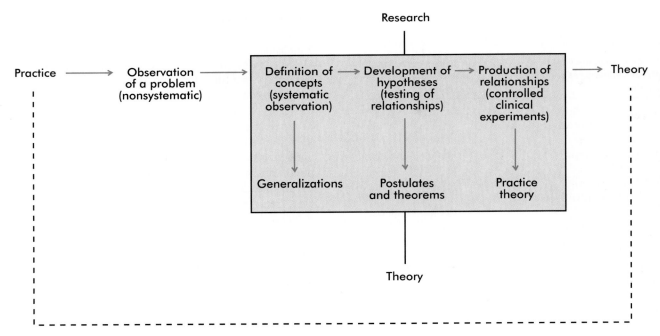

Fig. 10-7 Relationship between theory, practice, and research.
From O'Toole A: J *Psychosoc Nurs Ment Health Serv* 19:11, 1981.

Table 10-4   Nursing Research Participation Based on Education

Educational preparation	Research involvement
Associate Degree in Nursing	Help identify clinical problems in nursing practice; assist in data collection within a structured format; use research findings in practice with supervision
Baccalaureate Degree in Nursing	Identify clinical problems in need of research; help experienced investigators gain access to clinical sites; influence the selection of appropriate methods of data collection; participate in data collection and implementation of research findings
Master's Degree in Nursing	Collaborate in proposal development, data collection, data analysis, and interpretation; appraise the clinical relevance of research findings; provide leadership for integrating findings into practice
Doctoral education	Develop nursing knowledge through research and theory development; conduct funded independent research projects; develop and coordinate funded research projects; disseminate research findings to the scientific community

lated to nurses' advanced levels of education, although the authors suggested that research skills could be fostered through inservice education classes and individualized learning experiences.

Research in the area of psychiatry and psychiatric nursing is difficult for many reasons.[18] Problems such as sample size, outcome measurements, and the complexity of human behavior all compound the difficulties. It is also difficult to balance the rights of the individual against the desire to accomplish sound research. For example, consent to psychiatric research is complex. First, the researcher needs to consider whether the subject is able to consent and the degree to which it is an informed choice. Next is the issue of the treatment itself and whether it alters the subject's affect, perceptions, or ability to process information. The risks involved in psychiatric research must be carefully studied, and ethics must be maintained.

Research is sorely needed on the outcomes of psychi-

atric nursing intervention to determine its effectiveness and how psychiatric nurses compare with other mental health care providers.[10,14] Important data are being accumulated regarding the cost effectiveness of nursing interventions in acute care, chronic care, primary care, and health promotion. One controlled investigation conducted in England demonstrated that community psychiatric nurses' clinical and social care of neurotic patients was comparable with that provided by outpatient psychiatrists.[16] In addition, the patients assigned to the nurses reported greater consumer satisfaction and had higher rates of discharge. Finally, over the whole study period, the care provided by the psychiatric nurses was less expensive. Psychiatric nurses need to undertake and report similar research studies if this speciality area of practice is to survive and remain viable.

Research on psychiatric nursing has increased in the past decade, and it is obvious that nurses can construct sophisticated designs with both theoretical and practical importance. The clinical problems are numerous, and as nurses gain the skills and experience to validate their work scientifically, they can make a significant contribution to psychiatric theory and practice.

Resource Utilization

STANDARD VIII—RESOURCE UTILIZATION

The psychiatric–mental health nurse considers factors related to safety, effectiveness, and cost in planning and delivering client care.

▼ *Rationale*

The client is entitled to psychiatric–mental health care that is safe, effective, and affordable. As the cost of health care increases, treatment decisions must be made in such a way as to maximize resources and maintain quality of care. The psychiatric–mental health nurse seeks to provide cost-effective quality care by using the most appropriate resources and delegating care to the most appropriate, qualified health-care provider.

▼ *Nursing conditions*

Knowledge of the political and economic environment

Ability to evaluate costs versus benefits of treatment

Skill in negotiating and accessing resources

▼ *Nursing behaviors*

Fact-based decision making

Cost-effective allocation of resources

Patient advocacy on an individual and collective basis

▼ *Key elements*

Nurses play a critical role in integrating and coordinating health-care services

Nurses should be fiscally accountable for the care they provide

Resources should be allocated based on cost-benefit analyses and documented expected outcomes

Resource utilization may be one of the most important aspects of psychiatric nursing practice in the years to come. Discussing the costs and benefits of treatment options with patients, families, providers, and reimbursers will become increasingly important in an era of managed care (see Chapter 1). To fulfill this professional performance standard, psychiatric nurses need to request and obtain both cost and outcome information related to tests, consultations, evaluations, therapies, and continuum of care alternatives. Nurses will need to assume an active role in questioning, advising, and advocating for the most cost-effective use of resources.

Psychiatric nurses will also need to determine the most appropriate treatment setting for patients given the continuum of psychiatric care (see Chapters 31 and 32). Most recently the mental health reimbursement system has favored paying for inpatient and acute care. Reimbursement for preventive, early interventions and chronic care has been limited. With managed care, however, this trend is changing and nurses must be aware of all possible treatment options and the advantages and disadvantages of each.

It is also true that the mental health professions previously often acted on professional self-interest rather than on the public interest. This has been a disservice to patients and families of the mentally ill. The time has come for all mental health disciplines to work together in the development of service delivery models that are cost effective and contribute significantly to the quality of life of patients with psychiatric disorders.

Finally, one of the most critical resources in the mental health field is that of psychiatric manpower.[17] Because each team member has different competencies, a challenge for the mental health system will be to use the best that each discipline has to offer and to develop an integrated set of clinical services that will offer the highest quality care for psychiatric patients.

> Psychiatric nurses must become increasingly cost and outcome conscious. Identify three commonly ordered tests for psychiatric patients. Find out how much they cost and analyze how helpful they are in planning treatment strategies.

SUGGESTED CROSS-REFERENCES

SUMMARY

1. The standards of professional performance apply to self-regulation and accountability for practice that must be demonstrated by psychiatric nurses both individually and as a group. The standards also relate to professional autonomy and self-definition.

2. Psychiatric nurses need to participate actively in the formal organizational evaluation of overall patterns of care through a variety of quality improvement activities including systems, consumer, and clinical evaluation.

3. Performance appraisal involves administrative review of work performance and clinical supervision of nursing care.

4. Psychiatric nurses are expected to engage in a continual learning process to maintain currency with the latest information in the field.

5. Collegiality requires that psychiatric nurses view their nurse peers as collaborators in the caregiving process who are valued and respected for their unique contributions.

6. Ethical considerations combine with legal and therapeutic issues to affect all aspects of psychiatric nursing practice and require the use of ethical decision making in caring for patients.

7. Collaboration is the shared planning, decision making, problem solving, goal setting, and assumption of responsibilities by individuals who work together cooperatively and with open communication. Psychiatric nurses collaborate with patients, families, nurse colleagues, and members of the health-care team.

8. Research is an essential professional role activity for psychiatric nurses, and additional research is needed on the outcomes of psychiatric nursing intervention to determine its effectiveness.

9. Psychiatric nurses must also evaluate the most appropriate use of resources in the delivery of care. Issues of costs, benefits, outcomes, treatment setting, and appropriate use of mental health care providers must be considered.

REFERENCES

1. American Nurses' Association: *Code for nurses with interpretive statements*, Kansas City, Mo, 1985, The Association.
2. American Nurses' Association: *Credentialing in nursing*, Washington, DC, 1993, The Association.
3. American Nurses' Association: A *statement on psychiatric–mental health clinical nursing practice and standards of psychiatric–mental health clinical nursing practice*, Washington, DC, 1994, The Association.
4. Bloch S, Chodoff P: *Psychiatric ethics*, New York, 1991, Oxford University Press.
5. Curtin L: A proposed model for critical ethical analysis, *Nurs Forum* 17:12, 1978.
6. Ehrat K: The value of differentiated practice, *J Nurs Adm* 21:42, 1991.
7. Ekstein R, Wallerstein R: *The teaching and learning of psychotherapy*, New York, 1958, Basic Books.

8. Forchuk C: Ethical problems encountered by mental health nurses, Issues Ment Health Nurs 12:375, 1991.

9. Forsey L, Cleland V, Miller B: Job descriptions for differentiated nursing practice and differentiated pay, J Nurs Adm 23:33, 1993.

10. Foundation for Health Services Research: Health outcomes research: a primer, Washington, DC, 1993, The Association.

11. Goertzen I, ed: Differentiating nursing practice into the twenty-first century, Kansas City, Mo, 1991, American Academy of Nursing.

12. Glotz N, Johnsen G, Johnson R: Advancing clinical excellence: competency-based patient care, Nurs Manage 25:42, 1994.

13. Goode C et al: What kind of recognition do staff nurses want? Am J Nurs 1993:64, 1993.

14. Jennings B: Patient outcomes research: seizing the opportunity, Adv Nurs Sci 14:59, 1991.

15. Joint Commission on Accreditation of Healthcare Organizations: Accreditation manual for hospitals, Oakbrook Terrace, Ill, 1991, The Commission.

16. Mangen S et al: Cost-effectiveness of community psychiatric nurse or outpatient psychiatrist care of neurotic patients, Psychol Med 13:407, 1983.

17. Merwin E, Fox J: Cost-effective integration of mental health professions, Issues Ment Health Nurs 13:139, 1992.

18. Mirin S, Namerow M: Why study treatment outcome? Hosp Community Psychiatry 42:1007, 1991.

19. Moore R: Ethics in the practice of psychiatry: origins, functions, models, and enforcement, Am J Psychiatry 135:157, 1978.

20. O'Toole A: When the practical becomes theoretical, J Psychosoc Nurs Ment Health Serv 19:11, 1981.

21. Pesut D, Williams C: The nature of clinical supervision in psychiatric nursing: a survey of clinical nurse specialists, Arch Psychiatr Nurs Care 4:180, 1990.

22. Poster E, Betz C, Randell B: Psychiatric nurses' attitudes toward and involvement in nursing research, J Psychosoc Nurs Ment Health Serv 30:26, 1992.

23. Wake M: Nursing care delivery systems: status and vision, J Nurs Adm 20:47, 1990.

ANNOTATED SUGGESTED READINGS

Bloch S, Chodoff P: Psychiatric ethics, New York, 1991, Oxford University Press.
Excellent overview of ethical aspects of psychiatric treatment. Written for psychiatrists but of value to nurses as well.

*Bonnivier J: A peer supervision group: put countertransference to work, J Psychosoc Nurs Ment Health Serv 30:5, 1992.
Reports on the value of a peer countertransference supervision group in helping staff manage and use their countertransference therapeutically. Good discussion of countertransference—an important but often overlooked concept of practice.

Deremo D: Integrating professional values, quality practice, productivity, and reimbursement for nursing, Nurs Adm Q 14:9, 1989.

This article puts it all together and describes a practice model that results in a truly professional practice environment. More such examples are needed, particularly in psychiatric nursing settings.

*Evans M: Using a model to structure psychosocial nursing research, J Psychosoc Nurs Ment Health Serv 30:27, 1992.
Specifies a model that the author suggests could guide psychiatric nursing research across investigators, projects, and sites.

Foundation for Health Services Research: Health outcomes research: a primer, Washington, DC, 1993, The Association.
Basic overview of what constitutes outcomes research, how health status is measured, and who funds outcomes research.

*Glotz N, Johnsen G, Johnson R: Advancing clinical excellence: competency-based patient care, Nurs Manage 25:42, 1994.
Describes a competency-based program for psychiatric nurses and significant outcomes related to its implementation.

*Jennings B: Patient outcomes research: seizing the opportunity, Adv Nurs Sci 14:59, 1991.
Opportunities and challenges posed to nurses by patient-outcome research are addressed. Highly recommended for all nurses interested in outcomes research.

*Kane I, Fickley B: Correlating nursing care, nursing practice, and nursing performance standards, Perspect Psychiatr Care 28:27, 1992.
Shows how psychiatric nursing standards of practice, standards of care, and standards of performance can be integrated into job descriptions, performance appraisals, peer review, and quality management activities.

*McDaniel C: Ethical issues in restructuring of psychiatric services, Issues Mental Health Nurs 13:31, 1992.
Timely exploration of the often ignored ethical issues related to restructuring psychiatric services in an era of health-care reform; offers suggestions for retaining quality nursing care.

*McDonald S: An ethical dilemma: risk versus responsibility J Psychosoc Nurs Ment Health Serv 32:19, 1994.
Reports on the experience of nurses who spoke out when a hospital exploited certain psychiatric diagnoses by encouraging extended lengths of stay and restricting patients' rights. Should be read and discussed by all nurses.

*Poster E: Quality assurance and treatment outcome: a psychiatric nursing perspective. In Mirin S, Gossett J, Grob M, eds: Psychiatric treatment: advances in outcome research, Washington, DC, 1991, American Psychiatric Press.
This chapter describes the application of the quality assurance process in a psychiatric nursing setting and links it to the potential for outcome studies in the field.

*Slater J: Effecting personal effectiveness: assertiveness training for nurses, J Adv Nurs 15:337, 1990.
Discusses why it is difficult for nurses to act assertively and presents the process and content of a program designed for nurses on assertiveness training.

*White G: Ethical dilemmas in contemporary nursing practice, Washington, DC, 1993, American Nurses Publishing.
Uses case studies, three of which are particularly relevant to psychiatric nurses, to explore ethical dilemmas in practice.

*Nursing reference.

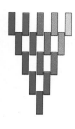

Continuum of Care

Continuum. What an interesting word. It means "a series of variations, or a sequence of things in regular order." As such, it is the perfect descriptor of the levels of contemporary psychiatric treatment. The continuum of psychiatric care allows nurses to use the full range of their skills and talents, often in new settings and innovative programs. Perhaps best of all, it provides patients, families, and communities with the "healing" ability to build competence, resilience, and health rather than merely to "Band-Aid" disability, illness, and disease. It therefore includes working with patients in crisis, acute, maintenance, and health-promotion stages of treatment. Such is the brave new world of psychiatric and mental health nursing.

In this unit you will learn about intervening with primary, secondary, and tertiary prevention activities. All nurses, regardless of their specialty area, need to know how to promote mental health, intervene with patients and families in crisis, and build rehabilitative functioning in those who have fallen ill. You will find that in the future you will use these skills more often than you might ever have imagined, and you will think back to this unit and the information it imparted with greater appreciation for the caregiving continuum.

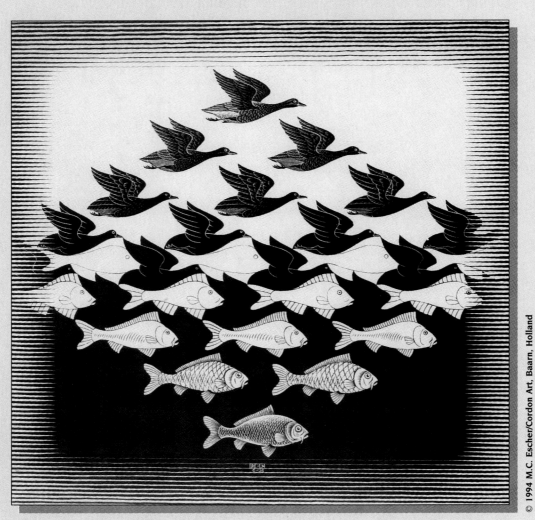

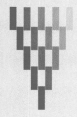

CHAPTER 11

Primary Mental Health Prevention

GAIL W. STUART

What is this thing called health? Simply a state in which the individual happens transiently to be perfectly adapted to his environment. Obviously, such states cannot be common, for the environment is in constant flux.

H.L. Mencken: *The American Mercury, March* 1930

LEARNING OBJECTIVES

After studying this chapter the student should be able to:

▼ Define primary, secondary, and tertiary prevention
▼ Compare and contrast the epidemiological, behavioral, and nursing paradigms of primary prevention
▼ Assess the vulnerability of various groups to developing maladaptive coping responses
▼ Describe the levels of intervention and activities related to the following primary prevention nursing interventions: health education, environmental change, and supporting social systems
▼ Assess the importance of evaluation of the nursing process when applied to primary prevention

TOPICAL OUTLINE

Conceptualizing Primary Prevention
    Epidemiological Prevention Paradigm
    Behavioral Prevention Paradigm
    Nursing Prevention Paradigm
Assessment
Planning and Implementation
    Health Education
    Environmental Change
    Supporting Social Systems
Evaluation

Many people regard prevention of mental disorders as a desirable goal that should be actively pursued. Although this may seem obvious, in fact, the issues of prevention are complex and controversial. Caplan[6] discussed basic concepts underlying preventive mental health in his classic work, *Principles of Preventive Psychiatry*. He applies the three levels of preventive intervention from the public health model to mental illness and emotional disturbance.

1. **Primary prevention** is lowering the *incidence* of mental disorders or reducing the rate at which new cases of a disorder develop.
2. **Secondary prevention** involves reducing the *prevalence* of a disorder by reducing the number of existing cases. Secondary prevention activities include early case finding, screening, and prompt effective treatment.
3. **Tertiary prevention** activities attempt to reduce the *severity* of a disorder and associated disability through rehabilitative activities.

The major thrust in the United States has been in secondary prevention activities or the treatment of mental disorders. This is evident in the allocation of economic resources, the nature of caregiving organizations and institutions, and the activities of mental health professionals. For example, a 1991 survey of state mental health authorities focused on the extent to which primary prevention activities were conducted or supported at the state level. All 50 states responded: 7 reported significant involvement in prevention, 7 reported some involvement, and 36 reported none. The authors concluded that although some states are involved in significant prevention activities, relatively few states have made a real commitment to prevention.[12]

CONCEPTUALIZING PRIMARY PREVENTION

Although primary prevention is often described with such slogans as "An ounce of prevention is worth a pound of cure" or "Curing is costly—prevention, priceless," it is only recently emerging as a substantial force in the mental health movement. One of the reasons it is gaining momentum is because of health-care reform. As health and mental health care move toward capitated payment and managed care, there is a greater economic incentive to prevent illness rather than treat it. This may be one of the most positive outcomes of the health-care debate.

The reality of this change is evident in two recent reports. The first report was prepared by the National Mental Health Association and 17 national member organizations of the National Prevention Coalition. It recommends five preventive mental health interventions that should be included in a reformed health-care system:

1. Screening for developmental delays and mental health problems for children and adolescents as part of their regular checkups
2. Screening for mental health problems in adults as part of routine preventive examinations; for example, to screen for depression, anxiety, or potential suicide
3. Counseling for individuals and families in situations that place them at high risk for developing mental or emotional disorders
4. Home visits and other intensive interventions in high-risk situations involving stress and lack of social support for pregnant women and parents and infants, such as premature infants, low-income households, and teenage parents
5. Self-help groups to assist persons confronting health problems, mental health problems, or life situations of stress or change

The second report was issued by the Institute of Medicine in January 1994.[18] It concluded that research on the prevention of mental disorders can play an important role in alleviating the financial and social burdens imposed by these disorders. The report stated that, although little evidence exists that any specific mental disorder can be prevented, research aimed at reducing risk factors associated with a disorder should be conducted and rigorously evaluated.

The idea of promoting mental health in general is attractive. Promotion sounds optimistic and positive. It is consistent with the idea of self-help and being self-responsible for health. It implies changing human behavior and draws on a holistic approach to health. A continuing problem, however, with the strategy of promoting mental health is the vastness and vagueness of its goals. Theoretically, everything has implications for primary prevention, for reducing emotional disorders, and for strengthening and fostering mental health. Thus goals are often ill defined, and evaluation of promotion activities is difficult. Even if goals of a project can be identified and measured, their relation to long-term behavior is often questionable. For example, successful teaching of coping skills to schoolchildren may fulfill short-term goals, but what this precisely means for their mental health as adults may be unclear and unsupported by empirical evidence.

Another problem concerns the fuzziness of the concepts and definitions underlying the issues. For example, primary prevention programs may be aimed at an entire population or only at persons believed to be at high risk for developing a disorder. This depends on how primary prevention in general is viewed—is it disease prevention or health promotion? There also needs to be agreement on what is being promoted or prevented to best determine what action should be taken.

 The terms *health promotion* and *disease prevention* are often used interchangeably. In what ways do they overlap and how are they different?

Epidemiological Prevention Paradigm

There is basic disagreement on what is important in understanding and preventing mental disorders. One group of mental health professionals favors the genetic-biochemical explanation that each mental disease has a separate physical cause. The prevention model this group favors focuses narrowly on genetic counseling and on biochemical and brain research to discover the specific causes of mental illness. They argue that there is no real proof that social stresses cause mental illness and that the high rate of mental illness among the poor may be because disturbed people tend to "drift downward" from the upper and middle classes into poverty.

They suggest that primary prevention activities are best focused on illness prevention. Viewing mental illness as a disease in the medical model perspective allows the use of the classic, epidemiological paradigm in primary prevention. This paradigm consists of the following steps:

1. Identify a disease of sufficient importance to justify the development of a preventive intervention program. Develop reliable methods for its diagnosis so that people can be divided into groups according to whether they do or do not have the disease.

2. By a series of epidemiological and laboratory studies identify the most likely cause of that disease.

3. Launch and evaluate an experimental preventive intervention program based on the results of those studies.

This paradigm has been effective for a broad array of communicable diseases, such as smallpox, typhus, malaria, diphtheria, tuberculosis, rubella, and polio, and nutritional diseases, such as scurvy, pellagra, rickets, kwashiorkor, and endemic goiter. It has also proved useful in a variety of mental disorders caused by poisons, chemicals, licit or illicit drugs, electrolyte imbalances, and nutritional deficiencies. All these diseases have one thing in common. For each, there is a known necessary, although not always sufficient, causative agent.

 Identify one psychiatric disorder that would lend itself to the epidemiological prevention paradigm.

Behavioral Prevention Paradigm

A contrasting view of the causes and prevention of mental illness is presented by mental health professionals who support a social learning model. In this model mental disorders are believed to result from faulty early learning of social coping skills, from low levels of competence, from low self-esteem, and from poor support systems interacting with high levels of stress. This viewpoint stresses that mental disorders do not appear to have a single identified precondition and may have causative factors that are multiple, interactive, situational, and sociocultural in nature. They thus require that prevention of mental illness be thought of in a more behavioral way as the prevention of problems or maladaptive responses. This view calls for prevention of the following:

1. **Specific behaviors** that are self-defeating or harmful to others, such as poor or unhealthy habits, overeating, procrastinating, evasiveness, blaming others, and "setting the stage" to fail

2. **Role failures,** as a student, a parent, or an employee

3. **Relationship breakdowns** between husband and wife, parent and child, boss and employee, including detection and control of interpersonal "games" that are destructive

4. **Feeling overreactions,** such as panics, new situation anxiety, flights, and temper tantrums

5. **Psychological disabilities,** such as the social deterioration of a confined ill person, decompensation, "going to pieces," or falling into melancholia instead of experiencing normal grieving

With such a conceptualization, many of the services already given in the community by mental health and other helping agencies can be identified and publicly acknowledged as prevention efforts.

By defining problems in this way they can include both single-episode events, such as a divorce, or a long-standing condition, such as marital conflict. They can also reflect either an acute health problem or a chronic health problem. For example, the following categories of problems can arise from the abuse of alcohol:

1. Acute health problems, such as overdose or delirium tremens

2. Chronic health problems, such as cirrhosis of the liver

3. Casualties, such as accidents on the road, in the home, or elsewhere, and suicide

4. Violent crime and family abuse

5. Problems of demeanor, such as public drunkenness and use of alcohol by teenagers

6. Default of major social roles—work or school and family roles

7. Problems of feeling state—demoralization and depression and experienced loss of control

This is a new paradigm for primary prevention. It assumes that problems are multicausal, that everyone is vulnerable to stressful life events, and that any disability or problem may arise as a consequence of them. For example, four vulnerable persons can face a stressful life event—perhaps the collapse of their marriage or the loss of their job. One person may become severely depressed, the second may be involved in an automobile accident, the third may head down the road to alcoholism, and the fourth may develop a psychotic thought disorder or coronary artery disease. This behavioral paradigm does not search for a cause for each problem. Rather, it attempts to reduce the incidence of stressful life events as outlined in the following steps[4]:

1. Identify a stressful life event that appears to have undesirable consequences in a significant proportion of the population. Develop procedures for reliably identifying persons who have undergone or who are undergoing that stressful experience.

2. By traditional epidemiological and laboratory methods, study the consequences of that event and develop hypotheses related to how the nega-

Table 11-1 Developmental Stages and Tasks of the Individual and Family Unit

Erikson's stage of individual psychosocial development	Developmental task of the individual	Duvall's stage of the family life cycle	Developmental task of the family identified by Streff
Trust vs. mistrust (0-2 years)	Oral needs are of primary importance Adequate mothering is necessary to meet infant's needs Acquisition of hope	Premarital-married couple	Establishing relationship Defining mutual goals Developing intimacy Developing appropriate dependence, independence, interdependence patterns Establishing mutually satisfying relationship Negotiating boundaries of couple relationship and with individual's families of origin Discussing issue of childbearing Making decision to conceive
Autonomy vs. shame (1½-3 years)	Anal needs are of primary importance Father emerges as important figure Acquisition of will	Childbearing	Working out authority and responsibility issues Working out caretaker roles Having children Forming new unit Facilitating child's establishment of trust Acknowledging need for personal time and space while sharing with each other and child
Initiative vs. guilt (3-6 years)	Genital needs are of primary importance Family relationships contribute to early sense of responsibility and conscience Acquisition of purpose	Preschool	Continuing individual development as couple, parent, and family Experiencing changes in energy and time for individual and couple needs Promoting continued growth in each other and the relationship while encouraging child to develop autonomy and retain self-esteem Establishing own family tradition with each other and children without guilt related to breaks with traditions of families of origin
Industry vs. inferiority (6-12 years)	Active period of socialization for child during move from family into society Acquisition of competence	School age	One or both spouses establishing new roles in work settings or community or changes in child-rearing practices and gaining recognition for selves and children Children in school and after-school activities, relating with peers, self-esteem being enhanced or inhibited, and interfacing with activities in family
Identity vs. identity diffusion (13+ years)	Search for self, in which peers play important role Psychosocial moratorium is provided by society to aid adolescent Acquisition of fidelity	Teenage	Parents continue to develop roles in community and interests other than with children Children examine ways to experience freedom while expressing responsibility for actions Struggles evolve with parents as emancipation process proceeds Family's value system may be challenged Couple's relationship may be strong or weak, depending on how members respond to each other's needs
Intimacy vs. isolation (adulthood)	Characterized by increasing importance of human closeness and sexual fulfillment Acquisition of love	Launching career	Parents launching young adults with rituals marking rites of passage Change in relationship with children who are becoming adults and/or in new living situations; change in couple's relationship because of children's absence and increased time with one another

Table 11-1   Developmental Stages and Tasks of the Individual and Family Unit—cont'd.

Erikson's stage of individual psychosocial development	Developmental task of the individual	Duvall's stage of the family life cycle	Developmental task of the family identified by Streff
Generativity vs. self-absorption (middle-age)	Characterized by productivity, creativity, parental responsibility, and concern for new generation Acquisition of care	Middle-age parents	Energy channeled into guiding next generation via family or community activities, or couple may now be dealing with issues of aging of their own parents Children of middle-age parents may be adolescent
Integrity vs. despair (old age)	Characterized by unifying philosophy of life and more profound love for mankind Acquisition of wisdom	Aging family members	Persons have achieved satisfying relationships and feel sense of accomplishment and desire to continue to live fully until death instead of existing in state of despair Aging members are coping with bereavement and may not be living alone

tive consequences of the event might be reduced or eliminated.

3. Launch and evaluate experimental preventive intervention programs based on these hypotheses.

This paradigm shifts attention from nonspecific predisposing factors of mental illness to more discrete and identifiable precipitating stressors. These factors may be single-episode life events, such as loss of a job, or more long-term life event stressors, such as job dissatisfaction. Narrowing the focus of the study in this way limits the population at risk and uses financial and program resources more wisely.

 Analyze the problem of child abuse from the behavioral prevention paradigm.

Nursing Prevention Paradigm

Nurses can engage in primary prevention activities based on the stress adaptation model used in this text. It would involve the application of the nursing process with a focus on the primary prevention of maladaptive coping responses associated with an identified stressor. This would incorporate the following aspects:

1. **Assessment.** Identification of a stressor that precipitates maladaptive responses and a target or vulnerable population group that is at high risk in relationship to it
2. **Planning.** Elaboration of specific strategies of prevention and relevant social institutions and situations through which the strategies may be applied
3. **Implementation.** Application of selected nursing interventions aimed at decreasing maladaptive re-

sponses to the identified stressor and enhancing adaptation
4. **Evaluation.** Determining the effectiveness of the nursing interventions with regard to short- and long-term outcomes, use of resources, and comparison with other prevention strategies

The nursing process can thereby be used in a goal-directed way to decrease the incidence of mental illness and promote mental health among individuals, families, groups, and communities.

ASSESSMENT

Three types of preventive interventions based on target populations have been identified[18]:

1. *Universal:* targeted to the general population group without consideration of risk factors
2. *Selective:* targeted to individuals or groups with a significantly higher risk of developing a particular disorder
3. *Indicated:* targeted to high-risk individuals identified as having symptoms foreshadowing a specific mental disorder or biological markers indicating predisposition for the disorder

A knowledge of normal growth and development is essential for assessing a person's functioning, as well as for intervening with preventive nursing interventions. The nurse should be familiar with normative stages, tasks, and parameters to know what issues the person has faced in the past and what challenges lie ahead. In addition to understanding the individual's development, the nurse must know about the family cycle, since many nursing interventions are directed at the family, from mobilizing their support of a patient to modifying dysfunctional family patterns.

Table 11-1 summarizes the developmental stages of

the individual, using Erikson's theory[9] of psychosocial development and Duvall's stages[7] of the family life cycle. Streff[26] integrated Erikson's theory with Duvall's to define developmental tasks of the family paralleling those of the individual. This integrated approach allows life to be viewed as stages marked by critical developmental tasks. This helps the nurse identify potential future stressors for an individual or family. By understanding and anticipating these stressors, the nurse can implement effective preventive nursing care.

Although all people and all families face similar developmental tasks, not everyone adapts to them or copes with them positively. Individuals or groups in our society have additional stressors placed on them, inadequate coping resources, and fewer positive experiences to balance out their perceived stress. These people are thus particularly vulnerable or at high risk for developing maladaptive responses. It is extremely helpful if the nurse has an awareness of these vulnerable people. The increased sensitivity that results from this awareness will affect the nurse's assessment of both existing and potential problems and one's actual work with people from these high-risk groups. Nurses, as the largest group of health-care providers, can make a significant impact in promoting mental health if they would anticipate problems and commit their time and skill to preventing their occurrence.

Assessment in primary prevention therefore involves identifying groups of people who are vulnerable to developing mental disorders or who may display maladaptive coping responses to specific stressors or risk factors. To complete such an assessment, the nurse needs to draw on information generated from theory, research, and clinical practice.

The actual identification of vulnerable groups depends on the nurse's geography and life experiences, and not all individuals within these groups are at equal risk. What these groups do share, however, is the experience of a life event, stressor, or risk factor that represents a loss of some kind or places an excessive demand on one's ability to cope. The more clearly the subgroup can be defined, the more specifically the prevention strategies can be researched, identified, and implemented.

Can you identify three groups of people vulnerable to the development of psychiatric illness—one based on biological factors, one based on psychological factors, and one based on sociocultural factors?

Box 11-1

HEALTHY PEOPLE 2000 OBJECTIVES RELATED TO MENTAL HEALTH AND MENTAL DISORDERS

To reduce mental disorders by the year 2000, objectives target the following:
▼ Reducing suicide
▼ Reducing suicide attempts among children and adolescents
▼ Reducing mental disorders among adults
▼ Reducing adverse health effects from stress
▼ Increasing use of community support programs by people with mental disorders
▼ Increasing use of treatment by people with major depressive disorders
▼ Increasing the proportion of people who seek help for personal and emotional problems
▼ Reducing uncontrolled stress
▼ Increasing appropriate suicide prevention strategies in jails
▼ Increasing workplace stress management programs
▼ Increasing the number of states with established mutual help clearinghouses
▼ Increasing routine review of mental functioning by primary care providers for both children and adults

PLANNING AND IMPLEMENTATION

Under the sponsorship of the Public Health Service, a national incentive has been undertaken to promote health and prevent disease in this country. The *Healthy People* 2000 objectives related to mental health and mental disorder are listed in Box 11-1.[27] A number of potential measures have been identified to meet one of the objectives for the control of stress and violent behavior. These include education, service, and technological and legislative measures as identified in Box 11-2. This list provides the nurse with a good overview of the many areas appropriate for nursing intervention.

In addition, the stress adaptation model presented in Chapter 4 and represented in Fig. 11-1 is useful for the nurse in planning strategies for primary prevention. It suggests both target areas and types of activities that might be useful. If the overall nursing goal is to promote constructive coping mechanisms and maximize adaptive coping responses, then the model suggests that prevention strategies should be directed toward influencing predisposing factors, precipitating stressors, appraisal of stressors, and coping resources and mechanisms through the following interventions:

1. Health education
2. Environmental change
3. Supporting social systems

Box 11-2

POTENTIAL PRIMARY PREVENTION MEASURES FOR THE CONTROL OF STRESS AND VIOLENT BEHAVIOR

EDUCATION AND INFORMATION

▼ Increasing the public's awareness, through planned campaigns using the appropriate media, that stress can be an antecedent of illness and that stress management can be an important component of health

▼ Creating new educational pathways for developing enhanced professional skills in biobehavioral fields of medicine and public health

▼ Developing the capacities of health-care professionals in stress diagnosis and management

▼ Helping parents recognize and deal with stress

▼ Training secondary, elementary, and preschool teachers to include discussion of stress recognition and management in school health curricula

▼ Training of police in handling calls involving domestic and interpersonal disputes that would potentially lead to violent behavior

▼ Public education, especially for high-risk groups, on steps to take to reduce risks of rape

▼ Training all "helping" professionals regarding signs that indicate high risk for suicide

▼ Helping the public be aware of indicators of possible suicide

SERVICE

▼ Hotlines for people under acute stress (suicide, child abuse prevention)

▼ Stress management programs in workplaces

▼ Stress management programs targeted to adolescents, parents, and the elderly

▼ Stress appraisal analysis (self-administered or performed by a legitimate objective outside source)

▼ Professional and social support systems to assist in resolution of stressful life events, including mutual aid and self-help groups such as Reach for Recovery, child abusing parents, bereavement groups, single parent groups

▼ Information and counseling with regard to individually appropriate leisure and stress-reducing activities including exercise

▼ A variety of self-help relaxation and biofeedback techniques, which can be individualized in concert with a diversity of life-styles and work requirements

▼ Psychophysiological tests to aid in assisting employees who are having difficulty adjusting to their work and to their coworkers

▼ Support services for inevitable or necessary life change events—especially in relation to death, separation, job changes, and geographic relocation

▼ Domestic crisis teams to defuse domestic disputes

▼ Targeting the above measures to high-risk populations and individuals with low coping abilities

▼ Evaluating intervention efforts

▼ Follow-up services for persons who have attempted suicide

▼ Shelters for abused wives (and husbands)

▼ Training all health (and other human services—including educational) personnel to be alert to evidence of child abuse

TECHNOLOGY

▼ Actions by employers, labor, and government to reduce stress-creating work environments

▼ Reducing stressful aspects of the environment such as noise pollution and overcrowding

LEGISLATION AND REGULATION

▼ Activities to create employment opportunities for youth

▼ Action to limit the availability of handguns, to reduce homicides and suicides that occur during stressful periods

▼ Strengthening mandatory child abuse reporting laws

Modified from US Department of Health and Human Services: *Healthy people* 2000, Washington, DC, 1990, Public Health Service.

Because the process depicted in the model is a dynamic one, it is not possible to discretely link a particular strategy with a particular component of the model. Rather, the strategies can affect multiple aspects of a person's life. For example, an environmental change, such as changing jobs, can affect an individual's predisposition to stress, decrease the amount of stress, change the appraisal of the threat, and perhaps increase financial or social coping resources. This interactive effect can thus serve to justify the use of these prevention strategies for vulnerable groups.

Health Education

The health education strategy of primary prevention in mental health involves the strengthening of individuals and groups through **competence building.** It is based on the assumption that many maladaptive responses are the result of a lack of competence, that is, a lack of perceived control over one's own life, of effective coping strategies, and the lowered self-esteem that results. Competence building may be the single most important preventive strategy for dealing with individual and social issues in most communities. A competent indi-

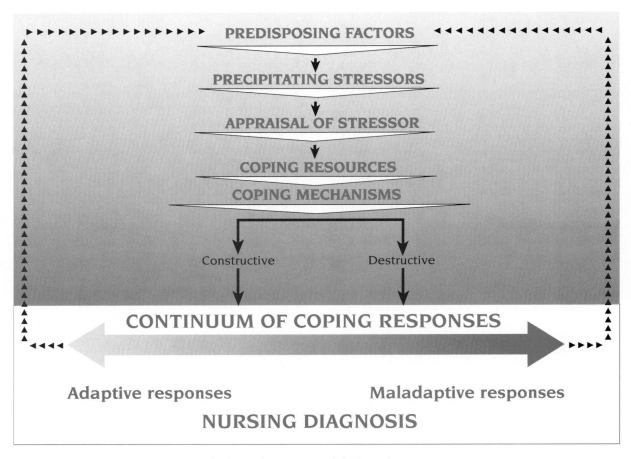

Fig. 11-1   A stress adaptation model of psychiatric nursing care.

vidual or community is aware of resources and alternatives, can make reasoned decisions about issues, and can cope adaptively with problems.

 How is the concept of competency similar to the concept of positive mental health?

Levels of Intervention. Health education or competence building can be viewed as having the following four aspects:

1. Increasing the individual's or group's awareness of issues and events related to health and illness. Awareness of normal developmental tasks and potential problems is fundamental.
2. Increasing understanding of the dimensions of potential stressors, possible outcomes (both adaptive and maladaptive), and alternative coping responses.
3. Increasing knowledge of where and how to acquire the needed resources. Many health professionals

assume this is common knowledge, although for many individuals it is not.
4. Increasing the actual abilities of the individual or group. This means improving or maximizing coping skills, such as problem-solving skills or interpersonal skills, tolerance of stress and frustration, motivation, hope, self-esteem, and power.

Programs and Activities. Mental health education can take place in any setting, can assume a formal or informal structure, can be directed toward individuals or groups, and can be related to predisposing factors or potential stressors.[23] Health education directed toward strengthening an individual's predisposition to stress can take various forms. Growth groups may be formed for parents that focus on parent-child relations, normal growth and development, or effective methods of child rearing.[15,16,22] Groups of children or adolescents can discuss peer relationships, sexuality, or potential problem areas, such as drug abuse or promiscuity. Employee groups can form to discuss career burnout and related issues. Or a more activity-centered educational program can be initiated, such as Outward

Bound, which helps the individual discover that step by step competence can be expanded to master new, unexpected, and potentially stressful situations in an adaptive way.

Probably the most common type of health education program implemented currently is one that aids the individual in coping with a specific potential stressor. Consider, for example, the impending stressor or risk factor of marital separation. Families about to experience marital separation are vulnerable to emotional problems, physical complaints, and increased use of health-care facilities. Children and adults about to experience this event may be offered educational and supportive group intervention aimed at enhancing their ability to cope. Education groups can similarly be offered to those experiencing retirement, bereavement, or any other stressful event (see Critical Thinking about Contemporary Issues).

Parent education classes are a well-known example of the type of anticipatory guidance that can be offered to high-risk groups. [13] Although raising children is considered a serious aspect of life, until recently little attention has been directed to the belief that effective parenting is not an innate ability. Whether nurses subscribe to a specific set of beliefs and strategies for parenting or choose an eclectic approach, the opportunities for promoting mental health abound. Possibly one of the most beneficial results of parent education is the acknowledgment that all parents become frustrated, angry, and ambivalent toward their children. Parent education goes beyond acknowledging feelings and includes learning and practicing alternative ways of interacting with children. During these classes situations are anticipated, and discussions focus on identifying potential crisis situations and dealing with them through simulated encounters such as role playing. Education for mental health can thus address the needs of both children and parents as family roles shift and respond to societal change.

Stigma. Finally, health education activities can be directed to the larger community. One way to do this is by changing the attitudes and behavior of health-care providers and consumers. This may involve activities related to dispelling myths and stereotypes associated with vulnerable groups, providing knowledge of normal parameters, increasing sensitivity to psychosocial factors affecting health and illness, and enhancing the ability to give sensitive, supportive, and humanistic health care.

A community-level strategy would be to provide public education on mental health issues and community resources. For example, a recent study documented that people with mental illnesses have the highest rate of negative portrayal on television. [1] Another study on

CRITICAL THINKING ABOUT CONTEMPORARY ISSUES

What is the Future for Children with Mentally Ill Parents?

Living with a mentally ill parent does not necessarily mean that the child will develop the disorder, but it does not make growing up any easier. Although the mechanisms for transmitting psychiatric illness across generations are controversial, many studies support the fact that parental illness affects children. For example, it has been noted that coping with a mentally ill parent may be more difficult than coping with parental loss. So too, these children feel a sense of psychological vulnerability and fear becoming ill themselves. The major research findings on this topic are as follows [14]:

▼ Children of mentally ill parents are at greater risk for psychiatric and developmental disorders than are children of well parents.

▼ The risk to children is greater if the mother rather than the father is the ill parent.

▼ In studies of depressed versus nondepressed groups, differences in the mother-child interaction are evident as early as 3 months' postpartum.

▼ Many children with emotionally disturbed parents do not become disordered themselves. The nature of the parent's illness, the child's genetic and constitutional make-up, the family's functional ability, and the availability of healthy attachment figures all play an important role in predicting the future mental health of the child.

The evidence suggests, therefore, that psychiatric nurses need to focus more attention on the children of mentally ill parents. [2] They should assess parenting problems whenever parents with children at home are hospitalized for psychiatric care. [14] They can also implement psychoeducational, preventive nursing interventions that will enhance mental health in high-risk children and families. [3] ▼

American's attitudes toward mental illness revealed that Americans do not consider themselves well informed about mental illness but do think they should know more. They are also reluctant to welcome a wide variety of mental health facilities into their communities. [5] Results of these studies suggest that misperceptions regarding vulnerable subgroups of the population need to be corrected. They are the result, in part, of the cultural stigma against mental illness that is prevalent in contemporary society.[10]

Stigma, in its original definition, meant a "scar left by a hot iron on the face of an evil doer." Stigma is now defined as a mark of disgrace that is used to identify and separate out those people whom society sees as deviant, sinful, or dangerous. For the psychiatrically ill, stigma is a barrier that separates them from society and keeps them apart from others. Patients and their families often report that the diagnosis of a mental illness is followed by increasing isolation and loneliness as family and friends retreat and withdraw. Patients feel rejected and feared by others, and their families are met by blame. Stigma against mental illness is clearly a reflection of the cultural biases of contemporary American society, biases that are shared by consumers and health-care providers alike.

The stigma, misunderstanding, and fear surrounding mental illness are related to both the agencies providing mental health services and the people receiving these services who are often elderly, poor or members of social minority groups. Unlike physical illness, which tends to evoke sympathy and the desire to help, mental disorders tend to disturb and repel people. Yet everyone encounters stress, and all people are subject to maladaptive coping responses. Mental health professionals can educate the public that health is a continuum and illness is caused by a complex combination of factors. In doing so, consumers may begin to understand that no one is immune from mental illness or emotional problems, and that the fear, anxiety, and even anger we feel about people who suffer these problems may merely reflect some of our own deepest fears and anxieties.

> Have you observed the stigma associated with psychiatric illness in your personal or professional life? If so, what steps have you taken or could you take to overcome it?

Environmental Change

Activities in primary prevention involving environmental change have a social setting focus. They require the modification of an individual's or group's immediate environment or the larger social system. They are particularly appropriate actions when the environment has placed new demands on the person, when it is not responding to the person's developmental needs, and when it provides a diminished level of positive reinforcement for the individual. The nursing literature gives evidence that this is not an area of primary prevention in which nurses have been actively involved.

For the individual, various types of environmental changes may prove to promote mental health, including changes in economic, work, housing, or family situations. **Economically,** there may be the location of resources for financial aid or assistance obtained in budgeting and managing of income. **Work** changes may include vocational testing, guidance, education, or retraining that can result in a change of jobs or careers. It may also mean that an adolescent, a homemaker, or an older adult may be placed in a new career. Changes in **housing** can involve moving to new quarters, which may mean leaving family and friends or returning to them, improvements in existing housing, or the addition or subtraction of coinhabitants, whether they are family, friends, or roommates. Environmental changes that may benefit the **family** include attaining child care facilities, enrolling in a nursery school, grade school, or camp, or obtaining access to recreational, social, religious, or community facilities.

The potential benefit of all of these changes should not be minimized or overlooked by mental health practitioners. They can promote mental health by increasing coping resources, modifying the nature of stressors, and increasing positive, rewarding, and self-enhancing experiences.

Organizations and Politics. Nurses can also effect environmental changes at a larger organizational and political level. One way is by influencing health-care structures and procedures. They might become involved in training community, nonprofessional caregivers to increase the social supports available to vulnerable groups. Another approach would be to stimulate support for women's issues related to mental health, such as through studying the psychology of women; dispelling sex-role stereotypes; promoting feminist therapy; sponsoring programs, conferences, and workshops on women's issues; and recruiting more women professionals into the mental health field.

Obviously, if nurses believe that their profession makes a valuable contribution to health promotion, they should document the cost-effectiveness and quality of nursing care, lobby for greater patient access by nurses, and seek adequate compensation and reimbursement for nursing services. Many of these goals can be obtained if nursing has greater participation in the decision-making structures of health-care institutions, such as hospital boards, advisory groups, health system agencies, and legislative bodies.

Within organizations, environmental change can be achieved through program consultation (see Chapter 33). Such consultation with a large corporation, for example, may lead to the formulation of more flexible retirement plans or a preretirement counseling program. Involvement in community planning and development can have an impact in many different areas. For instance, a community may be helped to meet the needs of the elderly for educational opportunities, recreational programs, and access to social support networks through telephone tielines or special transportation services. So too, the stress associated with environmental pollutants, such as chemicals and radiation, can be addressed.

Some environmental changes require involvement at the national level that may be directed toward the media's portrayal of violence, laws on drunk driving, gun control legislation, access to family planning services, advocating changes in child-rearing practices, including the provision of day-care centers, flex time and paternity leave, or the passage of equal rights legislation.

Of course, many attitudes in and areas of the broader social system are in need of change, including racism, sexism, ageism, poverty, inadequate housing, and problems with the educational system. The dilemma is that global problems such as these are too broad, too pervasive, and too diffuse to be adequately addressed, let alone resolved. For any prevention strategies to be successful in the future, it will be necessary to document the ways in which a particular group is vulnerable to a specific stressor, how the proposed prevention program will be beneficial and cost effective, and the degree to which it succeeded or failed.

What legislation in your state is being considered that pertains to mental health care? What is your position on it and how can you impact on its potential passage?

Supporting Social Systems

As a primary prevention strategy, supporting social systems is not an approach that attempts to remove or minimize the stressor or risk factor. Rather, its rationale is that of strengthening social supports as a way of buffering or cushioning the effects of a potentially stressful event (Box 11-3).[17] It is an important concept for all levels of prevention—primary, secondary, and tertiary—and it has implications for promoting health, helping people seek assistance earlier, supporting them in times of stress, and aiding the situation of the chronically mentally ill. Social support systems can be helpful in emphasizing the strengths of individuals and families and focusing on health rather than illness.[25]

Given the goal that social support systems should be maximized, how can this be achieved? First, how much

---

Box 11-3

SUPPORT SYSTEM ENHANCEMENT

DEFINITION

Facilitation of support to patient by family, friends, and community

ACTIVITIES

Assess psychological response to situation and availability of support system

Determine adequacy of existing social networks

Identify degree of family support

Identify degree of family financial support

Determine support systems currently used

Determine barriers to using support systems

Monitor current family situation

Encourage the patient to participate in social and community activities

Encourage relationships with persons who have common interests and goals

Refer to a self-help group as appropriate

Assess community resource adequacy to identify strengths and weaknesses

Refer to a community-based promotion/prevention/treatment/rehabilitation program as appropriate

Provide services in a caring and supportive manner

Involve family/significant others/friends in the care and planning

Explain to concerned others how they can help

From McCloskey J, Bulechek G: *Nursing interventions classification*, St Louis, 1992, Mosby.

social support a high-risk group needs has to be determined then compared with the amount of social support that is available. Although the question is straightforward, it is complicated by the fact that there are multiple determinants of each element. The need for social support is influenced by predisposing factors, the nature of the stressors, and the availability of other coping resources such as economic assets, individual abilities and skills, and defensive techniques. The availability of social supports is similarly influenced by predisposing factors such as age, sex, socioeconomic status, the nature of the stressor, and the characteristics of the environment. Acute episodic stressors tend to elicit more intense support, whereas in chronic problems, support resources tend to not persist. So too, changes or stressors viewed in a positive way by the individual's social network, such as the birth of a baby or a promotion, may elicit a great deal of support, whereas a negative event, such as a sudden death, may generate little support.

In addition, the quantity and type of social support that meets one need may not meet another. Research suggests that different characteristics of social support may be needed for different stresses. The match between the type and level of social support and the nature of the stressor is an important, but not entirely understood, one.

Types of Interventions. Even though many variables related to social support need further study, social support can still be used to design and implement interventions in primary prevention. Four particular types of interventions are possible.

First, social support patterns can be used to assess communities and neighborhoods to identify problem areas and high-risk groups. Not only will information about the quality of life be gained, but also the social isolation of a particular group might become apparent as well as central individuals whose aid may then be enlisted in developing community-based programs.

A second preventive intervention would be to improve linkages between community support systems and formal mental health services. Often mental health professionals are not aware of or comfortable with the existence or functioning of community support systems. To correct this, they should be taught the skills involved in using and mobilizing community resources and social support systems. All health-care providers need to recognize when patients need social support and to provide them with access to appropriate community support systems.

The third type of intervention is to strengthen natural, existing caregiving networks. Health professionals can provide information and support to the variety of informal caregivers in the community who serve a very important and somewhat different function than more formalized and organized support systems. Informal support systems provide the following:

1. A natural training ground for the development of problem-solving skills
2. A medium in which personal growth and development is based on repeated episodes of people learning to direct the process of change for themselves
3. A supportive milieu that capitalizes on the strength of existing ties among people in our communities, rather than fragmenting intact social units on the basis of diagnosed needs or specialized services

A fourth possible intervention may be to help the person or group develop, maintain, and use a network. The person may also be encouraged to consider network expansion. This might require health education strategies with the goal of competence building. Alternatively, the network can be influenced more directly. Network therapy involves assembling and mobilizing all the important members of the family's kin and friendship network. The focus is then on tightening social bonds

---

> **Box 11-4**
> ## CHARACTERISTICS OF SELF-HELP GROUPS
>
> Supportive and educational in nature rather than therapeutic
> Based on shared experiences and the fact that the individual is not alone
> Focus on a single life-disrupting event
> Purpose is to support personal responsibility and change
> Anonymous and confidential in nature
> Voluntary membership
> Members lead the group and implement principles of self-governance
> Nonprofit orientation

within the network and breaking dysfunctional patterns. For families who are isolated and whose networks are depleted, network members may not be available for such a strategy. In this case, arranging for the use of mutual support groups may be effective.

Informal Support Groups. Numerous informal support groups exist. They may include church groups, civic organizations, clubs, women's groups, or work and neighborhood supports. Self-help groups are becoming more common as members organize themselves to solve their own problems. The members all share a common experience, work together toward a common goal, and use their strengths to gain control over their lives. The processes involved in self-help groups are social affiliation, learning self-control, modeling methods to cope with stress, and acting to change the social environment. Characteristics of self-help groups are listed in Box 11-4.[24]

Self-help groups are familiar to the public through such groups as Alcoholics Anonymous, Weight Watchers, Parents Without Partners, Recovery, and Parents Anonymous. They have demonstrated their ability to help those people experiencing psychiatric problems,[11] as well as grief reactions, such as widows and parents of children who died of sudden infant death syndrome. Since self-help groups use a variety of methods and membership criteria, each group should be assessed individually for its general effectiveness and appropriateness for particular individuals and families.[8,19] Some areas for the nurse to assess before recommending involvement in a self-help group are presented in Box 11-5.[19]

Working with natural, informal support systems should be done cautiously, however, to minimize undesirable consequences. The nurse should attempt to cre-

---

Box 11-5

ASSESSMENT GUIDELINES FOR SELF-HELP GROUPS

QUESTIONS FOR THE GROUP

1. What is its purpose?
2. Who are the group members and leaders?
3. What are the beneficial aspects of the group?
4. For whom would the group not be suitable?
5. What problems are inherent in the group?
6. Is the group effective in preventing further emotional distress?

QUESTIONS FOR THE POTENTIAL MEMBER

1. How does the person feel about attending a self-help group?
2. How compatible is the group and the individual's approach to the problem?
3. How accessible is the group to the potential member?

From Newton G: *J Psychosoc Nurs Ment Health Serv* 22:27, 1984.

---

ate the least amount of disruption possible and not to suppress the natural repertoire of helping behaviors of the informal caregivers.

If an individual's social support is inadequate, interventions may need to be more direct. To determine what interventions are possible, Norbeck[20] suggests that the following questions be asked:

1. What is the capacity of the network to change?
   a. *Network structure.* Are there persons who can be brought into (or back into) the network?
   b. *Network functioning.* Can existing network members be assisted to provide the kind of support that is needed (e.g., allow talk about the pregnancy or about a loss)?
   c. *Network disruption.* Can policies be changed or resources employed to minimize network disruption (e.g., due to hospitalization at a distant tertiary care facility)?
2. Does the individual have the interpersonal skills and attitudes required to establish and maintain contact with network members?
3. Is the individual receptive to using existing self-help or support groups or to having contact with a person who has coped with a similar experience?
4. If help from the indigenous social support system cannot be made available or acceptable, exactly what support does this individual require to cope with the current stressors or illness?
5. What long-term help would be required to assist the individual to establish and maintain an adequate social support network?

Finally, it should be noted that, although supporting social supports is an effective intervention, it is not one that is limited to primary prevention activities. Rather, all nurses in all settings can use this strategy as a way of providing holistic care to maximize the health of individuals, families, and groups.

EVALUATION

When talking about primary prevention, there is a tendency to think in terms of the total elimination of men-

tal illness and stress. Yet these are not realistic goals and maintaining them can only discourage any possible action. Perhaps it is possible to set goals of the reduction in suffering and the enhancement of the capacity to cope. But even these may be unattainable, given that the environment is constantly changing and adaptation is an ongoing challenge. Rather, if the focus is directed toward specific problems of a vulnerable group in society, nursing activity becomes more concentrated and the chance of success increases.

Clearly a need exists for the evaluation of programs in primary prevention. In a world of shrinking resources, only those programs with proven effectiveness are likely to be supported in the future. It needs to be demonstrated that the prevention strategy used has both short-term and long-term effects that benefited the individual and society. Also, it is necessary to determine whether the specific strategy implemented was the one most effective, appropriate, and efficient. Considering alternative approaches and comparing outcomes are essential aspects of the evaluation process.

In the initial evaluation of primary prevention programs, close attention must be given to two points: (1) the program or intervention must be described in reproducible terms, and (2) the target of the intervention program must be stated. The following points should then be considered in evaluating particular primary prevention interventions or programs[21]:

1. *Efficacy.* Does the program or intervention do more good than harm among those who agree to it?
2. *Effectiveness.* Does the intervention do more good than harm to those to whom it is offered?
3. *Efficiency.* Is the intervention being made available to those who could benefit from it with optimal use of resources?
4. *Length and timing of intervention.* Is there any evidence about the optimal length or timing of an intervention program?
5. *Harmful effects.* Are there data to suggest that the interventions may have harmful effects perhaps re-

sulting from the unfavorable consequences of labeling?

6. *Screening programs.* Is there any evidence about the sensitivity, specificity, and predictive accuracy of the screening program?

7. *Possible high-risk groups.* Is there any evidence that the program would be more efficient if it were applied to those at increased risk for the disorder to be prevented?

8. *Economic analysis.* What are the results of the cost-benefit and cost-effectiveness analyses?

Although preventing all illness is not possible, preventing some particular problems is. But a number of barriers exist that make expansion of primary prevention activities difficult. When faced with a choice, the needs of the presently ill consistently take precedence over preventing problems in the future. This holds true for nurses, as well as for the larger society. Yet by being more visionary, both groups could benefit greatly. Nursing has long maintained its role in health education and supportive care. If it can document these actions and their effectiveness, it will demonstrate its value as a profession and its importance in promoting the well-being of society.

SUGGESTED CROSS-REFERENCES

SUMMARY

1. Caplan's three levels of preventive intervention were described. The major thrust in current psychiatric care is in secondary prevention, although primary prevention is beginning to evolve as a major force in the mental health movement.

2. A paradigm for primary prevention was presented that attempts to reduce the incidence of particular stressful life events for vulnerable groups, and it was applied to the nursing process.

3. Assessment in primary prevention was presented as the identification of groups of people who are vulnerable to developing mental disorders or maladaptive coping responses to specific stressors or risk factors.

4. Prevention strategies should be directed toward influencing predisposing factors, precipitating stressors, appraisal of stressors, and coping resources through the following interventions: health education, environmental change, and supporting social systems.

5. In evaluating preventive strategies, one needs to consider specific criteria and use a systematic rating scale of scientific evidence.

COMPETENT CARING
A CLINICAL EXEMPLAR OF A PSYCHIATRIC NURSE

Penelope Chase, MSN, MEd, RN, CS

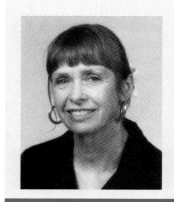

I was changing planes, having just left an inspiring psychiatric clinical nurse specialist conference in Florida, and was on my way to Boston to attend the reunion of my diploma nursing school. I was traveling alone and feeling safe from social interruptions. I was looking forward to some anonymity and a time to reflect and rest.

As I approached the check-in counter of the airport, I saw a young woman sitting nearby in the waiting area. The seats on either side of her were empty except for a soft knapsack on her left. She was wearing the loose-fitting cotton clothing and the nylon-strap sandals that college students often wear. She looked as if she were about to burst into tears or change her mind about being here and dash for the exit. I stopped in my tracks to observe her without being aware of deciding to do so. She turned her head with stiff, slightly jerky movements.

"Responding to internal stimuli," "seizure disorder," "hasn't taken her psychotropic medication" went through my professional mind, while "don't get involved" went through my personal mind, along with, "You're on vacation. Don't mess it up. Relax, you're not the only one who can help." So, I went ahead and checked in. I chose to wait in a seat in the row behind the young woman. "She may not be able to ask for help. I should assess further," my professional self reasoned. Maybe she's not alone. Maybe someone is traveling with her and will be back in a minute.

She compared her ticket information with the boarding announcement and sat back in her seat. A moment later, she shifted in her seat and put her hands over her face. It was then that I noticed that a man, somewhat older than she, seated two rows away and facing her was watching her intensely. My private self was afraid he might be a lonely traveler sizing up a vulnerable young woman that he could take advantage of. I intensified my vigil. I would be her advocate and protector.

I read a bit in my novel, keeping my peripheral vision and ears attuned in her direction. I had difficulty concentrating on my reading because I was constantly interrupted by imposing, opposing thoughts of "Do something" and "Let it be." At one point a uniformed airline employee passed near me on his way out the boarding door. I approached him and said, "I think there's a young lady in trouble here." "I'm a pilot," he replied. "The person you need to talk with is that gentleman at the counter." I wondered what I should do? If I were to say something, the young woman might be embarrassed, delayed, or asked to answer questions that might destroy whatever composure and dignity she was able to preserve. She had not indicated she needed any help . . . yet.

I was still deliberating when my flight was called. The young woman looked at her ticket, got up, and joined the line. I sat and waited until my row number was called. As the flight attendant checked the young woman's boarding pass, she looked carefully at the anguished face, then asked, "Are you okay"? The girl nodded. "Are you sure"? Another nod, but the flight attendant paused in her checking and turned briefly to watch as the girl began down the boarding ramp. It was then that I decided how to resolve my professional-helper's dilemma. I identified myself to the flight attendant as a psychiatric nurse and said that if there were an emergency, they could call on

me. "Oh, you noticed her, too," the woman smiled. "Thank you."

I had just gotten settled in my seat when the flight attendant approached me. "I pulled her up in the computer. It's an emergency flight—a death in the family." "Oh," I ventured, the underlying cause of the scenario suddenly becoming clearer in my mind. "Loss and grief are one of my specialties. I'd be happy to sit with her if she'd like, but only if she says she'd like someone with her." I suddenly remembered traveling 450 miles, mostly alone, to my younger brother's funeral.

Within a few minutes the flight attendant returned saying, "She said she'd like that." So, I took my purse and moved toward the back of the plane. As I approached her seat, the young woman looked up at me. I smiled, introduced myself by name, and said I was the person who would sit with her if that would be all right. She nodded assent, managed a wan smile, and said, "Thank you." I was trying to decide what my role would be. This was all happening rather quickly, yet somewhere in my gut or heart I knew it would be okay. I knew I wanted to stay in my role of a psychiatric nurse and a representative of my profession, and I was also aware that in a couple of hours our relationship would be ending. The time limit helped me focus on my goal of simply being available to her as a support.

Realizing that my seat partner was probably in the initial stage of shock in the grief process and thus lacked her usual coping skills, I decided to do a bit of framing for her. "The flight attendant told me you had a death in your family. I'm sorry," I said. "I'm a nurse who works with people who are going through losses. You could talk about it if you want to, or I could just sit here and read my book. It's up to you." I offered her two simple choices.

She sat silently, but with slightly changing facial expressions, and I thought she was getting ready to speak. I focused my attention softly on her and waited. "He wasn't supposed to die. He was going to have chemotherapy," she began. As her story unfolded, I listened, asked clarifying questions occasionally, and acknowledged her words and anguish. In between bits of content, I learned that she was being met by friends of the family and her sister at the airport with a subsequent 45-minute drive until she was in her hometown. At one point she said sadly, "Now he'll never see his grandchildren," and buried

Continued.

her head on my shoulder and sobbed for a little while. After a bit she said, "I think I need to sleep." That sounded like a good idea to me. As she slept, I evaluated what had unfolded and thought about where to go from here. I needed a plan for closure, for termination of the intervention.

I thought of how long she would have to stand in the aisle waiting to get off this big plane. I asked the flight attendant if there were some way the young woman could be one of the first passengers off the plane. We were moved to the first-class section near the door after she awoke. We talked briefly of how she wanted to depart. I let her know I was available to walk off the plane with her if she wanted and that I thought she could manage "just fine" without me,

as well. "I'll be alright," she said, giving me a hug as we stood up to disembark. "You don't know how much we appreciate this," the flight attendant said to me with sincere eye contact. I acknowledged her thanks. I motioned for my seat-mate to go ahead of me. As we approached the waiting area, I looked questioningly at her to see how she was managing. "I've got it," she said, and gave me the thumbs-up sign. I smiled and walked on.

I was met by two classmates and felt clear, reflective, and exhilarated. I felt that my clinical skills had positively influenced the outcome. I felt I had acted in a professionally responsible and caring manner. I felt good about being a psychiatric nurse. ▼

REFERENCES

1. American Federation of Television and Radio Artists and the Screen Actors Guild: *Women and minorities in television*, Pennsylvania, 1993, Annenberg School for Communication, University of Pennsylvania.
2. Atkins F: An uncertain future: children of mentally ill parents, J *Psychosoc Nurs Ment Health Serv* 30:13, 1992.
3. Beardslee W et al: Initial findings on preventive intervention for families with parental affective disorders, Am J *Psychiatry* 149:1335, 1992.
4. Bloom B: Prevention of mental disorders: recent advances in theory and practice, *Community Ment Health J* 15:179, 1979.
5. Borinstein A: Public attitudes toward persons with mental illness, *Health Affairs* Fall 1992, p 186.
6. Caplan G: *Principles of preventive psychiatry*, New York, 1964, Basic Book.
7. Duvall E: *Marriage and family development*, Philadelphia, 1977, JB Lippincott.
8. Emerick R: Self-help groups for former patients: relations with mental health professionals, H*osp Community Psychiatry* 41:401, 1990.
9. Erikson E: *Childhood and society*, New York, 1963, WW Norton.
10. Fink P, Tasman A: *Stigma and mental illness*, Washington, DC, 1992, American Psychiatric Press.
11. Galanter M: Zealous self-help groups as adjuncts to psychiatric treatment: a study of recovery, Am J *Psychiatry* 145:1248, 1988.
12. Goldston S: A survey of prevention activities in state mental health authorities, *Professional Psychology* 26:315, 1991.
13. Gorzka P, Blair C, Steckel A, Escallier L: Parenting: categories for anticipatory guidance, J *Child Psychiatr Nurs* 4:16, 1991.
14. Gross D: At risk: children of the mentally ill, J *Psychosoc Nurs Ment Health Serv* 27:14, 1989.
15. Killeen M, Smith C, Killinger P: Using Head Start centers

for teaching mental health promotion, J *Child Psychiatr Nurs* 3:79, 1990.
16. Marshall E, Buckner E, Powell K: Evaluation of a teen parent program designed to reduce child abuse and neglect and to strengthen families, J *Child Psychiatr Nurs* 4:96, 1991.
17. McCloskey J, Bulechek G: *Nursing interventions classification*, St Louis, 1992, Mosby.
18. Mrazek P, Haggerty R: *Reducing risks for mental disorders*, Washington, DC, 1994, National Academy Press.
19. Newton G: Self-help groups: can they help? J *Psychosoc Nurs Ment Health Serv* 22:27, 1984.
20. Norbeck J: Social support: a model for clinical research and application, *Adv Nurs Sci* 3:42, 1981.
21. Offord D: Primary prevention: aspects of program design and evaluation, J Am *Acad Child Psychiatry* 21:225, 1982.
22. Opie N, Slater P: Mental health needs of children in school, J *Child Psychiatr Nurs* 1:31, 1988.
23. Redman B: *The process of patient education*, St Louis, 1993, Mosby.
24. Roots L, Aaanes D: A conceptual framework for understanding self-help groups, H*osp Community Psychiatry* 43:379, 1992.
25. Stewart M: *Integrating social support in nursing*, Newbury Park, Calif, 1993, Sage.
26. Streff M: Examining family growth and development: a theoretical model, *Adv Nurs Sci* 3:61, 1981.
27. US Department of Health and Human Services: *Healthy people* 2000, Washington, DC, 1990, Public Health Service.

ANNOTATED SUGGESTED READINGS

Albee G, Joffee J, Dusenbury F: *Prevention, powerless, and politics: readings on social change*, Beverly Hills, Calif, 1988, Sage Publications.
    Argues that prevention will require social change and a redistribution of power.
Blumenkrantz D: *Fulfilling the promise of children's services: why primary prevention efforts fail and how they can succeed*, San Francisco, 1992, Jossey Bass.

Uses a series of stories to illustrate key concepts essential for the successful delivery of community-based primary care initiatives.

*Bushy A, Smith T: Lobbying: the hows and wherefores, Nurs Manage 21:39, 1990.

Describes how, by becoming politically active, nurses can influence change in the health-care system. Reviews the process of lobbying.

Fink P, Tasman A: *Stigma and mental illness*, Washington, DC, 1992, American Psychiatric Press.

Educates both professionals and the public of the pervasiveness of the stigmatization of mental illness.

*Gross D: At risk: children of the mentally ill, J *Psychosoc Nurs Ment Health Serv* 27:14, 1989.

Well-written discussion of the forgotten problem of children of the mentally ill with implications for preventive psychiatric nursing care.

Group for the Advancement of Psychiatry: *Psychiatric prevention and the family life cycle*, New York, 1989, Brunner/Mazel.

Identified risks at each family life cycle stage and provides specific risk-reduction techniques that are developmentally appropriate and designed to be implemented in a diversity of settings and by a range of family practitioners.

Price R, Cowen E, Lorion R, Ramos-McKay J: The search for effective prevention programs: what we learned along the way, Am J Orthopsych 59:49, 1989.

---

*Nursing reference.

Summarizes model prevention programs for high-risk groups throughout the life span. Program content is described, and implications for planning, implementing, and evaluating effective programs are discussed.

*Redman B: *The process of patient education*, St Louis, 1993, Mosby.

The definitive text on patient education. Should be on the book shelf of every nurse.

Roberts A, ed: *Contemporary perspectives on crisis intervention and prevention*, Englewood Cliffs, NJ, 1991, Prentice Hall.

Grounded discussion of primary and secondary prevention with implications for practice.

*Stewart M: *Integrating social support in nursing*, Newbury Park, Calif, 1993, Sage Publications.

Excellent discussion of the contributions nurses have made to understanding social support based on research and nursing theory.

*Welch M, Boyd M, Bell D: Education in primary prevention in psychiatric–mental health nursing for the baccalaureate student, International Nurs Rev 34:128, 1987.

Discusses how the concept of primary prevention can be taught to students of psychiatric nursing.

---

*Nursing reference.

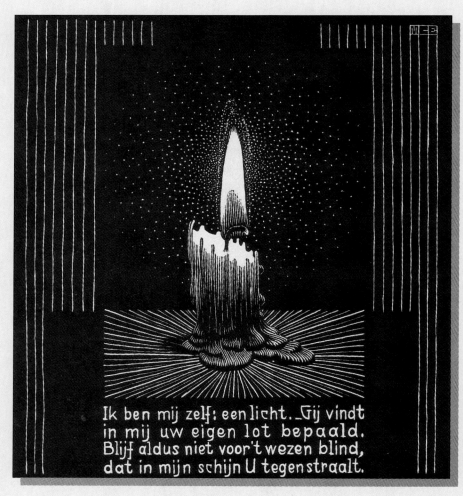

Ik ben mij zelf: een licht. Gij vindt
in mij uw eigen lot bepaald.
Blijf aldus niet voor't wezen blind,
dat in mijn schijn U tegenstraalt.

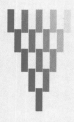

CHAPTER 12
Crisis Intervention

SANDRA E. BENTER

He knows not his own strength that hath not met adversity.

Francis Bacon: Of Fortune

Historically, those who studied and practiced preventive psychiatry used psychoanalytical concepts to develop crisis theory. They explored the possibility of intervening briefly during stressful periods to resolve problems in a healthy way. They observed the phases that people go through during stressful situations and studied the outcomes of the crises. Crisis intervention techniques were then identified for promoting healthy outcomes.

In 1944 Eric Lindemann[16] studied 101 patients who lost a relative during the course of psychiatric treatment, relatives of patients who died in the hospital, bereaved disaster victims (Coconut Grove fire) and their relatives, and relatives of members of the armed forces. He observed the course of normal grief and the symptoms of morbid grief reactions and thought that mental health workers could help free these individuals from their ties to the deceased. Lindemann also believed that the concept of intervention during bereavement could be applied to other stressful situations such as marriage and childbirth. He thought this could take place in the community and be patterned after a public health model so that many people could be reached. Lindemann, along with Gerald Caplan, set up a community mental health clinic in Massachusetts, where crisis intervention was first practiced as a brief, direct, and time-limited treatment strategy. It has since become an accepted and common intervention for nurses and other health-care providers.

CONTINUUM OF CRISIS RESPONSES
Adaptive and Maladaptive Crisis Responses

A **crisis** is a disturbance caused by a stressful event or a perceived threat to self. The person's usual way of coping becomes ineffective in dealing with the threat, causing anxiety. The threat, or precipitating event, can usually be identified. It may have occurred weeks or days ago, and it may or may not be linked (in the individual's eyes) to the crisis state. Precipitating events are perceived losses, threats of losses, or challenges.

After the precipitating event the person's anxiety rises and four phases of a crisis[5] emerge. In the first phase the anxiety activates the person's usual methods of coping. If these do not bring relief and there is inadequate support, the person moves to the second phase, which involves more anxiety because coping mechanisms have failed. In the third phase new coping mechanisms are tried or the threat is redefined so that old ones can work. Resolution of the problem therefore can occur in this phase. However, if resolution does not occur, the person goes on to the fourth phase in which the continuation of severe or panic levels of anxiety may lead to psychological disorganization. This is discussed in detail in Chapter 14.

In describing the phases of a crisis, it is important to consider the balancing factors identified by Aguilera[1] and shown in Fig. 12-1. These include the individual's perception of the event, situational supports, and coping mechanisms. Successful resolution of the crisis is more likely if the person has a realistic view of the event, if situational supports are available to help solve the problem, and if effective coping mechanisms are present.

The phases of a crisis and the impact of balancing factors are similar to the components of the stress adaptation model described in Chapter 4. However, by definition, crises are self-limiting. People in crisis are too upset to function at such a high level of anxiety indefinitely. A period of 6 weeks has been considered the time needed for resolution, whether it be a positive solution or a state of disorganization. However, some consider it unlikely that any specific time can be applied to all people undergoing crises.[2]

It is also important to recognize that periods of intense conflict can result in increased growth as seen in the continuum of crisis responses (Fig. 12-2). How the crisis is handled determines whether growth or disorganization will result. Growth comes from learning in new situations. People in crisis feel uncomfortable, often reach out for help, and accept help until they feel that their lives are back to normal. The fact that crises can lead to personal growth is important to remember when working with patients in crisis.

> Think of a crisis you have experienced. Do you feel that the way you handled it made you a better person in some way? If so, how?

Types of Crises

There are three types of crises: maturational, situational, and adventitious. Sometimes these crises can occur simultaneously. For example, an adolescent who is having difficulty adjusting to a change in role and body image (maturational crisis) may at the same time undergo the stress related to the death of a parent (situational crisis).

Maturational. Developmental psychology describes a series of steps that must be taken in growing toward maturity. During this process the transitional periods between stages can upset psychological equilibrium. These developmental stages are described in Chapter 11.

Maturational crises are developmental events requiring role changes. For example, successful progression

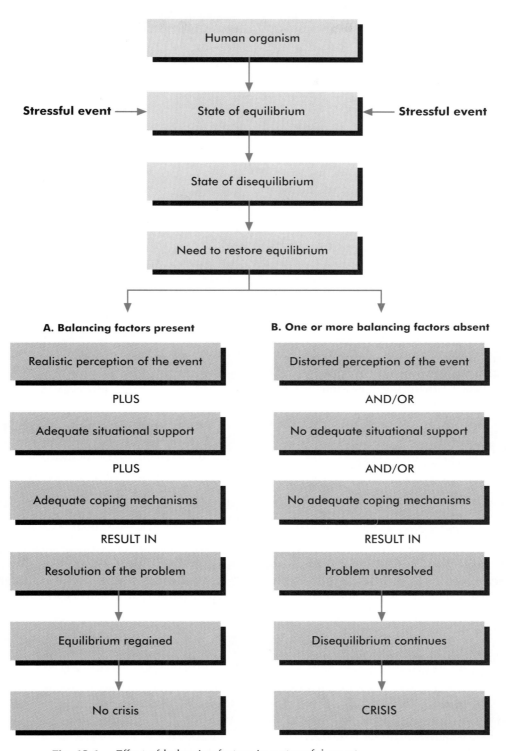

Fig. 12-1   Effect of balancing factors in a stressful event.
From Aguilera DC: *Crisis intervention: theory and methodology,* ed 7, St Louis, 1994, Mosby.

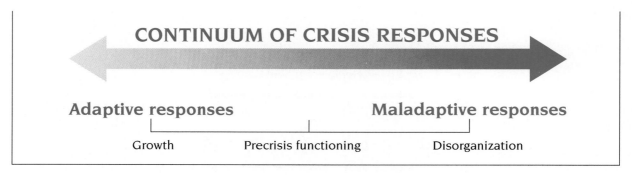

CONTINUUM OF CRISIS RESPONSES

Adaptive responses   Maladaptive responses

Growth   Precrisis functioning   Disorganization

Fig. 12-2   Continuum of crisis responses.

from early childhood to middle childhood requires the child to become socially involved with people outside the family. With the move from adolescence to adulthood, financial responsibility is expected. Both social and biological pressures to change can precipitate a crisis.

The nature and extent of the maturational crisis can be influenced by role models, interpersonal resources, and the ease of others in accepting the new role. Positive role models show the person how to act in the new role. Interpersonal resources encourage the trying out of new behaviors to achieve role changes. The ease of others in accepting the new role is also important. The greater the resistance of others, the more stress the person faces in making the changes.

Transitional periods during adolescence, parenthood, marriage, midlife, and retirement are key times for the onset of maturational crises. Some conflicts related to maturational crises are seen in the clinical examples that follow.

CLINICAL EXAMPLE

Ms. J was a 19-year-old black, single, unemployed woman who came to the mental health clinic a month after the birth of her first child. Ms. J complained of feeling depressed. Her symptoms included difficulty falling asleep, early morning awakening, crying spells, a poor appetite, difficulty in caring for the baby because of fatigue and apathy, and thoughts of wanting to hurt the baby. The patient lived with her parents and siblings and had never lived on her own. She had always been dependent on her mother to take care of her. Her mother worked, however, and the patient was totally responsible for her daughter's care each day. Also, Ms. J's mother was angry that she had had a child and often refused to care for the baby. The patient's boyfriend, who was the baby's father, had promised to marry her, but he had recently decided he was too young to handle the responsibility of a wife and child.

In summary, the young woman who had unmet dependency needs of her own was now a parent and had to meet the dependency needs of her infant. This precipitated a crisis for her.

Selected Nursing Diagnoses:
▼ Ineffective individual coping related to birth of a child as evidenced by feelings of depression
▼ Altered family processes related to birth of a grandchild as evidenced by lack of family support
▼ Altered parenting related to being a single mother as evidenced by thoughts of hurting her baby

CLINICAL EXAMPLE

Mr. R was a 67-year-old white, married pharmacist who came to the mental health clinic complaining of anxiety, depression, and insomnia. His symptoms had begun 2 weeks ago when his wife decided that they should move to a retirement community in Florida. He described his wife as a strong, willful woman who was also outgoing and charming and made friends easily. He considered himself a quiet, nervous person who was comfortable only with old friends and his two sons and their families. Mr. R, although at retirement age, had continued to work as a pharmacist, doing relief work for a drugstore chain when the regular pharmacists were absent. In moving to Florida, he would lose his pharmacist's license, which was valid only within his state of residence. He expressed difficulty in making the transition from a working person to a retired person. He had fears of becoming directionless and useless. He was anxious about leaving his sons and his friends. The possibility of both complete retirement and moving to another state precipitated his present distress.

Selected Nursing Diagnoses:
▼ Relocation stress syndrome related to pending retirement as evidenced by feelings of anxiety
▼ Altered family processes related to conflict about lifestyle changes as evidenced by inability to plan future

Situational. Situational crises occur when a life event upsets an individual's or a group's psychological equilibrium. Examples of situational crises include loss of a job, loss of a loved one, unwanted pregnancy, onset or worsening of a medical illness, divorce, school problems, and witnessing a crime.

The loss of a job can result in financial stress, feelings of inadequacy as a breadwinner, and marital conflict caused by a spouse's anger over the lost job. The loss of a loved one results in bereavement and can also cause financial stress, change in roles of family members, and loss of emotional support. Homelessness is another possible outcome of either the loss of a job or a loved one. The onset or worsening of a medical illness causes fear of the loss of a loved one. Again, financial stress and change in roles of family members often occur. Divorce is similar to the stress of the loss of a loved one, and there is the stress of dealing with the ex-spouse as well. An unwanted pregnancy is stressful because it requires decisions to be made about whether to complete the pregnancy or to abort it, and whether to keep the baby or place it for adoption. If the baby is to be kept, changes in life-style will be required. School problems can also lead to feelings of inadequacy. Parents often blame themselves or each other, and serious family conflict can result. Finally, being the victim of or witnessing a crime can cause feelings of helplessness, distrust of others, and guilt about causing or not stopping the crime.

Adventitious. Adventitious crises are accidental, uncommon, and unexpected events. Multiple losses with major environmental changes result. For example, fires, earthquakes, hurricanes, or floods, which disrupt entire communities, are adventitious crises (Fig. 12-3). Recent mass tragedies, which have become all too common, are also examples of adventitious crises and include group kidnappings (the taking of hostages), group killings in the workplace, airplane crashes, riots in cities, and the explosion of terrorist-planted bombs in crowded areas.

Unlike maturational and situational crises, adventitious crises do not occur in the lives of everyone. When they do occur, however, they challenge every coping mechanism because of the severity of the stress. During adventitious crises, mental health workers must reach larger numbers of people in crisis states. The multiple losses and major environmental changes that result from adventitious crises can be seen in the following situation.

At 5:04 PM on October 17, 1989, northern California was struck by an earthquake measuring 7.1 on the Richter scale. The epicenter was about 70 miles south of San Francisco, and the eruption extended north beyond San Francisco causing fatalities and severe damage to the marina area and Oakland's Cypress Structure. The economic impact from the earthquake

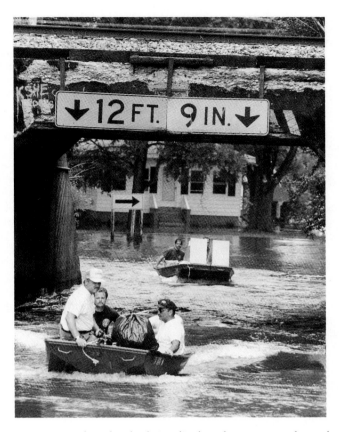

Fig. 12-3 The Flood of '93 displaced many people and caused millions of dollars worth of damage in many communities in the Midwest.

Photograph from High and mighty: the flood of '93, © 1993, St. Louis Post-Dispatch; Jim Rackwitz, photographer.

was estimated at $8.3 billion in direct losses. There were 62 deaths and 3000 injuries. Approximately 116,882 buildings were damaged, and 14,000 people were left homeless.[15]

Disaster-precipitated emotional problems often surface weeks or even months after the disaster. The symptoms usually occur in roughly five phases, which are described in Table 12-1.[10] If the reconstruction phase does not begin within 6 months after the disaster, the likelihood of lasting psychological problems is greatly increased. The severe psychological stress resulting from adventitious crises is described by Terr,[29] who studied 23 child kidnap victims:

In the town of Chowchilla, California, a school bus containing 26 children and a bus driver was stopped by three masked men and taken over at gunpoint. The captured children were driven around in boarded-over vans for 11 hours and were then transferred to a buried truck trailer. After 16 additional hours, two of the oldest boys dug them out. The children suffered from initial misperceptions, fears of further trauma, and hallucinations. Later they experienced posttraumatic play reenactment, personality changes, repeated dreams, fears of being kidnapped again, and a fear of common mundane experiences.

Table 12-1 Five Phases of Human Disaster Response

Phase	Response
Impact	Includes the event itself and is characterized by shock, panic, or extreme fear; the person's judgment and assessment of reality factors are very poor, and self-destructive behavior may be seen.
Heroic	A cooperative spirit exists between friends, neighbors, and emergency teams; constructive activity at this time can help to overcome feelings of anxiety and depression, but over-activity can lead to "burnout."
Honeymoon	Begins to appear 1 week to several months after the disaster; the need to help others is sustained, and the money, resources, and support received from various agencies allow life to begin again in the community; psychological and behavioral problems may be overlooked.
Disillusionment	Lasts from about 2 months to 1 year; a time of disappointment, resentment, frustration, and anger; victims often begin to compare their neighbors' plights with their own and may start to resent, envy, or show hostility toward others.
Reconstruction and reorganization	Individuals recognize that they must come to grips with their own problems; they begin to rebuild their homes, businesses, and lives in a constructive fashion; this period may last for years after the disaster.

Data from Frederick C, Garrison J: *Behav Today* 12:32, 1981.

 Some crises, such as obtaining a divorce, develop over time and are of longer duration. Other crises, such as an earthquake, are sudden and unexpected. How do you think the element of time affects the response to crisis?

Describe how sociocultural factors might affect a woman's decision whether or not to seek help after being raped.

Crisis Intervention

Aguilera[1] believes that crisis intervention can offer the immediate help that a person in crisis needs. It is an inexpensive, short-term therapy focused on solving the immediate problem, and it is usually limited to 6 weeks. The goal of crisis intervention is for the individual to return to a precrisis level of functioning. Often the person advances to a level of growth that is higher than the precrisis level because new ways of problem solving have been learned.

It is important for the nurse to remember that cultural attitudes strongly influence the communication and response style of the crisis worker. These attitudes are deeply ingrained in the processes of asking for, giving, and receiving help. They also affect the victimization experience, so it is essential to understand and respect the cultural values of the victims. Specific cultural factors to be considered in crisis intervention include the following[7]:

1. Migration and citizenship status
2. Gender and family roles
3. Religious belief systems
4. Child-rearing practices
5. Use of extended family and support systems

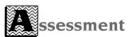ssessment

The first step of crisis intervention is assessment. During this phase, data regarding the nature of the crisis and its effect on the patient must be collected. It is from these data that a plan for intervention will be developed. During this phase the nurse begins to establish a positive working relationship with the patient. A number of specific areas should be assessed by the nurse. These are the balancing factors that are important in the development and resolution of a crisis and include the following:

1. Precipitating event or stressor
2. Patient's perception of the event or stressor
3. Nature and strength of the patient's support systems and coping resources
4. Patient's previous strengths and coping mechanisms

The components of the stress adaptation model that parallel the balancing factors in crisis intervention are highlighted in Fig. 12-4.

Behaviors

People in crisis experience many symptoms including those listed in Box 12-1. Sometimes these symp-

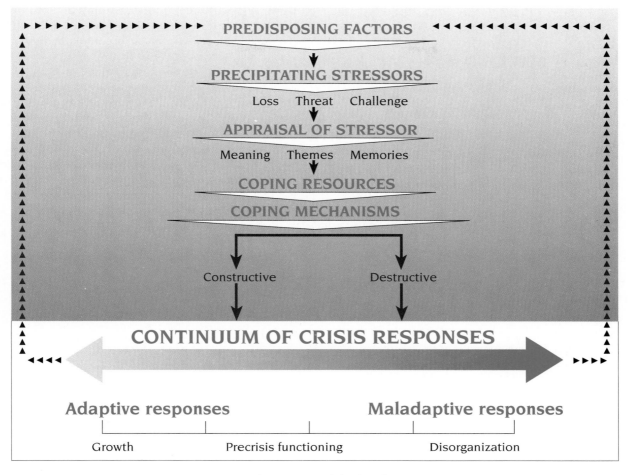

Fig. 12-4   A stress adaptation model related to crisis responses.

toms can cause further problems. For example, problems at work may lead to loss of a job, financial stress, and lowered self-esteem. Crises can also be complicated by old conflicts that can be brought out by the current problem, making crisis resolution more difficult.

Precipitating Event

To help identify the precipitating event, the nurse should explore the patient's needs, the events that threaten those needs, and the time at which symptoms appear. Four kinds of needs that have been identified are related to self-esteem, sexual role mastery, dependency, and biological function.[26] *Self-esteem* is achieved when the person attains successful social role experience. *Sexual role mastery* is achieved when the person attains vocational, sexual, and family role successes. *Dependency* is achieved when a satisfying interdependent relationship with others is attained. *Biological function* is

achieved when a person is safe and life is not threatened.

The nurse determines which needs are not being met by asking the patient to reflect on issues regarding self-image and self-esteem, on the areas of life that are considered a success, on the kinds of relationships with others, and on the degree of safety and security in life. The nurse looks for obstacles that might interfere with meeting the patient's needs. What recent experiences have been upsetting? What areas of life have had changes?

Coping patterns become ineffective and symptoms appear usually after the stressful incident. When did the patient begin to feel anxious? When did sleep disturbances begin? At what point in time did suicidal thoughts start? If symptoms began last Tuesday, ask what took place in the patient's life on Tuesday or Monday. As the patient connects life events with the breakdown in coping mechanisms, an understanding of the precipitating event can emerge.

Box 12-1

BEHAVIORS COMMONLY EXHIBITED AFTER A CRISIS

Anger	Headaches	Poor concentra-
Apathy	Helplessness	tion
Backaches	Hopelessness	Sadness
Boredom	Insomnia	School problems
Crying spells	Intrusive	Self-doubt
Diminished	thoughts	Shock
sexual drive	Irritability	Social withdrawal
Disbelief	Lability	Substance abuse
Fatigue	Nightmares	Suicidal thoughts
Flashbacks	Numbness	Survivor guilt
Forgetfulness	Overeating or	Work difficulties
	undereating	

Perception of the Event

The patient's perception or appraisal of the precipitating event is very important. What may seem trivial to the nurse may have great meaning to the patient. An overweight adolescent girl may have been the only girl in the class not invited to a dance. This may have threatened her self-esteem. A man with two unsuccessful marriages may have just been told by a girlfriend that she wants to end their relationship; this may have threatened his need for sexual role mastery. An emotionally isolated, friendless woman may have had car trouble and been unable to find someone to give her a ride to work. This may have threatened her dependency needs. A chronically ill man who has had a recent relapse of his illness may have had his need for biological function threatened.

Themes and surfacing memories of the patient give further clues to the precipitating event. Current issues of concern are often connected to past issues of concern. For example, a female patient who talks about the death of her father, which occurred 3 years ago, may, on questioning, reveal a recent loss of a relationship with a male. A patient who talks about feelings of inadequacy he had as a child because of poor school performance may, on questioning, reveal a recent experience in which his feelings of adequacy on his job were threatened. Since most crises involve losses or threats of losses, the theme of losses is a common one expressed. In assessment the nurse looks for a recent event that may be connected to an underlying theme.

Support Systems and Coping Resources

The patient's living situation and supports in the environment must be assessed. Does the patient live alone or with family or friends? With whom is the patient close, and who offers understanding and strength? Is there a supportive clergyman or friend? Assessing the patient's support system is important in determining who should come for the crisis therapy sessions. It may be decided that certain family members should come with the patient so that the family members' support can be strengthened. If the patient has few supports, participation in a crisis therapy group may be necessary so that the support of other group members can be elicited. Assessing the patient's coping resources is also vital in determining whether hospitalization would be more appropriate than outpatient crisis therapy. If there is a high degree of suicidal and homicidal risk along with weak outside resources, hospitalization may be a safer and more effective treatment.

 Identify people in your social system that you would turn to in a time of crisis. Compare your list with that of a friend.

Coping Mechanisms

Next, the nurse assesses the patient's strengths and previous coping mechanisms. How has the patient handled other crises? How were anxieties relieved? Did the patient talk out problems? Did the patient leave the usual surroundings for a period of time to think things out from another perspective? Was physical activity used to relieve tension? Did the patient find relief in crying? Besides exploring previous coping mechanisms, the nurse should also note the absence of other possible successful mechanisms.

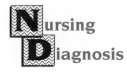

Nursing Diagnosis

Nursing diagnoses may be related to any aspect of the patient's life and can reflect the variety of nursing problems described in Chapters 14 to 24. The primary nursing diagnoses in crisis intervention are ineffective individual coping, ineffective family coping, altered family processes, and post-trauma response. Ineffective individual coping refers to the inability to ask for help, problem solve, or meet role expectations. Ineffective family coping exists when the family's economic or social well-being is threatened and supportive behaviors are not successful. Altered family processes describes a family system that cannot meet the physical or emotional needs of its members, has an inappropriate level or direction of energy, and is unable to adapt to traumatic

MEDICAL AND NURSING DIAGNOSES RELATED TO CRISIS RESPONSES

Related Medical Diagnoses (DSM-IV)*

Adjustment disorder with anxiety
Adjustment disorder with depressed mood
Adjustment disorder with disturbances of conduct
Adjustment disorder with mixed disturbance of emotions and conduct
Adjustment disorder with mixed anxiety and depressed mood
Posttraumatic stress disorder

Related Nursing Diagnoses (NANDA)†

Adjustment, impaired
Anxiety
‡**Coping, ineffective family: compromised**
‡**Coping, ineffective individual**
‡**Family process, altered**
Fear
Grieving, anticipatory
Growth and development, altered
Health maintenance, altered
Knowledge deficit
Parenting, altered
‡**Post-trauma response**
Rape trauma syndrome
Self-esteem disturbance
Social isolation
Spiritual distress

*From American Psychiatric Association: *Diagnostic and statistical manual for mental disorders*, ed 4, Washington, DC, 1994, The Association.
†From North American Nursing Diagnosis Association: NANDA *nursing diagnosis: definitions and classifications* 1992-1993, Philadelphia, 1992, The Association.
‡Primary nursing diagnosis for variations in sexual response.

experiences constructively. Post-trauma response is a sustained painful response to an overwhelming traumatic event. Nursing diagnoses related to the range of possible maladaptive crisis responses are identified along with related medical diagnoses in the Medical and Nursing Diagnoses.

Related Medical Diagnoses

Many patients who require crisis intervention fall under the DSM-IV category of adjustment disorders. These are short-term maladaptive reactions to a stressor that impair social functioning. They are less severe than other psychiatric disorders and are particularly responsive to crisis intervention.

Posttraumatic stress disorder (PTSD) is a type of anxiety disorder that is also often treated by crisis intervention.[13] If not treated early, this disorder can become chronic.[3,8] Two populations that often experience PTSD are trauma victims and war veterans. For example, a national study of Vietnam War veterans found that over one third of the men and one fourth of the women developed PTSD sometime during their lifetime.[14] Another group of people likely to suffer from PTSD are the victims of trauma (see Critical Thinking about Contemporary Issues); this includes rape and abuse victims, crime victims, and those who witness traumatic events. Their long-term adjustment should ideally follow four stages[4]:

1. Recovery
2. Avoidance
3. Reconsideration
4. Adjustment

In recovery victims realize that they are safe. In avoidance they try not to think about their experiences so that they do not have to face overwhelming feelings. In reconsideration they begin to reflect on their experiences and deal with their thoughts and feelings. Finally, having successfully reflected, they enter the stage of adjustment. Immediate psychological help following through these stages may prevent PTSD from becoming a chronic disorder.

Examples of complete NANDA nursing diagnoses related to crisis responses and the essential features of related DSM-IV diagnoses are presented in the Detailed Diagnoses box.

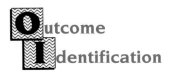

Outcome Identification

The expected outcome when working with a person who has experienced a crisis is:

The patient will recover from the crisis event and return to a precrisis level of functioning.

DETAILED DIAGNOSES
RELATED TO CRISIS RESPONSES

NANDA Diagnosis Stem	Examples of Complete Diagnosis
Coping, ineffective individual	Ineffective individual coping related to child's illness evidenced by limited ability to concentrate and psychomotor agitation.
	Ineffective individual coping related to daughter's death evidenced by inability to recall events pertaining to the car accident.
Coping, ineffective family	Ineffective family coping, compromised, related to separation from husband evidenced by excessive dependency on friends and preoccupation with having husband return home.
	Ineffective family coping, compromised, related to wife's cancer diagnosis evidenced by feelings of grief, fear, and guilt.
Family process, altered	Altered family process related to move to a new town evidenced by social withdrawal and rejection of help from others.
	Altered family process related to marriage of daughter evidenced by unclear family boundaries and distorted communication patterns.
Post-trauma response	Post-trauma response related to witnessing a violent robbery evidenced by nightmares and verbalization of survival guilt.

DSM-IV Diagnosis	Essential Features*
Adjustment disorder	A maladaptive reaction to an identifiable psychosocial stressor that occurs within 3 months of the stressor's onset but has not persisted from more than 6 months; behaviors include impairment in social functioning or symptoms of an excessive reaction to the stressor.
Adjustment disorder with anxiety	Nervousness, worry, jitteriness
Adjustment disorder with depressed mood	Tearfulness or hopelessness
Adjustment disorder with disturbances of conduct	Violation of others' rights or of major age-appropriate societal norms and rules
Adjustment disorder with mixed disturbance of emotions and conduct	Emotional features and disturbance of conduct
Adjustment disorder with mixed anxiety and depressed mood	Combination of depression and anxiety and other disorders
Posttraumatic stress disorder	Development of characteristic symptoms following a psychologically traumatic event that is generally outside the range of usual human experience; symptoms include reexperiencing the event, reduced involvement with the world, distressing dreams of the event, and a variety of anxious and depressed behaviors.

*Adapted from American Psychiatric Association: *Diagnostic and statistical manual for mental disorders*, ed 4, Washington, DC, The Association.

CRITICAL THINKING ABOUT CONTEMPORARY ISSUES

Do Battered Women Fit the DSM-IV Diagnosis of Posttraumatic Stress Disorder (PTSD)?

Battered women experience serious threats and injuries that may result in death. Women living in ongoing abusive relationships are exposed to chronic daily stress in addition to repeated, acute acts of violence. These women may display a wide variety of physiological and psychological reactions that are characteristic of PTSD including re-experiencing of the traumatic event, numbness, avoidance, and hypervigilance. However, do they fit the DSM-IV diagnosis of PTSD?

Much of the literature that supports PTSD as a framework for working with battered women is based on anecdotal reports or clinical observations and experiences. There is little empirical evidence available on the relationship between battered women and PTSD. In addition, many of the behaviors seen in battered women, such as low self-esteem, depression, and self-blame, are not prominent symptoms of PTSD. Woods and Campbell[32] suggest that additional research needs to be conducted on the relationship between battering and the subsequent development of PTSD. They believe that at this time it cannot be assumed that all abused women should be diagnosed with PTSD, that criteria need to be applied carefully to individual cases, and that other possible diagnoses should be considered. ▼

A more ambitious expected outcome would be for the patient to recover from the crisis event to a higher than precrisis level of functioning and improved quality of life.

This overall objective can be made more specific by identifying short-term goals. Some of these may include the following:

1. The patient will describe the crisis event.
2. The patient will explore feelings and emotions related to the event.
3. The patient will discuss ways in which stressful events have been handled in the past.
4. The patient will identify alternative solutions or ways of coping with the crisis situation.
5. The patient will implement one of the possible solutions.
6. The patient will report satisfaction with coping abilities and level of functioning.

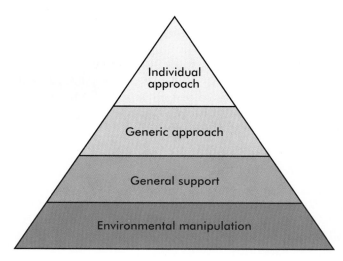

Fig. 12-5   Levels of crisis intervention.

Planning

The next step of crisis intervention is planning; the previously collected data are analyzed and specific interventions are proposed. Dynamics underlying the present crisis are formulated from the information about the precipitating event. Alternative solutions to the problem are explored, and steps for achieving the solutions are identified. The nurse decides which environmental supports to engage or strengthen and how to do this, as well as which of the patient's coping mechanisms to develop and which to strengthen.

Implementation

Interventions can take place on many levels using a variety of techniques. Shields[21] has described four levels of crisis intervention that represent a hierarchy from the most basic to the most complex (Fig. 12-5). Each level incorporates the interventions of the preceding level, and the progressive order indicates that the nurse needs additional knowledge and skill for high-level interventions. It is often helpful to consult with others when deciding which approach to use.

Environmental Manipulation

Environmental manipulation includes interventions that directly change the patient's physical or interpersonal situation. These interventions provide situational support or remove stress. For example, a patient who is having trouble coping with her six children may temporarily send several of the children to their grandparents' house. In this situation some stress is reduced. Similarly, a patient having difficulty on his job may take a week of sick leave so that he can be removed temporarily from that stress. A patient who lives alone may move in with his closest sibling for several days. Likewise, involving the patient in family or group crisis therapy provides environmental manipulation for the purpose of providing support.

General Support

General support includes interventions that convey the feeling that the nurse is on the patient's side and will be a helping person. The nurse uses warmth, acceptance, empathy, caring, and reassurance to provide this type of support.

Generic Approach

The generic approach is designed to reach high-risk individuals and large groups as quickly as possible. It applies a specific method to all individuals faced with a similar type of crisis. The course of the particular type of crisis is previously studied and mapped out. The intervention is then set up to ensure that the course of the crisis results of an adaptive response.

Grief is an example of a crisis with a known pattern that can be treated by the generic approach. Helping the patient to overcome ties to the deceased and find new patterns of rewarding interaction may effectively resolve the grief. Applying this specific intervention to people experiencing grief, especially with a high-risk group such as families of local disaster victims, is an example of the generic approach.

Another example of the generic approach is the use of **debriefing.** Originally a military concept, debriefing can be used as a therapeutic intervention to help individuals or groups recall events and clarify traumatic experiences. It attempts to place the traumatic event in perspective, allows the individual to relive the event in a factual way, and helps to prevent the maladaptive responses that may result if the trauma is suppressed.

Individual Approach

The individual approach is a type of crisis intervention similar to the diagnosis and treatment of a specific problem in a specific patient. The nurse must understand the specific patient's psychodynamics that led to the present crisis and must use the intervention that is most likely to help the patient develop an adaptive response to the crisis.[18] This type of crisis intervention can be effective with all types of crises. It is particularly useful in combined situational and maturational crises. The individual approach is also beneficial when symptoms

include homicidal and suicidal risk. The individual approach should also be applied if the course of the crisis cannot be determined and to crises that have not responded to the generic approach.

 How might each level of crisis intervention be used in a high school after a star player of the football team has just committed suicide?

Techniques

The nurse uses techniques that are active, focal, and explorative to carry out the interventions. The intervention must be aimed at achieving quick resolution. The nurse also must be active in guiding the crisis intervention through its various steps. A passive approach is inappropriate because of the time limitations of the crisis situation.

The nurse should be creative and flexible, trying many different techniques. Some of these include abreaction, clarification, suggestion, manipulation, reinforcement of behavior, support of defenses, raising self-esteem, and exploration of solutions.[19] A brief description of these techniques is presented.

Abreaction is the release of feelings that takes place as the patient talks about emotionally charged areas. As feelings about the events are realized, tension is reduced. Abreaction is often used in crisis intervention. The nurse encourages abreaction by soliciting the patient's feelings about the specific situation, recent events, and significant people involved in the particular crisis. The nurse asks open-ended questions and repeats the patient's words so that more feelings are expressed. The nurse does not discourage crying or angry outbursts but rather sees them as a positive release of feelings. Only when feelings seem out of control, such as in extreme rage or despondency, should the nurse discourage abreaction and help the patient concentrate on thinking rather than feeling. For example, if a patient angrily talks of wanting to kill a specific person, it is better to shift the focus to a discussion of the consequences of carrying out the act rather than to encourage free expression of the angry feelings.

Clarification is used when the nurse helps the patient to identify the relationship between events, behaviors, and feelings. For example, helping a patient see that it was after he was passed over for a promotion that he thought he was too sick to go to work is clarification. Clarification helps the patient gain a better understanding of feelings and how they lead to the development of a crisis.

Suggestion is influencing a person to accept an idea

or belief. In crisis intervention the patient is influenced to see the nurse as a confident, calm, hopeful, empathic person who can help. By believing the nurse can help, the patient may feel more optimistic, less anxious, and may want to please the nurse by getting better.

Manipulation is a technique in which the nurse uses patients' emotions, wishes, or values to their benefit in the therapeutic process. Like suggestion, manipulation is a way of influencing the patient. For example, the nurse may want to point out to the patient who prides himself on his independence that he is responsible for much of the work of solving his problem.

Reinforcement of behavior occurs when healthy, adaptive behavior of the patient is reinforced by the nurse who strengthens positive responses made by the patient be agreeing with or complimenting those responses. For example, when a patient who has passively allowed himself to be criticized by his boss states that he asserted himself in a discussion with his boss, the nurse can tell him she is pleased with his assertiveness.

Support of defenses occurs when the nurse encourages the use of healthy defenses and discourages those that are maladaptive. Defense mechanisms are used to cope with stressful situations and to maintain self-esteem and ego integrity. When defenses deny, falsify, or distort reality to the point that the person cannot deal effectively with reality, they are maladaptive. The nurse should encourage the patient to use adaptive defenses and discourage those that are maladaptive. For example, when a patient denies the fact that her husband wants a separation despite the fact that he has told her so, the nurse can point out that she is not facing facts and dealing realistically with the problem. This is an example of discouraging the maladaptive use of the defense mechanism of denial. If a patient who is furious with his boss writes a letter to his boss's supervisor rather than assaulting his boss, the nurse should encourage the adaptive use of the defense mechanism of sublimation.

In crisis intervention, defenses are not attacked but rather are more gently encouraged or discouraged. When defenses are attacked, the patient cannot maintain self-esteem and ego integrity. There is also not enough time in crisis intervention to replace the attacked defenses with new ones. Returning the patient to a previous level of functioning is the goal of crisis intervention, not the restructuring of defenses.

Raising self-esteem is a particularly important technique. The patient in a crisis feels helpless and may be overwhelmed with feelings of inadequacy. The fact that the patient has found it necessary to seek outside help may further increase feelings of inadequacy. The nurse should help the patient regain feelings of self-worth by communicating confidence that the patient can participate actively in finding solutions to problems. The nurse

---

Box 12-2

TECHNIQUES OF CRISIS INTERVENTION

Technique: **Abreaction**
Definition: The release of feelings that takes place as the patient talks about emotionally charged areas
Example: "Tell me about how you have been feeling since you lost your job."

Technique: **Clarification**
Definition: Encouraging the patient to express more clearly the relationship between certain events
Example: "I've noticed that after you have an argument with your husband you become sick and can't leave your bed."

Technique: **Suggestion**
Definition: Influencing an individual to accept an idea or belief, particularly the belief that the nurse can help and that the individual will feel better
Example: "Many other people have found it helpful to talk about this and I think you will too."

Technique: **Manipulation**
Definition: Using the patient's emotions, wishes, or values to benefit the patient in the therapeutic process
Example: "You seem to be very committed to your marriage and I think that you will work through these issues and have a stronger relationship in the end."

Technique: **Reinforcement of behavior**
Definition: Giving the patient positive responses to adaptive behavior
Example: "That's the first time you were able to defend yourself with your boss and it went very well. I'm so pleased that you were able to do it."

Technique: **Support of defenses**
Definition: Encouraging the use of healthy, adaptive defenses and discouraging those that are unhealthy or maladaptive
Example: "Going for a bicycle ride when you were so angry was very helpful, since when you returned you and your wife were able to talk things through."

Technique: **Raising self-esteem**
Definition: Helping the patient to regain feelings of self-worth
Example: "You are a very strong person to be able to manage the family all this time. I think you will be able to handle this situation too."

Technique: **Exploration of solutions**
Definition: Examining alternative ways of solving the immediate problem
Example: "You seem to know many people in the computer field. Couldn't you contact some of them to see if they might know of available jobs?"

should also convey that the patient is a worthwhile person by listening to and accepting the patient's feelings, being respectful, and praising help-seeking efforts.

Exploration of solutions is essential because crisis intervention is geared toward solving the immediate crisis. The nurse and patient actively explore solutions to the crisis. Answers that the patient had not thought of before may become apparent during conversations with the nurse as anxiety decreases. For example, a patient who has lost his job and has not been able to find a new one may become aware of the fact that he knows many people in his field of work whom he could contact to get information regarding the job market and possible openings.

These crisis intervention techniques are summarized in Box 12-2. In addition to using these techniques, Morley, Messick, and Aguilera[18] listed attitudes that are essential for the crisis worker to have. The crisis worker should see this work as the treatment of choice with per-

sons in crisis rather than a second-best treatment. Assessment of the present problem should be viewed as necessary for treatment, but complete diagnostic assessment is unnecessary. The goal and time limitations of crisis intervention should be kept in mind constantly, and unrelated material should not be explored. An active directive role must be taken, and flexibility of approach is essential. The Nursing Care Plan Summary describes interventions for working with individuals and families with ineffective coping responses.

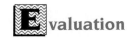 **valuation**

The last phase of crisis intervention is evaluation, when the nurse and patient evaluate whether the intervention resulted in a positive resolution of the crisis. Specific questions the nurse might ask include the following:

NURSING CARE PLAN SUMMARY
Coping Responses

Nursing Diagnosis: Ineffective coping (individual or family)

Expected Outcome: The patient will recover from the crisis event and return to a precrisis level of functioning.

Short-term Goals	Interventions	Rationale
The patient/family will describe the crisis event.	Invite patient to talk. Encourage ventilation of feelings. Communicate concern, empathy, and calm control.	Providing an atmosphere of support allows the patient to reach out for help and regain feelings of self-worth.
The patient/family will explore feelings and behaviors related to the crisis event.	Ask about the precipitating event. Determine precrisis level of functioning. Obtain patient's perception of the stress. Assess supports, resources, and usual coping mechanisms. Inquire about immediate future needs. Prioritize needs.	To plan nursing care, it is essential that the nurse understand the patient's perception of the crisis and its impact.
The patient/family will examine possible coping mechanisms.	Ask what coping mechanisms have been tried. Determine what the patient is capable of at this time. Suggest alternative coping strategies including environmental change, outside support, etc.	Crisis intervention is geared toward solving the problem. The nurse can suggest solutions that the patient had not considered.
The patient/family will implement one of the identified coping strategies.	Set specific short-term goals. Assist patient in implementing new coping strategies. Reinforce adaptive behavior. Support the use of healthy defenses.	The nurse should take an active role in mobilizing resources and reinforcing adaptive actions.
The patient/family will report satisfaction with coping responses and level of functioning.	Review the crisis experience with the patient. Identify positive aspects and strategies. Discuss ways these may be generalized to confront future life crises.	Crisis can be growth-producing if these skills are applied to future life situations.

1. Has the expected outcome been achieved, and has the patient returned to the precrisis level of functioning?
2. Have the needs of the patient that were threatened by the event been met?
3. Have the patient's symptoms decreased or been resolved?
4. Does the patient have adequate support systems and coping resources on which to rely?
5. Is the patient using constructive coping mechanisms?
6. Is the patient demonstrating adaptive crisis responses?
7. Does the patient need to be referred for additional treatment?

The nurse and patient should also review the changes that have occurred. The nurse should give credit for successful changes to patients so that they can realize their effectiveness and understand that what they learned from a crisis may help in coping with future crises. If the goals have not been met, the patient and nurse can return to the first step, assessment, and continue through the phases again. At the end of the evaluation process, if the nurse and patient believe referral for additional professional help would be useful, the referral should be made as quickly as possible.

All of the phases of crisis intervention are presented in the case study below.

SETTINGS FOR CRISIS INTERVENTION

Nurses work in many settings in which they see individuals in crisis. Medical hospitalizations are stressful for patients and their families and are often precipitating causes of crises.[25] The patient who becomes demanding or withdrawn or the wife who becomes bothersome to the nursing staff is a possible candidate for crisis intervention. The diagnosis of an illness, the limitations imposed on activities, and the changes in body image because of surgery can all be viewed as losses or threats that may precipitate a situational crisis. Simply the stress of being dependent on nurses for care can precipitate a crisis for the hospitalized patient.

Nurses who work in obstetric, pediatric, geriatric, or adolescent settings often observe patients or family members undergoing maturational crises. The anxious new mother, the acting-out adolescent, and the newly retired depressed patient are all possible candidates for crisis therapy. If physical illness is an added stress during maturational turning points, the patient is at an even greater risk. Emergency room settings are also flooded with crisis cases. People who attempt suicide, psychosomatic patients, and crime and accident victims are all possible candidates for crisis intervention. If the nurse is not in a position to work with the patient on an ongoing basis, a referral should be made.

Community health nurses work with patients in their own environments and can often spot and intervene in family crises. The child who refuses to go to school, the man who refuses to learn how to give himself an insulin injection, and the family with a member dying at home are possible candidates for crisis intervention. Community health nurses are also in an ideal position to evaluate high-risk families such as those with new babies, ill members, recent deaths, and a history of difficulty coping.

Finally, nurses in community mental health centers, departments of psychiatry, and managed care clinics also may see patients in crisis, such as those experiencing depression, anxiety, marital conflict, suicidal thoughts, illicit drug use, and traumatic responses. Crisis intervention can be implemented in any setting and should be a competency skill of all nurses, regardless of specialty area.

CASE STUDY

▼ ASSESSMENT

Mr. A was a 39-year-old, medium-built, casually dressed black man who was referred to the mental health clinic by his primary care provider. The patient came to the center alone. The nurse working with Mr. A collected the following data.

The patient worked in a large naval shipyard that was recently scheduled for closing. It was laying off many workers and reassigning others. One month earlier Mr. A was assigned to an area where he had difficulty 2 years ago. The foreman, the patient believed, was harassing him as he had done previously. Two weeks ago the patient got angry at the foreman and had thoughts of killing him. Instead, Mr. A became dizzy and his head ached. He requested medical attention but was refused. He then "passed out" and was taken by ambulance to the dispensary. Since that time Mr. A had a comprehensive physical examination and was found to be in excellent health. He was prescribed diazepam (Valium) on an as-needed basis, which was only slightly helpful. He returned to work for 2 days this week but again felt "sick."

Mr. A complained of being depressed, nervous, and tense. He was not sleeping well, was irritable with his wife and children, and was preoccupied with angry feelings toward his foreman. He denied suicidal thoughts but admitted that he felt like killing the foreman. He quickly added that he would really never do anything like that.

He appeared to have good comprehension, above average intelligence, adequate memory, and some paranoid ideation related to the foreman at work. His thought processes were organized, and there was no evidence of a perceptual disorder. Ego boundary disturbance was evident in the patient's paranoid thoughts. It seemed that the foreman was, in fact, a difficult man to get along with. However, the description of personal harassment seemed distorted.

Mr. A was raised by his parents. His father was "boss" and beat him and his siblings often. His mother was quiet and always agreed with his father. The patient had a younger brother and sister and an older sister. The patient and his brother had always been close. The two of them had stopped their father's beatings by ganging up on him and "psyching him out." As a child, Mr. A hung around with a "tough crowd" and fought frequently. He believed that he could physically overpower others but tried to keep out of trouble by talking to people rather than fighting.

Mr. A had no previous psychiatric history. His physical health was excellent and he was taking no medication. He had a tenth grade education, and his work record up to this time was good. His interests included bowling and other sports. He had been married for 17 years and had three daughters ages 16, 13, and 9. Mr. A stated that he had a good relationship with his wife and daughters and that both his wife and his brother were strong supports for him.

His usual means of coping were talking calmly with the threatening party and working hard on his job, at home, and in leisure activities. These coping mechanisms failed to work for him at this time but they had been successful in the past. He had no arrest record and was able to think through his actions rather than act impulsively. Mr. A showed strong motivation for working on his problem. He was reaching out for help and was able to form a therapeutic relationship with the nurse. Although his wife and brother were supportive, he felt no supports at work.

▼ NURSING DIAGNOSIS

Mr. A was in a situational crisis. The threat or precipitating stress was his transfer to a former boss. The patient's need for sexual role mastery was not being met, since he was not feeling successful at his job. Soon after the transfer, Mr. A's usual means of coping became ineffective and he experienced increased anxiety.

His nursing diagnosis was ineffective individual coping related to changes at work as evidenced by physical complaints of dizziness and tension. His DSM-IV diagnosis was adjustment disorder with mixed anxiety and depressed mood.

▼ OUTCOME IDENTIFICATION AND PLANNING

The expected outcome of treatment was for Mr. A to return to his precrisis level of functioning. If possible, he could reach a level above, having learned new methods of problem solving. The patient showed good potential for growth, and the nurse made a contract with him for crisis intervention. Mutually identified short-term goals included:
1. Mr. A will explore his thoughts and feelings about recent work events.
2. Mr. A will describe coping mechanisms that have been successful for him in the past.
3. Mr. A will identify three new ways of coping with work stress.
4. Mr. A will implement two of the new coping strategies.
5. Mr. A will be free of symptoms and function well at work.

▼ IMPLEMENTATION

The level of intervention used by the nurse was the **individual approach,** which includes the generic approach, general support, and environmental manipulation.

Environmental manipulation involved having the patient remain home from work temporarily. Letters were written by the nurse to his employer explaining Mr. A's absence in general terms. Mr. A was encouraged to talk to his wife about his difficulties so that she could understand his anxiety and provide emotional support.

General support was given by the nurse, who provided an atmosphere of reassurance, nonjudgmental caring, warmth, empathy, and optimism. Mr. A was encouraged to talk freely about the problem, and the nurse assured him that his problem was one that could be solved and that he would be feeling better soon.

The **generic approach** was used to decrease the patient's anxiety and guide him through the steps of problem solving. Levels of anxiety were assessed, and ways of reducing anxiety and helping the patient tolerate moderate anxiety were identified. The patient was encouraged to use his anxiety constructively to solve his problem and develop new coping mechanisms.

The **individual approach** was used in assessing and treating the specific problems of Mr. A who was strongly sensitive to mistreatment as a result of early childhood experiences. His emotional response was to strike out physically, as his father had struck out at him. Intellectually, Mr. A knew this would be disastrous, and his conflict was solved by becoming sick and passing out so that he could not assault his boss. Mr. A's intense anger was recognized and a high priority was placed on channeling the anger in a positive direction.

The first two meetings were used for data gathering and establishing a positive therapeutic relationship. Through the use of **abreaction** the patient ventilated angry feelings but did not concentrate on wanting to kill his boss. The nurse used **clarification** to help the patient begin to understand the precipitating event and its effect on him. **Suggestion** was used to allow the patient to see the nurse as one who can help. The nurse told the patient the problem could be worked out by the two of them and that he would soon be feeling better. Mr. A decided to contact several people at work to obtain information about transferring to another department and filing a formal complaint against the foreman. The patient and nurse therefore were **exploring solutions.** The nurse **reinforced** the patient's use of problem solving by telling him his ideas about alternative solutions were good ones. Throughout these and other sessions the nurse **raised his self-esteem** by communicating her confidence that he could find solutions to his problems. She listened to and accepted his feelings and treated him with respect. By contacting others at work, the patient also found some supportive individuals at work.

During the third session the patient described an incident in which he became furious at a worker in an automobile repair shop. The repairs on the patient's car were never right, and the patient kept returning the car there. The patient shoved the worker but limited his physical assault to that. He then felt nervous and jittery. The patient had previously expressed pride in his ability to control his angry feelings and not physically strike out at others. **Manipulation** was used by telling the patient he showed control in stopping the assault before it had become a full-blown fight and he could continue to exhibit this ability. During this session, also, the patient spoke of old, angry feelings toward his father. Some of this ventilation was allowed, but soon thereafter the focus was guided back to the present crisis.

In the fourth session the patient reported no episode of uncontrollable anger. He still put much emphasis, however, on being harassed by others. The nurse questioned the fact that others were out to intentionally harass the patient. Mr. A's defenses were not attacked, but his gross use of projection was discouraged. In the fifth session the patient reported that a car tried to run him off the road. At a red traffic light the patient spoke calmly to the driver and the driver apologized. The nurse **reinforced this behavior** and **supported his use of sublimation as a defense.** Discussion of termination of the therapy was begun.

In the sixth session Mr. A said that things were going well at work and that he would soon be going to a different department. He also talked about a course he had begun at a community college. He showed no evidence of anxiety, depression, or paranoia and thought he didn't need to come back to the mental health clinic.

▼ EVALUATION

The interventions resulted in an adaptive resolution of the crisis. The patient's need for sexual role mastery was being met. He was once again comfortable and successful at work. His symptoms of anxiety, paranoia, dizziness, headaches, passing out, and homicidal thoughts had ended. He no longer felt harassed. His original coping mechanisms were again effective. He was talking calmly to people he was having difficulty with, and he was again working hard in a goal-oriented way (i.e., a college course). He had learned new methods of coping, which included talking about his feelings to significant others, following administrative or official avenues of protest, and seeking support. The patient and nurse discussed how Mr. A could use the methods of problem solving he had learned from the experience to help cope with future problems. The expected outcome, return to the precrisis level of functioning, had been attained.

It was also recommended to the patient that he engage in psychotherapy so that he could deal with the old angers that continued to interfere with his life. Mr. A refused the recommendation at this time and stated he would contact the clinic if he changed his mind. ▼

MODALITIES OF CRISIS INTERVENTION

Recently, new community-based crisis intervention modalities have been developed. They are based on the philosophy that the health-care team must be aggressive and go out to the patients rather than wait for the patients to come to them. Nurses working in these modalities intervene in a variety of community settings, ranging from patients' homes to street corners.

Mobile Crisis Programs

Mobile crisis teams provide front-line interdisciplinary crisis intervention to individuals, families, and communities. The nurse who is a member of a mobile crisis team may respond to a desperate individual threatening to jump off a bridge in a suicide attempt, an angry individual who is becoming violent toward family members at home, or a frightened individual who has barricaded himself in an office building. By diffusing the immediate crisis situation, lives can be saved, incarcerations and hospitalizations can be avoided, and individuals can be stabilized.

Mobile crisis programs throughout the country vary somewhat in the services they provide and the procedures they use. However, they are usually able to provide on-site assessment, crisis management, treatment, referral, and educational services to patients, families, law enforcement officers, and the community at large. They are thus able to ensure mental health care for even the most underserved populations efficiently and cost effectively. Most important, the cost effectiveness of their services is defined by savings in monetary, human, and ethical terms.[27,33,34]

Group Work

Crisis groups follow the same steps that individual intervention follows. The nurse and group help the patient solve the problem and reinforce the patient's new problem-solving behavior. The nurse's role in the group is active, focal, and present oriented. The group follows the nurse's example and uses similar therapeutic techniques. The group acts as a support system for the patient and is therefore of particular benefit to socially isolated individuals. Often the way the patient functions in the group will suggest the faulty coping pattern that is responsible for the patient's current problem. For example, a patient's interaction with group members may show that he does not appear to listen to anything said by others. This same patient may be in a crisis because his girlfriend left him because she thought he did not care about her thoughts and feelings. The nurse can comment on the faulty coping behavior seen in the group and encourage group discussion about it.

Most crisis groups focus on individuals who have common traits or stressors. Carter and Brooks[6] described a time-limited school-based group for friends of an adolescent suicide victim. They suggest that the most significant aspects of the group work were the ventilation of feelings and the support for healthy future responses. Stewart and colleagues[24] described a cognitive social support group that included both didactic and experiential learning activities for adolescents affected by Hurricane Hugo. Brown[4] reported on a hospital-based crisis support group that facilitated grieving following a pregnancy loss. The women and their families shared feelings and received information and support. Other crisis groups have been conducted for families of critically ill patients[12,20] and for men accompanying women seeking abortions.[11]

Nurses practicing on acute psychiatric units can use crisis intervention in working with patients and families to prepare for discharge and prevent rehospitalization. With the shortened lengths of hospital stays, crisis in-

tervention is often the treatment of choice. The hospitalization itself may be viewed as an environmental manipulation and part of the crisis intervention.

Telephone Contacts

Crisis intervention is sometimes practiced by telephone rather than through face-to-face contacts. Nurses working for hot lines or those who answer emergency telephone calls may find themselves practicing crisis intervention without visual cues. Referrals for face-to-face contact should be made, but often, because of the patient's unwillingness or inability to cooperate, the telephone remains the only contact. Listening skills must therefore be emphasized in the nurse's role. Most emergency telephone services have extensive training programs to teach this specialized type of crisis intervention. Manuals written for the crisis worker include content such as suicide-potential rating scales, community resources, drug information, guidelines for helping the caller discuss concerns, and advice on understanding the limitations of the crisis worker's role.[17]

Disaster Response

As part of the community, nurses are called on when adventitious crises strike the community. Floods, earthquakes, airplane crashes, fires, nuclear accidents, and other natural and unnatural disasters precipitate large numbers of crises. Frederick and Garrison[10] have described a "service model" in which mental health workers in the immediate postdisaster period should go to places where victims are likely to gather, such as morgues, hospitals, and shelters. Later, if Federal Disaster Assistance Centers are established, mental health workers may assist in the centers. Rather than waiting for people to publicly identify themselves as persons who are unable to cope with stress, it is suggested that the mental health workers work with the American Red Cross, talk to people waiting in lines to apply for assistance, go door-to-door, or, at a relocation site, ask people how they are managing their affairs and explore their reactions to stress.

> Nurses are frequently called on to help out in times of disaster. What special needs might nurses have in situations where they are both victims and caregivers?

Experts in the field of disaster response suggest that organized plans for crisis response be developed and practiced during nondisaster times. For example, one county organized its crisis intervention and disaster services into those that are clinic based, school based, disaster-service based, and ad hoc.[22] The combination of services used depended on the type of disastrous event. For example, the county's community crisis intervention team provided timely services in a school setting following an adolescent's suicide. If the event had been a natural disaster, a comprehensive on-site family community service would have been initiated.

Nurses providing crisis therapy during large disasters would use the generic approach to crisis intervention so that as many individuals as possible can receive help in a short amount of time. Tragedies such as group kidnappings and group killings in communities may affect fewer people and may at times require the individual approach. The nurse may choose to work with families or groups rather than individuals during adventitious crises so that individuals can gain support from others in their family or community who are undergoing stresses similar to theirs.

A good example of mental health professionals helping victims of an adventitious crisis occurred in Kansas City, Missouri, in the days and weeks following the crash of the overhead walkways at the Hyatt Hotel. Eight mental health centers in the Kansas City metropolitan area joined to help care for the emotional sufferings of the individuals involved. The centers formed an unofficial coalition and prepared a joint press release describing the many aspects of the grieving process and publicizing the services that they would offer to the survivors of those killed at the hotel—the injured, the observers, and the rescue workers. The services were of three kinds. First, all the centers offered phone counseling and support groups free of charge. Second, special services were planned, such as a grief workshop that was attended by about 200 people who had been at the crash scene. Other related seminars were also held. Third, the centers and media worked together to let the general public know about other resources and services as these became available and to reassure people that their strong reactions to the tragedy were normal.

Recently, attention has been focused on helping the helpers in disasters. Health and mental health professionals who are victims of disasters as well as providers of care during disasters often feel overwhelmed with stress.[31] These care providers describe feelings of concern for both their patients and their own families.[15] Crisis intervention strategies for the caregivers are essential. For example, Stuart and Huggins[28] described the actions that psychiatric nurse administrators took to care for their psychiatric nursing staff, and Stanley[23] reported on a hospital-wide crisis stabilization program that provided large group debriefing and small group follow-up sessions for all nursing staff after Hurricane Hugo devastated South Carolina in 1989. Walker and Gatzert-Snyder[30] described the use of debriefing and support groups following the San Francisco earthquake.

Hospital nurses who cared for victims of the 1993 New York World Trade Center explosion also held group meetings in which they vented their feelings about the tragedy.

Health Education

Although health education can take place during the entire crisis intervention process, it is emphasized during the evaluation phase. At this time the patient's anxiety has decreased, and so better use can be made of cognitive abilities. The nurse and patient summarize the course of the crisis and the intervention to teach the patient how to avoid other similar crises. For example, the nurse helps the patient to identify the feelings, thoughts, and behaviors experienced as anxiety rose following the stressful event. The nurse explains that if these feelings, thoughts, and behaviors are again experienced, the patient should immediately become aware of being stressed and take steps to prevent the anxiety from increasing. The nurse then teaches the patient ways to use these newly learned coping mechanisms in future situations.

Nurses are also involved in identifying individuals who are at high risk for developing crises and in teaching coping strategies to avoid the development of the crises. For example, coping strategies that can be taught include how to request information, access resources, and obtain support.

The public is also in need of education so that they can identify those needing crisis services, be aware of available services, change their attitudes so that people will feel free to seek services, and obtain information about how others deal with potential crisis-producing problems. For example, a mother who learns about reactions to rape may identify her daughter as a rape victim. She then may take her daughter to the nearest rape crisis center. The mother, in encouraging her daughter to go to the crisis center, tells her daughter that rape is not the fault of the victim, thus enabling her daughter to change her attitude about the rape and feel positive about obtaining outside help. At the center the mother may be given a pamphlet that describes how to help rape victims, which she shares with friends so that they can cope quickly and effectively if their loved ones are raped.

> Explain how conducting a group on stress management for critical care nurses is an example of health education as crisis intervention.

The nurse educates the public by participating in programs in the media, by leading or participating in educational groups in the community, and by taking every opportunity to advertise crisis services. For instance, if a nurse is a member of a church group that has developed crisis services, the availability of these services should be shared with the child's school staff and the parent-teacher association. Nurses, as health-care professionals, have a great opportunity to provide health education and crisis intervention to individuals, families, and communities, thus preventing mental illness and promoting mental health.

SUGGESTED CROSS-REFERENCES

SUMMARY

1. A crisis is a disturbance resulting from a perceived threat that challenges the individual's usual coping mechanisms. Crises are a time of increased vulnerability, but they can also stimulate growth. There are three types of crises: maturational, situational, and adventitious.

2. Crisis intervention is a brief, active therapy with the goal of returning the individual to a precrisis level of functioning.

3. In assessing a patient, the nurse should identify the patient's behaviors, precipitating event, perception of the event, support systems and coping resources, and previous strengths and coping mechanisms.

4. Primary nursing diagnoses in crisis intervention are ineffective individual coping, ineffective family coping, altered family processes, and post-trauma response.

5. Primary DSM-IV diagnoses are categorized as adjustment disorders or anxiety disorders, which include posttraumatic stress disorder.

6. The expected outcome of nursing care is that the patient will recover from the crisis event and return to a precrisis level of functioning.

7. Levels of crisis intervention include environmental manipulation, general support, generic approach, and individual approach.

8. The nurse and patient should consider the following factors in evaluating nursing care: the patient's level of functioning, symptoms, coping resources, coping mechanisms, evidence of adaptive coping responses, and need for referral for further treatment.

9. Crisis intervention can be implemented in any setting including hospitals, clinics, community health centers, and the home. It should be a competency skill of all nurses.

10. New modalities of crisis intervention include mobile crisis programs, group work, telephone contacts, disaster response, and health education.

COMPETENT CARING
A CLINICAL EXEMPLAR OF A PSYCHIATRIC NURSE

Beth Maree, MSN, RN, CS

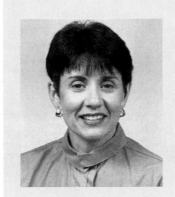

The mental health center setting presents many challenges, but few are broader in scope and higher in intensity than what I experienced while working there. My client, S, was a 28-year-old, married, unemployed woman with a 4-year-old son. The marriage was interracial, and her husband, 32 years her senior, was terminally ill with cancer. His disease had progressed to the point that he was unable to provide for the family either financially or emotionally. S found herself, for the first time, responsible for the family but without the necessary skills or resources.

At our first meeting, S was an emergency "walk-in" with complaints of anxiety, sadness, tearfulness, lack of appetite, poor impulse control, ambivalent feelings, helplessness, and hopelessness. Upon initial assessment, it was identified that her father was an alcoholic who had been physically abusive to her, her mother, and her siblings. Her mother had fled the home, leaving the children with the father. Both parents later remarried, and S lived with her mother and stepfather, who also was an alcoholic. She experienced much emotional trauma during her youth and reported having difficulty in dealing with the eventual deaths of her parents and her stepfather. She had been only minimally involved with her siblings, since they were unhappy with the choices she had made in her life. Her identified source of support was her husband, who had promised "to always care for her." S spoke haltingly and was obviously in great distress. During the assessment, she shared that she had abused her own child when he was 6 months old, and she feared losing control again under such extreme stress. This was the precipitating factor for seeking help. S expressed a need to be cared for herself and an inability to cope with the demands of her son and her terminally ill husband.

I knew that much care would be needed for this patient and her family system. I decided that crisis intervention would be my primary strategy to ensure the family's safety. This first meeting was critical for obtaining an accurate assessment, establishing a sound rapport, and developing a plan of action. From here on it would be important for me to maintain a nonjudgmental approach, display empathy, validate concerns, and gain cooperation in establishing safety and ensuring her ongoing involvement in treatment. This could be difficult given the circumstances.

I offered positive reinforcement to S for her courage in admitting past abusive behavior and her recognition of its possible recurrence. The responsibility of reporting information related to abuse was explained to her and framed in a nonpunitive, protective manner. Her reaction of anger and fear was expected and accepted. She was encouraged to ventilate these feelings. In addition, her expectations of help were discussed and consequences of inadequate actions were explored.

S was able to accept the need to mobilize all available forms of assistance for her and her family as quickly as possible. The Department of Social Services was notified during the first meeting, and a caseworker was assigned to assess the home situation. With help, S was able to identify behavioral cues and situations that evoked her feelings of rage and hopelessness that often led to impulsive acts. She was able to contract for safety until her follow-up appointment and was provided with verbal and written instructions for emergency contacts via the mental health center and Department of Social Services' 24-hour phone lines.

S also agreed to ongoing treatment. The targeted problem areas were grief reaction associated with the progressive loss of her husband, combined with few effective coping and parenting skills, dependency issues, and low self-esteem. She had a poor social support network and required mobilization and coordination of many agencies, programs, and professionals to meet her needs and those of her family. In addition to the protective services offered by the Department of Social Services, I enlisted help from the following agencies and professionals:

▼ The mental health center psychiatrist for psychiatric evaluation and follow-up
▼ The patient's medical doctor, with her permission
▼ Family services for formalized parenting classes providing both information and a supportive peer group
▼ Hospice for provision of daily nursing care visits to the husband and teaching S about his case
▼ The youth division of the mental health center to provide evaluation and treatment for her son
▼ Vocational rehabilitation for skill development and exploration of employment opportunities

I also continued as her nurse clinician for 6 months of crisis intervention. The care I provided during our sessions remained largely supportive and educative. S, with a safety net of resources, began to work on grief and loss issues and related these to feelings of rejection and abandonment from her family of origin. She was allowed to progress through the phases of grief and to develop insight and personal growth at her own pace. Slowly, S began to identify her strengths and set goals. Together we formed a partnership to accomplish these goals with collaboration from the many services now involved in her treatment. My role as coordinator, facilitator, educator, and advocate was to assist S in achieving success toward meeting her goals and improving her self-esteem. In this case the importance of the patient as a human being with dignity and worth was reinforced, and the relationship of the individual to the family and the community was never more apparent.

Termination was the last critical task of our relationship; in this case the termination was twofold. First, her husband died with S at his bedside. She notified me, and support was offered at her request with my quiet presence at his funeral. A home visit was arranged shortly afterward to evaluate her adjust

Continued

ment to her husband's death. Second, due to a change in position, I was no longer able to serve as her clinician. Before I was transferred, S was able to meet her new clinician and establish some rapport with her. This transition went very smoothly, and S became an active, participating member in a strong therapy group. Months later I received a follow-up letter from her in which she expressed a new vision for herself that included assuming responsibility for providing a future for herself and her son. My goal of providing S with a sense of hope and a framework that would support her was accomplished. Looking back on it, I still feel good about what I was able to accomplish as a psychiatric nurse. ▼

REFERENCES

1. Aguilera DC: *Crisis intervention: theory and methodology*, ed 7, St Louis, 1994, Mosby.
2. Auerbach SM: Crisis intervention research: methodological considerations and some recent findings. In Cohen W, Claiborn WL, Specter GA, eds: *Crisis intervention*, New York, 1983, Human Sciences Press.
3. Benbenishty R: Combat stress reaction and changes in military medical profile, *Mil Med* 156:68, 1991.
4. Brown Y: The crisis of pregnancy loss: a team approach to support, *Birth* 19:82, 1991.
5. Caplan G: *Principles of preventive psychiatry*, New York, 1964, Basic Books.
6. Carter BF, Brooks A: Suicide postvention: crisis or opportunity? *School Counselor* 37:378, 1990.
7. Cohen R: Training mental health professionals to work with families in diverse cultural contexts. In Austin L, ed: *Responding to disaster: a guide for mental health professionals*, Washington, DC, 1992, American Psychiatric Press.
8. Davidson J et al: A diagnostic and family study of posttraumatic stress syndrome, *Am J Psychiatry* 142:1, 1985.
9. Figley CR, Leventman, eds: *Strangers at home: Vietnam veterans since the war*, New York, 1990, Brunner/Mazel.
10. Frederick C, Garrison J: Disaster and mental health: an overview, *Behav Today* 12:32, 1981.
11. Gordon RH: Efficacy of a group crisis counseling program for men who accompany women seeking abortions, *Am J Community Psychol* 6:239, 1978.
12. Halm MA: Effect of support groups on anxiety of family members during critical illness, *Heart Lung* 19:62, 1990.
13. Horowitz M: Stress-response syndromes: a review of posttraumatic and adjustment disorders, *Hosp Community Psychiatry* 37:241, 1986.
14. Kulka RA, Schlenger WE, Fairbank JA, Hough R, Jordan BK, Marmar CR, et al: The National Vietnam Veterans Readjustment Study: contractual report of findings. In *Trauma and the Vietnam war generation*, New York, 1990, Brunner/Mazel.
15. Laube-Morgan J: The professional's psychological response in disaster: implications for practice, *J Psychosoc Nurs Ment Health Serv* 30:17, 1992.
16. Lindemann E: Symptomatology and management of acute grief, *Am J Psychiatry* 101:141, 1944.
17. Mills P: *Crisis intervention resource manual*, Vermillion, SD, 1973, Educational Research and Service Center.
18. Morley WE, Messick JM, Aguilera DC: Crisis paradigms of intervention, *J Psychiatr Nurs* 5:537, 1967.
19. Rusk TN: Opportunity and technique in crisis psychiatry, *Compr Psychiatry* 12:249, 1971.
20. Schigoda MG, Hook ML: "Take heart . . ." developing support sessions for families of acutely ill cardiac patients, *AACN Clin Issues Crit Care Nurs* 2:299, 1991.
21. Shields L: Crisis intervention: implications for the nurse, *J Psychiatr Nurs* 13:37, 1975.
22. Silver T, Goldstein H: A collaborative model of a county crisis intervention team: the Lake County experience, *Community Ment Health J* 28:249, 1992.
23. Stanley SR: When the disaster is over: helping the healers to mend, *J Psychosoc Nurs Ment Health Serv* 28:13, 1990.
24. Stewart J et al: Group protocol to mitigate disaster stress and enhance social support in adolescents exposed to Hurricane Hugo, *Issues Ment Health Nurs* 13:105, 1992.
25. Strain JJ, Grossman S: *Psychological care of the mentally ill*, New York, 1975, Appleton-Century-Crofts.
26. Strickler M, LaSor B: Concepts of loss in crisis intervention, *Ment Hygiene* 54:302, 1970.
27. Stroul BA: *Profiles of psychiatric crisis response systems*, Rockville, Md, 1991, Community Support Program, NIMH.
28. Stuart G, Huggins E: Carring for the caretakers in times of disaster, *J Child Adolesc Psychiatr Nurs* 3:144, 1990.
29. Terr LC: Psychic trauma in children: observations following the Chowchilla school bus kidnapping, *Am J Psychiatry* 138:14, 1981.
30. Walker V, Gatzert-Snyder S: When disaster strikes: the concern of staff nurses, *J Psychosoc Nurs* 29:9, 1991.
31. Waters K, Selander J, Stuart G: Psychological adaptation of nurses post-disaster, *Issues Ment Health Nurs* 13:177, 1992.
32. Woods S, Campbell J: Posttraumatic stress in battered women: does the diagnosis fit? *Issues Ment Health Nurs* 14:173, 1993.
33. Zealberg JJ, Christie SS, Puckett JA, McAlhany D, Durban M: A mobile crisis program: collaboration between emergency psychiatric services and police, *Hosp Community Psychiatry* 43:6, 1992.
34. Zealberg JJ, Santos AB, Fisher RK: Benefits of a mobile crisis program, *Hosp Community Psychiatry* 44:16, 1993.

ANNOTATED SUGGESTED READINGS

*Aguilera DC: *Crisis intervention: theory and methodology*, ed 7, St Louis, 1994, Mosby.
Detailed and thorough presentation of crisis theory and methods.

*Nursing reference.

Austin L, ed: *Responding to disaster: a guide for mental health professionals,* Washington, DC, 1992, American Psychiatric Press.
Collection of clinical accounts and clearly presented overview of disaster interventions with firsthand and practical descriptions.

*Blair D, Hildreth N: PTSD and the Vietnam veteran: the battle for treatment, J *Psychosoc Nurs Ment Health Serv* 29:15, 1991.
Excellent discussion of PTSD and problems with its application to the Vietnam veteran, including special circumstances of the Vietnam conflict.

*Clark M, Friedman D: Pulling together: building a community debriefing team, J *Psychosoc Nurs Ment Health Serv* 30:27, 1992.
Describes building a debriefing team and the postdisaster debriefing process—excellent nursing strategies.

Dazord A, Gerin P, Iahns J: Pretreatment and process measures in crisis intervention as predictors of outcome, *Psychother Res* 1:135, 1991.
Reports on a crisis intervention outcomes study that relates patient and treatment characteristics to outcomes 1 and 2 years later. Good example of research in the field.

*Fisher H: Psychiatric crises: making the most of an emergency room visit, J *Psychosoc Nurs Ment Health Serv* 27:4, 1989.
Addresses techniques for intervening with patients who present in emergency rooms with psychiatric crises. Clear and very helpful.

*Hoff LS: *People in crisis: understanding and helping,* Menlo Park, Calif, 1989, Addison-Wesley.
Presents theory and practice of crisis intervention stressing the social and cultural context.

Horowitz M: Stress-response syndromes: a review of posttraumatic and adjustment disorders, *Hosp Community Psychiatry* 37:241, 1986.
Excellent review of the symptoms, phases, diagnosis, processing of stressful events, and treatment of PTSD.

*Laube-Morgan J: The professional's psychological response in disaster: implications for practice, J *Psychosoc Nurs Ment Health Serv* 30:17, 1992.
Describes victims' psychological response in disaster with attention to victims who are health-care workers assisting other victims.

Roberts A: *Crisis intervention handbook,* Belmont, Calif, 1990, Wadsworth.
Clearly examines the application of crisis theory and the crisis model in child and family, emergency health, mental health, and private practice settings.

*Samter J, Fitzgerald M, Braudaway C, et al: Debriefing: from military origin to therapeutic application, J *Psychosoc Nurs Ment Health Serv* 31:23, 1993.
Describes both individual and group debriefing with Operation Desert Storm/Shield participants.

*Stewart J, Hardin S, Weinrich S, et al: Group protocol to mitigate disaster stress and enhance social support in adolescents exposed to Hurricane Hugo, *Issues Ment Health Nurs* 13:105, 1992.
Reports on the structure, content, process, rationale, and cost of a cognitive social support group for adolescents exposed to the stress of Hurricane Hugo.

*Stuart G, Huggins E: Caring for the caretakers in time of disaster, J *Child Adolesc Psychiatr Nurs* 3:144, 1990.
Unique firsthand report of how psychiatric nurse administrators supported and cared for their nursing staff during Hurricane Hugo.

Zealburg J, Christie S, Puckett J, et al: A mobile crisis program: collaboration between emergency psychiatric services and police, *Hosp Community Psychiatry* 43:612, 1992.
Linkages between mobile crisis programs and police departments are identified with two case studies.

---

*Nursing reference.

---

*Nursing reference.

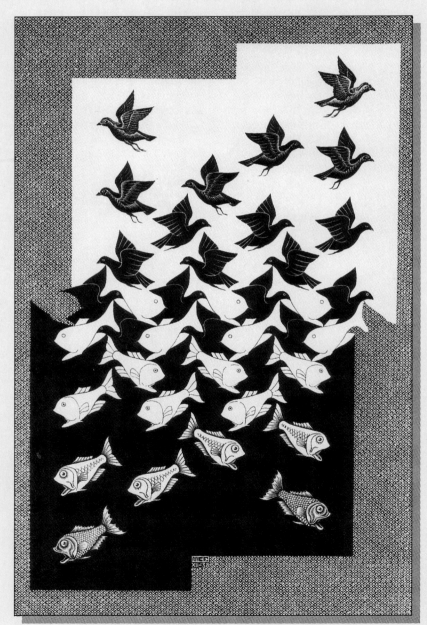

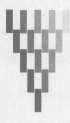

CHAPTER 13
Psychiatric Rehabilitation

SANDRA J. SUNDEEN

Of equality—as if it harm'd me giving others the same chances and rights as myself—as if it were not indispensable to my own rights that others possess the same.

Walt Whitman: *Thought*

The public health model of prevention identifies **tertiary prevention** as the limitation of disability related to an episode of illness. The National Mental Health Advisory Council has addressed the services needed to prevent disability in people who have serious and persistent mental illnesses. "With any illness, but especially with these disorders that endure and disable people, providing the right medication is essential, but not enough. A full range of services attending to rehabilitation, independent living, and enhanced quality of life is needed. Finding ways to improve the standard of care, and ways to provide it through better organization and financing of services is a compelling public health need."[29]

Any episode of illness may involve lasting change in a person's level of functioning. An individual who has been seriously ill is more likely to have problems living productively in the community. Hospitalization is especially disruptive, and it is often difficult to adjust after discharge. Nurses who work in institutional settings must be aware of the total range of patient care needs both during and after hospitalization. Tertiary prevention usually begins before discharge from the hospital. Caplan[9] says the goal of tertiary prevention is to reduce the rate of maladaptive functioning related to mental disorder in a community. Although concepts of tertiary prevention can be applied to anyone who has experienced an episode of illness, they are particularly relevant to those with serious and persistent mental illnesses, sometimes called *chronic mental illness*. Because of the stigma associated with the term *chronic*, *serious mental illness* is used in this chapter.

It has been estimated that between 2 and 4 million Americans have serious mental illnesses.[29] Nurses care for people who have serious mental illnesses in a variety of settings: private and public psychiatric hospitals, psychiatric and medical-surgical units in general hospitals, emergency rooms, community-based treatment and rehabilitation programs, and patients' homes. As patients alternate between community-based and hospital-based care, nurses in all settings share responsibility for their care. Knowledge of the special needs and characteristics of this population is important for all nurses.

REHABILITATION

Tertiary prevention is carried out by the performance of activities identified as **rehabilitation.** This is the process of helping the person return to the highest possible level of functioning. The goal is to teach "individuals disabled by mental illness to work and live independently, to overcome blocks in both opportunity and motivation, and to follow regimens of living likely to maintain or restore the highest possible level of well-being."[29] In addition, many patients need help developing new skills and finding ways to overcome functional deficits.

Tertiary prevention was largely ignored until community mental health programs were initiated in the 1960s. The development of effective new treatments allowed mental health care providers to think about the future with patients who were about to reenter the community. Medication and psychotherapy, in particular, assisted patients in developing positive interpersonal relationships. Hospitalization was not needed for some patients who were able to function in the community with the help of intensive intervention.

A new interest in the civil rights of psychiatric patients increased the importance of psychiatric rehabilitation. The right to treatment in the least restrictive setting was established (see Chapter 8). This resulted in reassessment of patients in hospitals, some of whom had been there for many years. It soon became obvious that many people who were returning to communities lacked the skills needed for daily life. Community support resources were inadequate. Scandals occurred as discharged psychiatric patients were discovered in shabby boarding houses, soup kitchens, and skid row. Many became victims of crime because they lacked the skills to protect themselves. Many returned to the hospital for brief admissions, creating a revolving door between the hospital and the community. Others became inmates of other kinds of institutions, especially jails and nursing homes, as they demonstrated their inability to cope or were unable to gain access to needed services.

Anthony[3] has applied the World Health Organization classification of the consequences of disease to psychiatric rehabilitation. According to this model, impairment represents the direct effects of the illness, and disability and disadvantage are related to its consequences (Table 13-1).

In addition, the following five principles have been identified related to psychiatric rehabilitation[39]:

1. Goals should focus on improving quality of life as identified by the patient and family.
2. Rehabilitation takes place in partnership with the disabled person.
3. Individual differences must be recognized and respected.
4. Rehabilitation must adjust to the changes that people experience over time.
5. Rehabilitation really encompasses all of the services that people need to live successfully in the community.

Table 13-1 The Rehabilitation Model For Severe Mental Illness

	Stages		
	Impairment	**Disability**	**Disadvantage**
Definitions	Any loss or abnormality of psychological, physiological, or anatomical structure or function	Any restriction or lack of ability to perform an activity and/or role in the manner or within the range considered normal for a human being (resulting from an impairment)	A lack of opportunity for a given individual that limits or prevents the fulfillment of a role that is normal (depending on age, sex, social, or cultural factors) for that individual (resulting from an impairment and/or a disability)
Examples	Hallucinations, delusions, depression	Lack of work adjustment skills, social skills, or ADL* skills, which restricts one's residential, educational, vocational, and social roles	Discrimination and poverty, which contribute to unemployment and homelessness

From Anthony WA, Cohen MD, Farkas MD: *Psychiatric rehabilitation*, Boston, 1990, Boston University, Center for Psychiatric Rehabilitation.
*ADL, Activities of daily living.

Compare and contrast the principles of psychiatric rehabilitation with your knowledge of physical rehabilitation. How do the principles affect nursing intervention?

The process of moving long-term hospital patients to the community is called **deinstitutionalization.** For this process to succeed, patients need an array of services addressing needs for shelter, safety, social relationships, working, and learning. Mental health treatment services range from traditional outpatient clinics to mobile outreach and crisis intervention programs. Rehabilitation services also are offered in a variety of settings.

Rehabilitative psychiatric nursing must be studied in the contexts of the patient and social system. This requires the nurse to focus on three elements: the individual, the family, and the community. The nursing care of people with serious mental illnesses are considered related to these three elements and the activities of assessment, intervention, and evaluation.

ASSESSMENT
The Individual

Assessment of the need for rehabilitation begins with the initial contact between the nurse and the patient. A comprehensive psychiatric nursing assessment, as described in Chapters 5, 6, 7, and 9, provides information that enables the nurse to help the patient achieve maximum possible functioning. Nurses are expected to identify and reinforce strengths as one means of assisting the patient to cope. This is basic to the concept of rehabilitation. Thus good nursing care is really rehabilitative nursing care.

The stress adaptation model (Fig. 13-1) may be applied within the context of rehabilitative nursing practice. It is important for the nurse to identify stressors that may interfere with the patient's adjustment to a health-promoting life-style. Nurses need to be aware of patients' perceptions of their experiences. It is also essential to validate each person's response to significant life changes.

When conducting an initial assessment, the nurse needs to think beyond the limits of the patient care set-

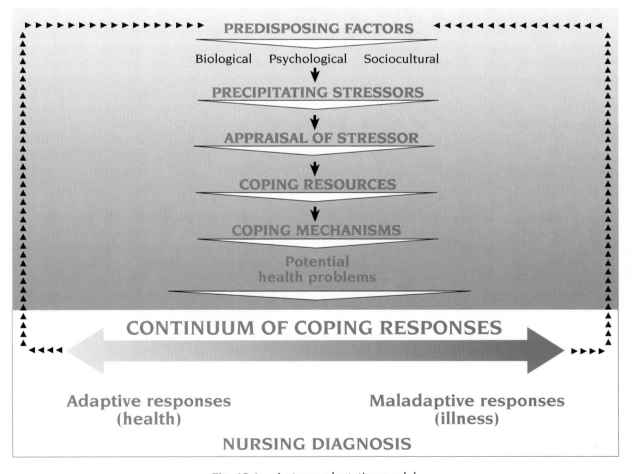

Fig. 13-1   A stress adaptation model.

ting and try to anticipate the patient's other contacts with the health-care system. In hospitals this process of discharge planning is expected. Nurses in community settings should also expect patients to progress to other levels of care. Although some people will need long-term outpatient care, others will be discharged from psychiatric care.

Characteristics of Serious Mental Illness. People who have serious mental illnesses are likely to have both primary and secondary symptoms. Primary symptoms are directly caused by the illness. For example, hallucinations and delusions are primary symptoms of schizophrenia, and elation and hyperactivity are primary symptoms of bipolar disorder. Secondary symptoms such as apathy and social isolation are caused by the person's response to the illness or its treatment. They are associated with the disability of the illness. Symptoms related to specific mental disorders are described in Chapters 14 through 24.

Behaviors related to primary symptoms may violate social norms and standards of conduct and be considered deviant. This leads to a social interactive process whereby society protects itself from the person's norm violation.[21] An example of this is community opposition to the establishment of group homes. As this social interactive process unfolds, individuals increasingly identify themselves as "mentally ill." They begin to relate to society in terms of this identity rather than of others, such as wife, mother, husband, father, or worker. The person's acceptance of mentally ill status and adjustment to society in terms of this role are accompanied by the secondary symptoms of serious mental illness. In contrast, public health epidemiologists study the "natural history" of physical and mental diseases. According to the public health model, individuals show increasing symptoms of functional impairment and disability as they move through the four stages of chronic illness. These are described in Table 13-2.

Behaviors Related to Serious Mental Illness. Surveys have revealed that people with serious mental illnesses are generally not employed, are less educated, less likely to be involved in close relationships, and more likely to live in poverty than their peers.[17,28] The exact causes of these characteristics have yet to be identified. Some could be related to primary and secondary symptoms or disabilities of the illness and others to society's reaction to the mentally ill person, referred to by Bachrach[5] as "tertiary disability." Attitudes that could contribute to tertiary disability are illustrated by the list of myths about people with mental illness compiled by the National Institutes of Mental Health (Table 13-3). None of these myths is true, but they are commonly believed and lead to stigma. This often prevents people with mental illnesses from gaining access to needed services and opportunities.

Copy the list of myths about mental illness and discuss them with a group of people who have little personal experience with mental illness. Then discuss the list with a small group of people who have a serious mental illness. Compare and contrast the responses of the two groups.

ACTIVITIES OF DAILY LIVING. Activities of daily living (ADL) applied to serious mental illness means the skills that are necessary to live independently, such as housekeeping, shopping, food preparation, money management, and personal hygiene. A major goal of psychosocial rehabilitation is to assist the person to develop independent living skills. A national survey of members of the National Alliance for the Mentally Ill (NAMI), a family advocacy group, revealed that 23% of their seriously mentally ill family members need help with ADL.[43]

INTERPERSONAL RELATIONS. People who have serious mental illnesses are often described as apathetic, withdrawn, and socially isolated. The existence of interpersonal problems is supported by the very low number of marriages in this population.[17] Previously, it was assumed that relationship problems were a result of prolonged institutional life, which did not encourage close

Table 13-2   Stages of the Natural History of Chronic Illness

Stage	Characteristics
Susceptibility	Exposure to environmental, biological, behavioral, and emotional risk factors
Presymptomatic disease	No overt symptoms of disease; pathological changes begin; risk factors intensify; behaviors increasing susceptibility solidify and become patterns
Clinical disease	Anatomical and functional changes occur; presence of recognizable disease symptoms
Disability	Disease symptoms increase; anatomical and functional changes produce reduction in activity; impairment of instrumental or expressive function

Modified from Anderson S, Bauwens E: *Chronic health problems: concepts and application*, St Louis, 1981, Mosby.

Table 13-3   Myths and Facts about People with Mental Illnesses

Myths	Facts
A person who has been mentally ill can never be normal.	Mental illness is often temporary or episodic. Former mentally ill patients deserve to be judged on their own merits.
Even if some mentally ill persons return to normal, chronically mentally ill people remain different—in fact, crazy.	Many people who have chronic mental illnesses have been hospitalized for a long time. After discharge, they must continue to take medication. The combination of the illness and medication side effects may cause them to look or act strange, but the longer they are in the community the more they look like everyone else.
If people who recover from other illnesses can cope on their own, recovered mental patients should be able to do so, too.	Most people who have been through a disabling illness, mental or physical, need rehabilitation. For mentally ill people this is focused on social support.
Persons with mental illness are unpredictable.	Although some mentally ill people are impulsive and unpredictable when they are actively ill, most are consistent in their behavior when recovered.
Those with schizophrenia or other severe mental disorders must be really crazy.	With appropriate treatment, people who have severe mental disorders tend to be calm and reliable.
Mentally ill persons are dangerous.	Patients who have come through mental illness and have returned to the community are apt, if anything, to be anxious, timid, and passive. They rarely present a danger to the public.
Recovered mentally ill patients are surely potentially dangerous. They could go berserk at any time.	Most people who are mentally ill never went "berserk" in the first place. Mentally ill patients are more likely to be depressed and withdrawn than wild and aggressive. Most relapses develop gradually.
Anyone who has had shock treatment must *really* be in a bad way.	Shock treatment (electroconvulsive therapy, or ECT) is an effective treatment for serious depression. There is no reason to assume that someone who has received this therapy is sicker than others.
When you learn a person has been mentally ill, you have learned the most important thing about his or her personality.	Every type of disturbance is different in every patient. A recovered patient needs to be viewed as an individual rather than as an anonymous member of a stereotyped group.
You can't talk to someone who has been mentally ill.	Most recovered people who have had mental illnesses are rational and intelligent. Even people with current illnesses are likely to be rational in many ways.
If a former mentally ill patient has a really bad history there isn't much hope.	Some people may be ill for many years before they receive effective treatment or their condition improves for other reasons. Once recovered, they may remain well for the rest of their lives.
A former mentally ill patient is bound to make a second-rate employee.	Many recovered patients make excellent employees. Some people who are subject to relapses may need to work in a flexible situation.
Perhaps recovered mentally ill patients can work successfully at low-level jobs, but they aren't suited for really important or responsible positions.	The career potentials of recovered mentally ill patients, as with anyone else, depend on the person's talents, abilities, experience, motivation, and health status.
Recovered mentally ill patients have a tough row to hoe, but there's not much that can be done about it.	The way *we* act toward former mentally ill patients can make all the difference.

From The National Institutes of Mental Health: *The 14 worst myths about recovered mental patients*, DHHS Pub No (ADM) 88-1391, Washington, DC, 1988, DHHS.

friendships. As more is learned about the nature of neurobiological disorders, it is becoming apparent that these difficulties are more closely related to the primary symptoms of the illness. For instance, depression causes apathy and withdrawal; schizophrenia leads to problems in perceiving and processing communications from others. These behaviors create serious problems in establishing close relationships.

LOW SELF-ESTEEM. Self-esteem is the feeling of self-worth or regard for oneself. It is difficult to maintain high self-esteem when an individual is aware of low achievement related to cultural expectations. Lack of ability to maintain employment, live independently, marry, and have children all contribute to low self-esteem. People who have serious mental illnesses often feel cheated of the life experiences they expected to enjoy before they became ill. They feel inadequate, especially if they believe that their illness is the result of a personality flaw rather than a physiological brain disorder.

One mental health professional who also has a serious mental illness describes her experience of being diagnosed with schizophrenia during adolescence[12]:

I was told I had a disease that was like diabetes, and if I continued to take neuroleptic medications for the rest of my life and avoided stress, I might be able to cope. I remember that as these words were spoken to me by my psychiatrist it felt as if my whole teenage world—in which I aspired to dreams of being a valued person in valued roles, of playing lacrosse for the U.S. Women's Team or maybe joining the Peace Corps—began to crumble and shatter. It felt as if these parts of my identity were being stripped from me. I was beginning to undergo that radically dehumanizing and devaluing transformation from being a person to being an illness; from being Pat Deegan to being 'a schizophrenic.'

MOTIVATION. For many seriously mentally ill persons, success and greater competence result in increased anxiety causing regression rather than in pride and continued progress. Patients attribute their uneasiness with success to fear that it will lead to higher expectations of others that they may not be able to attain. Fear of failure often results in reluctance to try new experiences. This may be perceived by others as lack of motivation. Apparent lack of motivation may also be caused by low energy. This can be related to the biological effect of the illness or to medication. In this case the person may want to be more active but is physically unable.

STRENGTHS. Rehabilitation depends on the control of illness, as well as on the development of health potential by mobilizing strengths. A strength is an ability, skill, or interest that an individual has used before. An emphasis on strengths provides hope that improved functioning is possible. Strengths may be related to recreational and leisure activities, work skills, educational accomplishments, self-care skills, special interests, talents and abilities, and positive interpersonal relationships. Seriously mentally ill people often need help in defining their skills, abilities and interests as strengths. Low self-esteem may lead them to believe that they only have problems, no strengths.

NONADHERENCE. Lack of adherence to prescribed treatment is often cited as a behavior of people who have serious mental illnesses. Failure to take medication is a frequent cause of rehospitalization. It is important to assess the reasons for nonadherence. There may be a lack of understanding of the reason for the treatment regimen. Sometimes the person wants to comply but needs assistance such as transportation to clinic appointments or advice about obtaining a medical assistance card. Some patients do not like the side effects of their medication. They may lack the assertiveness to tell the prescriber about their discomfort. The nurse can assist patients with this by rehearsing what to say before the appointment or accompanying them to provide support. Teaching patients to write notes about care providers' instructions and to keep lists of questions for the provider may also increase adherence.

Living Skills Assessment. The nursing assessment of a patient who has a serious mental illness should include an analysis of the person's community living skills. Some of the assessment tools presented in Chapter 6 are relevant, in particular those related to cognitive functioning and activities of daily living. Anthony[2] has developed a matrix (Table 13-4) of the skills required for successful functioning in the community. He describes the physical, emotional, and intellectual components of the skills needed for living, learning, and working. The nurse may use these examples in working with the patient to identify strengths, establish goals, and set priorities for skill development. Such a model provides a rational basis for assessing the patient's readiness to function productively in the community. It also provides objective information that can be shared with other mental health care providers.

The daily "hassles" experienced by people with serious mental illness have also been studied.[40] Daily "hassles" refer to "concerns, worries, or events that disrupt a person's well-being and daily life." The most frequently reported and severe hassles were concerns about money, loneliness, boredom, crime, past, present, and future accomplishments, oral and written communication problems, and physical health.

Table 13-4 Potential Skilled Activities Needed to Achieve the Goal of Psychiatric Rehabilitation

Physical	Emotional	Intellectual
LIVING SKILLS		
Personal hygiene	Human relations	Money management
Physical fitness	Self-control	Use of community resources
Use of public transportation	Selective reward	Goal setting
Cooking	Stigma reduction	Problem development
Shopping	Problem solving	
Cleaning	Conversational skills	
Sports participation		
Using recreational facilities		
LEARNING SKILLS		
Being quiet	Speech making	Reading
Paying attention	Question asking	Writing
Staying seated	Volunteering answers	Arithmetic
Observing	Following directions	Study skills
Punctuality	Asking for directions	Hobby activities
	Listening	Typing
WORKING SKILLS		
Punctuality	Job interviewing	Job qualifying
Use of job tools	Job decision making	Job seeking
Job strength	Human relations	Specific job tasks
Job transportation	Self-control	
Specific job tasks	Job keeping	
	Specific job tasks	

From Anthony WA: *Principles of psychiatric rehabilitation*, Baltimore, 1980, University Park Press.

Specific Populations

YOUNG ADULTS WITH SERIOUS MENTAL ILLNESS. The young patient, generally between the ages of 18 and 35, differs in important ways from seriously mentally ill people who are older. Many of these differences can be traced to deinstitutionalization and an increased emphasis on community-based care. Generally, younger patients have not experienced long psychiatric hospitalizations. For them, short hospital stays at times of crisis or acute exacerbation of symptoms have alternated with care in the community. The personal adaptations necessary for this pattern are different from those needed for long-term hospitalization.

Alternating between hospital and community life, young patients compare themselves with others of their age and expect their lives to be similar to those of their peers. They expect that they should marry, have children, and work. Inability to meet these role expectations and limited ability to cope with community living may lead to abuse of alcohol and drugs or suicidal behavior. Because they do not see themselves as patients, they have little motivation to become involved in treatment or rehabilitation programs or to take medication.

Because their illness interferes with voluntary treatment and ongoing participation in a therapeutic rela-

tionship, younger patients are more likely to enter the mental health system through hospital emergency rooms or the legal system. Younger patients may seek help voluntarily or at the insistence of family or friends during times of personal or family crisis. Behavior resulting from poor impulse control is often the precipitating event. Many of these patients enter the mental health system through involvement with the law for offenses such as "minor property damage" and "petty assault."

Young patients often become angry in response to their illnesses and often times are sarcastic and argumentative. The nurse should recognize the possibility of representing the success that has been denied to the patient, especially if the nurse and patient are close in age. In this case, anger is related to the situation, not the person. Another factor that commonly contributes to anger and acting out behavior by these patients is concurrent substance abuse. Living in the community offers opportunities to experiment with drugs, which is often appealing to the young person because it facilitates interaction with peers. Unfortunately the interaction of the abused substance, medications, and the biological disorder associated with the illness can have serious consequences. Substance abuse and the problem of dual diagnosis are discussed in Chapter 22.

CRITICAL THINKING ABOUT CONTEMPORARY ISSUES

What Are the Obligations of Society and the Mental Health Care System To Provide Psychiatric Treatment for Homeless People Who Have Serious Mental Illnesses?

There is an ongoing debate about the provision of mental health services for approximately one third of the homeless population who have a serious mental illness. The primary questions are whether there are resources available to provide the complex array of services needed by this population, and if there are not enough resources whether the homeless mentally ill should be forced to enter institutional programs.

Homeless mentally ill people tend to cluster in urban areas that have many other disadvantaged groups competing for scarce social and health-care services. Mental health treatment for these patients requires extensive outreach and major changes in traditional patterns of service delivery. Additionally, many service providers do not feel equipped to meet the needs of the homeless mentally ill. When the general public comes into contact with these people, they are often annoyed or embarrassed by their behavior. These factors combine to create pressure to remove homeless mentally ill people from the streets. The proposed solution is usually some form of involuntary reinstitutionalization, perhaps at a lower level of care than the hospital.

Opponents[13,27] to this approach cite civil liberties including the right to treatment in the least restrictive setting. Consumer advocates have worked long and hard to secure these rights. They fear that a return to acceptance of long-term institutional stays would result in a return to the neglect of mentally ill people. Some suggest that people should have a choice of their living conditions, including homelessness. Others question whether the problem is a lack of resources for services or a refusal to prioritize the needs of a group of people who have little political clout and few who are willing to fight for them.

Proponents of creating involuntary services include some family members and some service providers.[19,47] Families worry about the health and safety of their ill members who are living on the streets. The concept of "asylum" as a place of safety and shelter has been proposed as a way to provide for the needs of these people. Those who would remove the homeless to other settings acknowledge that this is not an ideal solution but believe that it is more humane than leaving people who are often vulnerable to exploitation without assistance. They are pessimistic that resources for community services will be available in the near future. They believe that society is neglecting its responsibility by allowing people who have impaired judgment and decision-making abilities to refuse to be helped. As professionals and citizens, nurses need to consider these issues and form their own opinions. ▼

HOMELESS PEOPLE WITH SERIOUS MENTAL ILLNESS. The media have linked deinstitutionalization with homelessness, which leads to the impression that most of the approximately 600,000 homeless people in the United States are mentally ill. Government estimates report that the number of homeless mentally ill is closer to one third, or 200,000 people.[13] This is still a substantial number and represents a particularly challenging population. Homeless people are difficult to reach and less likely to be involved with community resources. They are often, but not always, alienated from their families. They frequently distrust service systems and providers. Traditional mental health services have been particularly unsuccessful at working with this population because of a lack of flexibility and inability to focus on the patients' priorities. The response of the community is often to demand removal of the homeless, preferably to an institution. This has led to active debate among policymakers and mental health professionals (see Critical Thinking about Contemporary Issues).

The Family

The image of isolated chronically mentally ill people who return to a community where they have no connections has been widely publicized. However, most mentally ill people are involved with their families and will have frequent contact with family members while they are in the community. It has been reported that approximately 65% of people who have mental illnesses live with their families.[16] Therefore family resources must be assessed when a rehabilitation plan is being developed. Health-care providers and patients' families have often been adversaries. The family may be viewed by the providers as the cause of the problem or resistant to the treatment plan. Family members have a right to provide input to the treatment plan. They can identify potential problem areas and enhance the patient's compliance with the plan.

Components of Family Assessment. The nurse who assesses the family as part of a rehabilitation plan should include the following areas:

1. Family structure, including developmental stage, roles, responsibilities, norms, and values
2. Family attitudes toward the mentally ill member
3. The emotional climate of the family (e.g., fearful, angry, depressed, anxious, calm)
4. The social supports that are available to the family, including extended family, friends, financial support, religious involvement, and community contacts
5. Past family experiences with mental health services
6. The family's understanding of the patient's problem and the plan of care

Some of this information may be obtained from the social worker. However, it is the nurse's responsibility to be available to the family. This includes regular planned contacts with the family and inclusion of the family as part of the treatment team.

Family Burden. The presence of a mentally ill member affects the entire family. The impact of a family member's mental illness is often referred to as **family burden.** Maurin and Boyd[24] reviewed the literature on burden. They differentiate between *burden* and *distress*. D*istress* refers to the impact of all of the pressures of life on a family member, whereas *burden* is limited to the impact of the relative who has a mental illness. Burden may be objective or subjective. Objective burden is related to the patient's behavior, role performance, adverse effects on the family, need for support, and the financial costs of the illness. Subjective burden is the individual's own feeling of being burdened; it is individual and not consistently related to the elements of objective burden. For instance, a patient may lack ambition and remain in a dependent role well into adulthood. Family members that value success and upward mobility would be likely to feel more subjective burden related to this situation than members who are comfortable with nurturing and supporting someone. By assessing family burden, the nurse can work with the family to identify concerns with which they would like help.

Parker[33] is a nurse who is also very active in the National Alliance for the Mentally Ill. She has identified several categories of family response to mental illness. These are useful when assessing subjective burden.

▼ **Grief** is common and is related to the loss of the person they knew before the illness, as well as loss of the future that they expected to share with the ill family member. Because serious mental illness is usually cyclical, grief tends to be recurrent; it subsides during remission and returns during exacerbations. This is especially difficult for families to handle. In addi-

tion, social support systems may not recognize or respond to their need because of discomfort with the situation or the related stigma. Family members often feel guilty about the relative's illness. Unfortunately some theorists of mental illness have reinforced this guilt by blaming family members, especially mothers, for the illness. Although this is becoming less common, guilt still occurs. It is common for those who are close to a person with any serious illness to wonder if they could have done something to prevent it. For instance, spouses of heart attack victims may think they could have prevented it if they had not encouraged such patients to shovel snow. Similarly, relatives of a depressed person may believe that they could have prevented the depression if they had not shared their own worries with the patient. In neither of these situations did relatives cause the illnesses, but they feel guilt because of their interpretation of the situation. Another source of guilt for relatives of people with mental illness is the need at times to set limits on the patient's behavior. For instance, the family of a patient who is physically abusive may need to arrange involuntary hospitalization if the mentally ill member becomes dangerous to them.

▼ **Anger** may be directed toward the patient, but it is more often felt toward other family members, mental health care providers, or the entire system. Anger within the family relates to differing perceptions of the patient and varied ideas about how to manage the illness. Prolonged stress results in irritability that is often taken out on those to whom one is closest. Anger at the system frequently is justified because it is related to deficiencies in the accessibility or acceptability of services.

▼ Families' realization that they are dealing with a long-term recurrent illness leads to a feeling of **powerlessness** and **fear.** Most people believe that the health-care system should cure illnesses. When this is impossible, they feel powerless and frustrated. This understanding can also result in fear about the future of the ill family member and for themselves. Powerlessness and fear are especially troublesome for parents who are aging and worried about care arrangements for their mentally ill child when they can no longer provide care. Some families also fear ill members who may be dangerous because of the symptoms of the illness.

Social Support Needs. Norbeck and her colleagues[31] have studied families' needs for social support. They identified four categories of support needs. These are presented in Table 13-5 and can be used by the nurse as a guide for assessing family needs.

Although much of the exploration of family concerns

Table 13-5 Support Needs Expressed by Family Caregivers

EMOTIONAL SUPPORT

Acceptance	Absence of stigmatization; acceptance of the caregiver despite being related to a mentally ill patient
Commitment	Demonstrating to the caregiver a commitment to the well-being of the patient, or sharing the burden of caregiving if only through being in contact with the caregiver
Social involvement	Social contacts and companionship for the caregiver
Affective	Showing love and caring for the caregiver, including concern for his or her well-being (with qualities of sympathy, compassion, and occasionally true empathy)
Mutuality	Reciprocity in supportive exchanges

FEEDBACK SUPPORT

Affirmation	Validation of the actions, feelings, and decisions associated with the caregiving role
Listening	Active listening by the support person, provision of a sounding board, and allowing for unburdening by the caregiver
Talking	The opportunity to talk with another person (without the quality of active listening, emotional presence, or the feeling of unburdening)

INFORMATIONAL OR COGNITIVE SUPPORT

Illness information	Information about the patient's illness, care, or supervision
Behavior management	Information about behavior management strategies
Coping	Advice about personal coping strategies for the caregiver
Decision	Help in the decision-making process around caregiving issues and offering solutions
Perspective	Supportive interactions that give the caregiver a new perspective about caregiving or about the caregiving situation

INSTRUMENTAL SUPPORT

Resources	Help in locating resources, negotiating systems, or advocating for needs
Respite	Provision of time-off for the caregiver and support for meeting the caregiver's own needs
Care-help	Provision of help with the actual tasks of caregiving, including physical care assistance and monitoring activities (watching the behavior of the patient and setting limits)
Backup	Help is available when needed, including financial help
Household	Help with such home activities as repairs, grocery shopping, or housecleaning

From Norbeck J, Chafetz L, Skodol-Wilson H, Weiss SJ: *Nurs Res* 40:208, 1991.

has focused on parents, sibling needs have also been studied. In one study[20] siblings of schizophrenic individuals identified the following concerns:

1. A need for more information about the illness, especially prognosis
2. Interest in meeting with other siblings of people with schizophrenia
3. A need for help in learning to communicate with their ill sibling

Nurses can play an important role in offering family members opportunities to discuss their concerns and in taking action to meet their needs whenever possible.

You are approached by the parent of a hospitalized young adult patient who has a serious mental illness. The family is upset because the discharge plan is to refer the patient to a community program that has not been helpful in the past. What nursing interventions would you suggest in this case?

The Community

The community greatly influences rehabilitation of its mentally ill members. Mental health professionals have a unique role in the community because they are community members and advocates for mentally ill people and their families at the same time. Care providers, including nurses, can and should assume a leadership role in assessing the adequacy and effectiveness of existing community resources and in recommending changes.

Nurses in all settings must be familiar with the community agencies that provide services to people who have mental illnesses. Most communities have a social and medical services directory that can be consulted for basic information such as location, type, and cost of the services provided. Most agencies serve people who come from a particular geographical area such as one part of a city or, in a rural area, one or several counties. As nurses gain experience, they will become familiar with other agencies that provide services for the same people. Nurses should pay attention to patients' evaluations of the agencies from which they receive services.

This information helps to identify agencies that are responsive and helpful as opposed to those that are difficult for patients to approach. Howie the Harp,[18] an advocate for services to homeless mentally ill people and who was once homeless and mentally ill, has described consumer priorities for mental health services. They include independent living, freedom to choose, and low-income, decent, permanent housing connected to support services.

Personal contact with community agencies can be very useful as part of a community assessment. This may be achieved by making an appointment with an agency staff member. However, a more realistic picture of an agency's services can be obtained by going to the agency with someone who is requesting services. The nurse will see how the agency responds to the patient and how the patient handles personal affairs in the community. The nurse can also provide emotional support if the patient is insecure in a new situation. Nurses should introduce themselves to the staff of the agency and explain that they, as well as the patient, would like to learn more about the services. Collaborative relationships between mental health care providers and community agencies are essential if rehabilitation is to succeed.

A wide range of community services must be available to patients. Those that are directed toward basic needs include provisions for shelter; food, clothing, and household management; income and financial support; meaningful activities; and mobility and transportation. Other services provide for special needs that may differ from one person to the next such as general medical services, mental health services, habilitation and rehabilitation programs, vocational services, and social services. A third group of services have the purpose of coordinating the system. These include patient identification and outreach, individual assessment and service planning, case management, advocacy and community organization, community information, and education and support. Information like this is valuable to those who are advocating for the allocation of additional resources for mental health care.

PLANNING AND IMPLEMENTATION
The Individual

Treatment planning and intervention in rehabilitative psychiatric nursing focuses on fostering independence by maximizing the person's strengths. This is directly parallel to the nurse's role in physical rehabilitation. It differs from nursing care that is given to patients when they are acutely ill. During acute illness, people require a nurturing approach. The nurse must provide for all of the basic life functions that the person is unable to manage. However, the relationship becomes less dependent as patients grow stronger and are able to care for themselves. Residual functional deficits may remain. The nurse and patient must then work together to find ways for the patient to overcome any remaining impaired areas of functioning.

Developing Strengths and Potentials. The development of the seriously mentally ill person's strengths and potentials is important. Nursing interventions that develop strengths and potentials can help patients develop independent living skills, interpersonal relationships, and coping resources, and thus help meet their special needs. Ultimately, the expected outcome of such interventions is change in the patient's self-concept and an increase in self-esteem. The negative self-concept and low self-esteem that characterize people who have serious mental illnesses interfere with their ability to see themselves as individuals with strengths and potentials. Through experiences of adequacy, self-concept can be altered and self-esteem increased. One intervention that helps patients alter their negative self-perceptions is for nurses to describe their perception of patients' strengths. Nursing interventions in which patients become aware of their strengths fall into two categories: those that occur spontaneously and those that are planned. The following clinical example illustrates a nurse's use of spontaneously occurring situations to increase awareness of strengths.

CLINICAL EXAMPLE

Theresa, a woman in her fifties, had been in and out of psychiatric hospitals for 30 years and had been living in a supervised apartment in the community for 1 year. Theresa shared the apartment with two roommates. She was a talented musician and had her own baby grand piano. Despite her love for classical music, she played only the "oldies and goodies" her roommates preferred. She said that she didn't want to upset her roommates by practicing classical music. She was afraid that if she brought the issue out in the open she might get so upset she would hurt someone. She offered as evidence the numerous times she'd been placed in seclusion rooms for violent behavior. Clearly, keeping peace was her priority.

The nurse and Theresa discussed her strengths as a peacemaker, as well as ways in which she might calmly express her own needs to her roommates. The nurse offered to be with Theresa during the discussion. Declining the nurse's offer, Theresa said that even though she was somewhat anxious, she had a clearer understanding of the abilities she had to use in the situation, and she wanted to try to "pick up" for herself in a situation of interpersonal conflict. She carried out her plan and expressed surprise that her roommates accepted her need and quickly arranged 2 hours a day for her to practice. As she told of her success, Theresa smiled, saying she wondered what would have happened if she had tried expressing her needs many months earlier.

Cindy, in her early twenties, had recently moved into the supervised apartment with Theresa and one other roommate. Cindy arrived at the day treatment program crying because she had fainted while at her nursing home job the evening before. She felt that in addition to having been embarrassed, she had failed to live up to the trust invested in her by the director of the nursing home. She had decided to quit her job.

The nurse explored with Cindy the meaning of these events in terms of her many strengths in caring for others. Her sensitivity to anticipated criticism and rejection from the director was related to the same sensitivity that allowed her to respond creatively to others' needs. Cindy, at this point, firmly stated that the job was important to her sense of being needed. The nurse encouraged her to call the nursing home, express both her embarrassment and sense of failure, yet state that she wanted to continue working there. Cindy made the phone call with the nurse present for support. Her pleasure at finding out the job was still hers, that she was not viewed unfavorably by the director of nursing, and her sense of personal achievement at having taken a risk and won were so visible and contagious that the other patients staged an impromptu celebration.

Selected Nursing Diagnoses:
▼ *Theresa:* Impaired social interaction related to fear of aggressive impulses as evidenced by social inhibition
▼ *Cindy:* Chronic low self-esteem related to fear of rejection as evidenced by feelings of inadequacy

Community-Based Services. Supporting people who have serious mental illnesses in community settings requires the development of a wide array of community support programs. Some of these are rehabilitation centers, housing services, employment opportunities, education, crisis intervention and outreach, and case management. When these services are provided, it has been demonstrated that people who would have spent much of their time in the hospital can live successfully in the community. One longitudinal study found that 75% of a group of former state hospital patients remained in the community 11 years after discharge.[32] Although some required hospital stays during that time, these totaled only 2.6% of the study period. All but one of the patients preferred community life to hospitalization.

REHABILITATION PROGRAMS. Psychiatric rehabilitation programs (also referred to as *psychosocial rehabilitation*) were rare before the 1970s. They were developed in response to the plight of people who had been discharged

from state mental hospitals lacking the skills and resources needed to live independently in the community. These programs are diverse with each developing services related to the needs of its consumers and the philosophy of its consumers and staff. In general they are based on the principles of rehabilitation that were described earlier in this chapter. Several models are presented here as an overview of some of the psychiatric rehabilitation approaches that have been found to be effective.

Fountain House. Fountain House, in New York City, was established in the late 1940s by a group of former state mental hospital patients. It began as a consumer-operated program, but a decade later employed a professional staff. Many of the current psychiatric rehabilitation programs are built on the Fountain House model. Fountain House functions as a club in which patients are members. The usual hierarchical distinctions between staff (the healthy) and patients (the ill) do not exist. It is a place where members care about each other and pool their resources and abilities as they work toward increasing independence. Thus Fountain House combats loneliness and isolation while providing a variety of living and work situations that require differing levels of functional ability.

The first month at Fountain House is a residential phase, and members are taught skills necessary for apartment living. Fountain House owns and leases apartments that have staff on call, although not in residence. These supervised apartments allow individuals to make a gradual transition to independent living in the community.

Fountain House runs several businesses providing a protected environment in which members can develop self-confidence and job skills. Progressing to a more complex work situation, Fountain House has creatively arranged for transitional employment placements, called TEPs. Recognizing that job interviews are tremendously stressful, staff, rather than members, seek out and contract with businesses for jobs. The jobs are assigned to Fountain House rather than to individuals. Staff assign a member to a transitional employment position for as long as needed. The employer is promised that if members are unable to manage the job or do not show up, Fountain House staff will work in their place. Fountain House members, who share responsibility for a job with staff, can assume increasing responsibility as they are able to handle it. A TEP can easily be transferred from a member who is ready for a more complex work experience to a member who needs a TEP. Furthermore, employers are satisfied because the quality of work is guaranteed.

Ronald Peterson, a veteran of 10 years of residence in a state hospital, speaks poignantly of the loneliness and isolation he felt when he left the state hospital to live alone in a small hotel room. Since he had no job, knew no one, and lived on welfare, it never occurred to him that things could be any different. He said, "You take what you can get. There is no choice."[35] Eventually becoming a staff member of Fountain House, Peterson spoke for many persons trying to adjust to community living when he described the wish for a place where one belongs and is needed.

> I think the greatest need is to have a place to go where you are expected each day, a place where you can be with people like yourself and do things that mean something to yourself and others . . . you have to remember that many of us did a lot of things in the hospital. If given a chance we can do lots of things in the community—if we have places to go and can be with people who need us to contribute, to take part, to help, and who notice when we're not present and do something about it.[35]

Training in Community Living. The Training in Community Living program attempts to keep patients in their own homes in the community.[42] This program was developed in Madison, Wisconsin, to provide services to former state hospital patients. It has served as a model for community-based programs throughout the United States. In this model when a person is in crisis and may need hospital admission, a substitute intervention is implemented. Staff are assigned to remain with the person in the community, providing support and assistance. Nurses accompany patients as they perform their usual activities. This real-world experience with the patient enables the nurse to accurately assess the skills that the person needs to learn. The nurse and patient mutually agree on realistic goals. Staff contact is decreased as the patient functions more independently. When patients live with their families, families may also receive counseling and guidance in assisting patients.

Community Bound. Malone[23] described Community Bound, a rehabilitation program for seriously mentally ill people in Austin, Texas. She identified several concepts that contributed to the rehabilitation of the patients. These are summarized in Table 13-6.

Consumer-run services. Many of the former mental hospital patients (consumers) who founded Fountain House became dissatisfied with the program after it came under the control of professionals and left. There continues to be a strong feeling among some consumers that psychosocial rehabilitation programs are not truly responsive to their needs unless they are consumer controlled. In recent years there has been slow but steady growth of new consumer-run programs in many communities. Some of these are drop-in centers that provide peer support and a safe place to be, whereas others offer a full range of rehabilitative services.

Chamberlin,[11] a former mental health services con-

Table 13-6   Concepts Related to Rehabilitation

Concept	Characteristics
Survival skills	Community living skills including housekeeping, money management, and shopping; socialization skills including manners, assertiveness, and vocational skills
Cooperation	Ability to obey rules and participate in a structured program
Hanging out	Informal socialization with others; development of friendships
Checking up	Staff ensuring that things are going well
Backing	Helping someone deal with community agencies
Supplementing	Providing material resources such as food or clothing

Adapted from Malone J: *Issues Ment Health Nurs* 10:121, 1989.

sumer, has described service models that claim to decrease staff/patient differentiation.

Partnership model. Participants in this type of program are told that they are partners. However, there is still a clear distinction between caregivers and receivers. Chamberlin refers to these as "alternatives in name only." Fountain House is an example of a partnership model program. It is run by professionals and, according to Chamberlin, looks and functions like an institution. She further criticizes the apparent assumption that all ex-patients are like the severely disabled people on whom the program focuses.

Supportive model. In the supportive model membership is open to all who want mutual support. Ex-patients and those who have never been hospitalized are equal. It is believed that any person can sometimes be in need of help and sometimes be able to provide help to others. Professionals are excluded, except to promote community support or funding.

Separatist model. In the separatist model ex-patients support each other and run the service. All others are excluded. It is believed that anyone who has never experienced the psychiatric patient role will interfere with the consciousness-raising process and will have stereotyped attitudes.

Chamberlin believes very strongly that alternative treatment programs should be run by consumers. Successful programs also include other elements. They must address needs identified by the members, and participation must be voluntary. There should be options to participate in all or part of the total program. Help is provided either by members to members or by others whom they select. Consumers are responsible for the administrative direction of the program, and they determine criteria for membership. Finally, the program is mainly accountable to the members. Strict confidentiality is maintained, but all information related to treatment is made available to the person.

What is your response to Chamberlin's assertion that consumers should run alternative treatment programs? Discuss positive and negative implications.

RESIDENTIAL SERVICES. Housing is consistently identified as a critical element of successful psychiatric rehabilitation services. Appropriate housing must be safe, affordable, and acceptable to the consumer. Early housing programs tended to focus on existing supervised living situations, such as foster care. There was little oversight of these programs, and exploitation of patients was not uncommon. More recently an array of housing options has been developed under the leadership of consumers and psychiatric rehabilitation professionals.

Group homes and supervised apartments are the predominant types of housing for seriously mentally ill people. Most incorporate some form of rehabilitation programming along with housing. Staff supervision ranges from intensive 24-hour awake staffing to telephone consultation, based on the consumer's level of need. Although these programs are a distinct improvement on foster care, there are also drawbacks. Most housing programs focus on providing a "normal" community living experience but fall short of this goal. Supervision needs may lead to organization of housing around levels of care, sometimes requiring consumers to move if their needs become more or less intensive. This can be very disruptive. Consumers rarely have a choice of housemates and they hardly ever lease or own the house in their own names. This type of housing program structure also leads to clustering of group homes or supervised apartments, reinforcing stigmatization and triggering community apprehension.

Some traditional residential programs are now evolving into "supported housing" programs. This concept has been developed by Carling and his associates[10] at the Center for Community Change through Housing and Support in Burlington, Vermont. Housing is conceptualized as a basic service that should mirror the housing choices of others in the community. It is permanent and under the control of the resident. Housing program staff assist consumers to find affordable housing of their choice. If people decide to live together it is also their choice. Staff may introduce consumers to each other, but they decide whether or not to establish a household. Mental health and rehabilitative services are flexible and designed to assist the person to live successfully in the community. Some supported housing programs are part of comprehensive psychiatric rehabilitation programs and are an element of a broader "supportive living" approach. In this case staff intervention is directed not only at maintaining the person in housing but also at assisting the consumer to become fully involved in community life to the extent that the person chooses. A "personal future planning" process assists the consumer to identify goals, preferences, and the important people who can assist in accomplishing these.

Studies of consumer preference have supported the supportive living approach.[44] In a review of 43 consumer preference surveys, it was consistently found that consumers preferred having their own house or apartment, living alone or with a significant other, and did not want to live with another consumer of mental health services. A study of consumers in one supportive housing program found that personal empowerment and instrumental role involvement were improved after at least 5 months in the program. Social support and involvement in decision making were particularly important to the consumers.[25]

VOCATIONAL SERVICES. Many psychiatric rehabilitation programs provide vocational rehabilitation services. Prevocational training usually begins within the program itself. Members may be organized into work teams around the activities needed to keep the program running, usually clerical, food service, and maintenance tasks. Aside from the development of marketable work skills, the goal of these programs is to foster good work habits. Some members continue indefinitely in prevocational services. Others may move into temporary employment placements such as those developed at Fountain House. The final stage of vocational rehabilitation is finding competitive employment. Some consumers use vocational services successfully to achieve this goal. Box 13-1 lists six principles to be considered related to vocational rehabilitation of people who have serious mental illnesses.[4]

Although mental health service providers have supported the idea of vocational rehabilitation, they have been reluctant and sometimes actively opposed to hiring consumers themselves. If they do, it is often as a janitor, housekeeper, or groundskeeper. Consumers have begun to assert their unique qualifications as counselors and case managers. They have been successfully employed in this role and have achieved good outcomes for themselves and those to whom they provide services.[41]

Besio and Mahler[6] have reported the results of a survey about the benefits and problems resulting from employing consumer staff in supported housing services. Benefits to service recipients included more positive

Box 13-1

PRINCIPLES OF VOCATIONAL REHABILITATION

▼ Vocational services must be integrated with other rehabilitation services.

▼ There must be an array of vocational options and provision for changes in career goals.

▼ Support and backup services must be provided at the work site.

▼ Job expectations must be realistic, neither too high nor too low.

▼ Compensation should be adequate and should not interfere with ongoing benefits (e.g., food stamps and medical assistance).

▼ Program development must be based on the realities of the community context related to economic and political considerations.

From Bachrach LL: *Am J Psychiatr* 149:1455, 1992.

staff-recipient relationships, better knowledge of resources and ways to overcome barriers, advocacy, and role modeling. Problems for recipients included concerns about confidentiality and lack of consumer staff training. For the consumer staff, benefits included improved self-esteem, vocational skill development, and increased income. Stress management and the impact of job stress on their mental illness were problems for the consumer staff. The organization benefited from increased sensitivity to consumers and awareness of consumer capabilities by nonconsumer staff, improvement in the relevance of services, and the availability of a pool of good employees. Organizational problems included distrust and stigmatization of consumer staff by their nonconsumer co-workers and the need to accommodate disability-related behaviors. They also reported a benefit to the community related to improvement in the image of people with mental illnesses.

EDUCATIONAL SERVICES. Many people with serious mental illnesses have not completed formal education through high school or beyond because of the effects of the illness. Rehabilitation programs often offer remedial education related to vocational services. Education that is offered in a supportive environment can increase self-esteem, improve job qualifications, and encourage some consumers to pursue higher education.

CRISIS INTERVENTION AND OUTREACH SERVICES. These services are integral parts of a comprehensive community support system. Crisis intervention is described in Chapter 12 and mental health outreach in Chapter 32.

Nursing Interventions. Rehabilitative psychiatric nursing tries to maximize the person's strengths and minimize weaknesses. The nursing care plan should be organized around very specific behavioral goals that are based on a comprehensive assessment of the person's living skills. These goals should build on those that are developed during the acute phase of the illness. This part of the nursing care plan may be labeled the *discharge plan* in an inpatient treatment setting. Discharge plans should also be developed in community settings. This will remind the nurse and patient that the expected outcome of nursing care is independent functioning. Even patients who need long-term medication can usually receive maintenance prescriptions from their family physician as part of their general health-care program. This helps to put the mental illness into perspective as a chronic health problem that is not so different from other chronic problems the person might have.

The nurse and patient must decide together on the desired level of functioning. If the patient is unwilling to take on activities that the nurse thinks would be helpful, it is important to discover why. Sometimes nurses try to push a patient ahead too rapidly. Behavior that has developed gradually over time cannot be changed quickly. Learning new behavior patterns and giving up old ones is frightening and causes anxiety. The nurse must be sure that the patient's coping skills are adequate to deal with the stress of growth. Feedback must be requested to be sure that the rehabilitation plan continues to address the patient's needs. Sometimes the plan assumes greater importance than the patient. The nurse must prevent this.

PSYCHOEDUCATION. Several theorists have suggested educational approaches to assist with rehabilitation. This type of intervention is called **psychoeducation.** Goldman[14] defines psychoeducation as "education or training of a person with a psychiatric disorder in subject areas that serve the goals of treatment and rehabilitation, for example, enhancing the person's acceptance of his illness, promoting active cooperation with treatment and rehabilitation, and strengthening the coping skills that compensate for deficiencies caused by the disorder." He adds that patient education must be provided by a qualified person and should be part of the treatment plan.

 Review a book intended for mental health consumers. Critique it in terms of accuracy, practical advice, and emotional tone. Ask a consumer or a family member of a consumer to review the book. Compare your critiques.

Psychoeducation in the context of a rehabilitative approach often focuses on **social skills training,** which assists the learner to acquire behaviors that will support community living (see Chapter 28). Ideally, social skills training begins while the patient is in the hospital. This is particularly important for those who have been hospitalized for extended periods of time. Boyd and her colleagues[7] have described a social skills training project for long-term inpatients. It focused on self-maintenance, social functioning, and community living skills. Patients were assigned to small groups based on their level of functioning. The program did result in measurable skills improvement.

The effectiveness of social skills training has been investigated. One study[45] found that a structured social skills training program resulted in patient improvement that was maintained for at least a year. This successful program incorporated videotapes, role-playing, practice, and homework assignments centered around practical problems, such as medication management or obtaining social services, that individuals might encounter in the community.

Buckwalter and Kerfoot[8] identified several topics that can help the patient avoid rehospitalization. These are presented in the Patient Education plan below. A patient education program such as this can be used in hospital or community settings. Specific content can be planned to meet the needs of a patient or a group. Consumers are growing to expect health teaching as a part of professional service. Nurses are the best-equipped health-care providers to offer this service.

PATIENT EDUCATION PLAN
COPING WITH PSYCHIATRIC ILLNESS

Content	Instructional activities	Evaluation
Identify and describe common psychiatric diagnoses	Provide handouts outlining behaviors Discuss coping behaviors Assign homework from lay literature Compare mental illness to physical illness	Patient recognizes characteristics of the diagnosis Patient distinguishes between cure and coping
Describe the role of stress in contributing to psychiatric disorders	Sensitize the patient to signs of increased stress Define stress as a test of coping skills Teach relaxation exercises	Patient verbalizes level of stress Patient performs relaxation exercises and describes a reduction in perceived stress
Assist to gain a sense of control by recognizing personal pattern of signs and symptoms	Provide feedback when symptomatic behavior occurs Instruct patient to keep a diary of behavior and to identify symptoms	Patient consistently labels symptoms and seeks professional help when necessary
Development of social skills to enable participation in vocational and recreational activities	Role play social interaction in a variety of situations Field trips to community activities Supervised vocational training in real work settings	Patient participates in progressively more independent social and work activities
Identify and describe community support systems	Provide a list of community support programs, including self-help groups, mental health-care agencies, and social agencies Invite representatives of programs to speak to patient group Escort to first agency contact	Patient selects community programs that offer needed resources Patient becomes able to access agency independently
Describe and discuss psychoactive medications	Instruct about actions, side effects, and contraindications to common psychoactive medications Distribute handouts describing the patient's medications Suggest systems to help patient remember when to take medication and how much	Patient describes characteristics of prescribed medications Patient reports effects of prescribed medications Patient takes medication as prescribed

Modified from Buckwalter KC, Kerfoot KM: J *Psychosoc Nurs Ment Health Serv* 20:15, 1982.

SOCIAL SUPPORT. The role of nurses relative to social support groups has been described by Norbeck.[30] She relates the following assumptions about social support:

1. Supportive relationships are needed by people to manage everyday role demands and to cope with life changes and unusual stressors.
2. A network of social relationships forms the context for the giving and receiving of social support.
3. Social network relationships are relatively stable over time, especially those that are the individual's primary ties.
4. To be supportive, a relationship should be basically healthy, not pathological.
5. The quantity and type of support needed depend on the characteristics of the individual and the nature of the situation.
6. The quantity and type of support available also depend on the characteristics of the individual and the situation.

CASE MANAGEMENT. Case management services are essential for integration of the total array of psychiatric rehabilitation services. The role of nurses in case management is discussed in Chapter 32.

The Family

Family support is very important to the successful rehabilitation of a mentally ill person. The mental illness of a member is often a shock and a source of great stress to the family. Nurses are in a favorable position to help families cope with the stress and adapt to changes in the family structure. Pfeiffer and Mostek[36] have identified three categories of programs for families of people with serious mental illnesses: empowerment, treatment, and educational. Empowerment and educational programs are discussed here. Family treatment is presented in Chapter 30.

Empowerment. Walsh,[46] a parent of an adult child who has schizophrenia, has suggested several common trouble spots in family life. Learning ways to handle these troublesome areas empowers the family by giving them a sense of control over their lives. The problem areas include the following:

1. Disrupted communications
2. Mechanics of everyday life, including the need for privacy and control over personal space, keeping a regular schedule, television usage, money management, and grooming
3. Responding to hallucinations, delusions, and odd behavior, particularly coping with violent or suicidal threats
4. Alcohol and drug use

5. Need for relatives to remember to take care of themselves

This last area of concern identified by Walsh is frequently ignored by family members and professionals alike. She recommends the following ways to accomplish this:

1. Accept the fact of a mentally ill family member.
2. Plan a self-care program.
3. Continue to pursue personal activities and interests.
4. Get involved with organizations such as self-help groups or churches.
5. Avoid the advice and opinions of those who have not lived with a schizophrenic.
6. Remember that happiness is possible.
7. Stop blaming yourself.

Reviewing this list gives the nurse some understanding of the pain and stress that is experienced by the family of a mentally ill person.

Families and mental health care providers sometimes become engaged in power struggles related to the care of the mentally ill family member. This interferes with their ability to work as a team. Several helpful approaches to families have been identified.[15] The first is to allow the family members to express their feelings about the patient's illness and how it relates to their lives. The next task is to provide the information that families need to participate in decision making. One nursing study found that siblings were often the relayers of information in the family, while nurses were rarely identified as sources of information.[22] Families have feelings related to the member's illness. These may include relief that the member is receiving help, guilt over hospitalizing the member, fear about what will happen in the future, and depression if the member does not respond well to treatment. Another task is to assist them to deal with these feelings. Families may try to cope with the member's mental illness by denying the seriousness of the problem, by being overcontrolling, or by withdrawing. A task of the nurse is to identify the coping method that is being used and assess its helpfulness. Finally, the nurse must help the family learn to balance their own needs with those of the patient. Because nurses are usually viewed as supportive and helpful, they are in a good position to be sensitive to the needs of families and address them. Ways that professionals can share power with families are summarized in Box 13-2.[48]

Family Education. Family education has become a primary nursing intervention when providing rehabilitative services to relatives of seriously mentally ill people. Nurses have established workshops for family members that have been well received and have helped families

Table 13-7   Overview of the Family Intervention Process

Phases	Goals	Techniques
Phase I	Connection with the family and enlistment of cooperation with program	Joining
		Establishment of treatment contract
	Decrease of guilt, emotionality, and negative reactions to the illness	Discussion of crisis history and feelings about the patient and the illness
	Reduction of family stress	Empathy
		Specific practical suggestions that mobilize concerns into effective coping mechanisms
Phase II	Increased understanding of illness and patient's needs by family	Multiple family education and discussion
Survival skills workshop		Concrete data on schizophrenia
	Continued reduction of family stress	Concrete management suggestions
	Deisolation—enhancement of social networks	Basic communication skills
Phase III	Patient maintenance in community	Reinforcement of boundaries (generational and interpersonal)
Reentry and application	Strengthening of marital/parental coalition	
	Increased family tolerance for low-level dysfunctional behaviors	Task assignments
		Low-key problem solving
	Decreased and gradual resumption of responsibility by patient	
Phase IV	Reintegration into normal roles in community systems (work, school)	Infrequent maintenance sessions
Maintenance		Traditional or exploratory family therapy techniques
	Increased effectiveness of general family processes	

From Anderson CM, Hogarty GE, Reiss DJ: *Schizophr Bull* 6:495, 1980.

cope with the challenges presented by the mental illness.[26,34]

A four-phase process for intervention with the families of schizophrenic patients is summarized in Table 13-7. Intervention using the model should not be attempted without advanced education at the graduate level. However, nurses can be very helpful if they try to understand family needs and reinforce family coping mechanisms.

 If you were responsible for developing a nursing program for psychiatric rehabilitation, what would it be like? Describe the setting, the program, its goals, and the roles of staff and patients.

The Community

There are several ways that nurses can intervene in the community to encourage the establishment of tertiary prevention programs. Among these are health education, membership in advocacy groups, networking, and political action. It has been noted that stigma decreases with increased formal education. Most nurses have a strong background and a firm belief in health education. Mental health education in the community provides a real opportunity to have an impact on the experience of patients as community members. Greater understanding of the behaviors and needs of the mentally ill could increase community acceptance, leading to the development of better services. Thus nurses should take advantage of opportunities to speak to community groups about mental health.

Psychiatric nurses can also perform a valuable service by educating their co-workers and professional colleagues about current research related to serious mental illnesses. Although it is seldom discussed, significant stigmatizing attitudes toward mentally ill people exist in the professional community. These attitudes are then transmitted to the general public. Professionals have even taken the lead in opposing the establishment of group homes in their neighborhoods. Well-informed nurses can make mental health care workers aware of their prejudices and assist them to change their behavior.

Membership by nurses in community advocacy groups can also be helpful. Nurses can join forces with other professional and lay people who share concerns about the care of the mentally ill. The National Mental Health Association is the largest advocacy group that addresses mental health issues. Members of this organization have been useful in drawing attention to the needs of mentally ill people and in supporting positive legislation at the federal and state levels. They monitor the effectiveness of the mental health care system. Nurses can provide useful input to this part of their activities.

Nurses can also promote working relationships among advocacy groups, professional organizations, self-help groups, and concerned citizens. With limited funding available and health-care costs escalating, the formation of coalitions is essential to lobby for the allocation of resources to mental health care. Psychiatric nurses have taken a leadership role in coalitions to influence reforms in the American health-care system.

The activities of community-wide networks are frequently directed toward the political system. Aside from allocation of money and other resources, the nature of mental health care in a community is strongly influenced by the political structure of that community. As described in Chapter 8, legal issues have a great effect on mental health care delivery. Nurses need to be aware of and involved in the political process. They should communicate directly with their legislators at all levels, sharing their interests and concerns. Politicians are well aware of the need to respond to the priorities of their constituents.

Nurses can also become more directly involved in the political system. They can run for office and support other nurses who are legislators. Nurses are often invaluable members of appointed boards and commissions having to do with health care. Their knowledge can be shared with others who are planning community health-care systems. These voluntary activities are time consuming, but they can have great impact on the health care system. Community-level policies can either inhibit or facilitate direct care efforts. Active involvement in professional organizations often leads to productive and rewarding community activities. There is a great sense of satisfaction to be derived from selling a community on a new idea and seeing it become a reality.

Obtain a copy of a bill considered by your state legislature that is relevant to psychiatric rehabilitation. Explain the effect that this legislation would have on the mental health care system, including the potential effect on nursing practice.

EVALUATION

Evaluation of psychiatric rehabilitation services usually takes place at the levels of the impact on the patient and family and the effectiveness of the community service system.

Patient Evaluation

Evaluation of the services provided to patients and family members must focus on the achievement of the expected outcomes of the intervention. Most psychiatric rehabilitation programs rely on both objective and subjective measures of outcome. Objective measures are generally related to the following questions:

▼ Is the person living in housing of personal choice?
▼ Have days of hospitalization in the last year decreased?
▼ How many emergency room visits has the person made?
▼ How many days in the last year have been spent in a transitional employment placement? In competitive employment?
▼ How often does the person have contact with family members? Who are they?
▼ Can the person identify people to provide support in a crisis?
▼ Is the person involved in community activities?
▼ Is the person enrolled in an adult education course? In an academic education program?

The answers to questions such as these are compared with the individual rehabilitation plans, providing a picture of the success of the services received. They should be discussed with program participants and their families as a basis for further planning.

Subjective measures of effectiveness include periodic discussions with patients and families about the

COMPETENT CARING
A CLINICAL EXEMPLAR OF A PSYCHIATRIC NURSE

Iona Bradley, RN, C

Ms. C was one of the first patients in my mobile treatment caseload. She had had multiple admissions to the state hospital. Her psychiatric diagnosis was bipolar disorder. The referral to this new program was made in an attempt to assist her to spend more time in the community. We have now been working together for 6 years. Soon after I met her I realized that there were several nursing problems that I would need to address. She had a history of poor compliance with her medications. She was also diabetic and not good about following her prescribed diet. Because of her diabetes, she had a neurogenic bladder for which an indwelling catheter had been inserted. She was not managing her catheter care very well.

She had been living with an abusive alcoholic boyfriend. Although she knew that this was not a good situation for her, she was unable to break away from him. Her conditional release from the hospital required her to live in supervised housing. This forced her to distance herself from him. A stable living situation also enabled me to observe her behavior over time. I discovered that her bipolar cycle involved manic episodes every 21 days. Knowing this, I could work with her to schedule her life to accommodate her cycle. For instance, she is not pressured to attend her daytime psychosocial rehabilitation program during the manic phase. I also observed a relationship between the manic phase of her bipolar disorder and her diabetes. While manic, she craves sweets and is unable to control her carbohydrate intake. I have worked with the residential staff to remove as many sweets as possible from the house when her manic phase is due to happen. If she does eat sweets she becomes irritable and agitated. Since all of her caregivers are aware of this, she is supported until she regains her stable state.

It took a long time to gain Ms. C's trust. I had to demonstrate over and over that I really cared about her. Once she was able to trust me, I was able to focus on some of her physical nursing care needs. Her urinary catheter was a major inconvenience. She didn't always secure the collection bag well and sometimes it would be found around her ankle. In the past, her boyfriend had pulled it out. With a great deal of support, she agreed to the insertion of a suprapubic catheter. This was easier for her to care for and she has even regained some bladder tone. Her diabetes is becoming more fragile. It is expected that she will need to take insulin in the near future. I have found that pharmacy students are available to monitor medication use in the home for patients who are having problems with self-administration or compliance. I have referred Ms. C to that program. I am also teaching the residential staff about meal planning and nutritious diets.

A long-term relationship like this is rewarding but also challenging. Ms. C and I have shared important life experiences. This has led to a closeness that is not a friendship, but is deeper than I have experienced with patients in other settings. I have become a part of her life. I have participated in the realization by her and her boyfriend that they cannot live together. I have had the opportunity to help both of them recognize and deal with their feelings. I feel good that they were able to remain friends while gaining a realistic view of their relationship.

I have learned that working in the community means that the psychiatric nurse has to attend to all of the patient's needs, not just the psychiatric needs. In fact, sometimes the psychiatric needs are not the most important. I have dealt with medical needs, fi-nancial needs, needs for housing, and relationship needs. It has been a growth experience for me to be Ms. C's nurse as she has begun to cope with her many problems. It has been very satisfying to be a part of her progress and her road to health. ▼

progress of rehabilitation. Staff members share their observations about the person's response to the program and also invite feedback from the consumers. Many programs also conduct regular consumer satisfaction surveys. More recently, consumers have been employed as advocates to seek information about consumer dissatisfaction and present complaints to program administrators.

Program Evaluation

Program evaluation is conducted to inform administrators about the relevance and cost effectiveness of the services that they offer. It is often required by funding, regulatory, and licensure agencies to confirm that public mental health dollars are being spent wisely.

Consumers should be involved in program evaluation. Pratt and Gill[37] described an evaluation program that empowers people who have serious mental illnesses by involving them in program evaluation. First, they educate the consumers about current research on mental illness by giving them journal articles to read and conducting discussion groups. Having been informed about what they should expect from a rehabilitation program, they are asked to evaluate the effectiveness of their own program. A third part of this process prepares the consumers to conduct public education programs about serious mental illness. This process improves the individual's self-esteem and provides a sense of control over the services that are received.

National surveys of program effectiveness provide valuable information to policy-makers, as well as groups of providers about which approaches have been successful. One such study focused on housing. It asked about the types of programs that were available, the services that they offered, and the qualifications of the staff.[38] They found rapid growth in numbers of programs but little choice of types of housing in most states. They also found that few staff in housing programs had any professional training, many having very little training at all. This is an issue that should be of great concern to nurses.

Program evaluation is evolving as program funders and the general public demand greater accountability from service providers. Community advisory boards, legislators, and consumer advocates are all recognizing the importance of reviewing the effectiveness of individual programs and service systems. As comprehensive community-based service systems for people with serious mental illnesses continue to grow, evaluation approaches will provide direction.

SUGGESTED CROSS-REFERENCES

SUMMARY

1. Rehabilitation is the tertiary prevention process of helping the person who has a serious mental illness return to the highest possible level of functioning.

2. Assessment related to rehabilitative psychiatric nursing focuses on the individual, the family, and the community. Individual assessment is based on knowledge of the characteristics of serious mental illnesses. Behaviors that are assessed include activities of daily living, interpersonal relations, self-esteem, motivation, strengths, and compliance. Specific populations of concern include young adults who have serious mental illnesses and homeless mentally ill people. Family assessment focuses particularly on family burden and social support needs.

3. Planning and implementation of rehabilitative psychiatric nursing care with individuals consist of developing strengths and potentials, supporting involvement in community-based services, psychoeducation, social support, and case management. Family intervention is built on empowerment and focuses on education. Nurses intervene at the community level by serving as advocates for mental health services and fighting stigma.

4. Evaluation takes place at the patient and program levels.

REFERENCES

1. Anderson CM, Hogarty GE, Reiss DJ: Family treatment of adult schizophrenic patients: a psychoeducational approach, *Schizophr Bull* 6:490, 1980.
2. Anthony WA: *The principles of psychiatric rehabilitation*, Baltimore, 1980, University Park Press.
3. Anthony WA: Psychiatric rehabilitation: key issues and future policy, *Health Aff* 11:164, 1992.
4. Bachrach LL: Perspectives on work and rehabilitation, *Hosp Community Psychiatr* 42:890, 1991.
5. Bachrach LL: Psychosocial rehabilitation and psychiatry in the care of long-term patients, *Am J Psychiatr* 149:1455, 1992.
6. Besio SW, Mahler J: Benefits and challenges of using consumer staff in supported housing services, *Hosp Community Psychiatr* 44:490, 1993.
7. Boyd MA, Morris MM, Turner M, Little J: For those left behind: an educational inpatient rehabilitation program, *J Psychosoc Nurs Ment Health Serv* 29:24, 1991.
8. Buckwalter KC, Kerfoot KM: Teaching patients self care: a critical aspect of psychiatric discharge planning, *J Psychosoc Nurs Ment Health Serv* 20:15, 1982.
9. Caplan G: *Principles of preventive psychiatry*, New York, 1964, Basic Books.
10. Carling PJ: Housing and supports for persons with mental illness: emerging approaches to research and practice, *Hosp Community Psychiatry* 44:439, 1993.
11. Chamberlin J: *On our own*, New York, 1978, McGraw-Hill.
12. Deegan PE: Recovering our sense of value after being labeled mentally ill, *J Psychosoc Nurs Ment Health Serv* 31:7, 1993.
13. Federal Task Force on Homelessness and Severe Mental Illness: *Outcasts on Main Street*, Washington, DC, 1992, Interagency Council on the Homeless.
14. Goldman CR: Toward a definition of psychoeducation, *Hosp Community Psychiatr* 36:666, 1988.
15. Grunebaum J, Friedman H: Building collaborative relationships with families of the mentally ill, *Hosp Community Psychiatr* 39:1183, 1988.
16. Hatfield AB: Families as caregivers: a historical perspective. In Hatfield AB, Lefley HP, eds: *Families of the mentally ill: coping and adaptation*, New York, 1987, The Guilford Press.
17. Hazel KL, Herman SE, Mowbray CT: Characteristics of seriously mentally ill adults in a public mental health system, *Hosp Community Psychiatr* 42:518, 1991.
18. Howie the Harp: Taking a new approach to independent living, *Hosp Community Psychiatr* 44:413, 1993.
19. Lamb HR: Will we save the homeless mentally ill? *Am J Psychiatr* 147:649, 1990.
20. Landeen J et al: Needs of well siblings of persons with schizophrenia, *Hosp Community Psychiatr* 43:266, 1992.
21. Lemert E: Secondary deviance and role conceptions. In Farrell R, Swigert V, eds: *Social deviance*, New York, 1975, JB Lippincott.
22. Main MC, Gerace LM, Camillari D: Information sharing concerning schizophrenia in a family member, *Arch Psychiatr Nurs* 7:147, 1993.
23. Malone J: Concepts for the rehabilitation of the long-term mentally ill in the community, *Issues Ment Health Nurs* 10:121, 1989.
24. Maurin JT, Boyd CB: Burden of mental illness on the family: a critical review, *Arch Psychiatr Nurs* 4:99, 1990.
25. McCarthy J, Nelson G: An evaluation of supportive housing for current and former psychiatric patients, *Hosp Community Psychiatr* 42:1254, 1991.
26. Moller M, Wer J: Simultaneous patient/family education regarding schizophrenia: the Nebraska model, *Arch Psychiatr Nurs* 3:332, 1989.
27. Mossman D, Perlin ML: Psychiatry and the homeless mentally ill: a reply to Dr. Lamb, *Am J Psychiatr* 149:951, 1992.
28. Mulkern V, Manderscheid R: Characteristics of community support program clients in 1980 and 1984, *Hosp Community Psychiatr* 40:165, 1989.
29. National Mental Health Advisory Council: *Caring for people with severe mental disorders: a national plan of research to improve services*, Washington, DC, 1991, NIMH.
30. Norbeck JS: The use of social support in clinical practice, *J Psychosoc Nurs Ment Health Serv* 20:22, 1982.
31. Norbeck J, Chafetz L, Skodol-Wilson H, Weiss SJ: Social support needs of family caregivers of psychiatric patients from three age groups, *Nurs Res* 40:208, 1991.
32. Okin RL, Pearsall D: Patients' perceptions of their quality of life 11 years after discharge from a state hospital, *Hosp Community Psychiatr* 44:236, 1993.
33. Parker BA: Living with mental illness: the family as caregiver, *J Psychosoc Nurs Ment Health Serv* 31:19, 1993.
34. Peternelj-Taylor CA, Hartley VL: Living with mental illness: professional/family collaboration, *J Psychosoc Nurs Ment Health Serv* 31:23, 1993.
35. Peterson R: What are the needs of chronic mental patients? In Talbott J, ed: *The chronic mental patient: problems, solutions, and recommendations for a public policy*, Washington, DC, 1978, The American Psychiatric Association.
36. Pfeiffer EJ, Mostek M: Services for families of people with mental illness, *Hosp Community Psychiatr* 42:262, 1991.
37. Pratt CW, Gill KJ: Sharing research knowledge to empower people who are chronically mentally ill, *Psychosoc Res J* 13:75, 1990.
38. Randolph FL, Ridgway P, Carling PJ: Residential programs for persons with severe mental illness: a nationwide survey of state-affiliated agencies, *Hosp Community Psychiatr* 42:1111, 1991.
39. Sartorius N: Rehabilitation and quality of life, *Hosp Community Psychiatr* 43:1180, 1992.
40. Segal SP, VanderVoort DJ: Daily hassles of persons with severe mental illness, *Hosp Community Psychiatr* 44:276, 1993.
41. Sherman PS, Porter R: Mental health consumers as case management aides, *Hosp Community Psychiatr* 42:494, 1991.
42. Stein LI, Test MA: An alternative to mental hospital treatment. In Stein LI, Test MA, eds: *Alternatives to mental hospital treatment*, New York, 1978, Plenum Press.
43. Steinwachs DM, Kasper JD, Skinner EA: Patterns of use and costs among severely mentally ill people, *Health Aff* 11:178, 1992.
44. Tanzman B: An overview of surveys of mental health consumers' preferences for housing and support services, *Hosp Community Psychiatr* 44:450, 1993.

45. Wallace CJ et al: Effectiveness and replicability of modules for teaching social and instrumental skills to the severely mentally ill, *Am J Psychiatr* 149:654, 1992.

46. Walsh M: *Schizophrenia: straight talk for families and friends*, New York, 1985, William Morrow.

47. Wasow M: The need for asylum revisited, *Hosp Community Psychiatr* 44:207, 1993.

48. Zipple AM, Spaniol L: Current educational and supportive models of family intervention. In Hatfield AB, Lefley HP, eds: *Families of the mentally ill: coping and adaptation*, New York, 1987, The Guilford Press.

ANNOTATED SUGGESTED READINGS

Backlar P: *The family face of schizophrenia: practical counsel from America's leading experts*, New York, 1994, GP Putnam's Sons.

This is an excellent resource for nurses and families alike. Its unique format presents a family story followed by commentary by an expert regarding that problem.

*Bawden EL: Reaching out to the chronically mentally ill homeless, *J Psychosoc Nurs Ment Health Serv* 28:6, 1990.

Case histories demonstrate nursing approaches that have been effective in working with the homeless mentally ill population. Especially useful for nurses who do community outreach.

*Bryson KK, Naqvi A, Callahan P, Fontenot D: Brief admission program: an alliance of inpatient care and outpatient case management, *J Psychosoc Nurs Ment Health Serv* 28:19, 1990.

Describes the nurse's role in maintaining continuity of care for seriously mentally ill patients who require brief hospital admissions.

Deegan PE: Recovering our sense of value after being labeled mentally ill, *J Psychosoc Nurs Ment Health Serv* 31:7, 1993.

All psychiatric nurses should read this former patient's thoughts about the mental health care system and the stigmatizing effect of labeling. She addresses the article to herself at the age of 17, when she first was diagnosed with a mental illness, and gives advice to her younger self.

*Dibner LA, Murphy JS: Nurse entrepreneurs, *J Psychosoc Nurs Ment Health Serv* 29:30, 1991.

Description of nurses' experience in developing and operating a supervised apartment program for people discharged from a state hospital.

Hatfield AB, Lefley HP: Families of the mentally ill: coping and adaptation, New York, 1987, The Guilford Press.

Valuable resource for all mental health service providers. A comprehensive overview of family issues and concerns.

Hatfield AB, Lefley HP: *Surviving mental illness: stress, coping, and adaptation*, New York, 1993, The Guilford Press.

A presentation of the experience of serious mental illness presented from the patient's perspective.

*Hochberger JM, Fisher-James L: A discharge group for chronically mentally ill: easing the way, *J Psychosoc Nurs Ment Health Serv* 30:25, 1992.

A nurse and social worker team describe a psychoeducational approach that they developed to assist long-term inpatients to prepare for discharge.

*Mann NA et al: Psychosocial rehabilitation in schizophrenia: beginnings in acute hospitalization, *Arch Psychiatr Nurs* 7:154, 1993.

Describes a social skills training program conducted by nurses that is planned to address the needs of schizophrenic patients during short-term acute hospitalizations. Examples of training materials are provided.

Susko MA, ed: *Cry of the invisible*, Baltimore, 1991, The Conservatory Press.

Anthology of creative writings, art, and autobiographical vignettes created by "the homeless and survivors of psychiatric hospitals." Demonstrates the many strengths of people who have serious mental illnesses.

Walsh M: *Schizophrenia: straight talk for families and friends*, New York, 1985, William Morrow.

An excellent presentation of the impact of schizophrenia on the family. Includes much information and advice, including a list of rehabilitation resources.

*Wilkinson L: A collaborative model: ambulatory pharmacotherapy for chronic psychiatric patients, *J Psychosoc Nurs Ment Health Serv* 29:26, 1991.

Example of a collaboration among nurse, patient, family, and psychiatrist to assist patients to use their medication to help them function in community settings.

*Worley NK, Lowery BJ: Linkages between community mental health centers and public mental hospitals, *Nurs Res* 40:298, 1991.

Example of service system research that identifies strengths and weaknesses in interagency relationships. Demonstrates that nurse researchers can play an important role in providing information that can influence mental health policy decisions.

*Nursing reference.

*Nursing reference.

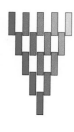

Applying Principles in Nursing Practice

Have you always thought that most people with psychiatric problems were suffering from schizophrenia? Did you ever suspect that one of your friends or family members had an emotional or psychiatric problem but dismissed the idea as impossible? Have you ever worried about the barometer of your own mental health but felt embarrassed to discuss it? If you have answered "yes" to any of these questions, then you are in for an awakening. The fact is that one out of six Americans experience some type of psychiatric problem. Most of these problems are not what nurses commonly think of as a "psychiatric illness." But anxiety disorders, mood disorders, and substance use disorders are by far the most common of psychiatric disorders, and they are experienced by people more often than many physical illnesses. They are disabling disorders that cause people significant distress, yet they are often underdiagnosed and undertreated. These facts are more than interesting. They suggest that a wide variety of educational and treatment strategies are needed by health-care professionals to address these issues.

In this unit you will explore the adaptive and maladaptive coping responses used by people experiencing stress. Some of what you read will surprise you; some of it will concern you; and it is hoped that most of it will intrigue you. It is important that you understand, however, that these psychiatric problems are a common part of the human experience. As such, each and every one of them merits the careful study and consideration of nurses just like yourself.

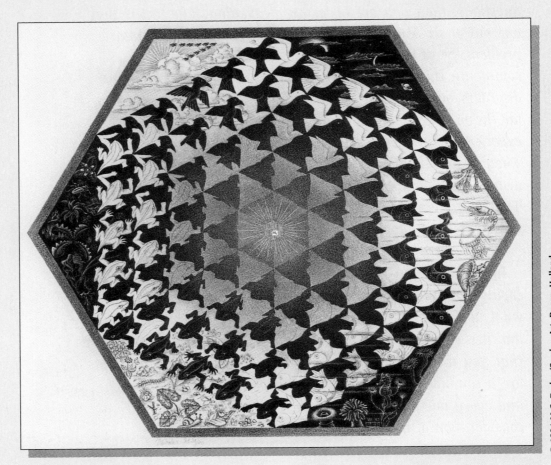

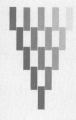

CHAPTER 14

Anxiety Responses and Anxiety Disorders

GAIL W. STUART

. . . . The fears we know are of not knowing . . . It is getting late. Shall we ever be asked for? Are we simply not wanted at all?

W.H. Auden: *The Age of Anxiety*

LEARNING OBJECTIVES

After studying this chapter the student should be able to:

▼ Describe the continuum of adaptive and maladaptive anxiety responses
▼ Identify behaviors associated with anxiety responses
▼ Analyze predisposing factors and precipitating stressors related to anxiety responses
▼ Describe coping resources and coping mechanisms related to anxiety responses
▼ Formulate nursing diagnoses for patients related to anxiety responses
▼ Assess the relationship between nursing diagnoses and medical diagnoses related to anxiety responses
▼ Identify expected outcomes and short-term nursing goals for patients related to anxiety responses
▼ Develop a patient education plan to promote adaptive anxiety responses
▼ Analyze nursing interventions for patients related to anxiety responses
▼ Evaluate nursing care for patients related to anxiety responses

TOPICAL OUTLINE

During the past 20 years, anxiety, a pervasive aspect of contemporary life, has been the subject of more than 500 articles or books. Between 10% and 25% of the population of the United States suffers from an anxiety disorder.[20] Anxiety has always existed, however, and belongs to no particular era or culture. It derives from the Greek root meaning "to press tight." *Anxious* is related to the Latin term *angere*, which means "to strangle," and "to distress."

Although the concept of anxiety is timeless, its great impact on human life has been realized only recently. Every aspect of human endeavor is affected by anxiety. It resembles the term *anger*, when defined as "grief" or "trouble." It is also related to *anguish*, which is described as "acute pain, suffering, or distress." It involves one's body, perceptions of self, and relationships with others, making it a foundational concept in the study of psychiatric nursing and human behavior.

CONTINUUM OF ANXIETY RESPONSES

May[15] defines anxiety as "diffuse apprehension that is vague in nature and associated with feelings of uncertainty and helplessness." Feelings of isolation, alienation, and insecurity are also present. The person perceives that the core of one's personality is being threatened. Experiences provoking anxiety begin in infancy and continue throughout life. They end with the fear of the greatest unknown, death.

Defining Characteristics

Anxiety is an emotion and a subjective individual experience. It is an energy and therefore cannot be observed directly. A nurse infers that a patient is anxious based on certain behaviors. The nurse needs to validate this with the patient. Also, anxiety is an emotion without a specific object. It is provoked by the unknown and precedes all new experiences such as entering school, starting a new job, or giving birth to a child.

This characteristic of anxiety differentiates it from fear. **Fear** is an individual ideation with a specific source or object that the person can identify and describe. Fear involves the *intellectual appraisal* of a threatening stimulus; anxiety involves the *emotional response* to that appraisal. A person generally fears a set of circumstances that may occur at some point in the future. A fear is caused by physical or psychological exposure to a threatening situation. Fear produces anxiety. The two emotions are differentiated in speech; we speak of *having* a fear but of *being* anxious.

Anxiety is communicated interpersonally. If a nurse is talking with a patient who is anxious, within a short time the nurse will also experience feelings of anxiety. Similarly, if a nurse is anxious in a particular situation, this will be readily communicated to the patient. The contagious nature of anxiety can therefore have positive and negative effects on the therapeutic relationship. The nurse must carefully monitor these effects. It is also important to remember that anxiety is part of everyday life. It is basic to the human condition and provides a valuable warning system to the individual. In fact, the capacity to be anxious is necessary for survival.

The crux of anxiety is preservation of self. Anxiety occurs as a result of a threat to a person's selfhood, self-esteem, or identity. It results from a threat to something central to one's personality and essential to one's existence and security. It may be connected with the fear of punishment, disapproval, withdrawal of love, disruption of a relationship, isolation, or loss of body functioning. Anxiety is experienced when the values a person identifies with existence are threatened. Culture is related to anxiety because culture can influence the values the individual considers most important. Underlying every fear is the anxiety of losing one's own being.

This is the frightening element. However, a person can meet the anxiety and grow from it to the extent that the person's values are stronger than the threat.

All people therefore need a balance between courage and anxiety to preserve themselves, fulfill their beings, and affirm their existence. It is only by moving through anxiety-creating experiences that a person achieves self-realization. As May[15] summarizes it, "the positive aspects of selfhood develop as the individual confronts, moves through, and overcomes anxiety-creating experiences."

 Name two situations that provoke anxiety in you. Compare these to two situations that stimulate fear in you.

Levels of Anxiety

Peplau[19] identified four levels of anxiety and described their effects on the individual (Fig. 14-1):

1. **Mild anxiety** is associated with the tension of day-to-day living. During this stage the person is alert and the perceptual field is increased. The person sees, hears, and grasps more than previously. This kind of anxiety can motivate learning and can produce growth and creativity.
2. **Moderate anxiety,** in which the person focuses only on immediate concerns, involves the narrowing of the perceptual field as the person sees, hears, and grasps less. The person blocks out selected areas but can attend to more if directed to do so.
3. **Severe anxiety** is marked by a significant reduction in the perceptual field. The person tends to focus on a specific detail and not think about anything else. All behavior is aimed at relieving anxiety, and much direction is needed to focus on another area.
4. **Panic** is associated with awe, dread, and terror. At this stage details are blown out of proportion. Because of a complete loss of control, the person is unable to do things even with direction. Panic involves the disorganization of the personality. A person can no longer function as an organized human being. There is increased motor activity, decreased ability to relate to others, distorted perceptions, and loss of rational thought.[17] Panic is a frightening and paralyzing experience. The person in panic is unable to communicate or function effectively. This level of anxiety cannot persist indefinitely because it is incompatible with life. A

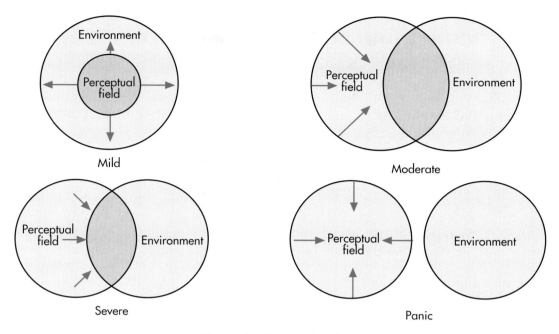

Fig. 14-1 Levels of anxiety.

prolonged period of panic would result in exhaustion and death.

The nurse will be able to identify which level of anxiety a patient is experiencing by the behaviors observed. Fig. 14-2 shows the range of anxiety responses from the most adaptive response of anticipation to the most maladaptive response of panic. The patient's level of anxiety and its position on the continuum of coping responses will be relevant to the nursing diagnosis. The type of intervention the nurse implements will be based on these factors.

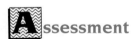ssessment

Behaviors

Anxiety can be expressed directly through physiological and behavioral changes or indirectly through the formation of symptoms or coping mechanisms developed as a defense against anxiety. The nature of the behaviors displayed by the patient depends on the level of anxiety. The intensity of the behaviors will increase with increasing anxiety.

In describing anxiety's effects on **physiological responses,** mild and moderate anxiety heighten the person's capacities. Conversely, severe and panic levels paralyze or overwork capacities and structures. The physiological responses associated with anxiety are primarily mediated through the autonomic nervous system. This involves the internal adjustment of the body

without a conscious or voluntary effort. Two types of autonomic responses exist:

1. The sympathetic, which activate body processes
2. The parasympathetic, which conserve body responses

Studies support the predominance of the sympathetic reaction. This reaction prepares the body to deal with an emergency situation by either a "fight" or a "flight" reaction. When the cortex of the brain perceives a threat, it sends a stimulus down the sympathetic branch of the autonomic nervous system to the adrenal glands. Because of a release of epinephrine, respiration deepens, the heart beats more rapidly, and arterial pressure rises. Blood is shifted away from the stomach and intestines to the heart, central nervous system, and muscle. Glycogenolysis is accelerated, and the blood glucose level rises. For some individuals, however, the parasympathetic reaction may coexist or predominate and produce somewhat opposite effects. Other physiological reactions may also be evident. The variety of physiological responses to anxiety that the nurse may observe in patients are summarized in Box 14-1.

Psychomotor manifestations, or **behavioral responses,** are also observed in the anxious patient. Their effects have both personal and interpersonal aspects. High levels of anxiety affect coordination, involuntary movements, and responsiveness and can also act as disruptive forces in human relationships. In an interpersonal situation anxiety can warn a person to withdraw from a situation where discomfort is anticipated. The anxious patient typically withdraws and decreases inter-

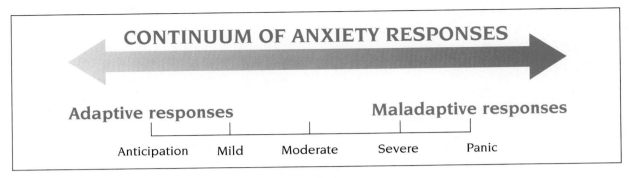

Fig. 14-2   Continuum of anxiety responses.

personal involvement. The possible behavioral responses the nurse might observe are presented in Box 14-1.

Mental, or intellectual, functioning is also affected by anxiety. **Cognitive responses** the patient might display when experiencing anxiety are described in Box 14-1.

Finally, the nurse will be able to assess a patient's emotional reactions, or **affective responses,** to anxiety by the subjective description of the patient's personal experience. Frequently, patients describe themselves as "tense, jittery, on edge, jumpy, worried, or restless." One patient described feelings in the following way: "I'm expecting something terribly bad to happen, but I don't know what. I'm afraid, but I don't know why. I guess you can call it a generalized bad feeling." All these phrases are expressions of apprehension and overalertness. It seems clear that the person interprets his anxiety as a kind of warning sign. Additional affective responses are listed in Box 14-1.

Anxiety is an unpleasant and uncomfortable experience that most people try to avoid. They frequently try to replace anxiety with a more tolerable feeling. Pure anxiety is rarely seen. Anxiety is usually observed in combination with other emotions. Patients might describe feelings of anger, boredom, contempt, depression, irritation, worthlessness, jealousy, self-depreciation, suspiciousness, sadness, or helplessness. This makes it difficult for the nurse to discriminate between anxiety and depression, for instance, because the patient's descriptions may be similar.

Close ties exist between anxiety, depression, guilt, and hostility. These emotions often function reciprocally; one feeling acts to generate and reinforce the others. The relationship between anxiety and hostility is particularly close. The pain experienced with anxiety frequently causes anger and resentment toward those thought to be responsible. These feelings of hostility in turn increase anxiety.

This cycle is evident in the case of a dependent and insecure wife who was very attached to her husband. She expressed numerous vague fears. In exploring her feelings, she also expressed great hostility toward him and their relationship. This symbolized her helplessness and increased her feelings of weakness. Verbalizing these angry feelings further increased her anxiety and unresolved conflict.

Thus anxiety is frequently expressed through anger, and a tense and anxious person is more likely to become angry.

> Think of a patient you cared for recently who appeared to be angry or critical. Could this have been the patient's way of dealing with anxiety? If so, how would your nursing interventions have been different?

Predisposing Factors

Anxiety is a prime factor in the development of the personality and formation of individual character traits. Because of its importance, various theories of the origin of anxiety have been developed.

Psychoanalytic View. Freud initiated the study of anxiety. In the beginning Freud regarded anxiety as a purely physiological reaction to a person's chronic inability to reach an orgasm in sexual relations. He believed that unexpressed sexual energy was converted into anxiety. Alleviation of anxiety therefore merely required improved sexual technique. Not until 30 years later did he see the importance of anxiety for a theory of personality development.[8,9]

His later viewpoint included two types of anxiety—primary and subsequent. Primary anxiety, the "traumatic" state, begins in the infant as a result of the sudden stimulation and trauma of birth. Anxiety continues with the possibility that hunger and thirst might not be satisfied. Primary anxiety therefore is a state of tension or a drive produced by external causes. The environment

Box 14-1

PHYSIOLOGICAL, BEHAVIORAL, COGNITIVE, AND AFFECTIVE RESPONSES TO ANXIETY

PHYSIOLOGICAL		BEHAVIORAL	COGNITIVE	AFFECTIVE
Cardiovascular	**Neuromuscular**	Restlessness	Impaired attention	Edginess
		Physical tension	Poor concentration	Impatience
Palpitations	Increased reflexes	Tremors	Forgetfulness	Uneasiness
Heart racing	Startle reaction	Startle reaction	Errors in judgment	Tension
Increased blood pressure	Eyelid twitching	Rapid speech	Preoccupation	Nervousness
Faintness*	Insomnia	Lack of coordination	Blocking of thoughts	Fear
Actual fainting*	Tremors	Accident proneness	Decreased perceptual	Fright
Decreased blood pressure*	Rigidity	Interpersonal withdrawal	field	Alarm
Decreased pulse rate*	Fidgeting	Inhibition	Reduced creativity	Terror
	Pacing	Flight	Diminished productivity	Jitteriness
Respiratory	Strained face	Avoidance	Confusion	Jumpiness
	Generalized weakness	Hyperventilation	Hypervigilance	
Rapid breathing	Wobbly legs		Self-consciousness	
Shortness of breath	Clumsy movement		Loss of objectivity	
Pressure on chest			Fear of losing control	
Shallow breathing	**Urinary Tract**		Frightening visual images	
Lump in throat			Fear of injury or death	
Choking sensation	Pressure to urinate*			
Gasping	Frequency of urination*			
Gastrointestinal	**Skin**			
Loss of appetite	Face flushed			
Revulsion toward food	Localized sweating			
Abdominal discomfort	(palms)			
Abdominal pain*	Itching			
Nausea*	Hot and cold spells			
Heartburn*	Face pale			
Diarrhea*	Generalized sweating			

*Parasympathetic response.

is capable of threatening as well as satisfying. This implicit threat predisposes the individual to anxiety in later life.

With increased age and ego development, a new kind of anxiety arises. Freud viewed this subsequent anxiety as the emotional conflict that takes place between two elements of the personality—the id and the superego. The id represents instinctual drives and primitive impulses. The superego reflects conscience and culturally acquired restrictions. The ego, or I, tries to mediate the demands of these two clashing elements. Freud therefore suggested that one major function of anxiety was to warn the person that the ego was in danger of being overtaken.

Interpersonal View. Sullivan[22] disagreed with Freud. He believed that anxiety could not arise until the organism had some awareness of its environment. He believed that anxiety originated in the early bond between the infant and mother. Through this close emotional bond, anxiety is first conveyed by the mother to the infant. The infant responds as if he and his mother were one unit. As the child grows older, he sees this discom-

fort as a result of his own actions. He believes that his mother either approves or disapproves of his behavior. In addition, developmental traumas such as separations and losses can lead to specific vulnerabilities.[7] Sullivan believed that anxiety in later life arises when a person perceives he will be viewed unfavorably or will lose the love of a person he values.

Sullivan identified two other aspects of anxiety that are important in the nurse-patient relationship. The first is that a mild or moderate level of anxiety is frequently expressed as anger. The second is that areas in the personality marked by anxiety often become the areas of significant growth. This can result when the individual learns to deal with anxiety constructively, as in a therapeutic relationship.

An individual's level of self-esteem is also an important factor related to anxiety. A person who is easily threatened or has a low level of self-esteem is more susceptible to anxiety. This is evident in students with test anxiety. Anxiety is high because they doubt they can succeed. This may have nothing to do with their actual abilities or how much they studied. The anxiety is caused only by their perception of their ability, which reflects their self-concept. They may be well prepared for the examination, but their severe level of anxiety reduces their perceptual field significantly. They may omit, misinterpret, or distort the meaning of the test items. They may even block out all their previous studying. The result will be poor grade, which will reinforce their poor perception of self.

Behavioral View. Some behavioral theorists propose that anxiety is a product of frustration caused by anything that interferes with attaining a desired goal. An example of an external frustration for young people might be the loss of a job. Many of their goals may be potentially blocked, such as financial security, pride in work, and perception of self as family provider. An internal frustration is evidenced by young college graduates who set unrealistically high career goals and are frustrated by job offers of a clerical or apprentice nature. In this case their view of self is being threatened by their unrealistic goals. They are likely to experience feelings of failure, insignificance, and mounting anxiety.

Other experimental psychologists regard anxiety as a drive that is learned because of an innate desire to avoid pain. They believe that anxiety begins with the attachment of pain to a particular stimulus. If the reaction is strong enough, it may become generalized to similar objects and situations. Learning theorists believe that individuals who have been exposed in early life to intense fears are more likely to be anxious in later life. In this respect, parental influences are important. Children who see their parents respond with anxiety to every minor stress soon develop a similar pattern. Paradoxically, if parents are completely unmoved by potentially stressful situations, children feel alone and lack emotional support from their families. The appropriate emotional response of parents gives children security and helps them learn constructive coping methods of their own.

Anxiety is also theorized to arise through conflict, which is defined as the clashing of two opposing interests. The person experiences two competing drives and must choose between them. A reciprocal relationship exists between conflict and anxiety. Conflict produces anxiety, and anxiety increase the perception of conflict by producing feelings of helplessness. Dollard and Miller[5] view conflict as deriving from two tendencies: approach and avoidance. Approach is the tendency to do something or move toward something. Avoidance is the opposite tendency—not to do something or not to move toward something. The authors identify four kinds of conflict (Fig. 14-3).

1. **Approach-approach,** in which the individual is motivated to pursue two equally desirable but incompatible goals. This type of conflict seldom produces anxiety.
2. **Approach-avoidance,** in which the individual wishes to both pursue and avoid the same goal.

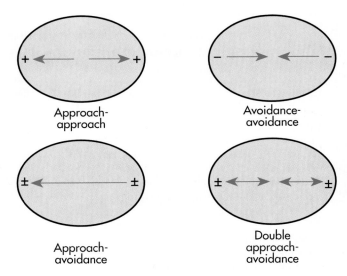

Fig. 14-3   Types of conflict.

The patient who wants to express anger but feels great anxiety and fear in doing so experiences this type of conflict. Another example is the ambitious business executive who must compromise values of honesty and loyalty to be promoted.

3. **Avoidance-avoidance** in which the person must choose between two undesirable goals. Since neither alternative seems beneficial, this is a difficult choice usually accompanied by much anxiety.
4. **Double approach-avoidance,** in which the person can see both desirable and undesirable aspects of both alternatives. This is the kind of conflict experienced by a person living with the pain of one's social and emotional life and destructive coping patterns. The alternative is to seek psychiatric help and expose oneself to the threat and potential pain of the therapy process. Double approach-avoidance conflict feelings are frequently described as *ambivalence.*

In summarizing their theory, Dollard and Miller stress the importance of conditioning early in life. However, little is known about how most complex learned drives are acquired or what permits one person to easily resolve a conflict while another is plunged into a tumultuous emotional state.

 Think of an example of each of the four kinds of conflict you have experienced in your life.

Family Studies. Epidemiological and family studies show that anxiety disorders clearly run in families and that they are common and of different types.[3,12] Anxiety disorders can overlap, as do anxiety disorders and depression. Individuals with one anxiety disorder are more

---

Box 14-2
MEDICAL DISORDERS ASSOCIATED WITH ANXIETY

CARDIOVASCULAR/RESPIRATORY

Asthma
Cardiac arrhythmias
Chronic obstructive pulmonary disease
Congestive heart failure
Coronary insufficiency
Hyperdynamic beta-adrenergic state
Hypertension
Hyperventilation syndrome
Hypoxia, embolus, infections

ENDOCRINOLOGICAL

Carcinoid
Cushing's syndrome
Hyperthyroidism
Hypoglycemia
Hypoparathyroidisms
Hypothyroidism
Menopause
Pheochromocytoma
Premenstrual syndrome

NEUROLOGICAL

Collagen vascular disease
Epilepsy
Huntington's disease
Multiple sclerosis
Organic brain syndrome—delirium, dementia
Vestibular dysfunction
Wilson's disease

SUBSTANCE RELATED
Intoxications

Anticholinergic drugs
Aspirin
Caffeine
Cocaine
Hallucinogens including phencyclidine ("angel dust")
Steroids
Sympathomimetics
THC

Withdrawal syndromes

Alcohol
Narcotics
Sedative hypnotics

---

likely to develop another or to experience a major depression within their lifetime. It has been estimated that only about a quarter of those with anxiety disorders receive treatment. However, these persons are high users of health-care facilities, as they seek treatment for the various symptoms caused by anxiety such as chest pain, palpitations, dizziness, and shortness of breath.

Biological Basis. Basic science advances in understanding anxiety have been considerable in recent years.[11] Some of the most recent developments are described in Chapter 5. For example, investigators have learned that the brain contains specific receptors for benzodiazepines and that these receptors probably help to regulate anxiety. The discovery of benzodiazepine receptors has prompted a search for naturally occurring brain substances that bond to them. The inhibitory neuroregulator gamma-aminobutyric acid (GABA), which is enhanced by the benzodiazepines, also may play a major role in biological mechanisms relating to anxiety, as may the endorphins. Although the theory is still controversial, some investigators believe that an area deep in the brain may have a key role in certain forms of anxiety. This area, called the *locus ceruleus*, is known to be important in several behaviors. Rigorous studies of drugs that either relieve or produce anxiety should help pro-

vide additional information regarding the biological basis for anxiety disorders.

It has also been shown that an individual's general health has a great effect on predisposition to anxiety. Anxiety may accompany some physical disorders such as those listed in Box 14-2. Coping mechanisms may also be impaired by toxic influences, dietary deficiencies, reduced blood supply, hormonal changes, and other physical causes. In addition, symptoms from some physical disorders may mimic or exacerbate anxiety.

Similarly, fatigue increases irritability and feelings of anxiety. It appears that fatigue caused by nervous factors predisposes the individual to a greater degree of anxiety than does fatigue caused by purely physical causes. Thus fatigue may actually be an early symptom of anxiety. Patients complaining of nervous fatigue may already be suffering from moderate anxiety and be more susceptible to future stress situations.

Precipitating Stressors

Given these numerous theories about the origin of anxiety, what kinds of events might precipitate feelings of anxiety? Precipitating stressors can be grouped into two categories: threats to physical integrity and threats to self-system.

Threats to Physical Integrity. These threats suggest impending physiological disability or decreased capacity to perform the activities of daily living. They may include both internal and external sources. External sources may include exposure to viral and bacterial infection, environmental pollutants, safety hazards, lack of adequate housing, food, or clothing, and traumatic injury. Internal sources may include the failure of physiological mechanisms such as the heart, immune system, or temperature regulation. The normal biological changes that can occur with pregnancy and failure to participate in preventive health practices are other internal sources. Pain is often the first indication that physical integrity is being threatened. It creates anxiety that often motivates the person to seek health care.

Threats to Self-System. Threats in this second category are pervasive. They imply harm to a person's identity, self-esteem, and integrated social functioning. Both external and internal sources can threaten self-esteem. External sources may include the loss of a valued person through death, divorce, or relocation, a change in job status, an ethical dilemma, and social or cultural group pressures. Internal sources may include interpersonal difficulties at home or at work or assuming a new role, such as parent, student, or employee. In addition, many of the threats to physical integrity previously mentioned also threaten self-esteem, since the mind-body relationship is an intimate and overlapping one.

This distinction of categories is only theoretical. The person responds to all stressors, whatever their nature and origin, as an integrated whole. No specific event will be as equally stressful to all individuals or even to the same individual at different times.

An Integrative Model. A true understanding of anxiety requires integration of knowledge from all the various points of view (Fig. 14-4). Akiskal[1] has proposed a model that integrates data from psychoanalytical, interpersonal, behavioral, genetic, and biological perspectives. This multicausal model provides a useful frame of reference for the nurse. It is holistic in nature and encourages the assessment of behaviors and perceptions in developing appropriate nursing interventions. It also suggests a variety of causative factors and stresses the interrelationship among them in explaining present behavior. It proposes that anxiety disorders can best be understood as an integration of the factors listed in Box 14-3.

Coping Resources

The individual can cope with stress and anxiety by mobilizing coping resources in the environment. These may include a variety of intrapersonal, interpersonal, and so-

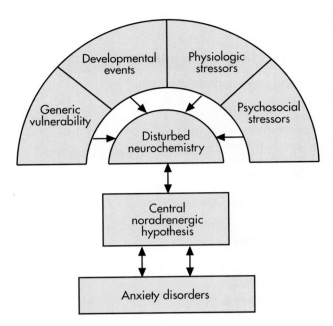

Fig. 14-4 Unified model of anxiety disorders.

Box 14-3

FACTORS IN A UNIFIED MODEL OF ANXIETY DISORDERS

▼ There is a built-in neurobiological substance that prepares the individual to cope with danger.
▼ Evolution has affected this substance in such a way that stimuli threatening to survival are selectively avoided.
▼ Individuals may be born with a central autonomous nervous system that is overly sensitive to stimuli that are generally harmless.
▼ Childhood and adult learning experiences may ultimately determine the extent, severity, and nature of the situations that will evoke anxiety.
▼ Chronic inability to cope with dangerous situations adaptively could increase the tendency to respond with anxiety.
▼ The cognitive functions might permit continual focusing on anxiety reactions, so the mere anticipation of aversive stimuli would provoke anxiety.
▼ Such a person might be more vulnerable to insecurities, especially if intelligent and introspective.

---

cial factors. Such coping resources as economic assets, problem-solving abilities, social supports, and cultural beliefs can help the person integrate stressful experiences and adopt successful coping strategies. They can also help the individual find meaning in the experience and suggest alternative strategies for mediating stressful events.

How might a person's religious or spiritual belief system serve as a resource in coping with a moderate level of anxiety?

Coping Mechanisms

As the level of anxiety increases to the severe and panic levels, the behaviors displayed become more intense and injurious to the individual. People seek to avoid anxiety and the circumstances that produce it. When experiencing anxiety, the individual uses various coping mechanisms to try to relieve it (see A Patient Speaks). The inability to cope with anxiety constructively is a primary cause of pathological behavior. To neutralize, deny, or counteract anxiety, the individual develops patterns of coping. The pattern used to cope with mild anxiety dominates when anxiety becomes more intense. Anxiety plays a major role in the psychogenesis of emotional illness, since many symptoms of illness develop as attempted defenses against anxiety.

 A PATIENT SPEAKS

It's hard to describe just what it feels like. You know something isn't right. Most people don't have to check their doors five or six times before they go to bed. Most people aren't afraid to be near children or feel like they have to count their money over and over again before they can put it back in their wallet. But that's the way my life has been ever since I was a little girl.

Of course I realized I needed help, and so I saw a number of different professionals. With one psychologist we discussed every aspect of my childhood and my earliest memories of life. Unfortunately I finished that therapy still counting everything around me. Next I went to a physician, but he told me that I was just nervous about getting married and things would get better with time. They didn't. Then my mother suggested I go to the University and see someone. That's where I met the psychiatric nurse who did a number of things I'll always remember. First she put me at ease and clearly told me that I wasn't crazy. Then she told me that what I had was obsessive-compulsive disorder and gave me lots of great books and information for me to read. Finally, she told me that it was a treatable illness and together we devised a treatment plan. It included both medication and behavioral therapy and wow what a difference! I'm sure glad that I was persistent, but I'm even more glad that there are caring professionals out there who can really help. ▼

The nurse needs to be familiar with the coping mechanisms people use when experiencing the various levels of anxiety. For **mild anxiety,** the anxiety caused by the tension of day-to-day living, there are several coping mechanisms including crying, sleeping, eating, yawning, laughing, cursing, physical exercise, and daydreaming. Oral behavior, such as smoking and drinking, is another means of coping with mild anxiety. When dealing with other people, the individual copes with low levels of anxiety through superficiality, lack of eye contact, use of clichés, and limited self-disclosure. People can also protect themselves from anxiety by assuming comfortable roles and limiting close relationships to those with values similar to their own. Mild levels of anxiety are often handled without conscious thought, and their effects can be easily minimized.

Moderate, severe, and **panic** levels of anxiety, however, pose greater threats to the ego. They require more energy to cope with the threat. These coping mechanisms can be categorized as task-oriented and ego-oriented reactions.

Task-oriented Reactions. Task-oriented reactions are thoughtful, deliberate attempts to solve problems, resolve conflicts, and gratify needs. They are aimed at realistically meeting the demands of a stress situation that has been objectively appraised. They are consciously directed and action oriented. These reactions can include attack, withdrawal, and compromise.

In **attack behavior** a person attempts to remove or overcome obstacles to satisfy a need. There are many possible ways of attacking problems, and this type of reaction may be destructive or constructive. Destructive patterns are usually accompanied by great feelings of anger and hostility. These feelings may be expressed by negative or aggressive behavior that violates the rights, property, and well-being of others. Constructive patterns reflect a problem-solving approach. They are evident in self-assertive behaviors that respect the rights of others.

Withdrawal behavior may be expressed physically or psychologically. Physically, withdrawal involves removing oneself from the source of the threat. This can apply to biological stressors, such as smoke-filled rooms, exposure to irradiation, or contact with contagious diseases. An individual can also withdraw in various psychological ways, such as by admitting defeat, becoming apathetic, or lowering aspirations. As with attack, this type of reaction may be constructive or destructive. When it isolates the individual from others and interferes with the ability to work, the reaction creates additional problems.

Compromise is necessary in situations that cannot be resolved through either attack or withdrawal. This involves changing usual ways of operating, substituting goals, or sacrificing aspects of personal needs. Compromise reactions are usually constructive and are frequently employed in approach-approach and avoidance-avoidance situations. Occasionally, however, the person realizes with time that the compromise is not acceptable; a solution must then be renegotiated or a different coping mechanism adopted.

The capacity for task-oriented reactions and effective problem solving is greatly influenced by the person's expectation of at least partial success. This in turn will depend on remembering past successes in similar situations. On this basis it is possible to go forward and deal with the current stressful situation. Perseverance in problem solving also depends on the person's expectation of a certain level of pain and discomfort and on the belief in being capable of tolerating the problem. Here lies the balance between courage and anxiety.

 What coping mechanisms do you use when you are mildly, moderately, and severely anxious? How adaptive or maladaptive are they?

Ego-oriented Reactions. Task-oriented reactions are not always successful in coping with stressful situations. Consequently, ego-oriented reactions are often used to protect the self. These reactions, also called **ego defense mechanisms,** are the first line of psychic defense. Everyone uses defense mechanisms, and they frequently help people cope successfully with mild and moderate levels of anxiety. They protect the person from feelings of inadequacy and worthlessness and prevent awareness of anxiety. They can be used to such an extreme degree, however, that they distort reality, interfere with interpersonal relationships, and limit the ability to work productively. This results in ego disintegration instead of self-integrity.

As coping mechanisms, they have certain drawbacks. First, ego-oriented reactions operate on relatively unconscious levels. The person has little awareness of what is happening and little control over events. Second, they involve a degree of self-deception and reality distortion. Therefore they usually do not help the individual to cope with the problem realistically. Table 14-1 lists some of the more common ego defense mechanisms.

When discussing ego-oriented reactions, or defense mechanisms, it is important to note that individuals frequently monitor their own level of emotional tolerance and the need to use ego defenses. This idea is supported by Elliott,[6] who believes denial in particular may effectively allay anxiety immediately following a stressful event. She believes that if denial is gradually eliminated as the stress begins to subside, the person may better adapt to the new situation.

The evaluation of whether the patient's use of certain defense mechanisms is adaptive or maladaptive involves four issues:

1. The accurate recognition of the patient's use of the defense mechanism by the nurse.
2. The degree to which the defense mechanism is used. Does it imply a high degree of personality disorganization? Is the person unresponsive to facts about his life situation?
3. The degree to which use of the defense mechanism impedes the patient's progress toward regained health.
4. The reason the patient used the ego defense mechanism.

The nurse will better understand the patient and plan more effective nursing care after considering these areas.

If the ego defense mechanisms fail and the level of anxiety remains high, the person must use exaggerated and inappropriate coping mechanisms. These coping patterns are maladaptive responses that may appear deviant or abnormal to others. They include the many hidden, unconscious, and devious pathways in which the effects of anxiety are converted psychologically.

Obviously, many coping mechanisms are available to the individual for minimizing anxiety. Some of these defense mechanisms appear to be essential for all human beings to maintain emotional stability. The exact nature and number of the defenses used by the individual strongly influence the personality pattern. When these defenses are overused or used unsuccessfully, they cause many physiological and psychological symptoms commonly associated with emotional illness.

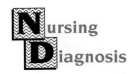 ursing Diagnosis

The nurse who has adequately assessed a patient and uses a conceptual model for understanding anxiety will be able to formulate a nursing diagnosis based on the patient's position on the continuum of anxiety responses (Fig. 14-5). The nurse will review the objective data collected, as well as the subjective responses of the patient to questions and statements and the patient's history. The nurse's personal response to the patient will also be important, since anxiety is readily communicated interpersonally.

To formulate a nursing diagnosis, the nurse must determine the quality and quantity of the anxiety experienced by the patient (see Critical Thinking about Con-

Table 14-1   Ego Defense Mechanisms

Defense mechanism	Example	Defense mechanism	Example
Compensation: Process by which a person makes up for a perceived deficiency by strongly emphasizing a feature that he regards as an asset.	A businessman perceives his small physical stature negatively. He tries to overcome this by being aggressive, forceful, and controlling in business dealings.	**Projection:** Attributing one's thoughts or impulses to another person. Through this process one can attribute intolerable wishes, emotional feelings, or motivations to another person.	A young woman who denies she has sexual feelings about a coworker accuses him without basis of being a "flirt" and says he is trying to seduce her.
Denial: Avoidance of disagreeable realities by ignoring or refusing to recognize them; probably simplest and most primitive of all defense mechanisms.	Mrs. P has just been told that her breast biopsy indicates a malignancy. When her husband visits her that evening, she tells him that no one has discussed the laboratory results with her.	**Rationalization:** Offering a socially acceptable or apparently logical explanation to justify or make acceptable otherwise unacceptable impulses, feelings, behaviors, and motives.	John fails an examination and complains that the lectures were not well organized or clearly presented.
Displacement: Shift of emotion from a person or object to another usually neutral or less dangerous person or object.	A 4-year-old boy is angry because he has just been punished by his mother for drawing on his bedroom walls. He begins to play "war" with his soldier toys and has them battle and fight with each other.	**Reaction formation:** Development of conscious attitudes and behavior patterns that are opposite to what one really feels or would like to do.	A married woman who feels attracted to one of her husband's friends treats him rudely.
Dissociation: The separation of any group of mental or behavioral processes from the rest of the person's consciousness or identity.	A man is brought to the emergency room by the police and is unable to explain who he is and where he lives or works.	**Regression:** Retreat in face of stress to behavior characteristic of any earlier level of development.	Four-year-old Nicole, who has been toilet trained for over a year, begins to wet her pants again when her new baby brother is brought home from the hospital.
Identification: Process by which a person tries to become like someone he admires by taking on thoughts, mannerisms, or tastes of that individual.	Sally, 15 years old, has her hair styled similarly to her young English teacher whom she admires.	**Repression:** Involuntary exclusion of a painful or conflictual thought, impulse, or memory from awareness. It is the primary ego defense, and other mechanisms tend to reinforce it.	Mr. R does not recall hitting his wife when she was pregnant.
Intellectualization: Excessive reasoning or logic is used to avoid experiencng disturbing feelings.	A woman avoids dealing with her anxiety in shopping malls by explaining that she is saving the frivolous waste of time and money by not going into them.	**Splitting:** Viewing people and situations as either all good or all bad. Failure to integrate the positive and negative qualities of oneself.	A friend tells you that you are the most wonderful person in the world one day, and how much she hates you the next day.
		Sublimation: Acceptance of a socially approved substitute goal for a drive whose normal channel of expression is blocked.	Ed has an impulsive and physically aggressive nature. He tries out for the football team and becomes a star tackle.
Introjection: Intense type of identification in which a person incorporates qualities or values of another person or group into his own ego structure. It is one of the earliest mechanisms of the child; important in formation of conscience.	Eight-year-old Jimmy tells his 3-year-old sister, "Don't scribble in your book of nursery rhymes. Just look at the pretty pictures," thus expressing his parents' values to his little sister.	**Suppression:** A process often listed as a defense mechanism but really a conscious counterpart of repression. It is intentional exclusion of material from consciousness. At times, it may lead to subsequent repression.	A young man at work finds he is thinking so much about his date that evening that it is interfering with his work. He decides to put it out of his mind until he leaves the office for the day.
Isolation: Splitting off of emotional components of a thought, which may be temporary or long term.	A second-year medical student dissects a cadaver for her anatomy course without being disturbed by thoughts of death.	**Undoing:** Act or communication that partially negates a previous one; primitive defense mechanism.	Larry makes a passionate declaration of love to Sue on a date. On their next meeting he treats her formally and distantly.

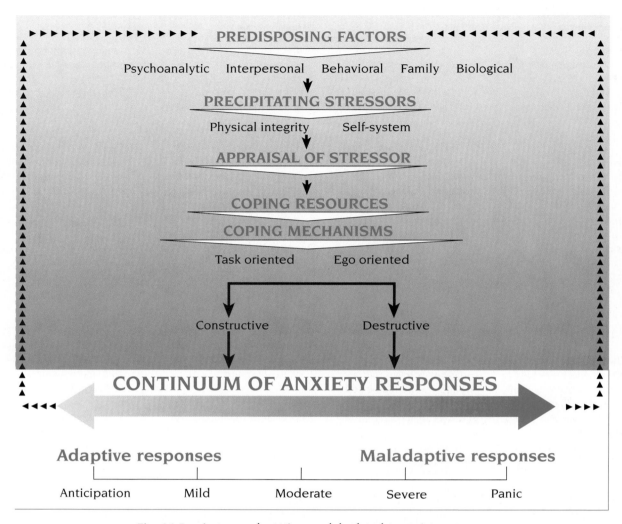

Fig. 14-5   A stress adaptation model related to anxiety responses.

temporary Issues). In considering the quality of the anxiety, the nurse might question the appropriateness of the patient's response to the perceived threat. Is it warranted and adaptive or irrational? A problem may exist if the response is out of proportion to the threat. This would indicate that the patient's cognitive appraisal of the threat is unrealistic. The quantity of the reaction is the next consideration in determining the level of anxiety. When anxiety reaches the severe and panic levels, it indicates that the conflict is increasingly problematic for the patient.

The nurse also needs to explore how the patient is coping with the anxiety. Constructive coping mechanisms are protective responses that consciously confront the threat. Destructive coping mechanisms involve repression into the unconscious. They tend to be ineffective, inadequate, disorganized, inappropriate, and exaggerated. They may be evident in bizarre behavior or symptom formation.

Finally, the nurse needs to determine the overall effect of the anxiety on the individual. Is it stimulating growth? Or is it interfering with effective living and life satisfaction? Is it enhancing one's sense of self? Or is it depersonalizing and despiritizing? Whenever possible, the patient should be included in identifying problem areas. This may not always be feasible, however, particularly if the patient's anxiety level is at the severe or panic level.

There are three primary NANDA nursing diagnoses concerned with anxiety responses: anxiety, ineffective coping, and fear. Many additional nursing problems may also be identified from the way the patient's anxiety reciprocally influences interpersonal relationships, self-concept, cognitive functioning, physiological status, and other aspects of life.[14] The identification of nursing problems should be as complete as possible to ensure an adequate plan of care and implementation. Nursing diagnoses related to the range of possible maladaptive

CRITICAL THINKING ABOUT CONTEMPORARY ISSUES

Is the Anxiety Experienced by a Patient before Surgery the Same as the Anxiety Experienced by a Patient with an Anxiety Disorder?

This question raises the controversy of whether the domain of psychiatric nursing practice is "psychosocial" or "psychiatric." Clearly the nursing diagnosis of anxiety is used frequently in all areas of nursing practice. Research studies in nursing diagnosis indicate that anxiety is one of the most commonly occurring diagnoses.[23] The issue is whether the etiology, descriptors, and treatment of anxiety differ based on whether it is a primary or a secondary problem. Some argue that the difference is primarily a matter of degree. Others contend that some of the anxiety disorders, such as panic disorder, agoraphobia, and obsessive-compulsive disorder, have a genetic and biochemical component that must be considered when designing treatment strategies.

In reality, this question is much like that of which came first, the chicken or the egg. The integrative model of anxiety suggests that the answer is complex and multidimensional.[1] So too, treatment strategies need to incorporate biological, cognitive, and behavioral interventions to be truly effective. Regardless of how this question is answered, it is clear that psychiatric nurses have much to learn to move beyond support and reassurance to psychopharmacology, behavioral treatment, and cognitive restructuring when intervening in maladaptive anxiety responses. ▼

of anxiety. Psychotic individuals feel they are "breaking into pieces." The anxiety of psychosis is not just fear of failure or fear of being unable to cope with the threatening situation. It is the fear that the failure will reveal defeat in the "process of living" and failure in the "process of being."

In addition to differentiating between neurotic and psychotic anxiety responses, the nurse will need to discriminate between anxiety and depression. These frequently overlap because anxious patients are often depressed and depressed patients are often anxious.[23] For example, both anxious and depressed patients share the following symptoms: sleep disturbances, appetite changes, nonspecific cardiopulmonary and gastrointestinal complaints, difficulty concentrating, irritability, and fatigue or lack of energy. Yet there are often discrete, if subtle, differences between the two groups. These are described in Box 14-6. Studies show that anxiety disorders occur twice as often in women as in men, and obsessive-compulsive disorder is about equally prevalent in women and men. No outstanding differences in the prevalence of anxiety disorders have been found on the basis of race, income, education, or rural versus urban dwelling.[20] Thus these disorders affect every aspect of the population. The essential features of the medical diagnoses related to anxiety responses are presented in the Detailed Diagnoses box on pp. 341-342.

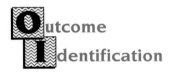

Outcome Identification

Goals such as "decrease anxiety" and "minimize anxiety" lack specific behaviors and evaluation criteria. These goals therefore are not particularly useful in guiding nursing care and evaluating its effectiveness. The expected outcome for patients with maladaptive anxiety responses is:

The patient will demonstrate adaptive ways of coping with stress. Short-term goals can then break this down into readily attainable steps. This allows the patient and nurse to see progress even if the ultimate goal still appears distant.

When the nursing diagnosis describes the patient's anxiety at the severe or panic levels, the highest-priority short-term goals should address lowering the anxiety level. Only after this has been achieved can additional progress be made. The reduced level of anxiety should be evident in a reduction of behaviors associated with the severe or panic levels. Following are examples of short-term goals for a particular patient.

After 4 days Mr. Jones will:
1. Attend and remain seated during all meetings

responses and related medical diagnoses are identified in the Medical and Nursing Diagnoses box on p. 340. The primary NANDA nursing diagnoses and examples of complete nursing diagnoses are presented in the Detailed Diagnoses box on pp. 341-342.

Related Medical Diagnoses

Many patients with mild or moderate anxiety have no medically diagnosed health problem. However, patients with more severe levels of anxiety usually have neurotic disorders that fall under the category of anxiety disorders in the DSM-IV.[2] A **neurosis** is a mental disorder characterized by anxiety that involves no distortion of reality. Neurotic disorders are maladaptive anxiety responses associated with moderate and severe levels of anxiety.

Psychosis, however, can emerge with the panic level

MEDICAL AND NURSING DIAGNOSES RELATED TO ANXIETY

Related Medical Diagnoses (DSM-IV)*

Panic disorder without agoraphobia
Panic disorder with agoraphobia
Agoraphobia without panic attacks
Specific phobia
Social phobia
Obsessive-compulsive disorder
Posttraumatic stress disorder
Acute stress disorder
Generalized anxiety disorder

Related Nursing Diagnoses (NANDA)†

Adjustment, impaired
‡**Anxiety**
Breathing pattern, ineffective
Communication, impaired verbal
‡**Coping, ineffective individual**
Diarrhea
‡**Fear**
Health maintenance, altered
Incontinence, stress
Injury, potential for
Nutrition, altered
Posttrauma response
Powerlessness
Self-esteem disturbance
Sensory/perceptual alterations
Sleep pattern disturbance
Social interaction, impaired
Social isolation
Thought processes, altered
Urinary elimination, altered patterns

*From American Psychiatric Association: *Diagnostic and statistical manual of mental disorders,* ed 4, Washington, DC, 1994, The Association.
†From North American Nursing Diagnosis Association: NANDA *nursing diagnoses: definitions and classifications* 1992-1993, Philadelphia, 1992, The Association.
‡Primary nursing diagnosis for anxiety.

2. Participate at least three times during each meeting
3. Discuss one topic for a minimum of 10 minutes when meeting with his nurse
4. Attend all occupational therapy sessions
5. Sleep a minimum of 6 hours a night

When these goals are met, the nurse can assume and validate that the patient's level of anxiety has been reduced. The nurse may then develop new short-term goals directed toward insight or relaxation therapy.

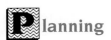 **lanning**

The main goal of the nurse working with anxious patients is not to free them totally from anxiety. Patients need to develop the capacity to tolerate mild anxiety and to use it consciously and constructively. In this way the self will become stronger and more integrated. As they learn from these experiences, they will move on in their development. Patients must also be convinced that the values to be gained in moving ahead are greater than those to be gained by escape. Anxiety can be con-

sidered a war between the threat and the values individuals identify with their existence. Maladaptive behavior means that the struggle is won by the threat. The constructive approach to anxiety means that the struggle is won by the person's values. Thus a general nursing goal is to help patients develop sound values. This does not mean that patients assume the nurse's values. Rather, the nurse works with patients to sort out their own values.

Anxiety can also be an important factor in the patient's decision to seek treatment. Since anxiety is undesirable, the individual will seek ways to reduce it. If the patient's coping mechanism or symptom does not minimize anxiety, the motivation for treatment will be increased. Conversely, anxiety about the therapeutic process can delay or prevent the individual from seeking treatment.

The patient should actively participate in planning treatment strategies. If the patient is actively involved in identifying relevant stressors and planning possible solutions, the success of the implementation phase will be maximized. Patients in extreme anxiety initially will not be able to participate in the problem-solving process. However, as soon as their anxiety is reduced, the

DETAILED DIAGNOSES
RELATED TO ANXIETY RESPONSES

NANDA Diagnosis Stem	Examples of Complete Diagnoses
Anxiety	Panic level of anxiety related to family rejection evidenced by confusion and impaired judgment.
	Severe anxiety related to sexual conflict evidenced by repetitive handwashing and recurrent thoughts of dirt and germs.
	Severe anxiety related to marital conflict evidenced by inability to leave the house.
	Moderate anxiety related to financial pressures evidenced by recurring episodes of abdominal pain and heartburn.
	Moderate anxiety related to assumption of motherhood role evidenced by inhibition and avoidance.
	Moderate anxiety related to poor school performance evidenced by excessive use of denial and rationalization.
Ineffective individual coping	Ineffective individual coping related to daughter's death evidenced by inability to recall events pertaining to the care accident.
	Ineffective individual coping related to child's illness evidenced by limited ability to concentrate and psychomotor agitation.
Fear	Fear related to impending surgery evidenced by generalized hostility to staff and restlessness.

DSM-IV Diagnoses	Essential Features*
Panic disorder without agoraphobia	Recurrent unexpected panic attacks (see Box 14-4) and at least one of the attacks has been followed by a month (or more) of: (a) persistent concern about having additional attacks; (b) worry about the implications of the attack or its consequences; or (c) a significant change in behavior related to the attacks. Also the absence of agoraphobia.
Panic disorder with agoraphobia	Meets the above criteria. In addition, the presence of agoraphobia, which is anxiety about being in places or situations from which escape might be difficult (or embarrassing) or in which help may not be available in the event of having an unexpected or situationally predisposed panic attack. Agoraphobic fears typically involve characteristic clusters of situations that include being outside the home alone; being in a crowd or standing in a line; being on a bridge; and traveling in a bus, train, or car. Agoraphobic situations are avoided, or else endured with marked distress or with anxiety about having a panic attack, or require the presence of a companion.
Agoraphobia without history of panic disorder	The presence of agoraphobia and has never met critiera for panic disorder.
Specific phobia	Marked and persistent fear that is excessive or unreasonable, cued by the presence or anticipation of a specific object or situation (e.g., flying, heights, animals, receiving an injection, seeing blood). Exposure to the phobic stimulus almost invariably provokes an immediate anxiety response. The person recognizes the fear is excessive, and the distress or avoidance interferes with the person's normal routine.
Social phobia	A marked and persistent fear of one or more social or performance situations in which the person is exposed to unfamiliar people or to possible scrutiny by others. The individual fears that he or she will act in a way (or show anxiety symptoms) that will be humiliating or embarrassing. Exposure to the feared situation almost invariably provokes anxiety. The person recognizes the fear is excessive, and the distress or avoidance interferes with the person's normal routine.

*Adapted from American Psychitric Association: *Diagnostic and statistical manual of mental disorders*, ed 4, Washington, DC, 1994, the Association.

Continued.

DETAILED DIAGNOSES
RELATED TO ANXIETY RESPONSES—cont'd

Obsessive-compulsive disorder	Either obsessions or compulsions (see Box 14-5) are recognized as excessive and interfere with the person's normal routine.
Posttraumatic stress disorder	The person has been exposed to a traumatic event in which both of the following have been present: (1) the person has experienced, witnessed, or been confronted with an event or events that involve actual or threatened death or serious injury, or a threat to the physical integrity of oneself or others. (2) the person's response involved intense fear, helplessness, or horror. The traumatic event is reexperienced, and there is an avoidance of stimuli associated with the trauma and a numbing of general responsiveness.
Acute stress disorder	Meets the above criteria for exposure to a traumatic event and experiences three of the following symptoms: sense of detachment, reduced awareness of one's surroundings, derealization, depersonalization, dissociated amnesia.
Generalized anxiety disorder	Excessive anxiety and worry, occurring more days than not for at least 6 months, about a number of events or activities. The person finds it difficult to control the worry and experiences at least three of the following six symptoms: restlessness or feeling keyed up or on edge, being easily fatigued, difficulty concentrating or mind going blank, irritability, muscle tension, sleep disturbance.

nurse should encourage their involvement. This will also reinforce that they are responsible for their own growth and personal development.

mplementation

Severe and Panic Levels of Anxiety

Establishing a Trusting Relationship. The patient with severe or panic levels of anxiety may be hospitalized. To reduce this patient's level of anxiety, most nursing actions are supportive and protective. Initially nurses need to establish an open, trusting relationship. Nurses should actively listen to patients and encourage them to discuss their feelings of anxiety, hostility, guilt, and frustration. Nurses should answer patients' questions directly and offer unconditional acceptance. Both their verbal and nonverbal communications should convey awareness of patients' feelings and acceptance of them. Nurses should remain available and respect use of personal space. A 6-foot distance in a small room may create the optimum condition for openness and discussion of fears. The more this distance is increased or decreased, the more anxious the patient may become.

Self-Awareness. Nurses' feelings are of particular importance when working with highly anxious patients. They may find themselves being unsympathetic, impa-

---

Box 14-4
PANIC ATTACK CRITERIA

A panic attack is a discrete period of intense fear or discomfort in which at least four of the following symptoms developed abruptly and reached a peak within 10 minutes:

1. Palpitations, pounding heart, or accelerated heart rate
2. Sweating
3. Trembling or shaking
4. Sensations of shortness of breath or smothering
5. Feeling of choking
6. Chest pain or discomfort
7. Nausea or abdominal distress
8. Feeling dizzy, unsteady, lightheaded, or faint
9. Derealization (feelings of unreality) or depersonalization (being detached from oneself)
10. Fear of losing control or going crazy
11. Fear of dying
12. Paresthesias (numbness or tingling sensations)
13. Chills or hot flushes

---

tient, and frustrated. These are common feelings of reciprocal anxiety that nurses should be aware of and accept. If nurses are alert to the development of anxiety in themselves, they can learn from it and use it therapeutically. For example, it may indicate some important emotional issue that the patient is unable to identify

---

Box 14-5

OBSESSIONS AND COMPULSIONS CRITERIA

OBSESSIONS

1. Recurrent and persistent thoughts, impulses, or images that are experienced at some time during the disturbance as intrusive and inappropriate and cause marked anxiety or distress
2. The thoughts, impulses, or images are not simply excessive worries about real-life problems
3. The person attempts to ignore or suppress such thoughts or impulses or to neutralize them with some other thought or action
4. The person recognizes that the obsessional thought, impulses, or images are a product of one's own mind

COMPULSIONS

1. Repetitive behaviors (e.g., hand washing, ordering, checking) or mental acts (e.g, praying, counting, repeating words silently) that the person feels driven to perform in response to an obsession or according to rules that must be applied rigidly
2. The behaviors or mental acts are aimed at preventing or reducing distress or preventing some dreaded event or situation; however, these behaviors or mental acts either are not connected in a realistic way with what they are designed to neutralize or prevent or are clearly excessive

---

Box 14-6

DIFFERENCES BETWEEN ANXIETY AND DEPRESSION

ANXIETY

Predominantly fearful or apprehensive
Difficulty falling asleep (initial insomnia)
Phobic avoidance behavior
Rapid pulse and psychomotor hyperactivity
Breathing disturbances
Tremors and palpitations
Sweating and hot or cold spells
Faintness, light-headedness, dizziness
Depersonalization (feeling detached from one's body)
Derealization (feeling that one's environment is strange, unreal, or unfamiliar)
Negative appraisals are selective and specific and do not include all areas of life
Sees some prospects for the future
Does not regard defects or mistakes as irrevocable
Uncertain in negative evaluations
Predicts that only certain events may go badly

DEPRESSION

Predominantly sad or hopeless with feelings of despair
Early morning awakening (late insomnia) or hypersomnia
Diurnal variation (feels worse in the morning)
Slowed speech and thought processes
Delayed response time
Psychomotor retardation (agitation may also occur)
Loss of interest in usual activities
Inability to experience pleasure
Thoughts of death or suicide
Negative appraisals are pervasive, global, and exclusive
Sees the future as blank and has given up all hope
Regards mistakes as beyond redemption
Absolute in negative evaluations
Global view that nothing will turn out right

---

and verbalize, or it may reflect a conflict within the nurse that is interfering with the ability to be therapeutic. Nurses should therefore be alert to the signs of anxiety in themselves, accept them, and attempt to explore their cause. The nurse may ask the following questions:

▼ What is threatening me?
▼ Is this patient a source of reflected esteem for me?
▼ Have I failed to live up to what I imagine is the patient's ideal?
▼ Am I comparing myself to a peer or another health professional?
▼ Is the patient's area of conflict one that I have not resolved in myself?

▼ Is my anxiety related to something that will or may happen in the future? Is my patient's conflict really one of my own that I am projecting?

If nurses deny their own anxiety, it can have detrimental effects on the nurse-patient relationship. Because of their own anxiety, nurses may be unable to differentiate between levels of anxiety in others. They may also transfer their fears and frustrations to patients, thus compounding their problem. Finally, nurses who are anxious will arouse defenses in other patients and staff that will severely interfere with their therapeutic usefulness. Nurses should strive to accept their patients' anxiety without reciprocal anxiety by continually clarifying their own feelings and role, as indicated in the following clinical example.

CLINICAL EXAMPLE

Ms. R was a 35-year-old married woman and mother of three children, ages 4, 6, and 9. She was a full-time housewife and mother. Her husband was a salesman and spent about two nights each week out of town. She came to the clinic complaining of severe headaches that "come upon me very suddenly and are so terrible that I have to go to bed. The only thing that helps is for me to lie down in a dark and absolutely quiet room." She said that these headaches were becoming a real problem for everyone in the family, and her husband told her that she "just had to get over them and get things back to normal."

Mr. W, a psychiatric nurse, offered to see Ms. R in therapy once a week. After 4 weeks, he was asked to present his evaluation, treatment plans, and progress report to the clinic staff at their regular weekly team conference. Mr. W began his presentation by stating, "This case is really a tough nut to crack. I'll start with the progress report and say that there is none because I can't seem to get past all the complaining this patient does!" He then went on to discuss his evaluation and treatment plan in depth. It became obvious to the other members of the staff that Mr. W saw his patient as a woman who was not living up to her roles and responsibilities. He defended Ms. R's husband even though the husband has refused to come to the sessions with his wife. When the psychiatrist asked about the possibility of a medication evaluation for Ms. R, the nurse replied, "Everyone gets headaches. I don't think we should reward or reinforce this woman's complaints."

In reviewing this case the staff noted that Mr. W appeared to have problems relating empathically to his patient because of her particular set of problems and some of his own values and perceptions. Mr. W agreed with this and said he had thought of asking someone else to work with Ms. R. Mr. W's supervisor observed that the nurse had problems with this type of patient in the past, and a more constructive approach would be to increase his supervision on this case, focusing on the dynamics between the patient and nurse that were blocking learning and growth for both of them. Mr. W and his supervisor then set a time when they could begin to meet with this purpose in mind.

What clinical situations or patient problems raise your anxiety as a nurse?

Protecting the Patient. Another major area of intervention is protecting the patient and reassuring him of his safety. One way of decreasing patient anxiety is by allowing the patient to determine the amount of stress that can be handled at the time. Nurses should not force severely anxious patients into situations they are not able to handle. They should also not attack their coping mechanisms or try to strip them of these. Rather, nurses should attempt to protect patients' defenses. The coping mechanism or symptom is attempting to deal with an unconscious conflict. Usually patients do not understand why the symptom has developed or what they are gaining from it. They only know that the symptom relieves some of the intolerable anxiety and tension. If they are unable to release this anxiety, their tension mounts to the panic level and they could lose control. It is also important to remember that the severely anxious patient has not worked through the area of conflict and therefore has no alternatives or substitutes for present coping mechanisms.

This principle also applies to severe levels of anxiety, such as obsessive-compulsive reactions and phobias. Nurses should not initially interfere with the repetitive act or force patients to confront the phobic object. They should not ridicule the nature of their defense. Also, nurses should not attempt to argue with patients about it or reason them out of it. They need this coping mechanism to keep their anxiety within tolerable limits. Nurses must not reinforce the phobia, ritual, or physical complaint by focusing attention on it and talking about it a great deal. With time, however, nurses can place some limits on patients' behavior and attempt to help them find satisfaction with other aspects of life.

Modifying the Environment. If the patient is hospitalized, the nurse can consult with other members of the health team to identify anxiety-producing situations for the patient and attempt to reduce them. The nurse can set limits by assuming a quiet, calm manner and decreasing environmental stimulation. Limiting the patient's interaction with other patients will minimize the contagious aspects of anxiety. Supportive physical measures such as warm baths, massages, or whirlpool baths may also be helpful in decreasing a patient's anxiety.

Encouraging Activity. The nurse should encourage the patient's interest in activities. This limits the time available for destructive coping mechanisms and increases participation in and enjoyment of other aspects of life. Within the hospital setting the patient may become engaged in simple games, concrete tasks, or occupational or art therapy. The nurse can share some of these activities to provide support and reinforce socially productive behavior. The nurse might also schedule vigorous physical activities, such as walking, a sport, or an active hobby. This form of physical exercise helps to relieve anxiety because it provides an emotional release and directs the patient's attention outward. In one study, participation in a jogging program resulted in the reduction of anxiety for chronically distressed community patients. These gains were maintained 15 months after the completion of the study.[13]

Similar interventions can be implemented with the severely anxious patient who is not hospitalized. The nurse and patient can plan a daily schedule of activities that can be carried out in the community. Family members may be involved in the planning, since they can be very supportive in setting limits and stimulating outside activity (see A Family Speaks).

Some nursing interventions can be detrimental and increase anxiety in severely anxious patients. These include pressuring the patient to change prematurely, being judgmental and verbally disapproving of the patient's behaviors, and asking the patient a direct question that brings on defensiveness. Focusing in a critical way on the patient's anxious feelings with other patients present, lacking awareness of one's own behaviors and feelings, and withdrawing from the patient can also be detrimental to the anxious patient.

Medication. Nursing intervention may include the administration of antianxiety medications to the highly

anxious patient (Table 14-2). Because anxiety is a pervasive problem, large portions of the population take these drugs. Americans are now spending more than $500 million each year for drugs to relieve anxiety. Among these drugs, the benzodiazepines are the medication of choice in the management of anxiety and are the most widely prescribed drugs in the world. They have almost replaced the barbiturates in the treatment of anxiety because of their effectiveness and wide margin of safety. Use of these drugs in combination with alcohol, however, may result in a serious or even fatal sedative reaction. Antipsychotic drugs are frequently prescribed for those patients experiencing a panic level of anxiety of psychotic proportions.

Although some patients may need to take antianxiety drugs for extended periods these drugs should always be used in conjunction with nonpharmacological treatments. Potential dangers of these drugs include withdrawal syndrome side effects and addiction. It should be emphasized that psychopharmacology is not

A FAMILY SPEAKS

My daughter has obsessive-compulsive disorder (OCD). I didn't always know that, and I've spent many years of my life wondering what was wrong with her and if I were to blame. It's not easy living with someone who has an illness like that. At times it is just annoying. At other times it really makes you mad, and still other times you want to burst out laughing—but all that only makes it worse.

I think the one thing the family needs from the mental health care system is for health-care professionals to talk with them. The nurse who sees my daughter told me that I can call her with questions, and she explained all about OCD to my husband and me in great detail. Families want to help and support their members who are suffering, but how can we help if we don't know what to do? I used to try to physically stop my daughter from checking things. Then I told her how ridiculous it was. I even tried ignoring it for a while. How was I supposed to know what to do? Things are different now. We've all learned about this illness and how we can best help our daughter. After all, that's all we ever really wanted. ▼

TABLE 14-2
ANTIANXIETY DRUGS

Chemical class generic name (trade name)	Usual dosage range (mg/day)
ANTIANXIETY DRUGS	
Benzodiazepines	
Alprazolam (Xanax)	0.5-4
Chlordiazepoxide (Librium)	20-100
Chlorazepate (Tranxene)	7.5-60
Clonazepam (Klonopin)	1.5-2.0
Diazepam (Valium)	10-40
Halazepam (Paxipam)	80-160
Lorazepam (Ativan)	2-6
Oxazepam (Serax)	15-90
Prazepam (Centrax)	10-60
Antihistamines	
Diphenhydramine (Benadryl)	50
Hydroxyzine (Atarax)	100-300
Beta-adrenergic blocker	
Propranolol (Inderal)	10-40
Anxiolytic	
Buspirone (Buspar)	10-40
Imidazopyridine	
Zolpidem (Ambien)	10
TRICYCLIC ANTIDEPRESSANT DRUGS	
Chlomipramine (Anafranil)	50-200

a substitute for an ongoing therapeutic relationship. When used together, psychopharmacology can enhance the therapeutic relationship. Chemical control of painful symptoms allows the patient to direct attention to the conflicts underlying the anxiety. More detailed information on antianxiety and antipsychotic medications is presented in Chapter 25.

The Nursing Care Plan Summary summarizes the plan of care related to severe and panic levels of anxiety.

Moderate Level of Anxiety

The nursing interventions previously mentioned are supportive and directed toward the general short-term goal of reducing severe or panic-level anxiety. When the patient's anxiety is reduced to a moderate level, the nurse can begin helping with problem-solving efforts to cope with the stress. Long-term goals focus on helping the patient understand the cause of the anxiety and learn new ways of controlling it.

Education is an important aspect of promoting the

NURSING CARE PLAN SUMMARY
Severe and Panic Anxiety Responses

Nursing Diagnosis: Severe/panic level of anxiety

Expected Outcome: The patient will reduce anxiety to a moderate or mild level.

Short-term Goals	Interventions	Rationale
The patient will be protected from harm.	Initially accept and support, rather than attack, the patient's defenses. Acknowledge the reality of the pain associated with the patient's present coping mechanisms. Do not focus on the phobia, ritual, or physical complaint itself. Give feedback to the patient about behavior, stressors, appraisal of stressors, and coping resources. Reinforce the idea that physical health is related to emotional health and that this is an area that will need exploration in the future. In time, begin to place limits on the patient's maladaptive behavior in a supportive way.	Severe and panic levels of anxiety can be reduced by initially allowing the patient to determine the amount of stress that can be handled. If the patient is unable to release anxiety, tension may mount to the panic level and the patient may lose control. At this time the patient has no alternatives for present coping mechanisms.
The patient will experience fewer anxiety-provoking situations.	Assume a calm manner with the patient. Decrease environmental stimulation. Limit the patient's interaction with other patients to minimize the contagious aspects of anxiety. Identify and modify anxiety-provoking situations for the patient. Administer supportive physical measures, such as warm baths and massages.	The patient's behavior may be modified by altering the environment and the patient's interaction with it.
The patient will engage in a daily schedule of activities.	Initially share an activity with the patient to provide support and reinforce socially productive behavior. Provide for physical exercise of some type. Plan a schedule or list of activities that can be carried out daily. Involve family members and other support systems as much as possible.	By encouraging outside activities, the nurse limits the time the patient has available for destructive coping mechanisms while increasing participation in and enjoyment of other aspects of life.
The patient will experience relief from the symptoms of severe anxiety.	Administer medications that help reduce the patient's discomfort. Observe for medication side effects and initiate relevant health teaching.	The effect of a therapeutic relationship may be enhanced if the chemical control of symptoms allows the patient to direct attention to underlying conflicts.

patient's adaptive responses to anxiety. The nurse can identify relevant health teaching needs of each patient and then formulate an individualized teaching plan to meet those needs. Plans should be designed to increase patients' knowledge of their own predisposing and precipitating stressors, coping resources, and adaptive and maladaptive responses. Alternative coping strategies can be identified and explored. Health teaching should also address the beneficial aspects of mild levels of anxiety in motivating learning and producing growth and creativity.

The specific nursing interventions for a moderate level of anxiety were originally described by Peplau[18] and Burd[4] and reflect the problem-solving process. Short-term goals may be written for each step of this process. Goals include recognition of anxiety, insight into the anxiety, and coping with the threat. They incorporate principles and techniques of cognitive behavioral therapy (see Chapter 28) and can be implemented in any setting—psychiatric, community, or general hospital.[10,21]

Recognition of Anxiety. After analyzing the patient's behaviors and determining the level of anxiety, the nurse helps the patient to recognize anxiety by helping the patient explore underlying feelings with such questions as "Are you feeling anxious now?" or "Are you uncomfortable?" It is also helpful for the nurse to identify the patient's behavior and link it to the feeling of anxiety (e.g., "I noticed you smoked three cigarettes since we started talking about your sister. Are you feeling anxious?"). In this way the nurse acknowledges the patient's feeling, attempts to label it, encourages the patient to describe it further, and relates it to a specific behavioral pattern. The nurse is also validating inferences and assumptions with the patient.

The patient's goal, however, is often to avoid or negate anxiety and therefore might use any of the resistive approaches described in Box 14-7.[16] All these resistive approaches may create feelings of frustration, irritation, or reciprocal anxiety in the nurse, who must recognize personal feelings within and identify the patient's behavior pattern that might be causing them.

In attempting to deal with these patient defenses and intervene successfully, the importance of a trusting relationship becomes evident. If nurses establish themselves as warm, responsive listeners, give patients adequate time to respond, and are supportive of self-patient expressions, they will become less threatening. In helping patients recognize their anxiety, nurses should use open questions that move from nonthreatening topics to central issues of conflict. It may be helpful to vary the amount of anxiety to enhance the patient's motivation. In time, supportive confrontation may be used with the patient to address the repeated use of a particular resistive pattern. If, however, the patient's level of anxiety begins to rise rapidly, the nurse might choose to refocus the discussion to another topic.

Box 14-7

PATIENT RESISTANCES TO RECOGNIZING ANXIETY

1. **Screen symptoms.** The patient focuses attention on minor physical aliments to avoid acknowledging anxiety and conflict areas.
2. **Superior status position.** The patient attempts to control the interview by questioning the nurse's abilities or asserting the superiority of the patient's knowledge or experiences. The nurse should not respond emotionally to this approach nor accept the patient's challenge and compete, since this would only further avoid the issue of anxiety.
3. **Emotional seduction.** The patient attempts to manipulate the nurse and to elicit pity or sympathy.
4. **Superficiality.** The patient relates on a surface level and resists the nurse's attempts to explore underlying feelings or analyze issues.
5. **Circumlocution.** The patient gives the pretense of answering questions, but actually talks around the topic to avoid it.
6. **Amnesia.** This is a type of purposeful "forgetting" of a certain incident or event to avoid confronting and exploring it with the nurse.
7. **Denial.** The patient may use this approach only when discussing significant issues with the nurse or may generalize denial to all others, including self. The purpose is often to avoid humiliation.
8. **Intellectualization.** Patients who use this technique usually have some knowledge of psychology or medicine. They are able to express appropriate insights and analysis yet lack personal involvement in the problem they describe. They are not actually participating in the problem-solving process.
9. **Hostility.** The patient believes that offense is the best defense and therefore relates to others in an aggressive, defiant manner. The greatest danger in this situation is that the nurse will take this behavior personally and respond with anger. This serves to reinforce the patient's avoidance of his anxiety.
10. **Withdrawal.** The patient may resist the nurse by replying in vague, diffuse, indefinite, and remote ways.

Insight into the Anxiety. Once the patient is able to recognize anxiety, subsequent nursing interventions strive to expand the present context of the patient. The patient may be asked to describe the situations and interactions that immediately precede the increase in anxiety. Together the nurse and patient make inferences about the precipitating causes or biopsychosocial stressors.

The nurse then helps the patient see which values are being threatened by linking the threat with underlying causes, analyzing how the conflict developed, and relating the patient's present experiences to past ones. It is also important to explore how the patient reduced anxiety in the past and what kinds of actions produced relief.

Coping with the Threat. If previous coping responses have been adaptive and constructive, the patient should be encouraged to use them. If not, the nurse can point out their maladaptive effects and inform the patient that the present way of life appears unsatisfactory and distressing and that the patient is not attempting to improve the situation. The patient needs to assume responsibility for actions and realize that limi-

tations have been self-imposed. Other people must not be blamed. In this phase of intervention the nurse assumes an active role by interpreting, analyzing, confronting, and correlating cause and effect relationships. The nurse should proceed clearly so that the patient can follow while maintaining anxiety within appropriate limits. If the patient's anxiety becomes too severe, the nurse may change topics temporarily.

The nurse can help the patient in problem-solving efforts in various cognitive and behavioral ways (see Chapter 28). One way of helping the patient cope is to reevaluate the nature of the threat or stressor. Is it as bad as the patient perceives it? Is the cognitive appraisal realistic? Together they might discuss fears and feelings of inadequacy. Does the patient fear others are as critical, perfectionistic, and rejecting as the patient is of others? Is the conflict based in reality, or is it the result of unvalidated, isolated, and distorted thinking? By sharing fears with family members, peers, and staff, the patient frequently gains insight into such misperceptions.

Another approach is to help the patient modify behavior and learn new ways of coping with stress.[21] The nurse may act as a role model in this regard or engage

PATIENT EDUCATION PLAN
THE RELAXATION RESPONSE

Content	Instructional activities	Evaluation
Describe the characteristics and benefits of relaxation	Discuss physiological changes associated with relaxation and contrast these with the behaviors of anxiety	Patient identifies own responses to anxiety Patient describes elements of a relaxed state
Teach deep muscle relaxation through a sequence of tension-relaxation exercises	Engage the patient in the progressive procedure of tensing and relaxing voluntary muscles until the body as a whole is relaxed	Patient is able to tense and relax all muscle groups Patient identifies those muscles that become particularly tense
Discuss the relaxation procedure of meditation and its components	Describe the elements of meditation and assist the patient in using this technique	Patient selects a word or scene with pleasant connotations and engages in relaxed meditation
Assist in overcoming anxiety-provoking situations through systematic desensitization	With patient, construct a hierarchy of anxiety-provoking situations or scenes Through imagination or reality, work through these scenes using relaxation techniques	Patient identifies and ranks anxiety-provoking situations Patient exposes self to these situations while remaining in a relaxed state
Allow the rehearsing and practical use of relaxation in a safe environment	Role play stressful situations with the nurse or other patients	Patient becomes more comfortable with new behavior in a safe, supportive setting
Encourage patient to use relaxation techniques in life	Assign homework of using the relaxation response in everyday experiences Support success of patient	Patient uses relaxation response in life situations Patient is able to regulate anxiety response through use of relaxation techniques

NURSING CARE PLAN SUMMARY
Moderate Anxiety Responses

Nursing Diagnosis: Moderate level of anxiety

Expected Outcome: The patient will demonstrate adaptive ways of coping with stress.

Short-term Goals	Interventions	Rationale
The patient will identify and describe feelings of anxiety	Help the patient identify and describe underlying feelings Link the patient's behavior with such feelings Validate all inferences and assumptions with the patient Use open questions to move from nonthreatening topics to issues of conflict Vary the amount of anxiety to enhance the patient's motivation In time, supportive confrontation may be used judiciously	To adopt new coping responses, the patient first needs to be aware of feelings and to overcome conscious or unconscious denial and resistance
The patient will identify antecedents of anxiety	Help the patient describe the situations and interactions that immediately precede anxiety Review the patient's appraisal of the stressor, values being threatened, and the way in which the conflict developed Relate the patient's present experiences with relevant ones from the past	Once feelings of anxiety are recognized, the patient needs to understand their development, including precipitating stressors, appraisal of the stressor, and available resources
The patient will describe adaptive and maladaptive coping responses	Explore how the patient reduced anxiety in the past and what kinds of actions produced relief Point out the maladaptive and destructive effects of present coping responses Encourage the patient to use adaptive coping responses that were effective in the past Focus responsibility for change on the patient Actively help the patient correlate cause and effect relationships while maintaining anxiety within appropriate limits Assist the patient in reappraising the value, nature, and meaning of the stressor when appropriate	New adaptive coping responses can be learned through analyzing coping mechanisms used in the past, reappraising the stressor, using available resources, and accepting responsibility for change
The patient will implement two adaptive responses for coping with anxiety	Help the patient identify ways to restructure thoughts, modify behavior, use resources, and test new coping responses Encourage physical activity to discharge energy Include significant others as resources and social supports in helping the patient learn new coping responses Teach the patient relaxation exercises to increase control and self-reliance and reduce stress	One can also cope with stress by regulating the emotional distress that accompanies it through the use of stress management techniques

the patient in role playing. This can decrease anxiety about new responses to problem situations. One nursing function therefore is to teach the patient how aspects of mild anxiety can be constructive and growth producing. Physical activity should be encouraged as a way to discharge anxiety. Interpersonal resources such as family members or close friends should be incorporated into the nursing plan of care to provide the patient with support.

Frequently the cause for anxiety arises from an interpersonal conflict. In this case it is constructive to include the persons involved when analyzing the situation with the patient. In this way cause and effect relationships are more open to examination. Coping patterns can be examined in light of their effect on others, as well as on the patient.

Working through this problem-solving or reeducative process with the patient will take time, since it has to be accepted both intellectually and emotionally. Breaking previous behavioral patterns can be difficult. Nurses need to have a patient and consistent approach and continually reappraise their own anxiety.

Promote the Relaxation Response. In addition to problem solving, one can also cope with stress by regulating the emotional distress associated with it. Long-term goals directed toward helping the patient regulate emotional distress are supportive.

Relaxation can be taught individually, in small groups, or even in larger group settings. A Patient Education Plan for teaching the relaxation response is presented on p. 348. It is within the scope of nursing practice, requires no special equipment, and does not need a physician's supervision. As a group of interventions, relaxation can be implemented in various settings. A major benefit for patients is that after several training sessions, they can practice the techniques on their own. This puts the control in their hands and increases their self-reliance. Relaxation training is described in detail in Chapter 28. The Nursing Care Plan Summary for patients with moderate anxiety is presented on p. 349.

Evaluation

Evaluation is an ongoing process engaged in by the nurse and patient that is part of each phase of the nursing process. Even before begining to formulate the nursing diagnosis, the nurse should ask: "Did I critically observe my patient's physiological and psychomotor behaviors? Did I listen to my patient's subjective description of experience? Did I fail to see the relationships between my patient's expressed hostility or guilt and

underlying anxiety? Did I assess intellectual and social functioning?" After collecting the data, the nurse should analyze it. Was I able to identify the precipitating stressor for the patient? What was the patient's perception of the threat? How was this influenced by physical health, past experiences, and present feelings and needs? Did I correctly identify the patient's level of anxiety and validate it?

When using the criteria of adequacy, effectiveness, appropriateness, efficiency, and flexibility in evaluating the nursing goals and actions, the following questions can be raised:

▼ Were the planning, implementation, and evaluation mutual?

▼ Were goals and actions adequate in number and sufficiently specific to minimize the patient's level of anxiety?

▼ Were maladaptive responses reduced?

▼ Were new adaptive coping responses learned?

▼ Was the care plan reasonable in terms of time, energy, and expense?

▼ Was the nurse accepting of the patient and able to monitor personal anxiety throughout the relationship?

Answering these questions enables the nurse to review the total care provided. The nurse will also identify personal strengths and limitations in working with the anxious patient. Plans may then be made for overcoming the areas of limitation and further improving nursing care.

SUGGESTED CROSS-REFERENCES

A Stress Adaptation Model of Psychiatric Nursing Care	Chapter 4
Crisis Intervention	Chapter 12
Psychophysiological Responses and Somatoform and Sleep Disorders	Chapter 15
Psychopharmacology	Chapter 25
Cognitive Behavioral Therapy	Chapter 28

SUMMARY

1. Anxiety is diffuse apprehension that is vague and associated with feelings of uncertainty and helplessness. It is an emotion without an object that is subjective and communicated interpersonally. Levels of anxiety include mild, moderate, severe, and panic.

2. Patient behaviors related to anxiety include physiological, behavioral, cognitive, and affective responses.

3. Predisposing factors for anxiety responses are described from psychoanalytical, interpersonal, behavioral, family, and biological perspectives. Precipitating stressors include threats to physical integrity and self-system.

4. Coping mechanisms can be categorized as task-oriented reactions such as attack, withdrawal, and compromise, or ego-oriented reactions also known as defense mechanisms.
5. Primary NANDA diagnoses related to anxiety responses are anxiety, ineffective coping, and fear.
6. Primary DSM-IV diagnoses are categorized as anxiety disorders.
7. The expected outcome of nursing care for patients with maladaptive anxiety responses is that the patient will demonstrate adaptive ways of coping with stress.
8. Interventions include establishing a trusting relationship, self-awareness, protecting the patient, modifying the environment, encouraging activity, medication, and learning new ways to cope with stress.
9. The nurse should use the criteria of adequacy, effectiveness, appropriateness, efficiency, and flexibility in evaluating nursing care.

COMPETENT CARING
A CLINICAL EXEMPLAR OF A PSYCHIATRIC NURSE

Madelyn Myers, BS, RN

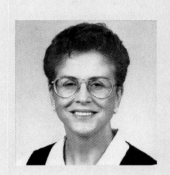

As the night shift charge nurse on an adult psychiatric unit, I learned the "graveyard shift" was anything but routine. On return to the unit after my days off, I was told that Mr. B's behavior had deteriorated in the last few days. Mr. B was a 68-year-old man with a diagnosis of organic brain syndrome secondary to alcohol abuse. He was unable to stay in bed for more than a few minutes at a time and he was at risk for falls due to his confusion and as a side effect of his tranquilizing medication. The previous nights the staff had found it necessary to contain Mr. B with soft restraints to keep him in bed and reduce the risk of his falling.

After shift report I made my nursing rounds, accounting for all patients and assessing the situation of the unit. Mr. B was obviously distraught and anxious. His first question to me was, "You're not going to rope me, are you?" I sat down to talk with Mr. B to reassure him and explain that it was time for him to get ready for bed. He refused to change his clothing, stating he just needed to walk around a little longer. I asked the therapeutic assistants if they would walk him around a while longer to try calming him down.

I went to the office to start verifying the day's orders, but found it impossible to get much done as Mr. B was calling me and coming to the nursing office to ask questions very frequently. The staff were also getting frustrated because he seemed very tired but would sit down for only a few minutes before he would jump up again. After I did a few more tasks, I relieved the staff member sitting with Mr. B. I was able to get Mr. B to lie down on his bed only after he saw me take the posey off the bed and out of the room. I watched him as he lay down and he seemed to doze off to sleep almost immediately. Then again just as quickly he awoke and started out of bed. He said, "Something is very wrong with me—I'm afraid I might die." We discussed his anxiety, and I reassured him that one of the staff would sit with him if that would make him feel more secure. He nodded in affirmation. I sat by his bedside. He fell asleep immediately and again repeated his previous pattern of awakening with a start, but this time he just looked over, saw me, and returned to sleep.

A short while later, one of the other staff came to relieve me. I shared with her my concern that Mr. B had been quite anxious and my plan was to sit at his bedside and gradually move the chair back until we were sitting just outside his room but still in his line of sight. This way, he would be reassured that staff were still close by and we could observe him if he tried to get out of bed. That night he actually slept 4 hours with only two brief awakenings. The previous nights he had only dozed for minutes at a time.

The next morning I spoke with the clinical nurse specialist on his team and relayed his fear of dying and of being "roped" with the posey. I shared with her the strategy we used of sitting with him and how he was able to sleep. The new plan of care was placed in his Kardex for all to follow. The next few nights we continued with our plan and each night Mr. B slept a little longer. He would even get changed into his pajamas before bed. He no longer started to "escalate" at bedtime. As he was sleeping better, Mr. B was also feeling better physically and his anxiety level de-

creased dramatically. He required less medication for his anxiety; thus he was much more stable on his feet, no longer at risk for falls. Mr. B's ability to perform his ADLs increased over the next week and he was able to return to his previous living situation.

Many of his symptoms seemed to have been from sleep deprivation, high levels of anxiety, and the untoward effects of tranquilizers. This rewarding experience was not an isolated event on the night shift. It seems many people sleep through the night and only see the shadows of the staff making rounds, but then there are others for whom the care they receive during these darkened hours makes a critical difference. ▼

REFERENCES

1. Akiskal H: Anxiety: definition, relationship to depression, and proposal for an integrative model. In Tuma A, Maser J, eds: *Anxiety and the anxiety disorders*, Hillsdale, NJ, 1985, Lawrence Erlbaum Associates Publishers.
2. American Psychiatric Association: *Diagnostic and statistical manual of mental disorders*, ed 4, Washington, DC, 1994, The Association.
3. Barloon D: Effects on children of having lived with a parent who has an anxiety disorder, *Issues Ment Health Nurs* 14:187, 1993.
4. Burd S: Effects of nursing intervention in anxiety of patients. In Burd SF, Marshall MA, eds: *Some clinical approaches to psychiatric nursing*, New York, 1963, Macmillan.
5. Dollard J, Miller N: *Personality and psychotherapy*, New York, 1950, McGraw-Hill.
6. Elliott S: Denial as an effective mechanism to allay anxiety following a stressful event, *J Psychiatr Nurs* 18:11, 1980.
7. Free N, Winget C, Whitman R: Separation anxiety in panic disorder, *Am J Psychiatry* 150:595, 1993.
8. Freud S: *Problem of anxiety*, New York, 1936, WW Norton.
9. Freud S: *A general introduction to psychoanalysis*, New York, 1969, Pocket Books.
10. Hallam R: *Counselling for anxiety problems*, Newbury Park, Calif, 1992, Sage Publications.
11. Hoehn-Saric R, McLeod D: *Biology of anxiety disorders*, Washington, DC, 1993, American Psychiatric Press.
12. Laraia M, Stuart G, Frye L, Lydiard R, Ballenger J: Childhood environment of women having panic disorder with agoraphobia, *J Anxiety Dis* 8:1, 1994.
13. Long B: Stress-management interventions: a 15-month follow-up of aerobic conditioning and stress innoculation training, *Cognitive Ther Res* 9:471, 1985.
14. Massion A, Warshaw M, Keller M: Quality of life and psychiatric morbidity in panic disorder and generalized anxiety disorder, *Am J Psychiatry* 150:600, 1993.
15. May R: *The meaning of anxiety*, New York, 1950, Ronald Press.
16. Meares A: *The management of the anxious patient*, Philadelphia, 1963, WB Saunders.
17. Oden G: Individual panic: elements and patterns. In Burd S, Marshall M, eds: *Some clinical approaches to psychiatric nursing*, New York, 1963, Macmillan.
18. Peplau H: Interpersonal techniques: the crux of psychiatric nursing, *Am J Nurs* 62:53, 1962.
19. Peplau H: A working definition of anxiety. In Burd S, Marshall M, eds: *Some clinical approaches to psychiatric nursing*, New York, 1963, Macmillan.
20. Robins L et al: Lifetime prevalence of specific psychiatric disorders in three sites, *Arch Gen Psychiatry* 41:949, 1984.
21. Suinn R: *Anxiety management training*, New York, 1990, Plenum Press.
22. Sullivan HS: *The interpersonal theory of psychiatry*, New York, 1953, WW Norton.
23. Whitley G: Anxiety: defining the diagnosis, *J Psychosoc Nurs Ment Health Serv* 27:7, 1989.

ANNOTATED SUGGESTED READINGS

*Barloon D: Effects on children of having lived with a parent who has an anxiety disorder, *Issues Ment Health Nurs* 14:187, 1993.

Describes the problems of children with a family history of anxiety disorders with implications for nursing care.

Calvocoressi L et al: Inpatient treatment of patients with severe obsessive-compulsive disorder, *Hosp Community Psychiatry* 44:1150, 1993.

Presents pharmacological, psychosocial, and behavioral management strategies for treating OCD patients on general psychiatric units. Useful for nursing staffs.

*Deakin H: The treatment of agoraphobia by nurse therapists: practice and training. In Gournay K, ed: *Agoraphobia: current perspectives on theory and treatment*, New York, 1989, Routledge.

Outlines the development of nurse behavior therapist training in England. Gives specific information on course design and core clinical skills.

---

*Nursing reference.

Hallam R: *Counselling for anxiety problems*, Newbury Park, Calif, 1992, Sage Publications.

Excellent, practical presentation of assessing and treating anxiety disorders. Highly recommended.

Klerman G et al: *Panic anxiety and its treatment*, Washington, DC, 1993, American Psychiatric Press.

Report of the APA task force that reviews the clinical findings regarding panic anxiety related to diagnosis, treatment, and future research.

*Laraia M: Biological correlates of panic disorder with agoraphobia: practice perspectives for nurses, Arch Psychiatr Nurs 5:373, 1991.

A concise, clear description of the latest biological theories pertaining to anxiety disorders, with implications for nursing practice and research.

*Laraia M, Stuart G, Best C: Behavioral treatment of panic-related disorders: a review, Arch Psychiatr Nurs 3:125, 1989.

Behavioral theories and therapy techniques for panic-related disorders. An excellent, inclusive article.

*Laraia M, Stuart G, Frye L, Lydiard R, Ballenger J: Childhood environment of women having panic disorder with agoraphobia, J Anxiety Dis 8:1, 1994.

Research conducted by nurses in an interdisciplinary team on the childhood environment of women with panic disorder.

*Simoni P: Obsessive-compulsive disorder: the effect of research on nursing care, J Psychosoc Nurs Ment Health Serv 29:19, 1991.

Reviews the etiology, neurobiology, and nursing care implications for OCD based on the latest research on the disorder.

*Tilley S, Weighill V: How nurse therapists assess and contribute to the management of alcohol and sedative drug use among anxious patients, J Adv Nurs 11:499, 1986.

Describes a nursing research study on patients with anxiety disorders and assessment of their substance use by nurse therapists. Implications for nursing education and practice are included.

Tillich P: *The courage to be*, New Haven, Conn, 1952, Yale University Press.

Addresses anxiety, its conquest, and the meaning of courage. A distinguished classic in the field.

Van Noppen B, Tortora M, Rasmussen S: Learning to live with obsessive-compulsive disorder, *Innovations and Research* 2:41, 1993.

Helpful reading for family members trying to cope with the demands of OCD. Important information that can be generalized for other psychiatric disorders.

*Waddell K, Demi A: Effectiveness of an intensive partial hospitalization program for treatment of anxiety disorders, Arch Psychiatr Nurs 7:2, 1993.

Reports on the effectiveness of a 5-week partial hospitalization program based on an integration of biological, cognitive, and behavioral theories.

Zetin M, Kramer M: Obsessive-compulsive disorder, *Hosp Community Psychiatry* 43:689, 1992.

Reviews studies on OCD and related disorders that respond to the new serotonergic antidepressants and behavioral therapy.

---

*Nursing reference.

---

*Nursing reference.

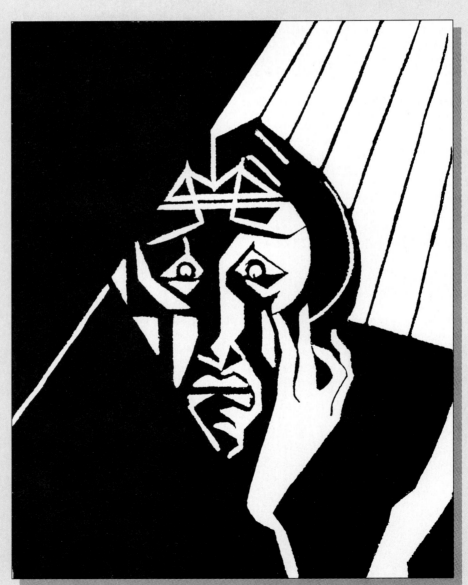

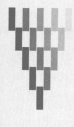

CHAPTER 15

Psychophysiological Responses and Somatoform and Sleep Disorders

GAIL W. STUART
SANDRA J. SUNDEEN

The cure of many diseases is unknown to the physicians of Hellas, because they disregard the whole, which ought to be studied also, for the part can never be well unless the whole is well.

Plato

LEARNING OBJECTIVES

After studying this chapter the student should be able to:

▼ Describe the continuum of adaptive and maladaptive psychophysiological responses

▼ Identify behaviors associated with psychophysiological responses

▼ Analyze predisposing factors and precipitating stressors related to psychophysiological responses

▼ Describe coping resources and coping mechanisms related to psychophysiological responses

▼ Formulate nursing diagnoses for patients related to psychophysiological responses

▼ Assess the relationship between nursing diagnoses and medical diagnoses related to psychophysiological responses

▼ Identify expected outcomes and short-term nursing goals for patients related to psychophysiological responses

▼ Develop a patient education plan to promote adaptive psychophysiological responses

▼ Analyze nursing interventions for patients related to psychophysiological responses

▼ Evaluate nursing care for patients related to psychophysiological responses

TOPICAL OUTLINE

Continuum of Psychophysiological Responses
Assessment
    Behaviors
    Predisposing Factors
    Precipitating Stressors
    Coping Resources
    Coping Mechanisms
Nursing Diagnosis
    Related Medical Diagnoses
Outcome Identification
Planning
Implementation
    Psychological Approaches
    Patient Education
    Physiological Support
Evaluation

Throughout history, philosophers and scientists have debated the nature and extent of the relationship between the mind (*psyche*) and body (*soma*). Recently, there has been a renewed interest in holistic health practices, based on the idea that mental processes influence physical well-being and vice versa. Research is attempting to identify the links between thoughts, feelings, and body functioning. Great interest has arisen about the role of the endocrine and immune systems in the development of psychophysiological disorders. Many believe that all illness has a psychophysiological component—that physical disorders have a psychological component and mental disorders a physical one.

CONTINUUM OF PSYCHOPHYSIOLOGICAL RESPONSES

Much of the current thinking about psychophysiological behavior is related to an increased understanding of the role of stress in human life. In 1929 Walter Cannon[9] published his landmark work, *Bodily Changes in Pain, Hunger, Fear and Rage*. Based on research on animal physiology, he described the "fight-or-flight" response. In response to Cannon's research, other investigators began to study physical responses to a variety of stressors, including psychological ones. For instance, in 1951 Wolf and colleagues[30] reported their research on the connection between stress and hypertension. They found that emotional arousal did lead to elevations in blood pressure.

Stress theory was significantly advanced when Hans Selye[26] published *The Stress of Life* in 1956. Selye described the stress response in detail, creating a greater understanding of the effect of stressful experiences on physical functioning. He identified a three-stage process of response to stress. This generalized response is called the general adaptation syndrome (GAS). These levels of response are:

1. **The alarm reaction.** This is the immediate response to a stressor that has not been eliminated in a localized area. Adrenocortical response mechanisms occur, resulting in behaviors associated with the fight-or-flight response.
2. **Stage of resistance.** There is some resistance to the stressor. The body adapts and functions at a lower than optimal level. This requires a greater than usual expenditure of energy for survival.
3. **Stage of exhaustion.** The adaptive mechanisms become worn out and fail. The negative effect of the stressor spreads to the entire organism. If the stressor is not removed or counteracted, death will ultimately result.

Selye's theory has aided investigators in psychophysiology as they attempt to identify more specific mental-physical interactions and interventions in stress responses.

Any experience believed by the individual to be stressful may stimulate a psychophysiological response. The stress does not have to be recognized consciously, and in fact, often it is not. If individuals recognize that they are under stress, they are often unable to connect the cognitive understanding of feeling stress with the physical symptoms of the psychophysiological disorder. Fig. 15-1 illustrates the range of possible psychophysiological responses to stress, based on Selye's theory.

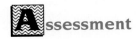 **ssessment**

Behaviors

Many behaviors are associated with psychophysiological disorders. Careful assessment is needed so that actual organic problems are defined and treated. This type of illness should never be dismissed as "only psychosomatic" or "all in one's head." Serious psychophysiological disorders can be fatal if not treated adequately.

Physiological. The primary behaviors observed with psychophysiological responses are the physical symp-

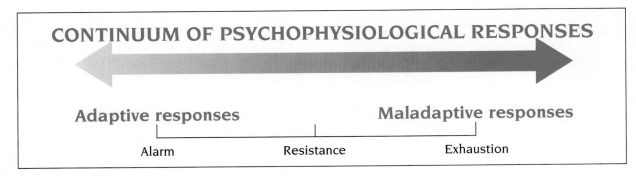

CONTINUUM OF PSYCHOPHYSIOLOGICAL RESPONSES

Adaptive responses   Maladaptive responses

Alarm   Resistance   Exhaustion

Fig. 15-1 Continuum of psychophysiological responses.

toms. These disruptions lead the person to seek health care. Psychological factors affecting the physical condition may involve any body part.[10] The most common organ systems involved are listed in Box 15-1. In addition, longer lengths of stay in the general hospital have been reported to be associated with greater psychological comorbidity, particularly depression, anxiety, and organicity.[25] Such research underscores the importance of linking physiological and psychological assessments.

The person is often reluctant to believe, however, that a physical problem may be related to psychological factors. In part, this occurs because being physically ill is more socially acceptable than having psychological problems. The situation is compounded because the pa-

tient really does have physical symptoms. Denial of the psychological component of the illness may lead to "doctor shopping." The patient searches for someone who will find an organic cause for the illness. This tendency to experience and communicate psychological distress in the form of physical symptoms and to seek help for them in general medical settings is a widespread clinical phenomenon that may involve up to 30% to 40% of medical patients.[13] The following clinical example illustrates this problem.

 ## CLINICAL EXAMPLE

Mr. R was a successful 42-year-old executive who had risen quickly to the top of his company. He worked long hours and had difficulty delegating any of his responsibilities. He set high standards for his employees and was believed to be insensitive to human concerns. He viewed himself as "tough," but fair." However, he had little sympathy for a worker who requested extra time off for personal business.

Mr. R was married but saw little of his family. He expected his wife and children to do their part to maintain his standing in the community by associating with "the right people." He seldom interacted with his children except to reprimand them if they disturbed his concentration while he was working. His wife reported that their sexual relationship was unsatisfying to her. Mr. R used it for physical release for himself but was not concerned about meeting her needs. She suspected that he was involved in an extramarital affair but did not want to endanger the marriage by confronting him.

Mr. R was expecting to be named to the board of directors on a prestigious philanthropic foundation. He anticipated that this would add to his social prominence in the community. Shortly before the announcement was to be made, his 14-year-old son was arrested in a drug raid in the lower middle class part of town. Mr. R did not get the appointment. He was furious with his son but dealt with his anger by withdrawing still more. One day at work, he experienced an episode of dizziness, followed by a severe headache. He attributed it to tension, took some aspirin, and continued to work. However, after several similar episodes, he decided to consult his family doctor. The physician arrived at a diagnosis of essential hypertension. He tried to discuss work, family, and social behavior with Mr. R but was frustrated by superficial responses. Although concerned about Mr. R's condition and stress level, the doctor gave in to Mr. R's demand for medication to lower his blood pressure. He also advised Mr. R to exercise and to find a relaxing activity.

Box 15-1

PHYSICAL CONDITIONS AFFECTED BY PSYCHOLOGICAL FACTORS

CARDIOVASCULAR

Migraine
Essential hypertension
Angina
Tension headaches

MUSCULOSKELETAL

Rheumatoid arthritis
Low back pain (idiopathic)

RESPIRATORY

Hyperventilation
Asthma

GASTROINTESTINAL

Anorexia nervosa
Peptic ulcer
Irritable bowel syndrome
Colitis
Obesity

SKIN

Neurodermatitis
Eczema
Psoriasis
Pruritis

GENITOURINARY

Impotence
Frigidity
Premenstrual syndrome

ENDOCRINOLOGICAL

Hyperthyroidism
Diabetes

Selected Nursing Diagnoses

▼ Impaired adjustment related to family and work stress as evidenced by denial and development of physical symptoms
▼ Altered family processes related to rigid role expectations as evidenced by withdrawal and lack of communication.

Mr R is typical of many people with stress-related psychophysiological disorders. He is reluctant to admit to a lack of control over his mind and body. He expects a magical cure that will let him follow his usual life-style without interruption. He will probably stop taking his medication as soon as he feels better. Distance from the stressor may allow him to function for a while without noticeable symptoms of his hypertension. Sooner or later, however, new stressors will lead to another dizzy spell, headaches, or possibly myocardial infarction or cerebrovascular accident.

Psychological. Some people have physical symptoms without any organic impairment. These are termed *somatoform disorders.* They include somatization disorder, in which the person has many physical complaints; conversion disorder, in which a loss or alteration of physical functioning occurs; hypochondriasis, the fear of or belief that one has an illness; body dysmorphic disorder, in which a person with a normal appearance is concerned about having a physical defect; and pain disorder, in which psychological factors play an important role in the onset, severity, or maintenance of the pain. The next clinical example is a case history of a person with a medical diagnosis of somatization disorder.

 CLINICAL EXAMPLE

Ms. O, a 28-year-old single woman, was admitted to the medical unit of a general hospital for a complete medical workup. When asked about her main problem during the nursing assessment, she replied, "I've never been very well. Even when I was a child I was sick a lot." Ms. O listed multiple complaints during the physical assessment. These included palpitations, dizzy spells, menstrual irregularity, painful menses, blurred vision, dysphagia, backache, pain in her knees and feet, and a variety of gastrointestinal symptoms including stomach pain, nausea, vomiting, diarrhea, flatulence, and intolerance to seafood, vegetables of the cabbage family, carbonated beverages, and eggs. Except for the food intolerances, none of the symptoms was constant. They occurred at random, making her fearful of going out of her home.

The psychosocial assessment revealed that Ms. O lived with her parents. She was the youngest of three children. Her siblings were living away from the parental home. She had graduated from high school but had poor grades because of her frequent absences. She had tried to work as a clerk in a retail store but was asked to leave because of absenteeism. She did not seem particularly bothered about the loss of her job. She had never tried to find other work, although she had been unemployed for 8 years. When asked how she spent her time, she said that she did some gardening and some housework when she felt well enough. However, she spent most of her time watching television.

Ms. O's parents visited her most of every day. Her mother asked whether she could spend the night in her daughter's room and was displeased when told no. The family had many complaints about the quality of the nursing care, most about failures to anticipate the patient's needs, Extensive diagnostic studies failed to reveal any organic basis for Ms. O's physical complaints. When informed that the problem was most likely psychological and advised to obtain psychotherapy, the family protested angrily and refused a referral to a psychiatric clinic. Ms. O was discharged and returned to her parent's home.

Selected Nursing Diagnoses:

▼ Ineffective denial related to physical and emotional health status as evidenced by repeated medical care visits and refusal to obtain psychiatric treatment
▼ Altered family processes related to mother-daughter dependency issues as evidence by excessive caretaking by mother and passivity of daughter

Ms. O shows the dependent behavior that is often typical of people with somatization disorder. Her many symptoms allowed her to be taken care of and to avoid the demands of adult responsibility. Her need to be cared for fit with her mother's need to nurture. Therefore she received little encouragement to give up her symptoms. A periodic hospital stay served to reinforce the seriousness of her problem. Secondary gain related to the gratification of dependency needs is a powerful deterrent to change in many patients.

Another type of somatoform disorder is the conversion disorder. Symptoms of some physical illness appear without any underlying organic cause. The organic symptom reduces the patient's anxiety and usually gives a clue to the conflict. For example, a patient who has an impulse to harm his domineering mother may develop paralysis of his arms and hands. The primary gain this patient receives is that he is unable to carry out his impulses. He also may experience secondary gain in the form of attention, manipulation of others, freedom from responsibilities, and economic benefits. Conversion symptoms might include the following:

1. Sensory symptoms, such as areas of numbness, blindness, or deafness
2. Motor symptoms, such as paralysis, tremors, or mutism
3. Visceral symptoms, such as urinary retention, headaches, or difficulty breathing

It is often difficult to diagnose this reaction. Other patient behaviors may be helpful. Often patients display little anxiety or concern about the conversion symptom and its resulting disability. The classic term to describe this lack of concern is *la belle indifference*. The patient also tends to seek attention in ways not limited to the actual symptom.

Hypochondriasis is another type of somatoform disorder. These individuals have an exaggerated concern with physical health that is not based on any real organic disorders. They fear presumed diseases and are not helped by reassurance. They also tend to seek out and use information about diseases to convince themselves that they are probably ill or about to become so. Unlike the conversion reaction, no actual loss or distortion of function occurs. Patients appear worried and anxious about their symptoms. This concern may be based on physical sensations overlooked by most people or on symptoms of a minor physical illness that the patient magnifies. This is frequently a chronic behavior pattern and is often accompanied by a history of visits to numerous physicians.

Hypochondriacal behavior is not related to a conscious decision. If a person decides to fake an illness, the behavior is called *malingering*. This is usually done to avoid responsibilities the person views as burdensome. Many otherwise healthy people malinger at one time or another. For instance, a person involved in an automobile accident may feign neck pain to receive insurance money. Frequently, the person exaggerates symptoms, is evasive, and tells contradictory stories about the illness.

Pain. Pain is a complex symptom consisting of a sensation underlying potential disease and an associated emotional state. Acute pain is a reflex biological response to injury. By definition, chronic pain consists of pain of a minimum of 6 months' duration. Somatoform pain disorder is a preoccupation with pain in the absence of physical disease to account for its intensity. It does not follow a neuroanatomical distribution. There may also be a close correlation between stress and conflict and the initiation or exacerbation of the pain.

Sleep. Sleep disturbances are common in the general population and among people with psychiatric disorders.[8,19] Insomnia is the most prevalent disorder. Up to 30% of the population have insomnia and seek help for it. Other behaviors include excessive daytime sleepiness, difficulty sleeping during desired sleep time, and unusual nocturnal events such as nightmares and sleepwalking. Sleep disorders are more common in the elderly.[5,7]

Sleep disorders are classified by the Association of Sleep Disorders Centers (ASDC) into four major groupings with considerable overlap[17]:

1. Disorders of initiating or maintaining sleep, also known as **insomnia.** Anxiety and depression are major causes of insomnia.
2. Disorders of excessive somnolence, also known as **hypersomnia.** This category includes narcolepsy, sleep apnea, and nocturnal movement disorders such as restless legs.
3. Disorders of the sleep-wake schedule, characterized by normal sleep but at the wrong time. These are transient disturbances associated with jet lag and work shift changes. They are usually self-limited and resolve as the body readjusts to a new sleep-wake schedule.[23]
4. Disorders associated with sleep stages, also known as **parasomnia.** This category includes conditions such as sleepwalking, night terrors, nightmares, and enuresis. These sleep problems are often experienced by children and can have a significant effect on functioning and well-being.[18]

The assessment of patients with sleep problems is multifaceted, involving a detailed history and medical and psychiatric examinations, extensive questionnaires, the use of sleep diaries or logs, and often psychological testing. Many patients are referred for formal sleep studies, which include all night polysomnography and physiological measures of daytime sleepiness.[16,24] Many members of the health-care team collaborate within sleep centers to deliver multidisciplinary care to patients with sleep-related disturbances.

Have you ever experienced a problem sleeping? Which ASCD grouping would your problem have fit into, and what did you do to relieve it?

Predisposing Factors

A number of biopsychosocial factors are believed to influence the individual's psychophysiological response to stress. Most of the specific relationships between physical and psychological processes are still not well described. Thus it is important for the nurse to consider all possibilities when assessing factors that might predispose the patient to a particular disorder.

Biological. It is thought by some that biological factors may predispose a person to psychophysiological illness. Endocrine activity has been noted to have an effect on the person's personality.[20] However, although efforts have been made to link specific hormones and emotions, little success has been achieved.

Genetic factors have also been considered.[6] It has been proposed that a biological tendency for particular psychophysiological responses could be inherited. This theory suggests that any prolonged stress can cause physiological changes, which result in a physical disorder. Each person has a "shock organ" that is genetically vulnerable to stress. Thus some patients may be prone to cardiac illness, whereas others may react with gastrointestinal distress or skin rashes. People who are chronically anxious or depressed are believed to have a greater vulnerability to psychophysiological illness.

Recent research on the biological factors causing psychophysiological illness has emerged within the field of **psychoneuroimmunology.**[22] It has been demonstrated that the immune response can be modified by behavior modification techniques. Researchers are now investigating the possibility of modifying the immune response in the treatment of autoimmune illnesses such as rheumatoid arthritis, systemic lupus erythematosus, myasthenia gravis, and pernicious anemia. Other related research is exploring the relationship between the immune system, stress, and cancer. It has been suspected that high stress, especially if prolonged, can decrease the immune system's ability to destroy neoplastic growths. Unfortunately, this is an extremely difficult area in which to conduct research. There has not been enough time to conduct prospective studies of this hypothesis. Retrospective studies are compromised by the person's stress response to the medical diagnosis, which makes it impossible to measure preexisting stress levels accurately.

Psychological. Philosophers and scientists have long speculated about the roles that personality and stress may play in the development of illness. In the 1930s and 1940s Flanders Dunbar[12] and Franz Alexander[3] developed personality profiles of those prone to several diseases including hypertension, coronary artery disease (CAD), cancer, ulcers, and rheumatoid arthritis. Research regarding their theories has evolved since their early work in the field.

Recent studies suggest that a negative affective style marked by depression, anxiety, and hostility may be associated with the development of such chronic diseases as asthma, headaches, ulcers, arthritis, and CAD.[15] The clearest evidence to date relates to the negative effects of chronic hostility on cardiovascular disease. More specifically, Type A behavior, which has been characterized by competitive drive, impatience, hostility, irritability, and aggressiveness, has been shown to predict both the physiological changes that are associated with CAD and the development of CAD itself. Type As are also more likely to have accidents, to die as a result of accidents or violence, to have migraine headaches, to smoke more, and to have higher levels of serum cholesterol. Thus Type A behavior appears to be a risk factor not only for cardiovascular disease but also for an array of other disorders. Finally, while such research suggests the possibility of a disease-prone personality, the exact nature of the relationship is unknown at present. For example, a negative emotional state may:

▼ Produce pathological physiological changes
▼ Lead people to practice faulty health behaviors
▼ Produce illness behavior but no underlying pathology
▼ Be associated with illness through other factors that are presently not known

Complementing the research on negative emotional states and disease is the increasing focus on the potentially protective role of positive emotional states. One idea regarding these traits is that of a "self-healing" personality, which is characterized by enthusiasm.[14] Self-healing, emotionally balanced people are believed to be alert, responsive, and energetic, although they may also be calm and conscientious. They are curious, secure, and constructive. Self-healing personalities also have a sense of continuous growth and resilience and an extra margin of emotional stability that can be called on when their capacities are challenged. Two other positive traits include optimism and perceived control. Optimists appear to have fewer physical symptoms and may show faster recoveries from illness. Belief in personal control, or *self-efficacy*, appears to affect the likelihood of developing illness by directly influencing the practice of health behaviors and by buffering individuals against the adverse effects of stress.

Think of people you know who always seem to be ill. What personality characteristics do they share? How do they compare with people you know who are hardly ever ill?

Sociocultural. It has been proposed that health, illness, and suffering are patterned by culture and realized as personal worlds of experience.[28] In this view psychophysiological illness derives from the relationships between body, psyche, and society (see Critical Thinking about Contemporary Issues). Illness is not seen as simply the natural unfolding of an exclusively biological process. Rather, its course is also influenced by sociocultural factors. The social course of illness is a concept with at least two meanings.[29]

The first is the idea that the severity of the person's symptoms is influenced by aspects of the social environment. This means that subjectively experienced distress can be increased or decreased by the nature and number of major and minor problems in the person's world, changes in the emotional climate of that world, or in the manner in which the ill person chooses to engage in social life.

In the second meaning the symptoms shape and structure the person's social world, as the illness, by its very presence, initiates a series of changes in the person's environment. The resulting chain of illness-related interpersonal events thus becomes a part of the

social course of the person's illness. This can be seen in the concept of the *sick role*, first described in the 1950s by Parsons. It proposes that being sick is a social role as well as a condition and that society places certain beliefs and expectations on the individual who falls ill.[21] These include:

1. The sick are allowed to be exempt from their usual social role responsibilities.
2. The sick are not seen as being responsible for being ill.
3. The sick are expected to want to get well.
4. The sick are expected to seek competent help and cooperate with the helper in trying to get well.

Although the premises of the sick role have been questioned in recent years, they do demonstrate the impact of sociocultural factors on the expression and resolution of psychophysiological responses.

CRITICAL THINKING ABOUT CONTEMPORARY ISSUES

Is Chronic Fatigue Syndrome a Culturally Sanctioned Form of Illness Behavior?

There has been much interest in the recently defined disorder of *chronic fatigue syndrome*, which is characterized by exhaustion or fatigue and marked reduction in activity and is correlated with a high prevalence of psychiatric disorders and psychophysiological symptoms secondary to stress.[1] This attention has been related to reports of its growing frequency, substantial morbidity, and unclear pathogenesis. This interest has also been fueled by debates about emotional factors related to the illness and questions as to whether it represents a discrete disorder.

Currently the diagnosis of chronic fatigue syndrome is more common among women. It has been proposed that it is related to the struggle of American culture with the expanding role of women and the mismatch between women's ambitions and social possibilities.[2] In contemporary society illness and the sick role are the only socially legitimate excuses for abandoning the workplace and the pursuit of achievement. Thus the diagnosis of chronic fatigue syndrome may provide a legitimate "medical" reason for a variety of psychophysiological responses, thereby allowing the individual to withdraw from situations that are intolerable because of illness rather than choice. This example of the cultural shaping of illness and disease further underscores society's preference for individuals to be diagnosed with a physical illness and thus the continued stigmatization of psychiatric illness and emotional distress. ▼

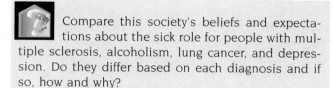

Compare this society's beliefs and expectations about the sick role for people with multiple sclerosis, alcoholism, lung cancer, and depression. Do they differ based on each diagnosis and if so, how and why?

Precipitating Stressors

Any experience that the individual interprets as stressful may lead to a psychophysiological response. Some of these are relatively mild and short-lived. Examples include diarrhea before an examination or a dry mouth when speaking before a large group of people. Sometimes the response is more serious and indicates a higher level of anxiety. For instance, a person might feel panicky and experience tachycardia when boarding an airplane. Because the psychophysiological disorder is an attempt to deal with anxiety, it is recommended that information on stressors related to anxiety (Chapter 14) be reviewed.

One type of stressor that has been shown to cause physical illness and even death is the loss of a significant interpersonal relationship. Siegel[27] has noted that "one of the most common precursors of cancer is a traumatic loss or a feeling of emptiness in one's life." An increased mortality rate has been found among recently widowed people. Similar observations have been made about people admitted to institutions such as nursing homes, who are separated from significant others. Children who have been separated from their mothers, especially if placed in an impersonal environment, also show a decline in physical health. The effect of a loss may cause both physical and psychological symptoms for an extended period of time. Illnesses and deaths related to loss of a loved person seem to represent the exhaustion phase of the general adaptation syndrome.

Sometimes a psychophysiological problem is a response to an accumulation of rather small stressors. A patient may find it difficult to identify one specific stressor that preceded a particular problem. Careful assessment may reveal a pattern of overwork and overcommitment or a series of seemingly minor events that all required extra effort. Most of the psychophysiological disorders come and go. This may be related to changes in the person's stress level. When the cumulative stress gets too high, the body "calls time out" by developing physical symptoms.

Coping Resources

One of the most important parts of promoting adaptive psychophysiological responses involves changing health habits. Those individuals who adopt positive health practices and good health measures can prevent the occurrence of a variety of biopsychosocial illnesses. Patient Education Plans that include coping skills training, such as the one presented below, can increase a person's knowledge about the effect on stress, reduce anxiety, increase a person's feelings of purpose and meaning in life, reduce pain and suffering, and improve coping abilities.

Social support from family, friends, and caregivers is also an important resource for adaptive psychophysiologic responses (see A Family Speaks). It may lower the likelihood of developing maladaptive responses, speed the recovery from illness, and reduce the distress and suffering that accompanies illness. Social support groups are another coping resource that can satisfy needs for social support that are unmet by family members and caregivers.

Coping Mechanisms

The psychophysiological disorders may be seen as attempts to cope with the anxiety associated with overwhelming stress. Unconsciously the person links the anxiety to the physical illness. Secondary gain then adds to the psychological relief experienced.

Several of the defense mechanisms described in Chapter 14 may be seen in psychophysiological disorders. *Repression* of feelings, conflicts, and unacceptable impulses often lead to physical symptoms. The maintenance of repression over long periods of time requires a great deal of psychic energy. As the system approaches a state of exhaustion, physical symptoms occur. When a psychological basis for illness is suggested, the patient denies it. This indicates the inability to handle the anxiety that would otherwise be released if the person admitted the psychic conflicts being repressed. The need for this defense should be respected.

Some individuals respond to psychophysiological ill-

PATIENT EDUCATION PLAN
TEACHING COPING STRATEGIES

Content	Instructional activities	Evaluation
Definition of stress	List feelings that indicate stress Discuss behaviors associated with elevated stress	The patient will identify behaviors associated with stressful situations
Recognition of stressful situations	Ask patients to describe situations they have experienced as stressful Role play the situation (with videotape if possible) Discuss stress-related behaviors observed and feelings experience	The patient will correctly identify a stressful experience
Description of common life stressors	Ask for a description of one situation that produces stress Conduct discussion about common elements of stressful experiences	The patient will identify stressful aspects of life
Identification of coping mechanisms	Review the role-played stressful situations Discuss alternative ways to cope with the stressors Role play at least one coping mechanism Provide feedback about the effectiveness of the selected coping mechanism	The patient will identify and practice alternative coping mechanisms The patient will select an appropriate coping mechanism when experiencing stress

A FAMILY SPEAKS

I worry about my husband. He drives himself so hard. I also feel guilty at times since I know he is doing it for me and the children. But I sure would like for him to slow down. Here's a good example of how things go in our house. Every year in the weeks before Christmas he works overtime to give us a little extra money. But then on Christmas Eve, without fail, his ulcer kicks up and we wind up spending part of each holiday in the hospital visiting him.

I know every family has problems and maybe ours aren't so bad. But then again maybe they are. This last Christmas our doctor recommended that we see a family therapist to discuss the situation. I want to go, but my husband says it's silly. Maybe this year for Christmas I'll ask him to give me that as my present and we'll finally have a really happy New Year. ▼

ness with *compensation*. They attempt to prove that they are actually healthy by being more active and exerting themselves physically even if told to rest. This coping style is typical of type A people, who need desperately to prove that they are in control of their bodies, not controlled by them. The opposite of this reaction is the person who uses *regression* as a coping mechanism. This individual becomes dependent and embraces the sick role to avoid responsibility and dealing with conflict.

Common to each of these coping mechanisms is the need not to confront the basic conflict that is leading to stress and anxiety. This need is so strong that premature attempts to convince the person of psychological conflicts may result in the substitution of a less adaptive coping mechanism for a more adaptive one. In extreme cases, if the person is stripped of all efforts to cope and not provided with a substitute, death can result, either from worsening of the organic disorder or from suicide.

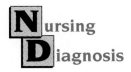

Nursing Diagnosis

The nursing diagnosis must reflect the complex biopsychosocial interaction that is the hallmark of psychophysiological disorders. The individual's effort to cope with stress-related anxiety may result in many somatic and emotional disorders. All the possible disruptions must be considered when formulating a complete nursing diagnosis.

The stress adaptation model (Fig. 15-2) may help in the diagnostic process. A thorough interview will reveal many of the predisposing factors and precipitating stressors present for the individual. The nurse must use good communication skills during the interview to enable sharing of the patient's experience as completely as possible. Areas of resistance and gaps in information should be noted as possible indicators of a conflict. These may be explored more completely as trust is established in the nurse-patient relationship. Questions related to life-style and usual activities may help identify precipitating stressors and coping behaviors. It is particularly important to elicit the patient's view of what is happening. This will provide valuable information about the patient's awareness of the relationship between mind and body. Nonverbal behaviors also give clues about the patient's concerns. Apparent lack of concern may reveal the use of denial suggestive of a conversion disorder.

As the diagnosis is formulated, the nurse must consider the individual's coping in the context of the stress response. Is the patient in a stage of alarm with many coping resources at hand? Or is the patient in the stage of resistance, using coping mechanisms but depleting personal energy resources? Has the patient reached the stage of exhaustion, needing intensive intervention to maintain life? The determination of the level of stress and coping being used influences the interventions initiated for patient care.

There are three primary nursing diagnoses for maladaptive psychophysiological responses. The first is impaired adjustment, a state in which the individual is unable to modify life-style in a manner consistent with a change in health status. The second is chronic pain, which is when an individual has pain that continues for more than 6 months. The third is sleep pattern disturbance, which is a disruption of sleep time that causes discomfort or interferes with desired life-style. Nursing diagnoses related to the range of possible maladaptive responses and related medical diagnoses are identified in the Medical and Nursing Diagnoses box on p. 365. The primary NANDA diagnoses and examples of complete nursing diagnoses are presented in the Detailed Diagnoses box on p. 366.

Related Medical Diagnoses

Medical disorders related to maladaptive psychophysiological responses are classified under the general categories of somatoform disorders, sleep disorders, and psychological factors affecting medical condition.[4] The specific medical diagnoses and their essential features that fall under each of these diagnostic classes in the DSM-IV are also described in the Detailed Diagnoses box.

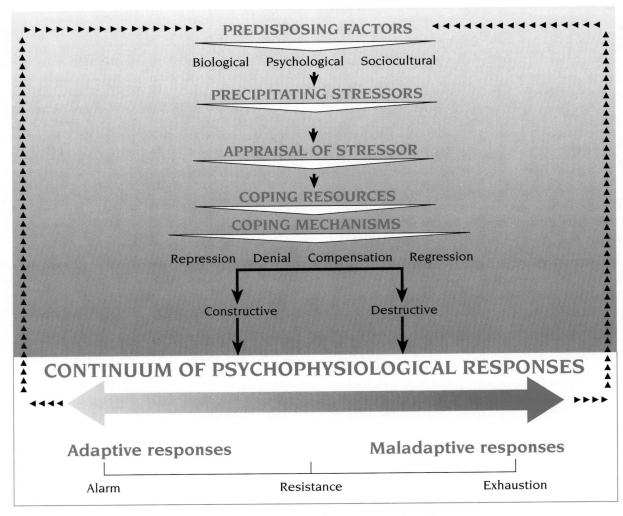

Fig. 15-2   A stress adaptation model related to psychophysiological responses.

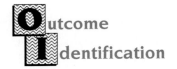
Outcome Identification

The expected outcome when working with a patient with maladaptive psychophysiological responses is:

The patient will express feelings verbally rather than through the development of physical symptoms.

This is a long-term goal, and some may never reach it. However, an increased level of self-awareness is beneficial and should be achievable to some extent by all patients. An improved ability to deal with conflict will reduce the patient's need to use repression and denial. This in turn will decrease stress and allow the patient to function with fewer episodes of physical illness. In addition, specific goals can also be set addressing problems related to pain and sleep.

The establishment of mutual goals with these patients is often a problem. The patient's primary goal is to ease the physical symptoms of the illness, often through medical or surgical treatment. Exploration of psychological conflicts is likely to be seen as unnecessary. This resistance is related to the need to maintain defenses against the extreme anxiety that has led to the illness. The nurse must identify common treatment goals. The nurse also wants the patient to obtain relief from physical symptoms. Many patients will receive medical or surgical treatment and related nursing care. At the same time, the nurse should try to build a trusting relationship so that the patient can begin to feel safe in exploring interpersonal conflicts and feelings.

Significant others must also be considered in developing the plan of care. It is important to explore their understanding of the patient's problem. They can be valuable allies in encouraging the patient to make a lifestyle change, if this is necessary. At the same time, the nurse must recognize that a change in one family mem-

MEDICAL AND NURSING DIAGNOSES RELATED TO PSYCHOPHYSIOLOGICAL ILLNESS

Related Medical Diagnoses (DSM-IV)*

Somatization disorder
Conversion disorder
Hypochondriasis
Body dysmorphic disorder
Pain disorder
Primary insomnia
Primary hypersomnia
Narcolepsy
Breathing—related sleep disorder
Circadian, rhythm sleep disorder
Psychological factors affecting medical conditions

Related Nursing Diagnoses (NANDA)†

‡Adjustment, impaired
Anxiety
Body image disturbance
Constipation
Coping, ineffective individual
Denial, ineffective
Diarrhea
Diversional activity deficit
Family processes, altered
Fear
Gas exchange, impaired
Health maintenance, altered
Hopelessness
Mobility, impaired physical
Nutrition, altered: less than body requirements
‡Pain, chronic
Powerlessness
Self-care deficits
Self-esteem, chronic low
Self-esteem disturbance
Self-esteem, situational low
Skin integrity, impaired
‡Sleep pattern disturbance
Social interaction, impaired
Social isolation
Spiritual distress

*From American Psychiatric Association: *Diagnostic and statistical manual of mental disorders*, ed 4, Washington, DC, 1994, The Association.
†From North American Nursing Diagnosis Association: NANDA *nursing diagnoses: definitions and classifications* 1992-1993, Philadelphia, 1992, The Association.
‡Primary nursing diagnosis for maladaptive psychophysiological responses.

ber requires a change in all the others. The family may be active participants in the patient's maladaptive behavioral style. In this case, goals should include addressing the family relationships with the patient.

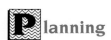

Planning

Care plans for these patients may be lengthy. The nurse must attend to all the patient's biopsychosocial needs. Most patients, while having needs in all areas, have their most urgent needs in a limited area of functioning. Physical disorders are usually disabling and may be life threatening. Psychosocial problems will hinder recovery from the physical illness and so must also be given immediate attention.

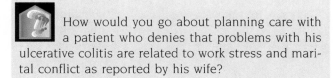

How would you go about planning care with a patient who denies that problems with his ulcerative colitis are related to work stress and marital conflict as reported by his wife?

 # Implementation

Patients with psychophysiological illnesses are most frequently seen in general hospital and outpatient settings. They usually seek health care because of symptoms related to physiological functioning. Only after a thorough medical examination can the role of psychosocial stressors in the disorder be evaluated. In some

DETAILED DIAGNOSES
RELATED TO PSYCHOPHYSIOLOGICAL RESPONSES

NANDA Diagnosis Stem	Examples of Complete Diagnosis
Impaired adjustment	Impaired adjustment related to fear of assuming adult responsibilities evidenced by multiple somatic complaints.
	Impaired adjustment related to inability to express hostile and competitive feelings evidenced by labile hypertension.
Chronic pain	Chronic pain related to marital conflict evidenced by back problems and protected gait.
	Chronic pain related to work pressures evidenced by reports of headaches and facial mask.
Sleep pattern disturbance	Sleep pattern disturbance related to financial and familial concerns evidenced by difficulty falling asleep and frequent awakening during the night.

DSM-IV Diagnosis	Essential Features*
Somatization disorder	A history of many physical complaints beginning before the age of 30, occurring over a period of several years, and resulting in treatment being sought or significant impairment in social or occupational functioning. The patient must display at least four pain symptoms, two gastrointestinal symptoms, one sexual symptom, and one symptom suggesting a neurological disorder.
Conversion disorder	One or more symptoms or deficits affecting voluntary motor or sensory function suggesting a neurological or general medical condition. Psychological factors are judged to be associated with the symptom or deficit because the initiation or exacerbation of the symptom or deficit is preceded by conflicts or other stressors. The symptom or deficit cannot be fully explained by a neurological or general medical condition and is not a culturally sanctioned behavior or experience.
Hypochondriasis	Preoccupation with fears of having, or ideas that one has, a serious disease based on the person's misinterpretation of bodily symptoms. The preoccupation persists despite appropriate medical evaluation and reassurance and has existed for at least 6 months. It causes clinically significant distress or impairment in functioning.
Body dysmorphic disorder	Preoccupation with an imagined or exaggerated defect in appearance that causes clinically significant distress or impairment in functioning.
Pain disorder	Pain in one or more anatomical sites is the predominant focus of the clinical presentation. It is of sufficient severity to warrant clinical attention and causes clinically significant distress or impairment in functioning. Psychological factors are judged to have an important role in the onset, severity, exacerbation, or maintenance of the pain.
Primary insomnia	Difficulty initiating or maintaining sleep, or nonrestorative sleep, for at least 1 month that causes clinically significant distress or impairment in functioning.
Primary hypersomnia	Excessive sleepiness for at least 1 month as evidence by either prolonged sleep episodes or daytime sleep episodes occurring almost daily that causes clinically significant distress or impairment in functioning.
Narcolepsy	Irresistible attacks of refreshing sleep occurring daily over at least 3 months with cataplexy (brief episodes of sudden bilateral loss of muscle tone) and hallucinations or sleep paralysis at the beginning or end of sleep episodes.
Breathing-related sleep disorder	Sleep disruption leading to excessive sleepiness or insomnia judged to be due to sleep apnea or central alveolar hypoventilation syndrome.
Circadian rhythm sleep disorder	Persistent or recurrent pattern of sleep disruption leading to excessive sleepiness or insomnia that is due to a mismatch between the sleep-wake schedule required by a person's environment and one's circadian sleep-wake pattern that causes clinically significant distress or impairment in functioning.
Psychological factors affecting medical condition	Presence of a medical condition in which psychological factors influence its cause, interfere with its treatment, constitute additional health risks for the individual, or elicit stress-related physiological responses that precipitate or exacerbate its symptoms.

*Adapted from American Psychiatric Association: *Diagnostic and statistical manual of mental disorders*, ed 4, Washington, DC, 1994, The Association.

cases a pathophysiological disruption requires physical nursing intervention. If the physical condition is life threatening, this intervention is given highest priority. For instance, a person with a bleeding ulcer needs intensive care to maintain life. However, once the physical crisis is past, the nurse can assist the patient in avoiding similar problems in the future.

Physical illnesses with psychosocial etiologies require psychiatric nursing approaches. Skilled and compassionate nursing care directed to the patient's physical needs is the first step in establishing the trusting relationship. A person who is in pain, bleeding, or covered with a rash is unable to discuss emotions or interpersonal relationships. The cardinal principle for patients with psychophysical disorders is to assess the patient's stress level and, whenever possible, act to reduce it. Stress and anxiety are at the root of the patient's problem. The nurse must care for immediate needs before addressing less obvious ones.

Psychological Approaches

The psychophysiological symptom defends the person from overwhelming anxiety. It provides some patients with a way to receive help and nurturance without admitting the need for it. Others are protected from expressing frightening aggressive or sexual impulses. Recognizing the defensive nature of the symptom, the nurse should never try to convince the patient that the problem is entirely psychological. Likewise, the attitude that the patient only needs to get life under control to get better is not therapeutic. The patient has not made a conscious choice to be hypertensive or to develop a conversion disorder. The dilemma of these disorders is that the patient consciously would like nothing more than to be cured but is unconsciously unable to give up the symptom. Conscious recognition of the psychological role of the symptom defeats its purpose and is therefore vigorously resisted. An example of this resistance is illustrated in the following clinical example.

CLINICAL EXAMPLE

Ms. W was a 20-year-old woman who was admitted to the general hospital with a history of sudden onset of blindness. There was no evidence of any pathophysiological process affecting her eyes. Assessment revealed that she had witnessed her father's suicide by gunshot at the age of 5, although she claimed to have no memory of this. Her boyfriend had recently been expressing suicidal thoughts to her.

It appeared that the blindness was a conversion reaction. To confirm the diagnosis, the physician decided to interview Ms. W while she was sedated with amobarbital sodium. The interview was videotaped. During the interview, Ms. W was able to see. She read the day's menu and told the time by looking at a clock across the room. She also described the incident with her father. However, when the sedation wore off, Ms. W was again blind. The decision was made to show her the videotape so that she would recognize the psychogenic nature of her blindness. As she watched the tape, she did indeed regain the ability to see. However, when it reached the part in which she described her father's suicide, she became deaf.

Selected Nursing Diagnoses:
▼ Ineffective denial related to early life events as evidenced by symptoms affecting sight and hearing
▼ Impaired social interaction related to boyfriend's depressive thoughts as evidence by development of physical symptoms

It is not unusual for a person with a conversion disorder to substitute another symptom if the original one is taken away. This happens because the basic conflict remains. The ego still needs to be defended from experiencing repressed anxiety. The patient really needs assistance in dealing with the conflict. When this is resolved, the symptom will disappear because there is no longer a need for it.

Great skill is needed to intervene therapeutically with patients with maladaptive psychophysiological responses. Psychological approaches include supportive therapy, insight therapy, group therapy, cognitive behavioral strategies, stress reduction, relaxation training, and psychopharmacology. The nurse should be supportive and available to talk with the patient and provide physical care (see A Patient Speaks).

The process of insight-oriented therapy for patients with psychophysiological disorders requires that the patient's underlying feelings be recognized and confronted supportively. As the patient becomes aware of anger, appropriate expression of it may be difficult. The nurse should accept the patient's attempts to express anger as healthy and provide feedback. Sometimes patients in this phase of therapy are labeled as hostile or demanding and avoided by nursing staff. This only reinforces their conviction that angry feelings are unacceptable.

The next step in therapy is to identify and explore the patient's defenses. The therapist proceeds very carefully, helping the patient discover and test new, more adaptive coping mechanisms as the dysfunctional ones are given up. The nurse can help by supporting the patient in using new behaviors. Spending time with the patient and appreciating the patient's positive qualities will help the patient build self-esteem and confidence. The

A PATIENT SPEAKS

All I want to do is to feel better. My husband tells me that I make up all these complaints, but who would want to be sick? It isn't any fun missing out on family and church events because you don't feel good. It isn't fun going to bed with a headache and waking up with back pain day after day after day. On the other hand, my doctors tell me that they can't find anything wrong. Now where does that leave me?

Right now I'm working with a nurse who is helping me to learn new habits that may help my physical condition. She has taught me how I can relax myself when I am tense and in pain. She has suggested some activities that I can start doing right now and is also reviewing with me situations and events that seem to trigger my physical problems. Will it help? I don't know, since we're just starting out, but I do know that she is at least one person that I can talk to and who supports me in my fight to feel like my old self again. ▼

---

nurse should be alert to signs of increased anxiety and report these immediately. The physical disorder may worsen if the therapy moves too rapidly. The therapist may decide to recommend changes in the environment to assist the patient in functioning more comfortable. If the patient must consider a job change or another change in life-style, the nurse can offer time to talk about alternatives.

Patients may also need help in explaining life-style change or changes in themselves to significant others. The family is a system, and a change in one component of the system requires adjustment in the other parts. For instance, a man who was very involved in his job and out several nights a week agreed to limit himself to 8-hour work days. This affected the rest of the family. Although his wife had protested for years that he spent too much time away from home, in reality she built her life around his schedule. She spent several evenings a week in other activities. If he were to be at home every evening, she would have to reevaluate her activities and decide whether she should go out or be with him. These are not easy decisions for family members to make.

It is important that any underlying feelings of resentment be revealed and discussed to prevent indirect expression, which would create a new stressor for the patient. Family therapy may be necessary if family members have been supporting the patient's disorder. For instance, families sometimes become adjusted to having a dependent member and unwittingly sabotage efforts to foster independence. Since

---

Box 15-2

SLEEP HYGIENE STRATEGIES

▼ Set a regular bedtime and wake-up time 7 days a week.

▼ Exercise daily to aid sleep initiation and maintenance; however, vigorous exercise too close to bedtime may make falling asleep difficult.

▼ Schedule time to wind down and relax before bed.

▼ Avoid worrying when trying to fall asleep.

▼ Guard against nighttime interruptions. Earplugs may help with a noisy partner. Heavy window shades help to screen out light. Create a comfortable bed.

▼ Maintain a cool temperature in the room. A warm bath or warm drink before bed helps some people fall asleep.

▼ Excessive hunger or fullness may interfere with sleep. Avoid large meals before bed. If hungry, a light carbohydrate snack may be helpful.

▼ Avoid caffeinated drinks, excessive fluid intake, stimulating drugs, and excessive alcohol in the evening and before bed.

▼ Excessive napping may make it difficult for some people to fall asleep at night.

▼ Do not eat, read, work, or watch television in bed. The bed and bedroom should be used only for sleep and sex.

▼ Maintain a reasonable weight. Excessive weight may result in daytime fatigue and sleep apnea.

▼ Get out of bed and engage in other activities if not able to fall asleep.

---

social support systems may help patients cope with their illnesses, the nurse may need to look for alternatives when the family is not supportive. Self-help groups often provide the needed social support. Group interventions have also been found to be helpful in decreasing overuse of health-care services by patients with somatoform disorders.[11]

Nurses must be aware that countertransference frequently occurs with these patients (see Chapter 2). It is easy to become impatient with a demanding patient who is not acutely ill when sicker patients also need nursing care. Reacting to this behavior by avoidance or anger only adds to the patient's anxiety and makes the situation worse. Clinical supervision by an experienced psychiatric nurse is highly recommended for nurses who work with these difficult patients. Frequent nursing care conferences are also helpful. If possible, a limited number of staff members should be assigned to the care of these patients. This fosters the development of a trusting relationship.

NURSING CARE PLAN SUMMARY
Maladaptive Psychophysiological Responses

Nursing Diagnosis: Impaired adjustment

Expected Outcome: The patient will express feelings verbally rather than through the development of physical symptoms.

Short-Term Goals	Interventions	Rationale
The patient will identify areas of stress and conflict and relate feelings, thoughts, and behaviors to them.	Assist patient in identifying stressful situations by reviewing events surrounding the development of physical symptoms. Facilitate the association among cognitions, feelings, and behaviors.	Inability to deal with intrapsychic conflict leads to anxiety and stress resulting in physiological dysfunction.
The patient will describe present defenses and evaluate whether they are adaptive or maladaptive.	Proceed slowly in analyzing defenses. Explore alternative coping behaviors with the patient.	Defenses should not be attacked; rather the nurse should support the positive exploration of the patient and suggest alternative responses.
The patient will adopt two new coping mechanisms to deal with stress.	Give patient positive feedback for new adaptive behaviors. Actively support patient in testing new coping mechanisms. Enlist the support of family and significant others to reinforce change.	Change requires time and positive reinforcement from others. Family members can be particularly important in promoting adaptive responses.
The patient will display a decrease in physical symptoms and greater biological integrity.	Teach the patient relaxation training. Encourage physical activity to reduce stress. Counsel the patient on diet and nutrition needs. Review the patient's sleep habits and promote good sleep hygiene practices.	Wellness requires a balance between biological and psychosocial needs. Interventions focused on the patient's physiological needs can help the patient restore biological integrity.

Patient Education

Health education is important in caring for the patient with a psychophysiological disorder. The patient with an organic pathologic condition usually needs instruction about medications, treatments, and life-style changes. The patient and family will need information about follow-up care and crisis management (see Chapter 12). In addition, patients should be offered education about ways to cope with anxiety and stress, as described in Chapter 14. Group classes on stress management may be productive. They may enable patients to share experiences and make suggestions to each other about coping behaviors. Former patients who have made successful life adjustments can also be effective teachers of coping strategies.

Do you think that patients with maladaptive psychophysiological responses will be more or less likely to comply with their treatment plan? How might you enhance their adherence?

Physiological Support

A variety of physiological treatments can also be implemented by the nurse. Relaxation training as described in Chapter 28 can be very helpful in promoting adaptive psychophysiological responses. Encouraging physical activity is also a positive way of promoting stress reduction. Ideally, it should be an activity that the patient enjoys and can share with others. Diet counseling may be helpful in building the person's resistance to stress and illness. Patients under stress should not over-use dietary stimulants, such as caffeine. They may need education about the elements of a healthful diet and help in planning balanced meals. A patient who has been relying on alcohol or drugs to cope with stress should be encouraged to find more adaptive coping mechanisms (see Chapter 22).

Finally the effective treatment of sleep disorders requires that the underlying cause of the sleep problem be identified. Drugs and alcohol frequently produce fragmented sleep, as do caffeinated beverages. Poor sleep hygiene habits may also be a problem, and the patient can be encouraged to engage in good sleep hygiene strategies (Box 15-2). Sedative medications can also be used to help induce sleep, but these drugs should be used for only a limited time because of the risk of dependence (see Chapter 25).

The Nursing Care Plan Summary for patients with maladaptive psychophysiological responses is presented on p. 369.

Evaluation

The evaluation of the nursing care of the patient with psychophysiological illness is based on the identified patient care goals. If goal achievement is not attained, the nurse must ask the following questions:

▼ Was the assessment complete enough to correctly identify the problem?

▼ Did the patient agree with the goal?

▼ Was enough time allowed for goal achievement?

▼ Was I skilled enough to carry out the desired intervention?

▼ Were there environmental constraints that affected goal accomplishment?

▼ Did additional stressors change the patient's ability to cope?

▼ Was the goal achievable for this patient?

▼ What alternative approaches should be tried?

It is very important that neither the patient nor the nurse interpret the lack of goal achievement as a failure. The nurse should try to look at it as a challenge and convey that attitude to the patient. It is not at all helpful to add failure to achieve a goal to the patient's collection of stressors. The care of these patients is exceedingly complex. The nurse may expect to modify the treatment

plan several times before finding a successful approach. The most important thing is to keep trying and to encourage the patient to persist in the effort to find health.

SUGGESTED CROSS-REFERENCES

SUMMARY

1. The continuum of possible psychophysiological responses to stress based on Selye's theory include the stages of alarm, resistance, and exhaustion.

2. Patient behaviors related to psychophysiological responses include physical conditions affected by psychological factors, psychological symptoms such as somatization, conversion, body dysmorphic and pain disorders, hypochondriasis, and sleep problems.

3. Predisposing factors are described from biological, psychological, and sociocultural perspectives. Precipitating stressors include any experience the individual interprets as stressful.

4. A variety of coping mechanisms are used in psychophysiological response such as repression, denial, compensation, and regression.

5. Primary NANDA nursing diagnoses for psychophysiological responses are impaired adjustment, chronic pain, and sleep pattern disturbance.

6. Primary DSM-IV diagnoses are categorized as somatoform disorders, sleep disorders, and psychological factors affecting medical condition.

7. The expected outcome of nursing care is that the patient will express feelings verbally rather than through the development of physical symptoms.

8. Interventions include psychological approaches, patient education, and physiological support.

9. The care of these patients is complex, and the nurse may expect to modify the treatment plan several times before finding a successful approach.

COMPETENT CARING
A CLINICAL EXEMPLAR OF A PSYCHIATRIC NURSE

Audrey Joseph, MSN, RN

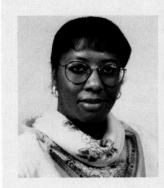

Often it is difficult for health-care professionals to communicate with their patients concerning psychosomatic illness. Also, the patient's denial or rejection of this diagnosis does not make this communication process any easier. Psychiatric staff and family members can get caught in the middle when primary care physicians fail to tell their patients that they need a psychiatric evaluation to rule out a psychosomatic illness. I know this from an experience I had that taught me much about psychiatric care.

I was working the evening shift as a staff nurse on an inpatient unit when Mrs. O, an elderly woman, presented herself on the unit for voluntary admission. She was well dressed and quite cheerful. Her medical history revealed that she had visited her family doctor and the emergency room weekly for the last 2 months. She had many diagnostic studies, the results of which were all negative. Mrs. O reported that she was referred by her family doctor for a diagnostic workup. A psychosocial assessment revealed that her husband had recently died and that she lived alone. The patient was allowed to become acclimated to the unit. Three days after admission, the staff explained to her why she was admitted. She became angry and left against medical advice.

About 3 weeks later Mrs. O's son arranged for her to be readmitted because she was constantly going to the emergency room and to her family doctor. She was angry with her son for having her admitted. To keep her in the hospital he told her that he would have her committed if it were necessary. Mrs. O on this admission was neatly dressed but looked tired. Her chief complaint was choking and a general infection throughout her body that was causing a vaginal discharge. Her family doctor still did not tell her that he could not find anything physically wrong with her. She was started on a regimen of antidepressant medication. During the 2 weeks she was in the hospital, she spent most of her time socializing with other patients. She was not interested in psychotherapy and did not develop a therapeutic alliance with the staff.

On her third admission, approximately 2 months later, Mrs. O's family doctor still had not told her that he thought she had a psychosomatic illness. At this time she was disheveled and looked physically ill. Mr. O spent most of the day in bed. She constantly complained of choking and a vaginal discharge. She admitted that she stopped taking the antidepressant medication right after discharge from the hospital. At this point she was angry with all her children and thought they were all against her. She could not understand why they would not accept the fact that she was physically ill. After 3 weeks of treatment Mrs. O was discharged home. Two years later I met Mrs. O in another psychiatric hospital where she was again admitted for treatment.

Clearly this is not a success story. In fact it taught me much about the problems of nonintegrated physical and psychiatric systems of care in which patients are treated as "parts" rather than "wholes." I also realized that I shared responsibility for not providing better care for Mr. O. To this day, she is often in my thoughts, and I now advocate for treating patients broadly within the context of their worldview rather than within the narrow realm our society defines as medical care. ▼

REFERENCES

1. Abbey S, Garfinkle P: Chronic fatigue syndrome and the psychiatrist, *Can J Psychiatry* 35:625, 1990.
2. Abbey S, Garfinkle P: Neurasthenia and chronic fatigue syndrome: the role of culture in the making of a diagnosis, *Am J Psychiatry* 148:1638, 1991.
3. Alexander F: *Psychosomatic medicine: its principles and application*, New York, 1950, WW Norton.
4. American Psychiatric Association: *Diagnostic and statistical manual*, ed 4, IV. Washington, DC, 1994, The Association
5. Bachman D: Sleep disorders with aging: evaluation and treatment, *Geriatrics* 47:53, 1992.
6. Barsky AJ: Somatoform disorders. In Kaplan HI, Sadock BJ, eds: *Comprehensive textbook of psychiatry*, ed 3, Baltimore, 1989, Williams & Wilkins.
7. Becker P, Jamieson A: Common sleep disorders in the elderly: diagnosis and treatment, *Geriatrics* 47:41, 1992.
8. Benca R, Obermeyer W, Thisted R, Gillin C: Sleep and psychiatric disorders, *Arch Gen Psychiatry* 49:651, 1992.
9. Cannon WB: *Bodily changes in pain, hunger, fear, and rage*, New York, 1929, Appleton-Century-Crofts.
10. Cassileth B, Drossman D: Psychosocial factors in gastrointestinal illness, *Psychother Psychosom* 59:131, 1993.
11. Corbin LJ et al: Somatoform disorders: how to reduce overutilization of health care services, *J Psychosoc Nurs Ment Health Serv* 26:31, 1988.
12. Dunbar F: *Psychosomatic diagnosis*, New York, 1943, Hoeber.
13. Fava G: The concept of psychosomatic disorder, *Psychother Psychosomatics* 58:1, 1992.
14. Friedman H: *The self-healing personality: why some people achieve health while others succumb to illness*, New York, 1991, Holt.
15. Friedman H, ed: *Hostility, coping, and health*, Washington, DC, 1992, American Psychological Association.
16. Johns M: A new method for measuring daytime sleepiness: the Epworth sleepiness scale, *Sleep* 14:540, 1991.
17. Lilie J, Lahmeyer H: Psychiatric management of sleep disorders, *Psychiatr Med* 9:245, 1991.
18. Mindell J: Sleep disorders in children, *Health Psychol* 12:151, 1993.
19. Nofzinger E, Buysse D, Reynolds C, Kupfer D: Sleep disorders related to another mental disorder: a DSM-IV literature review, *J Clin Psychiatry* 54:244, 1993.
20. Oken D: Current theoretical concepts in psychosomatic medicine. In Kaplan HI, Sadock BJ, eds: *Comprehensive textbook of psychiatry*, ed 5, Baltimore, 1989, Williams & Wilkins.
21. Parsons T: *The social system*, New York, 1951, The Free Press.
22. Plotnikoff N: *Stress and immunity*, Boca Raton, Fla, 1991, CRC Press.
23. Regestein Q, Monk T: Is the poor sleep of shift workers a disorder? *Am J Psychiatry* 148:1487, 1991.
24. Report of the Therapeutics and Technology Assessment Subcommittee of the American Academy of Neurology, *Neurology* 42:269, 1992.
25. Saravay S et al: Psychological comorbidity and length of stay in the general hospital, *Am J Psychiatry* 148:324, 1991.
26. Selye H: *The stress of life*, New York, 1956, McGraw-Hill.
27. Siegel BS: *Love, medicine, and miracles*, New York, 1986, Harper & Row.
28. Starck P, McGovern J, eds: *The hidden dimension of illness: human suffering*, New York, 1993, National League for Nursing.
29. Ware N, Kleinman A: Culture and somatic experience: the social course of illness in neurasthenia and chronic fatigue syndrome, *Psychosom Med* 54:546, 1992.
30. Wolf S et al: *Life stress and essential hypertension*, Baltimore, 1955, Williams & Wilkins.

ANNOTATED SUGGESTED READINGS

Becker P, Jamieson A: Common sleep disorders in the elderly: diagnosis and treatment, *Geriatrics* 47:41, 1992.
Reviews normal changes in sleep, sleep disorders, and treatment strategies for the elderly.
Cousins N: *Anatomy of an illness*, New York, 1979, WW Norton.
Account of the author's participation in own recovery from a potentially fatal illness through use of a stress management approach.
*Dossey B et al: *Holistic nursing: a handbook for practice*, Rockville, Md, 1988, Aspen Publishers.
Describes the holistic and healing traditions within nursing with clear descriptions on the use of relaxation, imagery, and music therapy.
Friedman H, VandenBos G: Disease-prone and self-healing personalities, *Hosp Community Psychiatry* 43:1177, 1992.
Excellent overview of knowledge to date about the effects of personality traits on physical health.
*Lewis MC: Attribution and illness, *J Psychosoc Nurs Ment Health Serv* 26:14, 1988.
Application of concepts of attribution related to the cause of illness in a study of patients with inflammatory bowel disease.
Lilie J, Lahmeyer H: Psychiatric management of sleep disorders, *Psychiatr Med* 9:245, 1991.
Excellent summary of basic sleep physiology and the characteristics and management of sleep disorders.
Lynch JJ: *The language of the heart*, New York, 1985, Basic Books, Inc.
Author's observations of patients who suffer from psychophysiological disorders and approaches to their treatment. Describes his partnership with a clinical nurse specialist who carries out much of the intervention.
Mindell J: Sleep disorders in children, *Health Psychol* 12:151, 1993.
Reviews sleep disorders experienced by children and presents future directions for research in this field.
Selye H: *The stress of life*, New York, 1956, McGraw-Hill.
Classic work setting forth the description of the stress response.
Sontag S: *Illness as metaphor*, New York, 1977, Vintage Books.
Small but thought-provoking book that uses the examples of tuberculosis and cancer to demonstrate the many meanings attributed to illness.
*Starck P, McGovern J (eds): *The hidden dimension of illness: human suffering*, New York, 1993, National League for Nursing Press.
Powerful book about the meaning and purpose of human suffering

---

*Nursing reference.

from the physical, psychological, sociological, and spiritiual perspective. Should be required reading for all health-care professionals.

Sullivan M: Integrated treatment of a woman with chronic hand pain, Hosp Community Psychiatry 42:474, 1991.

Case report of the integrated biopsychosocial treatment of a patient with chronic pain that included physical therapy, psychotherapy, pharmacotherapy, and vocational advocacy.

Tamm M: Models of health and disease, Br J Med Psychol 66:213, 1993.

Describes and analyzes six models of health and disease, five of which are holistic. Suggests that doctors, nurses, and patients look at health from partly different models.

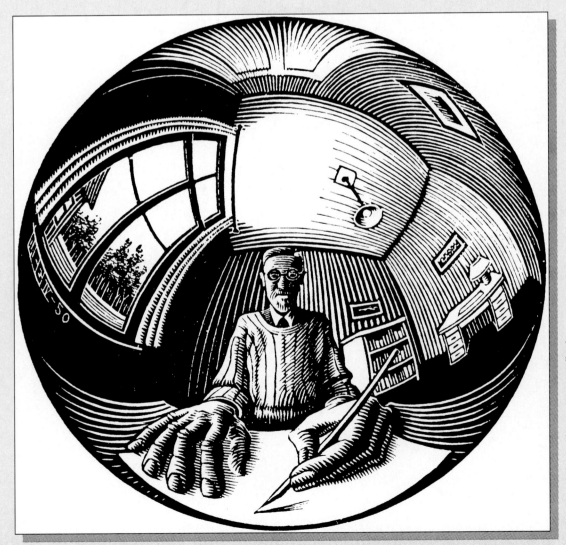

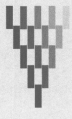

C H A P T E R   1 6
Self-Concept Responses and Dissociative Disorders

GAIL W. STUART

To venture causes anxiety, but not to venture, is to lose one's self. And to venture in the highest sense is precisely to be conscious of one's self.

Soren Kierkegaard

LEARNING OBJECTIVES

After studying this chapter the student should be able to:

▼ Describe the continuum of adaptive and maladaptive self-concept responses

▼ Identify behaviors associated with self-concept responses

▼ Analyze predisposing factors and precipitating stressors related to self-concept responses

▼ Describe coping resources and coping mechanisms related to self-concept responses

▼ Formulate nursing diagnoses for patients related to their self-concept responses

▼ Assess the relationship between nursing diagnoses and medical diagnoses related to self-concept responses

▼ Identify expected outcomes and short-term nursing goals for patients related to self-concept responses

▼ Develop a patient education plan to promote patients' adaptive self-concept responses

▼ Analyze nursing interventions for patients related to their self-concept responses

▼ Evaluate nursing care for patients related to their self-concept responses

TOPICAL OUTLINE

Continuum of Self-concept Responses
    Self-concept
    Body Image
    Self-ideal
    Self-esteem
    Role Performance
    Personal Identity
    Healthy Personality
Assessment
    Behaviors
    Predisposing Factors
    Precipitating Stressors
    Coping Resources
    Coping Mechanisms
Nursing Diagnosis
    Related Medical Diagnoses
Outcome Identification
Planning
Implementation
    Level 1—Expanded Self-awareness
    Level 2—Self-exploration
    Level 3—Self-evaluation
    Level 4—Realistic Planning
    Level 5—Commitment to Action
Evaluation

Of all human attributes, the self appears to be the most complex and most intangible. The concept of self is not clearly defined, has various meanings, and is used in many different ways. The self is the most real aspect of one's experience, however, and it is the frame of reference through which a person perceives, conceives, and evaluates one's world. **Self-concept** can be defined as all the notions, beliefs, and convictions that constitute an individual's self-knowledge and that influence relationships with others. It includes the individual's perceptions of personal characteristics and abilities, interactions with other people and the environment, values associated with experiences and objects, and goals and ideals.

Helping professionals of all backgrounds have increasingly come to view the self-concept as a critical and central element for the understanding of people and their behavior, and it is now the subject of an enormous body of theory and research. This inquiry has given rise to a theoretical school known as "self theory," which is based on the principle that human behavior is always meaningful and that individuals react to the world in terms of the way they perceive it. No two people have identical self-concepts. The self-concept emerges or is learned through each person's internal experiences, relationships with other people, and interactions with the outer world. Because it is the frame of reference through which the person interacts with the world, it is a powerful influence on human behavior. Self theorists believe it is impossible to understand a person fully or to predict behavior accurately without understanding the person's internal frame of reference. This involves sharing the person's perceptual world and view of the self. Thus understanding a patient's self-concept is a necessary component of all nursing care.

CONTINUUM OF SELF-CONCEPT RESPONSES

Self-concept

Developmental Influences. Although theories of self-concept development vary considerably, most theorists agree that the self-concept does not exist at birth. The self develops gradually as the infant recognizes and distinguishes others and begins to gain a sense of differentiation from others. The boundaries of the self are defined as the result of exploratory activity and experience with the person's own body. At first self-differentiation is slow, but with the development of language it accelerates. Language helps to clarify the concept of the self, and the child's own name is a major linguistic aid. The use of a proper name helps with the identification and perception of being an individual—someone special, unique, and independent. In general, language allows clear distinctions to be made between the self and the

rest of the world and the ability to symbolize and understand experiences. Once the infant has begun this process of differentiation from other people and the environment, the continued process of self-concept development is greatly benefited by the following:

▼ Interpersonal and cultural experiences that generate positive feelings and a sense of worth
▼ Perceived competence in areas valued by the individual and society
▼ Self-actualization, or the implementation and realization of a person's true potential

SIGNIFICANT OTHERS. The self-concept is learned in part through accumulated social contacts and experiences with other people. Sullivan[26] called this development "learning about self from the mirror of other people." What a person believes about himself is a function of his interpretation of how others see him, as inferred from their behavior toward him. His concept of self therefore rests partly on what he thinks others think of him. "Significant others" in the life of a child particularly affect the development of self-concept, and for a young child the most significant others are his parents who help him grow and react to his experiences. The family provides the individual with his earliest experiences of:

1. Feelings of adequacy or inadequacy
2. Feelings of acceptance or rejection
3. Opportunities for identification
4. Expectancies concerning acceptable goals, values, and behaviors

Research indicates that parental influence is strongest during early childhood and continues to have a significant impact through adolescence and young adulthood. Over time, however, the power and influence of friends and other adults increase, and they become significant others to the individual. Parents and immediate family members therefore are crucial to the initial development of the self-concept, and continuing development and change in self-perceptions are influenced by countless experiences with many other people.

Culture and socialization practices also affect self-concept and personality development. The dominant cultural patterns of the individual's environment give important clues to the sources of personality formation. General cultural patterns as well as cultural subdivisions, such as social class membership, have formative influences on the individual's view of self.

 What sociocultural factors had an impact on your self-concept as you were growing up? Which ones currently influence your self-concept?

SELF-PERCEPTIONS. A person's view of himself is not exclusively a collection of the views, expectations, and desires of others. Each person can observe his own behavior the same way that others do and form opinions about himself. One's perception of reality is selective, however, according to whether the experience is consistent with one's current concept of self. The way a person behaves is a result of how one perceives the situation, and it is not the event itself that elicits a specific response but rather the individual's subjective experience of the event. An individual's needs, values, and beliefs strongly influence perceptions. One more readily perceives that which is meaningful and consistent with present needs and personal values. Similarly, people behave in a manner consistent with what they believe to be true. In this case, a fact is not what is but what one believes to be true. Once perceptions are acquired and incorporated into one's self-system, they can be difficult to change. Ways exist to change perceptions, however, including modification of cognitive processes, exposure to drugs, sensory deprivation, and biochemical changes within the body.

As the self-concept develops, it brings a unique perspective of one's relationship with the world. A person with a weak or negative self-concept and who is unsure of himself is likely to have narrowed or distorted perceptions. Because he feels easily threatened, his anxiety level will rise quickly and he will become preoccupied with defending himself. In contrast, a person with a strong or positive self-concept can explore his world openly and honestly because he has a background of acceptance and success. Positive self-concepts result from positive experiences leading to perceived competence.

In conclusion, self-concept is a critical and central variable in human behavior. Individuals with positive self-concepts function more effectively. In contrast, negative self-concept is correlated with personal and social maladjustment. Fig. 16-1 describes the continuum of self-concept responses from the most adaptive state

of self-actualization to the most maladaptive response of depersonalization.

Because one's self-concept pervades every aspect of life, therapeutic interventions related to self-concept are a core element in psychiatric nursing. This requires an understanding of various components of the self, including body image, self-ideal, self-esteem, role, and identity, which are now briefly discussed.

Body Image

The concept of one's body is central to the concept of self. The body can be thought of as a capsule in which one is permanently enclosed and through which one interacts with the world. One lives with his body 24 hours a day from birth until death. It is the most material and visible part of the self, and, although it alone never accounts for one's entire sense of self, it remains a life-long anchor for self-awareness. An individual's attitude toward his body may mirror important aspects of his identity. A person's feelings that his body is big or small, attractive or unattractive, or weak or strong also reveal something about his self-concept. Numerous research studies have documented the close positive relationship between self-concept and body image. This association appears to exist both within American society and across other cultures.[5]

Body image can be defined as the sum of the conscious and unconscious attitudes the individual has toward his body. It includes present and past perceptions as well as feelings about size, function, appearance, and potential. Body image is a dynamic entity because it is continually being modified by new perceptions and experiences. It serves as a target or screen on which the person projects significant personal feelings, anxieties, and values.

Developmental Influences. One is not born with a body image. The infant receives input from his body but reacts to it in a global, undifferentiated way. As he

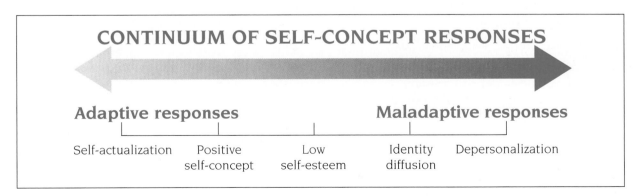

Fig. 16-1   Continuum of self-concept responses.

gradually explores parts of his body, receives sensory stimulation from others, and begins to manipulate the environment, he becomes aware of the separateness of his own body. In the development of body awareness, the external body, that is, the body that can be seen and felt, is easier to learn about and is discovered earlier than the inner body. This recognition grows out of pleasurable and painful experiences. Actually, pain becomes the dominant learning experience because pain sensory endings are distributed over the total surface of the body, whereas sensations of pleasure are concentrated in a few erotic zones. For the preschooler, the exploration of genitals and the discovery of anatomical differences between the sexes become especially important. The body occupies a middle position between the external world and the self as the agent of one's perceiving, thinking, and acting. The body can be viewed more externally and objectively than one's inner tensions, thoughts, and feelings. With increasing age there is a further differentiation of the self as a body and the self as a mind that can solve problems, make decisions, and experience feelings.

During adolescence the physical self is a focus of concern more than during any other period of life, except perhaps old age. Basic physical changes force the body into the adolescent's awareness. New sensations, features, and body proportions emerge. Height, weight, and physical strength increase, and the growth of secondary sex characteristics may be troublesome or embarrassing. Physical changes at adolescence also symbolize the end of childhood; maturity is just over the horizon. Adult proportions begin to emerge, but it is impossible to be certain of the nature, extent, or duration of changes still to come.

Early adulthood brings some stability to body change. For the healthy adult, the body experience is a moment-to-moment, highly flexible aspect of one's daily life pattern. The emerging adult needs to retain awareness of direct body sensation and blend it into all aspects of life. Many parts of one's body experience must become automatic responses, such as walking and breathing. Other aspects of the body experience must emerge as flexibly adjusted pleasures, such as eating, orgasm, and exercise.

Middle age brings new challenges as different body parts age at different rates. The individual realizes one's body is not functioning as well as it previously had. The later years of life accelerate the decline in physical abilities and can severely influence one's life-style and self-concept. As one's body image develops, extensions of the body become important, and anything that extends the effectiveness or control of one's body function can be called one's own. Clothes become identified closely with the body, and in the same way toys, tools, and possessions serve as extensions of the body and help to

widen one's sense of self. Still later, position and wealth serve similar functions.

When the individual values one's body and acts to preserve and protect it, the body image becomes the basis through which the bodies and possessions of others are also valued. Body image, appearance, and positive self-concept are related. Studies indicate that the more a person accepts and likes his body, the more secure and free from anxiety he feels. It has also been shown that people who accept their bodies are more likely to manifest high self-esteem than people who dislike their bodies.[14,16] Thus the concept of body image is a central one to understanding self theory, and the relationship between the two will have implications for developing and implementing nursing care. Problems related to body image are discussed in Chapter 23.

 What does it mean when one says that "a child lives in his body but an adult lives in his mind?"

Self-ideal

The **self-ideal** is the individual's perception of how one should behave based on certain personal standards. The standard may be either a carefully constructed image of the type of person one would like to be or merely a number of aspirations, goals, or values that one would like to achieve. The self-ideal creates self-expectations based in part on society's norms to which the person tries to conform. Formation of the self-ideal begins in childhood and is influenced by significant others who place certain demands or expectations on the child. With time, the child internalizes these expectations, and they form the basis of his own self-ideal. New self-ideals that may persist throughout life are taken on during adolescence, formed from identification with parents, teachers, and peers. In old age additional adjustments must be made that reflect diminishing physical strength and changing roles and responsibilities.

Various factors influence self-ideal. First, a person tends to set goals within a range determined by abilities. One does not ordinarily set a goal that is accomplished without any effort or that is entirely beyond one's abilities. Self-ideals are also influenced by cultural factors as the person compares his self-standards with those of peers. Other influencing factors include one's ambitions and the desire to excel and succeed, the need to be realistic, the desire to avoid failure, and feelings of anxiety and inferiority. Based on these factors, one's self-ideal may be clear and realistic and thus facilitate personal growth and relations with others, or it may be vague, unrealistic, and demanding. The adequately functioning individual, however, demonstrates congruence between one's perception of self and self-ideal. That is, he sees himself as being very similar to the person he wants to be.

In summary, self-ideals are important in maintaining mental health and balance. They serve as internal regulators and help a person maintain an even course in the face of conflicting or confusing circumstances. For mental health the self-ideal must neither be too high and demanding nor too vague and shadowy, yet it must be high enough to give continuous support to self-respect.

Self-esteem

Self-esteem is the individual's personal judgment of his own worth obtained by analyzing how well his behavior conforms to his self-ideal. The frequency with which his goals are achieved will directly result in feelings of superiority (high self-esteem) or inferiority (low self-esteem) (Fig. 16-2). If a person is repeatedly successful, he tends to feel superior, but if he fails to live up to his expectations, he feels inferior. High self-esteem is a feeling rooted in unconditional acceptance of self, despite mistakes, defeats, and failures, as an innately worthy and important being. It involves accepting complete responsibility for one's own life.

Self-esteem is derived from two primary sources: the self and others. It is first a function of being loved and of gaining the respect of others. Self-esteem is lowered when love is lost and when one fails to receive approval from others. Conversely, it is raised when love is regained and when one is applauded and praised. The origins of self-esteem can be traced to childhood and are based on acceptance, praise, and respect.[24] Coopersmith[9] described the four best ways to promote a child's self-esteem:

1. Providing him with success
2. Instilling ideals
3. Encouraging his aspirations
4. Helping him build defenses against attacks to his self-perceptions

These should provide the child with a feeling of significance, or success in being accepted and approved of by others; a feeling of competence, or an ability to cope effectively with life; and a feeling of power, or control over one's own destiny.

Self-esteem increases with age and is most threatened during adolescence, when concepts of self are being modified and many self-decisions need to be made. The adolescent has to choose an occupation and decide if he is good enough to succeed in a given career. He has to decide whether he is able to participate or is accepted in various social activities.

With adulthood the self-concept stabilizes, and maturity provides a clearer picture of self. The adult tends to be more self-accepting and less idealistic than the adolescent. He has learned to cope with many of his self-deficiencies and to maximize his self-strengths. Not all adults attain maturity; some continue to function as adolescents for many of their adult years.

In later life, self-esteem problems again arise because of the new challenges posed by menopause, retirement, loss of spouse, and physical disability. The impact of aging on self-esteem is also affected by the status of older people in American society. Being old in a society that values youth often leads to an assignment of low status and prejudicial attitudes toward old age and the

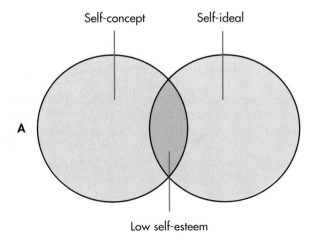

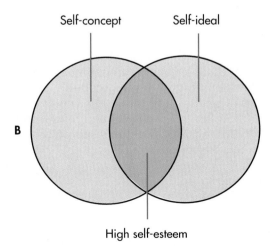

Fig. 16-2 **A,** Individual with a low level of self-esteem caused by a large discrepancy between self-concept and self-ideal. **B,** Person with a greater conformity of self-concept and self-ideal and therefore a person with a high level of self-esteem.

From Sundeen SJ et al: *Nurse-client interaction: implementing the nursing process,* ed 5, St Louis, 1993, Mosby.

aged themselves. The negative stereotypes of the elderly and the stigmatization that result can decrease self-esteem. Two other potential negative factors are the decreased social interaction of the elderly and the loss of control the elderly have over their environment, both of which can result in fewer opportunities for the elderly to validate and confirm their self-concepts.[27]

Research shows a clear relationship between self-reported physical health and self-esteem.[4] The report of a health problem, regardless of its type or severity, is associated with significantly lower self-esteem than is the report of no health problem. In contrast, high self-esteem has similarly been correlated with low anxiety, effective group functioning, and acceptance of others.[6] It is a prerequisite to self-actualization; once self-esteem is achieved, the individual is free to concentrate on achieving one's potential.

 Why do you think low self-esteem is associated with poor interpersonal relations and depressive states?

Role Performance

Roles are sets of socially expected behavior patterns associated with an individual's functioning in various social groups. Identity emerges from self-concept and is evident as role behavior. The individual assumes various roles that he attempts to integrate into one functional pattern. Because these roles overlap, an understanding of the person requires the nurse to see him in the context of the several roles he occupies. On the basis of his perception of role adequacy in the most "ego-involved" roles, the individual develops a level of self-esteem. High self-esteem results from roles that meet needs and are congruent with one's self-ideal. Many factors, including the following, influence an individual's adjustment to the role he occupies:

▼ The clarity of the behaviors appropriate to the role and his knowledge of specific role expectations
▼ The consistency of the response of significant others to his role
▼ The compatibility and complementarity of various roles
▼ The congruency of cultural norms and his own expectations for role behavior
▼ The separation of situations that would create incompatible role behaviors

Sex roles affect one's performance in other roles. They are particularly significant to family roles but permeate most others as well and are frequently the cause

of role conflict or disturbance. Another difficult problem faced by the individual growing up is that of emancipation from one's parents and establishment of an independent life. This primarily occurs during adolescence and early adulthood, when great ambiguity in role definitions occurs. The social roles of child and adolescent make it difficult to prepare oneself for adulthood. The child is not expected to be responsible; the adult is. The child is expected to be submissive; the adult dominant. The child is expected to be asexual; the adult is expected to be sexually mature and maintain intimate sexual relationships. However, few transitions or "rites of passage" exist to help the adolescent shift his role behavior. A final crisis is faced during old age, when role behavior must again be changed by aging parents. They rely on their children yet strive to balance their lives with a sense of independence and a high level of self-esteem. Role behavior is intimately related to self-concept and identity, and role disturbances frequently involve conflicts between independent and dependent functioning.

Personal Identity

The word identity is derived from the Latin root *idem*, meaning the same. It is the organizing principle of the personality. **Identity** is the awareness of "being oneself," as derived from self-observation and judgment. It is the synthesis of all self-representations into an organized whole and is not associated with any one accomplishment, object, attribute, or role.

Identity is different from self-concept in that it refers to a feeling of distinctness from others. It implies consciousness of oneself as an individual with a definite place in the general scheme of things. The person with a sense of identity feels integrated, not diffuse. When a person acts in accordance with his self-concept, his sense of identity is reinforced; when he acts in ways contrary to his self-concept, he experiences anxiety and apprehension. The person with a strong sense of identity sees himself as a unique individual.

Identity combines many conscious and unconscious elements. It connotes autonomy based on understanding of and confidence in self. In this sense autonomy arises from feelings of self-respect, competency, and mastery over one's destiny. Autonomy implies self-acceptance with a tendency toward self-assertion and self-expansion.

Developmental Influences. The concept of ego identity was developed by Erikson[12] and built within his formulation of the eight stages of human development. For each stage, Erikson describes a "psychosocial crisis" that must be resolved for further growth and personality development. Chapter 11 describes these developmental stages over the life span.

In adolescence the crisis of "identity versus identity diffusion" occurs. At no other phase of life are the promise of finding oneself and the threat of losing oneself so closely aligned. The adolescent's task is one of self-definition as he strives to integrate previous roles into a unique and reasonably consistent sense of self.

Important in achieving identity is the issue of sexuality, the image of oneself as a male or a female and convictions about what that implies. "What does it feel like to be a girl?" "Do I like being a boy?" The answers to these questions are built up gradually from infancy as the result of learned conceptions about males and females. Society's ideals of masculinity and femininity provide important standards for judging oneself as good, bad, inferior, superior, desirable, or undesirable. These ideals are passed down from generation to generation and become an important part of the culture that transmits expectations to males and females. If males are defined as superior, this idea becomes part of the self-image of both males and females. If passivity and obedience are feminine ideals in a society, most little girls will be taught to be unassertive and obedient.

In addition, much of one's identity is expressed in relationships with others. How a person relates to other people is a central personality characteristic. This presents a paradox in that everyone is a part of humanity yet each person is also separate from all others. Achieving identity is both the precursor to and the prerequisite for establishing an intimate interpersonal relationship. Research has shown that only after a stable sense of identity has been established can one engage in genuinely intimate, mature, and successful relationships.

Healthy Personality

It is possible to describe the healthy personality according to developmental theory and the dynamics of the self. This description may help give perspective to the many aspects of self previously discussed. An individual with a healthy personality would experience the characteristics listed in Table 16-1. An individual with these qualities is able to perceive himself and his world accurately. His insight into himself creates a feeling of harmony and inner peace.

 How do you compare with the qualities of a healthy personality listed in Table 16-1?

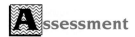

Assessment

Behaviors

Assessing the various components of a patient's self-concept will present a challenge to the nurse. Because self-concept is the cornerstone of the personality, it is intimately related to states of anxiety and depression, problems in relationships, acting out, and self-destructive behavior. All behavior is motivated by a desire to enhance, maintain, or defend the self; thus the nurse will have extensive information to evaluate. However, the nurse must delve beyond objective and observable behaviors to the patient's subjective and internal world. Only when the nurse explores this area will the patient's actions be given meaning.

The nurse can begin the assessment by observing the patient's appearance. Posture, cleanliness, makeup, and clothing provide data. The nurse might discuss the patient's appearance with him to determine his values related to body image. Observing or inquiring about his eating, sleeping, and hygiene patterns gives clues to his biological habits and tendencies toward self-care.

These initial observations should lead the nurse to ask, "What does my patient think about himself as a person?" The nurse might ask the patient to describe himself or how he feels about himself. What strengths does he think he has? What areas of weakness? What is his self-ideal? Does he conform to it? Does fulfillment of his self-ideal bring him satisfaction? Does he value his strengths? Does he view his weaknesses as important personality deficits, or are they relatively unimportant to his self-concept? What are his priorities? Is he a participant in life or an observer? Does he feel unified and self-directed or diffuse and other directed?

The nurse can then compare the patient's responses to his behavior, looking for inconsistencies or contradictions. How does he relate to other people? How does he respond to compliments and criticisms? The nurse can also examine one's own affective response to the patient. Is it one of hopelessness, despair, anger, or anxiety? The nurse's own response to the patient is often a good indication of the quality and depth of the patient's pain.

Associated with Low Self-esteem. Low self-esteem is a major problem for many people and can be expressed in moderate and severe levels of anxiety. It involves negative self-evaluations and is associated with feelings of being weak, helpless, hopeless, frightened, vulnerable, fragile, incomplete, worthless, and inadequate. Low self-esteem is a major component of depression, which acts as a form of punishment and anesthesia for the individual. Low self-esteem indicates self-

Table 16-1   Qualities of the Healthy Personality

Characteristic	Definition	Description
Positive and accurate body image	Body image is the sum of the conscious and unconscious attitudes the individual has toward one's body. It includes present and past perceptions, as well as feelings about size, function, appearance, and potential.	A healthy body awareness would be based on self-observation and appropriate concern for one's physical well-being.
Realistic self-ideal	Self-ideal is the individual's perception of how one should behave or the standard by which behavior is appraised.	An individual with a realistic self-ideal would have attainable life goals that are valuable and worth striving for.
Positive self-concept	Self-concept consists of all the aspects of the individual of which one is aware. It includes all self-perceptions that direct and influence behavior.	A positive self-concept implies that the individual expects to be successful in life. It includes the acceptance of the negative aspects of the self as part of the individual's personality. Such a person does not fear rejection, feels secure and accepted, faces life openly and realistically, and affirms his own existence.
High self-esteem	Self-esteem is the individual's personal judgment of his own worth, which is obtained by analyzing how well he matches up to his own standards and how well his performance compares with others. It evolves through a comparison of the individual's self-ideal and self-concept.	A person with high self-esteem views oneself as someone worthy of respect and dignity. He believes in his own self-worth and approaches life with aggressiveness and zest. The individual with a healthy personality is one who sees himself as very similar to the person he wants to be.
Satisfying role performance	Roles are sets of socially expected behavior patterns associated with an individual's functioning in various social groups.	The individual with a healthy personality can relate to others intimately and receives gratification from social and personal roles. Through open and honest communication he can trust others and enter into mutual and interdependent relationships.
Clear sense of identity	Identity is the integration of inner and outer demands in the individual's discovery of who one is and what one can become. It is the realization of personal consistency.	The person with a clear sense of identity experiences a unity of personality and perceives himself to be a unique individual. His "sense of self" gives his life direction and purpose.

rejection and self-hate, which may be a conscious or unconscious process expressed in direct or indirect ways.

Direct expressions of self-hate or low self-esteem may include any of the following:

1. **Self-criticism.** The patient has negative thinking and believes he is doomed to failure. Although the expressed purpose of the criticism may be self-improvement, there is no constructive value to it and the underlying goals is to demoralize oneself. This occurs when the individual places himself in a situation he cannot handle and then subjects himself to ridicule. He might describe himself as "stupid," "no good," or a "born loser." He views the normal stressors of life as impossible barriers and becomes preoccupied with self-pity.

2. **Self-diminution.** The minimizing of one's ability by avoiding, neglecting, or refusing to recognize one's real assets and strengths.

3. **Guilt and worrying.** Destructive activities by which the individual punishes himself. They may be expressed through nightmares, phobias, obsessions, or the reliving of painful memories and indiscretions. They indicate self-rejection.

4. **Physical manifestations.** These might include hypertension, psychosomatic illnesses, and the abuse of various substances, such as alcohol, drugs, tobacco, or food.

Box 16-1

BEHAVIORS ASSOCIATED WITH LOW SELF-ESTEEM

Criticism of self or others
Decreased productivity
Destructiveness toward others
Disruptions in relatedness
Exaggerated sense of self-importance
Feelings of inadequacy
Guilt
Irritability or excessive anger
Negative feelings about one's body
Perceived role strain

Pessimistic view of life
Physical complaints
Polarizing view of life
Rejection of personal capabilities
Self-destructiveness
Self-diminution
Social withdrawal
Substance abuse
Withdrawal from reality
Worrying

---

5. **Postponing decisions.** A high level of ambivalence or procrastination produces an increased sense of insecurity.

6. **Denying oneself pleasure.** The self-rejecting person feels the need to punish himself and expresses this through denying himself the things he finds desirable or pleasurable. This might be a career opportunity, a material object, or a desired relationship.

7. **Disturbed relationships.** The person may be cruel, demeaning, or exploitive with other people. This may be an overt or a passive-dependent pattern of relating, which indirectly exploits others. Another behavior included in this category is withdrawal or social isolation, which arises from feelings of worthlessness.

8. **Withdrawal from reality.** When anxiety resulting from self-rejection reaches severe or panic levels, the individual may dissociate and experience hallucinations, delusions, and feelings of suspicion, jealousy, or paranoia. Such withdrawal from reality may be a temporary coping mechanism or a long-term pattern indicating a profound problem of identity confusion.

9. **Self-destructiveness.** Self-hatred can be expressed through accident proneness or attempting dangerous feats. Extremely low levels of self-esteem can lead to the ultimate act of rejection, suicide.

10. **Other destructiveness.** People who have overwhelming consciences may choose to act out against society. This activity serves to paralyze their own self-hate and displaces or projects it on victims in their environment.

Indirect forms of self-hate complement and supplement the direct forms. They may be chronic patterns and difficult to change in therapy:

1. **Illusions and unrealistic goals.** Self-deception is the core element; the individual refuses to accept a limited here and now. Illusions increase the possibility of disappointment and further self-hate. The illusions or goals frequently involve money, love, power, prestige, marriage, sex, children, family, success, and parenthood. Examples of illusions are "If I were married, I would be happy" and "Money brings fulfillment." This indirect form of low self-esteem may make the person sensitive to criticism or overresponsive to flattery. It may also be evident in the defensive mechanisms of blaming others for one's failures and becoming hypercritical to create the illusion of superiority.

2. **Exaggerated sense of self.** The individual may also attempt to compensate by expressing an exaggerated opinion of his ability. He may continually boast, brag of his prowess and exploits, or claim possession of extraordinary talents. An extreme compensatory behavior for low esteem is grandiose thinking and related delusions. Another example is evident in the perfectionist. Such individuals strain toward impossible goals and measure their own worth entirely in terms of productivity and accomplishment.

3. **Boredom.** This involves the rejection of one's possibilities and capabilities. The individual may neglect or reject aspects of himself that have great potential for future growth.

4. **Polarizing view of life.** In this case the individual has a simplistic view of life in which everything is worst or best, wrong or right. He tends to have a closed belief system that acts as a defense against a threatening world. Ultimately this view of life will lead to confusion, disappointment, and alienation from others.

The behaviors associated with low self-esteem are described in the clinical example that follows and are summarized in Box 16-1.

CLINICAL EXAMPLE

Mrs. G was a 66-year-old woman admitted to the psychiatric hospital with a major depressive episode. She told the admitting nurse that "things have been building up for some time now" and she had been seeing a private psychiatrist for the past 6 months who suggested she enter the hospital. Mrs. G slowly recounted an extensive medical history with numerous gastrointestinal problems. These did not, however, significantly interfere with her functioning. She had been employed in a community college as a librarian until 18 months previously when she was forced to retire. Mrs. G said she had been married for 39 years and had two grown children who were married and lived out of state. Her husband worked as an accountant but had retired a month previously. She said that since her retirement she had felt "useless and lost and closed in by their apartment." She seldom left the apartment, however, and had lost contact with many of her friends. She said she worried a great deal about their financial situation, especially now that her husband was also retired. He has repeatedly reassured her that they have sufficient funds, but she cannot stop worrying about it. She said her children called her weekly, but she thought they did this only out of duty and were not "really interested" in her or her husband. She thought that if they did love her and were concerned about her, they would never have moved out of state.

Mrs. G said that she liked her job very much and thought she was good at it. A younger woman took her place at the library, and Mrs. G was very bitter when talking about her. She said that, little by little, this woman took over duties Mrs. G was responsible for and one day even cleaned out Mrs. G's desk and took it as her own. Since her retirement, she said "things have been going downhill steadily." She said she is not a good housewife and dislikes cooking. These tasks had become even more difficult since her husband retired because he is "always underfoot and criticizing what I do." In the past couple of weeks, she had had great difficulty sleeping, a decreased appetite, fatigue, and little interest in her personal appearance. She said it seemed that all she had to do was "wait around to die."

Selected Nursing Diagnoses:

▼ Self-esteem disturbance related to developmental transition as evidenced by self-criticism and lack of pleasure in life
▼ Altered role performance related to retirement as evidenced by feeling useless and failing to complete routine activities
▼ Social isolation related to low self-worth as evidenced by lack of contact with friends

In this clinical example, Mrs. G's favorable perception of self was closely related to her ability to work. Her retirement created role changes difficult to adapt to. This example points out the close relationship between feelings of low self-esteem and role strain. The situation was further compounded by her husband's retirement. Mrs. G's feelings of low self-esteem were evident in her self-criticism, refusal to recognize her own strengths, worrying, physical complaints, reduced social contacts, and unrealistic expectations of her family. Her diagnosis of major depressive episode was based on the severity of her feelings of self-depreciation, somatic problems, saddened emotional tone, history of losses, and absence of a manic episode.

Low self-esteem is also a major element of disturbed body image. The following clinical example illustrates the effect of the loss of a body part on a person's self-concept.

CLINICAL EXAMPLE

Mrs. M was an attractive 32-year-old married woman admitted to the general hospital for a total hysterectomy. Her history was presented in a nursing care conference because she was making many demands and the head nurse noticed that many of the staff were avoiding caring for her. Mrs. M had been married for 2 years and did not have any children. It was observed that Mr. M seldom visited his wife, although she spoke to him over the phone daily. Mrs. M complained that she was unable to sleep at night and often rang for the nurses with apparently minor requests. She appeared to have established a relationship with one of the evening nurses who was able to describe some of Mrs. M's concerns.

Mrs. M appeared to have a severe level of anxiety about her hysterectomy. She feared the effect of the surgery on her sexual desires, attractiveness, and ability to have intercourse and respond to her husband. Without her reproductive organs she said she felt "inadequate and no longer like a woman." She said that she and her husband always planned on having children, and she wondered if her husband might leave her in the future. She also feared that having the hysterectomy would cause her to lose her beauty and youth.

When the nursing staff became aware of Mrs. M's many fears and concerns, they were better able to understand her behavior and plan nursing care. They discussed with her the physiological implications of a hysterectomy and encouraged her to verbalize her feelings. Mr. M was not aware of his wife's concerns, and the nursing staff supported open discussions between them. As the staff were able to identify Mrs. M's concerns, they realized that some of their previous avoidance behavior resulted from their own fears and discomfort. The female nurses had identified with her as a patient, and the hysterectomy, in some ways, threatened their own concepts of self, body integrity, and sexual identity.

Selected Nursing Diagnoses:
▼ Body image disturbance related to hysterectomy as evidenced by expressed fears about her attractiveness and functioning as a woman
▼ Altered family processes related to lack of ability to bear children evidenced by limited communication with husband

Associated with Identity Diffusion.

Important behaviors that relate to identity diffusion include disruptions in relationships or problems of intimacy. The initial behavior may be withdrawal or distancing. If a person is experiencing an undefined identity, he may wish to ignore or destroy those people who threaten him. The problem is one of gaining intimacy, but it is reflected in isolation, denial, and withdrawal from others. Such patients lack empathy.

A contrasting behavior that may be evident is **personality fusing.** Erikson has pointed out that true intimacy involves a sense of mutuality, which implies a firm self-delineation of the partners and not a diffused merger of two people. If a person is struggling to cope with a weak or undefined identity, however, he may try to establish his sense of self by fusing or belonging to someone else. This may occur in formal relationships, intense friendships, or brief affairs, since each can be seen as a desperate attempt to outline one's own identity. This personality fusion, however, leads to a further loss of identity. Some of these behaviors are evident in this clinical example.

 ## CLINICAL EXAMPLE

Mrs. P was seen by a psychiatric nurse in the psychiatric outpatient department of a general hospital. She was a well-dressed 24-year-old woman who had numerous somatic complaints, including decreased appetite, frequent headaches, fatigue, and difficulty falling asleep. She reported she had no energy or interest in doing anything or being with people. She said she dreaded each day and felt abandoned and all alone.

She was married at the age of 17 to the only boy she ever dated in high school. He was 19 at the time and she "looked up to him tremendously." He established a successful career in the insurance business, and she stayed at home to care for the house. She described herself as "centering my whole world around him." Three months previously he had told her that he wanted a

separation and suggested she begin making a new life for herself. He said he intended to move out of the house at the end of the present month, but Mrs. P said she hoped he would not do that when he saw how much she loved and needed him.

Mrs. P also described feelings of being unloved and unlovable. She said she "felt empty inside" and "didn't really know who she was." She complained about her appearance and expressed much fear about living alone, finding a job, and getting along with people, especially men.

Selected Nursing Diagnoses:
▼ Personal identity disturbance related to impending separation as evidenced by feelings of loneliness and abandonment
▼ Self-esteem disturbance related to doubts about self and her own abilities as evidenced by expressed fears of living alone, finding a job, and getting along with people

Many of the behaviors displayed by Mrs. P reflect the problem of identity diffusion. She married at an early age before defining her own sense of self as an autonomous individual. Her only experience in a close relationship was with her husband, and she attempted to establish her own identity by living through his. Within the security of the marriage, she managed to avoid any self-analysis, but the impending separation brought forth her fears and self-doubts. She displayed a low level of self-esteem and an unresolved conflict between dependence and independence.

Personality fusion and problems with identity also have serious implications for the larger family system. Dysfunctional families are frequently characterized by a fusion of ego mass that may be evident in severe symptomatology by one or more family members. This may be expressed in some form of family violence or abuse (see Chapter 37) or in the scapegoating of one family member, who becomes the "diagnosed" or "symptomatic" psychiatric patient (see Chapter 30).

Individuals with identity diffusion often display weak gender identity or gender confusion. They may lack an historical-cultural basis of identity and thus display a peculiar lack of ethnicity. This is evident in their sense of history, cultural norms, group affiliations, object choices, life-style, and child-rearing practices. A related behavior is the absence of a moral code or of any genuine inner value. These behaviors characteristic of identity diffusion are summarized in Box 16-2.

Associated with Depersonalization.

A more maladaptive response to problems in identity involving withdrawal from reality occurs when the individual experiences panic levels of anxiety. This panic state pro-

---

Box 16-2

BEHAVIORS ASSOCIATED WITH IDENTITY DIFFUSION

Absence of moral code
Contradictory personality traits
Exploitative interpersonal relationships
Feelings of emptiness
Fluctuating feelings about self
Gender confusion
High degree of anxiety
Inability to empathize with others
Lack of authenticity
Problems of intimacy

---

duces a blocking off of awareness, a collapse in reality testing, and feelings of depersonalization and dissociation.[1] **Depersonalization** is a feeling of unreality in which one is unable to distinguish between inner and outer stimuli. It is, in essence, a true alienation from oneself. The individual has great difficulty distinguishing self from others, and one's body has an unreal or strange quality.

Depersonalization is the subjective experience of the partial or total disruption of one's ego and the disintegration and disorganization of one's self-concept. Because of this, it is the most frightening of human experiences. It develops as an outcome of uncertainties in human relationships. The individual has a not-loved feeling and, as a result of his failure to be loved, he fails to love himself. Depersonalization serves as a defense, but it is destructive because it masks and immobilizes anxiety without diminishing its intensity. It can occur in a variety of clinical illnesses, including depression, schizophrenia, manic states, and organic brain syndromes, and it represents the advanced state of ego breakdown associated with multiple personality disorder and psychotic states.

Many behaviors are associated with depersonalization.[23] Primarily, the patient experiences feelings of estrangement as though he were hiding something from himself. He experiences a lack of inner continuity and sameness and feels as if life is happening *to* him rather than his living by his own initiative. The patient may say that the world appears queer, dreamlike, or frightening. He may experience a loss of identity and express confusion regarding his own sexuality. He may describe related feelings of insecurity, inferiority, frustration, fear, hate, shame, and a loss of self-respect and be unable to derive a sense of accomplishment from any activity.

In depersonalization there may be a loss of impulse control and an absence of feeling and emotion that is manifested in impersonality, stiffness, formality, and rigidity in social situations. The individual may become lifeless and lack spontaneity and animation. He may plod through each day in a state of numbness and may respond to situations ordinarily eliciting emotion without characteristic love, hate, anxiety, or guilt. A heightened sense of isolation may mark his interpersonal relationships. The individual may become increasingly passive, as shown by withdrawing from social contacts, failing to assert himself, losing interest in his surroundings, and allowing others to make decisions for him.

Another sign of depersonalization is a disturbance in the individual's perception of time, space, and memory. He may become disoriented and be unable to recognize events as pertaining to yesterday or tomorrow or to plan his activities with reference to a schedule. A disturbance of memory may be characterized by aphasia, amnesia, or memory distortion. His thinking and judgment may be impaired and may reflect great confusion and distortion or focus on trivial details. Problems in information processing may be evident in visual hallucinations, and disturbed interpersonal relationships may be reflected in delusions, auditory hallucinations, and incongruent or idiosyncratic communication.

Another behavior associated with depersonalization is a confused or disturbed body image. The person may have a feeling of unreality about parts of his body. He may feel that his limbs are detached or that the size of his body parts is changed, or he is unable to tell where his body leaves off and the rest of the world begins. Some patients describe the feeling that they had stepped outside their bodies and were observing themselves as detached and foreign objects.

Finally, the person may exhibit dissociative behaviors related to **multiple personality disorder**,[11,25] which is the existence of distinct and separate personalities within the same person, each of which dominates the person's attitudes, behaviors, and self-view as though no other personality existed (see A Family Speaks). Because most patients with multiple personality disorder usually conceal their condition, there are only limited periods in their lives when they show overt symptoms that can be easily diagnosed. During these times, patients with multiple personality disorder often show subtle dissociative signs in their affects, thoughts, memories, behaviors, object relations, and transferences.[13] For this reason the use of a screening tool, such as the Dissociative Experiences Scale, may be helpful in identifying patients with multiple personality disorder.[2,8] The many behaviors associated with depersonalization and dissociation are summarized in Box 16-3. The next clinical example may further clarify these behaviors.

Box 16-3

BEHAVIORS ASSOCIATED WITH DEPERSONALIZATION

AFFECTIVE

Experiences loss of identity

Feelings of alienation from self

Feelings of insecurity, inferiority, fear, shame

Feelings of unreality

Heightened sense of isolation

Lack of sense of inner continuity

Unable to derive pleasure or a sense of accomplishment

PERCEPTUAL

Auditory and visual hallucinations

Confusion regarding one's sexuality

Difficulty distinguishing self from others

Disturbed body image

Experiences the world as dreamlike

COGNITIVE

Confusion

Disoriented to time

Distorted thinking

Disturbance of memory

Impaired judgment

Presence of separate personalities within the same person

BEHAVIORAL

Blunting of affect

Emotional passivity and nonresponsiveness

Incongruent or idiosyncratic communication

Lack of spontaneity and animation

Loss of impulse control

Loss of initiative and decision-making ability

Social withdrawal

A FAMILY SPEAKS

My wife has multiple personality disorder, and it feels like I'm living with several different people. One moment everything is great and the next thing I know she is in a frenzy or a state of rage. There are other problems, too. For example, things keep appearing in our household and no one knows where they came from, or I get calls at work from my wife telling me she is lost and doesn't know how she ended up there. At other times she tells me things and later denies she said them. Sometimes, people come up to my wife and talk like they know her, but she says she's never seen them before. And then there are days when she dresses up and acts just like our teenage daughter.

What is it like to live with someone with this illness? Well, it's unreal and very upsetting. Most of all, it's like living in a world of doubt and uncertainty. Who is this woman I married 12 years ago? What is she all about? What is she capable of doing? These are the questions I ask myself each night as I fall asleep. They are the same ones that go unanswered in the early morning hours as well. ▼

CLINICAL EXAMPLE

Mr. S was a 40-year-old man with no history of psychiatric hospitalization. Two months before his present admission, he was severely burned while on the job in a steel-making plant. He received second- and third-degree burns over his face, hands, chest, and back and was treated in the burn center of a large university hos-

pital. Three days before he was to be discharged from the burn unit, he experienced a psychotic episode. He reported hearing voices telling him to kill himself, and he was unable to recall any events surrounding the accident that produced his burns. He said he "felt his arms were withering away and his eyes were falling into his skull." He was unable to change the dressing on his burns even though he had done this previously. When looking at his arms or chest, his face remained impassive and he showed no emotion. He began to talk continuously about returning to work but was unable to identify how long he had been out on sick leave or the amount of time recommended by his physician for recovery.

With the onset of these symptoms, he was transferred from the burn unit to the psychiatric unit of the hospital. He remained socially isolated on the unit and refused to participate in ward meetings and group activities. At times he would wander into other patients' rooms and take pieces of their clothing. He would later be seen wearing this clothing, and the staff would intervene to return it to its owner.

Selected Nursing Diagnoses:

▼ Panic level of anxiety related to severe burn injuries as evidenced by confusion regarding identity, hearing voices, and reported body distortions

▼ Altered thought processes related to psychotic state as evidenced by confusion and disorientation

This example and the previous discussion show that the various feelings and perceptions associated with depersonalization represent extreme defenses against threats to self that do not serve to alleviate the anxiety and may add to it because of the frightening experience. The patient views his own behavior as foreign and sees himself as a strong, unknown, and unpredictable being whom he does not recognize. As both a participant and a spectator, he observes himself with great fear, since he is unable to control his own impulses. He cannot completely escape the pain of self-awareness. He therefore disowns his behavior, feelings, thoughts, and body and becomes alienated from his true self.

Predisposing Factors

Affecting Self-esteem.

Predisposing factors that originate in early childhood can contribute to problems with self-concept. Because the infant initially views himself as an extension of his parents, he is very responsive to both his parents' self-hate and any feelings of hatred toward himself. Parental rejection causes the child to be uncertain of himself and other human relationships. As a result of his failure to be loved, the child fails to love himself and is unable to reach out with love to others.

As he grows older, the child may experience lack of recognition and appreciation by parents and significant others. He may learn to feel inadequate because he is not encouraged to be independent, to think for himself, and to take responsibility for his own needs and actions. Overpossessiveness, overpermissiveness, or overcontrol, exercised by one or both parents, can nurture a feeling of unimportance and lack of esteem in the child. Harsh, demanding parents can set unreasonable standards, often raising them before the child has developed the ability to meet them. Parents may also subject their children to unreasonable, harsh criticism and inconsistent punishment. These actions can cause early frustration, defeatism, and a destructive sense of inadequacy and inferiority. Another factor in creating such feelings may be the rivalry or unsuccessful imitation of an extremely bright sibling or of a prominent parent, often generating a sense of hopelessness and inferiority. In addition, repeated defeats and failures can destroy self-worth. In this instance the failure in itself does not produce a sense of helplessness, but internalization of the failure as proof of personal incompetency does.

UNREALISTIC SELF-IDEALS. With age, additional factors emerge that can cause and perpetuate feelings of low self-esteem. The individual who lacks a sense of meaning and purpose in life also fails to accept responsibility for his own well-being. He becomes dependent on others, self-indulgent, and fails to develop his capabilities and potential. He denies himself the freedom to full expression, including the right to make mistakes and fail, and becomes impatient, harsh, and demanding with himself. He sets standards that cannot be met. Self-consciousness and observation then turn to self-contempt and self-defeat. This results in a further loss of self-trust.

These self-ideals or goals are often silent assumptions, and the person may not be immediately aware of them. They reflect high expectations and are unrealistic in relation to one's proved capacities. When the individual judges his performance by these unreasonable and inflexible standards, he cannot live up to his ideals and, as a result, experiences guilt and low self-esteem. Horney[15] has described these inner dictates as the "tyranny of the shoulds," and some of the common ones are identified in Box 16-4.

The person who overemphasizes these rules or ideals often makes, for example, the following series of deductions: "Everyone should love me . . . If he doesn't love me, I have failed . . . I have lost the only thing that really matters . . . I am unlovable . . . There is no point in going on . . . I am worthless." This inner punishment results in feelings of depression and despair because the demands on self are those no human being could fulfill. Slavishly striving for these ideals interferes with other activities, such as living a reasonably healthy life and having satisfying relationships with other people. These predisposing factors lay the groundwork for feelings of low self-esteem.

Affecting Role Performance

SEX ROLES. An important source of strain in contemporary America comes from values, beliefs, and behaviors about sex roles. Research demonstrates that soci-

---

Box 16-4

UNREALISTIC SELF-EXPECTATIONS: THE TYRANNY OF THE SHOULDS

▼ I should have the utmost generosity, considerateness, dignity, courage, and unselfishness.

▼ I should be the perfect lover, friend, parent, teacher, student, and spouse. Everyone should love me.

▼ I should be able to endure any hardship with equanimity.

▼ I should be able to find a quick solution to every problem.

▼ I should never feel hurt; I should always be happy and serene.

▼ I should know, understand, and foresee everything. I should be competent in all ways.

▼ I should always be spontaneous; I should always control my feelings.

▼ I should assert myself; I should never hurt anybody else.

▼ I should never be tired or get sick.

▼ I should always be at peak efficiency. I should not make mistakes.

From Horney K: *Neurosis and human growth*, New York, 1950, WW Norton.

ety continues to have clearly defined sex-role stereotypes for men and women. Women are perceived as relatively less competent, less independent, less objective, and less logical then men. Men are perceived as lacking interpersonal sensitivity, warmth, and expressiveness in comparison to women. Moreover, stereotyped masculine traits are more often perceived as desirable than are stereotyped feminine characteristics.

To the extent that these results reflect societal standards of sex-role behavior, both women and men are put in role conflict by the difference in the standards. If a woman adopts behaviors desirable for a man, she risks censure for her failure to be appropriately feminine; if she adopts behaviors designated as feminine, she is deficient in the values associated with masculinity. So, too, if a man adopts the behaviors specified as desirable for a woman, his masculinity and sexuality may be questioned and his contributions may be devalued or ignored; if he adopts the behaviors associated with masculinity, he risks alienating attributes of his personality associated with warmth, tenderness, and responsiveness. Thus when a woman steps out of her home, where her sex role has traditionally been defined and confined, and enters the world of work, she may expect to experience heightened role strain. Similarly, the man who arrives home from work in the evening may feel uncertain or in conflict about how he should relate to his school-age son, infant daughter, or working wife.

Role conflict and role ambiguity arise from the biological factors and social expectations set for men and women. Role overload can also occur for the woman who has numerous, often conflicting, roles imposed on her. Thus the interaction of marriage, parenting, and employment emerges as a likely source of role strain for women.

Compare the value the American, Japanese, and Arabic cultures place on feminine and masculine roles and traits.

WORK ROLES. Work does not imply, however, a singular social role. It is possible to distinguish between women who perceive their employment as careers and those who view their work as a job. Women are still in the minority of most high-status occupations and are clustered near the bottom in terms of professional status and financial reward. A study was conducted that compared conflict experienced by career and noncareer (job) women in relationship to the roles of worker, spouse, parent, and self as a self-actualizing person. Greater role conflict was reported by the job versus career group, particularly involving the parent versus self

and spouse versus self roles. The career group reported receiving significantly more life satisfaction from both work and self roles than the job group. This and other studies suggest that work viewed as desirable, valuable, and adequately compensated can bring greater life satisfaction.

The problem appears to be the lack of support for women performing multiple roles. This lack is reflected in payment received, willingness by other family members to share family tasks, and encouragement for the woman pursuing her own goals. At present in American society, women are socialized to seek an ideal that includes marriage, children, higher education, and satisfying work outside the home. They are increasingly expected to perform in both "feminine" and "masculine" spheres.

This situation has both positive and negative aspects. First, it can be argued that it merely replaces the traditional woman's role with another equally confining one. By valuing the new role, the traditional roles of wife and mother become devalued. Second, although women are expected to assume more "masculine" qualities, a corresponding trend for men to assume more "feminine" behaviors is not apparent. Third, the woman who seeks such an expanded role is faced with reconciling the often conflicting goals of work, marriage, homemaking, and parenting. Little organized support by society exists to aid the woman, however, and thus her task can be formidable or overwhelming.

Despite social and economic changes, there is often little sharing of tasks when men and women are both gainfully employed. Rather, most industrial societies have witnessed a gradual change in the obligations of women, who now perform a double, or "dual," role—outside employment and continued responsibility for home and children. The expectation exists that the woman will make the adjustments needed both at home and in her career, including housekeeping and managing; arranging meals, lessons, and appointments; entertaining; caring for the sick; and communicating with the family. There is also the traditional expectation that the wife will be the primary caretaker of the child and will subsume other activities to this end.

One might conclude, therefore, that sex and work roles will continue as a source of stress (1) until care of children, home, and career are viewed as equally valuable and important by both sexes and (2) until gender is regarded as irrelevant to the abilities, personalities, and activities of the individuals involved. Such a change in attitude should begin with nurses and other mental health clinicians who, by accepting the stereotyped views of society, indirectly increase role strain. The cause of mental health might be better served if psychiatric clinicians encouraged both men and women to maximize individual potential rather than adjust to existing restrictive sex roles.

Affecting Personal Identity. Constant parental intervention interferes with adolescent choices. In American culture this is related to the lack of a fixed limit to parental intervention. Parental distrust leads a child to wonder whether his own choices are correct and to feel guilty if he goes against parental ideas. Parental distrust implies belittlement because it devalues the child's opinions and leads to indecisiveness, impulsiveness, and acting out in an attempt to achieve some identity. When the parent does not trust the child, the child ultimately loses respect for the parent. It has been found that parents and children do not disagree on significant issues, such as war, peace, race, or religion. Instead, personal and narrow concerns—fads, dating, a party, the car, curfews, homework—create the conflict between parents and youth. Here parental intervention interferes with options and identity.

Peers also add to the problem of identity. The adolescent wants to belong, to feel needed and wanted. The peer group, with its rigid standards of behavior, gives him this feeling and provides a bridge between childhood and adulthood. The adolescent loses himself in the fads and the language of the group. However, the group is often a cruel testing ground that hurts as much as it helps. Taught to be competitive, the young person competes with his friends, "putting them down" to bring himself up. Membership in the peer group is brought at a high price; the adolescent must surrender much of his identity to belong. Often there is open destruction of self-esteem and insistence on conformity. In sexual relationships adolescents introduce further uncertainty into their lives, which can interfere with developing a stable self-concept.

Precipitating Stressors

Trauma. Specific problems with self-concept are initiated by almost any difficult situation to which the person does not have the capacity to adjust. Specifically, emotional trauma such as sexual and psychological abuse in childhood has been reported by most patients with multiple personality disorder.[19] This abuse, especially ongoing incest and sadistic or ritualistic abuse, is considered to be a major cause of this disorder. A small percentage of patients report no abuse but have experienced a trauma they perceive as life threatening to themselves or to someone else, such as a near-drowning or witnessing a violent crime. It is believed, however, that the chronic and pervasive dissociation present in multiple personality disorder usually results from prolonged exposure to abuse rather than from an isolated instance of trauma.

Role Strain. People who experience stress associated with expected roles are said to experience role strain. Role strain is the frustration felt when the person is torn in opposite directions or feels inadequate or unsuited to enact certain roles. As a general term, role strain incorporates the concepts of role conflict, role ambiguity, and role overload described in Table 16-2.

In the course of a lifetime a person faces numerous role transitions. These transitions may require the in-

Table 16-2 Concepts Related to Role Strain

Concept	Example
Role conflict occurs when a person is subjected to two or more contradictory expectations that cannot be met simultaneously. Conflict can arise because two needs, drives, or motives are incompatible, or because an internal need, drive, or motive opposes an external demand.	Role conflict is evident in family roles. Each adult brings to marriage a set of perceived family roles greatly influenced by his or her own upbringing. Often the individuals' perceptions may be contradictory and pose problems within the marriage.
Role ambiguity appears when shared specification set for an expected role are incomplete or insufficient to tell the individual what is desired or how to do it. This confusion regarding role expectations and appropriate behavior can be very stressful.	Adolescents are pressured to play different roles by their parents, the mass media, and their peers. They are expected to "earn their own keep" but are unable to find jobs in times of high unemployment and economic inflation. They are confused by the discrepancy between the morality practiced by society and the morality they learned as a child.
Role overload occurs when a person faces a role set that is too complex. The person lacks the physical, intellectual, emotional, or economic resources to perform the necessary role. Each of the roles may be making legitimate discrete demands, but together the expectations are overwhelming and perhaps impossible.	An example is the numerous roles of the contemporary woman—wife, cook, mother, employee, chauffeur, maid, lover, and so on.

corporation of new knowledge and alterations in behavior. There are three categories of role transitions[21]:

1. Developmental
2. Situational
3. Health-illness

Developmental transitions are normative changes associated with growth. Situational transitions involve the addition or subtraction of significant others, occurring through birth or death; an example is the change from nonparental to parental status. Health-illness transitions involve moving from a well state to an illness state. Each of these role transitions can precipitate a threat to the individual's self-concept.

DEVELOPMENTAL TRANSITIONS. Various developmental stages can precipitate threats to self-identity. Adolescence is perhaps the most critical, since it is a time of upheaval, change, anxiety, and insecurity. An adult's problems of identity are simpler than those of an adolescent. Maturity stabilizes self-concept and provides a firmer picture of self. A serious threat to identity in adulthood is cultural discontinuity. This occurs when a person moves from one cultural setting to another and experiences emotional upheaval. Faced with differing cultural standards, many people have difficulty maintaining their self-esteem. In addition, problems within the social structure, such as political upheavals, economic depression, and high unemployment, can pose threats to identity.

Cultural stressors confront a person in challenging personal values: conformity versus individuality, cowardice versus bravery, winning versus losing, career versus marriage, equality versus superiority, cooperation versus competition, dependence versus independence, intelligence versus feeling. Although these values are not necessarily opposite or mutually exclusive, they raise fundamental questions that the individual must resolve. Sexual identity can also be influenced by cultural pressures, which can control both the individual's expression of sexuality and how it fits into the individual's self-esteem. Definitions of acceptable approaches to both sexes, the values placed on virility and procreation as proof of virility, definitions of suitable sex partners, and values concerning marital fidelity may all be culturally determined.

In late maturity and in old age identity problems again arise. New problems and roles result from the process of aging and from the view of the elderly held by the more youthful members of society. Menopause, retirement, and increasing physical disability are problems for which the aging person must work out adaptive responses.

HEALTH-ILLNESS TRANSITIONS. Some stressors can cause disturbances in body image and related changes in self-concept. One threat is the loss of a major body part, such as an eye, breast, or leg. Disturbances also may occur following a surgical procedure in which the relationship of body parts is disturbed. The results of the surgical intervention may be either visible, as with a colostomy or gastrostomy, or invisible, as with a hysterectomy or gallbladder removal. Changes in body size, shape, and appearance can threaten the person's self-perceptions. These changes can result from rapid weight gain or loss, a skin infection, or even plastic surgery. Threats to body image can occur from a pathological process that causes changes in the structure or function of the body, such as arthritis, multiple sclerosis, Parkinson's disease, cancer, pneumonia, and heart disease. The failure of a body part, as experienced by the paraplegic or stroke victim, is particularly difficult to integrate into one's self-perceptions. The physical changes associated with normal growth and development may pose problems, as may some potentially threatening medical or nursing procedures, such as enemas, catheterizations, suctioning, radiation therapy, dilation and curettage, and organ transplantation.

All these stressors can pose a threat to body image, with resultant changes in self-esteem and role perception. Any threat to body integrity is interpreted as a threat to self. How the individual perceives the threat determines the coping mechanism used. Factors that influence the degree of threat to body image are listed in Table 16-3.

Finally, physiological stressors may also disturb a person's sense of reality, interfere with an accurate perception of the world, and threaten ego boundaries and identity. Such stressors include oxygen deprivation, hy-

Table 16-3 Factors Influencing Self-concept Based on Health-Illness Transitions

Factor	Question
Meaning of the threat for the individual	Does it threaten the person's ideal of youth or wholeness and decrease self-esteem?
Degree to which the person's pattern of adaptation is interrupted	Does it jeopardize the person's security and self-control?
Coping capacities and resources available	What is the response of significant others, and what help is offered?
Nature of the threat, extent of change, and rate at which it occurs	Is the change that of many small adjustments over time or a great and sudden adjustment?

perventilation, biochemical imbalances, severe fatigue, and sensory and emotional isolation. Alcohol, drugs, and other toxic substances may also produce self-concept distortions. Usually these stressors produce only temporary changes.

Whether the problem in self-concept is precipitated by psychological, sociological, or physiological stressors, the critical element is the patient's perception of the threat. When assessing pertinent behaviors and formulating a nursing diagnosis, the nurse must continue to validate observations and inferences to establish a mutual, therapeutic relationship with the patient.

> The incidence of breast cancer is rising in this country. What strategies are women using to promote adaptive self-concept responses to deal with this health problem?

Coping Resources

It is important that the nurse and patient review possible coping resources. All people, no matter how disturbing their behavior, have some areas of personal strength,[7] which might include the following:

- ▼ Sports and outdoor activities
- ▼ Hobbies and crafts
- ▼ Expressive arts
- ▼ Health and self-care
- ▼ Education or training
- ▼ Work, vocation, job, or position
- ▼ Special aptitudes
- ▼ Intelligence
- ▼ Imagination and creativity
- ▼ Interpersonal relationships

When the patient's positive aspects become evident, the nurse should share them with the patient to expand the patient's self-awareness and suggest possible areas for future intervention.

Coping Mechanisms

Short-term Defenses. An identity crisis may be resolved with either short-term or long-term coping mechanisms. These are used to ward off the anxiety and uncertainty of identity confusion. Logan[20] has described the following four categories of short-term defenses:

1. Activities that provide temporary escape from the identity crisis
2. Activities that provide temporary substitute identities
3. Activities that serve temporarily to strengthen or heighten a diffuse sense of self

4. Activities that represent short-term attempts to make an identity out of meaninglessness and identity diffusion—that try to assert that the meaning of life is meaningless itself

The first category of temporary escape includes any of several activities that seem to provide intense immediate experiences. These experiences so overwhelm the senses that the issue of identity literally does not exist because the person's entire being is occupied with "right now" sensations. Examples of this might include drug experiences, loud rock concerts, fast car and motorcycle riding, some forms of hard physical labor, exercise or sports, and even obsessive television watching.

The category of temporary substitute identity is derived from being a "joiner"; the identity of a club, group, team, movement, or gang may function as a basis for self-definition. The individual temporarily adopts the group definition as his own identity in a type of devotion to the larger entity. Temporary substitute identities can also be obtained by playing a certain role within a group, such as clown, bully, or chauffeur, or by purchasing objects that are marketed with ready-made identities. Thus a certain type of cologne, make of car, or article of dress implies built-in personalities the person can adopt as his own.

The third category of defenses involves "putting oneself up against something" to feel more intensely alive. This is evident in risk taking for its own sake, which creates a feeling of heroic bravado and notoriety. Competitive activities, such as sports, academic achievement, and popularity contests, can also fit into this category. The idea is that competition and comparison with an outsider more sharply define a sense of self. Another example of this is bigotry and prejudice. By adopting a bigoted stance toward some outgroup or scapegoat, the individual can temporarily strengthen self-esteem or ego integrity.

The final category helps to explain the fads that people indulge in with such fervor and that seem so meaningless to others. The sheer force of commitment to the fads is an attempt to transform them into something meaningful.

Long-term Defenses. Any of these short-term defenses may develop into a long-term one that will be evident in maladaptive behavior. Other resolutions or long-term defenses are also possible. A positive resolution or adaptive response produces an integrated ego identity and unified self, as previously described. Another type of long-term resolution has been identified as **identity foreclosure.** This occurs when individuals adopt "ready made" the type of identity desired by others without really coming to terms with their own desires, aspirations, or potential. This is a less desirable long-term resolution, as is adopting a deviant or negative identity.

A **negative identity** is one that is at odds with the values and expectations of society. Individual autonomy is perceived as being jeopardized, or social norms may not be valued. In this case the individual then attempts to define the self in a nonprescribed or antisocial manner. The choice of a negative identity represents an attempt to retain some mastery in a situation in which a positive identity does not seem possible or desirable. The person may be saying, "I would rather be somebody bad than nobody at all." The following clinical example describes the negative identity assumed by an adolescent with a medical diagnosis of "conduct disorder—undersocialized, aggressive."

 ## CLINICAL EXAMPLE

Ken was a 17-year-old boy referred to the local community mental health center by his high school nurse. She made the referral after attending a team conference at school concerning Ken's repeated behavioral problems. He had a history of aggressive and destructive behavior in school, poor peer relationships, and low academic performance. The school had suspended him on three occasions, and the result of the team conference was to expel him for the remainder of the school year.

Mr. P, a psychiatric nurse at the mental health center, established a contract to work with Ken and his family. He noted that Ken was an obese young man (112.5 kg [250 pounds]) who took little interest in his appearance. His dress was sloppy, his complexion unclean, and his hair oily. He sat slumped in the chair in a disinterested and slightly defiant posture.

As Ken talked about himself, he complained of many pressures he experienced in his part-time job at a local hardware store. He thought the work was too difficult and tiring and that he was qualified for better and more prestigious work. When asked for specifics, he could not identify another job in particular. He also expressed a great deal of harassment from his family. His mother and father had been married for 31 years, and he was the only child of the marriage. His mother worked part-time at a bakery, and his father was recently retired from his job as a supervisor at a local utility company, where he was highly regarded.

Ken said that his father "always had things for me to do." He described how his father signed him up for various team sports—baseball, basketball, football—without acknowledging how much Ken hated sports and how uncoordinated he was. His father also stressed good grades and "the necessity of college" for success in life. Ken described his mother as passive and polite and said he had little respect for her. He said his aggressive outbursts occurred both at home and at school—whenever he was frustrated. People reacted by staying out of his way. He said he never hurt anyone with his temper. He mostly destroyed property and objects.

Ken avoided the subject of peers but, when asked about friends, said he "hung out" with a couple of boys in the neighborhood. They were older than he was. Most had dropped out of high school and were employed in odd jobs. He denied drug use but said he drank heavily, especially on the weekends. He said he had no girlfriends and "wasn't interested in complicating my life with some broad."

Selected Nursing Diagnoses:
▼ Personal identity disturbance related to fear of failure as evidenced by aggressive and destructive behavior and poor school performance
▼ Altered family processes related to conflict with parents as evidenced by avoidance and lack of communication

Ken displays many of the behaviors characteristic of a negative identity. The nurse working with Ken explored his underlying feelings and self-perceptions. Great anger with his father began to surface, and Ken was able to verbalize it. Because he was the only son, he believed he was competing with his father and had to live up to his father's ideals. Ken feared failing in trying to adopt a positive identity and resented the identity his father was trying to impose on him. He thought he had no part in defining it and that it did not represent his real self.

Ego Defense Mechanisms. Patients with alterations in self-concept may use a variety of ego-oriented mechanisms to protect themselves from confronting their own inadequacies. However maladaptive, the defenses represent attempted solutions to inner problems and perceived deficiencies. Typical ego defense mechanisms include fantasy, dissociation, isolation, projection, displacement, splitting, turning anger against the self, and acting out.

Other, more damaging compensatory mechanisms can also be used to protect the self-esteem of the individual. When self-esteem is threatened, the individual chooses a behavior that will protect it. These include a variety of behaviors that may be characteristic of individual maladjustment or social deviance including the following:

Obesity	Delinquency
Anorexia	Crime
Promiscuity	Drug use
Chronic overworking	Family violence
Suicide	Incest

These are not adaptive coping responses, but they provide the individual with an excuse for failure. They all reflect a feeling of inferiority or lack of goal accomplishment.

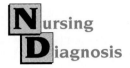

Nursing Diagnosis

Self-concept is a critical aspect of the individual's overall personality adjustment. Problems with self-concept are associated with feelings of anxiety, hostility, and guilt. These often create a circular, self-propagating process that ultimately results in maladaptive coping responses (Fig. 16-3).

Most individuals who express dissatisfaction with life, display deviant behavior, or have difficulty functioning in social or work situations have problems related to self-concept. The nature of the patient's problem, the degree of disruption, and the level of anxiety will be determined by the patient and nurse together on the basis of the behavioral or objective data the nurse has collected, as well as the patient's subjective responses and description.

The primary NANDA nursing diagnoses related to alterations in self-concept are body image disturbance; self-esteem disturbance; role performance, altered; and personal identity disturbance. Nursing diagnoses related to the range of possible maladaptive responses of the patient are identified in the Medical and Nursing Diagnoses box on p. 395.

Examples of complete nursing diagnoses related to self-concept are presented in the Detailed Diagnoses box on p. 396. However, alterations in self-concept affect all aspects of an individual's life. Therefore many additional nursing problems are expected to be identified by the nurse.

Related Medical Diagnoses

In practice, maladaptive responses indicating alterations in self-concept can be seen in a variety of people

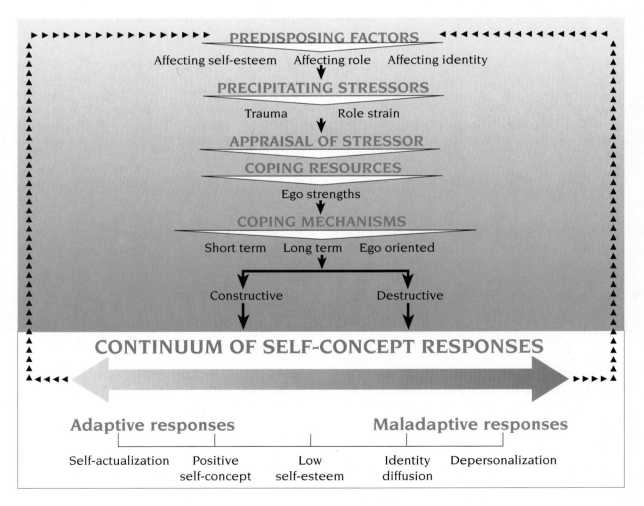

Fig. 16-3   A stress adaptation model related to self-concept responses.

experiencing threats to their physical integrity or self-system. These nursing diagnoses are not limited to the psychiatric setting and do not have a discrete category of medical diagnoses associated with them. Because they pertain to basic personality structure and feelings about oneself, they can emerge with many neurotic and psychotic disorders (see A Patient Speaks) and may be related to all the diagnostic categories identified in the DSM-IV,[3] since all these disorders ultimately reflect on one's view of self. Several specific medical diagnoses deserve particular attention, however, since their dominant features include alterations in self-concept. They are listed in the Medical and Nursing Diagnoses box below and include identity problem and dissociative identity disorder, also known as multiple personality disorder.

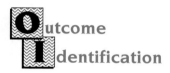

Outcome Identification

The expected outcome when working with a patient with a maladaptive self-concept response is:

The patient will obtain the maximum level of self-actualization to realize one's potential.

The nurse must move with the patient and assess the patient's readiness for growth within the therapeutic relationship. Together they formulate long-term goals that should reflect a positive resolution of the problem and of the stressor identified in the nursing diagnosis. Short-term goals should be as clear and explicit as possible. They should identify realistic steps that the patient can accomplish. In this way the patient's self-confidence will increase, and this will directly affect feelings of self-esteem. These goals should emphasize strengths instead of weaknesses. If they are mutually identified, they will serve to motivate the patient and help him assume increased responsibility for his own behavior. Following are examples of goals related to role performance:

Long-term
Mrs. P will resolve role conflict by achieving greater congruency between work and family roles.

Short-term
After 1 week:

1. Mrs. P will describe her responsibilities in both her work and home roles.
2. She will identify aspects of these roles that provide her with satisfaction.
3. She will identify areas of role incompatibility.

MEDICAL AND NURSING DIAGNOSES RELATED TO SELF-CONCEPT RESPONSES

Related Medical Diagnoses (DSM-IV)*

Identity problem
Dissociative amnesia
Dissociative fugue
Dissociative identity disorder (multiple personality disorder)
Depersonalization disorder

Related Nursing Diagnoses (NANDA)†

Adjustment, impaired
Anxiety
‡**Body image disturbance**
Communication, impaired verbal
Coping, ineffective individual
Grieving, dysfunctional
Hopelessness
‡**Personal identity disturbance**
Powerlessness
‡**Role performance, altered**
Self-care deficit
‡**Self-esteem disturbance**
Sensory-perceptual alteration
Sexuality patterns, altered
Social interaction, impaired
Social isolation
Spiritual distress
Thought processes, altered
Violence, potential for

*From American Psychiatric Association: *Diagnostic and statistical manual of mental disorders* ed 4, Washington, DC, 1994, The Association.
†From North American Nursing Diagnosis Association: NANDA *nursing diagnoses: definitions and classifications* 1992-1993, Philadelphia, 1992, The Association.
‡Primary nursing diagnosis for alterations in self-concept.

DETAILED DIAGNOSES
RELATED TO SELF-CONCEPT RESPONSES

NANDA Diagnosis Stem	Examples of Complete Diagnosis
Body image disturbance	Body image disturbance related to fear of becoming obese as evidenced by refusal to maintain body weight at normal limits
	Body image disturbance related to leukemia-chemotherapy as evidenced by negative feelings about one's body
	Body image disturbance related to cerebrovascular accident as evidenced by lack of acceptance of body limitations
Self-esteem disturbance	Self-esteem disturbance related to death of spouse as evidenced by withdrawal from others and feelings of hopelessness
	Self-esteem disturbance related to overly high self-ideals as evidenced by depressed mood and withdrawal from activities
Role performance, altered	Role performance, altered, related to incompatibility of newly assumed work and family roles as evidenced by self-criticism and feeling of inadequacy
	Role performance, altered, related to incongruency of cultural and self-role expectations about aging as evidenced by feelings of frustration and criticism of others
Personal identity disturbance	Personal identity disturbance related to unrealistic parental expectation as evidenced by running away from home
	Personal identity disturbance related to drug toxicity as evidenced by confusion and loss of impulse control.

DSM-IV Diagnosis	Essential Features*
Identity problem	Uncertainty about multiple issues relating to identity such as long-term goals, career choice, friendship patterns, sexual orientation and behavior, moral values, and group loyalties
Dissociative amnesia	The predominant disturbance is one or more episodes of inability to recall important personal information, usually of a traumatic or stressful nature, that is too extensive to be explained by ordinary forgetfulness.
Dissociative fugue	The predominant disturbance is sudden, unexpected travel away from home or one's customary place of work, with inability to recall one's past. Confusion about personal identity or assumption of a new identity.
Dissociative identity disorder (multiple personality disorder)	The presence of two or more distinct identities or personality states (each with its own relatively enduring pattern of perceiving, relating to, and thinking about the environment and self). At least two of these identities or personality states recurrently take control of the person's behavior. Inability to recall important personal information that is too extensive to be explained by ordinary forgetfulness.
Depersonalization disorder	Persistent or recurrent experiences of feeling detached from, and as if one is an outside observer of, one's mental processes or body (e.g., feeling like one is in a dream). During the depersonalization experience, reality testing remains intact. The depersonalization causes clinically significant distress or impairment in functioning.

*Adapted from The American Psychiatric Association: *Diagnostic and statistical manual of mental disorders*, ed 4, Washington, DC, 1994, The Association.

After 2 weeks:
1. She will describe three alternative ways of increasing the complementarity of the roles.
2. She will discuss the advantages and disadvantages of each alternative.

After 3 weeks:
1. She will take the necessary measures to implement one of the identified alternatives.

Following are examples of goals related to body image disturbance:

A PATIENT SPEAKS

Thoughts on Mental Illness

It came to me—so clear that I could not deny it,
the pain, the hurt, the anger—I am mentally ill.
I've tried to pretend that I'd get better
putting the hurt away—gutting out the pain
hoping it would eventually pass—yes,
eventually pass.
So I did therapy
I talked about what I had experienced,
Perceptual disturbances, they said.
I talked about what unrealness, the flatness—like card-
board.
Depersonalization, they said.
I talked about people making me nervous,
about staying to myself.
You must think rationally, do self-talk, change
your behaviors.
Take these drugs, they said
because I had heard a voice, or felt something
they had not.
I had psychotic symptoms—load her up on
Mellaril,
so what if she gets as fat as a pig—keep increasing
the dosage
Too fat? Load her up on Haldol.
But I'm not psychotic—
Oh, but you are schizo-affective, no—let's make
that borderline,
on second thought, maybe major depression
with psychotic features?
No, more like depersonalization disorder
Let's check for temporal lobe epilepsy,
what the hell, it isn't our money—why are you
complaining?
And the therapy goes on—I feel worse
The drugs don't work—
You're resistant to treatment
take some more drugs—they will help you feel
better
So I take the damn drugs—is one antidepressant any different from another? —how
much of the stuff can you take?
It doesn't do any good
how many times do I have to say that?
Why doesn't my doctor listen?
Why does she keep writing prescriptions for
more of the stuff?
Who is taking this stuff—me, or her? I should
know if it works.
I do therapy with the silicone people,
they who make no mistakes,
who are always clinically correct—always clean
nice people—but inside I am not clean.
I fear that I may be defective,
that some loose part may come undone and all will be
lost.

I'm so scared and I work overtime to find
something positive
something good to come out of all this chaos.
I don't think he understands
when I talk to my therapist I sometimes feel
cheap and shallow because I've bought the
time and I know he would not be talking to me
if I hadn't.
I feel frustrated because I've been trapped in
this sickness.
How can they feel the humiliation—the stigma
The ones so well—that they can heal?
Pain, Hurt, and Fear are subjectively private,
but even for me the loneliness is too much.
And so I ask the silicone people,
have you ever been afraid? Yes, they say.
But they don't feel the fear,
and they don't connect with the fear
But I feel it, and—I want the silicone folks to
feel it too.
I do not want to hurt by myself
I want someone to also feel the hurt
So all you silicone therapists—hear me:
to hurt when someone IS there but still is NOT,
is the worst kind of hurt of all—listen up. ▼

—Judy Mays

From South Carolina Self-Help Association Regarding Emotions: *Share the News*, Spring 1993.

Long-term

Mr. B will accept his modified body image after treatment with
chemotherapy for leukemia.

Short-term

After the first phase of chemotherapy:
1. He will identify the medications he is receiving.
2. He will describe the effect they have on his illness and
   related body systems.
3. He will express his feelings (e.g., anger, sadness) about
   his illness and therapy.
4. He will identify three positive aspects of his modified
   body image.

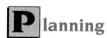lanning

Research indicates that patients with negative self-
concepts believe their illnesses have a greater negative
effect on their lives, have less hope and optimism about
the future, and are more anxious about their illnesses.
These findings support the need for effective nursing intervention related to problems with self-concept.

The nurse's focus is to help the individual understand
himself more fully and accurately so that he can direct
his own life in a more satisfying way. In a sense, nurs-

ing intervention concerns all that is involved in promoting the patient's self-realization. This means helping him strive toward a clearer, deeper experience of his feelings, wishes, and beliefs; toward a greater ability to tap his resources and use them for constructive ends; and toward a clearer perception of his direction in life, assuming responsibility for himself, his decisions, and his actions. It involves replacing repression with consciousness and unreality with reality. Sustaining, protecting, and enhancing the self results in increased self-esteem and self-acceptance. A positive therapeutic outcome results in greater self-direction, tolerance, flexibility, risk taking, and most important, a change in behavior.

Self-awareness is a crucial aspect in bringing about changes in self-concept, but people usually spend little time in introspection. Certain conditions or events, however, do stimulate self-awareness. This may occur when stimuli from the body are intensified, as in states of pain, fatigue, or anger, or when stimuli from the environment are decreased, as in sensory deprivation or states of isolation. Self-awareness may be triggered when something unexpected or extraordinary takes place, when the person has succeeded well or failed miserably, or when the person is confronted with himself by looking in a mirror, listening to his voice on a tape recorder, or reading an old letter. Special occasions, such as birthdays, anniversaries, New Year's Eve, or a death may stimulate introspection. It may also be initiated when others direct their attention to the person through conversation or touch.

Once the person begins to look at and analyze himself, changes in the self become possible. Frequently they are the result of feelings of failure, unhappiness, anxiety, inadequacy, doubt, or perceived discrepancies between one's concept of self and the demands of the environment or the expectations of others. Usually changes in the self occur only as a result of experiences and occur gradually. Occasionally, however, a change may take place suddenly. A traumatic experience may force a person to face that he is inadequate or out of step with his peers and that something drastic must be done. The nurse should take all these factors into consideration when planning nursing care.

Similarly, the family of origin is a source of many people's self-esteem. The key relationships for improving basic self-differentiation are those with parents and siblings, even in adulthood. These relationships involve the unresolved emotional fusion that influences many interactions. Adult contact with parents and siblings can correct misconceptions underlying low self-esteem and allow more positive beliefs. Learning to interact with family members with closeness, but without counterproductive forms of fusion and emotionality, can enable a more mature pattern to develop. Family relationships

would therefore be an appropriate focus for patient education. A Patient Education Plan using family systems is presented on p. 399. Chapter 30 has a more detailed discussion of family systems theory and family interventions.

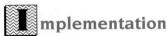

Implementation

The mutually identified goals can be reached by a problem-solving approach that focuses primarily on the present, removes much of the responsibility from the nurse, and actively engages the patient in working on personal difficulties. This approach increases the patient's self-confidence and self-esteem. It requires that the patient first develop insight into his problems and life situation and then take action to effect lasting behavioral changes. The nurse must thus incorporate both the responsive dimensions (insight oriented) and the action dimensions (action oriented) of the therapeutic relationship described in Chapter 2.

The focus of this approach is on the patient's cognitive appraisal of life, which may contain faulty perceptions, beliefs, and convictions. Awareness of feelings and emotions is also important, since they too may be subject to misconceptions. Often the patient's display of affect is a clue to significant problem areas. Only after examining the patient's cognitive appraisal of the situation and related feelings can one gain insight into the problem and bring about behavioral change. Adaptive behavior is based both on insight and on carrying out the solution to the initial problem.

There are principles of nursing care that are applicable to the various problems with self-concept. These principles are incorporated here within a problem-solving approach and are presented as progressive levels in the sequence in which they occur. They focus primarily on the level of the individual. They may, however, be implemented in conjunction with group- or family-level interventions, and the nurse is expected to include the patient's family, significant others, and community supports whenever possible. Such a mobilization of the patient's coping resources can have both preventive and curative effects.

Level 1—Expanded Self-awareness

A consistent picture of the self is necessary for security; to avoid anxiety, most people resist change. The ego resists change as a threat to its stability and integration. Furthermore, the closer a deviant perception of the self is to the core of the self-concept, the more difficult it is to change. In general, change in the self is easier when threat is absent. Threat forces a person to defend him-

PATIENT EDUCATION PLAN
FAMILY RELATIONSHIPS

Content	Instructional activities	Evaluation
Define the concept of self-differentiation within one's own family of origin	Discuss the differences between high and low levels of self-differentiation Ask the patient to identify level of functioning among own family members	Patient identifies functioning level in family of origin
Describe the characteristics of emotional fusion, emotional cutoff, and triangulation	Analyze types and patterns of family relationships Use paper and pencil to diagram family patterns	Patient describes interactional patterns within own family Patient identifies own roles and behavior
Discuss the role of symptom formation and symptom bearer in a family	Sensitize the patient to family dynamics and manifestations of stress Encourage communication with family of origin	Patient recognizes family contribution to the stress of individual members Patient contacts family members
Describe a family genogram and show how it is constructed	Use a blackboard to map out a family genogram Assign family genogram as homework	Patient obtains factual information about own family Patient constructs family genogram
Analyze need for objectivity and responsibility for changing one's own behavior and not that of others	Role-play interactions with various family members Encourage testing out new ways of interacting with family members	Patient demonstrates a higher level of differentiation in family of origin

self; perceptions are narrowed, and the person has difficulty forming new perceptions of himself (see Critical Thinking about Contemporary Issues).

To expand the patient's self-awareness and reduce the element of threat, the nurse should adopt an accepting attitude. Acceptance allows the patient the security and freedom to examine all aspects of himself as a total human being with positive and negative qualities. The basis of a therapeutic relationship will be established by listening to the patient with understanding, responding nonjudgmentally, expressing genuine interest, and conveying a sense of caring and sincerity. Creating a climate of acceptance allows previously denied experiences to be brought into consciousness and explored. This broadens the patient's concept of self and helps him to accept all aspects of his personality. It also indicates to him that he is a valued individual who is responsible for himself and is able to help himself. This is important because the nurse must work with whatever ego strength the patient possesses.

Most patients seen in clinics, the general hospital, and the community setting possess considerable ego strength. Hospitalized individuals, however, might have limited ego resources with which to work. Psychotic patients experiencing depersonalization and identity confusion often present difficult challenges for the nurse.

They tend to isolate themselves and withdraw from reality, so little ego strength is available for problem solving. For this type of patient, expanding self-awareness means first confirming the patient's identity. The nurse should attempt to provide supportive measures to decrease the panic level experienced by this patient. Additional interventions related to anxiety and psychotic states are described in Chapters 14 and 19.

The nurse can spend time with the patient in an undemanding way and approach him nonaggressively. Initially the nurse may accept the patient's need to remain nonverbal or attempt to clarify and understand his verbal communication even though it may be distorted or lack apparent logic. Attempts should be made to prevent the patient from isolating himself and establish a simple routine for him. If the patient displays bizarre behavior, such as inappropriate laughing or mannerisms, the nurse can set limits on his behavior. It is important to orient him frequently to reality and reinforce appropriate behavior.

The patient should be helped to increase the activities that provide positive experiences for him. This may involve the use of occupational therapy, recreational therapy, or activity groups because success at tasks and increased involvement with objects can increase self-esteem. Movement therapy or body ego technique pro-

CRITICAL THINKING ABOUT CONTEMPORARY ISSUES

What is the Recommended Treatment for Multiple Personality Disorder?

Reported cases of multiple personality disorder have increased dramatically in the last decade. Yet there is relatively little data on the preferred treatment of this illness. Most recommendations are made based on the experience of individual clinicians rather than on systematic research.

A recent study addressed the problem of the relative efficacy of treatment modalities currently used with patients with multiple personality disorder. The findings supported the primacy of psychotherapy and the moderate benefits of psychopharmacology with antidepressant and antianxiety agents.[22] The authors also reported that the length of treatment, frequency of treatment, and cost of treatment for this illness have major implications for the mental health care system. As a result of inadequate third-party funding and community resources, it is likely that many of these patients will be unable to obtain adequate treatment despite substantial morbidity, social impairment, and risk of continuing a cycle of abuse and violence into future generations. ▼

vides a goal-directed way to develop identity, body image, and ego structure. It is predominantly a nonverbal therapy because the emphasis is on movement and not on what the person says.

Depersonalization often leads to poor hygiene and an unkempt personal appearance. Nurses who are aware of their own value system regarding cleanliness and grooming can assist patients unable to care for themselves. They can use patience and repetition to establish health routines and can kindly but firmly encourage patients to care for themselves. Through verbal and nonverbal messages, nurses can encourage the patients to take pride in their appearance and reinforce any progress made. Another possible nursing intervention is photographic self-image confrontation. This involves taking photographs of patients and then discussing them. This intervention can provide a means for establishing a nurse-patient relationship and mutually exploring some aspects of the self.

Mutuality is often difficult to establish with a patient experiencing depersonalization. Initially the nurse will determine appropriate activities and incorporate the patient into them without asking for a response. Gradually, however, the nurse can expect greater participation and can involve the patient in decision making. Table

16-4 summarizes the nursing interventions appropriate to level 1.

Sometimes the nurse's attitudes or behaviors can block patients from expanding their self-awareness. This can be in the form of criticism, belittlement, condemnation, condescension, indifference, or insincerity. An impersonal attitude or ignoring the patient can decrease self-esteem. Excessive demands or direct challenges to self-concept can result in further withdrawal. Nurses should not allow patients to remain alone or inactive, attempt to shame them into improving their habits, or assume total care for them. If they avoid these behaviors and strive for acceptance, they remove themselves as a source of threat and encourage patients to lower their defenses. Patients are then prepared to undertake the next step in problem solving.

How do you think that the nurse's level of self-esteem affects nursing interventions in patient's self-concept responses?

Level 2—Self-exploration

At this level of intervention nurses encourage patients to examine feelings, behavior, beliefs, and thoughts, particularly in relationship to the current stressful situation. The cognitive behavioral strategies described in Chapter 28 are very useful at this time. Patients' feelings may be expressed verbally, nonverbally, symbolically, or directly. Acceptance continues to be important because when nurses accept the patients' feelings and thoughts, they are helping them to accept them as well. Nurses should facilitate the expression of strong emotions, such as anger, sadness, and guilt. In a sense, patients' emotions or affect serve as clues to inner thoughts and current behavior.

As the patient is helped to focus his attention on the meaning that experiences have for him, he is clarifying his perceptions and concept of himself and his relationship to the people and events around him. The nurse can elicit his perception of strengths and weaknesses and have him describe his self-ideal. He can be made aware of his self-criticisms. Jourard[17] has noted that many patients will experience a reduction in anxiety following the experience of full self-disclosure to an interested nurse. He believes patients withhold self-disclosure because of anxiety and the belief that no one is really interested in them.

It is important for nurses to accept and deal with their own feelings before becoming involved in the self-exploration of others. Self-awareness will limit the potential negative effects of countertransference in the re-

Table 16-4 Nursing Interventions in Alterations in Self-concept at Level 1
Goal—Expand the patient's self-awareness

Principle	Rationale	Nursing interventions
Establish an open, trusting relationship	Reduces the threat that the nurse poses to the patient and helps him to broaden and accept all aspects of his personality	Offer unconditional acceptance Listen to the patient Encourage discussion of thoughts and feelings Respond nonjudgmentally Convey to the patient that he is a valued individual who is responsible for himself and able to help himself
Work with whatever ego strength the patient possesses	Some degree of ego strength, such as the capacity for reality testing, self-control, or a degree of ego integration, is needed as a foundation for later nursing care	Identify the ego strength possessed by the patient Guidelines for the patient with limited ego resources are as follows: 1. Begin by confirming his identity 2. Provide support measures to reduce his panic level of anxiety 3. Approach him in an undemanding way 4. Accept and attempt to clarify any verbal or nonverbal communication 5. Prevent him from isolating himself 6. Establish a simple routine for him 7. Set limits on inappropriate behavior 8. Orient him to reality 9. Reinforce appropriate behavior 10. Gradually increase activities and tasks that provide positive experiences for him 11. Assist him in personal hygiene and grooming 12. Encourage the patient to care for himself
Maximize the patient's participation in the therapeutic relationship	Mutuality is necessary for the patient to assume ultimate responsibility for his own behavior and maladaptive coping responses	Gradually increase the patient's participation in decisions that affect his care Convey to the patient that he is a responsible individual

lationship. It will also allow nurses the freedom to demonstrate authentic behavior that, in turn, can be elicited and reinforced in the patient. Often patients will experience great difficulty in discussing or describing their feelings, possibly because society tends to discourage self-revelation or because some patients are honestly out of touch with their inner self. In these cases nurses can use themselves therapeutically by sharing feelings, verbalizing how they might feel in the situation, or mirroring their perception of patients' feelings. In this way nurses can help patients explore maladaptive thinking.

The nurse must be careful not to reinforce the patient's self-pity by responding with sympathy. Patients frequently deny any personal responsibility for their "plight," and they fail to see how their own behavior precipitates the problem about which they complain. Examples include patients who seek treatment because of things that happened *to* them, such as their wife left them, their husband beat them, or their boss fired them, and patients who seek help because of things that have *not* happened, such as not being happy or not having friends. These patients fail to see that they have a choice in life and that personal growth and satisfaction involve both risk and responsibility.

The nurse can clarify with the patient that he is not helpless or powerless. He is powerless when he sees himself as such and gives up control and responsibility for his behavior. Each person is responsible for his own behavior, including the things he decides to do or not to do. One must also accept responsibility for logical consequences. Only if a patient fully understands the implications of his actions and the scope of his choices can he set goals, explore alternatives, and effect change.

In stressing the importance of behavior, the nurse helps the patient see that he chooses to behave in certain ways. If the patient projects his problems onto the environment, the nurse can discuss with him the difficulty in changing other people and instead explore the possibilities of changing his own self. This means helping the patient realize that when he says, "I can't," he really means "I don't want to." The nurse should not give the impression that she has the power to change a patient's life. That power lies with the patient alone. The nurse can, however, help him to maximize his strengths, use available resources, and see that there is more to life than being involved with misery and pain.

Self-exploration need not take place solely within the one-to-one relationship. Family sessions and group meetings can help clarify how the individual appears to others.[8] These meetings can supplement the individual sessions with the patient, and similar nursing interventions can be applied within family or group therapy. Regardless of the setting, the nurse collects information on the patient's thinking about himself, logical or illogical reasoning, and reported or observed reactions. Interventions at this level should see the patient progress from denying or attributing contradictory feelings to the external situation, to recognizing a major conflict within himself (Table 16-5).

 Do you believe contemporary society encourages or discourages personal responsibility for behavior? Defend your point of view.

Level 3—Self-evaluation

This level involves hard work for the patient as he critically examines his own behavior, accepts the consequences for it, and judges whether it is the best possible choice. At this point, the problem should be clearly defined, and the patient should be helped to understand that his beliefs influence both his feelings and his behavior. Only by actively and systematically challenging his faulty beliefs and perceptions can he hope for change. Previously identified misperceptions and distortions should be evaluated. Irrational beliefs, such as the following, should be identified and analyzed:

▼ Everyone must love me.
▼ I must be competent and adequate in all ways.
▼ I am unable to control my own happiness and destiny.
▼ I should condemn myself for making mistakes.

▼ I am better off if I avoid responsibilities rather than trying to face them.
▼ I am controlled by my past and can never break free of it.
▼ If I worry about potential problems, my anxiety will prevent their occurrence.
▼ My life is a disaster if it doesn't work out exactly as I had planned.

The patient's hopelessness should be countered by exploring areas of realistic hope. It is important to point out the mature part of the patient's personality and contrast it to the childhood part that causes problems. The behaviors that interfere with effective functioning should be put in perspective; thus the patient can see that his maladaptive behavior is only a small part of his total personality.

Success and failure must be placed in perspective. Failures occur every moment of every day and are a natural consequence of human activity. As long as people strive to achieve, they will frequently not reach their goals. The only way to avoid failure is to do absolutely nothing. Failure may be caused by one's own mistakes; it may be a result of lack of motivation; or it may result from circumstances beyond one's control. Whatever the reason, failure is the unavoidable outcome of human effort. The problem arises when individuals are labeled or label themselves as failures. This is illogical and potentially destructive. As an inherent aspect of life, failure should be viewed either as a neutral concept or a positive one for the learning experience it has provided, rather than a negative one.

Unrealistic self-ideals, dependency patterns, and denial are all potential areas that can be analyzed. The patient can be helped to realize that all behavior and coping responses have positive and negative consequences. Contrasts can be drawn between behavior that is destructive, inhibitory, or sabotaging and behavior that is productive, enhancing, or growth producing. The patient must see that he acts in self-defeating ways because some "payoff" or personal gain is in it for him. The drawbacks or disadvantages to the patient's maladaptive coping responses will probably be well known to him. The payoffs, or secondary gains, may be more obscure and well repressed. Following are some frequently experienced payoffs:

▼ Procrastination
▼ Avoiding risks
▼ Retreating from the present
▼ Evading responsibility for one's actions
▼ Avoiding working or having to change

More specific payoffs should be identified by the nurse and patient together, relative to his particular problem. For example, possible secondary gains from being obese include having people feel sorry for you, having an excuse for not dating or being married, being the focus of dieting attention, or being easily recognized

Table 16-5 Nursing Interventions in Alterations in Self-concept at Level 2

Goal—Encourage the patient's self-exploration

Principle	Rationale	Nursing interventions
Assist the patient to accept his own feelings and thoughts	When nurses show interest in and accept the patient's feelings and thoughts, they are helping him to do so as well	Attend to and encourage the patient's expression of his emotions, beliefs, behavior, and thoughts—verbally, nonverbally, symbolically, or directly Use therapeutic communication skills and empathic responses Note his use of logical and illogical thinking and his reported and observed emotional responses
Help the patient to clarify his concept of self and his relationship to others through self-disclosure	Self-disclosure and understanding one's self-perceptions are prerequisites to bringing about future change; this may, in itself, produce a reduction in anxiety	Elicit his perception of self-strengths and weaknesses Assist him to describe his self-ideal Identify his self-criticisms Help him to describe how he believes he relates to other people and events
Be aware and have control of your own feelings	Self-awareness allows the nurse to model authentic behavior and limits the potential negative effects of countertransference in the relationship	Openness to and acceptance of one's own positive and negative feelings Therapeutic use of self by: 1. Sharing one's own feelings with the patient 2. Verbalizing how another might have felt 3. Mirroring one's perception of the patient's feelings
Respond empathically, not sympathetically, emphasizing that the power to change lies with the patient	Sympathy can reinforce the patient's self-pity; rather, the nurse should communicate that the patient's life situation is subject to his own control	Use empathic responses and monitor oneself for feelings of sympathy or pity Reaffirm to the patient that he is not helpless or powerless in the face of his problems Convey that the patient is responsible for his own behavior, including his choice of maladaptive or adaptive coping responses Discuss with him the scope of his choices, his areas of ego strength, and coping resources that are available Use the support systems of family and groups to facilitate the patient's self-exploration Assist the patient in recognizing the nature of his conflict and the maladaptive ways in which he tries to cope with it

and noticed when with other people. Possible secondary gains for an adult remaining dependent on his parents might include not having to make one's own decisions, having someone else to blame if things go wrong, being protected from risks and venturing out in the world, not establishing lasting intimate relationships, or not having to establish one's own identity, but rather adopting the values and goals of others. Such payoffs can be identified for each nursing diagnosis.

The nurse becomes more active at this level of intervention by confronting, interpreting, persuading, and challenging. The goal is to increase the patient's objectivity in dealing with stressors. For example, the nurse can show the patient that the negative and positive characteristics of people can be integrated. Thus the same person can nurture and gratify as well as anger and frustrate, since both negative and positive qualities coexist in the same person. In interpretation and confrontation, the nurse offers information that the patient may not have or does not recognize as relevant. Supportive confrontation may be particularly effective in calling to the patient's attention inconsistencies in words and actions. The climate of acceptance established by the nurse in level 1 and the empathic communication developed in level 2 provide a basis for confrontation in level 3. This groundwork is necessary to prevent premature confrontation, which can be destructive.

The nurse may use various aspects of role theory during this level of intervention including assisting the patient in role clarification, which is the gaining of knowledge, information, and cues needed to perform a role. It involves identification of behaviors, clarification of expectations, and specification of goals relative to the role, taking into consideration the influence of significant others and the context of the situation. The nurse can also encourage the patient to participate in any activity in which he can observe his own behavior. Role playing may be particularly effective in providing the patient with feedback and increasing his insight. Through it, he may be able to gain objectivity toward the irrationality and self-destructiveness of his self-criticisms.

The nurse-patient relationship provides a rich source of information for the patient. Within this relationship he is enacting and experiencing many of his problem areas, and the nurse can use this as a "study in miniature." The nurse can assist the patient in observing how he reacts in the one-to-one situation and share reactions with him to give him feedback on how he affects others and openly disclose some of her own feelings about the patient's behavior. The analysis and use of transference and countertransference reactions constitute the nurse's "therapeutic use of self." When a block arises within the relationship or anxiety is increased, the nurse should explore its meaning with the patient. The nurse should confront the problem and openly discuss it with him. This can also be done in family or group therapy sessions.

During this level of intervention the patient and nurse critically evaluate the patient's behavior (Table 16-6). Misperceptions, unrealistic goals, and distortions of reality are explored. This provides the patient with sufficient knowledge to progress to the next level of problem solving.

 Think of one of your less desirable habits. What payoff or personal gain does it provide you?

Level 4—Realistic Planning

The nurse and patient are now ready to formulate possible solutions or alternatives. This begins by investigating what solutions were attempted in the past and evaluating their effectiveness. When inconsistent perceptions are held by the individual, he is faced with several choices. He can change his perceptions and beliefs to bring them closer to a reality that cannot be changed. Alternately, he may seek to change his environment to bring it in line with what he believes. When his behavior is not consistent with his self-concept, he can change his behavior, change the beliefs underlying his self-concept so that they include his behavior, or change his self-ideal while leaving his self-concept intact.

At this time, all possible solutions should be openly discussed with the patient. Nurses must be careful not to use their influence to persuade the patient to do anything that represents their values rather than the patient's. The nurse should help him conceptualize his goals. If they are within his reach, his efforts can be supported. If the patient has conflicting goals, the nurse helps him identify which are more realistic or obtainable by discussing emotional and practical consequences.

The nurse can work with the patient in various ways. The patient may be encouraged to give up superhuman standards by which he judges his behavior. These standards may set him up for failure and create a pathological cyclical pattern. The patient may need to lower his self-ideal and limit his goals to what is humanly possible. He should be encouraged to renew involvement with life and enter new experiences for their growth potential.

Role rehearsal, role modeling, and role playing may be employed. In role rehearsal the person imagines how a particular situation might take place and how his role

Table 16-6 Nursing Interventions in Alterations in Self-concept at Level 3

Goal—Assist the patient's self-evaluation

Principle	Rationale	Nursing interventions
Help the patient to define the problem clearly	Only after the problem is accurately defined can alternative choices be proposed	Identify relevant stressors with the patient and his appraisal of them Clarify that the patient's beliefs influence both his feelings and behaviors Mutually identify faulty beliefs, misperceptions, distortions, illusions, and unrealistic goals Mutually identify areas of strength Place the concepts of success and failure in proper perspective Explore the patient's use of coping resources
Explore the patient's adaptive and maladaptive coping responses to his problem	It is then necessary to examine the coping choices the patient has made and evaluate both the positive and the negative consequences of them	Describe to the patient how all coping responses are freely chosen and have both positive and negative consequences Contrast adaptive and maladaptive responses Mutually identify the disadvantages of the patient's maladaptive coping responses Mutually identify the advantages, or payoffs, of the patient's maladaptive coping responses Discuss how these payoffs have perpetuated the maladaptive response Use a variety of therapeutic skills, such as the following: 1. Facilitative communication 2. Supportive confrontation 3. Role clarification 4. The transference and countertransference reactions occurring in the one-to-one relationship

might evolve. He mentally enacts his role and tries to anticipate the responses of significant others. Role rehearsal is important in anticipating and planning the course of future action. Role modeling occurs when the individual observes someone else playing a certain role so that he is able to understand and emulate those behaviors. The person he observes may be the nurse, a family member, a group member, or a peer. The nurse can be important in assisting the patient in his role learning by modeling the behavior that may pose problems for the patient, such as expression of feelings, specific socialization skills, or realistic self-expectations. Proceeding one step further, the nurse and patient may role-play certain situations to conceptualize alternative solutions.

Visualization can also be used to enhance self-esteem through goal setting.[10] Through the conscious programming of desired change with positive images,

expectations are molded. Strong, positive expectations can then become self-fulfilling. To use visualization, the nurse should:

1. Ask the patient to select a positive, specific goal, such as: "I will call a friend and suggest we go out together."
2. Help the patient to relax using a relaxation technique (see Chapter 28).
3. Have the patient repeat the goal phrase several times slowly.
4. Instruct the patient to close his eyes and visualize the goal written on a piece of paper.
5. Have the patient, while relaxed, imagine accomplishing the goal.

The patient should then describe how he feels when the desired goal is reached and how other people are responding to him. In this way the patient can be helped to gain positive control over his life.

Nursing actions at this level of intervention are summarized in Table 16-7. Ultimately the patient should decide on a plan that includes a clear definition of the change to be achieved. Converting a "talking decision" into an "action decision" is the final, but most important, step.

Level 5—Commitment to Action

The nurse assists the patient to become committed to his decision and then achieve his goals. The patient's development of self-awareness, self-understanding, and insight is not the ultimate desired outcome of the nursing therapeutic process. Insight alone does not make problems disappear or transform one's world in magical ways. Although a patient may have obtained a high level of insight, he may nevertheless continue to function at a minimum level. Such a patient may be able intellectually to discuss with great ease the nature of his problem and the contributing influences, but the problem continues to be unresolved. Some patients actually use their insights to resist moving forward and avoid the hard work involved in making behavioral changes. The value of having the patient gain insight and increase his self-understanding is that he can gain perspective on why he behaves the way he does and what must be done to break maladaptive patterns.

Providing opportunity for the patient to experience success becomes essential at this time. To help him commit himself to his goal, the nurse can relate to the patient how she sees him, correcting his own poor self-image. In this mirroring technique, the nurse can openly and honestly describe to the patient the healthy parts of his personality and how, by using these parts, he can achieve his goal. The nurse should reinforce his strengths or skills and provide him with opportunities to use them whenever possible.

Sometimes the lack of vocational or social skills may be a causative factor for low self-esteem. If so, nursing

Table 16-7 Nursing Interventions in Alterations in Self-concept at Level 4

Goal—Assist the patient in formulating a realistic plan of action

Principle	Rationale	Nursing interventions
Help the patient identify alternative solutions	Only when all possible alternatives have been evaluated can change be effected	Help the patient understand that he can only change himself, not others If the patient holds inconsistent perceptions, help him to see that he can change the following: 1. His beliefs or ideals to bring them closer to reality 2. His environment to make it consistent with his beliefs If his self-concept is not consistent with his behavior, he can change the following: 3. His behavior to conform to his self-concept 4. The beliefs underlying his self-concept to include his behavior 5. His self-ideal Mutually review how coping resources may be better used by the patient
Help the patient conceptualize his own realistic goals	Goal setting that includes a clear definition of the expected change is necessary	Encourage the patient to formulate his own (not the nurse's) goals Mutually discuss the emotional, practical, and reality-based consequences of each goal Help the patient clearly define the concrete change to be made Encourage the patient to enter new experiences for their growth potential Use role rehearsal, role modeling, role playing, and visualization when appropriate

intervention can be directed toward gaining vocational assistance for the patient. Group and family involvement may be instrumental in raising self-esteem. The experience of being accepted by others, the sense of belonging and being important to others, and the opportunity to develop interpersonal competence can all enhance self-esteem.

At this point the individual needs much support and positive reinforcement in effecting and maintaining change. For many patients, this will mean breaking chronic behavior patterns and exposing themselves to real risk. A person must actively maintain the processes learned to avoid slipping back to the previous behavior. Doing this is difficult and requires that the patient build on the progress he has made in the other levels. Successful change is a continuing process of modifying not only one's behavior but one's environment to help ensure that the change to new ways of behaving is permanent. Otherwise a relapse will occur.

The nurse serves as a transition between the pain of the past and the positive gratification of the future. Both nurse and patient must allow sufficient time for change. A significant period may be required for patterns that developed over months or years to be broken and new ones established. The nurse's role now becomes less active and directive and more confirming of the value, potential, and accomplishments of the patient. A Nursing Care Plan Summary for maladaptive self-concept responses is presented on p. 408.

Evaluation

Problems with self-concept are prominent in many psychological disorders. Changes in self-concept are accompanied by greater self-realization and self-acceptance and lead to behavioral changes and improved personality adjustment. To evaluate the success or failure of the nursing care given in this area, each phase of the nursing process should be reviewed and analyzed by the nurse and patient:

The nurse's assessment should include both the objective and the observable behaviors as well as the subjective perceptions of the patient.

▼ Did the nurse explore the patient's strengths and weaknesses and elicit his self-ideal?

▼ Was information obtained on his body image, feelings of self-esteem, role satisfaction, and sense of identity?

▼ Did the nurse compare responses to his behavior, and were any inconsistencies or contradictions identified?

▼ Was the nurse aware of personal affective response to the patient, and how did this affect the ability to be therapeutic?

The nurse should have adopted a problem-solving approach that placed responsibility for growth on the patient. The most fundamental nursing action should have been to create a climate of acceptance that confirmed the patient's identity and conveyed a sense of value or worth. In expanding the patient's self-awareness:

▼ How effective was the nurse in promoting full and pertinent self-disclosure?

▼ Was the nurse able to manifest authentic behavior in the relationship and share thoughts and reactions?

▼ What interventions were used, and which ones proved beneficial—validation, reflection, confrontation, suggestion, role clarification, role playing?

▼ Did the nurse progress on the basis of the patient's readiness and motivation?

▼ What was the outcome of the patient's cognitive analysis and exploration of feelings?

▼ Was he able to transfer his new perceptions into possible solutions or alternative behavior?

▼ Did they both allow sufficient time for changes to occur?

The degree of overall success achieved through nursing care can be determined by eliciting the patient's perception of his own growth and comparing his behavior to the healthy personality described in this chapter. Not everyone will achieve all these characteristics, but success has been achieved if the patient's potential has been maximized.

SUGGESTED CROSS-REFERENCES

Therapeutic Nurse-Patient Relationship	Chapter 2
A Stress Adaptation Model of Psychiatric Nursing Care	Chapter 4
Primary Mental Health Prevention	Chapter 11
Anxiety Responses and Anxiety Disorders	Chapter 14
Emotional Responses and Mood Disorders	Chapter 17
Neurobiological Responses and Schizophrenia and Psychotic Disorders	Chapter 19
Eating Regulation Responses and Eating Disorders	Chapter 23
Cognitive Behavioral Therapy	Chapter 28
Family Interventions	Chapter 30
Adolescent Psychiatric Nursing	Chapter 35

SUMMARY

1. The continuum of self-concept responses ranges from the most adaptive state of self-actualization to the most maladaptive response of depersonalization.

NURSING CARE PLAN SUMMARY
Maladaptive Self-Concept Responses

Nursing Diagnosis: Self-esteem disturbance

Expected Outcome: The patient will obtain the maximum level of self-actualization to realize one's potential.

Short-term Goal	Intervention	Rationale
The patient will establish a therapeutic relationship with the nurse.	Confirm the patient's identity. Provide supportive measures to decrease panic level of anxiety. Set limits on inappropriate behavior. Work with whatever ego strengths the patient possesses. Reinforce adaptive behavior.	Mutuality is necessary for the patient to assume responsibility for his behavior. Some degree of ego integrity is needed for later interventions.
The patient will express feelings, behaviors, and thoughts related to the present stressful situations.	Assist the patient to express and describe feelings and thoughts. Help the patient in identifying self-strengths and weaknesses, self-ideal, self-criticisms. Respond empathically emphasizing that the power to change lies within the patient.	Self-disclosure and understanding are necessary to bring about future change. The use of sympathy is not therapeutic because it can reinforce the patient's self-pity. Rather the nurse should communicate that the patient is in control.
The patient will evaluate the positive and negative consequences of his self-concept responses.	Identify relevant stressors and the patient's appraisal of them. Clarify faulty beliefs and cognitive distortions. Evaluate advantages and disadvantages of current coping responses.	Only after the problem is defined can alternative choices be examined. It is then necessary to evaluate the positive and negative consequences of current patterns.
The patient will identify one new goal and two adaptive coping responses.	Encourage the patient to formulate a new goal. Help the patient clearly define the change to be made. Use role rehearsal, role modeling, and visualization to practice the new behavior.	Only after alternatives have been explored can change be effected. Goal setting specifies the nature of the change and suggests possible new behavioral strategies.
The patient will implement the new adaptive self-concept responses.	Provide opportunity for the patient to experience success. Reinforce strengths, skills, and adaptive coping responses. Allow the patient sufficient time to change. Promote group and family involvement. Provide the appropriate amount of support and positive reinforcement for the patient to maintain progress and growth.	The ultimate goal in promoting the patient's insight is to have him replace the maladaptive coping responses with more adaptive ones.

Components of the self include body image, self-ideal, self-esteem, role, and identity.

2. Patient behaviors related to self-concept responses include low self-esteem, identity diffusion, and depersonalization.

3. Predisposing factors affecting self-concept responses are related to unrealistic self-ideals, sex and work roles, and challenges to personal identity. Precipitating stressors include role strain and developmental and health-illness transitions.

4. Coping resources focus on the patient's ego strengths, whereas coping mechanisms may be short- or long-term defenses and ego defense mechanisms.

5. Primary nursing diagnoses are body image disturbance, self-esteem disturbance, altered role performance, and personal identity disturbance.
6. Primary DSM-IV diagnoses are categorized as dissociative disorders and identity problem.
7. The expected outcome of nursing care is that the patient will obtain the maximum level of self-actualization to realize one's potential.

8. Interventions include assisting the patient in expanding self-awareness and engaging in self-exploration, self-evaluation, realistic planning, and commitment to action.
9. The degree of overall success achieved through nursing care can be determined by eliciting the patient's perception of his own growth and comparing his behavior to characteristics of a healthy personality.

COMPETENT CARING
A CLINICAL EXEMPLAR OF A PSYCHIATRIC NURSE

Monica Molloy, MSN, RN, CS

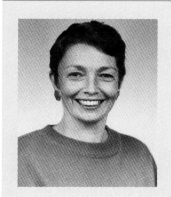

Last week one of my patients died.

I have been a nurse for 16 years. I have experienced patients' deaths—many different kinds of deaths, some of them seemingly senseless. I think particularly of young patients with head injuries from motorcycle or automobile accidents. But I understood those deaths. I understood the concept of accident. What I don't understand is the concept of murder.

In November, a woman was sitting apart from most of the members of a therapy group I colead with a graduate nursing student. I asked her why she didn't join the circle. She replied she was afraid the group didn't want her near them; she thought the odor of her cancer would offend them. When the women in the group responded that they hadn't noticed any odor, she seemed to accept the reassurance offered; but she continued to sit apart.

Last week that woman was murdered.

She was a homeless woman, one of the women that embarrass us as a society. She lived in the Family Center of the homeless shelter. I'll call her C. I first met her 2 years ago, when the group began. I remember one group in particular when she and another shelter guest talked about trust issues in the homeless community. Then she moved away. This past fall she returned to the shelter. In addition to neurofibromatosis, she now had cancer. She looked different; she had lost nearly 40 pounds. She had been discharged from a local hospital to the shelter. Despite her willingness to take a risk and to disclose her fears about the odor she thought she had to the group, she essentially remained alone and apart.

C's death has given me one more opportunity to examine what it is to practice psychiatric nursing in the community. When nurses practice in inpatient environments, one of our fundamental responsibilities is to ensure patient safety. Sometimes that safety is interpersonal, sometimes it is environmental. Among the homeless population, environmental safety is tenuous at best. One goal for the group intervention in the shelter community is to enable the women to use themselves and each other as resources to create their own safety zone. Somehow that didn't work with C.

The day after her death, the graduate nursing student and I spent some time with the women in the Family Center community. We went there to be with the women, to provide support. We also went there to grieve. And perhaps most of all, we went there to try to answer some questions for ourselves—the same questions all clinicians ask when a patient dies—did we miss some signs, could we have done something different?

C's death is mentioned in the group weekly now. New guests use her death to concretize their fears about being homeless, as a metaphor for their own alienation experience. Through her death C has left a mark on that group, and on that community. I don't understand the concept of murder any better. I do understand more about the concept of alienation. Acknowledging alienation is a first step to creating a sense of personal safety. It is fundamental to the practice of psychiatric nursing in the community. I learned that from C, and for that I will always be grateful. ▼

REFERENCES

1. Allen J: Dissociative processes: theoretical underpinnings of a working model for clinician and patient, *Bull Menninger Clin* 57:287, 1993.
2. Allen J, Smith W: Diagnosing dissociative disorders, *Bull Menninger Clin* 57:1993.
3. American Psychiatric Association: *Diagnostic and statistical manual of mental disorders*, ed 4, Washington, DC, 1994, The Association.
4. Antonucci T, Jackson J: Physical health and self-esteem, *Fam Community Health* 6:1, 1983.
5. Austin J, Champion V, Tzeng O: Cross-cultural relationships between self-concept and body image in high school boys, *Arch Psychiatr Nurs* 3:234, 1989.
6. Bednar R, Wells M, VandenBos G: Self-esteem: a concept of renewed clinical relevance, *Hosp Community Psychiatry* 42:123, 1991.
7. Burns D: Focusing on ego strengths, *Arch Psychiatr Nurs* 5:202, 1991.
8. Carlson E et al: Validity of the dissociative experiences scale in screening for multiple personality disorder: a multicenter study, *Am J Psychiatry* 150:1030, 1993.
9. Coopersmith S: *The antecedents of self-esteem*, San Francisco, 1967, WH Freeman.
10. Crouch M, Straub V: Enhancement of self-esteem in adults, *Fam Community Health* 6:65, 1983.
11. Curtin S: Recognizing multiple personality disorder, *J Psychosoc Nurs Ment Health Serv* 31:29, 1993.
12. Erikson E: *Childhood and society*, New York, 1963, WW Norton.
13. Franklin J: The diagnosis of multiple personality disorder based on subtle dissociative signs, *J Nerv Ment Dis* 178:4, 1990.
14. Hamachek D: *Encounters with the self*, New York, 1971, Holt, Rinehart & Winston.
15. Horney K: *Neurosis and human growth*, New York, 1950, WW Norton.
16. Jourard S: *Personal adjustment: an approach through the study of the health personality*, New York, 1963, Macmillan.
17. Jourard S: *The transparent self*, New York, 1971, Litton Educational.
18. Klose P, Tinius T: Confidence builders: a self-esteem group at an inpatient psychiatric hospital, *J Psychosoc Nurs Ment Health Serv* 30:5, 1992.
19. Kluft R, Fine C: *Clinical perspectives on multiple personality disorder*, Washington, DC, 1993, American Psychiatric Press.
20. Logan R: Identity diffusion and psychosocial defense mechanisms, *Adolescence* 13:503, 1978.
21. Meleis A: Role insufficiency and role supplementation: a conceptual framework, *Nurs Res* 24:264, 1975.
22. Putnam F, Lowenstein R: Treatment of multiple personality disorder: a survey of current practices, *Am J Psychiatry* 150:104, 1993.
23. Ross C, Joshi S, Currie R: Dissociative experiences in the general population: a factor analysis, *Hosp Community Psychiatry* 42:297, 1991.
24. Sieving R, Zirbel-Donisch S: Development and enhancement of self-esteem in children, *J Pediatr Health Care* 4:291, 1990.
25. Stafford L: Dissociation and multiple personality disorder: a challenge for psychosocial nurses, 31:15, 1993.
26. Sullivan HS: *The interpersonal theory of psychiatry*, New York, 1963, WW Norton.
27. Taft L: Self-esteem in later life: a nursing perspective, *Adv Nurs Science* 8:77, 1985.

ANNOTATED SUGGESTED READINGS

*Anderson G, Ross C: Strategies for working with a patient who has multiple personality disorder, *Arch Psychiatr Nurs* 2:236, 1988.

Uses the nursing process to organize treatment strategies in caring for the patient with multiple personality disorder. Practical and well written.

*Bonham P, Cheney A: Concept of self: a framework for nursing assessment. In Chinn P, ed: *Advances in nursing theory development*, Rockville, Md, 1983, Aspen.

Reviews the literature and proposes a nursing model for self-concept.

*Burns D: Focusing on ego strengths, *Arch Psychiatr Nurs* 5:202, 1991.

Examines the need for nurses to build ego strengths of patients and ensure their stable identity.

*Curtin S: Recognizing multiple personality disorder, *J Psychosoc Nurs Ment Health Serv* 31:29, 1993.

Excellent presentation of the behavioral, clinical, and physiological symptoms associated with multiple personality disorder.

Erikson E: *Identity: youth and crisis*, New York, 1968, WW Norton.

Describes the adolescent crisis of identity. Reviews stages of the life cycle and explores identity confusion through theory and case history.

Gara M, Rosenberg S, and Cohen B: Personal identity and the schizophrenic process: an integration, *Psychiatry* 50:267, 1987.

---

*Nursing reference.

Explores the relation between identity theory and the schizophrenic process. Also discusses the effects of medication in establishing a patient identity and preventing psychotic relapse. Advanced reading.

Grame C: Internal containment in the treatment of patients with dissociative disorders, *Bull Menninger Clin* 57:355, 1993.

Describes strategies nurses can use to help patients with dissociative disorders cope with life and work through past traumas. Illustrated by case examples.

*Kerr N: Ego competency: a framework for formulating the nursing care plan, *Perspect Psychiatr Care* 26:30, 1990.

Describes a model of psychiatric nursing care based on the patient's ego strengths and deficits. Worthwhile reading.

Kluft R, Fine C: Clinical perspectives on multiple personality disorder, Washington, DC, 1993, American Psychiatric Press.

Definitive text on psychotherapeutic approaches and case studies related to multiple personality disorders.

*Price B: A model for body-image care, *J Adv Nurs* 15:585, 1990.

Proposes a model of body image care based on five central concepts with practical implications for intervention.

Raimy V: *Misunderstandings of the self*, San Francisco, 1975, Jossey-Bass.

Premise is that misunderstandings of the self may be major hindrances to personal and social adjustment. Easy to read, and integrates sophisticated features of various psychotherapies that involve cognitive change.

Rogers C: On *becoming a person*, Boston, 1961, Houghton Mifflin.

Discusses personal growth from the individual's and therapist's point of view. Highly recommended.

*Sieving R, Zirbel-Donisch S: Development and enhancement of self-esteem in children, *J Pediatr Health Care* 4:291, 1990.

Describes effective communication techniques, discipline strategies, child-centered guidance, and methods to promote children's autonomy.

*Watson W: Who are we? low self-esteem and marital identity, *J Psychosoc Nurs Ment Health Serv* 28:15, 1990.

Presents a family systems approach to the problem of self-esteem in married women. Includes highlights of clinical sessions.[2]

---

*Nursing reference.

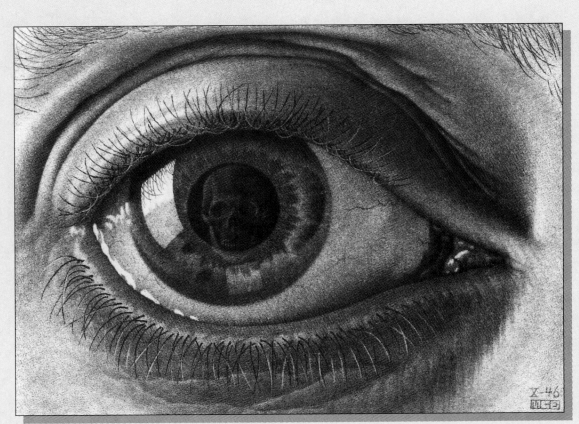

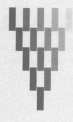

CHAPTER 17

Emotional Responses and Mood Disorders

GAIL W. STUART

Lying awake, calculating the future,
Trying to unweave, unwind, unravel
And piece together the past and the future,
Between midnight and dawn, when the
past is all deception,
The future futureless . . .

T.S. Eliot

LEARNING OBJECTIVES

After studying this chapter the student should be able to:

▼ Describe the continuum of adaptive and maladaptive emotional responses

▼ Discuss the epidemiology of mood disorders

▼ Identify behaviors associated with emotional responses

▼ Analyze predisposing factors and precipitating stressors related to emotional responses

▼ Describe coping resources and coping mechanisms related to emotional responses

▼ Formulate nursing diagnoses for patients related to their emotional responses

▼ Assess the relationship between nursing diagnoses and medical diagnoses related to emotional responses

▼ Identify expected outcomes and short-term nursing goals for patients related to emotional responses

▼ Develop a patient education plan to promote patients' adaptive emotional responses

▼ Analyze nursing interventions for patients related to their emotional responses

▼ Evaluate nursing care for patients related to their emotional responses

TOPICAL OUTLINE

Continuum of Emotional Responses
  Grief Reactions
  Depression
  Mania
Assessment
  Behaviors
  Predisposing Factors
  Precipitating Stressors
  Coping Resources
  Coping Mechanisms
Nursing Diagnosis
  Related Medical Diagnoses
Outcome Identification
Planning
Implementation
  Environmental Interventions
  Nurse-Patient Relationship
  Physiological Treatments
  Expressing Feelings
  Cognitive Strategies
  Behavioral Change
  Social Skills
  Mental Health Education
Evaluation

Variations or fluctuations in mood are a natural part of human existence. They indicate that a person is perceiving the world and responding to it. Extremes in mood have also been linked with extremes in human experience, such as creativity, madness, despair, ecstasy, romanticism, personal charisma, and interpersonal destructiveness. Moods have fascinated scientists, philosophers, and novelists alike, who romanticize, study, and exaggerate the possible links between mood, deep emotional experience, and talent.[23]

In this text, **mood** refers to a prolonged emotional state that influences the person's whole personality and life functioning. It pertains to prevailing and pervading emotion and is synonymous with the terms *feeling state* and *emotion*. As with other aspects of the personality, emotions or moods serve an adaptive role for the individual.

The four adaptive functions of emotions are social communication, physiological arousal, subjective awareness, and psychodynamic defense. The components of social communication, such as crying, posture, facial expression, and touch, promote early mother-child attachment and the formation of other interpersonal bonds. Depressive mood states also initiate physiological arousal involving the central nervous system, biogenic amines, and neuroendocrine systems. The subjective components of human emotions are believed to play important functions in goal setting and in the monitoring of current behavior, particularly in judging personal reality against internalized values and goals. Finally, the fourth adaptive function of emotion is in aiding psychodynamic defense on both conscious and unconscious levels.

CONTINUUM OF EMOTIONAL RESPONSES

Emotions such as fear, joy, anxiety, love, anger, sadness, and surprise are all normal aspects of the human condition. The problem arises in trying to evaluate when a person's mood or emotional state is maladaptive, abnormal, or unhealthy. Grief, for example, is a healthy, adaptive, separative process that attempts to overcome the stress of a loss. Grief work, or mourning, therefore, is not a pathological process; it is an adaptive response to a real stressor. The absence of grieving in the face of a loss is suggestive of maladaptation.

The continuum of of emotional responses is represented in Fig. 17-1. At the adaptive end is emotional responsiveness. This involves the person being affected by and being an active participant in both internal and external worlds. It implies an openness to and awareness of feelings. If used in such a way, feelings provide us with valuable learning experiences. They are barometers that give a person feedback about oneself and one's relationships, and they help a person function more effectively. Also adaptive in the face of stress is an uncomplicated grief reaction. Such a reaction implies that the person is facing the reality of the loss and is immersed in the work of grieving.

A maladaptive response would be the suppression of emotions. This may be evident as a denial of one's feelings, a detachment from them, or an internalization of all aspects of one's affective world. A transient suppression of feelings may at times be necessary to cope, such as in an initial response to a death or tragedy. Prolonged suppression of emotion, however, such as in delayed grief reaction, will ultimately interfere with effective functioning.

The most maladaptive emotional responses or severe mood disturbances can be recognized by their intensity, pervasiveness, persistence, and interference with usual social and physiological functioning. These characteristics apply to the severe clinical states of depression and mania, which complete the maladaptive end of the continuum of emotional responses.

Grief Reactions

Grief is the subjective state that follows loss. It is one of the most powerful emotional states of human experience and affects all aspects of a person's life. It forces

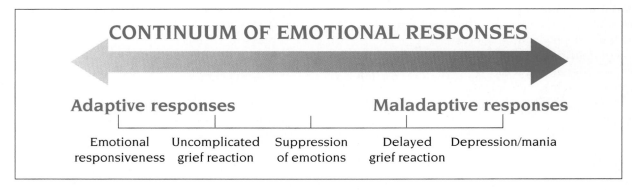

Fig. 17-1 Continuum of emotional responses.

the person to stop normal activities and to focus on present feelings and needs. Most often, it is the response to loss of a loved person through death or separation, but it also occurs following the loss of something tangible or intangible that is highly regarded. It may be a valued object, a cherished possession, an ideal, a job, or status. As a response to the loss of a loved one, grief is a universal reaction. As a person's interdependence on others grows, the chance increases of facing loss, separation, and death, which elicit intense feelings of grief. The capacity to form warm, satisfying relationships with others also makes a person vulnerable to sadness, despair, and grief when those relationships are terminated.

As a natural reaction to a life experience, grief is universal. It involves stress, pain, and suffering and an impairment of function that can last for days, weeks, or months. Thus the understanding of grief is of great importance because of its effect on both physical and emotional health.

The ability to experience grief is gradually formed in the course of normal development and is closely related to the capacity for developing meaningful object relationships. Grief responses may be either uncomplicated and adaptive or morbid and pathological. Uncomplicated grief runs a consistent course that is modified by the abruptness of the loss, the person's preparation for the event, and the significance of the lost object. It is a self-limited process of realization; it makes real the fact of the loss.

A maladaptive response to loss implies that something has prevented it from running its normal course. Two types of pathological grief reactions have been identified by Lindemann[35]—the delayed reaction and the distorted reaction. Depression is one type of a distorted grief reaction.

Persistent absence of any emotion may signal an undue delay in the work of mourning or a delayed grief reaction. The delay may occur in the beginning of the mourning process or become evident in a retarding of the process once it has begun, or both. The delay and rejection of grief may occasionally last for many years. The underlying emotions associated with the loss may be triggered by a deliberate recall of circumstances surrounding the loss or by a spontaneous occurrence in the patient's life. A classic example of this is the anniversary reaction in which the person experiences incomplete or abnormal mourning at the time of the loss, only to have the grieving response recur at anniversaries of the original loss.

Depression

The individual who does not mourn can experience a pathological grief reaction known as depression, or mel-
ancholia. It is an abnormal extension or overelaboration of sadness and grief. Depression is the oldest and most frequently described psychiatric illness. It has been described as early as 1500 BC, and it appears to be part of the human condition familiar to all yet mysterious to many. The term *depression* is used in a variety of ways. It can refer to a sign, symptom, syndrome, emotional state, reaction, disease, or clinical entity. In this chapter it is viewed as a clinical condition that is severe, maladaptive, and incapacitating.

Depression may range from mild and moderate states to severe states with or without psychotic features. Psychotic depression is relatively uncommon, however, accounting for less than 10% of all depressions. Major depression can begin at any age, although it usually begins in the midtwenties and thirties. Symptoms develop over days to weeks. Approximately one out of eight adults may experience major depression in their lifetime, and it affects 11.5 million people each year, 71% of whom are women. Approximately 15% of severely depressed patients commit suicide. Other complications include marital, parental, social, and vocational difficulties.

The lifetime risk for major depression is 7% to 12% for men and 20% to 30% for women. Women have nearly a twofold increase in risk with rates peaking between adolescence and early adulthood.[43,58] This difference holds true across cultures and continents (see Critical Thinking about Contemporary Issues).[30,33,54] Other risk factors include a history of depressive illness in first-degree relatives and a history of major depression.

Most untreated episodes of major depression last 6 to 24 months. While some people have only a single episode of major depression and return to presymptomatic functioning, it is estimated that over 50% of those who have such an episode will eventually have another, and 25% of patients will have chronic, recurrent depression.[13,59]

Depression often occurs along with other psychiatric illnesses (Table 17-1). Up to 43% of patients with major depressive disorders have histories of one or more non-mood psychiatric disorders. These statistics underscore the importance of this health problem and suggest the

Table 17-1 Comorbidity of Depression and Other Psychiatric Illness

	Major depressive disorder (%)	Dysthymic disorder (%)	Depression NOS (%)
Alcohol abuse	10	30	67
Drug abuse	19	30	26
Panic disorder	19	7	21
Obsessive-compulsive disorder	35	15	40

CRITICAL THINKING ABOUT CONTEMPORARY ISSUES

Is There a Difference in the Experience of Depression Between Black and White Women in American Society?

It has been suggested that black women's mental health is affected by their double minority status of being black and female within American society.[53] Yet the exact incidence of depression in black women is unclear because of controversy regarding misdiagnosis and lack of clinical research. Although it is known that black women report depression more often than black men, little is known about the sociodemographic indicators of risk and depressive symptoms.[25] The assumption that all women share similar experiences does not allow for differences to emerge regarding the diagnostic process, measurement tools, and successful treatment strategies for various cultural groups.[7]

It is clear that depression is an increasing problem for black women. These women are experiencing role changes and additional stressors. Depressed black women may perceive themselves as being devalued within society and may have fewer support systems to buffer stressful events. Depressive symptoms may graduate into clinical depression and thus further decrease the quality of life for black women. Psychiatric nurses can be instrumental in developing protocols and interventions that respond with cultural sensitivity to the psychological and physiological needs of depressed patients and thus improve their overall quality of life.[53] ▼

need for timely diagnosis and treatment. Unfortunately, only one third of all people with depression seek help, are accurately diagnosed and obtain appropriate treatment.

Research has also revealed the high incidence of depression among patients hospitalized for medical illnesses. These depressions are largely unrecognized and thus are untreated by health-care personnel. Depression is found in all severities of medical illness, although its intensity and frequency are higher in patients more severely ill. Available studies suggest that about one third of medical inpatients report mild or moderate symptoms of depression and up to one fourth may suffer from a depressive illness. Certain medical conditions are frequently associated with depression, especially cancer, stroke, epilepsy, multiple sclerosis, Parkinson's disease, cardiac disease, and a variety of endocrine disorders.

Thus research suggests depression is a common accompaniment of many major medical illnesses.

Depressive conditions are also highly prevalent in primary care settings. One out of five patients seeing a primary care practitioner has significant symptoms of depression. Yet only about one in 100 patients cites depression as a reason for the most recent visit, and health-care providers fail to diagnose major depression in their patients up to 50% of the time.[59] Finally, it has been estimated that depression cost the American economy $43.7 billion in worker absenteeism, lost productivity, and health care.[41]

A patient who just underwent cardiac surgery comes for a follow-up visit and tells the physician he is feeling depressed. He is told that depression is a normal response to cardiac illness and he will get over it in time. Do you agree with this? If not, what nursing actions are indicated?

Mania

In addition to a severely depressed disturbance of mood, manic episodes may also be experienced. These episodes, as with those of depression, can vary in intensity and accompanying level of anxiety from moderate manic states to severe and panic states with psychotic features. Basically, mania is characterized by a mood that is elevated, expansive, or irritable. **Hypomania** describes a clinical syndrome similar to, but not as severe as, that described by the terms *mania* or *manic episode*.

In the DSM-IV[3] the major affective disorders are separated into two subgroups—bipolar and depressive disorders—based on whether manic and depressive episodes are involved longitudinally (Table 17-2). In this classification major depression may involve a single episode or a recurrent depressive illness but without manic episodes. When there has been one or more manic episodes, with or without a major depressive episode, the category of bipolar I disorder is used. Bipolar I disorders are subdivided according to the symptoms of the current episode as manic, depressed, or mixed.

Thus a depressive episode with no manic episodes would be classified as a "depressive disorder." A depressive episode with previous or current manic episodes would be classified as a "bipolar disorder" or "manic depressive illness."

Although bipolar I affective disorders occur less often than depressive disorders, it is estimated that 0.6% to 0.88% of the adult population, or approximately 2 million Americans, suffer from bipolar disorder. Risk factors

Table 17-2 Classification of Mood (Affective) Disorders in DSM-IV* Relative to Depressive and Manic Episodes

	Depressive disorders		Bipolar I disorders		
	Single	Recurrent	Manic	Depressed	Mixed
Depressive episode	Yes	Yes	No	Yes–present	Yes–present
Manic episode	No	No	Yes–present	Yes–past	Yes–present

*American Psychiatric Association: *Diagnostic and statistical manual of mental disorders,* ed 4, Washington, DC, 1994, The Association.

are being female and having a family history of bipolar disorder. The data suggest that people under age 50 are at higher risk of a first attack, whereas those who already have the disorder face increased risk of a recurrent manic or depressive episode as they grow older.[16] Additional facts about depressive and bipolar disorders are presented in Box 17-1.

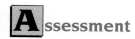 ssessment

Behaviors

Delayed Grief Reaction. Delayed grief reactions may be expressed by excessive hostility and grief, prolonged feelings of emptiness and numbness, an inability to weep or express emotions, low self-esteem, use of present tense instead of past when speaking of the loss, persistent dreams about the loss, retention of clothing of the deceased, an inability to visit the grave of the deceased, and the projection of living memories into an object held in place of the lost one. The following clinical example illustrates some of the behaviors associated with a delayed grief reaction.

 CLINICAL EXAMPLE

Mrs. G was a 38-year-old married woman with no history of depression. She came to the local community mental health center complaining of "severe throbbing headaches, difficulty falling asleep, fitful and disturbing dreams when asleep, and poor appetite." She said she felt "disgusted" with herself and "useless" to her family. She was living alone with her husband.

Her family history revealed she had three children—two boys and a girl. Her eldest son, age 20, was attending college out of state, and her daughter, age 19, was living with a girlfriend in the same city. Her youngest son was killed in an automobile accident 2 years ago when 15 years old. She described him as her "baby" and expressed much guilt for contributing to his death. She scolded herself for allowing him to drive to the seashore for the weekend with friends,

---

Box 17-1

FACTS ABOUT MOOD DISORDERS

MAJOR DEPRESSIVE DISORDER

Major depression is among the most common of all clinical problems encountered by primary care practitioners.

Major depression accounts for more bed days—people out of work and in bed—than any other "physical" disorder except for cardiovascular disorders, and it is more costly to the economy than chronic respiratory illness, diabetes, arthritis, or hypertension.

Psychotherapy alone helps some depressed patients, especially those with mild to moderate symptoms.

It can be treated successfully by antidepressant medications in 65% of cases.

"Success" rate of treatment increases to 85% when alternative or adjunctive medications are used or psychotherapy is combined with medications.

BIPOLAR DISORDER

Without modern treatments, patients typically spent one fourth of their adult life in the hospital and fully one half of their life disabled.

Effective medications (lithium and anticonvulsants for lithium-resistant patients), often used in combination with supportive psychotherapy, allow 75% to 80% of manic-depressive patients to lead essentially normal lives.

Lithium has saved the U.S. economy more than $40 billion since 1970: $13 billion in direct treatment costs and $27 billion in indirect costs.

---

and said she now worries a great deal about her other two children. She said she was trying to protect them from the dangers of the world, but they resented her advice and concern. On questioning by the nurse, Mrs. G reported that these feelings of sadness and guilt had emerged in the last month and seemed to be triggered by the graduation of her son's high school class.

Selected Nursing Diagnosis:

▼ Dysfunctional grieving related to son's death as evidenced by somatic complaints and feelings of sadness and guilt

In this example Mrs. G was experiencing a delayed grief reaction precipitated by the event of her deceased son's would-be graduation. She had failed to progress through mourning at her son's death and was beginning "grief work" at present.

Depression. The behaviors associated with depression vary. Sadness and slowness may predominate, or agitation may occur. The key element to a behavioral assessment is change—depressed individuals change their usual patterns and responses. Research indicates that individuals working through normal mourning respond to their loss with psychological symptoms often indistinguishable from depression, but accepted by them and by their environment as normal. In contrast, patients with depression experience their condition as a "change" unlike their usual self, which often leads them to seek help.

Many behaviors are associated with depression. These may be divided into affective, physiological, cognitive, and behavioral (Table 17-3). Obviously, some are contradictory and incompatible. The lists describe the spectrum of possible behaviors, and not all individuals experience all of them.[12]

The most common and central behavior is that of the depressive mood. This is not necessarily described by the patient as "depression" but as feeling sad, blue, down in the dumps, unhappy, or unable to enjoy life. Crying often occurs. On the other hand, some depressed persons do not cry and describe themselves as "beyond tears." The mood disturbance of the depressed patient resembles that of normal unhappiness multiplied in in-

tensity and pervasiveness. Another mood that often accompanies depression is anxiety—a sense of fear and intense worry. Both depression and anxiety may show diurnal variation, that is, a pattern whereby certain times of the day, such as morning or evening, are consistently worse or better.

Some patients may initially deny their anxious or depressed moods but identify a variety of somatic complaints. These might include gastrointestinal distress, chronic or intermittent pain, irritability, palpitations, dizziness, appetite change, lack of energy, change in sex drive, or sleep disturbances. The person often focuses on these symptoms because they are more socially acceptable than the profound feeling of sadness, inability to concentrate, or loss of pleasure in usual activities. In addition, the physical symptoms may help the person with depression explain why nothing is fun anymore. When patients have a range of somatic symptoms, the nurse should carefully evaluate these complaints but also return to the issues of mood and interest, thus considering the possible diagnosis of depression.

It may also be helpful for the nurse to be familiar with the subgroups of major depressive disorder. The common subgroups and clinical relevance of each are presented in Table 17-4.[13] These subgroups are not all-inclusive and may represent varying clinical expressions of the same illness over time, in different age groups, or in relation to specific precipitating stressors. Two of these subgroups merit special attention.

POSTPARTUM ONSET. Postpartum mood symptoms are divided into three categories based on severity: (1)

Table 17-3 Behaviors Associated with Depression

Affective	Physiological	Cognitive	Behavioral
Anger	Abdominal pain	Ambivalence	Aggressiveness
Anxiety	Anorexia	Confusion	Agitation
Apathy	Backache	Inability to concentrate	Alcoholism
Bitterness	Chest pain	Indecisiveness	Altered activity level
Dejection	Constipation	Loss of interest and	Drug addition
Denial of feelings	Dizziness	motivation	Intolerance
Despondency	Fatigue	Pessimism	Irritability
Guilt	Headache	Self-blame	Lack of spontaneity
Helplessness	Impotence	Self-depreciation	Overdependency
Hopelessness	Indigestion	Self-destructive	Poor personal hygiene
Loneliness	Insomnia	thoughts	Psychomotor retarda-
Low self-esteem	Lassitude	Uncertainty	tion
Sadness	Menstrual changes		Social isolation
Sense of personal	Nausea		Tearfulness
worthlessness	Overeating		Underachievement
	Sexual nonresponsive-		Withdrawal
	ness		
	Sleep disturbances		
	Vomiting		
	Weight change		

blues, (2) psychosis, and (3) depression.[28,52] **Postpartum blues** are brief episodes lasting 1 to 4 days of labile mood and tearfulness that occur in about 50% to 80% of women within 1 to 5 days of delivery. Treatment consists of reassurance and time to resolve this normal response. **Postpartum psychosis** can be divided into depressed and manic types. The incidence of postpartum psychosis is low, and the symptoms typically begin 2 to 3 days after delivery. The period of risk for developing postpartum psychosis is within the first month after delivery. The prognosis is good for acute postpartum psychosis. However, many patients subsequently develop a bipolar disorder. The recurrence rate is 33% to 51%. **Postpartum depression** may occur from 2 weeks to 12 months after delivery, but it usually does so within 6 months. The risk of postpartum depression is 10% to 15%, but the rate is higher for persons with a psychiatric history.

SEASONAL PATTERN. Seasonal affective disorder (SAD) is depression that comes with shortened daylight in winter and fall and that disappears during spring and summer. It is characterized by hypersomnia, lethargy and fatigue, increased anxiety, irritability, increased appetite with carbohydrate craving, and often weight gain.[39,45] It is believed to be related to abnormal melatonin metabolism. It has also been noted that there are two to three times as many people personally troubled by the winter recurrence of seasonal mood symptoms than there are those with behaviors severe enough to merit clinical diagnosis.

Conditions of light and darkness have often been noted to affect mood. Evaluate your environment for exposure to light. Compare it with a hospital environment.

SUICIDE. Finally, the potential for suicide should always be assessed in severe mood disturbances. Suicide

Table 17-4 Major Depressive Disorder Subgroups

Subgroup	Essential features	Diagnostic implications	Treatment implications	Prognostic implications
Psychotic	Hallucinations Delusions	More likely to become bipolar than nonpsychotic types May be misdiagnosed as schizophrenia	Antidepressant medication plus a neuroleptic is more effective than are antidepressants alone. ECT is very effective	Usually a recurrent illness Subsequent episodes are usually psychotic Psychotic subtypes run in families Mood-incongruent features have a poorer prognosis
Melancholic	Anhedonia Unreactive mood Severe vegetative symptoms	May be misdiagnosed as dementia More likely in older patients	Antidepressant medication is essential ECT is 90% effective.	If recurrent, consider maintenance medication
Atypical	Reactive mood Overeating/weight gain Oversleeping Rejection sensitivity Heavy limb sensation Fewer episodes	Common in younger patients May be misdiagnosed as personality disorder	TCAs may be less effective; MAOIs are preferred ?SSRIs preferred	Unclear
Seasonal	Onset, fall Offset, spring Recurrent	More frequent in non-equatorial latitudes Pattern occurs in major depressive and bipolar disorders	Medications have questionable efficacy Psychotherapy has questioanble efficacy Phototherapy is an option	Recurs
Postpartum psychosis/depression	Acute onset (<30 days) in postpartum period Severe, labile mood symptoms 1/1000 is psychotic form	Often heralds a bipolar disorder	Hospitalize Treat medically	50% chance of recurring in next postpartum period

From Depression Guideline Panel: *Depression in primary care*, vol 1, *Detection and diagnosis, Clinical practice guideline*, no 5, Rockville, Md, 1993, US Department of Health and Human Services, Public Health Service, Agency for Health Care Policy and Research, pub no 93-0550.
ECT, Electroconvulsive therapy; TCA, tricyclic antidepressant; MAOIs, monoamine oxidase inhibitors; SSRIs, selective serotonin reuptake inhibitors.

and other self-destructive behaviors are discussed in detail in Chapter 18. The intensity of anger, guilt, and worthlessness may precipitate suicidal thoughts, feelings, or gestures, as illustrated in the following clinical example.

 ## CLINICAL EXAMPLE

Mr. W was a 60-year-old man who lived alone. His son and daughter were married and lived in the same state. His wife died 2 years ago, and since that time his children had often asked him to move in with either of them. He had consistently refused to do this, believing that both he and his children needed privacy in their lives. Six months ago he was diagnosed as having advanced prostatic cancer with metastasis. After the diagnosis and because of increasing disability, he left his job and began to receive disability compensation. He visited his children and their families about twice a month and kept his regularly scheduled visits with the medical clinic. The nurses and physicians at the clinic noted he was "despondent and withdrawn" but viewed this as a normal reaction to his diagnosis and family history. No interventions were implemented based on his emotional needs. A week after attending the clinic for a routine, follow-up visit, he went to the cemetery where his wife was buried and at her gravestone shot himself in the head. A grounds keeper of the cemetery heard the shot, discovered what had happened, and called an ambulance. Mr. W was taken to the emergency room of the nearest hospital and, with prompt medical care, survived the suicide attempt.

Selected Nursing Diagnoses:

▼ Potential for self-directed violence related to feelings of depression as evidenced by gunshot to the head

▼ Hopelessness related to medical diagnosis of metastatic cancer as evidenced by withdrawal and despondency

This example dramatically emphasizes three important points. First, medical illness frequently involves a loss of function, body part, or appearance. Therefore all patients should be assessed for depression. Second, all people experiencing depression and despair have the potential for suicide. Third, nurses can intervene to support the grieving and mourning process whether it is uncomplicated or pathological. Nursing actions can be preventive, curative, or rehabilitative, based on the nursing assessment and diagnosis.

Mania. The essential feature of mania is a distinct period of intense psychophysiological activation. Some of the associated behaviors are given in Table 17-5. The predominant mood is elevated or irritable, accompanied by one or more of the following symptoms: hyperactivity, the undertaking of too many activities, lack of judgment in anticipating consequences, pressured speech, flight of ideas, distractibility, inflated self-esteem, and hypersexuality.

If the mood is elevated or euphoric, it is often infectious. Patients report feeling happy, unconcerned, carefree, and devoid of problems. Although such experiences would seem enviable, these affective moods are without any concern for reality or the feelings of others. The mood is often expansive, and some patients have extraordinary delusions about their power and importance. They characteristically involve themselves in seemingly senseless and risky enterprises.

Alternately, the mood may be irritable, especially when plans are thwarted. Patients can be contentious and provoked by seemingly harmless remarks. Self-

Table 17-5 Behaviors Associated with Mania

Affective	Physiological	Cognitive	Behavioral
Elation or euphoria	Dehydration	Ambitiousness	Aggressiveness
Expansiveness	Inadequate nutrition	Denial of realistic danger	Excessive spending of money
Humorous	Needs little sleep	Distractibility	Grandiose acts
Inflated self-esteem	Weight loss	Flight of ideas	Hyperactivity
Intolerance of criticism		Grandiosity	Increased motor activity
Lack of shame or guilt		Illusions	Irresponsibility
		Lack of judgment	Irritability or argumentativeness
		Loose associations	Poor personal grooming
			Provocativeness
			Sexual overactivity
			Social activity
			Verbosity

esteem is inflated during a manic episode, and, as activity level increases, feelings about the self become increasingly disturbed. Delusional grandiose symptoms are evident, and the patient is willing to undertake any project possible.

In contrast to depressed patients, manic patients are extremely self-confident, with an ego that knows no bounds; they are "on top of the world." Accompanying this magical omnipotence and supreme self-esteem is an equally inordinate lack of guilt and shame. Often they deny realistic danger. The patient's boundless energy, cunning, planning, scheming, and inability to forecast consequences frequently lead to irresponsible enterprises and excessive spending, as well as to misdemeanors of a sexual, aggressive, or possessive nature. In contrast to depressed patients, manic patients have heightened libidinal drives, with abounding energy and heightened sexual appetite. Characteristic physical changes are inadequate nutrition, partly because manic patients have no time to eat, and serious loss of weight related to their insomnia and overactivity. Extremely manic patients may be dehydrated and require prompt attention.

In addition to mood, speech is often disturbed. As mania intensifies, formal and logical speech is displaced by loud, rapid, and confusing language. As the activated state increases, speech becomes full of plays on words and irrelevancies that can increase to loosened associations and flight of ideas. Some of these behaviors are evident in the next clinical example.

 ## CLINICAL EXAMPLE

Mr. B was a 30-year-old single man who was admitted to the psychiatric unit of the local community hospital. He had been hospitalized 2 years ago for problems related to alcoholism. He was accompanied to the hospital by a friend who lived with him. His friend said that for the past 2 months Mr. B had been "running on ten cylinders instead of four." He slept and ate little and talked constantly, sometimes so fast that no one could understand what he was trying to say. He had redecorated his bedroom in the apartment twice and had gone into debt buying a new wardrobe. His friend brought him in because his behavior was becoming more erratic and his physical condition was failing.

The nurse who admitted Mr. B asked about his social relationships. He revealed that his girlfriend of 7 years had left him 6 months ago for another man. He said that initially he thought she would "see the light," but she had refused to see him since then. Mr. B said this "upset" him a little at the time, but he was sure it was "for the best and there were plenty other women out there just waiting for him."

Selected Nursing Diagnosis:
▼ Potential for self-directed violence related to interpersonal rejection as evidenced by agitated behavior and lack of self-care activities

Other behaviors found in mania include lability of mood with rapid shifts to brief depression. Such behavior accounts for those patients who have loosened associations and alternately laugh and cry. In addition, hallucinations of any type, ideas of reference, and frank delusions may be present with predominant feelings of guilt and thoughts of suicide. Manic episodes have a high tendency toward recurrence. Only about 25% of manic patients have just one episode, and almost all those with manic episodes also have depressive episodes. However, the duration and severity of the manic episodes vary, as do the intervals between relapses and recurrences.

All these clinical examples illustrate the interrelatedness of disturbances of mood with self-esteem and disrupted relationships. Multiple aspects of the individual's life are affected, including physical health. Hypertensive crises, irritable bowel syndromes, coronary occlusions, rheumatoid arthritis, migraine headaches, and various dermatological conditions can occur with severe mood disturbances.

Predisposing Factors

Genetics. There is wide agreement that both heredity and environment play an important role in severe mood disturbances. Both bipolar and major depressive disorders run in families, but evidence for heritability is higher for bipolar disorder.
▼ One parent with bipolar disorder—25% chance in child
▼ Two parents with bipolar disorder—50% to 75% chance in child
▼ One monozygotic twin bipolar—40% to 70% chance in other twin
▼ One dizygotic twin bipolar—about 20% chance in other twins
▼ One parent with depressive disorder—10% to 13% chance in child

Studies using only familial aggregations, however, do not necessarily demonstrate the role of genetics, since disturbances may be the result of nutritional, infectious, or psychological factors. Some studies using genetic markers such as color blindness suggest that bipolar affective disorder is transmitted by an X-linked dominant gene. Controversy surrounds the mode of genetic transmission in affective disorders, however, since the findings from other studies contradict this hypothesis. Most recent research suggests there are different forms of genetic transmission.

Other evidence includes the following:

1. An increased frequency of the illness in relatives of the patient compared with the general population
2. A greater concordance rate in monozygotic twins than in dizygotic twins
3. An increased frequency of psychiatric abnormalities in relatives of the affective disorder patient than in the general population
4. Onset of the illness at a characteristic age with no evidence of a precipitating event

Thus good evidence exists for the role of genetic factors in affective disturbances.[48] Studies continue in this important area.

Aggression-Turned-Inward Theory. The aggression-turned-inward theory of Freud views depression as the inward turning of the aggressive instinct, for some reason not directed at the appropriate object and accompanied by feelings of guilt. The process is initiated by the loss of an ambivalently loved object. The person feels angry and loving at the same time and is unable to express anger because it is considered inappropriate or irrational. Also, the person may have developed a pattern throughout life of containing feelings, especially those that are viewed negatively. Angry feelings are then directed inward. Freud believed that if a person went so far as to commit suicide, the act was a strike against the hated and loved object as well as against the self.

Although it is one of the most widely quoted theories of depression, little systematic evidence substantiates it. Some researchers have identified depressed patients who outwardly express anger and hostility. Furthermore, the redirection of hostility at outside objects has not been consistently correlated with clinical improvement. In some instances it may actually have negative effects on the patient's view of self and problem resolution. It should therefore be viewed as one possible theory of causation that is not applicable to all people.

Object Loss Theory. The object loss theory of depression refers to traumatic separation of the person from significant objects of attachment. Two issues are important to this theory: loss during childhood as a predisposing factor for adult depressions and separation in adult life as a precipitating stress.

The first issue proposes that a child has ordinarily formed a tie to a mother figure by 6 months of age, and once that tie is ruptured, the child experiences separation anxiety, grief, and mourning. Furthermore, this mourning in the early years frequently affects personality development and predisposes the child to psychiatric illness.

Evidence for this model was first reported by Spitz[49]

in 1942 when he described a deprivational reaction in infants separated from their mothers at age 6 to 12 months. The reaction was characterized by apprehension, crying, withdrawal, psychomotor slowing, dejection, stupor, insomnia, anorexia, and gross retardation in growth and development. This syndrome is called *anaclitic depression*. A similar separation reaction was described by Robertson and Robertson[44] and Bowlby[10] in older children. They identified three stages of response:

1. A "protest" stage in which the child appeared restless and tearful and searched for his mother
2. A "despair" stage of apathetic withdrawal
3. A "detachment" stage seen in some children who rejected their mothers on reunion

From a research point of view, the connection between early object loss and adult depression is complex. Robertson and Robertson[44] cast doubt on the universality of the responses described and suggest that appropriate mothering during the separation period can prevent their occurrence. Some studies indicate that depressive patients seem to experience more parental loss from death, separation, and other causes than do normal and other diagnostic groups. However, that factor alone does not seem sufficiently universal to account for all forms of depression. There is even discussion about the beneficial or immunizing effects of having successfully coped with an early loss in the development of resilience.

Personality Organization Theory. Another view of depression focuses on the major psychosocial variable of low self-esteem. The patient's self-concept is an underlying issue, whether expressed as dejection and depression or overcompensated with an air of supreme competence, as displayed in manic and hypomanic episodes. Threats to self-esteem arise from poor role performance, perceived low-level everyday functioning, and the absence of a clear self-identity.

Three forms of personality organization that could lead to depression have been identified.[4] One, based on the "dominant other," occurs because the patient has relied on an esteemed other for self-esteem. Satisfaction is experienced only through an intermediary. Clinging, passivity, manipulativeness, and avoidance of anger characterize the person with this type of depression. There is a noticeable lack of personal goals and a predominant focus on problems.

Another form of personality results when a person realizes that a desired, but unrealistic, goal may never be accomplished. This is the "dominant goal" type of depression. This person is usually seclusive, arrogant, and often obsessive. The person sets unrealistic goals and evaluates them with an all-or-nothing standard. An inordinate amount of time is spent in wishful thinking and introverted searches for meaning.

The third type of depression is manifested as a constant mode of feeling. These patients "inhibit any form of gratification because of strongly held taboos." They experience emptiness, hypochondriasis, pettiness in interpersonal relationships, and a harsh critical attitude toward themselves and others.

This view of depression looks at patients' belief systems in relation to their experiences. Even in the absence of an apparent precipitating stressor, their depression appears to be preceded by a severe blow to their self-esteem. It emphasizes the crucial position of self-concept in adaptation or maladaptation, and the importance of patients' appraisal of their life situation.

Cognitive Model. The cognitive model of Beck[8] proposes that people experience depression because their thinking is disturbed. He proposes that depression is a cognitive problem dominated by a negative evaluation of self, the world, and the future. This theory is in contrast to others that propose depressive feelings are primary and the negative thinking is secondary. Beck suggests that in the course of development certain experiences sensitize individuals and make them vulnerable to depression. The person also acquires a tendency to make extreme, absolute judgments; loss is viewed as irrevocable and indifference as total rejection.

The depression-prone person, according to this theory, is likely to explain an adverse event as a personal shortcoming. For example, the deserted husband believes "She left me because I'm unlovable," instead of considering the other possible alternatives, such as personality incompatibility, the wife's own problems, or her change of feelings toward him. As he focuses on his personal deficiencies, they expand to the point where they completely dominate his self-concept. He can think of himself only in a negative way and is unable to acknowledge his other abilities, achievements, and attributes. This negative set is reinforced when he interprets ambiguous or neutral experiences as additional proof of his deficiencies. Comparisons with other people further lower his self-esteem, and thus every encounter with others becomes a negative experience. His self-criticisms increase as he views himself as deserving of blame.

Depressed patients become dominated by pessimism; they expect future adversities and experience them as though they were happening in the present or had already occurred. Their predictions tend to be overgeneralized and extreme. Since they view the future as an extension of the present, they expect their failure to continue permanently. Thus pessimism dominates their activities, wishes, and future expectations.

Depressed individuals are capable of logical self-evaluation when not in a depressed mood or when only mildly depressed. When depression does occur, after some precipitating life stressors, the negative cognitive set makes its appearance. As depression develops and increases, the negative thinking increasingly replaces objective thinking.

Although the onset of the depression may appear sudden, it really develops over weeks, months, or even years, as each experience is interpreted as further evidence of failure. As a result of this "tunnel vision," depressed individuals become hypersensitive to experiences of loss and defeat and oblivious to experiences of success and pleasure. They have difficulty acknowledging anger, since they think they are responsible for, and deserving of, insults from others and problems in living. Along with low self-esteem, they experience apathy and indifference. They are drawn to a state of inactivity and withdraw from life. They lack all spontaneous desire and only wish to remain passive. Because they expect failure, they lack the ordinary energy to make an effort.

Suicidal wishes can be viewed as an extreme expression of the desire to escape. Suicidal patients see their life as filled with suffering, with no chance of improvement. Given this negative set, suicide seems a rational solution. It promises to end their misery and relieve their families of a burden, and they begin to believe that everyone would be better off if they were dead. The more they consider the alternative of suicide, the more desirable it may seem, and as their life becomes more hopeless and painful, their desires become stronger to end their life. Naturalistic, clinical, and experimental studies have provided substantial support for this model of depression.

 Relate the cognitive model of depression to the adage "mind over matter."

Learned Helplessness-Hopelessness Model. The learned helplessness-hopelessness model was first proposed by Seligman[47] in 1975. He defined helplessness as a "belief that no one will do anything to aid you" and hopelessness as a belief that neither "you nor anyone else can do anything." This theory proposes that it is not trauma per se that produces depression, but the belief that the individual has no control over the important outcomes in life and therefore refrains from adaptive responses. Learned helplessness is both a behavioral state and a personality trait of a person who believes that control has been lost over the reinforcers in the environment. These negative expectations lead to hopelessness, passivity, and an inability to assert oneself.

Seligman suggests that people resistant to depression have experienced mastery in life. Their childhood experiences proved that their actions were effective in producing gratification and removing annoyances. In contrast, those susceptible to depression have had lives devoid of mastery. Their experiences proved that they were helpless to influence their sources of suffering and gratification or they controlled too many reinforcers that did not allow for the development of their coping responses against failure.

In the past 20 years this model has undergone considerable revision. It was reformulated in 1978[2] and again in 1989.[1] The last revision produced the hopelessness theory of depression. This revision suggests that inferred negative consequences and negative characteristics about the self contribute to the formation of hopelessness and, in turn, the symptoms of hopelessness depression. Hopelessness theory now bears a strong similarity to Beck's cognitive model of depression previously described. The hopelessness model is also proposed as a sufficient, but not necessary, condition for depression. Other physiological and psychological factors can produce symptoms of depression in the absence of an expectation of uncontrollability. Finally, it must be emphasized that the model is still being empirically validated.

Behavioral Model. The behavioral model studied by Lewinsohn, Youngren, and Grosscup[34] is derived from a social learning theory framework in which the cause of depression is related to the person-behavior-environment interaction. Social learning theory assumes that psychological functioning can best be understood in terms of continuous reciprocal interactions among personal factors. These include cognitive processes, behavioral factors, and environmental factors, all operating as interdependent determinants of one another. The relative influences exerted by these interdependent factors differ in various settings and for different behaviors.

This theory views people as capable of exercising considerable control over their own behavior. They do not merely react to external influences. They select, organize, and transform incoming stimuli. Thus people are not viewed as powerless objects controlled by their environments, but neither are they absolutely free to do whatever they choose. Rather, people and their environment have a mutual effect on each other.

The concept of reinforcement is crucial to this view of depression. Person-environment interactions with positive outcomes provide positive reinforcement. Such interactions strengthen the person's behavior. Little or no rewarding interaction with the environment causes the person to feel sad or blue. Thus the key assumption in this model is that a low rate of positive reinforcement is the antecedent of depressive behaviors.

Two particular variables are important. One is that the individual may fail to provide appropriate responses to initiate positive reinforcement. The other is that the environment may fail to provide reinforcement and thus worsen the patient's condition. These variables are often apparent, since depressed patients have been shown to be deficient in the social skills needed to interact effectively. In turn, other people find the behavior of depressed individuals distancing, negative, or offensive and often avoid them as much as possible.

Depression is likely to occur if certain positively reinforcing events are absent; particularly those which fall into the following categories:
- ▼ Positive sexual experiences
- ▼ Rewarding social interaction
- ▼ Enjoyable outdoor activities
- ▼ Solitude
- ▼ Competence experiences

These may be described as "being sexually attractive," "being with friends," "being relaxed," "doing my job well," and "doing things my own way." Depression also occurs in the presence of certain punishing events, particularly those that fall into three categories:
- ▼ Marital or interpersonal discord
- ▼ Work or school hassles
- ▼ Receiving negative reactions from others

This model of depression emphasizes an active, rather than passive, approach to the person and relies heavily on an interactional view of personality. Treatment is aimed at assisting the person to increase the quantity and quality of positively reinforcing interactions and to decrease aversive interactions.

 How many positive reinforcing events have you experienced this month? How many punishing events? Relate these to your overall mood.

Biological Model. Another major area of research on depression involves a biological model, which explores chemical changes in the body during depressed states. The biology of depression is discussed in detail in Chapter 5. Whether these chemical changes cause depression or are a result of depression is not yet understood. However, significant abnormalities can be demonstrated in many body systems during a depressive illness. These include electrolyte disturbances, especially of sodium and potassium; neurophysiological alterations; dysfunction and faulty regulation of autonomic nervous system activity; adrenocortical, thyroid, and gonadal changes;

and neurochemical alterations in the neurotransmitters, especially in the biogenic amines, which serve as central nervous system and peripheral neurotransmitters. The biogenic amines include three catecholamines—dopamine, norepinephrine, and epinephrine—as well as serotonin and acetylcholine. From the early catecholamine theory to the theory of hypersensitive neurotransmitter receptors, most researchers agree that no single biochemical model adequately explains the affective disorders.[22]

ENDOCRINE DYSFUNCTION. The possibility of hormonal causes of depression has been considered for many years. Some symptoms of depression that suggest endocrine changes are decreased appetite, weight loss, insomnia, diminished sex drive, gastrointestinal disorders, and variations of mood. New assay techniques have recently detected alterations of hormone activity concurrent with depression. Mood changes have also been observed with a variety of endocrine disorders, including Cushing's disease, hyperthyroidism, and estrogen therapy. Further support for this theory is evident in the high incidence of depression during the postpartum period, when hormonal levels change.

Current study of neuroendocrine factors in affective disorders emphasize the disinhibition of the hypothalamic-pituitary-adrenal (HPA) axis and the hypothalamic-pituitary-thyroid (HPT) axis. Two tests based on the neuroendocrine theory and performed clinically may prove to be useful in diagnosing affective illnesses. The first is the corticotropin-releasing factor stimulation test that evaluates the pituitary's ability to respond to corticotropin-releasing hormone (CRH) and secrete sufficient amounts of adrenal corticotropin hormone (ACTH) to induce normal adrenal activity. The second test is the thyroid-releasing hormone (TRH) infusion test that differs from the CRH infusion by assessing the pituitary's ability to secrete sufficient amounts of thyroid-stimulating hormones (TSH) to produce normal thyroid activity. These tests may be helpful in differentiating unipolar from bipolar depression and mania from schizophrenic psychosis.

CORTISOL. Many depressed patients exhibit hypersecretion of cortisol; this has been used in the dexamethasone suppression test (DST) (dexamethasone is an exogenous steroid that suppresses the blood level of cortisol). The DST is based on the observation that, in patients with biological depression, late afternoon cortisol levels are not suppressed after a single dose of dexamethasone. However, many physical illnesses and some medications can interfere with the test results.

BIOLOGICAL RHYTHMS. Mood disorders are also typified by periodic variations in physiological and psycho-

logical functions. Affective illnesses are usually recurrent, with episodes often occurring and remitting spontaneously. Two subtypes of mood disorders are specifically cyclical in nature: rapid cycling bipolar disorder and depressive disorder with seasonal patterns.[9,38] In the first, cycles may be days, weeks, months, or years. In seasonal affective disorder, cycles occur annually at the same time each year, as individuals react to changes in environmental factors such as climate, latitude, or light.

People who are depressed or manic have certain characteristic changes in biological rhythms and related physiology. For instance, body temperature and certain hormones reach their peak earlier than normal; some depressed patients are more sensitive to the absence of sunlight than nondepressed persons; many depressed people describe circadian rhythm disturbances, such as diurnal variation and early morning awakening. All-night sleep studies of depressed patients show some basic abnormalities. Sleep problems associated with depression have to do with the timing of rapid eye movement (REM) sleep. The strongest finding is that REM sleep begins too early in the night (Fig. 17-2). It also lasts too long—up to twice as long as the first REM period in nondepressed individuals. This finding may help to explain why patients report feeling tired even after a night's sleep. There is also decreased total sleep time, an increased percentage of dream time, difficulty in falling asleep, and an increased number of spontaneous awakenings. These and other findings in the area of bio-

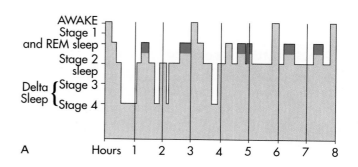

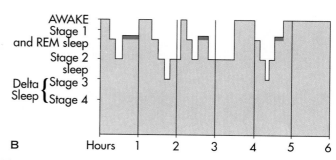

Fig. 17-2 **A,** Normal sleep architecture. **B,** Depressed sleep architecture.

logical rhythmicity may prove to be valuable diagnostic tools for depression.

Research on the biological model has been extensive and of high quality. It has lent support to a biological basis for mood disorders and suggested biological markers of clinical usefulness in diagnosis and treatment. The discovery of neuropharmacological abnormalities is neither surprising nor precludes psychological causes. Furthermore, a biochemical model based on one amine is undoubtedly an oversimplification. Research in this model of depression is conflicting at times. Sufficient evidence suggests that a variety of precipitating stressors can induce changes in biogenic amines. The neuropharmacological mechanisms investigated might form final common pathways for both psychological and biological causes. Some depressions might be caused primarily by neuropharmacological dysfunctions, resulting in reduced norepinephrine levels. Others might result from events whose psychological effect would presumably have similar neurophysiological phenomena, resulting in reduced release of norepinephrine. In other cases, both effects might apply, the life event tipping the balance more easily into depression because activity of the norepinephrine-producing system was already reduced. Some of the biological bases depression are shown in Fig. 17-3.

> Your pastor preaches about how depression results from "poor moral character" and "personal weakness." How would you respond?

Precipitating Stressors

Disturbances of mood are a specific response to stress. Two major types of stress exist. The first is the stress of major life events that is evident to other persons. The second type, the minor stress or irritations of daily life, may not be obvious to others. These are the small disappointments, frustrations, criticisms, and arguments that, when accumulated over time and in the absence of compensating positive events, produce a major and chronic negative impact. Stressors that may produce disturbances of mood include loss of attachment, major life events, roles, and physiological changes.

Loss of Attachment. Loss in adult life can precipitate depression. The loss may be real or imagined and may include the loss of love, a person, physical functioning, status, or self-esteem. Many losses take on importance because of their symbolic meaning, which makes the reactions to them appear out of proportion to reality. In this sense, even an apparently pleasurable event, such as moving to a new home, may involve the loss of old friends, warm memories, and neighborhood associations. Loss of hope is another significant stressor often overlooked. Because of the actual and symbolic elements involved in loss, the patient's perception takes on primary importance.

The individual is constantly experiencing losses and thus struggling with integrating them. The intensity of grief becomes meaningful only when the person understands earlier losses and separations. Persons reacting to a recent loss often behave as they did in previous separations. The intensity of the present reaction therefore becomes more understandable with the realization that the reaction is to earlier losses as well. By definition loss is negative, a deprivation. The ability to sustain, integrate, and recover from loss, however, is a sign of personal maturity and growth.

Uncomplicated grief reactions are the process of normal mourning or simple bereavement. Mourning includes a complex sequence of psychological processes. It is accompanied by anxiety, anger, pain, despair, and hope. The sequence is not a smooth, unvarying course, however; it is filled with turmoil, regressions, and potential problems. Certain factors have been identified that influence the outcome of mourning (Box 17-2).

These should be assessed by the nurse for each person experiencing a loss. Two of the factors—the nature of the relationship with the lost person or object and the mourner's perception of the preventability of the loss—have been identified as prime predictors of the intensity and duration of the bereavement. Concurrent crises, the circumstances of the loss, and a pathological relationship with the lost person or object are other factors that contribute to a failure to resolve grief.

INHIBITING FACTORS. Loss of a loved one is a major stressor for grief reactions. Most individuals resolve this loss through simple bereavement and do not experience pathological grief or depression. Various external and

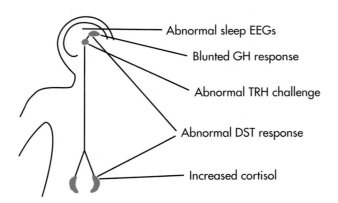

Fig. 17-3   Biologic factors related to depression.

internal factors, however, can inhibit mourning. An external factor may be the immersion of the mourner in practical, necessary tasks that accompany the loss but are not directly connected to the emotional fact of the loss. These tasks may include funeral arrangements, unfinished business of the deceased, or a search for immediate employment. All these tasks foster denial of the loss. Denial also may be encouraged by cultural norms that minimize or negate the finality of the loss. The American norm of "courage in the face of adversity" can prevent the mourner from an open display of grief.

Mourning may also be inhibited when the bereaved lack support from their social network. Nonsupportiveness suppresses grieving when significant others inhibit mourners' expression of sadness, anger, and guilt; block their review of the lost relationship; and attempt to orient them too quickly to the future. Finally, the widespread use of tranquilizers and antidepressant medications may suppress normal grief and encourage pathological reactions.

Internal factors that inhibit mourning are often fostered by a society that encourages the control and hiding of feelings. Crying, for example, may be seen as weakness, especially in men. Two emotions are particularly repressed in our society—grief and anger—and this may create many emotional problems. Another inhibitor is the belief that the quantity and quality of emotion is so unique it cannot be communicated. Both these factors lead to suppression of mourning.

In concluding this discussion of loss as a precipitating stressor, it is necessary to place it in proper perspective based on research. Some studies have failed to demonstrate a relationship between loss and depression. Other studies support the relationship but suggest that depression may be the cause of alienation and object loss, and not vice versa. Thus the following conclusions may be proposed:

1. Loss and separation events are possible precipitating stressors of depression.
2. Loss and separation are not present in all depressions.
3. Not all people who experience loss and separation will develop depressions.
4. Loss and separation are not specific to depression but may serve as precipitating events for a variety of psychiatric and medical illnesses.
5. Loss and separation may result from depression.

Life Events. Research conducted on life events and depression reveals that, on the average, depressed patients reported almost three times as many important life events during the 6 months before onset of clinical depressive episode as did normal subjects. The events included loss of self-esteem, interpersonal discord, socially undesirable occurrences, and major disruptions of life patterns. Those events perceived as undesirable were most often the precipitants of depression. Analysis of the data showed that exit events (separations and losses) more frequently than entrance events (additions and introductions) were followed by worsening of psychiatric symptoms, physical health changes, impairment of social role performance, and depressive illnesses in particular. The concept of exit events overlaps with the psychiatric concept of loss.

Certain types of events may also prove to be more important than others. For example, childhood physical and sexual abuse has been found to be associated with high depressive symptoms in women.[20] Similarly, Stuart and co-workers[51] researched the early childhood experiences of women with depression in comparison with women who were free of psychiatric diagnosis. They found that the depressed women experienced both parents as rejecting and perceived less warmth from their fathers; described less rational discussion in the resolution of family conflict; experienced significant separation anxiety as children; and grew up in households with more deaths and chronic physical illness. Nursing studies such as this one will assist nurses in understanding the personal world of the depressed person and organizing their observations regarding the depressed person's logic and thinking in a way that best promotes recovery.

Most psychiatric clinicians are convinced that a relationship does exist between stressful life events and depression. Some believe that life events play the primary role in depression; others limit the role of life events to that of contributing to the onset and timing of the acute

---

Box 17-2

FACTORS THAT INFLUENCE THE MOURNING PROCESS

Childhood experiences, especially the loss of significant others

Losses experienced later in life

Previous history of psychiatric illness, especially depression

Life crises before the loss

Nature of the relationship with the lost person or object, including kinship, strength of attachment, security of attachment, dependency-independency bonds, and intensity of ambivalence

Process of dying (when applicable), including age of deceased, timeliness, previous warnings, preparation for bereavement, expression of feelings, and preventability of the loss

Social support systems

Secondary stresses

Emergent life opportunities

episode. Any definitive conclusions, however, should be made with caution. All people experience stressful life events, but not all people become depressed. This suggests that specific events can contribute only partially to the development of depression.

Roles. It is possible to analyze social role stressors in detail. It becomes obvious in doing so that much of the literature focuses on women. This reflects the predominance of depression among women and the increasing interest in gender socialization processes and women's changing roles.[46] Role strain in marriage emerges as a major stressor related to depression for both men and women. In a classic study Gove[17] examined the rates of mental illness among married men and women. He found higher rates of mental illness for married women, whereas single, divorced, and widowed women have lower rates than men. From this he concluded that being married has a protective effect for males but a detrimental effect for females.

Another explanation for differing rates of mental illness, particularly depression, between men and women may be the role strain inherent in parenting. Additional research also shows that married career women have, or need, supportive husbands. The nature of this support, however, is not clearly described. Much of the literature on two-career families directly documents the additive nature of the mother's role, that is, the assumption of a career in addition to her domestic role.[21]

In a nursing research study, Woods[57] explored employment, family roles, and mental health in young married women. She found that the number of women's roles was not associated with poorer mental health and that no clear relationship existed between employment or parenting and mental health. She did find, however, that women who had traditional sex roles, little task-sharing support from a spouse, and little support from a confidant had poorer mental health than their counterparts. In addition, for women who were both spouse and parent, support from a confidant was most important. Task-sharing support was the most important for women who were employed but not parents. Nontraditional sex role norms had the most important protective effects for women who had multiple roles as spouse, employee, and mother. Clearly, the relationship between role strain and depression merits further exploration.

Describe how the early socialization of young girls in contemporary society might affect their cognitive and emotional coping responses. Compare this to the experiences of young boys.

Physiological Changes. Mood may also respond to drugs or a wide variety of physical illnesses (Table 17-6). Drug-induced depressions can follow treatment with antihypertensive drugs, particularly reserpine, and the abuse of addictive substances such as amphetamines, barbiturates, cocaine, and alcohol. Depression may also occur secondary to medical illnesses, for example, viral infections, nutritional deficiencies, endocrine disorders, anemias, and central nervous system disorders such as multiple sclerosis, tumors, and cerebrovascular disease. Most chronic debilitating illnesses, whether physical or psychiatric, are accompanied by depression.

The depressions of the elderly are particularly complex because the differential diagnosis often involves organic brain damage and clinical depression.[40] Diagnostic differentiation is complicated. Persons with early signs of senile brain changes, vascular disease, or other neurological diseases of aging may be more at risk for depression than the general population. In the United States there has been a tendency to overdiagnose arteriosclerosis and senility in persons over age 65, without recognizing that depression may manifest itself by a slowing of psychomotor activity. Lowered intellectual function and a loss of interest in sex, hobbies, and activities may be taken as signs of brain disease.

Mania can also be secondary to drugs, particularly steroids, amphetamines, and tricyclic antidepressants. It can be triggered by infections, neoplasms, and metabolic disturbances. The evidence that mania can result from pharmacological, structural, and metabolic disturbances suggests that mania, as with depression, is a clinical syndrome with multiple causes. The diversity of causes probably involves more than one pathophysiological pathway and challenges any one model of causation, whether biochemical, psychological, genetic, or structural.

Integrative Model. Debate continues throughout psychiatry over the nature of depression, that is, whether depression is a single illness with different signs and symptoms or whether several diseases exist. This discussion of the various models or theories of causation also suggests the controversies in psychiatric research and practice. Each theory contributes to an understanding of mood disturbances. Many of them overlap and interrelate. Recent research also clearly shows that there are multiple causes for mood disturbances. These involve an interactive effect among predisposing and precipitating factors that are biological and psychosocial in origin.[29] Thus a unitary theory is not possible, but perhaps a unified theory is. Table 17-7 summarizes these major theories on causation.

Whybrow, Akiskal, and McKinney[55] describe a unified model of mood disorders that integrates current con-

Table 17-6   Physical Illnesses and Drugs Associated with Depressive and Manic States

	Depression	Mania
Infectious	Influenza Viral hepatitis Infectious mononucleosis General paresis (tertiary syphilis) Tuberculosis	Influenza St. Louis encephalitis Q fever General paresis (tertiary syphilis)
Endocrine	Myxedema Cushing's disease Addison's disease Diabetes mellitus	Hyperthyroidism?
Neoplastic	Occult abdominal maligiancies (e.g., carcinoma of head of pancreas) Carcinoid Oat cell carcinoma	
Collagen	Systemic lupus erythematosus	Systemic lupus erythematosus Rheumatic chorea
Neurological	Multiple sclerosis Cerebral tumors Sleep apnea Dementia Parkinson's disease Nondominant temporal lobe lesions	Multiple sclerosis Diencephalic and third ventricular tumors
Cardiovascular	Stroke Coronary artery disease	
Nutritional	Pellagra Pernicious anemia	
Drugs	Steroidal contraceptives Reserpine Alpha-methyldopa Propranolol Glucocorticoids Cycloserine Physostigmine Alcohol Sedative-hypnotics Amphetamine withdrawal Benzodiazepines Neuroleptics	Steroids Levodopa Amphetamines Methylphenidate Cocaine Monoamine oxidase inhibitors Tricyclic antidepressants Thyroid hormones

ceptual models. They view depression as the interaction of three sets of variables at the chemical, experiential, and behavioral levels, with the diencephalon serving as the field of action. They propose that impairment in one of the variables affects the other two. Thus any one of the three variables can contribute to a depression and produce changes in the other two areas. For example, a chemical imbalance can result in distorted perceptions, or a major life change can cause a chemical imbalance. In this model, depressive illness is the interaction of various processes in those areas of the diencephalon modulating arousal, mood, motivation, and psychomotor functions. As depicted in Fig. 17-4, the form the illness takes depends on the following factors:

1. Genetic vulnerability—important, particularly in recurrent and manic-depressive illnesses
2. Developmental events—early object loss that may sensitize the individual to future stress, create negative cognitive sets, and result in learned helplessness
3. Physiological stressors—stimuli such as viral infections and childbirth that induce biochemical changes
4. Psychosocial stressors—stressful life events that overwhelm coping mechanisms

This integrative multicausal model presents a useful frame of reference for the nurse. It is holistic and encourages the assessment of behavior in developing

Table 17-7 Summary of Models of Causation of Severe Mood Disturbances

Model	Mechanism
Genetic	Transmission through hereditary and family history
Aggression turned inward	Turning of angry feelings inward against oneself
Object loss	Separation from loved one and disruption of attachment bond
Personality organization	Negative self-concept and low self-esteem influence belief system and appraisal of stressors
Cognitive	Hopelessness experienced because of negative cognitive set
Learned helplessness-hopelessness	Belief that responses are ineffectual and that reinforcers in the environment cannot be controlled
Behavioral	Loss of positive reinforcement in life
Biological	Impaired monoaminergic neurotransmission
Life stressors	Response to life stress from five possible sources: loss of attachment, major life events, roles, coping resources, and physiological changes
Integrative	Interaction of chemical, experiential, and behavioral variables acting on the diencephalon

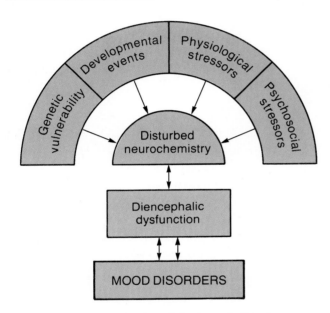

Fig. 17-4   Unified model of mood disorders.

nursing interventions. It also presents a variety of causative factors and stresses their interrelationship in explaining present behavior.

Coping Resources

Personal resources available to individuals include their socioeconomic status (income, occupation, social position, education), families (nuclear, extended), interpersonal networks, and the secondary organizations provided by the broader social environment (see A Family Speaks). The far-ranging effects of poverty, discrimination, inadequate housing, and social isolation cannot be ignored or taken lightly.

Research has clearly linked social support to depression. One study found subjective social support was

 A FAMILY SPEAKS

It's hard for me to imagine how life could be so bad that my beautiful and loving 22-year-old daughter couldn't get out of bed in the morning and cried most of the day. It all started when she quit college and returned home and told us about the biggest mistake she had made in her life. While at school, she accidentally got pregnant and then had an abortion. Since that event, she said she felt worthless, immoral, and extremely guilty.

We talked about it, and I suggested she get help. She saw two different mental health professionals but dropped out of therapy with each one after only a couple of visits. Then one of my friends recommended a nurse who specialized in working with women with depression. My daughter saw her twice a week initially, then once a week, and finally monthly. My daughter was able to open up to this nurse and together they worked at correcting my daughter's negative thoughts, feelings, and behaviors. She kept a diary and began to call friends and socialize.

Today, 8 months later, my daughter has a job and is going to college part-time in the evenings. Sometimes when I look at her, she seems like a different person to me—so much more grown up and mature. I'm sorry for her pain, but I know that now she is a stronger and wiser person for having endured it. ▾

most strongly associated with a positive outcome in depressive illness.[15] Another nursing study among older adults reported that poor physical health and lack of mastery, social resources, and economic resources were significant predictors of depression.[5] A final nursing study also linked depression with coping resources. Specifically, the four subgroups of social support, confidence, problem-solving ability, and tension reduction all showed a strong negative relationship with depression in hospitalized men and women.[19] Such research suggests the importance of nursing interventions that foster the person's ability to develop capacities for coping with life's disruptions. The risk factors for depression are listed in Box 17-3.

Coping Mechanisms

Uncomplicated grief reactions can be normal mourning or simple bereavement. Mourning includes all the psychological processes set in motion by the loss. Mourning begins with the introjection of the lost object. When grieving, the person's feelings are directed to a mental image of the loved one. Thus the mechanism of introjection serves as a buffering mechanism. Through reality testing, the individual realizes that the love object no longer exists, and then the emotional investment is withdrawn from it. The ultimate outcome is that reality wins out, but this is accomplished slowly over time. When the mourning work is completed, the ego becomes free to invest in new objects.

A delayed grief reaction uses the defense mechanisms of denial and suppression in an attempt to avoid intense distress. Specific defenses used to block mourning are repression, suppression, denial, and dissociation. Denial of the loss in depression results in profound feelings of guilt, anger, and despair that focus on the person's own unworthiness. Manic and hypomanic episodes occur more rarely than depressive states. Some believe that mania is a mirror image of depression and that, even though the behaviors are dissimilar, the dynamics and coping mechanisms are related. According to this view, manic behavior is a defense against depression, since the individual attempts to deny feelings of worthlessness and helplessness.

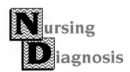 **Nursing Diagnosis**

The diagnosis of disturbances of mood depends on an understanding of many interrelated concepts, including anxiety and self-concept. One task of the nurse in formulating a diagnosis is to decide if the patient is experiencing primarily a state of anxiety (see Chapter 14) or depression. It is often difficult to distinguish between the two because they may coexist in one patient and are manifested by similar behaviors.

▼ The depressed patient is often slowed down in speech and movements.
▼ The anxious patient often responds normally or actively.

Box 17-3
RISK FACTORS FOR DEPRESSION

▼ Prior episodes of depression
▼ Family history of depression
▼ Prior suicide attempts
▼ Female gender
▼ Age of onset <40 years
▼ Postpartum period
▼ Medical comorbidity
▼ Lack of social support
▼ Stressful life events
▼ Personal history of sexual abuse
▼ Current substance abuse

▼ The depressed patient is reluctant to discuss problems or symptoms.
▼ The anxious patient is more likely to discuss symptoms and related topics.
▼ The depressed patient has decreased outside interests.
▼ The anxious patient usually retains interest in some things.
▼ The depressed patient has difficulty enjoying things.
▼ The anxious patient can enjoy some activities.
▼ The depressed patient usually feels worse in the morning or after sleep.
▼ The anxious patient usually feels worse in the evening and better after sleep or rest.
▼ The depressed patient usually has decreased appetite and enjoyment of food.
▼ The anxious patient usually eats intermittently and enjoys at least some foods.

Fig. 17-5 presents a stress adaptation model with the continuum of emotional responses. The maladaptive responses are a result of anxiety, hostility, self-devaluation, and guilt. This model suggests that nursing care will be centered around increasing self-esteem and encouraging expression of emotions.

The primary NANDA nursing diagnoses related to maladaptive emotional responses are dysfunctional grieving, hopelessness, powerlessness, spiritual distress, and potential for self-directed violence. Nursing diagnoses related to the range of possible maladaptive responses are identified in the Medical and Nursing Diagnoses box on p. 433. Examples of complete nursing diagnoses are presented in the Detailed Diagnoses box on p. 434.

 How does "spiritual distress" relate to mood disorders?

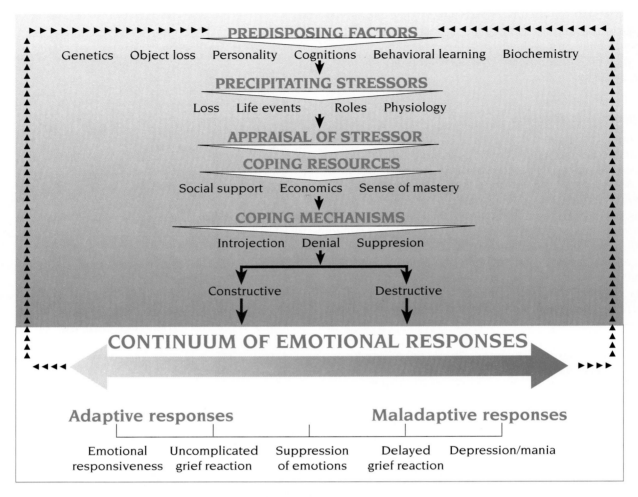

Fig. 17-5   A stress adaptation model related to emotional responses.

Related Medical Diagnoses

The psychiatric classification of affective disorders has largely reflected the controversies surrounding the nature, cause, and treatment of these disorders. Although these traditional labels are no longer used in the DSM-IV,[3] nurses know them because they may continue to have some research and clinical value.

One traditional distinction has been to separate patients into those with **psychotic versus neurotic affective states.** Unfortunately, these terms have acquired multiple meanings and have lost their precision in defining clinical or research practice. Another traditional distinction has been between **endogenous versus reactive, or exogenous, types of depression.** Endogenous depressions were believed to have resulted from early personality development and intrinsic biological processes, whereas exogenous, or reactive, types were believed to have occurred in response to external environmental stress, such as recent loss or disappoint-

ment. Research, however, has failed to verify these distinctions. Thus the psychotic-neurotic distinction and the endogenous-reactive dichotomy are better regarded as continuums along which patients may be placed. Most patients are intermediate on the continuum and few are at the extremes. Neither classification is used in the DSM-IV.

Another distinction has been made between **primary** and **secondary affective disorders** based on two criteria, chronology and the presence of associated illnesses. "Primary" affective disorders occur in patients who have been well or whose only previous episodes of psychiatric disease were mania or depression. "Secondary" affective disorders include feelings of sadness, inadequacy, and hopelessness that occur with another preexisting psychiatric disorder, such as anxiety reactions. It also includes symptoms secondary to medical illnesses.

A final distinction is the **bipolar-unipolar affective**

MEDICAL AND NURSING DIAGNOSES RELATED TO EMOTIONAL RESPONSES

RELATED MEDICAL DIAGNOSES (DSM-IV)*
Bipolar I disorder
Bipolar II disorder
Cyclothymic disorder
Major depressive disorder
Dysthymic disorder

RELATED NURSING DIAGNOSES (NANDA)†
Anxiety
Communication, impaired verbal
Coping, ineffective individual
Grieving, anticipatory
‡**Grieving, dysfunctional**
‡**Hopelessness**
Injury, potential for
Nutrition, altered
‡**Powerlessness**
Self-care deficit
Self-esteem disturbance
Sexual dysfunction
Sleep pattern disturbance
Social isolation
‡**Spiritual distress (distress of the human spirit)**
Thought processes, altered
‡**Violence, potential for self-directed**

*From American Psychiatric Association: *Diagnostic and statistical manual of mental disorders*, ed 4, Washington, DC, 1994, The Association.
†From North American Nursing Diagnosis Association: NANDA *nursing diagnoses: definitions and classifications* 1992-1993, Philadelphia, 1992, The Association.
‡Primary nursing diagnosis for disturbances in mood.

states. It proposes the separation of depressed patients with a history of manic episodes (the bipolar group) from those who have had only recurrent episodes of depression (the unipolar group). Among newer approaches, the bipolar-unipolar distinction has achieved considerable acceptance.[56]

Two major categories of mood or affective disorders are identified in the DSM-IV: bipolar disorders and depressive (unipolar) disorders (see the Medical and Nursing Diagnoses box above). The specific disorders are described in the Detailed Diagnoses box on p. 434. Diagnostic criteria for a major depressive episode and a manic episode are listed in Box 17-4.

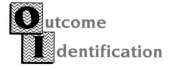

Outcome Identification

The expected outcome when working with a patient with a maladaptive emotional response is

The patient will be emotionally responsive and return to a pre-illness level of functioning.

Goals of nursing care for patients with severe mood disturbance have the following aims:

1. To allow for recognition and continuous expression of feelings, including denial, hopelessness, anger, guilt, blame, helplessness, regret, hope, and relief, within a supportive therapeutic atmosphere
2. To allow for gradual analysis of stressors while strengthening the patient's self-esteem
3. To increase the patient's sense of identity, control, awareness of choices, and responsibility for behavior
4. To encourage healthy interpersonal ties with others
5. To promote understanding of maladaptive emotions and to acquire adaptive coping responses to stressors

Specific short-term goals should be generated from behaviors of the patient, present areas of difficulty, and relevant stressors. Goal setting should involve a holistic view of the patient and the patient's world. Goals probably will need to be developed regarding the patient's self-concept, physical status, behavioral performance, expression of emotions, and relationships. All these areas can directly relate to the disturbance of mood. Patient participation in setting these goals can be a significant first step in helping patients to regain mastery over their life.

DETAILED DIAGNOSES
RELATED TO EMOTIONAL RESPONSES

NANDA DIAGNOSIS STEM	EXAMPLES OF COMPLETE DIAGNOSIS
Dysfunctional grieving	Dysfunctional grieving related to death of sister as evidenced by self-devaluation, sleep disturbance, and dejected mood
Hopelessness	Hopelessness related to loss of job as evidenced by feelings of despair and development of ulcerative colitis
Powerlessness	Powerlessness related to new role as parent as evidenced by apathy, uncertainty, and overdependency
Spiritual distress	Spiritual distress related to loss of child in utero as evidenced by self-blame, somatic complaints, and pessimism about the future
Potential for self-directed violence	Potential for self-directed violence related to rejection by boyfriend as evidenced by self-destructive acts

DSM-IV DIAGNOSIS	ESSENTIAL FEATURES*
Bipolar I disorder	Current or past experience of a manic episode, lasting at least 1 week, when one's mood was abnormally and persistently elevated, expansive, or irritable. The episode is sufficiently severe to cause extreme impairment in social or occupational functioning. Bipolar disorders may be classified as manic (limited to only manic episodes), depressed (a history of manic episodes with a current depressive episode), or mixed (a mixed presentation of both manic and depressive episodes).
Bipolar II disorder	Presence or history of one or more major depressive episodes and at least one hypomanic episode. There has never been a manic episode.
Cyclothymic disorder	A history of 2 years of hypomania in which the person experienced numerous periods with abnormally elevated, expansive, or irritable moods. These moods did not meet the criteria for a manic episode, and many periods of depressed mood did not meet the criteria of a major depressive episode.
Major depressive disorder	Presence of at least five symptoms during the same 2-week period, with one being either depressed mood or loss of interest or pleasure. Other symptoms might include weight loss, insomnia, psychomotor agitation or retardation, fatigue, feelings of worthlessness, diminished ability to think, and recurrent thoughts of death. Major depressions may be classified as single episode or recurrent.
Dysthymic disorder	At least 2 years of a usually depressed mood and at least one of the symptoms mentioned for major depression without meeting the criteria for a major depressive episode.

*Adapted from the American Psychatric Association: *Diagnostic and statistical manual of mental disorders*, ed 4, Washington, DC, 1994, The Association.

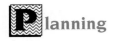

Planning

In planning care the nurse's priorities are the reduction and ultimate removal of the patient's maladaptive emotional responses, restoration of the patient's occupational and psychosocial functioning, improvement in the patient's quality of life, and minimization of the likelihood of relapse and recurrence. To achieve this, treatment consists of three phases: (1) acute, (2) continuation, and (3) maintenance (Fig 17-6).[32]

Acute Treatment Phase

The goal of acute treatment is to eliminate the symptoms. If patients improve with treatment, they are said to have had a **response**. A successful acute treatment brings patients back to an essentially symptom-free state and to a level of functioning comparable to before the illness. This phase usually lasts 6 to 12 weeks, and if patients are symptom-free at the end of that time, they are then in **remission.**

Box 17-4
DIAGNOSTIC CRITERIA FOR MAJOR DEPRESSION AND A MANIC EPISODE

MAJOR DEPRESSION

At least five of the following (including one of the first two) must be present most of the day, nearly daily, for at least 2 weeks:

1. **Depressed mood**
2. **Loss of interest or pleasure**
3. Weight loss or gain
4. Insomnia or hypersomnia
5. Psychomotor agitation or retardation
6. Fatigue or loss of energy
7. Feelings of worthlessness
8. Impaired concentration
9. Thoughts of death or suicide

MANIC EPISODE

At least three of the following must be present to a significant degree for at least 1 week:

1. Grandiosity
2. Decreased need for sleep
3. Pressured speech
4. Flight of ideas
5. Distractibility
6. Psychomotor agitation
7. Excessive involvement in pleasurable activities without regard for negative consequences

---

Continuation Treatment Phase

The goal of continuation treatment is to prevent **relapse,** which is the return of symptoms. The risk of relapse is very high in the first 4 to 6 months after recovery, and one of the greatest mistakes in the treatment of mood disorders is the failure to continue a successful treatment for a long enough time. This phase usually lasts 4 to 9 months.

Maintenance Treatment Phase

The goal of maintenance treatment is to prevent the **recurrence,** or return, of a new episode of illness. This concept is commonly accepted for bipolar illness, but it is a relatively new one for major depressive disorders. Nonetheless, a few research studies point out the effectiveness of maintenance therapy in preventing new episodes or lengthening the time interval between them.

Understanding the phases of treatment for mood disorders is critically important. The nurse should discuss them with the patient and family so that they may join in the therapeutic alliance and have clear expectations about the goals and course of treatment.

 Your patient tells you she stopped taking her medicine after 2 months because she was "feeling better." What would you tell her based on your understanding of the treatment phases of depression?

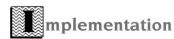mplementation

Maladaptive emotional responses may emerge at unpredicted moments, can vary in intensity from mild to severe, and can be transitory, recurrent, or more stable conditions. Episodes of depression and mania can occur in any setting and can arise in conjunction with existing medical problems. Also, the treatment of mood disturbances can take place in various settings—at home, at an outpatient department, or in a hospital. The choice of where the patient can be best treated depends on the severity of the illness, available support systems, and resources of the treatment center. In timing intervention, remember that help given when maladaptive patterns are developing is likely to be more acceptable and effective than help given after these patterns have been established. Thus early diagnosis and treatment are associated with more positive outcomes.

The nursing interventions that are described relative to severe mood disturbances are based on a unified, multicausal, and interactive model of affective disorders. Such a model dismisses the notion of one cause or one cure for the range of maladaptive emotional responses. Rather, it proposes that affective problems have many determinations and many dimensions that affect all aspects of a person's life. Thus a single approach to nursing care would be inadequate. Nursing interventions must instead reflect the complex nature of the model and address all maladaptive aspects of a person's life. Intervening in as many areas as possible should have the maximum effect in modifying maladaptive responses and alleviating severe mood disturbances. The ultimate aim of these nursing interventions is to teach the patient coping responses and increase the satisfaction gained from interaction with the world. Finally, these nursing actions can be implemented in any setting.

Environmental Interventions

Environmental interventions are useful when the patient's environment is highly dangerous, impoverished, aversive, or lacking in personal resources. In caring for the patient with a severe mood disorder, highest priority should be given to the potential for suicide. Hospitalization is definitely indicated when there is suicidal risk. In the presence of rapidly progressing symptoms and in the absence of support systems, hospitalization is strongly indicated. Nursing care in this case means protecting and assuring patients they will not be allowed to harm themselves. Specific interventions for suicidal patients are described in Chapter 18.

Depressed patients must always be assessed for possible suicide. They are at particular risk when they appear to be coming out of their depression, because they may then have the energy and opportunity to kill themselves. Acute manic states are also life threatening. These patients show poor judgment, excessive risk taking, and an inability to evaluate realistic danger and the consequences of their actions. In an acute manic episode, immediate measures must be instituted to prevent a fatal outcome.

Another environmental intervention involves changing the physical or social setting by assisting the patient to move to a new environment. Sometimes a change in the general pattern of living is indicated, such as a leave of absence from work, a different job, a new

peer group, or leaving a family setting. Changes such as these decrease the immediate stress and mobilize additional support.

Nurse-Patient Relationship

Depressed Patients. Depressed patients resist involvement through withdrawal and nonresponsiveness. Because of their negative views, they tend to remain isolated, verbalize little, think they are unworthy of help, and form dependent attachments.

In working with depressed patients nurses' approach should be quiet, warm, and accepting. They should demonstrate honesty, empathy, and compassion. Admittedly, it is not always easy to give warm, personal care to a person who is unresponsive and detached. The nurse may feel angry or resentful of the patient's helplessness or fear rejection. Patience and a belief in the potential of each person to grow and change are needed. If this is calmly communicated, both verbally and nonverbally, in time the patient may begin to respond.

Nurses should avoid assuming an overaggressive or lighthearted approach with the depressed individual. Comments such as "You have so much to live for," "Cheer up—things are sure to get better," or "You shouldn't feel so depressed" convey little understanding of and respect for the patient's feelings. They will create more distance and block the formation of a potential relationship. Also, nurses should not sympathize with the patient. Subjective overidentification by nurses can cause them to experience similar feelings of hopelessness and helplessness and can seriously limit therapy.

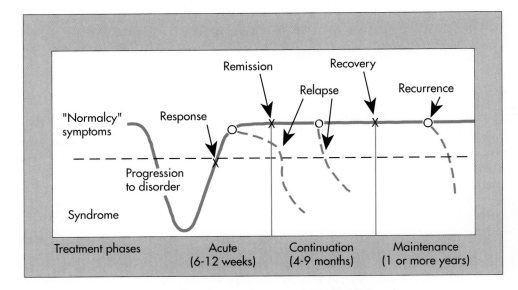

Fig. 17-6 The phases of treatment for mood disorders.
From Kupfer DJ: *J Clin Psychiatry* 52(suppl):28, 1991.

Rapport is best established with the depressed patient through shared time, even if the patient talks little, and through supportive companionship. The very presence of the nurse indicates belief that the patient is a valuable person. The nurse should adjust to the depressed patient's pace by speaking more slowly and allowing more time to respond. The patient should be addressed by name, talked with, and listened to. By studying the patient's life and interests, the nurse might select topics that lay the foundation for more meaningful discussions.

Manic Patients. In contrast, elated patients may be very talkative and need simple explanations and concise, truthful answers to questions. Although manic patients may appear willing to talk, they resist involvement through manipulation, testing limits, and superficiality. Their hyperactivity, short attention span, flight of ideas, poor judgment, lack of insight, and rapid mood swings all present special problems to the nursing staff.

Manic patients can be very disruptive to a unit and resist engagement in therapy. They may dominate group meetings or therapy sessions by their excessive talking and manipulate staff or patient groups. By identifying a vulnerable area in another person or a group's area of conflict, manic patients are able to exploit others. This provokes defensive and angry responses. Nurses are particularly susceptible to these feelings, since they often have the most contact with patients and the responsibility for coordinating and maintaining the psychiatric unit. When anger is generated, therapeutic care breaks down. Thus the maneuvers of manic patients serve as diversionary tactics. By alienating themselves, they can avoid exploring their own problems.

It is important for nurses to understand how manic patients are able to manipulate others and their reasons for doing so. The treatment plan for these patients should be thorough, well coordinated, and consistently implemented. Constructive limit setting on manic patients' behavior is an essential part of the plan. The entire treatment team must be consistent in their expectations of these patients, and progressive limits must be set as situations arise. Other patients may also be encouraged to carry out the agreed limits. Pressure applied by peers can sometimes be more effective than pressure applied by the staff. Frequent staff meetings are recommended to reduce faulty communication, share in understanding the manic patient's behavior, and ensure steady progress.

One goal of nursing care is ultimately to increase the patient's self-control, and this should be kept in mind when setting limits. Patients need to see that they can monitor their own behavior and that the staff is there to help them. Also, the nurse should point out that there are many positive aspects to their behavior. The ability

to be outgoing, expressive, and energetic are coping strengths that can be maximized.

Physiological Treatments

Physiological treatments include physical care, psychopharmacology, and somatic therapies. They begin with a thorough physical examination and health history to determine previous and current health problems and current treatments or medications that may be affecting the patient's mood. The indications for physiological treatment rather than or in addition to psychological treatment include symptoms that will respond to physiological measures, greater severity of illness, suicidal potential, and need for speed in recovery (Fig. 17-7).

In depression, physical well-being may be forgotten or the patient may not be capable of self-care activities. The more severe the depression, the more important is the physical care. For example, the nurse may need to monitor the diet of a patient who has no appetite and has lost weight. Staying with the patient during meals, arranging for preferred foods, and encouraging frequent small meals may be helpful. Recording intake and output and weighing the patient daily will help evaluate this need.

Sleep disturbances typically occur. It is best to plan activities according to each patient's energy levels; some feel best in the morning and others in the evening. A scheduled rest period may be helpful, but patients should not be encouraged to take frequent naps or remain in bed all day. Patients with depression experience less stage III and IV sleep, and since these stages depend on the period of wakefulness, napping may worsen sleep disturbances. For many patients, eating regularly, staying active during waking hours, and cutting back on caffeine (especially late in the day) may promote more normal sleep patterns.

The patient's appearance may be neglected and all movements slowed. Nurses may have to assist with

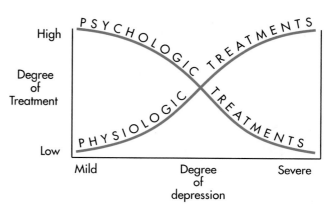

Fig. 17-7   Treatment indications for depression.

bathing or dressing. They should do this matter-of-factly, explaining that help is being offered because the patient is unable to do it independently right now. Cleanliness and interest in appearance can be noticed and praised. Nurses must allow patients to help themselves whenever possible. Often nurses might rush the patient or do a task themselves to save time, but this does not facilitate the patient's recovery and should be avoided.

Manic patients primarily need protection from themselves. They may be too busy to eat or take care of themselves. Eating problems can be handled in the same way as with depressed patients. Patients sleep little, so rest periods should be provided, along with baths, soft mu-

sic, and whirlpools. Manic patients may also need help in selecting clothes and carrying out hygiene. Setting limits and using firm actions are effective in physical care.

Psychopharmacology. Antidepressant medications are frequently administered to elevate the mood of the depressed patient. At this time no single drug has been found effective for all forms of depression.[43] There are three types of antidepressant drugs commonly used—tricyclics, nontricyclics, and monoamine oxidase (MAO) inhibitors (Table 17-8). Many consider lithium carbonate the drug of choice in the treatment of mania (Table 17-9). Some believe that it not only produces a remis-

TABLE 17-8
ANTIDEPRESSANT DRUGS

Chemical class generic name (trade name)	Usual dosage range (mg/day)	Available forms (mg)
TRICYCLIC DRUGS		
Tertiary (parent drug)		
Amitriptyline (Elavil, Endep)	50-300	tabs: 10, 25, 50, 75, 100, 150 inj: 10/ml
Doxepin (Adapin, Sinequan)	50-300	caps: 10, 25, 50, 75, 100, 125, 150 oral conc: 10/ml
Imipramine (SK-Pramine, Tofranil)	50-300	tabs: 10, 25, 50 caps: 75, 100, 125, 150 inj. 25/2 ml
Trimipramine (Surmontil)	50-300	caps: 25, 50, 100
Clomipramine (Anafranil)	50-250	tabs: 25, 50, 75
Secondary (metabolite)		
Desipramine (Norpramin, Pertofrane)	50-300	tabs; 25, 50, 75, 100, 150
Nortriptyline (Aventyl, Pamelor)	50-150	caps: 10, 25, 75 solution: 10/5 ml
Protriptyline (Vivactil)	15-60	tabs: 5, 10
NONTRICYCLIC DRUGS		
Amoxapine (Asendin)	50-600	tabs: 25, 50, 100, 150
Maprotiline (Ludiomil)	50-225*	tabs: 25, 50, 75
Trazodone (Desyrel)	50-600	tabs: 50, 100, 150
Bupropion (Wellbutrin)	50-600*	tabs: 50
SELECTIVE SEROTONIN REUPTAKE INHIBITORS		
Fluoxetine (Prozac)	20-80	caps: 10, 20
Sertraline (Zoloft)	50-200	tabs: 50, 100
Paroxetine (Paxil)	20-50	tabs: 20, 30
NONSELECTIVE UPTAKE INHIBITOR		
Venlafaxine (Effexor)	150-375	tabs: 25, 37.5, 50, 75, 100
MONOAMINE OXIDASE INHIBITORS		
Isocarboxazid (Marplan)	30-70	tabs: 10
Phenelzine (Nardil)	45-90	tabs: 15
Tranylcypromine (Parnate)	20-60	tabs: 10

*Antidepressants with a ceiling dose due to dose-related seizures.

sion of symptoms but also prevents recurrence. The overall success rate of drugs used to treat depressed patients is 60% to 80%.

Despite their success, antidepressant drugs have their limitations. Their therapeutic effects begin only after 2 to 6 weeks, and they have side effects that can deter some patients from maintenance. Thus patient education by the nurse is essential. Another major problem with some antidepressant medications is their toxicity. Tricyclics are lethal at high doses, which makes them particularly dangerous for people most in need of them—suicidal patients. In addition, antidepressant medications do not help everyone, and it is difficult to predict who will respond to which drug. Fortunately, those who do not benefit from one type frequently do well when switched to another. A more complete discussion of mood-stabilizing medications is presented in Chapter 25.

Somatic Therapies. Electroconvulsive therapy (ECT) is also used with depressed patients, particularly those with recurrent depressions and those resistant to drug therapy. ECT is regarded by many as a specific therapy for patients with severe depressions characterized by somatic delusions and delusional guilt, accompanied by a lack of interest in the world, suicidal ideation, and weight loss.

Sleep deprivation therapy may also be effective in treating depression.[31] Research indicates that depriving some depressed patients of a night's sleep will improve their clinical condition. How sleep deprivation works is not known, and the duration of improvement varies.

A final physiological treatment is that of phototherapy, or light therapy, in which patients are exposed to bright, artificial light for a specified amount of time each day. Phototherapy appears to be effective in the short-term treatment of patients with mild to moderate seasonal affective disorder (SAD). Each of these somatic therapies—electroconvulsive therapy, sleep deprivation,

Table 17-9   Lithium Preparations

Lithium salts (trade name)	Available forms (mg)
Lithium carbonate (generic)	150,300
Lithium carbonate	300
(Eskalith)	
(Lithotabs)	
(Lithane)	
(Lithonate)	
Lithium carbonate sustained release	
(Eskalith C-R)	450
(Lithobid)	300
Lithium citrate concentrate	
(Cibalith-S)	5 ml/300

and phototherapy—are described in detail in Chapter 26.

 What would you say to a patient who tells you that she doesn't want to take medicines for her depression because they are addictive?

Expressing Feelings

Affective interventions are necessary because patients with mood disturbances have difficulty identifying and expressing feelings. Feelings that are particularly problematic are hopelessness, sadness, anger, guilt, and anxiety. A range of interventions is available to the nurse in meeting patient needs in this area.

Intervening in emotions requires self-understanding by the nurse. Whether the interventions will be therapeutic depends greatly on the nurse's values regarding the various emotions, the nurse's emotional responsiveness, and the ability to offer genuine respect and nonjudgmental acceptance. Nurses must be able to experience feelings and express them if they expect to help patients.

Initially the nurse must express hope for depressed patients. They have a genuine need for repeated reassurance. The nurse can reinforce that depression is a self-limiting disorder and that the future will be better. This can be expressed calmly and simply. The intent is not to cheer the patient but to offer reassurance that, although recovery is a slow process involving weeks or months, the patient will feel progressively better. The nurse may acknowledge the patient's inability to take comfort from this reassurance. For the depressed, only the depression is real; past or future happiness is an illusion (see A Patient Speaks). By affirming belief in recovery, however, the nurse may make the patient's existence more tolerable.

This initial reassurance is a way of acknowledging the patient's pain and despair while also conveying a sense of hope in recovery. It is not the premature reassurance of "Don't worry—everything's going to be just fine." It is an openness to the patient's feelings and acknowledgment of them. This is a very important first step. It lets the patient see that the present state is not permanent. For the depressed patient who lacks time perspective, it directs thoughts beyond the present with genuine hopes for tomorrow.

Nursing actions in this area should convey that expressing feelings is normal and necessary. Blocking or repressing emotions is partly responsible for the patient's present pain. Nurses can help patients realize that their overwhelming feelings of dejection and worthlessness are defenses that prevent them from dealing

A PATIENT SPEAKS

In depression this faith in deliverance, in ultimate restoration, is absent. The pain is unrelenting, and what makes the condition intolerable is the foreknowledge that no remedy will come—not in a day, an hour, a month, or a minute. If there is mild relief, one knows that it is only temporary; more pain will follow. It is hopelessness even more than pain that crushes the soul. So the decision-making of daily life involves not, as in normal affairs, shifting from one annoying situation to another less annoying—or from discomfort to relative comfort, or from boredom to activity—but moving from pain to pain. One does not abandon, even briefly, one's bed of nails, but is attached to it wherever one goes. And this results in a striking experience—one which I have called, borrowing military terminology, the situation of the walking wounded. For in virtually any other serious sickness, a patient who felt similar devastation would be lying flat in bed, possibly sedated and hooked up to the tubes and wires of life-support systems, but at the very least in a posture of repose and in an isolated setting. His invalidism would be necessary, unquestioned, and honorably attained. However, the sufferer from depression has no such option and therefore finds himself, like a walking casualty of war, thrust into the most intolerable social and family situations. There he must, despite the anguish devouring his brain, present a face approximating the one that is associated with ordinary events and companionship. He must try to utter small talk, and be responsive to questions, and knowingly nod and frown and, God help him, even smile. But it is a fierce trial attempting to speak a few simple words.

William Styron: *Darkness visible*, New York, 1992, Vintage Books. ▼

---

with their problems. Encouraging a patient to express unpleasant or painful emotions can reduce their intensity and make the patient feel more alive and masterful. Thus nursing should be directed toward first helping the patient experience feelings and then express them. These actions are a prerequisite to interventions in the cognitive, behavioral, or social areas.

When the nurse accepts without criticism the anger, despair, or anxiety expressed by the patient, the patient sees that expressing feelings is not destructive or a sign of weakness. Sometimes, however, patients' expression of anger changes their cognitive set from self-blaming to blaming others. It may allow them to see themselves as more effective because it connotes power, superiority, and mastery. How this anger is expressed is important because aggressive behavior can be destructive and

serve to further isolate them. Many patients experiencing both depressive and manic emotional states have problems with expressing anger and need to learn assertive behavior. This important area of nursing intervention is explored in Chapter 27.

Relaxation techniques may also help both manic and depressed patients deal with their anxiety and tension and obtain more pleasure from life. Reducing anxiety to tolerable levels broadens the individual's perceptual field and allows the nurse to intervene in the cognitive and behavioral areas. Nursing actions to reduce anxiety are described in Chapters 14 and 28.

To successfully implement any of these nursing actions related to the patient's affective needs, the nurse must use a variety of communication skills (see Chapter 2). Particularly important are empathy skills, reflection of feeling, open-ended feeling-oriented questions, validation, self-disclosure, and confrontation. Feelings are the essence of empathy and thus make empathy an essential therapeutic quality. The various other communication skills must also focus on feelings rather than facts. The patient with a severe mood disturbance will challenge the nurse's therapeutic skills and stringently test the nurse's caring and commitment.

Cognitive Strategies

When intervening in the cognitive area, nurses have three major aims, which require that they begin with the patient's conceptualization of the problem:

1. To increase the patient's sense of control over goals and behavior
2. To increase the patient's self-esteem
3. To assist the patient in modifying negative thinking patterns

Depressed patients often see themselves as victims of their moods and environment. They do not view their behavior and their interpretation of events as possible causes of depression. They assume a passive stance and wait for someone or something to lift their mood. One task of the nurse, therefore, is to move patients beyond their limiting preoccupation to other aspects of their world that are related to it. To do this, the nurse must progress gradually. The first step is to help patients explore their feelings. This is followed by eliciting their view of the problem. In so doing, the nurse accepts the patient's perceptions but need not accept the patient's conclusions. Together they need to define the problem to give the patient a sense of control, a feeling of hope, and a realization that change may indeed be possible.

Nursing actions may then focus on modifying the patient's thinking. Depressed patients are noticeably dominated by negative thoughts. Often, despite a successful performance, the patient will view it negatively.

Cognitive changes may be brought about in a variety of ways as described in Chapter 28.

Frequently, negative thinking is an automatic process of which the patient is not even aware. The nurse can therefore assist patients in identifying their negative thoughts and decreasing them through thought interruption or substitution. Concurrently the patient can be encouraged to increase positive thinking by reviewing personal assets, strengths, accomplishments, and opportunities. Next the patient can be assisted in examining the accuracy of perceptions, logic, and conclusions. Misperceptions, distortions, and irrational beliefs become evident. The patient should be helped to move from unrealistic to realistic goals and to decrease the importance of unattainable goals. All these actions enhance the patient's self-understanding and increase self-esteem.[11] More detailed interventions related to alterations in self-concept, which are inherent in disturbances of mood, are explored in Chapter 16.

Also, because the depressed patient tends to be overwhelmed by despair, it is important to limit the amount of negative evaluation in which he engages. One way is to involve the patient in productive tasks or activities; another way is to increase the level of socialization. These benefit the patient in two complementary ways: they limit the time spent on brooding and self-criticism, and they provide positive reinforcement.

A final consideration is that the nurse realize the meaning, nature, and value the patient places on behavior and mood change. Most research has focused on the psychopathological nature of affective disorders. One study that explored the positive aspects found that patients with bipolar illnesses receive pronounced short- and long-term positive effects from their manic-depressive illness.[24] The patients reported short-, and long-term increases in productivity, creativity, sensitivity, social outgoingness, and sexual intensity. It is important for the nurse to understand these attributions. They suggest that disturbances of mood can produce powerful reinforcers of a maladaptive response and thus make change more difficult. For some patients, the positive consequences of an illness may outweigh their perception of negative consequences.

Behavioral Change

Successful behavior is a powerful antidepressant. This idea, however, seldom occurs to depressed patients, who use their despondent mood as a rationalization for inactivity. They instead believe that once their mood lifts, they will be productive again. Such an idea is consistent with a negative cognitive set and a sense of helplessness. However, inactivity prevents satisfaction and social recognition. Thus it reinforces a depressive state.

Nursing interventions therefore should focus on activating the patient in a realistic, goal-directed way. Directed activities, strategies, or homework assignments mutually determined by the nurse and patient can reveal alternative coping responses. Many depressed patients benefit from nursing actions that encourage them to redirect their self-preoccupation to interests in the outside world. The timing of these interventions is crucial. Patients should not be forced into activities initially. Also, they will not benefit from coming into contact with too many people too soon. Rather, the nurse should encourage activities gradually and suggest more involvement on the basis of patients' energy.

For severely depressed hospitalized patients, a structured daily program of activities can be beneficial. Because these patients lack motivation and direction, they are slow to initiate actions. The nurse should take into consideration the patient's tolerance to stress and probability of succeeding. The particular task should neither be too difficult nor too time consuming. Success tends to increase expectations of success, and failure tends to increase hopelessness.

Elated patients usually need little encouragement to become involved with others. Because of their short attention span and restless energy, however, they cannot deal with complicated projects. They need tasks that are simple and that can be completed quickly. They need room to move about and furnishings that do not overstimulate them.

The ability to accomplish tasks and be productive depends on various factors. First, expectations and goals should be small enough to ensure successful performance, relevant to their needs, and focused on positive activities. Box 17-5 presents a positive activities list with categories of rewarding or potentially rewarding activities.

Next, attention should be focused on the task at hand, not what has yet to be done or was done incorrectly in the past. Finally, positive reinforcement should be based on actual performance. If such an approach is used consistently over time, the nurse can expect the patient to demonstrate increasingly productive behavior.

Occupational and recreational tasks are usually easily identified by the nurse. These can be most valuable and are well represented in the positive activities list. Another source of accomplishment is movement and physical exercise. Jogging, walking, swimming, bicycling, and aerobics are popular forms of exercise that may be incorporated in a regular program of activity. They are beneficial because they improve the patient's physical condition and release emotions and tensions.

Box 17-5

LIST OF POSSIBLE POSITIVE ACTIVITIES

Planning something you will enjoy
Going on an outing (e.g., a walk, a shopping trip downtown, a picnic)
Going out for entertainment
Going on a trip
Going to meetings, lectures, classes
Attending a social gathering
Playing a sport or game
Spending time on a hobby or project
Entertaining yourself at home (e.g., reading, listening to music, watching TV)
Doing something just for yourself (e.g., buying something, cooking something, dressing comfortably)
Spending time just relaxing (e.g., thinking, sitting, napping, daydreaming)
Caring for yourself, making yourself attractive
Persisting at a difficult task
Completing a routine task or unpleasant task
Doing a job well
Cooperating with someone else on a common task
Doing something special for someone else, being generous, going out of your way
Seeking out people (e.g., calling, stopping by, making a date or appointment, going to a meeting)
Initiating conversation (e.g., at a store, party, or class)
Discussing an interesting or amusing topic
Expressing yourself openly, clearly, or frankly (e.g., opinion, criticism, anger)
Playing with children or animals
Complimenting or praising someone
Physically showing affection or love
Receiving praise, compliments, attention

 What physiological changes occur as a result of exercise. Relate these to what is currently known about the biology of depression.

Social Skills

Social factors play a major role in the causation, maintenance, and resolution of affective disorders, particularly depression. Socialization moderates depression by providing an experience incompatible with depressive withdrawal. It also provides increased self-esteem through the social reinforcers of approval, acceptance, recognition, and support.

A major problem is that patients with maladaptive emotional responses are less accomplished in social interaction. In addition, they may be avoided by others because of their self-absorption, pessimism, or elation. One nursing action to counteract this problem is to help patients improve their social skills. A Patient Education Plan for enhancing social skills is presented on p. 443. It involves sequential learning that includes the following:

1. Assessing the patient's social skills, supports, and interests
2. Reviewing existing and potential social resources available to the patient
3. Instructing and modeling effective social skills
4. Role playing and rehearsing troublesome social situations and interactions
5. Providing feedback and positive reinforcement of effective interpersonal skills
6. Encouraging the initiation of socialization in an expanded social arena

Number 6 often proves difficult for depressed patients, who report they are unable to meet new people and engage in an active social life. Thus increasing a patient's social activities is another area of nursing intervention. Involvement with others often is a result of shared activities. The nurse can work with the patient to identify recreational, career, cultural, religious, and personal interests and how to best pursue these interests through community groups, organizations, and clubs. Women's groups, single-parent groups, jogging clubs, church groups, and neighborhood associations are all opportunities. Although this may appear to be a relatively simple nursing intervention, it is often one that taxes the nurse's creativity and knowledge of resources.

Family Involvement. In addition to a one-to-one relationship, patients with maladaptive emotional responses can benefit from family and group work. For example, it has long been suggested that family relationships are critical to successful reentry of the hospitalized patient back into the community,[27] yet conventional discharge planning and aftercare models tend to neglect the family.

In family therapy, depression can be related to dependency, which may be contributed to and supported by other family members. The patient's sense of powerlessness in human relationships is examined in light of family patterns, and all members are expected to take responsibility for their share of the continuing pattern. The theory that friends and partners often reinforce and support the patient's depression has been well documented. When a person becomes depressed, much attention and secondary gain are usually received from others, who respond by being helpful, nurturing, or an-

PATIENT EDUCATION PLAN
ENHANCING SOCIAL SKILLS

Content	Instructional activities	Evaluation
Describe behaviors interfering with social interaction	Instruct the patient on corrective behaviors	Patient identifies problematic and more facilitative behaviors
Discuss components of social performance relevant to the patient's situation	Model effective interpersonal skills for the patient	Patient describes specific skills that could be acquired
Analyze the way in which the patient could incorporate these specific skills	Use role-play and guided practice to allow patient to test out these new behaviors	Patient shows beginning skill in assumed social behaviors
Encourage patient to test out new skills in other situations	Give the patient homework assignments to do in patient's natural environment	Patient discusses ability to complete the assigned tasks
Discuss generalization of new skills to other aspects of the patient's life and functioning	Give feedback, encouragement, and praise for newly acquired social skills and their generalization	Patient is able to integrate the new social behaviors in social interactions with others

noyed. When the patient acts in a nondepressed way, however, attention given is minimal. Therefore one goal of family therapy is to have the family reinforce adaptive, nondepressed behavior and ignore maladaptive depressive responses. Family interventions also are needed with manic patients, since the patient's behavior can have a significant impact on the family environment.

Group Treatment. Group therapy can also provide multiple benefits. Knowledge that others have ambivalence and sharing this guilt, as well as realistic sympathy and support of the group members, enable depressed patients to lessen guilt. They can thereby give up their maladaptive behavior patterns and develop more satisfying relationships. For example, a format for group treatment of women with major depressive illness can have as its overall aim to increase self-worth and self-esteem through identification with the group and awareness of personal strengths. The depressed women can:

1. Learn more about their individual behavior and relationships with others based on feedback from members and group process
2. Increase social support through group relatedness
3. Gain a heightened sense of identity, self-understanding, and control over their own lives
4. Realize that other people have problems similar to their own, which helps to reduce their sense of loneliness and isolation, thereby also decreasing feelings of hopelessness, helplessness, and powerlessness

5. Learn new ways to cope with stress from others in the group
6. More realistically modify their perceptions and expectations of self and others
7. Allow for the expression of feelings of hopelessness and frustration within the supportive context of the group

Other group interventions have also been described in the literature for bipolar patients[41] and for depressed women using cognitive behavioral strategies.[36]

Mental Health Education

A final but important aspect of nursing care related to maladaptive emotional responses is the provision of mental health education regarding the nature, extent, and treatments available for mood disorders.

Despite its prevalence, most people with a depressive illness do not seek treatment because many of them do not know that they have a treatable disease. As a result of this, in 1988 the National Institute of Mental Health (NIMH) initiated a national education campaign, called Depression/Awareness, Recognition, and Treatment (D/ART), about depressive illnesses. The campaign's goal is to reduce unnecessary suffering by encouraging people with depressive illness to get appropriate treatment. The D/ART campaign is directed toward providing health-care practitioners and the general public with the latest treatment information.[42]

Another important national initiative regarding depression was the publication of clinical practice guidelines on depression by the Agency for Health Care Policy and Research (AHCPR).[13,14] A patient's guide is also available to further help consumers. These educational materials are available to professionals and the public and provide the most current information regarding diagnostic and treatment issues.

Other strategies are also needed. For example, nurses in Arizona have implemented a mental health training program for primary care nurses that addresses primary and secondary prevention issues related to depression.[6] The program emphasized criteria for assessing depression, presented psychopharmacological and psychotherapeutic content, discussed care coordination among multiple agencies and providers, and addressed referral resources. Cultural and developmental issues for Native Americans, Mexican Americans, the elderly, and adolescents were highlighted. Another innovative strategy is the creation of a slide kit for nurses on detecting and treating depression from a nursing perspective.[50] This slide kit is available from Eli Lilly and can be used by nurses to educate students, practitioners, and consumers about this major public health problem and can be a positive learning resource.

Nursing care must also address the specific needs of patients and families for education regarding mood disorders. A psychoeducational approach to depression in women has been found to be effective in increasing their feelings of independence and self-confidence and assisting them to manage the stresses associated with being a woman in contemporary society.[37] The psychoeducational model can also be used with families who are a valuable resource in helping patients deal with their illness. The overall goal of such a program would be to improve patient and family functioning and decrease symptomatology by increasing a sense of self-worth and a sense of control for both patients and families. Specific information about the reciprocal impact of depression and family life can be outlined (Box 17-6) along with suggestions and strategies designed to aid family members in coping more effectively with mood disorders.[26]

In summary, the most important ideas that the nurse wishes to communicate through mental health education include the following:

▼ Mood disorders are a medical illness, not a character defect or weakness.

▼ Recovery is the rule, not the exception.

▼ Mood disorders are treatable illnesses, and an effective treatment can be found for almost all patients.

▼ The goal of intervention is to not just to get better, but to get and stay completely well.

A Nursing Care Plan Summary for patients with maladaptive emotional responses is presented on p. 446.

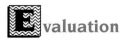 # **E**valuation

The effectiveness of nursing care is determined by changes in the patient's maladaptive emotional responses and the effect they have on present functioning. Problems related to self-concept and interpersonal relationships merge and overlap. Since all individuals experience life stress and related losses, the nurse can ask a fundamental question related to evaluation: "Did I assess my patient for problems in this area?"

Of particular significance are the many special aspects of transference and countertransference that may occur. The patient's heightened attachment and dependency behaviors and lowered defensiveness can lead to intense transference reactions that should be worked through. Themes of loss and fear of loss, control of emotions and lack of control, and ambivalence predominate. Termination of the nurse-patient relationship may be difficult, since the patient experiences it as another loss that requires mourning and integration.

Countertransference can be related to the nurse's own bereavements, attitudes about anger, guilt, sadness, and despair, the ability to confront these emotions openly and objectively, and most importantly, conflicts about death and loss. Difficulties with any of these issues can be evident in avoidance behavior, preoccupation with fantasies, blocking of feelings, or shortening of sessions. Nursing care will be more appropriate and effective if the nurse is aware of these issues and sensitive to personal feelings and conflicts regarding loss. Supervision and peer support groups can be of great help in this area.

SUMMARY

1. The continuum of emotional responses ranges from the most adaptive state of emotional responsiveness to the more maladaptive states of delayed grief reaction, depression, and mania.

Box 17-6

OUTLINE OF TOPICS FOR PATIENT-FAMILY PSYCHOEDUCATIONAL SESSIONS ON DEPRESSION

I. Defining depression
  A. Definitions and descriptions of depression and mania
  B. How depression differs from "the blues" we all experience (length of time it lasts, impact on mood, functioning, self-esteem, responsiveness to the environment)
  C. Possible causes: the stress adaptation model
II. Depression and the interpersonal environment
  A. What depression looks like: interpersonal difficulties
    1. Oversensitivity and self-preoccupation
    2. Unresponsiveness (to reassurance, support, feedback, sympathy)
    3. Behaviors that appear willful
    4. Apparent lack of caring for others, unrealistic expectations
    5. Apparent increased need to control relationships
    6. Inability to function at normal roles, tasks
  B. Negative interactional sequences
    1. Family attempts to help: coax, reassure, protect (potential for overinvolvement)
    2. Patient is unresponsive, family escalates attempts to help or withdraws
    3. Patient feels alienated, family becomes withdrawn, angry, or both
    4. Family feels guilty and returns to overprotective stance
    5. Patient feels unworthy, hopeless, infantilized
    6. Families burn out over time but remain caught in guilt/anger dilemma
    7. Alienation and/or overprotection

III. Treatments
  A. Psychotropic medication
  B. Psychotherapies
  C. Other treatments
IV. Coping with depression
  A. What to avoid
    1. Too rapid reassurance
    2. Taking comments literally
    3. Attempting to be constantly available and positive
    4. Allowing the disorder to dominate family life
  B. Creating a balance (neither overresponsive nor underresponsive)
    1. Recognition of multiple realities
    2. Distinguishing between the patient and the disorder
    3. Decreasing expectations temporarily
    4. Providing realistic support and reinforcement
    5. Avoiding unnecessary criticism (but providing feedback when necesssary)
    6. Communicating clearly and simply (proverbally)
    7. Providing activity, structure
  C. Taking care of self and family members other than the patient; skills for self-preservation
    1. Time out (away from patient)
    2. Avoiding martyrdom
    3. Accepting own negative feelings
    4. Minimizing the impact of the disorder
  D. Coping with special problems
    1. Suicide threats and attempts
    2. Medication
    3. Hospitalization
    4. Atypical responses

Adapted from Keitner G: *Depression and families: impact and treatment*, Washington, DC, 1990, American Psychiatric Press.

2. Patient behaviors related to emotional responses include delayed grief reaction, depression, and mania.

3. Predisposing factors affecting emotional responses include genetics, aggression turned inward, object loss, personality organization, cognition, learned helplessness-hopelessness, behavioral learning, and biochemistry. Precipitating stressors include loss of attachment, life events, roles, and physiological changes.

4. Coping resources focus on the patient's social and economic supports and a sense of personal mastery. Coping mechanisms include introjection, denial, and suppression.

5. Primary NANDA nursing diagnoses related to maladaptive emotional responses are dysfunctional grieving, hopelessness, powerlessness, spiritual distress, and potential for self-directed violence.

6. Primary DSM-IV diagnoses include bipolar I and II disorders, cyclothymic disorder, major depressive disorder, and dysthymic disorder.

7. The expected outcome of nursing care is that the patient will be emotionally responsive and return to preillness level of functioning.

8. Nursing interventions address environmental issues, nurse-patient relationship, physiological treatments, expressing feelings, cognitive strategies, behavioral change, social skills, and mental health education.

9. The effectiveness of nursing care is determined by changes in the patient's maladaptive emotional responses and the effect they have on present functioning. Supervision and peer support groups can be helpful to the nurse working with patients with mood disorders.

NURSING CARE PLAN SUMMARY
Maladaptive Emotional Responses

Nursing Diagnosis: Hopelessness

Expected Outcome: The patient will be emotionally responsive and return to preillness level of functioning.

Short-Term Goal	Intervention	Rationale
The patient's environment will be safe and protective.	Continually evaluate the patient's potential for suicide. Hospitalize the patient when there is a suicidal risk. Assist the patient to move to a new environment when appropriate (e.g., new job, peer group, family setting).	All patients with severe mood disturbances are at high risk for suicide; environmental changes can protect the patient, decrease the immediate stress, and mobilize additional resources.

The patient will establish a therapeutic relationship with the nurse.	Use a warm, accepting, empathic approach.
	Be aware of and in control of one's own feelings and reactions (e.g., anger, frustration, sympathy).
	With the depressed patient:
	   Establish rapport through shared time and supportive companionship
	   Allow the patient time to respond
	   Personalize care as a way of indicating the patient's value as a human being
	With the manic patient:
	   Give simple, truthful responses
	   Be alert to possible manipulation
	   Set constructive limits on negative behavior
	   Use a consistent approach by all health-team members
	   Maintain open communication and sharing of perceptions among team members
	   Reinforce the patient's self-control and positive aspects of patient behavior
		Both depressed and manic patients resist becoming involved in a therapeutic alliance; acceptance, persistence, and limit setting are necessary.

The patient will be physiologically stable and able to meet self-care needs.	Assist the patient to meet self-care needs, particularly in the areas of nutrition, sleep, and personal hygiene. Encourage the patient's independence whenever possible. Administer prescribed medications and somatic treatments.	Physiological changes occur in disturbances of mood; physical care and somatic therapies are required to overcome problems in this area.
The patient will be able to recognize and express emotions related to daily events.	Respond empathically with a focus on feelings rather than facts. Acknowledge the patient's pain and convey a sense of hope in recovery. Help the patient experience feelings and then express them. Assist the patient in the appropriate expression of anger.	Patients with severe mood disturbances have difficulty identifying and expressing feelings.

NURSING CARE PLAN SUMMARY—cont'd
Maladaptive Emotional Responses

Nursing Diagnosis: Hopelessness

Expected Outcome: The patient will be emotionally responsive and return to preillness level of functioning.

Short-Term Goal	Intervention	Rationale
The patient will evaluate thinking and correct faulty or negative thoughts.	Review the patient's conceptualization of the problem but do not necessarily accept conclusions. Identify the patient's negative thoughts and help to decrease them. Help increase positive thinking. Examine the accuracy of perceptions, logic, and conclusions. Identify misperceptions, distortions, and irrational beliefs. Help him move from unrealistic to realistic goals. Decrease the importance of unattainable goals. Limit the amount of negative personal evaluations the patient engages in.	This will help to increase sense of control over goals and behaviors, enhance self-esteem, and modify negative expectations.
The patient will implement two new behavioral coping strategies.	Assign appropriate action-oriented therapeutic tasks. Encourage activities gradually, escalating them as the patient's energy is mobilized. Provide a tangible, structured program when appropriate. Set goals that are realistic, relevant to the patient's needs and interests, and focused on positive activities. Focus on present activities, not past or future activities. Positively reinforce successful performance. Incorporate physical exercise in the patient's plan of care.	Successful behavioral performance counteracts feelings of helplessness and hopelessness.
The patient will describe rewarding social interactions.	Assess the patient's social skills, supports, and interests. Review existing and potential social resources. Instruct and model effective social skills. Use role playing and rehearsal of social interactions. Give feedback and positive reinforcement of effective interpersonal skills. Intervene with families to have them reinforce the patient's adaptive emotional responses. Support or engage in family and group therapy when appropriate.	Socialization is an experience incompatible with withdrawal and increases self-esteem through the social reinforcers of approval, acceptance, recognition, and support.

COMPETENT CARING
A CLINICAL EXEMPLAR OF A PSYCHIATRIC NURSE

Virginia A. Reuger, BSN, RN, C

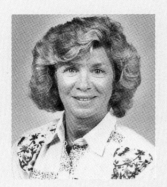

Sure, you read about therapeutic interactions in your nursing textbooks, but every person is not the same, so the only way you learn is by doing, by experiencing. Rarely in school do we have the time to become overinvolved with our patients. We are taught on our psychiatric rotation not to let the boundaries between self and others become blurred. Yet the dynamics of a therapeutic relationship are not real until we come face to face with the situation.

It happened to me, subtly, soon after I started working in a private psychiatric hospital. I was working as a staff nurse on the intensive care unit. I was assigned to the next admission. From the intake sheet, I could see it was another depressed, suicidal patient. But when R and her husband walked onto the unit, I was immediately drawn to her with a empathic feeling. She was tiny, frail looking; her face was thin and drawn. Her long, dark hair partially hid her face. She ignored introductions and stared at the floor. My initial challenge was to establish trust to open channels of communication, assess her suicide potential, and provide a secure environment. Her potential for self-harm was quite high. She was put on strict suicidal precautions. Initially, as I worked with R it required observations of her appearance, her gestures, and her interests, as well as nonverbal communication. I often had to make inferences, and I'd share these with her. I felt like she was testing the waters of trust. R would often wrap herself up in her pink blanket and rock back and forth during our interactions. I found myself wondering what she was thinking.

One day during our time together I asked her about how it felt to be depressed. For her, it was the beginning of self-disclosure. She was able to acknowledge her fear and pain and unmet needs. She talked about what it was like growing up in New York City, living in row houses that were rat infested. Her father worked at a bakery and sometimes their only food was the bread he would bring home. She had two brothers and two sisters. Eventually she told me her uncle and grandfather lived with them too. As she learned to trust me, she disclosed the sexual abuse she received from her uncle and grandfather. At times the details would become so vivid she would tremble as she cried. It is hard to express, but there was a sense that we were making contact.

We talked about her present life, her frigidity, her 6-year-old daughter, and the nightmares. She would often remark that her husband and daughter would be better off without her. She believed she could not have a "normal life." R was very bright and talented. She had many hobbies. We started concentrating on these things. I knew her self-esteem was low, and this was the start of some good work.

But being her primary nurse and assigned to her one-to-one daily made me realize I was becoming enmeshed in the situation. I went to my nurse manager for supervision. We discussed several options. I questioned whether I was helping her. I think sometimes nurses want to feel like omnipotent rescuers. I was not sure whether I was fostering independence or dependence. It was important to acknowledge my feelings to someone else openly, to discuss them, and then to move on. Even though I felt a bond, I had to help R find strength on her own. We discussed her upcoming discharge date; we talked about priorities and decisions she had made. We talked about good choices, bad choices, and no choices. She had suffered many setbacks, but she was making plans.

I remember staying late the day of her discharge to say goodbye. R sent me cards at the hospital, would drop gifts off at the admissions office for me, and once tried to reach me at home. It was difficult to not acknowledge these things; I wanted so much to talk to her. But I knew the boundaries of a therapeutic relationship, and I knew she would be fine. I did talk to her outpatient therapist, and he told me she had completed a course in sign language (during her stay we had a deaf elderly woman R became friends with), and she also was attending clown school, something she had always wanted to do—to make people laugh and feel good.

In psychiatric nursing it is important to remember that the art is to offer what you can without dictating the results while recognizing that you are not the only one to contribute to a person's health and happiness. This important lesson is what I learned from R. ▼

REFERENCES

1. Abramson L, Metalsky G, Alloy L: Hopelessness depression: a theory-based subtype of depression, *Psychol Rev* 96:358, 1989.
2. Abramson L, Seligman M, Teasdale J: Learned helplessness in humans: critique and reformulation, *J Abnorm Psychol* 87:49, 1978.
3. American Psychiatric Association: *Diagnostic and statistical manual of mental disorders*, ed 4, Washington, DC, 1994, The Association.
4. Arieti S, Bemporad J: The psychological organization of depression, *Am J Psychiatry* 137:1360, 1980.
5. Badger T: Physical health impairment and depression among older adults, *Image J Nurs Sch* 25:325, 1993.
6. Badger T, Cardea J, Biocca L, Mishel M: Assessment and management of depression: an imperative for community-based practice, *Arch Psychiatr Nurs* 4:235, 1990.
7. Barbee E: African-American women and depression: a review and critique of the literature, *Arch Psychiatr Nurs* 6:257, 1992.
8. Beck A et al: *Cognitive therapy of depression*, New York, 1979, The Guilford Press.
9. Betrus P, Elmore S: Seasonal affective disorder: Part 1. a review of the neural mechanisms for psychosocial nurses, *Arch Psychiatr Nurs* 5:367, 1991.
10. Bowlby J: Grief and mourning in infancy and early childhood, *Psychoanal Study Child* 15:9, 1960.
11. Campbell J: Treating depression in well older adults: use of diaries in cognitive therapy, *Issues Ment Health Nurs* 13:19, 1992.
12. Costello C: *Symptoms of depression*, New York, 1993, John Wiley & Sons.
13. Depression Guideline Panel: *Depression in primary care*, vol 1, *Detection and diagnosis*, Clinical practice guideline, no 5, Rockville, Md, 1993, US Department of Health and Human Services, Public Health Service, Agency for Health Care Policy and Research, pub no 93-0550.
14. Depression Guideline Panel: *Depression in primary care*, vol 2, *Treatment of major depression*, Clinical practice guideline, no 5, Rockville, Md, 1993, US Department of Health and Human Services, Public Health Service, Agency for Health Care Policy and Research, pub no 93-0551.
15. George L, Blazer D, Hughes D, Fowler N: Social support and the outcome of major depression, *Br J Psychiatry* 154:478, 1989.
16. Goodwin F, Jamison K: *Manic-depressive illness*, New York, 1990, Oxford University Press.
17. Gove W: The relationship between sex roles, marital status, and mental illness, *Soc Forces* 51:34, 1972.
18. Greenberg P et al: The economic burden of depression in 1990, *J Clin Psychiatry* 54:26, 1993.
19. Gulesserian B, Warren C: Coping resources of depressed patients, *Arch Psychiatr Nurs* 1:392, 1987.
20. Hall L, Sachs B, Rayens M, Lutenbacher M: Childhood physical and sexual abuse: their relationship with depressive symptoms in adulthood, *Image J Nurs Sch* 25:317, 1993.
21. Hare-Mustin R: Family change and gender differences: implications for theory and practice, *Fam Relations* 37:36, 1988.
22. Horton R, Katona C: *Biological aspects of affective disorders*, New York, 1991, Harcourt Brace Jovanovich.
23. Jamison K: *Touched with fire: manic-depressive illness and the artistic temperament*, New York, 1993, Free Press.
24. Jamison K et al: Clouds and silver linings: positive experiences associated with primary affective disorders, *Am J Psychiatry* 137:198, 1980.
25. Jones-Webb R, Snowden L: Symptoms of depression among blacks and whites, *Am J Public Health* 83:240, 1993.
26. Keitner G: *Depression and families: impact and treatment*, Washington, DC, 1990, American Psychiatric Press.
27. Keitner G, Miller I: Family functioning and major depression: an overview, *Am J Psychiatry* 147:1128, 1990.
28. Kendall-Tackett K, Kantor G: *Postpartum depression: a comprehensive approach for nurses*, Newbury Park, Calif, 1993, Sage.
29. Kendler K et al: The prediction of major depression in women: toward an integrated etiological model, *Am J Psychiatry* 150:1139, 1993.
30. Kessler R et al: Sex and depression in the national comorbidity survey I: lifetime prevalence, chronicity, and recurrence, *J Affect Disord* 29:85, 1993.
31. Kuhs H, Tolle R: Sleep deprivation therapy, *Biol Psychiatry* 29:1129, 1991.
32. Kupfer D: Long-term treatment of depression, *J Clin Psychiatry* 52(suppl):28, 1991.
33. Leon A, Klerman G, Wickramaratne P: Continuing female

predominance in depressive illness, *Am J Public Health* 83:754, 1993.

34. Lewinsohn P, Youngren M, Grosscup S: Reinforcement and depression. In Depue R, ed: *The psychobiology of the depressive disorders*, New York, 1979, Academic Press.

35. Lindemann E: Symptomatology and management of acute grief, *Am J Psychiatry* 101:141, 1944.

36. Maynard C: Comparison of effectiveness of group interventions for depression in women, *Arch Psychiatr Nurs* 7(5):277, 1993.

37. Maynard C: Psychoeducational approach to depression in women, *J Psychosoc Nurs Ment Health Serv* 31:9, 1993.

38. McEnany G: Psychobiological indices of bipolar mood disorder: future trends in nursing care, *Arch Psychiatr Nurs* 4:29, 1990.

39. Morin G: Seasonal affective disorder, the depression of winter: a literature review and description from a nursing perspective, *Arch Psychiatr Nurs* 4:182, 1990.

40. NIH Consensus Development Conference: *Diagnosis and treatment of depression in late life*, Rockville, Md, 1991, US Department of Health and Human Services, Public Health Service, NIH.

41. Pollack L: Improving relationships: groups for inpatients with bipolar disorder, *J Psychosoc Nurs Ment Health Serv* 28:17, 1990.

42. Regier D et al: The NIHM depression awareness, recognition, and treatment program: structure, aims, and scientific base, *Am J Psychiatry* 145:1351, 1988.

43. Richelson E: Treatment of acute depression, *Psychiatr Clin North Am* 16:461, 1993.

44. Robertson J, Robertson J: Young children in brief separation: a fresh look, *Psychoanal Study Child* 26:264, 1971.

45. Rosenthal N: *Winter blues: seasonal affective disorder*, New York, 1993, The Guilford Press.

46. Ruble D, Greulich F, Pomerantz E, Gochberg B: The role of gender-related processes in the development of sex differences in self-evaluation and depression, *J Affect Disord* 29:97, 1993.

47. Seligman M: *Helplessness: on depression, development and death*, San Francisco, 1975, WH Freeman.

48. Simmons-Alling S: Genetic implications for major affective disorders, *Arch Psychiatr Nurs* 4:67, 1990.

49. Spitz R: Anaclitic depression, *Psychoanal Study Child* 2:313, 1942.

50. Stuart G: Detection and treatment of depression: the nursing perspective, slide kit sponsored by Eli Lilly, Washington, DC, 1994, American Nurses' Foundation.

51. Stuart G et al: Early family experiences of women with bulimia and depression, Arch Psychiatr Nurs 4:43, 1990.

52. Ugarriza D: Postpartum affective disorders: incidence and treatment, *J Psychosoc Nurs Ment Health Serv* 30:29, 1992.

53. Warren B: Depression in African-American women, *J Psychosoc Nurs Ment Health Serv* 32:29, 1994.

54. Weissman M et al: Sex differences in rates of depression: cross-national perspectives, *J Affect Disord* 29:77, 1993.

55. Whybrow P, Akiskal H, McKinney W: *Mood disorders: toward a new psychobiology*, New York, 1984, Plenum Press.

56. Winokur G, Coryell W, Endicott J, Akiskal H: Further distinctions between manic-depressive illness (bipolar disorder) and primary depressive disorder (unipolar disorder), *Am J Psychiatry* 150:1176, 1993.

57. Woods N: Employment, family roles, and mental health in young married women, *Nurs Res* 34(1):4, 1985.

58. Work Group on Major Depressive Disorder: Practice guidelines for major depressive disorder in adults, *Am J Psychiatry* 150:1, 1993.

59. Zung W, Broadhead E, Roth M: Prevalence of depressive symptoms in primary care, *J Fam Pract* 37:337, 1993.

ANNOTATED SUGGESTED READINGS

*Affonso D: Postpartum depression: a nursing perspective on women's health and behaviors, *Image J Nurs Sch* 24:215, 1992.

Scholarly examination of postpartum depression from different disciplinary perspectives. Nursing's contributions are highlighted.

*Badger T, Cardea J, Biocca L, Mishel M: Assessment and management of depression: an imperative for community-based practice, *Arch Psychiatr Nurs*, 4:235, 1990.

Describes in detail an excellent mental health training program to increase primary care nurses' knowledge and skills about depression.

*Burnard P: Spiritual distress and the nursing response: Theoretical considerations and counseling skills, *J Adv Nurs* 12:377, 1987.

Examines the issues and practical skills involved in counseling people who fail to invest life with meaning. Good review of the literature on this topic.

Cappeliez P, Flynn R: *Depression and the social environment*, London, 1993, McGill-Queen's University Press.

Underscores the importance of the social environment in depression. Each chapter addresses a different population group in relation to this illness.

Copeland M: *The depression workbook*, Arlington, Va, 1991, National Alliance for the Mentally Ill.

Offers step-by-step guidance for taking responsibility including seeking care, building support systems, and increasing self-esteem. Written for consumers and families.

*Hauenstein E: Young women and depression, *Nurs Clin North Am* 26:601, 1991.

Reviews factors contributing to the high prevalence of affective disorders in women, the effect of this illness on them, and the unique contributions nurses can make.

*Kendall-Tackett K, Kantor G: *Postpartum depression: a comprehensive approach for nurses*, Newbury Park, Calif, 1993, Sage.

Clear, practical, and thorough review of the important clinical problem of postpartum depression. Highly recommended.

*Maynard C: Psychoeducational approach to depression in women, *J Psychosoc Nurs Ment Health Serv* 31:9, 1993.

Good example of an effective nursing intervention that could be replicated in other settings.

*Morin G: Seasonal affective disorder, the depression of winter: a literature review and description from a nursing perspective, *Arch Psychiatr Nurs* 4:182, 1990.

Good nursing article on diagnosing and intervening in SAD.

NIH Consensus Development Conference: *Diagnosis and treatment of depression in late life*, Rockville, Md, 1991, US Department of Health & Human Services, Public Health Service, NIH.

Best and most complete text on depression in the elderly.

*Rosenbaum J: Depression: viewed from a transcultural nursing theoretical perspective, *J Adv Nurs* 14:7, 1989.

---

*Nursing reference.

Depression is examined in the context of Leininger's theory of trans-cultural diversity. Implications for nursing care and research are included.

Rosenthal N: *Winter blues: seasonal affective disorder*, New York, 1993, The Guilford Press.

Most current and complete text on this clinical problem.

Schwartz A, Schwartz R: *Depression theories and treatments*, New York, 1993, Columbia University Press.

Written for the busy clinician, it presents a thorough but easy to un-derstand discussion of the many aspects of this complex problem area.

Seligman M: *Learned optimism*, New York, 1991, Alfred A. Knopf.

Blends scientific knowledge with practical advice on how to better un-derstand ourselves and change to be healthier and happier.

Styron W: *Darkness visible*, New York, 1992, Vintage Books.

First-person account of one man's experience of depression. Short, beautifully written, deeply moving, and very courageous.

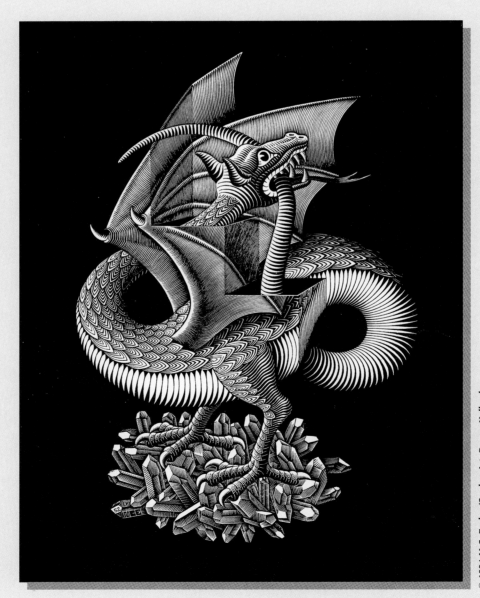

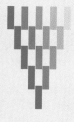

C H A P T E R   1 8

Self-Protective Responses and Suicidal Behavior

GAIL W. STUART
SANDRA J. SUNDEEN

Out, out brief candle!
Life's but a walking shadow, a poor player
That struts and frets his hour upon the stage
And then is heard no more. It is a tale
Told by an idiot, full of sound and fury,
Signifying nothing.

William Shakespeare: *Macbeth*, Act V

LEARNING OBJECTIVES

After studying this chapter the student should be able to:

▼ Describe the continuum of adaptive and maladaptive self-protective responses
▼ Discuss the epidemiology of suicide
▼ Identify behaviors associated with self-protective responses
▼ Analyze predisposing factors and precipitating stressors related to self-protective responses
▼ Describe coping resources and coping mechanisms related to self-protective responses
▼ Formulate nursing diagnoses for patients related to their self-protective responses
▼ Assess the relationship between nursing diagnoses and medical diagnoses related to self-protective responses
▼ Identify expected outcomes and short-term nursing goals for patients related to self-protective responses
▼ Develop a patient education plan to promote patients' adaptive self-protective responses
▼ Analyze nursing interventions for patients related to their self-protective responses
▼ Evaluate nursing care for patients related to their self-protective responses

TOPICAL OUTLINE

Continuum of Self-protective Responses
   Epidemiology of Suicide
Assessment
   Behaviors
   Predisposing Factors
   Precipitating Stressors
   Coping Resources
   Coping Mechanisms
Nursing Diagnosis
   Related Medical Diagnoses
Outcome Identification
Planning
Implementation
   Protection
   Contracting for Safety
   Increasing Self-esteem
   Regulating Emotions and Behaviors
   Mobilizing Social Support
   Mental Health Education
   Suicide Prevention
Evaluation

Life is characterized by risk. Individuals must choose the amount of potential danger to which they are willing to expose themselves. Sometimes these choices are conscious and rational. For instance, the elderly person who decides to stay in the house on an icy day has chosen not to risk falling and possibly fracturing a bone. Other risk-taking behavior is unconsciously determined. Soldiers who volunteer for a suicide mission are probably unaware of their motivation. If asked, they would probably cite patriotism or concern for comrades. Most people go through life accepting some risks as part of their daily routine while carefully avoiding others. Those who constantly take chances while driving may refuse to fly in an airplane because they feel unsafe.

Even though life is risky, most societies have a norm that defines the degree of danger to which persons may expose themselves. This norm varies according to age, gender, socioeconomic status, and occupation. In general, the very young, the old, and women are viewed as needing to be protected from harm. Great ambivalence is directed at those who engage in potentially self-destructive behavior. Some risk takers are admired, particularly athletes, military personnel, those with dangerous occupations, and those who place themselves in danger to help others. At the same time, feelings of admiration may be accompanied by fear and perplexity about the danger-seeking behavior. The varying attitudes toward cigarette smoking provide another example of cultural ambivalence. On one hand, smoking is viewed as mature behavior, denoting sophistication and social acceptability. On the other, it is seen as socially alienating, unhealthy, and inconsiderate of the needs of others.

CONTINUUM OF SELF-PROTECTIVE RESPONSES

Protection and survival are fundamental needs of all living things. A continuum of self-protecting responses would have self-enhancement as the most adaptive re-

sponse, while indirect self-destructive behavior, self-injury, and suicide would be maladaptive responses. Self-destructive behavior may thus range from subtle to overt.

Direct self-destructive behavior includes any form of suicidal activity, such as suicide threats, attempts, gestures, and completed suicide. The intent of this behavior is death, and the individual is aware of the desired outcome. Indirect self-destructive behavior is any activity detrimental to the person's physical well-being that potentially may result in death. However, the person may be unaware of this potential and deny it if confronted. Examples include eating disorders (see Chapter 23) and abuse of alcohol and drugs (see Chapter 22). Other examples include cigarette smoking, automobile accidents, gambling, criminal activity, socially deviant behavior, stress-seeking behavior, participation in high-risk sports, and noncompliance with medical treatment.

Theories of self-destructive behavior overlap with those of self-concept and disturbances in mood. Careful study of Chapters 16 and 17 will help the reader understand the behaviors discussed in this chapter. To think about or attempt destruction of the self, the person must have low self-regard. Low self-esteem leads to depression, which is always present in self-destructive behavior. The range of behaviors that includes self-protective responses is shown in Fig. 18-1.

The levels of behavior in the continuum may overlap. For instance, the girl who learns and excels at gymnastics is building her self-esteem and projecting a positive self-concept. However, if she tries stunts she is not prepared for and does not take safety measures, her behavior becomes self-injurious or indirectly self-destructive. Similarly, a diabetic man who has never complied completely with his prescribed diet and medication regimen may become discouraged and intentionally take an overdose of insulin. Thus the nurse must be alert to subtle shifts in the mood and behavior of patients when assessing maladaptive self-protective responses.

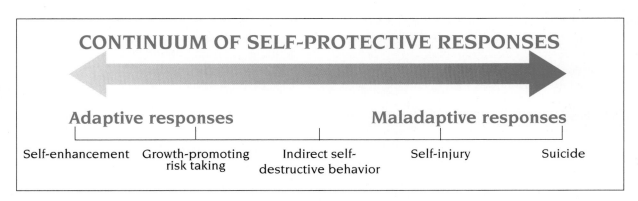

Fig. 18-1   Continuum of self-protective responses.

Epidemiology of Suicide

About 30,000 people complete the act of suicide each year, making it the eighth leading cause of death in the United States and the third leading killer of young people. The rate of suicide among youth has tripled in the past 30 years. The actual number of suicides may be two to three times higher because of the underreporting that occurs. In addition, many single motor car accidents and homicides are, in fact, suicides. In the world at least 1000 suicides occur each day, and 645,680 years of productive life are lost each year in the United States because of deaths by suicide. Of these, 71% occurred among white males, and white females accounted for another 19%. The United States now has one of the highest suicide rates for young men in the world, surpassing Japan and Sweden, countries long identified with high rates of suicide.[5]

Although the base rate of suicide has remained about the same for the past 20 years, the rate has soared for young people ages 15 to 24 and has increased by 25% for the elderly. The highest suicide rate for any group in this country is among people over age 65, especially among those between 75 to 85. Although this group constitutes 26% of the total U.S. population, it accounts for approximately 39% of deaths by suicide. White males over the age of 50 represent the greatest number of these deaths (Fig. 18-2).

Teen suicide in the United States is nearly five times as common among boys than girls. Suicide is also more common among whites than blacks at all ages. The overwhelming majority of completed suicides across the life cycle are committed by males. Well over half of these males shoot themselves, and the use of guns is increasing rapidly. Women attempt suicide three times as frequently as men, using potentially less lethal means, including medications and wrist slashing. However, one third of women who complete suicide and over half of those 15 to 29 years of age use guns.

Reports of suicide among young children are rare, but suicidal behavior is not. As many as 12,000 children, ages 5 to 14, may be hospitalized in this country every year for deliberate self-destructive acts.

 What factors might contribute to the high rate of suicide among white elderly males?

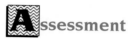ssessment

Behaviors

Noncompliance. It has been estimated that one half of patients do not comply with their health-care treatment plan. People who do not comply with recommended health-care activities are generally aware that they have chosen not to care for themselves. They usually have a reason for noncompliance, such as being asymptomatic, not being able to afford the treatment they need, not understanding the treatment, or not having time. Patients may also minimize the seriousness of their problems. Many chronic illnesses are characterized by long periods of stability, during which the person may not be aware of discomfort. This reinforces the noncompliant behavior.

Patients with chronic illnesses frequently search for health-care providers who will prescribe other, less disruptive treatment plans than the ones they are trying to avoid. They are susceptible to questionable practices such as miracle cures and faith healing in their search for the return of complete health. Patients who are receiving chemotherapy or radiation for cancer become frustrated with the side effects of the treatment. They are easily victimized by those who promote "cures" that involve no discomfort but have no scientifically proven effectiveness. The popular literature is constantly reporting miraculous new treatments for chronic diseases. Most of these lead to more suffering for those who become hopeful and are then disappointed.

The most prominent behavior associated with noncompliance is refusal to admit the seriousness of the health problem. This denial interferes with acceptance of treatment. At the same time, however, it protects the ego from the anxiety that recognition of impaired health will create. The greater the threat imposed by the illness, the greater the resistance to treatment. Many

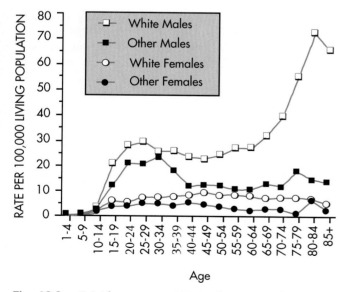

Fig. 18-2   Suicide rate per 100,000 living population, all ages, 1988.

chronic illnesses are associated with advancing age. Anxiety is increased because admission of illness also implies recognition of growing older. In a society that values youth, this behavior is not surprising.

An unfortunate aspect of noncompliance is that guilt about not following health-care recommendations may also interfere with obtaining regular care. Hypertensive persons who have not been taking their medication will be reluctant to have their blood pressure checked because an elevated reading will undermine their defensive system. If the medical system treats these people as children and chastises them for their behavior, they feel even guiltier and are more reluctant to seek routine health care.

Noncompliant people are also struggling for control. Serious illness is often seen as an attack on the person and a betrayal by the body. Patients need to reassert their control and prove that they are still the master of their fate. The diabetic who cheats on his diet is gambling that he still has control over his body and can resist his problem by will. Most chronically ill people need to test the limits of their control and the validity of the prescribed self-care regimen. The following clinical example illustrates the problem of noncompliance with a prescribed health-care regimen.

CLINICAL EXAMPLE

Ms. C was a 61-year-old, white married woman who had been in good health most of her life. She had three grown children who had left home and established their own families. She had been a homemaker since her marriage at age 19. She and her husband were both looking forward to his retirement in 6 months. They planned to buy a recreational vehicle and travel around the United States.

Ms. C visited the gynecologist regularly. She was very concerned about having annual Pap smears. Since she was receiving no other regular health care, the nurse practitioner who worked with this physician did a complete physical examination each time Ms. C was seen. On her most recent visit, laboratory studies revealed an elevated blood glucose level. She was then referred to an internist for a more thorough examination. Her diagnosis was diabetes mellitus, adult onset. Ms. C was told that her condition was not serious and could be controlled by diet. She was 20 pounds (9 kg) overweight and was advised that she needed to lose the excess weight. She was instructed about her diet, how to test her urine, and about possible complications of diabetes.

Ms. C was frightened about her condition but did not mention this because no one else seemed very concerned. At first, she was conscientious about following her diet and testing her urine. She felt very well and was proud when she lost 5 pounds. As time went on, Ms. C began to wonder if she was really so sick. She had never felt ill. On her husband's birthday, she fixed a special dinner and baked a cake. She decided she deserved a reward for "being good" and did not follow her diet. She anxiously tested her urine at bedtime and it was negative. Then her son and his family visited the C's for a week. She fixed all their favorite foods and ate with them. She still felt fine and decided she did not need to test her urine. When it was time for her next checkup, she postponed calling the physician. She was very busy preparing for retirement travel.

Selected Nursing Diagnosis:

▼ Noncompliance related to fear of the diagnosis of diabetes as evidenced by lack of adherence to medical treatment plan

 Do you think that noncompliance can ever be an adaptive response? Why or why not?

Self-injury. Society accepts some forms of self-injury as normal. Examples of culturally sanctioned forms include ear piercing, cosmetic eyebrow plucking, hair twisting, nail and hair clipping, and circumcision. Nail biting and tatoos fall on the outer limits of socially acceptable self-injury. Various terms have been used to describe self-injurious behavior: *self-abuse, self-directed aggression, self-harm, self-inflicted injury,* and *self-mutilation.* **Self-injury** can be defined as the act of deliberate harm to one's own body. The injury is done to oneself, without the aid of another person, and the injury is severe enough for tissue damage. Common forms of self-injurious behavior include cutting and burning the skin, banging head and limbs, picking at wounds, and chewing fingers.[25]

Many nurses mistake self-injury as potential suicide. In fact, these are two separate phenomena. Usually the lethality of self-injury is low, and patients who self-injure typically want relief from the tension they feel rather than to kill themselves. Self-injury is also different from other self-destructive behaviors, such as bingeing, drug abuse, smoking, and high-risk activities. Self-injury is a contained event that occurs in a short time span and with an awareness of the consequences of the act.

Self-injurious behavior may be categorized by the type of patient and clinical context in which the behavior occurs:

1. *Mentally retarded individuals.* Outward-directed aggression is common among the mentally retarded

and frequently coexists with self-injurious behavior.

2. *Psychotic patients.* Self-injuring acts among psychotic patients tend to be sporadic and often occur in response to command hallucinations or delusions.

3. *Prison populations.* Self-injury in prisons is difficult to assess because of poor documentation, drug use, and undiagnosed psychiatric disorders. Many self-injurious events among prisoners are suspected of being intentionally manipulative, designed to force transfer to a less restrictive facility.

4. *Character disorders,* particularly borderline personality disorder. This group is often young and female with a poor tolerance of anxiety and anger. They also include patients with eating disorders.

Suicidal Behavior. Suicidal behavior is usually divided into the categories of suicide threats, suicide attempts, and completed suicide. In addition, certain suicide attempts may be referred to as **suicide gestures.** The gesture is a suicide attempt directed toward the goal of receiving attention rather than actual destruction of the self. Use of this term is questionable. It implies that it is *only* an attention-seeking behavior and should not be taken seriously. This is not true. All suicidal behavior is serious, whatever the intent, and deserves the nurse's serious consideration. Therefore suicide gestures are included in the general category of suicide attempts.

The **suicide threat** may be veiled but usually occurs before overt suicidal activity takes place. The suicidal person may make a statement such as "Will you remember me when I'm gone?" or "Take care of my family for me." If taken in the context of recent stressors and the person's life situation, statements such as these may be ominous. Nonverbal communication frequently reveals the suicide threat. The person may give away prized possessions, make a will or funeral arrangements, or systematically withdraw from all friendships and social activities. Sometimes a person may make a direct verbal suicidal threat, but this occurs less often. The threat is an indication of the ambivalence that is usually present in the suicidal behavior. It represents the hope that someone will recognize the danger and rescue the person from self-destructive impulses. It may also be an effort to discover whether anyone cares enough to prevent the individual from self-harm.

Jourard[14] has presented an interesting analysis of suicidal behavior related to the wish for rescue. He believes that suicide is sometimes the result of an "invitation to die" extended by significant others. The invitation may be communicated by failure to respond to a suicide threat or, at times, even more directly. For instance, a woman was admitted to the hospital following the ingestion of iodine. She was severely depressed and highly suicidal. After a course of electroconvulsive therapy (ECT), she recovered and went home. The social history revealed that her husband was a tombstone carver. He reportedly had prepared a tombstone for his wife with only the date of death missing and kept it in a back room of their house. A few months after discharge the patient successfully committed suicide.

Suicide attempts include any self-directed actions taken by the individual that will lead to death if not interrupted. In the assessment of suicidal behavior, much emphasis is placed on the lethality of the method threatened or used. Although all suicide threats and attempts must be taken seriously, more vigorous and vigilant attention is indicated when the person is planning or tries a highly lethal means such as gunshot, hanging, or jumping. Less lethal means include carbon monoxide and drug overdose, which allow time for discovery once the suicidal action has been begun.

Assessment of the suicidal person also includes whether the person has made a specific plan and whether the means to carry out the plan are available. The most suicidal person is one who plans a violent death (e.g., gunshot to the head), has a specific plan (e.g., as soon as his wife goes shopping), and has the means readily available (e.g., a loaded gun in a desk drawer). This person is exhibiting little ambivalence about a suicide plan. On the other hand, the person who contemplates taking a bottle of aspirin if the situation at work does not improve soon is communicating an element of hope. This person is really asking for help in coping with a poor work situation. The following clinical example illustrates the behavior of a suicidal person.

 CLINICAL EXAMPLE

Mr. Y was a 52-year-old black man employed in the foundry of a large steel mill. He had worked for the company for 20 years. He lived in a rented room in a blue-collar neighborhood near the mill. Most of his neighbors were Appalachian white and southern black families who had moved to the community to work at the mill. There was an undercurrent of racial tension in the neighborhood, but Mr. Y was not involved in conflicts with his neighbors. He had separated from his wife before moving to the community and had no close friends or family. The separation resulted from his violent behavior related to drinking binges.

Mr. Y was seen by the occupational health nurse, Ms. G, when he came to the employee health clinic following a 6-week absence from work. He had been hospitalized for broken ribs and a concussion after he had been beaten and robbed by a gang of adolescents in an alley behind his home. Ms. G was familiar with this employee because he had been a participant in the company's Employee Assistance Program for alcoholics. When she saw him in the clinic, she immediately noted that he appeared depressed. His face was expressionless, his posture slumped, and he had lost weight. He appeared disheveled, which was a change from his usual neat appearance. He said he did not feel ready to return to work, but he had received a letter from the personnel office requesting that his condition be evaluated by the company's physician. His speech was slow and halting and so soft that he could barely be heard. He told Ms. G that he had a request to make of her. He knew from past conversations that she was an animal lover. He wanted her to take his pet dog because he did not feel able to care for it adequately, and the neighbors who kept it while he was in the hospital had neglected it.

Ms. G was very concerned about Mr. Y and asked him how he was spending his time. He said he kept the television on and he thought a lot. When asked, he said he felt "too shaky" to go outside unless he absolutely had to. He thought the boys who attacked him were still in the neighborhood. Ms. G asked if he had thought about harming himself. Mr. Y looked startled, then admitted that he saw no other solution to his problem. "It makes sense. I don't have anybody. If you take Rover, I can go." With further questioning, he admitted that he had a loaded revolver at home and planned to use it after he left the clinic. Ms. G realized that Mr. Y needed help immediately and initiated plans for hospitalization.

Selected Nursing Diagnoses:

▼ Potential for self-directed violence related to impoverished social environment as evidenced by intent to kill self with a gun

▼ Powerlessness related to recent neighborhood attack as evidenced by expressed feelings of despair and hopelessness

Completed suicide may take place after warning signs have been missed or ignored. Some people do not give any easily recognizable warning signs. Research done on completed suicide has of necessity been retrospective. However, it can be informative to interview survivors. This procedure is known as the *psychological autopsy*. It is a retrospective review of the individual's behavior for the time preceding the suicide. The information obtained can be used to better understand suicidal behavior and to enhance the effectiveness of primary prevention activities.

Significant others of suicidal people, including survivors, have many feelings about this behavior. An element of hostility exists in suicidal behavior. Frequently the message to significant others, stated or implied, is

"You should have cared more." At times, when the person survives the attempt, this message may be transmitted in a manipulative way. An example is the adolescent girl who discovers that her boyfriend is dating someone else and takes an overdose of over-the-counter sleeping pills. If she sets the scene so that she will almost inevitably be discovered and makes sure that her boyfriend hears of her behavior, she is behaving in a hostile, manipulative way. A remorseful response by the boyfriend would be reinforcing and increase the likelihood that the behavior will be repeated. It is important to treat these attempts seriously and help the patient develop healthier communication patterns. Persons who do not really intend to die may do so if they are not discovered in time.

When suicide is successful, the survivors are left with many feelings that they cannot communicate to the involved object, the dead person (see A Family Speaks). This may lead to an unresolved grief reaction and depression. Some suicide prevention centers have become involved in *postvention* to assist people to deal with this dilemma. Survivors are assisted either individually or in groups to express their feelings and work through their grief.

In summary, the suicidal patient may have many different clinical behaviors. Mood disturbances are frequently present, as are somatic complaints. It has been noted that hopelessness may be more important than depression in explaining suicidal ideation.[4] Nurses should take a careful medical and psychiatric history, paying specific attention to the mental status examina-

---

 A FAMILY SPEAKS

My husband died last year. He didn't commit suicide, but he took his own life just as surely as if he had pulled the trigger of a gun. Only his weapon was a cigarette. You see, 2 years ago his doctor discovered a cancer lesion on his lung. At that time my husband was told he needed to lose weight, cut down on his drinking, and most of all, stop smoking. But my husband wasn't a very good patient.

Sometimes I blame myself for not doing more. I nagged for a while, but that only seemed to make our marriage worse. My husband said that what he did with his life was his own choice and that his father had smoked all of his life and lived until he was 84. My husband died at age 62.

One good thing has come out of this tragedy, however. My son has stopped smoking and has vowed he will never touch another cigarette for as long as he lives. That small goodness gives me comfort and some sense of hope. ▼

tion described in Chapter 6 and the psychosocial history, and evaluate the patient for recent losses, life stresses, and substance use and abuse (see Critical Thinking about Contemporary Issues).

Contrary to common opinion, directly questioning the patient about suicidal thought and plans will not result in the patient taking suicidal actions. Rather, most people wish to be rescued and prevented from carrying out their self-destruction. Most patients will feel relieved to be asked about these feelings. One of the most important questions to be asked of suicidal patients is whether they think they can control their behavior and refrain from acting on their impulses. If patients cannot do this, immediate psychiatric hospitalization is indicated.

Finally, the nurse may find it helpful to use an assessment tool to explore self-protective responses. The Beck Scale for Suicide Ideation[3] and the Assessment of Suicide Potentiality[16] are two scales that address this area. Fig. 18-3 presents a nursing assessment tool de-

CRITICAL THINKING ABOUT CONTEMPORARY ISSUES

Are Health-Care Professionals "Missing" Suicidal Behavior in Their Patients?

It has been reported that 8 out of 10 patients who commit suicide have talked about it with someone before completing the act. Often the person they talk with is a health-care professional. The problem is that care providers frequently miss the signs and symptoms of depression and the subtle indicators of self-destructive intentions.

There is evidence, for example, that 30% of all people who complete and attempt suicide visit primary care physicians within 1 month before their attempt. Among the elderly, more than 80% give "warning clues" of their intent. Of those elderly who commit suicide, 75% are known to have visited their personal physician in the month before they took their life. In one study health-care professionals reported a surprisingly small amount of probing for depressive or suicidal symptoms, even when they were mentioned by the patient. Most interesting, those patients 55 and older who were possibly at the highest risk reported no health professional inquiries about suicidal thinking and perceived the least amount of attention or interest in their mental attitude.[10] It thus appears that much work needs to be done to alert health-care providers to the severity and extent of this problem and to assist them to better evaluate patients for potential self-destructive responses. ▼

veloped for this purpose by the Division of Psychiatric Nursing at the Medical University of South Carolina. Factors the nurse must consider in the assessment of the self-destructive patient are listed in Box 18-1.[5]

Predisposing Factors

No one theory adequately explains self-destructive responses or guides therapeutic intervention. Behavior theory suggests that self-injury is learned and reinforced in childhood or adolescence. In contrast, psychological theory focuses on significant defects in early stages of ego development. It suggests that self-destructive behavior may have its roots in early interpersonal trauma and that unmanaged anxiety may provoke continued episodes of self-injury.[23] Interpersonal theories propose that self-injury may result from interactions that leave the child feeling guilty and worthless. A history of abuse or incest may then precipitate self-destructiveness if negative perceptions have been internalized and acted upon and there is a lack of secure attachments. Other predisposing factors related to self-destructive behavior include the inability to communicate needs and feelings verbally, feelings of guilt, depression, and depersonalization, and fluctuating emotions.

Five domains of risk factors—psychiatric diagnosis, personality traits and disorders, psychosocial and environmental factors, genetic and familial variables, and biochemical factors—contribute to a theoretical biopsychosocial model for understanding self-destructive behavior over the life cycle.[6] Each of these domains, as shown in Fig. 18-4, increases the risk for suicide and helps explain why only some patients with particular psychiatric disorders attempt or complete suicide.

Psychiatric Diagnosis. More than 90% of adults who end their lives by suicide have an associated psychiatric illness. There are three broad psychiatric disorders that put individuals at particular risk for suicide:

▼ Affective disorders
▼ Substance abuse
▼ Schizophrenia

Recent studies suggest that patients with panic disorder also have increased risk of suicide, and adolescents who kill themselves tend to have depression and conduct disorders. In addition, a high percentage of these youth abused alcohol or drugs.[7]

Suicide is the most serious complication of affective disorders, with 15% of those with these illnesses ending their lives by suicide. Patients with bipolar disorder and psychotic depression are at greatest risk. Alcohol use is associated with 25% to 50% of suicides and is the second category of psychiatric illness related to suicide.[1] In patients with alcohol dependence, suicide frequently occurs late in the disease and is often related

Directions:
a. Assess each key factor and current admission precipitated by attempt.
b. Circle one (of three) descriptor for each factor which BEST describes the patient.
c. Add the points for each circled item plus current admission precipitated by suicide attempt to obtain the Total Score.
d. Add RN's subjective appraisal of risk score to Total Score.

Key Factors	High Risk (1:1)	Moderate Risk (q15min observation)	No Precautions
Contract for Safety	Unwilling to contract OR Unable to contract due to impaired reality testing (e.g., hallucinations, delusions, dementia, delirium, dissociation) 2	Contracts but is ambivalent and/or guarded 1	Reliably contracts for safety 0
Suicide Plan	Has plan with actual OR potential access to planned method 2	Has plan without access to planned method 1	No plan 0
Plan Lethality	Highly lethal plan (e.g., gun, hanging, jumping, carbon monoxide) 2	Low lethality of plan 1	Low lethality of plan (e.g., superficial scratching, head banging, pillow over face, biting, holding breath) 0
Elopement Risk	High elopement risk 2	Low elopement risk 1	No elopement risk 0
Suicidal Ideation	Constant suicidal thoughts 2	Intermittent or fleeting suicidal thoughts 1	No current suicidal thoughts 0
Attempt History	Past attempts of high lethality 2	Past attempts of low lethality 1	No previous attempts 0
Symptoms (circle those that apply) hopelessness helplessness anhedonia guilt/shame anger/rage impulsivity	5-6 symptoms present 2	3-4 symptoms present 1	0-2 symptoms present 0
Current Morbid Thoughts (e.g., reunion fantasies, preoccupation with death)	Constantly 2	Frequently 1	Rarely 0

Current Admission Precipitated by Suicide Attempt   Yes 2
    No 1

RN's Subjective Appraisal of Risk:
    Patient replies not trustworthy, several nonverbal cues   4
    Patient replies questionably, trustworthy, at least 1
    non-verbal cue   3
    Patient replies trustworthy   0

Scoring Key: High Risk Precautions   =   10 or more
           Moderate Risk Precautions   =   4-9
           No Precautions   =   0-3

Total Score   _____

Assessed by (RN):   _____

Date: _____

Time:

Fig. 18-3   Suicide/self-harm assessment.
Courtesy of Division of Psychiatric Nursing, Medical University of South Carolina.

to some interpersonal loss or the onset of medical complications. Schizophrenia, a disease that afflicts 1% of the population, carries a high incidence of suicide; 10% to 13% of patients with schizophrenia end their life by suicide.[9] The risk is greatest for those patients under age 40 who feel hopeless, are suicidal, fear mental disintegration, have made previous suicidal attempts, have a chronic or relapsing course to their illness, and do not comply with treatment.[8]

Personality Traits. The three aspects of personality that are most closely associated with increased risk of suicide are (1) hostility, (2) impulsivity, and (3) depression. These traits are important because they cross diagnostic groups. In addition, borderline personality disorder and antisocial personality disorder are also more highly correlated with suicidal behavior (see Chapter 20). The coexistence of antisocial and depressive symptoms appears to be a particularly lethal combination in

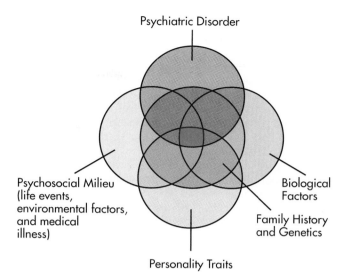

Fig. 18-4   Domains of risk factors for suicide.

Adapted from Blumental S, Kupfer D: *Suicide over the life cycle*, Washington, DC, 1990, American Psychiatric Press.

people are more socially withdrawn, have lower self-esteem, are less trusting of others, expect bad things to happen to them, feel powerless over their lives, and have a rigid and inflexible way of thinking.

How might the personality traits of hostility, impulsivity, and depression contribute to the development of substance abuse?

Psychosocial Milieu. This domain is concerned with social supports, life events, and chronic medical illnesses. Recent bereavement, separation or divorce, early loss, and decreased social supports are all important factors related to potential suicide.[21] Precipitants of suicidal behavior are often humiliating life events such as interpersonal problems, public embarrassment, loss of a job, or the threat of incarceration. In addition, evidence shows that knowing someone who attempted or committed suicide or exposure to suicide through the media may make an individual more vulnerable to self-destructive behavior. This appears to be a particularly important factor in cluster suicides (Box 18-2).

The strength of social supports is also important. It has been well documented that the strength and quality of these supports are important to the etiology of psychiatric problems, compliance with treatment, and response to therapeutic interventions. Finally, diseases with chronic and debilitating courses frequently precipitate self-destructive behavior. The prevalence of physical illness in suicides varies from 25% to 70% of cases and appears to be an important factor in 11% to 51%.

both adults and young people. The association between hostility and suicide stems from the notion proposed by Freud that the suicidal individual turns rage inward against the self. Other studies have found that suicidal

---

Box 18-2

EXAMPLE OF A CLUSTER SUICIDE

Between August and October of 1985, nine young men, ages 14 to 25, of the Shoshone tribe at Wind River, Wyoming (pop. 6000), killed themselves, all by hanging. This devastating rash of self-destruction is some 24 times in excess of the already-established high rate of suicide among Native American males in this age range. What happened at the Wind River reservation? Apart from obvious elements of suggestion and imitation, we may never completely know. The young men themselves left essentially no clues, and no evidence could be found of a suicide pact among them.

A plausible construction is that Wind River was host to a lethal concentration of the same problems that beset many Native American tribal societies and that impact especially on their young males: marginal status in the larger American society; a dearth of discernable opportunities to "break out" of a stark and bleak existence; rampant unemployment; erosion of ambition in the face of bureaucratically administered "welfare"; and searing boredom, from which available escape are largely limited to watching television and getting drunk. To these can be added, we surmise, the cruel realization of how far this fall has been for the descendants of the proud warriors who once ruled the continent.

In response to this crisis, tribal elders designed an intervention program emphasizing tribal history, tradition, and the revival of certain Native American healing rituals. The youth attended in large numbers, and the wave of suicides subsided.

Adapted from *Time*, October 21, 1985.

Among those disorders most frequently associated with suicide are cancer, Huntington's chorea, epilepsy, musculoskeletal disorders, peptic ulcer disease, and HIV/AIDS.

Family History. A family history of suicide is a significant risk factor for self-destructive behavior. Explanations for this association include identification with and imitation of a family member who has committed suicide, family stress, and transmission of genetic factors. Families of suicide victims have a significantly higher rate of suicide than do families with members who are nonsuicidally psychiatrically ill. In addition, monozygotic twins have a higher concordance rate for suicide than dizygotic twins. It will be important to distinguish the contribution of a family history of suicide from a family history of affective disorder to better identify high-risk groups for clinical intervention.

Biochemical Factors. Biologically, data suggest that serotonergically, opiatergically, and dopaminergically mediated processes may be implicated in self-destructive behavior.[17,20] Studies have found a common biochemical association between aggression, impulsivity, and reduced serotonergic function. Some research suggests that the finding of decreased serotonin in violent suicide attempters may increase the risk of completed suicide as much as tenfold. Studies of other transmitter receptors are in progress to further define the biochemical changes that occur in people with self-destructive behavior.

 Do you believe suicide is a fundamental human freedom and should be allowed by society? Why or why not?

Precipitating Stressors

Self-destructive behavior may result from almost any stress the individual feels as overwhelming. Stressors are somewhat individualized, as is the person's ability to tolerate stress. All self-destructive behaviors may be seen as attempts to escape from uncomfortable or intolerable life situations. Anxiety is therefore central to self-destructive behavior.

The anxiety associated with a deliberate attempt at self-destruction is overwhelming. It is difficult to imagine if it has not been experienced. Most people cringe from contemplating their own deaths, much less initiating self-destruction. Self-death is experienced differently from the death of another, since self-death literally cannot be experienced. In a sense, those who destroy themselves actually destroy everything else *but* themselves.

In contrast, people engaged in gradual self-destructive behavior tend to deny their eventual deaths, usually believing that they can assume control at any time. This fantasy of being able to control, although it alleviates anxiety, also helps to perpetuate the behavior. When the sense of self-worth is extremely low, self-destructive behavior reaches its peak. At this point, suicidal behavior is likely. Suicide implies a loss of the ability to value the self at all. Box 18-3 summarizes the risk factors for suicide.[11]

Coping Resources

Patients with chronic, painful, or life-threatening illnesses may engage in self-destructive behavior. Frequently these people consciously choose to kill themselves. Quality of life becomes an issue that overrides quantity of life. An ethical dilemma may arise for nurses who become aware of the patient's choice to engage in

---

Box 18-3

SUICIDE RISK FACTORS

PSYCHOSOCIAL AND CLINICAL

Hopelessness
Caucasian race
Male gender
Advanced age
Living alone

HISTORY

Prior suicide attempts
Family history of suicide attempts
Family history of substance abuse

DIAGNOSTIC

General medical illnesses
Psychosis
Substance abuse

---

this behavior. There are no easy answers to the question of how to resolve this conflict. Nurses must do so according to their own belief system.

Self-destructive behavior may be related to many social and cultural factors. Durkheim,[12] in his pioneer study of suicidal behavior, identified three subcategories of suicide, based on the individual's motivation:

1. *Egoistic suicide* results from the individual being poorly integrated into society.
2. *Altruistic suicide* results from obedience to customs and habit.
3. *Anomic suicide* results when society is unable to regulate the individual.

Durkheim believed the structure of society has a great influence on the individual. Society may either help or sustain individuals or lead them to self-destruction (see A Patient Speaks).

Social isolation may lead to loneliness and increase the person's vulnerability to suicide. People who are actively involved with others in their communities are more able to tolerate stress. Those who lose the ability to participate in social activities are more likely to turn to self-destructive behavior. Religious involvement is particularly supportive to many people during difficult times.

Coping Mechanisms

A patient may use a variety of coping mechanisms to deal with self-destructive feelings, including denial, rationalization, and regression. In addition the patient might display magical thinking. These coping mechanisms may be standing between the person and self-

 A PATIENT SPEAKS

The following are notes left by patients who committed suicide.

▼ Please forgive me and please forget me. I'll always love you. All I have was yours. No one ever did more for me than you; oh please pray for me, please.

▼ To Whom It May Concern,
   I, Mary Smith, being of sound mind, do this day make my last will as follows—I bequeath my rings, diamond and black opal to my daughter-in-law, Doris Jones, and any other of my personal belongings she might wish. What money I have in my savings account and my checking account goes to my dear father, as he won't have me to help him. To my husband, Ed Smith, I leave my furniture and car.

▼ I hate you and all of your family and I hope you never have peace of mind. I hope I haunt this house as long as you live here and I wish you all the bad luck in the world.

▼ Dear Daddy:
   Please don't grieve for me or feel that you did something wrong, you didn't. I'll leave this life loving you and remembering the world's greatest father.
   I'm sorry to cause you more heartache, but the reason I can't live anymore is because I'm afraid. Afraid of facing my life alone without love. No one ever knew how alone I am. No one ever stood by me when I needed help. No one brushed away the tears I cried for "help" and no one heard. I love you Daddy, Jeannie. ▼

---

destruction. They are defending the person from strong emotional responses to life events that are a serious threat to the ego. If they are removed, underlying depression will become overt and may lead to suicidal behavior.

Suicidal behavior indicates the imminent failure of the coping mechanisms. A suicidal threat may be a last-ditch effort to get enough help to be able to cope. Completed suicide represents the total failure of adaptive coping mechanisms.

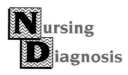 **Nursing Diagnosis**

When considering the nursing diagnosis of self-destructive behavior, the nurse must incorporate information about the seriousness and immediacy of the

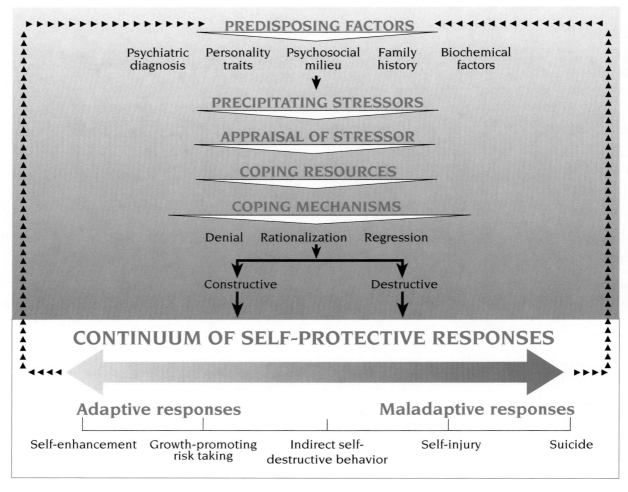

Fig. 18-5   A stress adaptation model related to self-protective responses.

patient's harmful activity. The nurse must consider the information obtained in the assessment to identify accurately the patient's need for nursing intervention (Fig. 18-5). Validation of the nursing diagnosis with the patient is needed. However, denial is a prominent defense with most self-destructive disorders. The patient may not be able to agree with a statement that confronts this behavior. The primary concern is to communicate, through the diagnosis, the level of protection needed by the patient. In the case of self-destructive behavior, caution is recommended in determining the level of risk. It is better to respond to the patient more intensively than to allow serious injury to occur.

Primary NANDA nursing diagnoses related to maladaptive self-protective responses are high risk for self-mutilation, noncompliance, and potential for self-directed violence. Because of the nature of the disorders associated with self-destructive behavior, other nursing diagnoses are frequently applied in the nurs-

ing care of these patients. Nursing diagnoses related to the range of possible maladaptive responses of the patient are listed in the Medical and Nursing Diagnoses box on p. 465. Examples of complete nursing diagnoses related to self-protective responses are presented in the Detailed Diagnoses box on p. 466.

Related Medical Diagnoses

Suicidal behavior is not identified as a separate diagnostic category in DSM-IV.[2] Several medical diagnostic classifications of the DSM-IV include actual or potential self-destructive behavior among their defining criteria. The medical diagnoses in which this behavior is listed as possible include bipolar disorder, major depression, noncompliance with treatment, schizophrenia, and substance use disorders. Their essential features are described in the Detailed Diagnoses box on p. 466.

MEDICAL AND NURSING DIAGNOSES RELATED TO SELF-PROTECTIVE RESPONSES

Related Medical Diagnoses (DSM-IV)*	Related Nursing Diagnoses (NANDA)†
Bipolar disorder	Adjustment, impaired
Major depressive disorder	Anxiety
Noncompliance with treatment	Body image disturbance
Schizophrenia	Coping, family-ineffective: compromised
Substance use disorders	Coping, ineffective individual
	Denial, ineffective
	Fluid volume deficit, potential
	‡**High risk for self-mutilation**
	‡**Noncompliance**
	Nutrition, altered: less than body requirements
	Nutrition, altered: more than body requirements
	Self-esteem disturbance
	Spiritual distress
	‡**Violence, potential for: self-directed**

*From American Psychiatric Association: *Diagnostic and statistical manual of mental disorders*, ed 4, Washington, DC, 1994, The Association.
†From North American Nursing Diagnosis Association: NANDA *nursing diagnoses: definitions and classifications* 1992-1993, Philadelphia, 1992, The Association.
‡Primary nursing diagnosis for self-destructive behavior.

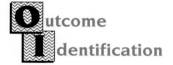

Outcome Identification

The expected outcome when working with a patient with maladaptive self-protection responses is:

The patient will not physically harm oneself.

Careful setting of priorities is necessary with the self-destructive patient. Highest priority should be given to goals related to preservation of life. The nurse must identify goals related to immediately life-threatening behavior. For example, the actively suicidal person must first be prevented from acting on impulses. Later, the nurse can attend to development of insight into the suicidal behavior and substitution of healthy coping mechanisms.

In dealing with self-destructive behavior, the nurse and the patient may appear to have incompatible goals. Suicidal patients may resist attempts to protect them and may actively try to evade their observers. However, most of these patients have some ambivalence. The nurse, in setting positive, life-preserving goals, is appealing to the healthy part of the person's self that wants to survive and be better able to cope with life. The very act of seeking help is an expression of this healthy aspect of the personality. The positive attitude of the nurse in setting constructive goals conveys a sense of hope to a patient who may be feeling hopeless.

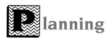

Planning

The nursing care plan for the person with self-destructive behavior must focus first on protecting the patient from harm. In addition, the plan must address the factors that contributed to the patient's dangerous behavior. The planning process also involves providing the patient with education about the specific illness. A Patient Education Plan for a patient who is noncompliant with medical treatment is on p. 467.

Implementation

Common elements exist in nursing intervention with all patients who exhibit self-destructive behavior. First, nurses must consider their own response to people who are trying to harm themselves. It can be difficult for a person who is happy and involved in life to imagine the depth of despair that leads to suicidal impulses or the lack of caring for the self that results in physically, psychologically, and socially damaging behavior, even if not immediately lethal. On the other hand, nurses who are depressed and dissatisfied with their own life may be threatened by interacting with patients who are more upset because they may fear similar consequences for

DETAILED DIAGNOSES
RELATED TO SELF-PROTECTIVE RESPONSES

NANDA Diagnosis Stem	Examples of Complete Diagnosis
High risk for self-mutilation	High risk for self-mutilation related to feelings of tension and worthlessness as evidenced by cutting of arms and legs
	High risk for self-mutilation related to command hallucinations as evidenced by dissection of calf
Noncompliance	Noncompliance with taking antihypertensive medication related to asymptomatic behavior as evidenced by unchanged elevation of blood pressure
	Noncompliance with 1800 calorie per day diabetic diet related to denial of illness as evidenced by gain of 10 pounds since last clinic visit
Potential for self-directed violence	Potential for self-directed violence related to loss of spouse as evidenced by purchase of a gun and discussions of death
	Potential for self-directed violence related to phencyclidine (PCP) abuse as evidenced by extreme psychotic disorganization and lack of body boundaries

DSM-IV Diagnosis	Essential Features*
Bipolar disorder	Presence of a manic episode and no past depressive episodes (see Chapter 17 for detail)
Major depressive disorder	The presence of at least five symptoms nearly everyday during the same 2-week period, with one being either depressed mood or loss of interest or pleasure (see Chapter 17 for details)
Noncompliance with treatment	Noncompliance with an important aspect of the treatment for a mental disorder or a general medical condition
Schizophrenia	Presence of two or more of the following symptoms for a 1-month period: delusions, hallucinations, disorganized speech, disorganized behavior, negative symptoms (see Chapter 19 for details)
Substance use disorders	Presence of substance dependence or substance abuse (see Chapter 22 for details)

*Adapted from the American Psychiatric Association: *Diagnostic and statistical manual of mental disorders*, ed 4, Washington, DC, 1994, The Association.

themselves. These nurses may also overidentify with the patient, which limits their ability to help the patient. There is a tendency to assume that the patient's and the nurse's situations are exactly alike, whereas in reality this is probably not so. A therapeutic approach is empathic and nonjudgmental, with limitation of subjective responses through awareness of one's own attitudes.

The reactions of nurses to long-term work with suicidal individuals have been studied, and four stages of reaction have been identified.[13]

1. *Stage of naiveté.* In the first exposure to suicidal behavior, nurses experience feelings of "shock, lack of understanding, avoidance, and denial."

2. *Stage of recognition.* The forced confrontation of these feelings leads to the next feeling cycle of "fear, anxiety, hopelessness, and confusion."

3. *Stage of responsibility.* Nurses experience conflict over the need to protect the patient combined with realization of their limitations to control the behavior of another person. The feelings associated with this stage are "responsibility, guilt, and anger."

4. *Stage of individual choice.* Nurses achieve a realistic understanding of the patient's responsibility for his own life. Nurses accept the possibility of losing a suicidal patient.

The recognition of patients' ultimate responsibility for determining their own fate does not imply a fatalis-

PATIENT EDUCATION PLAN
COMPLIANCE COUNSELING

Content	Instructional activities	Evaluation
Assess patient's knowledge of self-care activities	Ask patient to describe usual diet, exercise, and medication patterns.	Patient describes usual behavior.
	Validate whether described behaviors match self-care instruction received in the past.	Patient repeats previous directions.
Identify areas in which patient behavior differs from healthy self-care practices	Describe healthy self-care behavior to patient; provide written, patient education materials; encourage patient to describe reasons for not performing recommended self-care.	Patient discusses problems in compliance.
Discuss alternative approaches to self-care	Assist patient to identify alternative self-care behaviors that would be more acceptable. Enable patient to talk about feelings related to illness and treatment regimen.	Patient decides on different approach and shares feelings related to illness.
Agree on a reward for compliant behavior	Ask patient how he would reward himself for taking good care of himself.	Patient identifies reward.
Reinforcement	Praise patient for making a commitment to a healthier life-style.	Patient recognizes renewed commitment to self-care.

tic or unconcerned attitude by nurses. All possible efforts are made to protect patients and to motivate them to choose life. Nurses should align themselves with patients' wish to live and then assist them to be responsible for their own behavior. However, nurses must understand that some patients will choose death despite their best efforts to intervene. For the emotional health of nurses, they must recognize when this has happened. It has been reported that nurses take from 2 to 10 years to reach the stage of individual choice.[13]

 A friend tells you that suicidal patients are intent on dying and will ultimately succeed despite all intervention. How would you respond?

Protection

The highest priority nursing activity with self-destructive patients is to protect them from inflicting further harm on themselves and, if suicidal, from killing themselves. The message of protection is conveyed to patients verbally and nonverbally.

Verbally, patients are informed of the nurse's intention not to allow harm to come to the patient. To the suicidal patient the nurse might say, "I understand that you are feeling impulses to harm yourself. I will be here with you to help you control those impulses. I will do whatever is necessary to protect you. I'd like to talk with you about how you are feeling whenever you feel able to share that with me."

The nonverbal communications should reinforce and agree with the verbal. Obviously, dangerous objects such as belts, sharp implements, glass, and matches should be taken from the suicidal patient. It is impossible to make an environment perfectly safe. Even walls and floors can cause injury if patients throw themselves against them. However, the removal of dangerous objects gives a message of concern. One-to-one observation of the suicidal individual also communicates caring. This observation should be carried out with sensitivity, the nurse neither hovering over nor remaining aloof from the patient. The patient's nonverbal cues can guide the one-to-one interaction. It is important to remain alert until the mental health team and the patient agree that the self-destructive crisis is over. Suicidal patients may appear to be feeling much better immediately before making an attempt. This is attributed to the feeling of relief experienced when the decision has been made and the plans finalized. Nurses have been fooled by this behavior pattern, relaxing their vigilance, only to have patients kill themselves when they are allowed to be alone for a moment.

Contracting for Safety

An important aspect of protecting the patient involves coming to an agreement about the nature of the therapeutic relationship. This can involve the use of contracts in which the patient agrees not to inflict self-harm for a specified period of time. The patient further agrees that the clinician will be contacted should the patient be tempted to act on self-destructive impulses. The patient also agrees to give to others any possibly lethal articles such as guns or pills. Hospitalization is indicated if the patient is not willing to agree to these terms. If seen as an outpatient, the patient and clinician need names and telephone numbers to cover any emergencies. Finally, supportive others should also be involved in the contracting process. Families and friends are important allies in managing a suicidal patient.

After a trustworthy contract has been made, the nurse can then implement some additional steps to ensure the patient's safety. First, the patient should be supervised at all times. The patient should never be left alone. Second, the nurse can monitor any medications the patient may be receiving. For example, many of the antidepressants are fatal in overdose. This suggests that the patient should have only a few days' supply if treated as an outpatient. The nurse should note that the tricyclic antidepressants are associated with a higher rate of death in the event of overdose than the newer SSRI antidepressants[15] and that the benzodiazepines may disinhibit a patient, resulting in less control over self-destructive impulses (see Chapter 25).

Your depressed patient has been prescribed a tricyclic antidepressant because it is less expensive than other antidepressants. However, she lives in a rural area and cannot have the prescription filled every few days. You are worried about potential overdose. What alternatives can you identify?

Increasing Self-esteem

Self-destructive people have low self-esteem. The nurse may intervene by treating the patient as someone deserving of attention and concern. Positive attributes of the patient should be recognized with genuine praise. An attempt to make up reasons to praise the patient is usually recognized as artificial and lowers the patient's self-esteem. The message is that the patient is so bad that one has to search for positive characteristics. When getting to know the patient, the nurse should be alert to strengths that can be built on to provide the patient with positive experiences. Chapter 16 describes in de-tail interventions the nurse can use to enhance a patient's self-esteem.

Regulating Emotions and Behaviors

Nursing care should also be directed toward helping patients become aware of their feelings, label them, and express them appropriately. Anger is often a difficult feeling for these patients. The angry patient must be helped to deal constructively with anger through anger management skills. These are described in Chapter 27. Anxiety can also be overwhelming. Chapter 14 discusses anxiety-reducing interventions.

It may be helpful to assist patients with self-destructive responses to explore the predisposing and precipitating factors influencing their behavior. Once the acute crisis is over, the nurse can help the patient understand high-risk times and triggers, the feelings that get stimulated, dysfunctional thinking patterns, and resultant maladaptive coping responses. Plans can then be made to test out new coping mechanisms. For instance, during times of stress, the patient can[19]:

▼ Increase involvement with others
▼ Initiate a physical activity
▼ Engage in relaxation and tension-reducing activities
▼ Process feelings by talking with someone or writing in a journal

These and other examples of cognitive behavioral strategies that the nurse can implement are described in Chapter 28.

Mobilizing Social Support

Frequently, self-destructive behavior reflects a lack of both internal and external resources. Mobilization of social support systems is an important aspect of nursing intervention. Significant others probably have many feelings about the patient's self-destructive behavior. They need an opportunity to express their feelings and make realistic plans for the future. Family members must be made aware of control issues and helped to encourage self-control of the behavior by the patient. Both the patient and the family may need assistance in seeing that caring can be expressed by fostering self-care, as well as by providing care. Families of suicidal patients may be frightened of future suicidal activity. They need to be aware of behavioral clues to suicide and of community resources that can assist with crises. Suicidal behavior frequently recurs. False reassurance should be avoided. A better approach is to foster improved communication patterns and an ability to cope in the family. The nurse may help people sort out their feelings and frequently may want to refer significant others for individual intervention or family therapy.

If a patient commits suicide, it is important to intervene with the survivors who may be at risk for suicidal behavior. Van Dongen[24] has described approaches to work with survivors. They need someone who can listen to them and let them know that their feelings are not abnormal. They need to be able to discuss their beliefs about why the death occurred and assisted to find some meaning in the experience. Family members should be encouraged to support one another. Survivors are often stigmatized and may need assistance in dealing with this.

Community resources may also be important for the long-term care of the self-destructive person. Self-help groups may provide the recovering patient with needed peer support. Family therapy may assist in the reintegration of a family group that has been disrupted by the patient's recent experiences. Public health nurses, clergy, and other community-based helping people can provide the patient and family with day-to-day support. The nurse may be active in explaining resources to the patient and in initiating referrals to other agencies.

Mental Health Education

Patient education is another important aspect of nursing intervention. Education needs to be timed carefully. Patient readiness is essential if behavior change is to result. Patients who are noncompliant with prescribed health-care regimens may not understand the nature of their problem. Knowledge should be assessed and appropriate teaching initiated. Many patients are willing to participate in self-care if it makes sense to them. Teaching ways to monitor health status may also be helpful. For example, if hypertensive patients learn to check their blood pressure, they can learn to associate their health-care activities with their physiological response.

Patients following medication regimens, such as psychotropic medication for the previously suicidal patient, should know the prescribed dosage, frequency, and side effects. Information about how to handle any future crises should be provided to the patient. If the nurse has explained the possible reason for the patient's behavior, this may be reinforced at termination of the relationship to help the patient integrate the experience into his self-concept. Helping a patient to work through self-destructive behavior can be an extremely rewarding aspect of psychiatric nursing.

Suicide Prevention

Finally, nurses need to be aware of several important primary prevention strategies that may help to prevent suicide. These are listed in Box 18-4. Educational measures and suicide curricula in schools are other helpful

---

Box 18-4

SUICIDE PREVENTION STRATEGIES

▼ Gun control and decreased availability of lethal weapons

▼ Limitations on the sale and availability of alcohol and drugs

▼ Increased public and professional awareness about depression and suicide

▼ Less attention and reinforcement of suicidal behavior in the media

▼ Establishment of community-based crisis intervention clinics

▼ Campaigns to decrease the stigma associated with psychiatric care

▼ Increased insurance benefits for psychiatric and substance abuse disorders

---

interventions. These programs try to break down taboos about suicide and provide descriptions of the symptoms of depression to students, teachers, and parents.[18,22] The development of "at-risk" clinics in communities may also be helpful in preventing suicide. Such clinics might offer expert clinical assessment and treatment combined with strong community links, increased social supports, family education, and hotlines staffed with mental health professionals. In addition, education of the public and health-care providers is needed to increase knowledge about the early warning signs of self-destructive behavior and implement effective treatment strategies. A Nursing Care Plan Summary for patients with maladaptive self-protective responses is presented on p. 470.

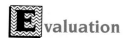 valuation

Evaluation of the nursing care of the self-destructive patient requires careful daily monitoring of the patient's behavior. Involvement of patients in evaluation of their progress can provide reinforcement and an incentive to work toward a goal. Modifications of the care plan are frequently necessary as patients reveal more of themselves and their needs to the nurse. As soon as possible, patients should participate in the planning, evaluation, and modification process.

Unfortunately, self-destructive behavior tends to recur. Nurses sometimes become discouraged and angry with patients who return again and again with the same behavior. When this occurs, nurses may be caught in the trap of feeling responsible for patient behavior. Nurses who have given the best nursing care possible have done as much as they can for the patient. It is impos-

NURSING CARE PLAN SUMMARY
Maladaptive Self-Protective Responses

Nursing Diagnosis: Potential for self-directed violence

Expected Outcome: The patient will not physically harm oneself.

Short-term Goal	Intervention	Rationale
The patient will not engage in self-injury activities.	Observe closely Remove harmful objects Provide a safe environment Provide for basic physiological needs Contract for safety if appropriate Monitor medications	Highest priority is given to life-saving patient care activities. The patient's behavior must be supervised until self-control is adequate for safety.
The patient will identify positive aspects of oneself.	Identify patient's strengths Encourage the patient to participate in activities that he likes and does well Encourage good hygiene and grooming Foster healthy interpersonal relationships	Self-destructive behavior reflects underlying depression related to low self-esteem and anger directed inward.
The patient will implement two adaptive self-protective responses.	Facilitate the awareness, labeling, and expression of feelings Assist the patient to recognize unhealthy coping mechanisms Identify alternative means of coping Reward healthy coping behaviors	Maladaptive coping mechanisms must be replaced with healthy ones to manage stress and anxiety.
The patient will identify two social support resources that can be helpful.	Assist significant others to communicate constructively with the patient Promote healthy family relationships Identify relevant community resources Initiate referrals to community resources	Social isolation leads to low self-esteem and depression, perpetuating self-destructive behavior.
The patient will be able to describe the treatment plan and its rationale.	Involve patient and significant others in care planning Explain characteristics of identified health care needs, nursing care needs, medical diagnosis, and recommended treatment and medications Elicit response to nursing care plan Modify plan based on patient feedback	Understanding of and participation in health-care planning enhance compliance.

sible to change the total life situation for the patient. The nurse can only help to identify alternative behaviors and provide encouragement for change. If the patient returns, the nursing process must begin again with an attitude of hope that this time the patient will learn and grow more and be better able to live a satisfying life.

SUGGESTED CROSS-REFERENCES

SUMMARY

1. The continuum of self-protective responses ranges from the most adaptive state of self-enhancement to the maladaptive responses of indirect self-destructive behavior, self-injury, and suicide.
2. Self-destructive behaviors may range from subtle to overt and include noncompliance with medical treatment plan, self-injury, and suicidal behavior.
3. Predisposing factors affecting self-protective responses include psychiatric diagnosis, personality traits, psychosocial milieu, family history, and biochemical factors. Precipitating stressors may be any stress the individual perceives as overwhelming.
4. Coping resources focus on social support systems, and coping mechanisms may include denial, rationalization, and regression.
5. Primary nursing diagnoses are high risk for self-mutilation, noncompliance, and potential for self-directed violence.
6. Suicide is not identified as a separate diagnostic category in the DSM-IV. Medical diagnostic classifications of the DSM-IV that include actual or potential self-destructive behavior are bipolar disorder, major depression, schizophrenia, and substance use disorder.
7. The expected outcome of nursing care is that the patient will not physically harm oneself.
8. Nursing interventions include protecting the patient, contracting for safety, increasing self-esteem, regulating emotions and behaviors, mobilizing social support, mental health education, and suicide prevention.
9. Evaluating nursing care requires daily monitoring of the patient's behavior. The nurse must also not become discouraged if self-destructive behavior recurs, and instead should approach the patient with the hope that this time the patient will grow and be better able to live a satisfying life.

COMPETENT CARING
CLINICAL EXEMPLAR OF A PSYCHIATRIC NURSE

Philip Macaione, BS, RN

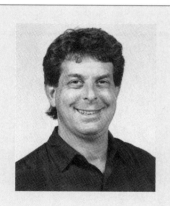

After 18 years of acute care nursing practice with a specialty in ICU, ER, and trauma nursing, I sought a new challenge and began psychiatric nursing practice. Having had the opportunity to associate professionally with hundreds of patients over the years who were experiencing critical and life-threatening situations, I felt well equipped to deal with psychiatric emergencies, until that seemingly "routine" day shift on an inpatient adult unit.

Ms. W had been committed to our unit as a dual-diagnosis patient. She was re ferred from our local county emergency room. She had been found near-stuporous, wandering the city streets and was thought to be homeless. She was a heroin and cocaine addict, as well as an alcoholic. She also suffered from multiple personality disorder, anxiety disorder, major depression, and schizotypical disorder. She was 6'2" and more than 300 pounds. Her hospital course over the previous 2 weeks was highlighted by her continued acting-out behaviors. These included disrupting the milieu, verbal, physical, and sexual threats to others, seeking the medication of other patients, noncompliance with her treatment plan, and defiance of unit rules and policies. Needless to say, she was a nursing challenge and required a firm, consistent approach by the staff and a constant vigil over her behavior.

One morning her behavior deteriorated to the point where staff intervened by placing her in scrubs and escorting her to the seclusion room to maintain her safety and that of the other patients. I explained to her that during this "time out" I would help her to begin processing her behavior and identify more effective coping strategies. I gave her a PRN medication for her agitation and anxiety and suggested she begin writing her thoughts and feelings down in her journal. After

Continued.

about a half hour, she verbally contracted for safety, seemed aware of her actions, and was resting quietly on her mattress. She also expressed that she was "feeling much better now" and thanked me for my help. I decided to put her on 15-minute checks but leave her in open-door seclusion until we agreed that she was ready to return to the milieu. I remember thinking, "Wow, I did a good job with this patient, and she is really making progress."

After years of nursing practice I notice that I have developed a sixth sense when I intuit that something is just not right. On the surface Ms. W seemed to be in control, but my sixth sense drew me back to the seclusion room only minutes after I had left her. As I walked into the room I did a double take and thought to myself "this can't be happening." Unfortunately, it was. Ms. W had managed, in the moments that had elapsed since I had left her side, to tear up her journal into small pieces, place the scraps between her legs and ignite them with a cigarette lighter we later discovered she had hidden in her vagina. She was madly waving the fire between her legs to produce more flames. Her scrub pants and mattress were now on fire.

At this point I just reacted. I ran to her, pulled away the mattress, patted down the flames on her pants, and yelled for help. The smoke alarm had gone off, and within seconds other staff arrived. I instructed them to remove the patient to the safety of the corridor and give the patient first aid. This was no easy task given the patient's size and level of agitation. I then activated the fire procedure, grabbed the fire extinguisher, and returned to the seclusion room. By now the smoke was thick, but I pulled the pin of the fire extinguisher, aimed, and released the foam. Within seconds, the fire was extinguished. The fire department had now arrived and moved in to deal with the smoldering mattress. Ms. W suffered no injuries and was discharged to a boarding house about 1 week later.

I learned a great deal from this incident and think I am a better nurse because of it. The staff response and teamwork in reacting to this crisis were extraordinary. I also think that the many years of critical decision-making opportunities afforded me throughout my nursing practice made me well equipped to handle this "seemingly" routine shift on our unit. Most of all, I have a greater appreciation and respect for the sixth sense of nurses, which may be the mark of truly competent nursing care. ▼

REFERENCES

1. Adams D: Suicidal behavior and history of substance abuse, *Am J Drug Alcohol Abuse* 18:343, 1992.
2. American Psychiatric Association: *Diagnostic and statistic manual of mental disorders*, ed 4, Washington, DC, 1994, The Association.
3. Beck A, Steer R: *Manual for the Beck hopelessness scale*, San Antonio, 1991, Psychological Corp.
4. Beck A, Steer R, Beck J, Newman C: Hopelessness, depression, suicidal ideation, and clinical diagnosis of depression, *Suicide Life Threat Behav* 23:139, 1993.
5. Blumenthal S: An overview and synopsis of risk factors, assessment, and treatment of suicidal patients over the life cycle. In Blumenthal S, Kupfer D: *Suicide over the life cycle*, Washington, DC, 1990, American Psychiatric Press.
6. Blumenthal S, Kupfer D: Generalizable treatment strategies for suicidal behavior, *Ann NY Acad Sci* 487:327, 1986.
7. Brent D et al: Psychiatric risk factors for adolescent suicide: a case-control study, *J Am Acad Child Adolesc Psychiatry* 32:521, 1993.
8. Caldwell C, Gottesman I: Schizophrenia—a high-risk factor for suicide: clues to risk reduction, *Suicide Life Threat Behav* 22:479, 1992.
9. Cohen L, Test M, Brown R: Suicide and schizophrenia: data from a prospective community treatment study, *Am J Psychiatry* 147:602, 1990.
10. Coombs D et al: Presuicide attempt communications between parasuicides and consulted caregivers, *Suicide Life Threat Behav* 22:289, 1992.
11. Depression Guideline Panel: *Depression in primary care: detection, diagnosis, and treatment: quick reference guide for clinicians*, no 5, Rockville, Md, 1993, US Department of Health and Human Services, Public Health Service, Agency for Health Care Policy and Research.
12. Durkheim E: *Suicide*, New York, 1951, The Free Press. Translated by JA Spaulding and G Simpson.
13. Hamel-Bissell BP: Suicidal casework: assessing nurses' reactions, *J Psychosoc Nurs Ment Health Serv* 23:20, 1985.
14. Jourard S: Suicide: an invitation to die, *Am J Nurs* 70:269, 1980.
15. Kapur S, Mieczkowski T, Mann J: Antidepressant medications and the relative risk of suicide attempt and suicide, *JAMA* 268:3441, 1992.
16. Los Angeles Suicide Prevention Center: *Assessment of suicidal potentiality*, Los Angeles, The Center.
17. Mann J, Arango V: Integration of neurobiology and psychopathology in a unified model of suicidal behavior, *J Clin Psychopharmacol* 12:2S, 1992.
18. Orbach I, Bar-Joseph H: The impact of a suicide prevention program for adolescents on suicidal tendencies, hopelessness, ego identity, and coping, *Suicide and Life Threat Behav* 23:120, 1993.

19. Pawlicki C, Gaumer C: Nursing care of the self-mutilating patient, *Bull Menninger Clin* 57:380, 1993.

20. Pitchot W, Hansenne M, Moreno A, Ansseau M: Suicidal behavior and growth hormone response to apomorphine test, *Biol Psychiatry* 31:1213, 1992.

21. Rich C et al: Suicide, stressors, and the life cycle, *Am J Psychiatry* 148:524, 1991.

22. Shaffer D: Preventing suicide in young people, *Innovations & Research* 2:3, 1993.

23. Van der Kolk B, Perry J, Herman J: Childhood origins of self-destructive behavior, *Am J Psychiatry* 148:1665, 1991.

24. Van Dongen C: The legacy of suicide, *J Psychosoc Nurs Ment Health Serv* 26:8, 1988.

25. Winchel R, Stanley M: Self-injurious behavior: a review of the behavior and biology of self-mutilation, *Am J Psychiatry* 148:306, 1991.

ANNOTATED SUGGESTED READINGS

Blumenthal S, Kupfer D: *Suicide over the life cycle*, Washington, DC, 1990, American Psychiatric Press.

One of the best and most comprehensive texts on the many aspects of suicide.

Canetto S: Gender and suicide in the elderly, *Suicide Life Threat Behav* 22:80, 1992.

Thought-provoking discussion of why elderly women are less likely to be suicidal than men. Integrates sociocultural aspects of suicidal behavior with suggestions for prevention.

*Cugino A et al: Searching for a pattern: repeat suicide attempts, *J Psychosoc Nurs Ment Health Serv* 30:23, 1992.

Reports on nursing research examining repeat suicide attempters.

*Jourard S: Suicide: an invitation to die, *Am J Nurs* 70:269, 1970.

Connects family process to suicidal behavior. Leads the reader to consider the broader social system, which usually affects the identified patient's behavior.

*Neville D, Barnes S: The suicidal phone call, *J Psychosoc Nurs Ment Health Serv* 23:14, 1985.

Discusses issues related to interacting with a suicidal person on the telephone, recommending information that should be collected, and helpful and unhelpful responses. Emphasizes the need for peer support of the telephone counselor.

Niswander GD, Casey TM, Humphrey JA: *A panorama of suicide*, Springfield, Ill, 1973, Charles C Thomas.

Presents a fascinating collection of psychological autopsies. Adds depth to one's understanding of the many facets of suicidal behavior.

*Pawlicki C, Gaumer C: Nursing care of the self-mutilating patient, *Bull Menninger Clinic* 57:380, 1993.

Excellent summary of nursing interventions for working with the difficult patient population of self-mutilators. Clear and practical.

Robinson R: *Survivors of suicide*, Santa Monica, Calif, 1989, IBS Press.

Excellent book directed toward the lay audience. Addresses facts about suicide, the experiences of survivors, and ways to help a suicidal person.

Rosowsky E: Suicidal behavior in the nursing home and a post-suicide intervention, *Am J Psychother* 47:127, 1993.

Uses a case presentation to explore suicide among the elderly in nursing homes including risk factors and postsuicide interventions. Highly recommended.

*Sebree R, Popkess-Vawter S: Self-injury concept formation: nursing diagnosis development, *Perspect Psychiatr Care* 27:27, 1991.

Reviews a historical perspective of self-injury behaviors, defines the phenomena, and outlines appropriate nursing interventions.

*Stanitis MA, Ryan J: Noncompliance: an unacceptable diagnosis? *Am J Nurs* 82:941, 1982.

Challenges the acceptability of the nursing diagnosis of noncompliance, pointing out that this is a value-laden term that may result in the development of negative attitudes toward the patient. Also questions whether compliance with a medical regimen is always a positive behavior. Could be assigned as a stimulus for group discussion.

*Valente S: Deliberate self-injury: management in a psychiatric setting, *J Psychosoc Nurs Ment Health Serv* 29:19, 1991.

Excellent overview of the etiology, assessment, and treatment of patients who self-injure.

White-Bowden S: *Everything to live for*, New York, 1985, Pocket Books.

A mother's account and analysis of her teenage son's suicide. Recommended for nurses and parents. Contains excellent advice related to prevention.

Winchel R, Stanley M: Self-injurious behavior: a review of the behavior and biology of self-mutilation, *Am J Psychiatry* 148:306, 1991.

Synthesizes current knowledge on self-mutilating behavior. For the advanced student.

*Nursing reference.

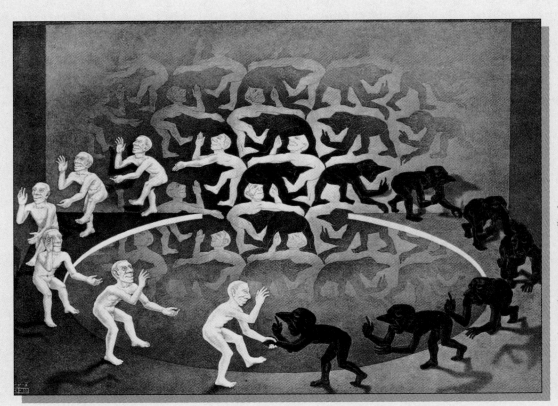

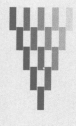

CHAPTER 19

Neurobiological Responses and Schizophrenia and Psychotic Disorders

MARY D. MOLLER
MILLENE F. MURPHY

How do I get away
Away from you—voices?
How do I leave you
behind me forever?
You who echo my feelings
haunt my thoughts
and ravage my
    nights . . .
How do I get away from
you?

I sing at the top
of my voice
and still I hear you.
I talk loud and
listen to people
and still I hear you.
Is there a me without
    you?

No, the answer comes
loud and clear,
there is no me without you.
As long as I have feelings
you will be my echo.
As long as I have thoughts
you will be the ghost.
As long as there is night
you will be in the darkness.

Sharon LeClaire

LEARNING OBJECTIVES

After studying this chapter the student should be able to:

▼ Describe the continuum of adaptive and maladaptive neurobiological responses
▼ Discuss the prevalence of schizophrenia and other psychotic disorders
▼ Identify behaviors associated with maladaptive neurobiological responses
▼ Analyze predisposing factors and precipitating stressors related to maladaptive neurobiological responses
▼ Describe coping resources and coping mechanisms related to maladaptive neurobiological responses
▼ Formulate nursing diagnoses for patients related to maladaptive neurobiological responses
▼ Assess the relationship between nursing diagnoses and medical diagnoses related to maladaptive neurobiological responses
▼ Identify expected outcomes and short-term nursing goals for patients related to maladaptive neurobiological responses
▼ Develop a family education plan to promote adaptive neurobiological responses
▼ Analyze nursing interventions for patients related to maladaptive neurobiological responses
▼ Evaluate nursing care for patients related to maladaptive neurobiological responses

TOPICAL OUTLINE

Continuum of Neurobiological Responses
Assessment
    Behaviors
    Predisposing Factors
    Precipitating Stressors
    Coping Resources
    Coping Mechanisms
Nursing Diagnosis
    Related Medical Diagnoses
Outcome Identification
Planning
    Murphy Wellness Model
Implementation
    Interventions Related to Instability
    Interventions Related to Stability
    Interventions Related to Actualization
Evaluation

Psychiatric nurses often are most challenged when providing nursing care to patients with maladaptive neurobiological responses such as schizophrenia and other psychotic disorders. The behaviors associated with these disruptions are difficult to understand and sometimes frightening. Patients who experience psychoses are also frightened by their experiences. They are usually unable to form close interpersonal relationships because of the demands of the illness for their attention and energy. Caring nurses must strive to make contact with psychotic patients and assist them to overcome or adapt to the effects of the illness. A Patient Speaks describes an individual's experience of psychosis.[10]

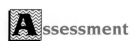 Read the patient's description of psychosis a second time. Focus on identifying the feelings that might be associated with these experiences.

CONTINUUM OF NEUROBIOLOGICAL RESPONSES

The symptoms of psychosis are clustered within five major categories of brain function: cognition, perception, emotion, behavior, and socialization, which is also referred to as relational. Fig. 19-1 presents the continuum of responses related to neurobiological functioning.

Assessment

About 2 million people in the United States suffer from schizophrenia during the course of their lifetime.[40] Schizophrenia is a chronic illness that is five times more common than multiple sclerosis; six times more common than insulin-dependent diabetes; sixty times more common than muscular dystrophy; and eighty times more common than Huntington's disease.[46] Overall spending for the care of patients with schizophrenia is estimated to exceed $25 billion. In three out of four cases it begins between the ages of 17 and 25, robbing its victims of their most productive young adult years. This adds an additional cost of $48 billion annually in lost productivity. Twenty-five percent of individuals with schizophrenia will never recover, and 50% will have disabling symptoms throughout much of their lives. The fear of relapse is disruptive to the lives of the patient and the family. One out of four patients with schizophrenia will attempt suicide, and 10% complete suicide in the first 10 years of the illness.[1]

A PATIENT SPEAKS

Psychosis is real. Its main feature is a loss of consciousness of the self in such a way that I can no longer discern my relationship to the reality that my body is in. This would not be destructive, except that I have done it inadvertently; I have done it without consciousness and have not provided for my body. My body, then, goes on without me. It wanders aimlessly and does not know to keep warm in the cold. It does not know how to avoid attack by violence. It does not know to protect itself from fire and deep water and the traffic that races down the highway.

My brain comes up with fantastical ideas about who I might be, since I am not there to tell it. Perhaps I am the Queen of Hearts, or a messenger from another planet, or even Jesus Christ himself. And why not? My brain distorts the reality of the senses: Is this burner hot, or cold? Is this coat wet or dry? Is this chair a chair, or, what exactly is this anyway, and for that matter, what in the world are you?

Maybe bugs are jumping out of my mind and onto that wall over there. Maybe there's a current coming up from the earth and into my feet and trying to pull me in. My brain can think of every kind of combination and definition, every kind of idea that it can put together, for it has a nearly infinite number of choices. It has all it has ever experienced, all the sounds, all the sights, all the sensations, all the dreams, all the fantasies, all the nightmares.

My brain chooses its manifestation according to what emotions were available to it when I was in charge. Only I am not there to add my discernment, my wisdom, and my awareness according to what I have learned. My brain goes haywire then. It has no person to guide it, no captain, no helm, and no rudder. It has no fingers at the keyboard. It wanders through its innerspace like the steel ball that is thrown into nothing and bounces at random from arbitrarily placed spots in the pinball machine.

What is this I, then, that is gone, and where did it go? It is consciousness. It is awareness. It is the presence of the I in me. It is ego. It is my separation. It is the part in me that tells me the difference between me and the world. It is the I-ness of me that holds me upright like a spine and says, "You will not fall into this tree, or this song, or this ocean of water or air, and it will not fall into you. The I that is gone is the intelligence that says I am me, and you are you." ▼

From Corday R: *Psychosis, the inner experience,* Boulder, Colo, 1991, Common Loon Productions.

Behaviors

Attempts at defining psychosis are varied and often related to the theoretical orientation of the person who is making the definition. Typically, psychosis has been defined within the context of a patient's perception of

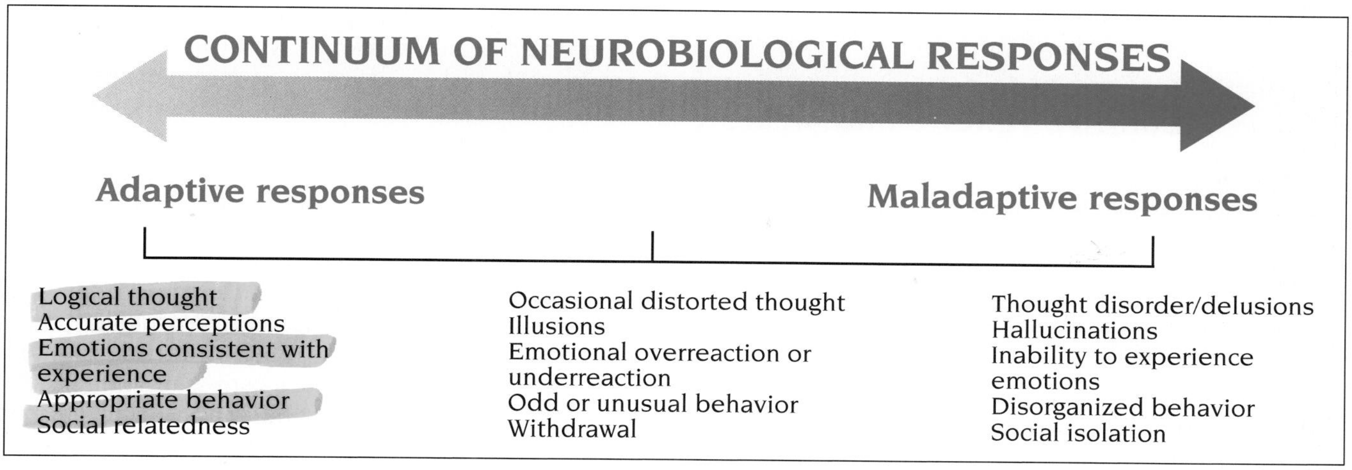

CONTINUUM OF NEUROBIOLOGICAL RESPONSES

Adaptive responses

Maladaptive responses

Logical thought	Occasional distorted thought	Thought disorder/delusions
Accurate perceptions	Illusions	Hallucinations
Emotions consistent with experience	Emotional overreaction or underreaction	Inability to experience emotions
Appropriate behavior	Odd or unusual behavior	Disorganized behavior
Social relatedness	Withdrawal	Social isolation

Fig. 19-1   Continuum of neurobiological responses.

reality and the resulting behavior. This has led to a bias toward treatment focused on reorienting the person to the "correct" reality.

Schizophrenia is an illness that results in psychotic behavior. It is actually one of a group of related disorders[3,4,41] that are heterogeneous in pathophysiology, predisposing factors, precipitating stressors, and related behaviors. Other psychotic disorders include schizoaffective disorder, delusional disorder, brief psychotic disorder, shared psychotic disorder (folie à deux), psychotic disorder due to a general medical condition, and substance-induced psychotic disorder.[2]

The term **schizophrenia** was introduced in 1911 by the Swiss psychiatrist, Bleuler. He observed that the schizophrenias were sometimes progressive, at times intermittent, and could stop or recede at any stage, although they did have a tendency toward deterioration. He believed that the schizophrenias were multidimensional and organic in nature. He also believed that these illnesses were strongly influenced and could be shaped by psychological factors.

The word *schizophrenia* is a combination of two Greek words, *schizein*, "to split," and *phren*, "mind." Bleuler's reference was not to a "split personality," which refers to having separate identities, but to his belief that a split occurred between the cognitive and emotional aspects of the personality. Confusion about the meaning of the term *schizophrenia* continues to exist today.

Bleuler also identified two major groups of behaviors related to schizophrenia. Primary symptoms are classically referred to as "The 4 A's." These are disturbances related to:

▼ *Associations*
▼ *Affect*
▼ *Ambivalence*
▼ *Autistic thinking*

Additional "A's" include:

▼ Attention defects
▼ Disturbances of activity

Secondary symptoms that can also occur include hallucinations, delusions, ideas of reference, and memory disturbances.

Finally, a nursing assessment of behaviors related to schizophrenia and other psychotic disorders relies heavily on findings from the mental status examination, which is described in detail in Chapter 6.

Cognition. Cognition is the act or process of knowing. It involves activities of awareness and judgment that enable the brain to process information in a way that ensures accuracy, storage, and retrieval. People with schizophrenia are sometimes unable to produce complex logical thoughts and express coherent sentences because the neurotransmissions travelling through the brain's malfunctioning information processing system are accelerated, delayed, or blocked. Behaviors related to problems in information processing associated with schizophrenia are often referred to as cognitive deficits. They include problems with all aspects of memory, attention, form and organization of speech (formal thought disorder), decision making, and thought content (delusions) (Box 19-1).

Information processing depends on anatomical and neurophysiological brain processes as well as prior learning. It involves organizing sensory input into behavioral responses. Sensory input is screened according to the individual's world view and the focus of the person's attention (Fig. 19-2).

World view is also referred to as a "cognitive map" that influences which stimuli receive attention as well as the perceptual organization and meaning of the stimuli.[43] This has a direct influence on behavior. Each person's cognitive map is formed during the developmental process and continues to be changed by learn-

Box 19-1

PROBLEMS IN COGNITIVE FUNCTIONING

MEMORY

Difficulty accessing and using stored memory
Impaired short-term/long-term memory

ATTENTION

Inability to maintain attention
Poor concentration
Distractibility

FORM AND ORGANIZATION OF SPEECH (FORMAL THOUGHT DISORDER)

Loose associations
Tangentiality
Incoherence/word salad/neologism
Illogicality
Circumstantiality
Pressured/distractible speech

DECISION MAKING

Failure to abstract
Indecisiveness
Lack of insight
Impaired judgment
Illogical thinking
Lack of planning skill
Inability to initiate tasks

THOUGHT CONTENT

Delusions
  Paranoid
  Grandiose
  Religious
  Somatic
  Nihilistic
Bizarre delusions
  Thought broadcasting
  Thought insertion
  Thought control

When information processing is distorted, an individual's cognitive map, or world view, is very different from that of others in one's environment. People with schizophrenia generally tend to have a world view that has been altered due to brain deficits. However, interferences with cognitive function often keep people with schizophrenia from realizing that their ideas and behavior are different from others. This is particularly evident in their self-perception of worth and abilities. They have a tendency to dramatically overestimate or underestimate their own capability. Hospitalization is often viewed as a sign that others are trying to eliminate the presence of the person with schizophrenia. The increased brain dysfunction during an acute episode makes it difficult for the patient to realize the need for assistance.

Memory is the retention or storage of knowledge learned about the world. Additional information about memory and its assessment can be found in Chapters 5, 6, and 21. Behaviors associated with schizophrenia that are related to memory problems include forgetfulness, disinterest, and lack of compliance. It is critical for the nurse to understand the frustration this symptom causes for patients. They commonly seek validation of the correctness of task accomplishment, frequently ask if it is time to attend a group function or go to an appointment, and ask permission to make a telephone call just to verify if they remember phone numbers. Often, because staff fail to recognize a symptom versus a "manipulative behavior," patients receive restrictions. When people with schizophrenia repeatedly ask the same question, request to know what time it is, or ask how to get somewhere, it is important for the nurse to simply provide the requested information in a kind and matter-of-fact manner that does not cause embarrassment or decrease the person's self-worth.

Attention is the ability to focus on one activity in a sustained, concentrated manner. Disrupted attention is an impairment in the ability to attend, observe, and concentrate on external reality. Inability to concentrate is almost always related to disrupted attention. Disturbances in attention are common in schizophrenia and include difficulty completing tasks, difficulty concentrating on work, and easy distractibility. Easy distractibility refers to a patient's attention being drawn easily to unimportant or irrelevant external stimuli such as noises, books out of order on a bookshelf, or people passing by. In addition, the patient who is experiencing auditory hallucinations often has problems with attention.

These impairments are not constant and frequently shift depending on the brain activity required. This generates much frustration for all involved in managing schizophrenia, especially the patient, who often verbalizes frustration about inability to complete tasks because "my mind is always wandering." The nurse needs

ing and life experiences. The more flexible the map is, the greater the change that occurs. It is through this map that individuals perceive the world and how the world affects them.

Describe how your cognitive map (world view) differs from a person of the opposite sex, an older generation, another race, and another socioeconomic class. What is the result of these differences?

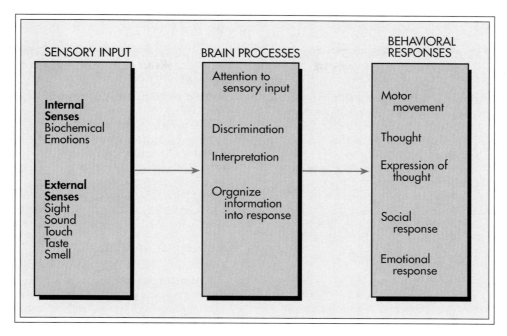

SENSORY INPUT

Internal Senses
Biochemical
Emotions

External Senses
Sight
Sound
Touch
Taste
Smell

BRAIN PROCESSES

Attention to sensory input

Discrimination

Interpretation

Organize information into response

BEHAVIORAL RESPONSES

Motor movement

Thought

Expression of thought

Social response

Emotional response

Fig. 19-2   Brain information processing.

to be aware of this problem and be prepared to redirect the patient back to the task at hand. The nurse will also need to repeat directions frequently in short, simple phrases.

> The parents of a young man who has schizophrenia tell you that they are frustrated by their son's unwillingness to return to work. Based on your understanding of the cognitive disorders that occur related to schizophrenia, how would you respond to them?

Malfunctions in information processing produce other disturbances in thinking that interfere with coherent communication. **Form and organization of speech** problems may include loose associations, word salad, tangentiality, illogicality, circumstantiality, pressure of speech, poverty of speech, distractible speech, and clanging. These behaviors are described in Chapter 6. Box 19-2 presents examples of nurse-patient dialogues that reflect behaviors in the form and organization of speech related to psychotic disorders.

Recognizing that speech is a reflection of cognitive processing helps the nurse appreciate the considerable difficulties a person with schizophrenia has in communicating needs clearly. The nurse will need to focus attention and use active listening to understand the patient. The nurse who is making an honest attempt to

identify and clarify patient wants does not need to be afraid of offending the patient by seeking to understand. It is essential to remember that the patient is sincerely trying to answer, no matter how difficult, weird, or bizarre the answer is. The nursing responsibility is to identify one or two key verbal or nonverbal responses and seek validation. This will most likely be achieved through simple trial and error.

Decision making means arriving at a solution or making a choice. Components of decision making include insight, judgment, logic, decisiveness, planning, ability to carry out decisions that have been made, and abstract thought. Lack of insight is probably one of the greatest problems occurring in schizophrenia, since patients generally do not believe that they are ill or different in any way. Unfortunately many clinicians confuse lack of insight with denial and treat people who have schizophrenia as if their symptoms were willful and within conscious control.

Faulty logic is often identified through the speech of people with schizophrenia who display the behaviors of thought disorder. When there are cognitive deficits in decision making, the patient makes decisions based on erroneous inferences, yet cannot understand that the judgment was faulty. Other people with schizophrenia are simply unable to reach a decision. For them, life is difficult at best. They wrestle with even simple decisions such as which coffee cup to use. Plans based on faulty decision making will not serve the intended purpose. This symptom creates much of the frustration related to schizophrenia. Initiating responses to follow-through on

---

Box 19-2

FORM AND CONTENT OF SPEECH RELATED TO PSYCHOTIC DISORDERS

LOOSE ASSOCIATIONS

Nurse: "Do you have enough money to buy that candy bar?"

Patient: "I have a real yen for chocolate. The Japanese have all the yen and have taken all our money and marked it. You know, you have to be careful of the Marxists because they are friends with the Swiss and they have all the cheese and all the watches and that means they have taken all the time. The worst thing about Swiss cheese is all the holes. People have to be careful about falling into holes."

Nurse: "It sounds like you are worried about your money."

Patient: "Yes, I have it all here in my wallet and you can't have it and the bank can't have it either."

INCOHERENCE

Nurse: "What does your family like to do at Christmas?"

Patient: "I believe they took Christmas from the Russians to get all the cars into the ocean and make jello. You could go and get the Christmas but you couldn't do it because the keylars have the fan."

TANGENTIALITY

Nurse: "I'm interested in learning more about your landscape paintings."

Patient: "My interest in art goes back to my parents who lived on a farm in Indiana. They had lots of haystacks, kind of like they do in Ohio, but you know, the hay is different colors in different states so that gave me the ability to paint so many different colors of yellow. Some people don't really like bright yellow hay, but I do. If I make the hay really bright yellow, then I make the barns a dull red, because barns really shouldn't be painted with bright red paint. Bright red should be saved for fire engines and fire hydrants and stop signs.

ILLOGICAL SPEECH

Nurse: "Do you think your medicine is helping you think more clearly?"

Patient: "I used to think my medicine helped me think. But I realized that it was me who took the medicine, so it wasn't the medicine that helped me think. Medicine can't think, don't you realize that? Maybe you should take some medicine to help you think better. But if you do, I would have to give it to you because it is the fact I took it myself that my thinking is better, so, no, I don't think the medicine is helping me think better."

DISTRACTIBLE SPEECH

Nurse: "I would like to talk with you about your understanding of schizophrenia."

Patient: "I know it's got something to do with my brain. What perfume are you wearing? It must be from France. Is that where that picture was taken? Your hair is different than when that picture was taken. Was that about 4 years ago?"

CLANG ASSOCIATIONS

Patient: "I got a new shirt but the buttons become loose. Do you suppose Lucifer's buttons become lucent or are they lucid like Lucy's?"

POVERTY OF CONTENT OF SPEECH

Nurse: "Do you want to go to the grocery store?"

Patient: "Yeah, uh huh, well what would I do with the, uh, the stuff that is over there on top of it? Do they, uh, have the, the, you know, the thing to do it with the wheels on the floor. I, uh, guess they should let me."

---

decisions is also a problem for people who have schizophrenia. Often this is mistaken as loss of motivation. Motivation involves having a desire as opposed to having the ability to follow through. People with schizophrenia typically have difficulty initiating tasks of any kind because of other problems related to components of decision making.

Concrete thinking typically replaces abstract thought in schizophrenia, particularly during acute episodes. It is indicated by the absence of abstracting abilities and by several key indicators. Patients often have difficulty with multiple-stage commands. In other words, if the nurse approaches the patient and presents the daily schedule and gives directions about the time and place of group and occupational therapies, the information is not all processed and the brain perceives an overload. The patient will probably miss one or more of the directions.

Another example of concrete thinking is difficulty with time management. Persons with schizophrenia describe this behavior as "trying to tell time with clocks that have no minute or second hands." Recognition of this is critical to understand why patients are late or miss events and appointments altogether. This may create fear in patients who have to be alone for long periods of time or for patients living alone who are required to be places at specific times. Some patients have developed clever ways to determine time, such as getting watches with built-in alarms and monitoring certain television programs.

Difficulty managing money is another result of concrete thinking. People with schizophrenia often lose their ability to understand the concept of dollars and cents and are exploited by other people. The patient may agree to purchase items without having enough money just because they see some money in their wallets. They may not remember to pay for items they get in a store or leave a restaurant without paying for the meal. Unfortunately, many nonhospitalized patients get into legal trouble because of this cognitive problem.

Literal interpretation of words and symbols is one of the most problematic behaviors related to concrete thinking. People with schizophrenia have difficulty abstracting the English language. Patients' descriptions of literal interpretation are presented in the following four clinical examples.

CLINICAL EXAMPLE

"I was standing in the medication line and the nurse asked me to take my pills. So I took the medicine cup and held it in my hand. The nurse asked me again to take my pills and I didn't know what to do. She began to lose her patience as I stood there holding the medicine cup. She then told me to put the pills in my mouth and to swallow them with the water she handed me. I could follow each of the instructions and eventually "took my pills'."

An example of literal interpretation of symbols is described by this patient:

"It took me at least 15 minutes to walk down the street because I stopped every time the light changed from green to red. I didn't understand that the traffic signal was only for cars."

Sometimes this problem advances to the point where the patient interprets a metaphor literally, as described in this example:

"I remembered the expression 'step on a crack and break your mother's back.' One day I was walking down the street and stepped on a crack in the sidewalk. That same day my mother had fallen off a step stool after getting a can of soup from the kitchen cupboard and fractured two vertebrae in her back. For 9 months I believed that I had caused this accident to happen."

This is also called *magical thinking*.

Nursing implications regarding patient teaching for the person experiencing concrete thinking are profound. Consider this example:

A nurse was instructed to collect a sterile urine specimen from a newly admitted male patient. The patient exhibited terror and strongly resisted completing the procedure. When the nurse gently questioned him why he was so frightened, he replied, "I don't want to become sterile."

The role of the nurse is to assist with decision making in a nonpunitive, supportive manner, recognizing these symptoms represent neurological disabilities over which the patient has little control. The nurse functions in a rehabilitative role and needs to provide information as clearly and concretely as possible. The language used should involve simple words in short phrases that are easy to understand. The nurse also needs to seek validation regarding how instructions were heard to clarify confusion and misunderstanding by the patient.

> It is important to involve the patient in a collaborative process of planning nursing care. Describe how you would accomplish this if the patient has cognitive problems that interfere with decision-making ability.

Content of thought is the last problem in cognitive functioning and includes the presence of delusions. A delusion is a personal belief based on an incorrect inference of external reality. One of the mind's primary functions is to produce thoughts. Thoughts provide a sense of identity. They rarely begin as the logical product we consider a thought. Thoughts are produced as a result of intricate processes that involve screening and filtering internal and external stimuli and use multiple feedback loops in the brain's structural units and between hemispheres. Recognizing the complexity of this process helps the nurse appreciate the unyielding way in which a person defends personal beliefs.

Recalling the cognitive deficits already described helps the nurse understand why the person with schizophrenia sometimes has different beliefs from others. It is also important to realize that a delusion does not always last. It is common for a belief to be fixed for only a few weeks or few months, particularly in the less severe forms of schizophrenia. Many patients have reported the relief they experienced when they realized the belief was actually a delusion, just a symptom, not the actual truth.

The inability of the brain to process data accurately can result in paranoid, grandiose, religious, nihilistic, and somatic delusions. The delusions can be complicated further by thought withdrawal, thought insertion, thought control, or thought broadcasting. Types of delusions are described in Chapter 6.

Delusions represent an elaborate interplay between brain physiology, current environmental stimuli, and the person's frame of reference regarding the world. Delusions have several characteristics that must be identified before effective interventions can be planned. Delusions can become intertwined with hallucinations. They may be a simple, mixed up thought or pervade the person's entire cognitive process. They can represent a complete thought or only a portion of an idea. Delusions may be systematized, which means they are restricted to a specific area of belief such as family or religion, or nonsystematized, meaning they extend into many areas of a person's life, so new people and new information are incorporated into the delusion.

Perception. Perception refers to identification and initial interpretation of a stimulus based on information received through the five senses of sight, sound, taste, touch, and smell. Remembering the complex interplay of brain functions among brain stem, diencephalon, and cortex for each of the five senses, it is important to recognize that perceptual problems are often the first symptoms in many brain illnesses. Hallucinations and illusions are perceptual distortions that occur in maladaptive neurobiological responses. Although hallucinations are most commonly associated with schizophrenia, only 70% of people with this illness experience them. They can also occur in a manic or depressive illness, as well as in delirium. It is essential to stress that hallucinations and illusions can occur in *any* illness that disrupts brain function. Hallucinations arise from any of the five senses. They are described in Table 19-1.

 A young woman is hospitalized in a forensic psychiatric unit because she attempted to kill her preschool children. She says her dead mother's voice told her to do this because the devil would get them unless they were in heaven with her. Is this a delusion, a hallucination, or both? Would knowing the woman's sociocultural background influence your response? Why or why not?

Another category of perceptual behaviors involves **sensory integration** and includes pain recognition, stereogenesis, graphesthesia, right/left recognition, and recognition and perception of faces. Symptoms related to these occur frequently in schizophrenia yet often are assessed inaccurately within a behavioral instead of a perceptual context. Sensory integration disruptions often lead to deliberate acts of self-harm, as described in this clinical example.

CLINICAL EXAMPLE

During an initial physical assessment a nurse noted numerous superficial scars on the left arm of a young woman who had just completed an 8-week education program regarding symptom management in schizophrenia. The nurse asked the patient to "tell me about those scars," to which the patient replied: "Before I knew it was okay to talk about my symptoms I often lost sensation in my left arm and hand and thought my arm was poisoned or dead. I tried to determine if I was alive or not. I could see myself walking and see and feel my right arm, so I thought I was probably alive but I didn't know for sure, so I used to take a knife and poke tiny holes in my skin. I couldn't feel the knife yet I saw blood. It was when I saw the blood that I knew I was still alive."

Selected Nursing Diagnoses:
▼ Altered sensory perception, tactile, related to disrupted sensory integration as evidenced by explanation of scars on right arm
▼ High risk for self-mutilation related to perceptual disturbance as evidenced by scars from past episodes of cutting right arm

The concept of pain and pain recognition has been well studied. Knowing that the parietal lobe is the major site of pain recognition helps the nurse to see this as a neurobiologically based symptom. Visceral pain recognition involves integration of stimuli from the spinal cord through the brain stem, diencephalon, and cortex using intricate feedback circuits. People with schizophrenia generally have poor visceral pain recognition and need to have an in-depth assessment of physical complaints as described by the patient in the next clinical example.

CLINICAL EXAMPLE

"I told my case manager that I had a stomach ache, some diarrhea, and vomiting and felt like I had the flu. I had a fever, so she took me to the doctor, who said I probably had the flu and should just go home and rest. After a few days I got real sick and had to be taken to the emergency room, where they discovered my appendix had ruptured, and I had to have a very long and complicated surgery."

It is not uncommon for persons with schizophrenia to think they have a bad cold and have it diagnosed as pneumonia. Unfortunately the physical needs of psychiatric patients are often disregarded.

Stereogenesis and graphesthesia are included in standard neurological examinations under the category *soft signs*, meaning they represent a neurological deficit in an undetermined location but are consistent with brain injury to the frontal or parietal lobes. These terms

Table 19-1 Sensory Modalities Involved in Hallucinations

Sense	Characteristics	Observable Behaviors
Auditory	Hearing noises or sounds most commonly in the form of voices Sounds that range from a simple noise or voice, to a voice talking about the patient, to complete conversations between two or more people about the person who is hallucinating Audible thoughts in which the patient hears voices that are speaking what the patient is thinking and commands that tell the patient to do something, sometimes harmful or dangerous	Moving eyes back and forth as if looking to see who or what is talking Listening intently to another person who is not speaking or to an inanimate object such as a piece of furniture Engaging in conversation with an inanimate object or with an invisible person Moving mouth as if speaking or responding to a sound
Visual	Visual stimuli in the form of flashes of light, geometric figures, cartoon figures, and/or elaborate and complex scenes or visions Visions can be pleasant or terrifying, as in seeing monsters	Suddenly appearing startled, frightened, or terrified by another person, an inanimate object, or by no apparent stimulus Suddenly running into another room
Olfactory	Putrid, foul, and rancid smells of a repulsive nature such as blood, urine, or feces; occasionally the odors can be pleasant Olfactory hallucinations are typically associated with stroke, tumor, seizures, and the dementias	Wrinkling nose as if smelling something horrible Smelling parts of the body Smelling the air while walking toward another person Responding to an odor with terror, as in smelling fire or blood Throwing a blanket or pouring water on another person as if putting out a fire
Gustatory	Putrid, foul, and rancid tastes of a repulsive nature such as blood, urine, or feces	Spitting out food or a beverage Refusing to eat, drink, or take medications Suddenly leaving the dinner table
Tactile	Experiencing pain or discomfort with no apparent stimuli Feeling electrical sensations coming from the ground, inanimate objects, or other people	Slapping self as if putting out a fire Jumping up and down on the floor as if avoiding pain or other stimuli to the feet
Cenesthetic	Feeling body functions such as blood pulsing through veins and arteries, food digesting, or urine forming	Verbalizing and/or obsessing about body processes Refusing to complete a task that may require a part of the body that patient believes is not working
Kinesthetic	Sensation of movement while standing motionless	Steadying oneself while grabbing onto furniture

refer to the ability to identify objects by touch. Stereogenesis is the ability to recognize an object only by touch, such as reaching into a paper bag filled with objects and identifying a key. Graphesthesia is the recognition of letters "drawn" on the skin, for example, recognizing the letters C-A-T "drawn" on one's back. Problems in these functions contribute to difficulty with fine motor actions of the hand, and the patient may appear clumsy. Problems with right/left discrimination also contribute to lack of coordination and ability to carry out directions involving right and left.

Misidentification and perception of faces can contribute to behaviors such as fear, aggressiveness, withdrawal from interactions, and hostility. This symptom involves self-recognition as well and often is present when patients refuse to look in a mirror or avoid eye contact.

When perceptions are altered, concurrent symptoms in cognitive functions are common. Studies have shown that 90% of people who experience hallucinations also have delusions, whereas only 35% who experience delusions also have hallucinations. Approximately 20% of patients have mixed sensory hallucinations, usually auditory and visual.

Environmental factors can stimulate hallucinations. In general, objects that are reflective or have the potential to cause glare such as television screens, photos not in nonglare frames, and fluorescent lights can contribute to visual hallucinations. Auditory hallucinations can be caused by excessive noise and by sensory deprivation. The nurse needs to be acutely aware of environmental stimuli and the patient's response or lack of response. Patients may withdraw from sensory stimuli in an attempt to decrease sensory responses.

Emotion. In psychiatry emotions are described in terms of mood and affect (see Chapter 6). **Mood** is defined as an extensive and sustained feeling tone that can be experienced for a few hours or for years and can noticeably affect the person's world view. (Chapter 17 includes a complete description of mood and mood disorders.) **Affect** refers to behaviors such as hand and body movements, facial expression, and pitch of voice that can be observed when a person is expressing and experiencing feelings and emotions. Terms related to affect include *broad, restricted, blunted, flat,* and *inappropriate.* What is considered normal varies greatly among cultures. *Broad* and *restricted* are usually considered within the range of normal, whereas *blunted, flat,* and *inappropriate* represent symptoms. Disorders of affect refer to expression of emotion, not the experience of emotion. Patients describe affective symptoms in the following examples:

"I remember trying to smile for 3 years, but my face didn't work."

"My face was as stiff as your fingers would be if you tied them to popsicle sticks for 3 months and then tried to use them to thread a needle."

Patients describe tremendous frustration with these affective symptoms because others assume they do not experience any emotion. These descriptions demonstrate why patients are commonly misjudged as appearing bored, disinterested, and unmotivated.

Emotion refers to moods and affects that are connected to specific ideas. Emotions are generated from an interplay of neural activity among the hypothalamus, amygdala, hippocampus, and the higher cortex centers such as the association cortices. The hypothalamus, in addition to its hormonal functions, is also the emotional coordinating center. Emotions can be hyperexpressed or hypoexpressed in an incongruent manner. Individuals with schizophrenia commonly are seen with symptoms of hypoexpression. Some patients express the perception that they no longer have any feelings. Problems of emotion usually seen in schizophrenia include alexithymia, apathy, anhedonia, and a decreased ability to feel intimacy and closeness:

▼ **Alexithymia:** difficulty naming and describing emotions

▼ **Apathy:** lack of feelings, emotions, interests, or concern

▼ **Anhedonia:** inability or decreased ability to experience pleasure, joy, intimacy, and closeness

In addition to problems with emotions and affect, people with schizophrenia can also have mood disorders. A full-blown depression may develop in up to 60%

of persons with schizophrenia.[3] A diagnosis of schizoaffective disorder is given to the patient who meets the diagnostic criteria for schizophrenia as well as one or both of the major mood disorders of bipolar disorder and major depression.

Understanding the effect that brain malfunctions can have on the emotions and affect of the person with schizophrenia is important for promoting constructive communication and problem solving. It is important to recognize that persons living with brain illnesses are often uncanny in their ability to sense the emotions of others, yet they may have difficulty identifying the emotion that they have perceived. This creates special problems in caring for the patient.

Caregivers also frequently confuse feelings that are a direct result of brain malfunction and those that are an indirect product of social difficulties resulting from illness. Examples of feelings that are a direct result of brain malfunction include paranoid hostility and emotional flattening. An example of feelings that are an indirect product of social difficulties caused by illness is frustration over not being able to achieve one's potential. When patients and caregivers have difficulty identifying and connecting with feelings and emotions, barriers in communication usually occur.

Movement and Behavior. Definition of "normal" behavior is based on culture, age appropriateness, and social acceptability. Maladaptive neurobiological responses cause behaviors that are odd, unsightly, confusing, difficult to manage, and puzzling to others. With exploration, many behaviors can be explained. Some make perfect sense in the context of information provided by the patient.

Describe unusual behaviors that you have observed in patients with maladaptive neurobiological responses. Were you able to discover the reason for the behavior? Can you think of possible explanations for: Wearing several layers of clothing in very hot weather? Refusing to bathe? Hugging oneself and rocking?

Maladaptive movements associated with schizophrenia include catatonia, extrapyramidal side effects of psychotropic medications, abnormal eye movements, grimacing, apraxia/echopraxia, abnormal gait, and mannerisms. *Catatonia* represents a stuporous state in which the individual may require complete physical nursing care, similar to that for a comatose patient, sometimes interspersed with unpredictable outbursts of aggressive behavior. (Extrapyramidal side effects of psychotropic medication are described in Chapter 25.) Grimacing refers to abnormal facial movements that are beyond the patient's control and are not due to psychotropic medications. Abnormal eye movements include difficulty following a moving target, absence or avoidance of eye contact, decreased or rapid eye blinking, and frequent staring. These are common ocular motor symptoms found in 40% to 80% of people with schizophrenia.

Apraxia is difficulty carrying out a purposeful, organized task that is somewhat complex such as dressing or completing multiple-stage commands. *Echopraxia* is defined as purposeless imitation of movements by other people. This symptom may not always be purposeless but can illustrate a delusion, as described by the patient in the following clinical example.

 ## CLINICAL EXAMPLE

"I thought the nurse was my mirror and I had to do what the mirror showed me, so I copied everything she did. As long as I could see her I could feel connected to myself and my surroundings, but she didn't understand how important it was for me to be around her and watch what she did. Of course I couldn't explain what was happening to me at the time because I was psychotic, so she put me in seclusion and restraints."

Selected Nursing Diagnosis:

▼ Altered thought processes related to maladaptive information processing as evidenced by belief that the nurse was a mirror

Staggering, intentional stepping, and walking with the toes touching the ground first are features of abnormal gait that are frequently found in individuals with schizophrenia. Mannerisms involve gestures that seem contrived and are not appropriate to the situation, such as stopping in the middle of a sentence to whirl two fingers around.

Maladaptive behaviors in schizophrenia include deteriorated appearance, lack of persistence at work or school, avolition, repetitive or stereotyped behavior, aggression and agitation, and negativism. Deterioration in appearance includes disheveled and dirty clothes, sloppy and unkempt appearance, poor or absent personal grooming, and lack of personal hygiene. This is often the first set of symptoms to occur and is a signal to the family that something is happening to their loved one. Accompanying deterioration in appearance is lack of persistence at work or school. As problems in brain function begin to appear, the cognitive skills once available seem to "short circuit" and the person can no longer perform routine tasks. As deterioration continues

the person begins to experience avolition, which means lack of energy and drive. This is primarily because of the brain changes that may be occurring rapidly and secondarily to frustration with the inability to accomplish tasks that required little effort in the past. Unfortunately, it is at this point that most people with schizophrenia are mislabeled as lazy, disinterested, and unmotivated.

As deterioration continues, individuals often engage in repetitive or stereotyped behaviors. These appear similar to obsessive-compulsive behavior but are related to a private meaning rather than to thoughts. Examples include having to eat foods in a certain way, wearing only certain clothes, walking four steps forward and one step back, or being able to drink only half a glass of water at a time.

Aggression, agitation, and the potential for violence unfortunately are often used to describe the typical person with schizophrenia. The person with schizophrenia generally is the victim rather than the aggressor. However, people experiencing psychoses are sometimes violent, especially when their illness is out of control. Agitation is common for anyone who is living with a chronic illness for which there is no cure. It is important to identify and document those situations that seem to be triggers for agitated behavior (refer to Chapter 27). People who have schizophrenia tend to become agitated when there is performance anxiety, particularly related to carrying out tasks that previously posed no difficulty or threat to self-esteem. Abnormal movements and behaviors in schizophrenia are summarized in Box 19-3.

Relatedness. Socialization is defined as the ability to form cooperative and interdependent relationships with others. This was placed last among the five major brain functions because problems with the others must be understood to appreciate the relational consequences of maladaptive neurobiological responses. Social problems are often the major source of concern to families and health-care providers because these tangible effects of illness are often more prominent than the symptoms related to cognition and perception.

Social problems may result from the illness directly or indirectly. Direct effects occur when symptoms prevent the individual from socializing within accepted sociocultural norms, or when brain function deteriorates to the point of there being no motivation. Regardless, the result is social withdrawal and isolation from life's activities. Behaviors directly causing these problems include inability to communicate coherently, loss of drive and interest, deterioration of social skills and personal hygiene, and paranoia.

Indirect effects on socialization are secondary consequences of the illness. An example is low self-esteem related to poor academic and social achievement compared with siblings and peers. Significant social discom-

---

Box 19-3

ABNORMAL MOVEMENTS AND BEHAVIORS IN SCHIZOPHRENIA

MOVEMENTS

Catatonia, waxy flexibility, posturing
Extrapyramidal side effects of psychotropic medications
Abnormal eye movements
Grimacing
Apraxia/echopraxia
Abnormal gait
Mannerisms

BEHAVIORS

Appearance
Aggression/agitation/violence
Repetitive or stereotyped behavior
Avolition
Impersistence at work or school

---

fort and further social isolation may result. Specific problems related to the development of socialization and relationships include social inappropriateness, disinterest in recreational activities, gender identity confusion, and stigma-related withdrawal by friends, families, and peers.

Social inappropriateness relates directly to cognitive deficits and results in behaviors such as suddenly beginning loud, evangelistic prayer in public, toileting in public, standing in the middle of a street trying to direct traffic, dressing bizarrely, and engaging in intimate conversation with total strangers. Social inappropriateness often involves bizarre sexual behavior such as public masturbation, running nude in the street, or making inappropriate sexual advances. Sometimes bizarre sexual behavior is related to gender identity confusion. It is not uncommon, particularly with temporal lobe involvement, for people with schizophrenia to be unable to recognize their genitalia as their own. This often is the reason for sudden undressing and what appears to be public masturbation, when it actually may be a patient's futile attempt at reality testing.

Stigma also presents major obstacles to developing relationships. Stigma, which literally means mark of shame, is a major cause of the social isolation of the person with schizophrenia. Stigma often spreads to the whole family, who may be having their own schizophrenia-related social problems stemming from embarrassment about having the illness in the family. They may avoid talking about it, or if they do want to talk they may not know how. Stigma and rejection encountered in the community and from members of the extended family may discourage them from talking. Family members may feel like social outcasts for having this illness in the family. One family member explained: "For the rest of my life I will be dealing not only with the heartbreak of my brother's illness, but with negative response, stigma, and ignorance in my home town that will affect me deeply. I know, because the last 10 years of it already has been sheer hell."

Describe your own attitudes and behaviors and those of your peers that are stigmatizing toward people who have maladaptive neurobiological responses and their families.

Predisposing Factors

Biological. Behaviors related to maladaptive neurobiological responses have been described in writing and art since biblical times. Causes proposed for these strange behaviors ranged from demon possession, bad blood, and witchcraft, to the full moon. Fortunately, modern science is now identifying many clues to the actual causes of these disorders. (Biological factors related to schizophrenia are discussed in detail in Chapter 5.)

The brain abnormalities causing maladaptive neurobiological responses are only beginning to be understood. The majority of what is known today has been discovered by research stemming from advances in brain imaging. Brain imaging studies indicate that virtually all areas of the brain are involved in persons with schizophrenia; however psychotic behaviors are most likely to be related to lesions in the frontal, temporal, and limbic regions (Fig. 19-3). Studies have suggested that the prefrontal cortex and the limbic cortex never fully develop in the brains of patients with schizophrenia. Positron emission tomography studies have confirmed that blood flow to the prefrontal and limbic cortical regions is consistently dysfunctional in patients with schizophrenia.[50] These findings presented a fundamental problem in understanding the dopamine (DA) connection in schizophrenia, as it had been believed that dopamine neurons did not exist in the prefrontal cortex. With the recent discovery of the D4 receptor, researchers have identified the role of the prefrontal and limbic cortices in the regulation of stress-related dopamine activity.

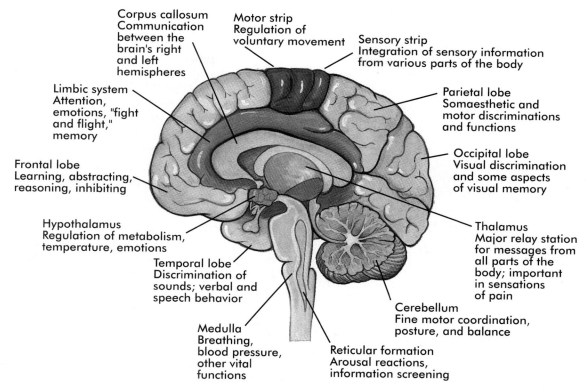

Fig. 19-3   Structure and function of the brain.

Neurons in the prefrontal cortex are particularly important for memory. A decrease in the numbers of these specific neurons may be the cause of loose associations. Memory-guided responses and sensory responses should be the same but are altered in schizophrenia. The resulting deficit is seen in the absence of 'working memory,' or the bringing of stored information to conscious awareness.

Other biological models suggest the importance of prenatal, perinatal, neonatal, and childhood neurological factors. Several researchers have proposed that schizophrenia is acquired in late fetal development or in the perinatal period.[5,39] These findings suggest that symptoms of schizophrenia may be caused by changes in the structure of brain tissue and failure of certain neuronal cells to migrate to their ultimate location.

Finally, family studies involving twins and adopted children historically have served as the basis of research designs attempting to identify a genetic cause for schizophrenia. In these studies, identical twins who were separated at birth with at least one adopted were found to have higher rates of schizophrenia in both twins than occurred in nonidentical pairs of siblings. Current research, however, focuses on families with a high incidence of schizophrenia and is moving toward locating specific susceptibility genes through gene-mapping techniques. Rigorous family studies have clearly shown that schizophrenia aggregates in families,

although little is known about the mode or what it is that is transmitted through genes. Current genetic research is focusing on several areas: (1) how many genes are there? (2) how common are they? and (3) what are their individual effects?[23] (Additional information about genetic transmission of schizophrenia is presented in Chapter 5.)

Psychological. In the past, in the absence of identified biological causes for schizophrenia, psychological, sociological, and environmental influences became the focus. For most of the twentieth century schizophrenia has been viewed as an illness that was caused partly by the family and partly by some individual character flaw. The mother was believed to be anxious, overprotective, or cold and unfeeling; the father was distant or overbearing. Marital conflict and families that stayed together for the sake of the children were blamed. There were theories describing a "schizophrenogenic" mother and theories that described how communicating in double messages could "double bind" a person into developing schizophrenia.

Schizophrenia was also viewed by some as failure to accomplish an early stage of psychosocial development. For example, an infant's inability to form a trusting relationship could lead to a lifetime of intrapsychic conflict. Schizophrenia was seen as the most severe example of inability to cope with stress. Disturbances in identity, inability to attach to a love object, and inability to control basic drives also served as key theories.

It is critically important for psychiatric nurses to realize, however, that with the psychobiological discoveries of recent years, most of these psychodynamic theories have found little scientific support. In addition, they can have a very negative impact on patient-family alliances with nurses and other mental health care professionals.

The "schizophrenogenic" mother was described as one who gave her child conflicting and confusing messages about their relationship, resulting in schizophrenia. How would this theory affect the mothers of people with schizophrenia, their relationships with their ill children, and their relationships with care providers?

Sociocultural. Some theorists proposed that poverty, society, and cultural disharmony could cause schizophrenia or that individuals chose to become schizophrenic to cope with the insanity of the modern world. Others proposed that schizophrenia was caused by living in the city or living in isolation in the country. Although accumulated stress related to environmental factors is likely to contribute to the onset of schizophrenia and to relapses, neurobiological findings point to other causes for the primary development of psychotic disorders.

Precipitating Stressors

Biological. Interference in a brain feedback loop that regulates the amount of information that can be processed at a given time has been identified as one possible biological stressor. Normal information processing occurs in a predetermined series of neural activities. Visual and auditory stimuli are initially screened and filtered by the thalamus and sent for processing by the frontal lobe. If too much information is sent at once, or if the information is faulty, the frontal lobe sends an overload message to the basal ganglia. The basal ganglia in turn send a message to the thalamus to slow down transmissions to the frontal lobe.[44] The decreased function already present in the frontal lobe impairs the ability of this feedback loop to perform. There is less ability to regulate the basal ganglia, and ultimately, the message to slow down transmissions to the frontal lobe never occurs. The result is information-processing overload and the neurobiological responses described in the beginning of this chapter.

Another possible biological stressor is the abnormal gating mechanisms that may occur in schizophrenia.[6]

Gating is an electrical process involving electrolytes. It refers to inhibitory and excitatory nerve action potentials and the feedback occurring within the nervous system related to completed nerve transmissions. Decreased gating is demonstrated by a person's inability to selectively attend to stimuli. For example, at a baseball game the individual with schizophrenia would be unable to differentiate the noise from the crowd, the organ, the team, or the public address system. Normally, when individuals hear a loud noise they become startled; however, when the noise is repeated, there is a decreased startle response. For example, if you hear a neighbor setting off firecrackers on the Fourth of July you become startled. When you hear a second explosion, you are generally less startled. The person with schizophrenia is just as startled the second time, and maybe even more than the first. This inability to "gate" a noise stimulus causes individuals to become frightened in crowds or wherever there is increased noise.[7]

Environmental Stress. There is no scientific research indicating that stress causes schizophrenia. However, studies of relapse and symptom exacerbation provide evidence that stress and problems with coping may predict the return of symptoms.[20,28] The stress-diathesis model described by Liberman and colleagues[26] states that schizophrenic symptoms develop based on the relationship between the amount of stress that a person experiences and an internal stress tolerance threshold. This is an important model because it integrates biological, psychological, and sociocultural factors in explaining the development of schizophrenia.

Symptom Triggers. Finally, precursors and stimuli often precede a new episode of the illness. The word *trigger* is used to describe these stressors. Common triggers of neurobiological responses related to health, environment, and attitudes and behaviors are listed in Table 19-2.

Coping Resources

Coping skills tend to be learned from parents. Children and young adults with schizophrenia need to be actively taught these skills because they have difficulty internalizing them from observation compared with individuals with more normal brain function. Family resources such as parental understanding of the illness, finances, availability of time and energy, and ability to provide ongoing support influence the course of illness.

It is important to remember that the mix of disabilities and resources that are present in a particular patient is related to the type and location of the brain dysfunction. Thus it is essential to assess mental status carefully to identify the person's strengths. For instance,

Table 19-2   Neurobiological Response Symptom Triggers

Health	Environment	Attitudes/behaviors
Poor nutrition	Hostile/critical environment	"Poor me" (low self-concept)
Lack of sleep	Housing difficulties (unsatisfactory housing)	"Hopeless" (lack of self-confidence)
Out of balance circadian rhythms	Pressure to perform (loss of independent living)	"I'm a failure" (loss of motivation to use skills)
Fatigue	Changes in life events, daily patterns of activity	"Lack of control" (demoralization)
Infection		Feeling overpowered by symptoms
Central nervous system drugs	Stress (lack of survival skills)	"No one likes me" (unable to meet spiritual needs)
Impaired cause-and-effect reasoning	Interpersonal difficulties, disruptions in interpersonal relationships	Looks/acts different from others who are of the same age, culture
Impaired information processing	Loneliness (social isolation, lack of social support)	Poor social skills
Lack of exercise	Missed environmental cues	Aggressive behavior
Behavioral disorder	Job pressures (poor occupation skills)	Violent behavior
Mood abnormalities	Poor social skills	Poor medication management
Moderate to high levels of anxiety	Poverty	Poor symptom management
	Lack of transportation (resources)	
	Inability to get/keep a job	

some people with maladaptive neurobiological responses are highly intelligent but unable to express themselves well. Others may be artistically talented but not skilled at verbal communication. Exploring these areas of strength assists the nurse in planning appropriate, individualized nursing interventions.

Coping Mechanisms

Patients behave in ways that are efforts to protect themselves from the frightening experiences caused by their illnesses. Regression occurs related to information processing problems and expenditure of large amounts of energy in efforts to manage anxiety, leaving little for activities of daily living. Projection represents an effort to explain confusing perceptions by assigning responsibility to someone or something. Withdrawal is related to problems establishing trust and preoccupation with internal experiences. Families often express denial when they first learn of their relative's diagnosis. This is the same as the denial that occurs whenever one receives information that causes fear and anxiety. It allows the person to gather internal and external resources and adapt to the stressor gradually.

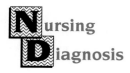

Nursing Diagnosis

In formulating the nursing diagnosis the nurse should review the complete nursing assessment as illustrated

in the stress adaptation model (Fig. 19-4). Nursing diagnoses take into account the functional level, stressors, and support systems of the patient and should be prioritized according to the level of wellness. The unstable patient will be given high priority with diagnoses related to safety needs. It is important for the nurse to diagnose relapse potential accurately to intervene before psychotic symptoms become dominant and the patient has a relapse that could last for months. The focus of diagnosis for the patient who is in the stable level of wellness is preventing relapse, facilitating habilitation, and identifying components of actualization. To reach the actualized level of wellness requires the patient to identify the desired quality of life and to outline steps needed to develop self-potential. Nursing diagnoses associated with maladaptive neurobiological responses are presented in the Medical and Nursing Diagnoses box on p. 491. Primary NANDA nursing diagnoses and examples of complete nursing diagnoses are presented in the Detailed Diagnoses box on pp. 492-493.

Related Medical Diagnoses

The medical diagnoses associated with maladaptive neurobiological responses include the schizophrenias, schizophreniform disorder, schizoaffective disorder, delusional disorder, brief psychotic disorder, and shared psychotic disorder. These diagnoses and related essential features are presented in the Detailed Diagnoses box.

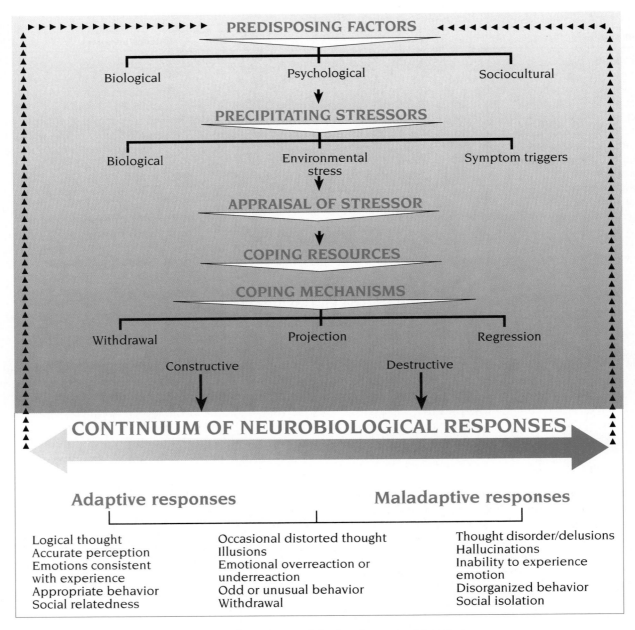

Fig. 19-4 A stress adaptation model related to neurobiological responses.

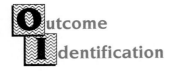

Outcome Identification

The expected outcome of patient care for this population is:

The patient will live, learn, and work at a maximum possible level of success as defined by the individual.

Prevention of relapse and early intervention are key components of a successful outcome. Relapse is defined as "the return of symptoms severe enough to interfere with activities of daily living."[38] It can be prevented only by thorough, ongoing symptom monitoring.[19,42] Planning therapeutic interventions depends on goals developed related to diagnosis and level of wellness.

Short-term goals would identify the steps that will lead the patient to successfully accomplish the expected outcome. Examples include:

1. The patient will initiate conversation with at least one person of choice daily.
2. The patient will participate in medication education group.
3. The patient will identify medications and describe the prescribed dose, expected effects, possible

MEDICAL AND NURSING DIAGNOSES RELATED TO MALADAPTIVE NEUROBIOLOGICAL RESPONSES

Related Medical Diagnoses (DSM-IV)*	Related Nursing Diagnoses NANDA†
Schizophrenia	Adjustment, impaired
Paranoid type	Anxiety
Disorganized type	‡Communication, impaired verbal
Catatonic type	Coping, family: potential for growth
Undifferentiated type	Coping, ineffective family: compromised
Residual type	Coping, ineffective individual
Schizophreniform disorder	Personal identity disturbance
Schizoaffective disorder	Role performance, altered
Delusional disorder	Self-care deficit (bathing/hygiene, dressing/grooming)
Brief psychotic disorder	Self-esteem disturbance
Shared psychotic disorder	‡Sensory/perceptual alterations (specify)
	‡Social interaction, impaired
	‡Social isolation
	‡Thought processes, altered
	Caregiver role strain, high risk for

*From American Psychiatric Association: *Diagnostic and statistical manual of mental disorders*, ed 4, Washington, DC, 1994, The Association.
†From North American Nursing Diagnosis Association: NANDA *nursing diagnoses: definitions and classifications* 1992-1993, Philadelphia, 1992, The Association.
‡Primary nursing diagnosis for maladaptive neurobiological responses.

side effects, and actions to take if questions arise for each.

4. The patient will describe preferred living situation following hospital discharge.
5. The patient will practice community living skills, such as food preparation, housekeeping, care of clothing, money management, and use of public transportation.

Planning

When the person's illness is unstable, care is often given in a hospital. The overall goal is to assist the individual to reach stability while establishing a foundation for habilitation. Because of the many, complex psychosocial needs of patients with maladaptive neurobiological responses, planning for discharge begins with admission. All patient resources must be studied. The family resources are particularly important, since families are the providers of care for at least 65% of patients with schizophrenia.[18] Federal law requires that patients and, with patients' permission, family members be present at treatment planning meetings. This facilitates a smooth transition from the hospital to home. Recognizing the burden that families experience in caring for loved ones with schizophrenia,[16] families must decide what resources they are willing and able to use to assist the

patient. These resources may include time, energy, knowledge, and money. The discharge plan needs to be based on the reality of available resources.

Care of the patient in the stable phase of wellness occurs at home or in another community setting. The focus of the stable phase is to assist with habilitation. The process of habilitation begins with learning to identify symptom triggers and prodromal symptoms. Prodromal symptoms are the first to occur at the beginning of an illness. Successful habilitation involves the identification of symptom management techniques that reduce the potential for relapse and maintain stability. Additional information about the rehabilitation of people with maladaptive neurobiological responses is included in Chapter 13.

When stability has been attained, the actualization phase begins. The ultimate goal of actualization is to collaboratively develop and implement symptom management techniques that prevent relapse. When patients and families recognize that relapse prevention is possible, they become empowered and can enjoy a quality of life that places the individual rather than the illness in control.

The Murphy Wellness Model

The Murphy wellness model (Fig. 19-5) provides a framework for planning nursing care for patients who have schizophrenia and other psychotic illnesses with peri-

DETAILED DIAGNOSES
RELATED TO MALADAPTIVE NEUROBIOLOGICAL RESPONSES

NANDA Diagnosis Stem	Examples of Complete Diagnosis
Impaired verbal communication	Impaired verbal communication related to formal thought disorder as evidenced by loose associations
Sensory/perceptual alteration (specify)	Sensory/perceptual alteration (auditory) related to physiological brain dysfunction as evidenced by verbal reports of "hearing voices that say bad things about me"
Social isolation	Social isolation related to inadequate social skills as evidenced by inappropriate sexual advances toward members of both sexes
Altered thought processes	Altered thought processes as related to physiological brain dysfunction as evidenced by stated belief that staff members are really actors who were hired by parents to watch him

DSM-IV Diagnosis	Essential Features*
Schizophrenia	At least two of the following, each present for a significant portion of time during a 1-month period: ▼ Delusions ▼ Hallucinations ▼ Disorganized speech ▼ Grossly disorganized or catatonic behavior ▼ Negative symptoms For a significant portion of the time since the onset of the disturbance, one or more major areas of functioning such as work, interpersonal relations, or self-care is markedly below the level achieved prior to the onset. Continuous signs of the disturbance persist for at least 6 months.
Paranoid type	Preoccupation with one or more delusions or frequent auditory hallucinations
Disorganized type	All of the following are prominent: disorganized speech, disorganized behavior, flat or inappropriate affect, and does not meet the criteria for catatonic type.
Catatonic type	At least two of the following dominate the clinical picture: motoric immobility as evidenced by catalepsy or stupor; excessive motor activity; extreme negativism or mutism; peculiarities of voluntary movement as evidenced by posturing, stereotyped movements, prominent mannerisms, or prominent grimacing; echolalia or echopraxia.
Undifferentiated type	Symptoms meeting the first general criteria for schizophrenia are present, but criteria for other types are not met.
Residual type	Criteria for schizophrenia are not met, nor are those for any other subtype. There is continuing evidence of the disturbance, indicated by negative symptoms or attenuated presence of two or more symptoms included in the general criteria.

*Adapted from the American Psychiatric Association: *Diagnostic and statistical manual of mental disorders*, ed 4, Washington, DC, 1994, The Association.

DETAILED DIAGNOSES
RELATED TO MALADAPTIVE NEUROBIOLOGICAL RESPONSES—cont'd

DSM-IV Diagnosis—cont'd	Essential Features—cont'd
Schizophreniform disorder	Meets criteria for schizophrenia and an episode lasts at least 1 month but less than 6 months. Specify "with" or "without" good prognostic features based on at least two of the following: onset of prominent psychotic symptoms within 4 weeks of first noticeable change in behavior or functioning; confusion or perplexity at the height of the psychosis; good premorbid social and occupational functioning; and absence of blunted or flat affect.
Schizoaffective disorder	An interrupted period of illness including a major depressive episode or manic episode concurrent with symptoms of schizophrenia. During the same period of illness, there have been delusions or hallucinations for at least 2 weeks in the absence of prominent mood symptoms. Symptoms of a mood episode are present during a substantial part of the illness.
Delusional disorder	Nonbizarre delusions (i.e., situations that could occur, such as being followed, poisoned, or having a disease) lasting at least a month. Has never met criteria for schizophrenia. Apart from the impact of the delusion, functioning and behavior are not markedly affected.
Brief psychotic disorder	Presence of at least one of the following: delusions, hallucinations, disorganized speech, or grossly disorganized or catatonic behavior. (Behaviors are not culturally sanctioned.) Duration between 1 day and 1 month, with eventual return to premorbid functioning. The presence (brief reactive) or absence of marked stressors should be noted, as should onset within 4 weeks postpartum.
Shared psychotic disorder (folie à deux)	A delusion develops in an individual in the context of a close relationship with someone who already has a delusion. The delusions of the people involved are similar in content.

ods of remission and potential for relapse. It is useful because it empowers individuals to self-manage these illnesses over time and enjoy a more productive life in the community.

Wellness. Wellness is a broader concept than health. It involves every aspect of living including how one functions in society. Wellness includes the interaction of health, environmental factors, attitudes and behavior in a way that enables individuals to attain a satisfactory quality of life as they define it. There are three levels of wellness that may be experienced by patients with

schizophrenia: unstable, stable, and actualized. **Instability** occurs when health, environmental factors, or attitudes and behavior are compromised so that the person's emotional, physical, cognitive, or social functioning is threatened. Relapse occurs as the balance tips from stable to unstable. **Stability** requires a balance of health, environmental factors, and attitudes and behavior so the patient can function within age and developmental norms with minimal help from others. **Actualization** is the ability to function at the highest level of potential, facilitating a satisfactory quality of life as defined by the person. It includes the freedom to function

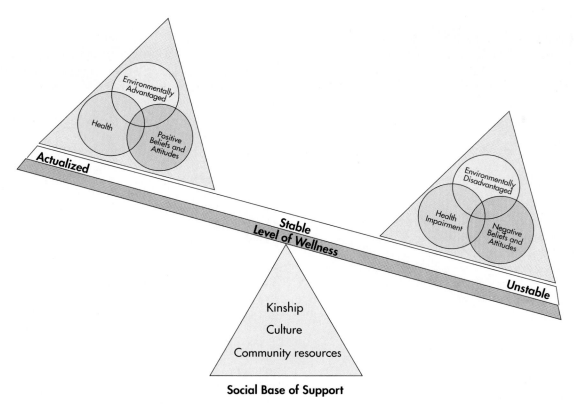

Fig. 19-5 Murphy wellness model for patients with schizophrenia and other psychotic illnesses.
Copyright 1992 Millene Freeman Murphy.

in the social setting of one's choice according to one's developmental level and abilities. Other important concepts of this model include health, environment, attitudes and behavior, and social support.

Health. Health is the ability of all body systems to function in a way that is compatible with life and the individual's social role. Disruption in any aspect of health moves the individual toward instability. Health includes the function of the entire body including information processing ability in relation to age and developmental level. Schizophrenia and other psychoses interfere with information processing, causing alterations in health, changes in attitudes and behavior, and difficulty in environmental interactions. Basic requirements for health are adequate nutrition, a balance of rest and activity, and sufficient exercise. Alterations in information processing and lack of energy make it difficult for the individual with schizophrenia to achieve these basic requirements.

Environment. Environment includes learning opportunities, life skills, socioeconomic status, transportation resources, employment, living arrangements, and interpersonal relationships. A supportive environment facilitates wellness, whereas a hostile environment pushes

the individual toward instability. Opportunities to develop life skills vary with the environment, information processing ability of the individual, and resources of the community and family. Life skills encompass activities of daily living, personal hygiene, meal preparation, caring for a residence, money management, and accessing appropriate community resources.

Interpersonal relationships and social behavior are influenced by brain maturity and the integration of neurobiological responses. The need to be accepted and understood by others also influences how the person views relationships. Issues related to feelings of power, control, and acceptance can restrict feelings about relationships and the ability to negotiate differences.

Attitudes and Behavior. Attitudes and behavior are the observable outcomes of information processing. They include such concepts as self-concept, ability to use knowledge, moral development, incorporation of self and societal values and norms into a world view, health management, spiritual satisfaction, and the way the person acts. Attitudes that foster dependency and "poor me" are in conflict with individual empowerment. Behaviors that facilitate movement toward desirable outcomes indicate a sense of personal empowerment.

Social Support. Social support is the base of the model and serves as the fulcrum upon which rests the ability to balance health, environment, and attitudes and behaviors.[48] The concepts of culture, kinship, and community resources are the components of the fulcrum that facilitate or hinder habilitation. Habilitation is defined as education or training to function in society at a level that is higher than that before the illness. Integration into the community is an important part of habilitation. An individual who associates with supportive, accepting people with adequate coping skills learns culturally acceptable behaviors.

mplementation

Intervention modalities encompass the full range of psychosocial and psychobiological treatments and must include the patient, family, and caretaker if possible. The modality chosen should be based on predisposing factors, precipitating stressors, coping resources, mechanisms and responses, and the patient's level of wellness.

Interventions Related to Instability

Unstable neurobiological responses require constant observation and monitoring of health, behavior, and attitudes. Nursing interventions in this phase should focus on restoration of adaptive neurobiological responses while providing for the safety and well-being of the patient. Box 19-4 describes patient goals and nursing interventions for patients with schizophrenia or other psychotic disorders and an unstable level of wellness.

Managing Delusions. Patients cope with delusions in several ways. Some adapt by learning to live with them. Others deny the presence of these troublesome symptoms. Still others seek to understand the symptom and become empowered to manage delusions when they occur. The art of communicating with individuals who have delusions requires the development of trust. Patients with cognitive disorders have difficulty processing language; therefore the beginning of trust is more readily accomplished through nonverbal communication. Patients with delusions perceive the environment as much more stimulating than others do. It is essential for the nurse to approach the patient with calmness, empathy, and gentle eye contact. Patients report they can literally "feel the vibrations" of others and can "sense if the nurse is with me or against me." Once trust is established, the use of clear, direct, and simple statements becomes significant in communicating with individuals who have delusions.

Box 19-4

NURSING INTERVENTIONS FOR PATIENTS WITH SCHIZOPHRENIA AND AN UNSTABLE LEVEL OF WELLNESS

Goal: To prevent death or injury until a stable level of wellness is reached.

Time to achieve goal: Varies with individual and effectiveness of intervention. May take a few hours to several days depending on level of illness and effectiveness of interventions. Takes longer if chemical substance use is involved.

HEALTH

Assess and monitor health status
Administer and monitor prn and scheduled medications
Identify symptoms of relapse
Identify factors that increase symptoms
Monitor for withdrawal from drugs or alcohol
Assist to manage delusions and hallucinations
Allow for sufficient rest for brain responses to stabilize

ENVIRONMENT

Provide a safe, protective, quiet environment
Reduce stress/pressure to perform
Reduce environmental factors that increase paranoid ideation
Allow to verbalize fears, concerns
Reduce factors that are bothering or upsetting
Provide supportive care
Use clear, concise, concrete communications
Facilitate communication with significant others

ATTITUDES/BEHAVIOR

Monitor behavior
Assess/monitor risk to self and others
Assist with activities of daily living as needed
Assist with anxiety management
Assist with anger management
Assist with problem solving; simplify decision making

SOCIAL SUPPORT

Assist to feel acceptable
Assist to access appropriate treatment resources
Assist to maintain dignity

Describe nonverbal nursing approaches that would foster the development of trust between a nurse and a delusional patient.

These patients are keenly sensitive to rejection. When they sense anxiety and avoidance in the nurse they of-

Box 19-5

STRATEGIES FOR WORKING WITH DELUSIONS

Establish a trusting, interpersonal relationship

Do not reason, argue, or challenge the delusion. Attempting to disprove the delusion is not helpful.

Assure the person that it is safe and no harm will come.

Do not leave the person alone; use openness and honesty at all times.

Encourage the person to verbalize feelings of anxiety, fear, and insecurity; offer concern and protection to prevent injury to self or others.

Convey acceptance of the need for the false belief. Talking about the delusion during the experience lends it reality. It is more helpful to talk about the experiences that may have triggered the delusion.

Center on the patient as a person, rather than on the need to control symptoms.

Remain calm.

Identify the content and type of delusion

Assist in understanding the patient and the purpose the delusion serves.

Clarify any confusion of the verbalization by asking what the patient is saying.

If you do not attempt to clarify confusion, the result may be even greater confusion, anxiety, and reaffirmed delusion.

Identify the presence of a central topic.

Identify the presence of a central feeling tone.

Investigate the meaning of the delusion

Assess areas in the person's life that can no longer be managed, controlled, or participated in.

Assess the concrete ways the delusion interferes with functioning or may explain "malfunctioning" to the person.

Ask whether the person has taken action based on the delusion.

Without agreeing or arguing, question the logic or reasoning behind the delusion.

Assess the intensity, frequency, and duration of the delusion

Fleeting delusions are able to be worked with in a short time frame.

Fixed delusions that have endured over a long time may have to be temporarily avoided to prevent them from becoming stumbling blocks in the relationship.

Does the person always greet you with the delusion? If so, just quietly listen and then give direction for the task at hand.

If it appears the individual cannot stop talking about the delusion, ask gently if the patient recalls what you have been doing and that it's time to resume that activity.

If the patient is very intent on telling you the delusion, just quietly listen until there is no need to discuss it any further. Remember, it is helpful to give the person reassurance during the delusion that as a person the patient is 'okay.'

Identify what triggered the delusion

Assess for a change in the person's ability to manage activities of daily living, since delusions can be triggered by minor changes such as alterations in the daily schedule. Anything that is potentially disruptive to the person can trigger delusions.

Place the delusion in a time frame

Identify all the components of the delusion by placing it in time and sequence.

Identify current major stresses

Assess if the person is under exaggerated stress (e.g., financial, family, or job difficulties).

Correlate the onset of the delusion with the onset of the stress

Help the patient connect the false beliefs to times of increased anxiety; if the person is able to interrupt escalating anxiety, delusional thinking may be prevented.

If the patient asks directly if you believe the delusion, respect that this is the patient's experience

Always present reality to the patient who is delusional, without invalidating one's perceptions.

Reinforce and focus on reality.

Talk about real events and real people using real situations to divert the patient away from a long, rambling conversation.

Identify emotional needs the delusion may be meeting

Respond to the underlying feelings rather than the illogical nature of the delusion. This will encourage discussion of fears, anxieties, and anger without assuming the delusion is right. The person generally attaches the emotional tone of the first experience of the delusion to each successive experience with that particular delusion.

Use the process of the conversation rather than the content by reflecting the feeling back to the patient.

Meet the needs the delusion fulfills

Promote activities that require attention, physical skill, or action. When a person's energy is diverted, pathological thinking is interrupted. Satisfying activities will help the person give up time used in delusional thinking.

Recognize healthy aspects of the patient's personality, this will help the patient to doubt delusional perceptions.

Structure situations so that it is difficult to spend time in a delusional system, this encourages alternative methods of meeting needs.

Once the delusion is understood, avoid and discourage repetitious talk of the delusion

Encourage person to accept responsibility for own behavior.

Give some measure of control regarding daily activities and decision making.

Involve the family when at all possible.

ten feel annoyed, inadequate, hopeless, and like a failure. Sensing rejection by health-care professionals can also lead to anger on the part of the patient. If patients perceive the nurse is "going along with the delusion," it becomes confusing, particularly if they sense that the nurse is trying to get their cooperation.

The nurse should not attempt a logical explanation of the delusion, because it will not be possible to identify one. Only the patient understands the logic behind the delusion and is not able to express it until after the delusion has reached conscious awareness. On gaining insight into the illness and illness symptoms the patient is able to differentiate experiences with delusions from those that are reality based. In the meantime the nurse should not underestimate the power of a delusion and the patient's inability to differentiate the delusion from reality.

It is normal for the nurse to feel confused by a delusion. The nurse must carefully assess the content of the delusion without appearing to probe. It is also important to assess the context and environmental triggers for the delusional experience. If at all possible, the nurse needs to avoid becoming incorporated into the delusion. This is difficult, however, if the nurse has achieved a trusting relationship with the patient because people who are significant to the patient in reality may also become part of the delusional world.

Box 19-5 identifies strategies helpful in working with the patient who is delusional, and Box 19-6 identifies barriers to intervening. The intervention plan must be followed exactly by the entire treatment team. If the nurse resorts to "trying anything" to gain compliance, care will be inconsistent and will create an even more chaotic environment for the individual who already has great difficulty identifying reality.

Managing Hallucinations. Approximately 70% of hallucinations are auditory, 20% are visual, and the remaining 10% are gustatory, tactile, olfactory, kinesthetic, or cenesthetic. Therapeutic nursing interventions for hallucinations involve understanding the characteristics of the hallucination and identifying the related anxiety level. Table 19-3 describes intensity levels, characteristics, and observable behaviors commonly associated with hallucinations.

The goal of intervention with patients who are hallucinating is to assist them to increase awareness of these symptoms so that they can distinguish between the world of psychosis and the world experienced by others. The first step toward achieving this goal is facilitative communication. Unfortunately, patients experiencing these symptoms are frequently laughed at, made fun of, belittled, and ignored when these symptoms emerge.

Learning about a person's hallucinations helps avoid the roadblocks to communication these symptoms can

---

Box 19-6

BARRIERS TO SUCCESSFUL INTERVENTION FOR DELUSIONS

Becoming anxious and avoiding the person

Anxiety leads to annoyance, anger, a sense of hopelessness and failure, feelings of inadequacy, and potential laughing at the patient.

Reinforcing the delusion

Do not "go along" with the delusion, especially to get the cooperation of the patient.

Attempting to prove the person is wrong

Do not attempt a logical explanation.

Setting unrealistic goals

Do not underestimate the power of a delusion and the patient's need for it.

Becoming incorporated into the delusional system

This will cause great confusion for the person and make it impossible to establish boundaries of the therapeutic relationship.

Failing to clarify confusion surrounding the delusion

By not clearly understanding the complexity and many intricacies of the delusion, the delusion will become more elaborate.

Being inconsistent in intervention

The intervention plan must be firmly adhered to; if you resort to "trying anything," approaches will become inconsistent and the person less able to identify reality.

Seeing the delusion first and the person second

Avoid saying "the person who thinks he's being poisoned."

---

create when unrecognized. Left unattended, hallucinations will continue and may escalate. Nurses may become so involved in planning what to say that they forget about the importance of listening. Listening and observing are the keys to successful intervention with the person who is hallucinating.

Hallucinations are very real to the person having them, just as dreams during sleep are very real. The hallucinating individual may have no way to determine whether these perceptions are real or not. It usually does not even occur to the person to verify the experience. An analogy might be hearing an ordinary weather report on the radio and not thinking to question whether the voice is from a real person or not. Inability to perceive reality accurately can make life difficult for pa-

Table 19-3 Levels of Intensity of Hallucinations

Level	Characteristics	Observable patient behaviors
Stage I: Comforting **Moderate level of anxiety** Hallucination is generally of a pleasant nature.	The hallucinator experiences intense emotions such as anxiety, loneliness, guilt, and fear and tries to focus on comforting thoughts to relieve anxiety. The individual recognizes that thoughts and sensory experiences are within conscious control if the anxiety is managed. **Nonpsychotic**	Grinning or laughter that seems inappropriate Moving lips without making any sounds Rapid eye movements Slowed verbal responses as if preoccupied Silent and preoccupied
Stage II: Condemning **Severe level of anxiety** Hallucination generally becomes repulsive.	Sensory experience of any of the identified senses is repulsive and frightening. The hallucinator begins to feel a loss of control and may attempt to distance self from the perceived source. Individual may feel embarrassed by the sensory experience and withdraw from others. **Nonpsychotic**	Increased autonomic nervous system signs of anxiety such as increased heart rate, respiration, and blood pressure Attention span begins to narrow Preoccupied with sensory experience and may lose ability to differentiate hallucination from reality
Stage III: Controlling **Severe level of anxiety** Sensory experiences become omnipotent.	Hallucinator gives up trying to combat the experience and gives in to it. Content of hallucination may become appealing. Individual may experience loneliness if sensory experience ends. **Psychotic**	Directions given by the hallucination will be followed, rather than objected to Difficulty relating to others Attention span of only a few seconds or minutes Physical symptoms of severe anxiety such as perspiring, tremors, inability to follow directions
Stage IV: Conquering **Panic level of anxiety** Generally becomes elaborate and interwoven with delusions.	Sensory experiences may become threatening if individual doesn't follow commands. Hallucinations may last for hours or days if there is no therapeutic intervention. **Psychotic**	Terror-stricken behaviors such as panic Strong potential for suicide or homicide Physical activity that reflects content of hallucination such as violence, agitation, withdrawal, or catatonia Unable to respond to complex directions Unable to respond to more than one person

tients. Hallucinations, therefore, can be considered problems needing a solution. This is best accomplished when the person can talk freely about the hallucinations. Nurses also need to be able to talk about hallucinations because they are useful indicators of the current level of symptoms in ongoing monitoring of a psychotic illness. To facilitate monitoring, the patient needs to be comfortable telling the nurse about symptoms.

Patients often learn not to discuss their unusual experiences with anyone because they have received negative responses from others who think their ideas are strange. The experience of hallucinations can be especially troublesome for the patient who does not have anyone to talk to about them. Being able to talk about one's hallucinations is a greatly reassuring and self-validating experience. This discussion can take place only in an atmosphere of genuine interest and concern.

For those who have never experienced a hallucination, it can be difficult to understand that the person has no control over it. Individuals with true psychosis have no direct voluntary control over the brain malfunction that causes hallucinations. This means that they cannot just will them away. Ignoring hallucinations may increase the confusion of the already chaotic brain filled with delusional ideas and disjointed thoughts. If the individual is left alone to sort out reality without the input of trusted health-care providers the symptoms may overwhelm available coping resources. Interactive discussion of hallucinations is a vital element in the development of reality testing skills. Communicating right at the time of the hallucination is particularly helpful. Honesty, genuineness, and openness are the foundation for effective communication during hallucinations.

Modulation of sensory stimulation to an optimal level is another useful technique for helping the individual minimize the perceptual confusion. Some patients do well with minimal environmental stimulation, whereas others find that noise and distraction help to drown out the hallucinations. It is essential to find out how the patient has previously managed hallucinations.

Command hallucinations are a special type of hallucination that are potentially dangerous. They may lead an individual to perform harmful acts such as cutting off a body part or striking out at someone at the instruction of voices. Fear caused by these often frightening hallucinations can also generate dangerous behaviors such as jumping out a window. Because of the potential seriousness of this symptom, the need to intervene becomes crucial.

Intervening during the acute phase of hallucinations requires patience and the ability to spend time with the patient. Patients have identified four basic principles that are helpful during the this phase: maintain eye contact, speak simply in a slightly louder voice than usual, call the patient by name, and use touch.[33] Basically the patient needs sensory validation to override the abnormal sensory processes that are occurring in the brain. Unfortunately, traditional interventions focus on isolating the patient. Isolating an individual during this time of intense sensory confusion often serves to reinforce the psychosis.

Because schizophrenia is a chronic illness, less intense hallucinations often occur on a daily basis. Box 19-7 outlines interventions useful for patients after the acute phase has passed. As with delusions, consistency is the essential ingredient to a successful intervention plan.

Psychopharmacology. The new wave of psychopharmacology described in Chapter 25 promises to improve patient response to antipsychotic medications. Drugs that are more site and symptom specific and provide a better response with fewer side effects will ultimately also improve patient adherence. Phenothiazines and phenothiazine derivatives currently provide some measure of symptom relief for 80% of patients.[22] The atypical phenothiazine, clozapine, assists approximately 30% of the 20% not responding to the traditional antipsychotics.[22] Risperidone is a new atypical antipsychotic drug that promises to be as effective as clozapine but without the life-threatening side effects. Table 19-4 summarizes the medications most often prescribed for maladaptive neurobiological responses.

Interventions Related to Stability

Nursing interventions that focus on teaching self-management of symptoms as well as identifying symptoms indicative of relapse are most useful in this level of wellness. Patient teaching should involve caregivers whenever possible (see A Family Speaks).[36] Behavioral interventions that teach patients skills for coping with psychotic symptoms include cognitive reframing regarding the cause of symptoms, gaining control over symptoms, and behavioral coping strategies.[12] In addition, patients and families should be taught the stages of relapse as a means to move toward the actualization level of wellness.

A FAMILY SPEAKS

When our daughter, Sue, was in college, she began to change quite suddenly. She had been almost a perfect child. She got good grades all the way through high school, and we never worried that she would get into trouble. In fact, we used to feel sorry for our friends who suspected that their children were experimenting with drugs and sex, hanging out with wild friends, and failing at school.

What a shock it was when we visited Sue and she had completely changed. Her room was a mess. She was wearing sloppy clothes and obviously needed a bath. When we asked what was wrong, she denied there was a problem and then became angry and refused to say anything more to us at all. When we got home, we called a counselor at the college, who told us that Sue was about to flunk out. She had not been attending classes, and other students had been reporting that she was "living in her own world."

We returned to the college to take our daughter home. We immediately took her to a psychiatrist who said that she was schizophrenic and referred her to a hospital. We were frightened, confused, and depressed. We had little understanding of schizophrenia, except that it is a terrible disease that people never recover from and they usually end up in a hospital forever. We also felt guilty that we had perhaps failed Sue in some way. What a relief it was to talk with her primary nurse. She immediately scheduled us for a family education group that met at the hospital. Every time that she was working when we visited, she made sure to spend time so that we could ask questions, and we had a million of them. Most important, she told us about the Alliance for the Mentally Ill. It was so reassuring to meet and talk with other family members who knew what we were going through. We know now that our daughter may never achieve the potential that we thought she once had, but she can lead a productive life. We continue to learn with her about how that will happen for her. ▼

Box 19-7
STRATEGIES FOR WORKING WITH HALLUCINATIONS

Establish a trusting, interpersonal relationship

Express feelings in an open, honest and direct manner. You will elicit the behavior you emit—if you are frightened, the individual will be frightened. Have as consistent a routine as possible. Be patient, show acceptance, and listen. Remember the individual is experiencing anxiety, fear, loneliness, low self-esteem, and the brain is not processing stimuli accurately.

Assess for symptoms of a hallucination

Look at and listen to the person for clues the hallucination is in the beginning level of intensity. Be patient and listen when the patient is ready to talk.

Focus on the symptom and ask the person to describe what is happening

The goal is to empower the person by helping to understand the symptoms experienced or demonstrated. This helps the person gain control of the illness, seek help, and hopefully prevent the hallucination from reaching a greater level of intensity. Be patient and use active listening techniques.

Identify if drugs and/or alcohol have been used

Determine if the person is using street drugs or alcohol. You need to teach that this is extremely dangerous, and a general rule of thumb is that one beer will act like a six-pack. Many persons turn to illicit drugs or alcohol as a coping mechanism or as a quick means to manage symptom intensity. The combination of brain disease and drugs or alcohol may cause irreparable harm and promote a long relapse.

If asked, point out simply that you are not experiencing the same stimuli

The goal is to guide the person through the experience and let them know what is actually happening in the environment. Do not argue about what is not occurring. When a hallucination occurs, do not leave the individual alone.

Help the person describe and compare the present and recently past hallucination

You need to find out what the person is seeing, hearing, tasting, touching, or smelling to begin to discover if a pattern exists. Encourage the person to remember when hallucinations first began. This process is similar to taking a nursing history for any other symptom.

Encourage the person to observe and describe thoughts, feelings, and actions, both present and past, as they relate to the hallucination

Frequently, people with schizophrenia appear to be able to "turn their symptoms on and off." Many have learned how to survive this illness by covering up symptoms to appear normal. It takes tremendous energy and concentration to control the illness. If you listen for at least 15 minutes, the person will usually be able to talk about their cognitive and perceptual symptoms and provide clues to the underlying psychosis.

Help the person describe needs that may be reflected in the content of the hallucination

Emotional needs can be grouped into four categories: (1) ability to express anger, (2) having power and control of decisions that affect daily life, (3) feeling egosyntonic with human sexuality, and (4) experiencing positive self-esteem. If one or more of these needs are not met, people will experience emotional distress. Try to step into the shoes of an individual with brain disease who is already impaired in the ability to accurately interpret reality. Then, add the effects of extra stress of unmet needs. For survival of the self, hallucinations may partially reflect these unmet needs.

Help the person identify if there is a correlation between the hallucination and the needs it may be reflecting

Focus on the unmet emotional need the person may be experiencing and discuss if there is a relationship to the appearance of hallucinations. Encourage the person to keep a chart or calendar of when hallucinations occur and how long they last in an effort to identify the trigger.

Suggest and reinforce the use of interpersonal relationships in meeting the need

It is important to find one individual who will give honest feedback to help the person sort out reality from the hallucination. This individual must be readily accessible to the individual. Remember that anxiety reduction is the key intervention to interrupting hallucinations.

Identify how other symptoms of psychosis have affected the person's ability to carry out activities of daily living

Share your concerns and provide feedback regarding the person's general coping responses. Use the symptom management assessment tool to help the person feel more in control of the illness. By assisting the person with symptom identification and recognition of the effect of symptoms on activities of daily living, self-esteem will be increased, anger will be diffused, and the person will feel in control of symptoms instead of feeling that the symptoms are in control.

*Adapted from Clack J: An interpersonal technique for handling hallucinations. In *Nursing care of the disoriented patient*, monograph 13, Kansas City, Mo, 1962, American Nurses' Association.

TABLE 19-4
ANTIPSYCHOTIC DRUGS

Chemical class subtype generic name (trade name)	Drug dosage: equivalence (mg)	Usual maintenance dosage range (mg/day)	Available forms (mg)
PHENOTHIAZINES			
Aliphatic type Chlorpromazine (Thorazine)	100	300-1400	tabs: 10, 25, 50, 100, 200 time released: 30, 75, 150, 200 caps: 300 syrup: 10/5 ml conc: 30/ml; 100/ml supp: 25, 100 inj: 25/ml
Piperidine type Thioridazine (Mellaril)	100	300-800*	tabs: 10, 15, 25, 50, 100, 150, 200 conc: 30/ml, 100/ml susp: 25/5 ml, 100/5 ml
Mesoridazine (Serentil)	50	100-500	tabs: 10, 25, 50, 100 conc: 25/ml inj: 25/ml
Piperazine type Perphenazine (Trilafon)	10	8-64	tabs: 2, 4, 8, 16 conc: 16/5 ml inj: 5/ml
Trifluoperazine (Stelazine)	5	10-80	tabs: 1, 2, 5, 10 conc: 10/ml inj: 2/ml
Fluphenazine (Prolixin)	2	5-40	tabs: 0.25, 1, 2.5, 5, 10 conc: 5/ml elix: 0.5/5 ml
THIOXANTHENE			
Thiothixene (Navane)	4-5	10-60	caps: 1, 2, 5, 10, 20 conc: 5/ml inj: 2/ml, powder 5/ml
BUTYROPHENONE			
Haloperidol (Haldol)	2	5-100	tabs: 0.5, 1, 2, 5, 10, 20 conc: 2/ml inj: 50/ml
DIBENZOXAZEPINE			
Loxapine (Loxitane)	15	50-250	caps: 5, 10, 25, 50 conc: 25/ml inj: 50/ml
DIHYDROINDOLONE			
Molindone (Moban)	10-15	25-250	tabs: 5, 10, 25, 50, 100 conc: 20/ml
ATYPICAL			
Clozapine (Clozaril)	100	300-600	tabs: 25, 100 7-day pack
Risperidone (Risperdal)	—	4-6	tabs: 1, 2, 3, 4

*Upper limit to avoid retinopathy.

Stages of Relapse. Five stages of relapse have been identified, scientifically replicated,[13,14] and validated by consumers and families.[34] It is important to recognize that the first two do not involve symptoms that indicate psychosis. This is relevant because this is the crucial time to intervene. In the first two stages the patient will be able to seek and use feedback constructively.

Stage one is referred to as **overextension.** In this stage the patient complains of feeling overwhelmed. Symptoms of anxiety are intensified and great energy is used to overcome them. Patients describe feeling overloaded, being unable to concentrate on or complete tasks, and a tendency to forget words in the middle of sentences. Other symptoms of overextension include expending increasing mental efforts to perform usual activities, decreasing performance efficiency, and easy distractibility.

Stage two is referred to as **restricted consciousness.** The previous symptoms of anxiety are replaced by symptoms of depression. The depression is more intense than usual daily mood variations. There are added dimensions of appearing bored, apathetic, obsessional, and phobic. Somatization may occur. The patient seems to withdraw from everyday events and limit external stimulation as a means to protect against the upcoming loss of control.

The first appearance of psychotic features occurs in stage three, **disinhibition.** Symptoms may resemble those of hypomania and usually include the emergence of hallucinations and delusions that the patient no longer is able to control. Previously successful defense mechanisms tend to break down.

In stage four, **psychotic disorganization**, clearly psychotic symptoms occur. Hallucinations and delusions intensify and the patient ultimately loses control. This stage is characterized by three distinct phases:

▼ The patient no longer recognizes familiar environments or people and may accuse family members of being impostors. Extreme agitation is possible. This phase is referred to as *destructuring of the external world.*

▼ The patient loses personal identity and may refer to the self in the third person. This subphase is referred to as *destructuring of the self.*

▼ *Total fragmentation* is the total loss of the ability to differentiate reality from psychosis and may be referred to as *loudly psychotic.* The patient experiences complete loss of control. Hospitalization is usually required at this point, and family members may have to enlist law enforcement officers to take the patient to the hospital. When this happens it is extremely devastating and embarrassing to both the patient and the family.

Stage five, **psychotic resolution,** usually occurs in the hospital. The patient is generally medicated and still experiencing psychosis, but the symptoms are "quiet." The person may appear to follow instructions in a robotic manner and often looks dazed. Unfortunately many patients are discharged in this stage because they are compliant or they no longer have insurance benefits.

 Identify ways that you would approach a patient and family regarding the need for a change in the treatment plan at each stage of the relapse process. Why is it important to identify relapse as soon as possible?

Docherty and colleagues[13] discovered that for most patients the process of recompensation involves the reversal of these five stages in a rather systematic fashion. This research has tremendous implications for teaching. When psychotic disorganization predictably reappears, patients, providers, and family members often believe a new episode has begun instead of understanding that the current episode is remitting. The recompensation phase can take much longer than decompensation, and there is often a tendency to rehospitalize the patient. An inappropriate rehospitalization will only return the patient to an unstable phase, deepen the psychosis, reinforce to the patient that the illness has taken control, and further decrease self-esteem. A most helpful intervention is to explain this process and for family members or residential staff to have someone available to be with the patient when the "loudly psychotic" symptoms return. Generally there is a period of chaos that will pass after 3 to 4 days.

An example of how well patients can recognize their symptoms compared with staff and families is described in the following clinical example.

CLINICAL EXAMPLE

During a class on relapse and symptom management, a patient was asked what symptoms caused a return to the hospital. The patient responded, "It was my red dots." When asked to explain he said, "I see red dots all the time, but when they change in a way that I can no longer tell the difference between *my* red dots, brake lights of the car in front of me, or stop lights, I know it's time to go back to the hospital for a medication check." A staff member said, "So that's why you are always staring at the exit sign, because it's red?" The patient nodded, and the staff member continued with, "So why didn't you tell us?" The patient simply said, "You didn't ask."[34]

This example clearly demonstrates the need not only to teach patients about symptoms indicative of relapse, but also to ask what they already know about their own symptoms.

Managing Relapse. The key to managing relapse is awareness of the onset of behaviors indicating relapse. About 70% of patients and 93% of families are able to notice symptoms of illness recurrence.[21] Almost all patients (98%) know when symptoms are intensifying.[39] These and other studies also identify a prodromal phase before relapse.[45]

Prodromal phase is defined as the length of time between the onset of symptoms and the need for treatment. Herz[20] identified that only 7% to 8% of patients and 11% of families reported full relapse in less than 24 hours after symptom onset, whereas 50% of patients and more than 66% of families indicated that the prodromal period lasted more than a week. With the majority of patients and families indicating a prodromal period longer than 1 week, it is essential that nurses collaborate with the patient, family, and residential staff regarding the onset of relapse.

Identifying and managing symptoms help to effectively decrease the number and severity of relapses. Teaching this to patients and families is a cost-effective intervention that can provide control over one's life and decrease the number or length of hospitalizations.

The Moller-Murphy symptom management assessment tool (MM-SMAT)[38] can be used for the patient to self-report symptoms, difficulties in activities of daily living, problems with medications, and ways of managing symptoms. Once patients can validate their experiences they are empowered to manage symptoms rather than have the symptoms rule their lives.

> In what ways is self-assessment of symptoms an empowering experience for patients? How might it positively affect the nurse-patient relationship?

When assessing symptom stability of any chronic illness, it is important to evaluate if daily symptoms are better, about the same, or worse than usual. Some patients with schizophrenia have psychotic symptoms daily yet are able to maintain a stable level of wellness and carry out activities of daily living. Relapse for these patients is usually indicated by an increase in symptom intensity.

The nurse conducting discharge teaching or working in an outpatient or residential setting needs to stress the lengthy recuperation process with special emphasis on the sedative qualities of the medication used to prevent relapse. When families and residential supervisors who do not understand the length of time needed for recuperation complain that the patient just wants to sit around, smoke, and watch television, the nurse is encouraged to provide information. This clinical example provides an example of this behavior.

CLINICAL EXAMPLE

A 26-year-old man with a medical diagnosis of schizophrenia who experienced a lengthy relapse was discharged from the acute care setting and admitted to a residential group home affiliated with a local mental health center. He was later asked to leave both community-based treatment programs because of not being able to actively engage in the required therapies. He was discharged to the care of his parents, who were to motivate him to take his medications and engage him in some type of therapy eventually leading to a job. The parents were active in the Alliance for the Mentally Ill. After months of frustration the local chapter conducted a program on relapse, and the parents learned about the lengthy rehabilitation period required. They were encouraged to see that their son ate well and kept up daily hygienic practices, to stop trying to force him to go out, and to start supporting his basic needs based on the wellness model. After 6 months he said one day that he wanted to enter a sporting activity at which he had previously excelled. He was encouraged to practice and entered the competition. After that positive experience he was able to reenter life within the limits of his neurobiological responses.

Selected Nursing Diagnoses:

▼ Social isolation related to low energy during recovery as evidenced by resistance to involvement in activities

▼ Caregiver role strain related to parents' unrealistic expectations for rapid recovery as evidenced by positive response to education about relapse and recovery

Anxiety and depression are often overlooked as major contributors to behavior causing poor health-related practices of individuals with schizophrenia. Common observable behaviors related to anxiety include pacing, restlessness, irritability, quickness to anger, or withdrawal. The high incidence of suicide in people with schizophrenia mandates the importance of assessing lethality, potential dangerousness toward self, and risk of leaving treatment against medical advice. Because of impaired information processing, patients should also be assessed for potential dangerousness to others.

Finally, a variety of symptom management techniques have been found useful by patients. Box 19-8 categorizes these techniques. Patients who have found other symptom management techniques should be encouraged to use them as long as the technique is not harmful to self or others.

Overall principles that assist the nurse to implement teaching regarding symptom management with increased effectiveness include developing a trusting relationship and believing in the patient's ability to recognize relapse. The nurse also facilitates rehabilitation and the actualization level of wellness by educating both patient and family. Interventions should be made in a collaborative partnership with the patient. It is important to listen carefully to the patient describe experiences and assess the level of information processing during each interaction.

The following six steps can serve as a guide to the teaching of effective symptom management techniques:
1. Identify problem symptoms
2. Identify current symptom management techniques
3. Identify specific support systems
4. Discuss additional symptom management techniques
5. Eliminate nonproductive symptom management
6. Develop new symptom management plan

The nurse can help guide the patient in developing successful symptom management by selecting symptom management techniques that are easily available, have a potential for positive response, are acceptable to the patient, are not potentially harmful to self or others, and promote socially acceptable behaviors.

Relapse and Medications.
The most common causes of relapse relate in some way to medications. Unfortunately, one of the first things that often occurs in assessing relapse is blaming the patient for not taking medications. The nurse should realize that relapse is likely to occur whether the patient is taking medications or not, particularly if the patient has poor health practices. There will be a distinct difference, however, in the onset, quality, and length of relapse based on compliance to the treatment regimen.[29]

Caffeine and nicotine consumption can affect the action of psychotropic medications (see Critical Thinking about Contemporary Issues). Prediction of the success of any medication is impossible if the patient consumes alcoholic beverages or uses illegal street drugs. Research on a variety of ethnic groups has also determined that enzyme variations among population groups cause medications to act and metabolize differently in individuals of different backgrounds.[27]

Studies consistently show that without medication, people with schizophrenia relapse at a rate of 60% to 70% within the first years of diagnosis. For those who are faithful to the medication regimen, the relapse rate is approximately 40%, but drops to 15.7% with a combination of medications, group education, and support.[30] This statistic has tremendous implications for the role of patient education.

Patients who are compliant yet still relapse tend to have rapid onset of mood-related symptoms and recover quickly with minimal or no change in their antipsychotic medications. These patients usually volunteer for treat-

---

Box 19-8
SYMPTOM MANAGEMENT CATEGORIES AND TECHNIQUES

CATEGORY I: DISTRACTION

Talking with friends
Listening to music or dancing
Prayer
Watching television
Working
Writing
Going for a walk or a ride

CATEGORY III: HELP SEEKING

Going to the hospital or mental health clinic
Talking with a health-care professional
Seeking the support of a family member

CATEGORY V: ISOLATION

Going to bed
Staying home

CATEGORY II: FIGHTING BACK

Positive self-talk
Positive thinking
Yelling at the voices
Not paying attention to the thoughts
Avoiding situations that increase symptoms

CATEGORY IV: ATTEMPTS TO FEEL BETTER

Eating
Taking a bath or shower
Hugging a pillow or stuffed animal
Using medication/relaxation

CRITICAL THINKING ABOUT CONTEMPORARY ISSUES

Should Inpatient and Residential Mental Health Care Facilities Be Caffeine and Nicotine Free?

Many patients are faithful to their treatment regimen but, because of a daily intake of over 250 mg of caffeine, experience a decrease in effectiveness of most antipsychotic and antianxiety drugs as well as lithium.[24] In addition, a nicotine intake of more than 10 to 20 cigarettes daily dramatically decreases the effectiveness of antipsychotic drugs.[17] Because of research on the effects of nicotine and caffeine on maladaptive neurobiological responses and the effectiveness of medications, many inpatient psychiatric units have eliminated use of these substances. Smoking has also been banned because of the direct and indirect impact on health.

This represents a major change in psychiatric settings. In the recent past, coffee and cigarettes were an important part of the inpatient culture. Cigarettes, in particular, were used as rewards in token economy behavioral management plans. Patients often measured the course of the day from one smoke break to the next. Given this history of reinforcement of these habits, some believe that it is cruel to deprive chronically hospitalized people of one of their few pleasures. Others believe that these restrictions are not in keeping with the philosophy of individual choice and the value that adults should make their own health-related decisions.

Limits on smoking and caffeine are supported based on the obligation of a health-care program to promote healthful behavior. It is emphasized that careful attention should be paid to patient education and programs that assist with withdrawal. An issue that needs more attention is the impact on a newly admitted person of sudden withdrawal from these substances. Nurses need to assess preadmission use of caffeine and nicotine carefully. The impact of withdrawal needs to be considered when evaluating response to medications. In addition, the nurse should be aware of the possibility of withdrawal symptoms, help the patient understand them, and obtain orders for medications when necessary. ▼

ment and are generally able to trace the onset of their relapse to an identifiable stressor. Nonadherent patients tend to have gradual onset of relapse with prominent psychotic features and generally enter treatment through an involuntary hospital commitment. They usually require a longer hospitalization and a change in medication. Typically they cannot trace the onset of the relapse to any specific trigger.[29]

Even with support, education, and adherence to the treatment regimen relapse still occurs. This emphasizes the need for ongoing symptom monitoring and identification of factors leading to nonadherence. Cooperative medication management can be fostered by including the patient as an equal partner in treatment.[11] This only occurs when the patient is taught about the effects and side effects of the medication and staff and family are sensitive to feedback from the patient about how the medication makes him feel.

Even with education, medication nonadherence still occurs. In a study of 253 psychiatric inpatients interviewed on the day of discharge from a short hospital stay, more than half did not know the name and dosage of the psychiatric medications prescribed for them or why they were supposed to take them[9]; 68% of the patients knew the names of all their psychiatric medications, but only 53% knew when to take them. These results are surprising because all patients had attended both group and individual medication instruction classes during the hospitalization. When considering the cognitive symptoms occurring during an acute episode of schizophrenia the results become less surprising and implications for ongoing, postdischarge medication instruction become quite clear. Box 19-9 identifies additional nursing interventions useful in working with patients with schizophrenia and other psychotic disorders who are in the stable level of wellness.

Interventions Related to Actualization

Teaching at the actualization level focuses on prevention of relapse and symptom management to facilitate early intervention. Patient teaching methods that involve simple, clear, and concrete instructions including repetition and return demonstrations are the most helpful.[35,47]

One of the keys to preventing relapse includes identification of symptom triggers and strategies for managing them. Box 19-10 summarizes nursing interventions to prevent relapse.

Box 19-11 identifies nursing interventions for patients with schizophrenia and other psychotic disorders and the actualized level of wellness.

Once patients have reached the actualized level of wellness, relatives often do not know how to react to more autonomous functioning and need as much teaching and support as the patient.[32] Recent studies have

---

Box 19-9

NURSING INTERVENTIONS FOR PATIENTS WITH SCHIZOPHRENIA AND A STABLE LEVEL OF WELLNESS

Goal: To maintain a stable level of wellness, recognize early signs of relapse, and facilitate habilitation.

Time to achieve goal: Varies with individual ability and effectiveness of intervention. Generally takes several months to several years depending on level of illness, preillness level of function, and response to interventions. Time is shortened with effective family/community support. Time is lengthened if chemical substance use is involved or if person has difficulty accepting diagnosis.

HEALTH

Teach health management: hygiene, health care, nutrition, sleep/rest patterns, exercise
Educate regarding diagnosis
Educate about treatment options
Assist with medication management
Assist to identify effective, acceptable treatment plan
Teach identification and management of symptoms
Teach relapse planning and prevention
Identify symptom triggers
Assist with avoidance of substance abuse
Teach and assist with preventing sensory overload
Teach and assist with preventing sensory isolation

ENVIRONMENT

Assist family members to cope
Facilitate effective communication and relationships with significant others including family
Encourage and assist with developing life skills including activities of daily living
Encourage to use resources to develop job skills
Assist to identify and cope with environment triggers

ATTITUDES/BEHAVIOR

Empower individuals to use own agency
Assist to learn and use problem solving skills
Encourage individual to manage own illness
Assist to maintain appropriate level of responsibility for own behavior
Assist to develop behaviors that are congruent with culture and environment

SOCIAL SUPPORT

Assist to establish kinship support
Assist to integrate into the community
Assist with accessing appropriate community resources
Assist with defining important culture values
Assist with planning to meet spiritual needs

Box 19-10

NURSING INTERVENTIONS TO PREVENT RELAPSE

Identify symptoms that signal relapse
Identify symptom triggers
Select symptom management techniques
Identify coping strategies for symptom triggers
Identify support system for future relapse
Document action plan in written form and file with key support people
Facilitate integration into family and community

---

also indicated that psychotherapy may be helpful in the rehabilitative phase of recovery as patients face and deal with the neurobiological deficits that often become apparent to them only then.[49,51] The focus of the psychotherapy is usually supportive and nonconfrontational in nature.

Many families make comments such as, "When we learned our son's diagnosis was schizophrenia, it was like he had died." Given this response, it is understandable that schizophrenia remains a closely held secret in many households. These attitudes often prevent families from effectively coping with schizophrenia.

Many strange and unhelpful ideas about communicating with persons with schizophrenia and their families have been dispensed by well-meaning advice-givers and mental health professionals. In the past, parents have been counseled not to discuss the illness with their child nor to try to intervene in their lives in any way. Some parents have even been advised to stop all communication with their ill family member and have no further contact for "therapeutic" reasons.

The situation may be complicated by wrongful advice from health professionals who tell parents or imply to them that they caused or perpetuated the illness. Parental guilt stemming from self-blame caused by this type of misinformation further blocks communication within the family. Parents find themselves at a loss about how to talk with their ill child, and perhaps even fear him. Clearly this situation does not help parents face the many problems they encounter when placed in the additional roles of case manager, residential supervisor, and legal guardian.

An equally complicated role of negotiator between the assigned case manager, guardian, and an adult child also falls to parents. No one knows an individual better

---

Box 19-11

NURSING INTERVENTIONS FOR PATIENTS WITH SCHIZOPHRENIA AND AN ACTUALIZED LEVEL OF WELLNESS

Goal: To reach one's potential and achieve a satisfactory quality of life as defined by the individual.

Time to achieve goal: This is a life process. Personal goals and desires are altered with age, life circumstances, and current ability level.

HEALTH

Education related to skills/abilities individual wants to develop
Education regarding health maintenance
Allow for activities to meet spiritual needs
Counseling
Assist to better cope with health triggers
Adapt teaching and interventions to level of cognitive functioning

ENVIRONMENT

Work/vocational rehabilitation
Assist with interpersonal skill improvement
Facilitate integration into community
Assist to better cope with environmental triggers

ATTITUDES/BEHAVIOR

Assist individual to define what "actualization" is for them
Assist to better cope with attitude/behavior triggers
Reframe concept of chronic illness
Develop satisfying leisure activities
Assist to cope with stigma
Develop process to define and redefine values

SOCIAL SUPPORT

Assist to effectively access appropriate community resources
Assist to effectively use kinship support
Choose which culture practices to participate in
Choose activities to meet spiritual needs
Gradually reduce health care involvement as individual becomes more capable of managing own life

---

than the family, but it can be emotionally painful and draining to be a loving, nurturing, advocating parent in one situation; a treatment-enforcing case manager in another; or residential supervisor to an outside case manager in yet another.

Introduction of simultaneous patient/family teaching regarding ongoing symptom management and medication compliance is useful at this stage of habilitation. Patient and family education may also dispel myths and provide suggestions for improving communication between and among members of the treatment team and

the family. This form of education was developed by psychiatric clinical nurse specialists in 1985 and has been successfully implemented with over 1500 individuals.[34,36] A facilitator training program was implemented in 1991, and over 30 people have begun implementing the program in the United States and Canada.[34] This program requires advanced group skills and is not recommended for beginning psychiatric nurses. However, the curriculum is provided in the Family Education Plan on p. 508 to provide information about recommended content.[37]

When the actualization level of wellness has been maintained, communication in the family changes. Instead of blaming each other, the family, including siblings, learns to reach out and involve the member with schizophrenia in a collaborative relationship. A Nursing Care Plan Summary for the patient with maladaptive neurobiological responses is presented on pp. 509 and 510.

 valuation

Evaluation of the nursing care provided to patients who have maladaptive neurobiological responses is based on input from the patient and family. Because these are serious, long-term illnesses, care is often episodic. Relapse should not be interpreted as a failure of the nursing intervention but should be considered in the context of the patient's life situation at the time.

To evaluate the nursing intervention, the following questions may be asked:

▼ Is the patient able to describe the behaviors that characterize the onset of a relapse?

▼ Is the patient able to identify and describe the medications prescribed, reason for taking them, frequency of taking them, and possible side effects?

▼ Does the patient participate in relationships with other people at a level that is comfortable?

▼ Is the patient's family aware of the characteristics of the illness and able to participate in a supportive relationship with the patient?

▼ Are the patient and family informed about available community resources such as rehabilitation programs, mental health care providers, educational programs, and support groups, and do they use them?

SUMMARY

1. Maladaptive neurobiological responses are related to disruptions in brain functioning and affect the areas of cognition, perception, emotion, behavior,

FAMILY EDUCATION PLAN
UNDERSTANDING THE WORLD OF PSYCHOSIS

Content	Instructional activities	Evaluation
Describe psychosis	Introduce participants and leaders State purpose of group Define terminology associated with psychosis	The participant will describe the characteristics of psychosis.
Identify the causes of psychotic disorders	Present theories of psychotic disorders Use audiovisual aids to explain brain anatomy, brain biochemistry, and major neurotransmitters	The participant will discuss the relationship between brain anatomy, brain biochemistry, and major neurotransmitters and the development of psychosis.
Define schizophrenia according to medical diagnostic criteria	Lead a discussion of the medical diagnostic criteria for schizophrenia	The participant will describe the medical diagnostic criteria for schizophrenia.
Describe the relationship between anxiety and psychotic disorders	Present types and stages of anxiety Discuss steps in reducing and resolving anxiety	The participant will identify and describe the stages of anxiety and ways to reduce or resolve it.
Analyze the impact of living with hallucinations	Describe the characteristics of hallucinations Demonstrate ways to communicate with someone who is hallucinating Show film, *The World of the Schizophrenic* (Sandoz)	The participant will demonstrate effective ways to communicate with a person who has hallucinations.
Analyze the impact of living with delusions	Describe types of delusions Demonstrate ways to communicate with someone who has delusions Discuss interventions for delusions	The participant will demonstrate effective ways to communicate with a person who has delusions.
Discuss the use of psychotropic medications and the role of nutrition	Provide and explain handouts describing the characteristics of psychotropic medications that are prescribed for schizophrenia Discuss special nutritional needs with medications	The participant will identify and describe the characteristics of medications prescribed for self/family member and discuss the role of nutrition related to the medication.
Describe the characteristics of relapse and the role of compliance with the therapeutic regimen	Assist the participants to describe their own experiences with relapse Discuss symptom management techniques and the importance of complying with the therapeutic regimen	The participant will describe behaviors that indicate an impending relapse and discuss the importance of symptom management and compliance with the therapeutic regimen.
Analyze behaviors that promote wellness	Discuss the components of wellness Relate wellness to the elements of symptom management	The participant will analyze the effect of maintaining a state of wellness on the occurrence of symptoms.
Discuss ways to cope with everyday living with psychosis	Lead a group discussion focused on the daily problems of living with psychosis and coping behaviors Propose ways to create a low stress environment	The participant will describe ways to modify life-style to create a low stress environment.

NURSING CARE PLAN SUMMARY
Maladaptive Neurobiological Responses

Nursing Diagnosis: Altered thought processes

Expected Outcome: The patient will live, learn, and work at a maximum possible level of success as defined by the individual.

Short-term Goals	Interventions	Rationale
The patient will participate in brief, regularly scheduled meetings with the nurse.	Initiate a nurse-patient relationship contract mutually agreed on by nurse and patient Schedule brief (5-10 minute), frequent contacts with the patient Consistently approach the patient at the scheduled time Extend length of sessions gradually based on patient's agreement	The establishment of a trusting relationship is fundamental to developing open communication. A patient with altered thought processes cannot tolerate extended, intrusive interactions and functions best in a structured environment.
The patient will describe delusions and other altered thought processes.	Demonstrate attitude of caring and concern Validate the meaning of communications with the patient Assist the patient to identify the difference between reality and internal thought processes	Patients are very sensitive to others' responses to their symptoms. A respectful, interested approach will enable the patient to discuss unusual and frightening thoughts. Identification of reality by a trusted person is helpful.
The patient will identify and describe the effect of brain disease on thought processes.	Provide information about causes of psychoses Discuss the relationship between the patient's behaviors and brain function Involve significant others in educational sessions	Understanding of the physiological basis for altered thought processes assists the patient to recognize symptoms and to feel in control of the illness. Significant others can provide support and experience less stigma if they are informed about the illness.
The patient will identify signs of impending relapse and describe actions to take to prevent relapse.	Assist patient and significant others to identify behaviors related to altered thought processes that indicate threatened relapse Identify community resources and mutually plan actions directed toward prevention of relapse	Relapse can be predicted if the patient and family are alert to warning signs. Early intervention allows the patient to be in control of the course of the illness. Family members can be helpful in assisting the patient to identify symptoms and providing support for seeking assistance.
The patient will describe symptom management techniques that are helpful in living with altered thought processes.	Describe symptom management techniques that other patients have used Ask the patient to describe techniques used to manage symptoms Encourage the patient to take control of the illness by using symptom management techniques	Many patients with psychoses continue to have delusions after the acute phase of the illness has passed. Patients can function better if they learn ways to manage the symptom.

NURSING CARE PLAN SUMMARY—cont'd
Maladaptive Neurobiological Responses

Nursing Diagnosis: Social isolation

Expected Outcome: The patient will live, learn, and work at a maximum possible level of success as defined by the individual.

Short-term Goals	Interventions	Rationale
The patient will engage in a trusting relationship with the nurse.	Initiate a nurse-patient relationship contract mutually agreed on by nurse and patient Establish mutual goals related to social interaction Establish trust by consistently meeting the elements of the plan and engaging in open and honest communication	Patients who have maladaptive neurobiological responses often have difficulty trusting others. Difficulty with information processing causes problems interpreting the communication of others.
The patient will discuss personal goals related to social interaction.	Encourage the patient to describe current relationship patterns Discuss past relationship experiences Identify problems associated with social interaction Explore goals	The patient may be unaware of the characteristics of mutually satisfying interpersonal relationships. Honest feedback from the nurse can assist the patient to identify the reasons for past problems. Knowledge of the patient's relationship goals leads to the development of realistic behavioral change.
The patient will identify behaviors that interfere with social relationships.	Share observations about the patient's behavior in social situations	Identification of problematic behavior helps the patient and nurse target changes.
The patient will practice alternative social behaviors with the nurse.	Discuss possible behavioral changes that will facilitate the establishment of social relationships Role play alternative behaviors Provide feedback	Practice will assist the patient to gain comfort with new behaviors. Feedback provides reinforcement for successful behavioral change.
The patient will select one person and practice social interaction skills.	Discuss experience of practicing new behavior with another person Discuss ways of maintaining a relationship	The patient will need ongoing feedback and support related to maintaining behavioral change.

and relatedness. Adaptive neurobiological responses include logical thought, accurate perceptions, emotions consistent with experiences, behavior consistent with cultural norms, and relatedness. Maladaptive neurobiological responses include thought disorder (delusions), misperceptions (hallucinations), inability to experience emotions, bizarre behavior, and social isolation.

2. The behaviors associated with maladaptive neurobiological responses include cognitive, perceptual, emotional, behavioral, and relational responses.

3. Predisposing factors for maladaptive neurobiologi-

cal responses are described from biological, psychological, and sociocultural perspectives. Precipitating stressors include biological characteristics, environmental stress, and symptom triggers.

4. Coping resources are individualized and depend on the nature and extent of the neurobiological disruption. Family resources are very important. Coping mechanisms may include regression, projection, and withdrawal and represent the person's attempt to control the illness.

5. Primary NANDA nursing diagnoses are impaired verbal communication, sensory/perceptual alter-

ations, impaired social interaction, social isolation, and altered thought processes.

6. Primary DSM-IV diagnoses are schizophrenia, schizophreniform disorder, schizoaffective disorder, delusional disorder, brief psychotic disorder, and shared psychotic disorder.

7. The expected outcome of nursing care is that the patient will live, learn, and work at a maximum possible level of success as defined by the individual.

8. The nursing care plan must be based on an understanding of the patient's disabilities, strengths, and preferences. Patient and family education about symptom management and relapse prevention is a critical element of the plan.

9. Primary nursing interventions for patients with maladaptive neurobiological responses include intervention in delusions, intervention with hallucinations, medication management, and patient and family education about symptom management and relapse.

10. Evaluation is based on the patient's satisfaction with the level of functioning and on the ability to communicate either improvement or impending relapse.

SUGGESTED CROSS-REFERENCES

COMPETENT CARING
A CLINICAL EXEMPLAR OF A PSYCHIATRIC NURSE

Melody Sewell, MSN, RN

I had the unique opportunity to broaden my skills as a psychiatric nurse by working with J, a psychotic patient. I learned invaluable lessons in patience and acceptance as I watched the thought processes of this young man unfold. He also taught me important lessons in caring during the period we built our therapeutic relationship.

J was a well-groomed, handsome 26-year-old white man with a 9-year history of paranoid schizophrenia. He displayed an intense facial expression. He was admitted to our 22-bed adult psychiatric unit for a second time within the year. Although he had a high level of functioning, he neglected to acknowledge his limits. This was evidenced by his working in excess of 60 hours per week in landscaping for the previous 6 months. The patient had been followed up on an outpatient basis monthly since his discharge last year. The psychiatrist working with him noted increasing symptoms of paranoia exacerbated by job-related stress.

J was admitted to the unit with a marked weight loss, guarded affect, and minimal interaction. Reiterating that, "I need to get back to my job—the bills must be paid," he verbalized the importance of maintaining his independence from his parents and retaining his employment and apartment. He was on the unit 1 week. A pending discharge date was set for 2 days hence in spite of his minimal disclosure and apparent lack of progress. As his nurse I was concerned he would return to the same environmental demands and deteriorate further if our treatment was not effective. This might also increase his risk for rehospitalization, which would further threaten his self-esteem and feelings of independence.

When I arrived at work, another patient reported to me that J was tearful, verbalizing feelings of helplessness and worthlessness. From my perspective he clearly was not ready for discharge without prompt constructive intervention. I realized that this would be difficult, however, because he withdrew from almost all interaction.

I approached J, providing a quiet, comfortable area free from distractions and allowing for privacy. Verbalizing my observation of his red and swollen eyes, he immediately responded: "I wear contacts." I provided an atmosphere of trust, building on my rapport with him that dated back to his previous hospitalization, and continued to offer myself in a nonjudgmental manner, encouraging him to explore issues that were perpetuating internal conflicts. This time my intervention worked. His once-guarded affect softened as tears filled his eyes.

He spoke of job-related stressors, his need to maintain independence from his parents, and his desire to provide for himself without government financial assistance. He elaborated on his feelings of failure as a son. When further explored, issues of his father's difficulty accepting the limitations associated with the mental illness of his "only son" became apparent. J explored this and realized that he had to accept responsibility for his own actions and provide boundaries for himself to maintain his sense of independence. To do so, he could no longer overextend himself and be able to maintain good functioning.

When encouraged to continue talking, he verbalized concerns regarding his sexuality. He greatly desired companionship but realized the chronicity of his illness. Painfully exploring the insight of his diminished ability to provide financially for a family, he cried. I empathized with his pain but also confirmed that he was a sexual being with options. At the end of our discussion, we established concrete steps to implement upon discharge. One of these included finding a job with fewer physical and time demands. He also expressed his gratitude to me, since he could now see that his symptoms had prevented any constructive interactions or positive outcomes previously.

Throughout the discussion with J I maintained an atmosphere of mutual interaction. He vacillated between intervals of tearfulness and guarded behavior, expressing that our interaction was uncomfortable for him at times. I also observed occasional twitching of his thumbs, which I assessed for possible extrapyramidal symptoms.

J was discharged with plans to implement the changes we had discussed. He expressed hope, admitting that he had previously thought of leaving the hospital and "travelling around the country to get away from everything and just see where I might end up." Now, with some pertinent education coupled with concrete steps to guide him, he was leaving the hospital with a sense of direction and hopeful intentions for his life.

Through a comprehensive care approach and expressed respect for my patient, J and I were able to mutually set attainable goals for his discharge, allowing him to leave the hospital with a sense of control and hope. I think about him often, especially on my hectic and sometimes discouraging days in psychiatric nursing, and quietly smile knowing the difference one nurse can make. ▼

REFERENCES

1. Allebeck P, Wistedt B: Mortality in schizophrenia, *Arch Gen Psychiatry* 43:650, 1986.
2. American Psychiatric Association: *Diagnostic and statistical manual of mental disorders*, ed 4, Washington, DC, 1994, The Association.
3. Andreasen N, Black D: *Introductory textbook of psychiatry*, Washington, DC, 1991, American Psychiatric Press.
4. Andreasen NC, Carpenter WT: Diagnosis and classification of schizophrenia, *Schizophr Bull* 19:199, 1993.
5. Benes F: Neurobiological investigations in the cingulate cortex of the schizophrenic brain, *Schizophr Bull* 19:537, 1993.
6. Braff D: New brain structural abnormalities in schizophrenia. Paper presented at the annual meeting of the National Alliance for the Mentally Ill, Miami, July 24, 1993.
7. Braff D: Information processing and attention dysfunctions in schizophrenia, *Schizophr Bull* 19:233, 1993.
8. Breslin N: Treatment of schizophrenia: current practice and future promise, *Hosp Community Psychiatry* 43:877, 1992.
9. Clary C, Dever A, Schweizer E: Psychiatric inpatients' knowledge of medication at hospital discharge, *Hosp Community Psychiatry* 43:140, 1992.
10. Corday R: *Psychosis, the inner experience*, Boulder, Colo, 1991, Common Loon Productions.
11. Corrigan P, Liberman RP, Engel J: From noncompliance to collaboration in the treatment of schizophrenia, *Hosp Community Psychiatry* 41:1203, 1990.
12. Corrigan P, Storzbach D: Behavioral interventions for alleviating psychotic symptoms, *Hosp Community Psychiatry* 44:341, 1993.
13. Docherty JP, Van Kammen DP, Siris SG: Stages of onset of schizophrenic psychoses, *Am J Psychiatry* 135:420, 1978.
14. Donlon P, Blacker K: Stages of schizophrenic decompensation and reintegration, *J Nerv Ment Dis* 157:200, 1973.
15. Dzurec L: How do they see themselves: self-perception and functioning for people with chronic schizophrenia, *J Psychosoc Nurs Ment Health Serv* 28:10, 1990.
16. Francel C, Conn V, Gray D: Families' perceptions of burden of care for chronic mentally ill relatives, *Hosp Community Psychiatry* 39:1296, 1988.
17. Goff D, Henderson D, Amico E: Cigarette smoking in schizophrenia: relationship to psychopathology and medication side effects, *Am J Psychiatry* 149:1189, 1992.
18. Goldman H: Mental illness and family burden: a public health perspective, *Hosp Community Psychiatry* 33:557, 1982.
19. Hamera E, Peterson K, Young L, Schaumloffel M: Symptom monitoring in schizophrenia: potential for enhancing self-care, *Arch Psychiatr Nurs* 7:324, 1993.
20. Herz M: Recognizing and preventing relapse in patients with schizophrenia, *Hosp Community Psychiatry* 35:344, 1984.
21. Herz M, Melville C: Relapse in schizophrenia, *Am J Psychiatry* 137:801, 1980.
22. Kane J, Honigfeld GL, Singer J, Meltzer H: Clozapine for the treatment-resistant schizophrenic, *Arch Gen Psychiatry* 45:785, 1988.
23. Kendler K, Diehl S: The genetics of schizophrenia: a current, genetic-epidemiologic perspective, *Schizophr Bull* 19:261, 1993.
24. Kirmer D: Caffeine use and abuse in psychiatric patients, *J Psychosoc Nurs Ment Health Serv* 26:20, 1988.
25. Lego S: *The American handbook of psychiatric nursing*, Philadelphia, 1984, JB Lippincott.
26. Liberman RP et al: The nature and problem of schizophrenia. In Bellack AS, ed: *Schizophrenia: treatment, management, and rehabilitation*, New York, 1984, Grune & Stratton.
27. Lin K, Poland R, Nakasaki G: *Psychopharmacology and psychobiology of ethnicity*, Washington, DC, 1993, American Psychiatric Press.
28. McCandless-Glimcher L et al: Use of symptoms by schizophrenics to monitor and regulate their illness, *Hosp Community Psychiatry* 37:929, 1986.
29. McEvoy J, Howe A, Hogarty G: Differences in the nature of relapse and subsequent inpatient course between medication-compliant and noncompliant schizophrenic patients, *J Nerv Ment Dis* 172:412, 1984.
30. McFarlane W et al: From research to clinical practice: dissemination of New York State's family psychoeducation project, *Hosp Community Psychiatry* 44:265, 1993.
31. Mann N et al: Psychosocial rehabilitation in schizophrenia: beginnings in acute hospitalization, *Arch Psychiatr Nurs* 7:154, 1993.

32. Mason S, Gingerich S, Siris S: Patients' and caregivers' adaptation to improvement in schizophrenia, *Hosp Community Psychiatry* 41:541, 1990.

33. Moller M: *Understanding and communicating with a person who is hallucinating*, videotape and study guide, Omaha, Neb, 1989, NurSeminars.

34. Moller M: *Understanding relapse: managing the symptoms of schizophrenia*, videotape and study guide, Omaha, Neb, 1991, NurSeminars.

35. Moller M, Wer J: Family identified health education needs regarding schizophrenia. In Malone J, ed: *Schizophrenia: handbook for clinical care*, Thorofare, NJ, 1992, Slack.

36. Moller M, Wer J: Simultaneous patient/family education regarding schizophrenia: the Nebraska model, *Arch Psychiatr Nurs* 3:332, 1989.

37. Moller M, Wer J, Murphy M: *How to enter the world of psychosis . . . . a consumer/family perspective, participant manual*, Nine Mile Falls, Wash, 1994, The Center for Patient and Family Mental Health Education.

38. Murphy M, Moller M: Relapse management in neurobiological disorders: The Moller-Murphy symptom management assessment tool, *Arch Psychiatr Nurs* 7:226, 1993.

39. Nasrallah H: The neuropsychiatry of schizophrenia. In Yudofsky S, Hales R, eds: *Textbook of neuropsychiatry*, ed 2, Washington, DC, 1991, The American Psychiatric Press.

40. National Foundation for Brain Research: *The care of disorders of the brain*, Washington, DC, 1992, The Foundation.

41. North C: Current concepts of schizophrenia, *Compr Ther* 15:8, 1989.

42. O'Connor F: Symptom monitoring for relapse prevention in schizophrenia, *Arch Psychiatr Nurs* 5:193, 1992.

43. Peck MS: *The road less traveled*, New York, 1978, Simon & Schuster.

44. Siegel B et al: Cortical-striatal-thalamic circuits and brain glucose metabolic activity in 70 unmedicated male schizophrenia patients, *Am J Psychiatr* 150:1325, 1993.

45. Subotnik K, Nuechterlein K: Prodromal signs and symptoms of schizophrenic relapse, *J Abnorm Psychol* 97:405, 1988.

46. Torrey EF: *Surviving schizophrenia: a family manual*, New York, 1988, Harper & Row.

47. Tratnack S, Harmon R: Taking the mystery out of mental illness: a patient education program. In Malone J, ed: *Schizophrenia: handbook for clinical care*, Thorofare, NJ, 1992, Slack.

48. Trevarthen C: Growth in education of the hemispheres. In Trevarthen C, ed: *Brain circuits and functions of the mind: essays in honor of Roger W. Sperry*, New York, 1990, Cambridge Press.

49. Wasylenki D: Psychotherapy of schizophrenia revisited, *Hosp Community Psychiatry* 43:123, 1992.

50. Weinberger D: A connectionist approach to the prefrontal cortex, *J Neuropsychiatry* 5:241, 1993.

51. Zahniser J, Coursey R, Hershberger K: Individual psychotherapy with schizophrenic outpatients in the public mental health system, *Hosp Community Psychiatry* 42:906, 1991.

ANNOTATED SUGGESTED READINGS

Backlar P: *The family face of schizophrenia*, New York, 1994, GP Putnam's Sons.

Collection of family stories with commentary by mental health professionals who work with people who have schizophrenia. It is useful for families and provides nurses with insight regarding the family's point of view.

Breslin NA: Treatment of schizophrenia: current practice and future promise, *Hosp Community Psychiatry* 43:877, 1992.

Review of the status of treatment of schizophrenia, including pharmacotherapy and psychotherapy.

Dixon L et al: Drug abuse in schizophrenic patients: clinical correlates and reasons for use, *Am J Psychiatry* 148:224, 1991.

Study that found that 50% of schizophrenic patients had abused drugs at some time. It was also determined that the drug-abusing patients were higher functioning at the time of discharge than patients who had not abused drugs.

*Hamera EK, Peterson KA, Young LM, Schaumloffel MM: Symptom monitoring in schizophrenia: potential for enhancing self-care, *Arch Psychiatr Nurs* 6:324, 1992.

Nursing study that identified indicators of impending relapse, categorized as psychotic, depressive, and anxiety based.

*Houseman C: The paranoid person: a biopsychosicial perspective, *Arch Psychiatr Nurs* 4:177, 1990.

Discusses the phenomenon of paranoia related to all aspects of the individual's functioning from the brain to the culture in which one lives.

*Hunter EP, Storat B: Psychosocial triggers of relapse in persons with chronic mental illness: a pilot study, *Issues Mentl Health Nurs* 15:67, 1994.

Pilot study in which five patients were interviewed regarding events preceding their hospital admission. In each case, the patient was able to identify a stressful event (toxic trigger) that led to relapse.

*Jacobs P, Bobek SC: Sexual needs of the schizophrenic client: *Perspect Psychiatr Care* 27:15, 1991.

Discusses the effects of schizophrenia on sexuality and recommends nursing interventions that will assist the patient to understand and meet sexual needs.

*Kane CF, DiMartino E, Jimenez M: A comparison of short-term psychoeducational and support groups for relatives coping with chronic schizophrenia, *Arch Psychiatr Nurs* 4:343, 1990.

Nursing study that compared two types of group intervention for relatives of schizophrenic patients.

*Mann NA et al: Psychosocial rehabilitation in schizophrenia: beginnings in acute hospitalization, *Arch Psychiatr Nurs* 7:154, 1993.

Describes a structured nursing program focused on rehabilitative interventions for schizophrenic patients in an acute psychiatric inpatient setting. Includes examples of patient education materials that have been developed.

*Mulaik JS: Noncompliance with medication regimens in severely and persistently mentally ill schizophrenic patients, *Issues Ment Health Nurs* 13:219, 1992.

Study based on the health belief model concluded that the patients studied failed to take medications because they did not believe that they needed them.

*O'Connor FW: Symptom monitoring for relapse prevention in schizophrenia, *Arch Psychiatr Nurs* 5:193, 1991.

Presents an approach to symptom monitoring that is based on the stress-vulnerability model of schizophrenia. Includes implications for patient and family education.

Olfson M, Glick ID, Mechanic D: Inpatient treatment of schizophrenia in general hospitals, *Hosp Community Psychiatry* 44:40, 1993.

Discusses interventions that are useful when treating schizophrenic patients in a short-term inpatient setting. Includes suggestions about interpersonal approaches, medication, family involvement, and discharge planning.

*Puskar KR et al: Psychiatric nursing management of medication-free psychotic patients, *Arch Psychiatr Nurs* 4:78, 1990.

Description of nursing interventions for psychotic patients who are being treated in a research unit and are not taking medication during some phases of the research.

---

*Nursing reference.

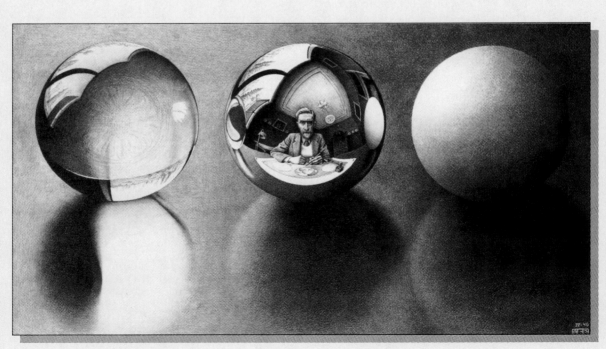

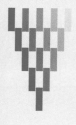

CHAPTER 20
Social Responses and Personality Disorders

CAROL PERLIN

The emptiness caused by dissatisfaction with mere achievement and the help-lessness that results when the channels of relation break down have brought forth a loneliness of soul such as never existed before.

Karl Jaspers: *Existenzphilosophie*

LEARNING OBJECTIVES

After studying this chapter the student should be able to:

▼ Describe the continuum of adaptive and maladaptive social responses
▼ Identify behaviors associated with social responses
▼ Analyze predisposing factors and precipitating stressors related to social responses
▼ Describe coping resources and coping mechanisms related to social responses
▼ Formulate nursing diagnoses for patients related to social responses
▼ Assess the relationship between nursing diagnoses and medical diagnoses related to social responses
▼ Identify expected outcomes and short-term nursing goals for patients related to social responses
▼ Develop a patient education plan to promote patients' adaptive social responses
▼ Analyze nursing interventions for patients related to social responses
▼ Evaluate nursing care for patients related to social responses

TOPICAL OUTLINE

Continuum of Social Responses
   Adaptive and Maladaptive Responses
   Development Through the Life Cycle
Assessment
   Behaviors
   Predisposing Factors
   Precipitating Stressors
   Coping Resources
   Coping Mechanisms
Nursing Diagnosis
   Related Medical Diagnoses
Outcome Identification
Planning
Implementation
   Establishing a Therapeutic Relationship
   Family Involvement
   Milieu Therapy
   Limit Setting and Structure
   Protection from Self-Harm
   Focusing on Strengths
   Behavioral Strategies
Evaluation

To find satisfaction in life, people must be able to establish positive interpersonal relationships. Individuals who are involved in such relationships experience closeness to each other while keeping their separate identities. This type of closeness is called *intimacy* and is characterized by being sensitive to the other person's needs.[34] There is also mutual validation of personal worth in these relationships. Rogers[28] has described other characteristics of healthy relatedness, including open communication of feelings, acceptance of the other person as valued and separate, and empathic understanding. In a similar way, friendships are "voluntary, primary, enduring, possible across the life span, . . .with no fixed legal or social norms, with limits, and with a reciprocal quality of exchange that includes intimacy and love."[3]

To become deeply involved with another person, an individual must be willing to risk revealing private thoughts and feelings. This can be frightening, especially if a person has had past difficulty sharing feelings with other people. Fear of exposing private feelings often makes people reluctant to become involved in intimate relationships. Individuals who have extreme difficulty in relating closely to others may have behaviors that are characteristic of the medical diagnostic category of personality disorders. This includes the diagnoses of borderline, antisocial, and narcissistic personality disorder, among others. These people often lack emotional depth and have limited authentic commitments in their lives. They may repeatedly provoke rejection by others while at the same time they are fearful of this rejection. Thus they sabotage their conscious efforts to achieve their goals and live productively. This brings about ultimate self-defeat and the living out of a "failure script."[26,35]

 Based on your experiences, compare family, friends, and nurse-patient relationships. Describe how they are alike and different.

CONTINUUM OF SOCIAL RESPONSES

Every person has the potential to be involved in many levels of relationships, from intimacy to casual contacts. Intimate and interdependent relationships provide security and instill the self-confidence necessary to cope with the demands of daily life. A lack of intimacy with family members and friends leaves only superficial encounters, taking away many of life's most meaningful experiences. The support of significant others frees energy for involvement with social groups, work groups, and the community. Mature adults can be involved at all these

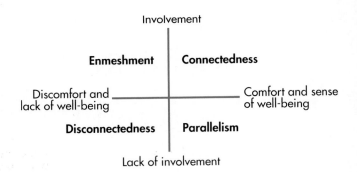

Fig. 20-1 States of relatedness.
From Hagerty BMK, Lynch-Sauer J, Patusky KL, Bouwsema M: *Image* 25:291, 1993.

levels and feel satisfied with the quality of their relationships with others.[11]

The concept of relatedness has been analyzed and described. Hagerty and associates[12] have identified four states of relatedness depending on the dimensions of involvement or lack of involvement and comfort and sense of well-being or discomfort and lack of well-being (Fig. 20-1). The state of connectedness indicates that the person is actively involved in satisfying relationships. Disconnectedness relates to a lack of involvement that is not satisfactory to the person. Parallelism refers to a lack of involvement that is comfortable for the person. Enmeshment occurs when the person is involved in relationships but is uncomfortable because of this. Competencies have been identified related to connectedness and disconnectedness. Connectedness involves high levels of belonging, mutuality, reciprocity and synchrony; the reverse is true for disconnectedness.

Adaptive and Maladaptive Responses

Within a relationship the participants usually develop a continuum of dependent and independent behavior. Ideally, these behaviors are balanced, which is described as interdependence. The interdependent person can decide when to rely on others and experience the caring that may be felt with dependency, and when it is appropriate to be independent. An interdependent person can let another be dependent or independent without needing to control that person's behavior. All individuals are responsible for controlling their own behavior while receiving support and help from significant others as needed. Adaptive social responses therefore include the ability to tolerate solitude and the expression of autonomy, mutuality, and interdependence.

Interpersonal relationship behaviors may be represented on a continuum that ranges from healthy interdependent interactions to those involving no real contact with other people (Fig. 20-2). At the midpoint of the continuum, a person experiences loneliness, with-

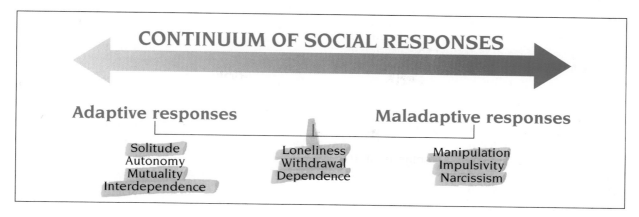

Fig. 20-2 Continuum of social responses.

drawal, and dependence. The maladaptive end of the continuum reflects the dominance of manipulation, impulsiveness, and narcissism. Patients with the medical diagnosis of borderline personality disorder, antisocial personality disorder, or narcissistic personality disorder function at the maladaptive end and have a variety of problems with relatedness. These often upset their relationships in the family, on the job, and in the social arena.

Development Through the Life Cycle

Infancy. From birth until 3 months the infant does not perceive physical separation between self and the mothering person. Although physical differentiation occurs at about 3 months, psychological differentiation does not begin until 18 months. This period between 3 and 18 months is the symbiotic stage of development.[20] The infant is completely dependent on others. Trust develops as needs are met consistently and predictably. The infant experiences the environment as unconditionally loving, nurturing, and accepting. Feelings of near omnipotence and positive self-worth result from the infant's complete dependence on an environment that is good and loving. This creates a capacity for empathic understanding in future interpersonal relationships.[8]

Preschool Years. Masterson[20] calls the period between 18 months and 3 years of age the separation-individuation stage. Separation defines and includes all the experiences, events, and developmental achievements that promote self-differentiation and a sense of being separate and unique. Individuation refers to the evolution of the child's internal psychological structure and growing sense of separateness, wholeness, and capability.[26] The toddler ventures away from the mothering person to explore the environment. During this phase, a sense of object constancy develops. This means that the child knows that a valued person or object continues to exist when it cannot be directly perceived. Games such as peek-a-boo teach object constancy. At the beginning of the separation-individuation process, the child seeks the parents' reassurance, support, and encouragement. If the response to autonomous behavior is positive and reinforcing, there is a foundation for building a solid sense of self and future relationships characterized by interdependence, commitment, and a capacity for interpersonal growth.

Childhood. Studies suggest that the internal development of morality and empathic feelings occur between the ages of 6 and 10 years.[25] During this period a supportive environment that encourages the budding sense of self fosters development of a positive, adaptive self-concept. Conflict occurs as adults set limits on behavior, often frustrating the child's efforts toward independence. Loving, consistent limit setting, however, communicates caring and helps the child develop interdependence. The older child adopts the parents' guidelines for behavior and a value system begins to appear. In school the child begins to learn cooperation, competition, and compromise. Peer relationships and approval of adults from outside the family, such as teachers, scout leaders, and friends' parents become important.

Preadolescence and Adolescence. By preadolescence the individual becomes involved in an intimate relationship with a friend of the same sex, a "best friend." This relationship involves sharing. It offers another chance to clarify values and recognize differences in people. This is usually a very dependent relationship. There are often active efforts to exclude others. However, as adolescence develops, the dependence on a close friend of the same sex usually yields to a dependent heterosexual relationship. While young people are involved in these dependent relationships with peers, they are asserting independence from their parents.

Friends support each other in this struggle, which often includes rebellious behavior. Parents can help the adolescent grow by consistent limit setting and a caring tolerance of rebellious outbursts. Another step toward mature interdependence is taken as the person learns to balance parental demands and peer group pressures.

Young Adulthood. Adolescence ends when the person is self-sufficient and maintains interdependent relationships with parents and peers. Decision-making is independent, taking the advice and opinions of others into account. The person may marry and begin a new family unit. Occupational plans are made and a career begun. The mature person demonstrates self-awareness by balancing dependent and independent behavior. Others are allowed to be dependent or independent as appropriate. Being sensitive to and accepting the feelings and needs of oneself and others is critical to this level of mature functioning. Interpersonal relationships are characterized by mutuality.

Middle Adulthood. Parenting and adult friendships test the person's ability to foster independence in others. Some dependence on the other person must be given up to allow that person to grow. Children gradually separate from parents, and friends may move away or drift apart. The mature person must be self-reliant and find new supports. Pleasure can be found in the development of an interdependent relationship with children as they grow. Decreased dependent demands by children creates freedom that can be used for new activities.

Late Adulthood. Change continues during late adulthood. Losses occur, such as the physical changes of aging, the death of parents, loss of occupation through retirement, and later the deaths of friends and one's spouse. The need for relatedness must still be satisfied. The mature person grieves over these losses and recognizes that others can help resolve the grief. However, new possibilities arise, even with a loss. Old friends and relatives cannot be replaced, but new relationships can develop. Grandchildren may become important to the grandparent, who may delight in spending time with them that was never available for children. The aging person may also find a sense of relatedness to the culture as a whole. Life has deeper meaning in relation to the individual's perception of personal accomplishments and contributions to the welfare of society. The mature older person can accept whatever increase in dependence is necessary but also retain as much independence as possible. Even loss of physical health does not necessarily force the person to give up all independence. The ability to maintain mature relatedness throughout life enhances self-esteem.

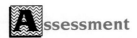

Assessment

Behaviors

The behaviors observed in maladaptive social responses represent the person's attempt to cope with anxiety related to loneliness, fear, anger, shame, guilt, and insecurity. Frequently occurring responses include manipulation, narcissism, and impulsivity.

Manipulation. People who use manipulative behaviors present a particularly difficult nursing problem. They treat others as objects, as illustrated in the following clinical example.

CLINICAL EXAMPLE

Mr. Y was a 20-year-old single man who was committed to an inpatient psychiatric unit by a judge for a psychiatric evaluation. He had been charged with sale of illicit drugs, statutory rape of his 15-year-old pregnant girlfriend, and contributing to the delinquency of a minor. He had been arrested on the grounds of a junior high school, where he was selling PCP and barbiturates to a group of young teenagers.

In jail Mr. Y had been observed to be "crazy" by the guards. He paced his cell, chanted, and threw his food on the floor. Because of this behavior, the judge agreed to order a psychiatric evaluation. On arrival at the psychiatric unit Mr. Y continued to behave in the same manner. However, his behavior did not seem typical of psychosis. There was no evidence of hallucinations or disorders of thought or affect. When unaware that he was observed, Mr. Y seemed relaxed and was noted at one time to be talking with another patient. By the day after admission he seemed to be free of his symptoms. At this point the staff began to describe him as a "nice guy." He complimented female staff members and behaved toward them in a pleasantly seductive manner. He was respectful to the physicians and agreed to abide by all the rules. He was helpful with other patients. In group meetings he admitted that he had behaved badly in the past and described how he had been led astray by his friends. He said he became involved in drugs because he wanted to be "one of the gang" and he needed money so he "had to" start selling drugs. By the end of his first week in the hospital he had received the sympathy of all the other patients and the staff.

Nine days after admission, following visiting hours, it was noted that Mr. Y and two other patients looked lethargic. Their speech was slurred, and their gaits ataxic. The nursing staff immediately collected urine and blood specimens for toxicological analysis. The unit was searched for hidden drugs, but none were found. The results of the toxicology screening tests were positive for barbiturates. Suspicion was immediately focused on Mr. Y, since the other patients involved were young adolescents with no history of drug abuse. When confronted, Mr. Y seemed amazed that he could be suspected and pointed out his past behavior as a model patient. He admitted that he had behaved strangely and wondered if someone had "slipped" him some drugs. He was convincing but was warned that if he was involved in any way with drugs, he would be sent directly back to jail.

Mr. Y began to pressure the physicians for their decision on his ability to be held responsible for his actions. He seemed to be actively engaged in therapy and promised to continue with outpatient treatment if recommended for probation. He also convinced his family of his good intentions, and they agreed to allow him to move into their house. On the basis of these indications of positive behavioral change, Mr. Y did receive a recommendation for probation, which was carried out by the judge.

Three months after discharge from the hospital, Mr. Y and a friend were arrested for operating a PCP-manufacturing laboratory in a friend's garage.

Selected Nursing Diagnoses:
▼ Impaired social interaction related to need for control as evidenced by illegal behavior and treating people like objects
▼ Defensive coping related to inability to identify relationship problems as evidenced by manipulation of others

There is usually little motivation to change because manipulative behavior often has rewards for the person, facilitating the accomplishment of a desired goal. The manipulator is goal-oriented or self-oriented, not other-oriented. However, this person is skilled at giving the impression of involvement with others. In this clinical example Mr. Y was able to gain the confidence of the staff. He knew he needed to do this to have support in court. This is typical of a person with the medical diagnosis of antisocial personality disorder.

The manipulative person is unaware of a lack of relatedness and assumes that all interpersonal relationships are formed to take advantage of others. This person cannot imagine an intimate, sharing relationship. The manipulator believes in maintaining control at all times to avoid being controlled. Shostrom[30] sees this issue of controlling or being controlled as central to manipulative behavior. He notes that manipulative behavior can also be positive, if it is used for positive purposes.

Patients with the medical diagnosis of borderline personality disorder are often manipulative. Borderline patients are believed to be manipulative because of a problem in psychosocial development. This results in their inability to participate in mature interpersonal relationships. This is illustrated in the next clinical example.

 CLINICAL EXAMPLE

Ms. S is a 23-year-old woman who was admitted to a general hospital psychiatric unit. She had lacerated her wrists superficially three times during the week before admission. Each time she cut herself, she had telephoned her therapist, a psychiatric clinical nurse specialist. Because her therapist was about to leave for vacation and she was concerned about the safety of Ms. S, the nurse decided to hospitalize her.

On admission Ms. S appeared mildly depressed. She gave the impression of a guilty child who had been punished. She denied any current self-destructive thoughts. During the physical assessment, the nurse noted that there were many scars on the patient's body. When asked about these, she claimed she was abused as a child. Her therapist's records described the scars as the result of much self-mutilation since the age of 16. This had been her main reason for seeking therapy. There was also a history of sexual promiscuity.

Ms. S described herself as a failure, stating that she had "the best parents in the world, but they did not get the daughter they deserve." She said she was a drifter who had never been able to settle on a career, a lifestyle, or any consistent friends. She didn't know who or what she was. When asked how she felt, she responded, "Most of the time, I don't feel anything, just empty." She had no signs of psychosis.

Ms. S was placed on constant observation to prevent further cutting. All sharp objects were removed from her room. At first she was very cooperative and superficially friendly to other patients. Because of her smooth adjustment, constant observation was discontinued after 3 days. She was also given a schedule of activities and informed that she was responsible for following it. The next day, an X-Acto knife was missing from the activities therapy room. Ms. S was found in the bathroom, bleeding from several small cuts on her ankles. This sequence was repeated several times. Each time the constant observation was discontinued, she would find a sharp object and cut herself.

She was also very labile emotionally. She had unpredictable outbursts of anger, similar to temper tantrums. However, these outbursts passed as quickly as they came, never lasting more than a few minutes. She also began to categorize the staff as "good guys and bad guys." When she was with staff members she liked, she was pleasant, complimenting them on their kind and understanding attitudes toward her. With staff she disliked, she was sullen and uncooperative, comparing them unfavorably to the others. Eventually the staff began to bicker about her care, some believing she was spoiled and others that she was neglected.

Ms. S remained in the hospital during her therapist's absence. When the therapist returned, Ms. S refused to see her. The frequency of angry outbursts increased dramatically. However, following frequent visits from her therapist, Ms. S began to request discharge. Behavioral criteria for discharge were set, including no self-mutilation and no temper tantrums. She met the criteria and was discharged back to outpatient treatment.

Selected Nursing Diagnoses:

▼ High risk for self-mutilation related to anxiety about her nurse-therapist's vacation as evidenced by lacerating her wrists

▼ Self-esteem disturbance related to unclear goals and expectations as evidenced by describing herself as a failure

▼ Impaired social interaction related to inability to tolerate close relationships as evidenced by splitting staff into "good guys" and "bad guys"

The diagnosis of borderline personality disorder is more frequently given to female patients. Some have questioned whether this is evidence of sex role stereotyping.[31,37] Gunderson[10] describes the behaviors characteristic of the borderline personality (Box 20-1).

Masterson[20] also notes the borderline person's failure to achieve object constancy during the separation-

---

Box 20-1

BEHAVIORAL CHARACTERISTICS OF BORDERLINE PERSONALITY DISORDER

▼ Interpersonal relationships are both intense and unstable.

▼ Interpersonal behavior is characterized by devaluation, manipulation, dependency, and masochism.

▼ Manipulative suicide attempts are designed to ensure rescue by significant others.

▼ An unstable sense of self leads to failure to develop a sense of object constancy and a fear of abandonment. These contribute to fear of aloneness.

▼ Negative affects, including anger, sustained psychological discomfort, and depression, reflect a basic sense of "badness."

▼ Occasional psychotic experiences are characterized by paranoia, regression, and dissociation.

▼ Impulsiveness occurs, with episodes of substance abuse and promiscuity.

▼ A history of low achievement is present.

---

individuation stage of psychosocial development. Because of this, the person relates to another as a series of disconnected parts rather than as a whole. The borderline person cannot recall the image of someone who is absent. He is not able to mourn the loss of another person. When someone fails to meet the borderline person's needs, the relationship is likely to end.

Individuals who fail to complete separation from the mother and develop autonomy in childhood often repeat this developmental crisis at adolescence. Behaviors characteristic of this phase include the following:

▼ Clinging

▼ Depression accompanied by rage and defended by acting out or neurotic behavior

▼ Detachment and withdrawal

Many of these behaviors can be seen in the preceding clinical example. Because of their inability to become involved in reciprocal interpersonal relationships and the related manipulativeness, these patients are frustrating for nursing staff. It must be remembered that their behavior is not consciously planned but is a defense against a fear of loneliness.

Narcissism. The term *narcissism* comes from the Greek myth of Narcissus, who fell in love with his own reflection in the waters of a spring and died. The flower that bears his name sprang up at the site of his death.

Many successful people are narcissistic. Acting, modeling, professional sports, and politics are usually attractive occupations to people with this personality trait. In these contexts self-centeredness is usually expected and therefore not a problem. However, problems do occur when the person never gains the status that they think they deserve or when they lose status. The frustration caused by lack or loss of recognition may be expressed as anger, depression, substance abuse, or other maladaptive behaviors.

Individuals with the medical diagnosis of narcissistic personality disorder have persistently fragile self-esteem, driving them to search constantly for praise, appreciation, and admiration. The clinical example that follows demonstrates narcissistic entitlement, which describes an egocentric attitude, envy, and rage when others are seen as either critical or not supportive.[18]

 ## CLINICAL EXAMPLE

Ms. T, the psychiatric clinical nurse specialist, was called to the emergency room to see Mr. F. He was accompanied by his wife. The nurse knew from the intake form that Mr. F was a 44-year-old man with no psychiatric history. His chief complaint was that he had gone into a "blind rage" when he had an argument with his wife earlier in the evening and he had punched her in the arm.

He was frightened by his loss of control and said that he felt like a failure. Both Mr. and Ms. F denied any history of violence, although Mr. F said that his first marriage ended "because of my anger."

Mr. F appeared quite anxious; he was tapping his foot and wringing his hands, and he avoided eye contact with Ms. T. After a short time, however, he became more verbal, and he willingly explained what had led to the "blow up." He had been self-employed for the past 10 years and had been "highly successful," expanding his company nationally. He told Ms. T that his father was a "multimillionaire" and that he had been on his way to exceeding his father's wealth. It seemed important to impress Ms. T by dropping the names of well-known people whom he described as his friends.

Ms. F angrily interrupted him, saying "that's important to you—who you know and how it looks." Ms. F then explained that business began slipping 2 years ago. Despite several profitable years, he had never invested or saved money. When sales fell, instead of cutting expenses and downsizing the company, he continued to live lavishly, making extravagant purchases. It was this situation that led to their argument. When Ms. F accused her husband of taking them to the brink of financial collapse, he went into a rage and punched her.

Ms. F began sobbing, and Mr. F seemed not to notice. He said he felt like his life was falling apart and that he must be the failure his father always said he was. He angrily referred to his "rich brother," who, in his father's eyes, was the perfect son. He became tearful, and Ms. F then turned to her husband attempting to provide support and reassurance.

Selected Nursing Diagnoses:

▼ Impaired social interaction related to need for approval by others as evidenced by attempts to impress others and inability to respond to wife's distress

▼ High risk for violence directed at others related to impulsivity as evidenced by acts engaged in during "blind rage"

▼ Altered family processes related to inconsistency between goals of husband and wife as evidenced by wife's reaction to patient's description of his problem

▼ Defensive coping related to fear of failure as evidenced by bragging and name-dropping

▼ Chronic low self-esteem related to perceived lack of caring and approval from father as evidenced by stated need to exceed his father's success and description of self as "a failure" in his father's eyes

Narcissism and impulsivity often go together. This was demonstrated in the previous clinical example, in which Mr. F's impulsiveness was shown by his extravagance, inability to establish and follow a life plan, failure to learn by experience, poor judgment, and unreliability.

The major behaviors related to maladaptive social re-

sponses are listed in Table 20-1. Individual patients frequently experience combinations of these behaviors. The nurse must be able to identify the complex behavior that any person may exhibit when confronted with high levels of stress and anxiety. In some cases a usual mode of behavior, such as manipulation, may be exaggerated or combined with a change in behavior. For instance, manipulative persons may withdraw when confronted by their manipulations and may be rejected by those they have been trying to manipulate. In other instances the behavior resulting from stress may be different from the individual's usual style of relatedness. A person who is usually outgoing may withdraw when under great stress. It is helpful to include a description of the patient's usual interpersonal relationships in the nursing assessment. This provides a baseline of behavior for that person against which the nurse measures the patient's progress.

Predisposing Factors

A variety of factors—within the individual, between the individual and significant others, and environmental—may lead to maladaptive social responses. Although much research has been done on disorders that affect interpersonal relationships, there are no specific conclusions about their causes. A combination of factors probably is involved. The nurse must recognize this and explore all relevant areas during the nursing assessment.

Developmental Factors. The capacity for relatedness results from a developmental process. Anything that interferes with that process decreases the person's ability to develop healthy interpersonal relationships. Parents who were deprived of caring as children may not know how to meet this need in their own children. Lack of attention or stimulation by the parent deprives an in-

Table 20-1   Behaviors Related to Maladaptive Social Responses

Behavior	Characteristics
Manipulation	Others are treated as objects
	Relationships center around control issues
	Person is self-oriented or goal-oriented, not other-oriented
Narcissism	Fragile self-esteem
	Constant seeking of praise and admiration
	Egocentric attitude
	Envy
	Rage when others are not supportive
Impulsivity	Inability to plan
	Inability to learn from experience
	Poor judgment
	Unreliability

fant of a sense of security. This results in failure to establish basic trust. The person may develop a suspicious attitude toward others continuing throughout life. The quality of parenting is also important. A child may be well fed and receive perfect physical care but without any communication of parental caring. A child who is treated as an object may become an adult who treats others as objects. Security may be found in material possessions rather than from caring relationships. Early experiences of maternal deprivation may also lead to depression in the child, as demonstrated in the studies of Spitz.[33]

> Describe aspects of contemporary American culture that are likely to negatively affect child-raising practices. What are the implications for mental health services? What preventive activities would be helpful?

Some people believe that borderline and narcissistic personality disorders result from a developmental arrest that occurs during the separation-individuation phase. That is, persons with these medical diagnoses experience various degrees of failure to separate and individuate from the parent. This makes it difficult to achieve awareness and acceptance of oneself as a separate, distinct individual, sometimes lasting throughout life.

Many persons with maladaptive social responses are enmeshed in a family system that obstructs further development and makes change difficult and hazardous. One family theory relates borderline and narcissistic development to the role structure of the family. It proposes that these families operate with the unspoken ground rule that independence and separation from the family imply rejection of family values. The parents often reenact their own developmental conflicts through their children, and role reversals (for example, parent as child) occur frequently.[32] Features of these families include various degrees of restrictiveness from the extrafamilial world, absence of clear-cut lines of authority, confusion of parental executive and nurturing roles, blurred generational boundaries, generations of family patterns in which individuals are labeled as good and bad, and the generational transmission of irrational forms of thinking and relating.[15]

Current thinking suggests two factors that may promote the development of antisocial behavior: (1) having an alcoholic parent and (2) being abused as a child. Children of alcoholic parents are more likely to be aggressive as a result of dysfunctional family dynamics characterized by a predominance of anger and other negative affects.[24] The nurse needs to assess the nature of family interactions, as well as gather information related to possible child abuse and alcohol abuse as part of a comprehensive data collection. Child abuse is discussed in Chapter 37 and alcoholism in Chapter 22.

Biological Factors. Growing evidence suggests that the development of the major personality disorders is determined by environmental factors that interact with biological factors such as lack of anxiety tolerance, aggressiveness, and genetic vulnerability to certain affects.[19] Twin studies of the relative effects of heredity and environment on the development of personality disorders conclude that these disorders occur on a continuum with normal personality traits.[18] Abnormal behaviors, except those related to attachment and dependency, showed a strong genetic component. There is also support for the theory that behavioral disorders occur when a person with a strong genetic predisposition experiences unusual life stress. It has also been suggested that the syndromes of minimal brain dysfunction and episodic dyscontrol are possible causes of borderline psychopathology and that the development of narcissistic personality disorder is influenced by hereditary factors.[21]

Genetic influences may also be significant factors in the primary bonding failure related to antisocial personalities.[2,26] Lewis et al.'s[17] study of children who later commit murder identified the prevalence of psychotic symptoms, major neurological impairment, psychotic first-degree relatives, violent acts witnessed during childhood, and severe physical abuse, thus strongly emphasizing the role of both biological and psychosocial factors in antisocial behavior. Furthermore, Grove et al.'s[9] study of monozygotic twins presents convincing evidence that antisocial behavior is heritable. Heath and Martin[13] explored environmental and genetic influences on the development of antisocial behavior. They found that genetic factors determine a general disposition to psychopathology, whereas family factors influence the development of hostility, tough-mindedness, and antisocial behaviors.

Finally, there is some evidence that a subgroup of patients with borderline personality disorder have biological abnormalities similar to those found in mood disorders.[4] This is as yet inconclusive. There is a possibility that dopaminergic function may contribute to the transient psychotic symptoms experienced by some borderline patients. Some studies have found an inverse relationship between serotonin and aggressive or suicidal behavior. These findings are suggestive of multiple biochemical disruptions related to maladaptive social responses. Further research is needed to clarify the role of the neurotransmitters in the development of personality disorders.

Sociocultural Factors. Sociocultural factors can also influence the person's ability to establish and maintain relatedness. Many forces in American culture make the individual feel isolated and lonely. Friendships are often short term because of the mobility involved in many occupations. Family relationships are more distant as adult children move away and see their parents only occasionally. Friends are often closer than siblings.

Warren[36] has developed the following criteria for social isolation:

▼ *Stigmatized environment.* The person is labeled as different, is aware of this, and is hesitant, unwilling, or does not know how to participate in social interactions.

▼ *Societal indifference.* The person experiences loneliness or lacks close, personal relationships.

▼ *Personal-societal disconnection.* Society reacts to the stigmatized person by denying access to close interpersonal relationships.

▼ *Personal powerlessness.* Society's rejection causes individuals to believe they are powerless to control their lives.

Involuntary social isolation also affects the disabled and chronically ill of any age. People with terminal illnesses or disfiguring disorders are frequently stigmatized and avoided by others. This is also true for people with long-term psychiatric problems. Although an effort has been made to decrease chronic institutionalization, many strongly resist integrating disabled people into the community. This involuntary isolation may result in a variety of maladaptive social responses as the person tries to cope with loneliness.

Immigration continues to be a reality in the United States and many other parts of the world. As people move into entirely different cultures, they may feel alienated and frightened about customs they do not understand. Sometimes immigrants form separate communities to preserve their traditions. These close-knit communities help to meet relationship needs but create barriers to broader community participation. Unfortunately, they also focus attention on the group, often attracting discriminatory behavior. Characteristics that relate to immigrant groups also apply to other cultural groups that adopt norms, behaviors, and value systems that differ from the mainstream, such as Native Americans and Orthodox Jews.

Closeness is the ideal in American culture. At the same time, people are given the message that they need to be careful in deciding whom to trust. This can cause confusion and a feeling of insecurity. Rising crime rates cause fear and reluctance to risk closeness or contact with strangers. Some urban residents, particularly the elderly, become prisoners in their homes, experiencing loneliness and the associated behaviors.

Precipitating Stressors

Maladaptive social responses are the result of experiences that influence the person's emotional growth. In most instances a series of life events predisposes a person to have interpersonal relationship problems. Many people cope with their interpersonal problems and say they are reasonably satisfied with their relationships. However, additional stress can cause a somewhat satisfying interpersonal life to become disrupted. Response to stressors is highly individual, and the nurse should remember that the person experiences an increase in anxiety as a result of the stressor. This is at the root of the behavioral disruption.

The mature person who can participate in healthy interpersonal relationships is still vulnerable to the effects of psychological stress. Either a series of losses or a single significant loss may lead to problems in establishing future intimate relationships. The pain of a loss can be so great that the person avoids future involvements rather than risk more pain. This response is more likely if the person had difficulty with developmental tasks pertinent to relatedness. Losses of significant others may cause difficulty with future relationships, but other types of losses may do the same. For example, the loss of a job decreases a person's self-esteem. This can also result in future withdrawal and problems with relatedness unless the person has a well-established interpersonal support system.

Sociocultural Stressors. Stressors leading to interpersonal relationship difficulties may be sociocultural. For instance, there can be instability in the family unit. Divorces are common. Mobility has broken up the extended family, depriving people of all ages of an important support system. Less contact occurs between the generations. Tradition, which provides a powerful link with the past and a sense of identity, is less observable when the family is fragmented. Interest in ethnicity and "roots" may reflect the efforts of isolated people to associate themselves with a specific identity. The many stresses on the family have made it more difficult for family members to accomplish the developmental tasks related to intimacy.

Nurses who work in general hospitals frequently encounter patients with maladaptive social responses. Even a reasonably well-adjusted person may have difficulty maintaining a satisfying level of intimacy while hospitalized. The patient's feeling of isolation is enhanced by the impersonal hospital environment. Sometimes patients need to be isolated because of infection, or in the psychiatric setting to control behavior. They are then susceptible to the effects of sensory deprivation. Creative nursing care is needed to lessen this problem. For instance, a patient who is in isolation for infection control could be given a schedule of times when staff will be present. This should include time to talk. Family members should be encouraged to visit, telephone, and share current activities. On the other hand, sensory overload may be a problem for patients in critical care units. This can also lead to loneliness and separation from others.

Psychological Stressors. Many psychological theories have been proposed to explain problems in establishing and maintaining satisfying relationships. It is known that high anxiety levels result in impaired ability to relate to others. A combination of prolonged or intense anxiety with limited coping ability is believed to cause severe relationship problems.

It has been suggested that the person with borderline personality disorder is likely to experience an incapacitating level of anxiety in response to life events that represent increased autonomy and separation, (e.g., high school or college graduation, going away to camp, marriage, birth of a child, employment, job promotion). The person who has narcissistic personality disorder tends to experience high anxiety, causing relationship difficulties, when the significant other no longer adequately nourishes the person's fragile self-esteem. These relationships often move through predictable stages:

▼ Idealization and overvaluation →
▼ Disappointment when unrealistic needs for maintaining self-esteem are not met →
▼ Rationalization and devaluation →
▼ Rejection of the other person based on "narcissistic injury"

Typically, these people go through life repeating this pattern—on the job, in marriages, and in friendships.

Coping Resources

When a person is having problems with interpersonal relationships, it is important for the nurse to assess the person's coping resources. For many people, when one relationship is troublesome or lost, others are available to offer support and reassurance. Those who have broad networks of family and friends have many resources to draw upon when they need assistance. Sometimes they need encouragement to reach out for help.

Some people do not have readily available human supports but have other ways of managing interpersonal problems. Pets can be an important way of expressing relatedness. Isolated elderly people often focus their need to give and receive affection on a dog or cat. Sometimes a person who is troubled about a relationship will use creative ways to express feelings. Use of expressive media such as art, music, or writing allows the individual to explore and resolve an upsetting experience.

Others are helped by reading, looking at art, dancing, or listening to music.

 Identify a novel, a popular song, or a work of art that would have meaning for a person who is trying to cope with an interpersonal loss.

Coping Mechanisms

Behaviors associated with maladaptive social responses are attempts to cope with anxiety related to threatened or actual loneliness. However, they are not healthy and sometimes have the unintended effect of driving people farther away. Thus the person is always caught in the approach-avoidance conflict of the need-fear dilemma, searching for some degree of human contact on the one hand and pushing people away on the other.

Manipulative people view other people as objects. Their defenses protect them from potential psychological pain related to the loss of a significant other. Reid[25] has described the defenses used by the individual with antisocial personality disorder as projection and splitting. ***Projection*** places responsibility for antisocial behavior outside of oneself. For instance, a patient may rationalize using drugs by saying, "Everybody I know uses cocaine. Why shouldn't I?" ***Splitting*** is characteristic of individuals with borderline and narcissistic personality disorders as well. Gunderson[10] defines splitting as the inability to integrate the good and bad aspects of oneself and of objects. An object is anything outside of the self, animate or inanimate, to which the person has an attachment. An object could be a parent, a friend, or a teddy bear. Characteristics of splitting include the following:

▼ Alternately expressing opposite sides of a conflict while appearing unconcerned about the contradiction
▼ Inconsistent lack of impulse control with periodic expression of primitive impulses and no concurrent anxiety
▼ Dividing perceptions of objects (people and things) into "all good" and "all bad"
▼ Fluctuation between "all good" and "all bad" perceptions

Masterson[20] adds several other defense mechanisms characteristic of individuals with borderline personality disorder. These include acting out, reaction formation, obsessive-compulsive mechanisms, projection, isolation, detachment, and withdrawal of affect. Danziger[5] has identified another set of coping mechanisms related to the borderline personality. In addition to splitting, she includes the following:

▼ Denial of responsibility for acting out behavior and denial of painful or threatening feelings
▼ Devaluation of another, which makes the borderline person appear good by contrast
▼ Idealization of positive traits of others, which when combined with identification, results in good feelings
▼ Projective identification, in which the borderline person projects various parts of oneself onto different individuals.

Projective identification is a complex defense mechanism that deserves further explanation. When the borderline patient projects parts of oneself onto others, these people are often not consciously aware of this. However, they may begin to behave like the projected parts. For example, a patient projects onto a nurse cruel, punishing parts of oneself. The projection reverberates with something in the nurse that had been submerged, and the nurse will tend to react to the patient in a cruel, punishing manner. Likewise, staff who have received idealized projected parts of the patient will tend to respond in an overly involved, protective, indulgent manner.[15] An example of projective identification is demonstrated by Ms. T in the following clinical example.

 ## CLINICAL EXAMPLE

A nurse, Ms. M, was describing her relationship with a borderline patient, Ms. T, who had been on the unit for approximately 2 weeks. She explained that Ms. T had become negativistic and increasingly demanding to the point that her demands had no bounds. For the past week Ms. T had been referring to Ms. M as "Nurse Ratchett." If that was not difficult enough, Ms. T was also telling new patients on the unit about what a tyrant Ms. M was. Further inquiry made it clear that soon after Ms. T had cast Ms. M into "Nurse Ratchett's" role, she started to react to the patient far more rigidly than was typical for her. Indeed, most of her interactions with Ms. T were now focused on policy adherence and strict limit setting. Although outside of her awareness, Ms. M was on her way to repeating a script straight out of the movie, *One Flew Over the Cuckoo's Nest.*

Selected Nursing Diagnosis:
▼ Self-esteem disturbance related to use of the defense mechanism of splitting as evidenced by need to belittle the nurse

Finally, the defense mechanisms of splitting and projective identification help explain why different staff members often see the same patient in very different ways, as illustrated in Fig. 20-3.

 Compare the processes of empathic understanding and projective identification.

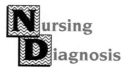 # Nursing Diagnosis

When diagnosing maladaptive social responses, the nurse should consider the extent and nature of maladaptive behaviors, coping mechanisms, and the predisposing factors and precipitating stressors leading to the behaviors. The nursing diagnoses should be thorough and reflect in-depth understanding of the patient's life situation. The nurse may formulate a nursing diagnosis by using the stress adaptation model developed by Stuart (Fig. 20-4) as a guide. When usual adaptive mechanisms fail, the patient exhibits symptomatic behaviors. Nursing diagnoses associated with maladaptive social responses and related medical diagnoses are presented in the Medical and Nursing Diagnoses box on p. 530. Primary NANDA diagnoses and examples of complete nursing diagnoses are presented in the Detailed Diagnoses box on pp. 531 and 532.

Related Medical Diagnoses

Medical diagnoses related to maladaptive social responses are categorized as personality disorders. Personality disorders are defined as "mental disorders in which personality traits are inflexible and maladaptive and cause either significant impairment in social or occupational functioning, or cause subjective distress."[14] Personality is composed of temperament, which is inherited, and character, which is learned.

In general the distinguishing characteristics of the personality disorders are that they are:
▼ Chronic and long-standing
▼ Not based on a sound personality structure
▼ Difficult to change
The borderline, antisocial, and narcissistic personality disorders are described in the Detailed Diagnoses box.

 Describe one of your own personality traits that is due to temperament and one that is due to character.

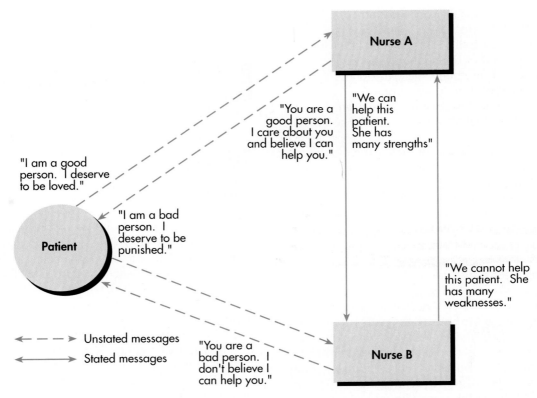

Fig. 20-3   Projective identification and splitting affects patient-to-nurse and nurse-to-nurse communication.

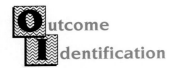

Outcome Identification

The expected outcome for nursing care of the patient with maladaptive social responses is:

The patient will obtain maximum interpersonal satisfaction by establishing and maintaining self-enhancing relationships with others.

Short-term goals are more specific to the individual's problems. They may progress from simpler to more complex changes in behavior.

It can be difficult to set mutual nursing care goals with a patient who has problems with relatedness. This is partly because mutuality must be based on a strong nurse-patient relationship. It is difficult to develop a strong relationship with a patient who fears intimacy. In addition, setting a goal implies a commitment to change. Many patients who have maladaptive social responses are reluctant to commit themselves to change. Since most of these behavioral problems also serve as

coping mechanisms, there is additional resistance to change.

For these reasons, even though it is desirable to have the patient's full participation, it may be necessary for the nurse to set initial goals. To overcome a problem with relatedness, the person must be involved with others. At first, the other person may be the nurse, but eventually others will take the nurse's place.

Short-term goals with these patients may focus on reducing acting-out behaviors and modifying specific communication patterns. Examples include the following:

▼ The patient will use verbal communication as an alternative to acting-out.

▼ The patient will verbally identify angry feelings when they occur during a one-to-one interaction.

These goals need to be developed with the patient's active participation.

Learning to relate more directly and openly causes anxiety. Therefore the patient's ability to tolerate anxiety must be considered when setting goals. Increasing the anxiety level before the patient has increased coping ability and environmental supports may reinforce use of maladaptive coping behaviors.

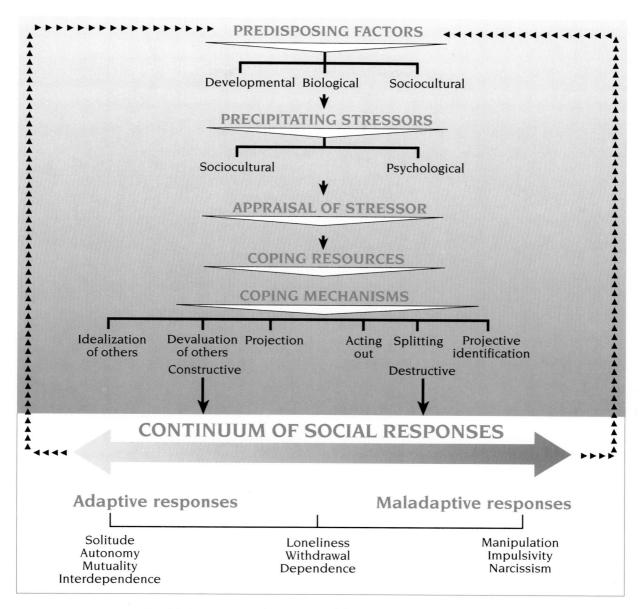

PREDISPOSING FACTORS

Developmental Biological   Sociocultural

PRECIPITATING STRESSORS

Sociocultural   Psychological

APPRAISAL OF STRESSOR

COPING RESOURCES

COPING MECHANISMS

| Idealization of others | Devaluation of others | Projection | Acting out | Splitting | Projective identification |

Constructive   Destructive

CONTINUUM OF SOCIAL RESPONSES

Adaptive responses   Maladaptive responses

Solitude	Loneliness	Manipulation
Autonomy	Withdrawal	Impulsivity
Mutuality	Dependence	Narcissism
Interdependence		

Fig. 20-4   A stress adaptation model related to social responses.

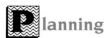lanning

The nursing care plan provides a guide for intervention and promotes consistency among the various nursing staff members who provide care to the patient. This is particularly important when working with patients with maladaptive social responses. Planning also includes attending to the patient's educational needs. A Patient Education Plan for modifying impulsive behavior is presented on p. 533. However, it is the nurse's responsibility to assist patients and their families to understand the nature and treatment of any of the disorders that cause maladaptive social responses.

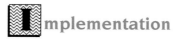mplementation

Establishing a Therapeutic Relationship

No matter what type of maladaptive social response the patient is experiencing, nursing care is based on accessibility. The nurse must be physically present with the

MEDICAL AND NURSING DIAGNOSES RELATED TO MALADAPTIVE SOCIAL RESPONSES

Related Medical Diagnoses (DSM-IV)*

Antisocial personality disorder
Borderline personality disorder
Narcissistic personality disorder

Related Nursing Diagnoses (NANDA)†

Adjustment, impaired
Anxiety
Coping, ineffective family
Coping, ineffective individual
Family processes, altered
‡**Personal identity disturbance**
Role performance, altered
‡**Self-esteem disturbance**
‡**Self-mutilation, high risk for**
‡**Social interaction, impaired**
Social isolation
Thought processes, altered
‡**Violence, high risk for:**
  Self-directed
  Directed at others

*From American Psychiatric Association: *Diagnostic and statistical manual of mental disorders,* ed 4, 1994, The Association.
†From North American Nursing Diagnosis Association: NANDA *nursing diagnoses: definitions and classifications* 1992-1993, Philadelphia, 1992, The Association.
‡Primary nursing diagnosis for maladaptive social responses.

patient regularly so that there is an opportunity for interaction. There must also be psychological accessibility. This means that the nurse shows interest in the patient. The nurse tries to understand the patient by clarifying meanings and validating perceptions. The nurse is also empathic. If the nurse-patient relationship is a healthy one, the patient can learn how to find satisfaction in other human relationships (see A Patient Speaks on p. 530).

Family Involvement

Since intimate relationships are always affected by maladaptive social responses, significant others must be involved in the plan of care (see A Family Speaks on p. 534). This is especially important for manipulative patients who often shift attention away from themselves by creating conflict between the family and the staff. For instance, the patient may complain to family members about poor nursing care. At the same time the patient may be telling the staff about mistreatment by the family. Staff and family are then in conflict. Attention is distracted from the patient, who avoids the discomfort of self-examination. When the staff finally realizes what is happening, the result is usually anger at the patient. Nurses should be aware of this tendency and avoid a punitive response. When manipulative patients are hospitalized, this behavior occurs many times. The patient returns home, still relating to others as objects.

 How would you assist family members to participate in the treatment of a person with a personality disorder?

Milieu Therapy

Because it is difficult and takes a long time to change maladaptive social responses, most patients are treated in the community. However, sometimes hospitalization is needed. For instance, the person with a borderline personality disorder may be self-destructive, or the antisocial person may require a structured environment with limit setting.

The milieu can very effectively provide patients with an opportunity to gain insight into their behavior. Aside from staff limit setting, patients with maladaptive social responses learn from other patients about how much acting-out will be tolerated. The patient responds well to a therapeutic milieu in which mature, responsible behavior is expected. Milieu work with these patients is most effective if it focuses on the following:

▼ Realistic expectations
▼ The process of decision making
▼ The process of interactional behaviors and the here and now

DETAILED DIAGNOSES
RELATED TO MALADAPTIVE SOCIAL RESPONSES

NANDA Diagnosis Stem	**Examples of Complete Diagnosis**
Personal identity disturbance	Personal identity disturbance related to early developmental arrest as evidenced by difficulty defining self boundaries
Self-esteem disturbance	Self-esteem disturbance related to physical abuse during childhood as evidenced by verbalized unhappiness with personal accomplishments
High risk for self-mutilation	High risk for self-mutilation related to fear of rejection as evidenced by cutting self following visits from parents
Impaired social interaction	Impaired social interaction related to rejection of sociocultural values as evidenced by stated belief that rules do not pertain to self
High risk for violence: self-directed	High risk for self-directed violence related to need to punish self as evidenced by repeated burning of hands and feet when criticized
High risk for violence: directed at others	High risk for violence directed at others related to use of projection as evidenced by blaming, argumentativeness, and recent purchase of a handgun

DSM-IV Diagnosis	**Essential Features***
Borderline personality disorder	Unstable mood, interpersonal relationships, and self-image and marked impulsivity beginning by early adulthood and present in various contexts. Indicated by five or more of the following characteristic behaviors: frantic efforts to avoid real or imagined abandonment; unstable relationships characterized by alternating idealization and devaluation; identity disturbance with unstable self-image or sense of self; impulsivity in at least two areas that are self-damaging; labile affect due to marked reactivity of mood; chronic feelings of emptiness; problems expressing anger appropriately; recurrent suicidal or self-mutilating behavior; and transient, stress-related paranoid ideation or severe dissociative symptoms
Antisocial personality disorder	Current age at least 18 years old and evidence of conduct disorder with onset before age 15. A pervasive pattern of disregard for and violation of the rights of others occurring since age 15, indicated by three or more of the following characteristic behaviors: irresponsibility indicated by a poor work record or failure to meet financial obligations; disregard for social norms indicated by repeated arrests; aggressiveness indicated by repeated fights or assaults; financial irresponsibility, impulsivity, or failure to plan ahead; deceitfulness, indicated by lying, use of aliases or conning others; recklessness; lacks remorse for harmful behavior indicated by indifference or rationalization of behavior

Adapted from the American Psychiatric Association: *Diagnostic and Statistical manual of mental disorders*, ed 4, Washington, DC, 1994, The Association.

Continued.

<table>
<tr><td colspan="2" style="text-align:center">DETAILED DIAGNOSES
RELATED TO MALADAPTIVE SOCIAL RESPONSES—cont'd</td></tr>
<tr><td>DSM-IV Diagnosis—cont'd</td><td>Essential Features—cont'd</td></tr>
<tr><td>Narcissistic personality disorder</td><td>A pervasive pattern of grandiosity, lack of empathy, and need for admiration, beginning by early adulthood, as indicated by at least five of the following: a grandiose sense of self-importance; belief that oneself is "special" and unique and should relate only to other special or high-status people; arrogant, haughty behaviors or attitudes; exploitation of others; inability to recognize or identify with feelings of others; sense of entitlement; envy; preoccupation with grandiose fantasies; and need for excessive admiration</td></tr>
</table>

Kernberg and Haran[16] recommend the following nursing roles in caring for the hospitalized borderline patient:

▼ Provide a structured environment
▼ Serve as an emotional sounding board
▼ Clarify and diagnose conflicts

Consistent clinical supervision is also very important, since countertransference is usually an issue when caring for these patients (see Chapter 2). Positive countertransference by some staff members, and negative by others, leads to splitting and staff conflict. Whenever these behavioral patterns emerge while there is a manipulative patient on the psychiatric unit, the staff must examine their level of involvement with the patient.[23]

Reid[25] addresses countertransference issues related to the antisocial patient. Countertransference feelings may include impulses to rescue, support, hurt, admire, identify with, or accept compliments from the patient. The principles of milieu treatment for antisocial patients include the following[25]:

▼ Establish control with no option to escape involvement
▼ Provide an experienced, consistent staff
▼ Implement a strict hierarchical structure with rules that are firm, not necessarily fair, and rigidly interpreted
▼ Provide support while the patient learns to experience painful feelings

Limit Setting and Structure

The way the nurse approaches limit setting can make the difference between a productive hospital experience and one that is either nonproductive or counterproductive. Angry, punitive limit setting confirms the patient's expectations. Suppressive and rigid limits create obstacles to self-exploration and therapeutic change. This approach also confirms the patient's belief of having little

or no control over life situations. It is essential that the nurse not view limits as a way of controlling the patient.

For example, a patient with antisocial personality structure engages in physically aggressive acting-out behavior. One way of dealing with this might be to emphasize the need for medications and to tighten up restrictions. The treatment team might also issue an ultimatum, such as "One more similar episode, and we're going to have to transfer you to another hospital." A more positive way of approaching the situation could be: "I can't understand why you're putting the team in the position of having to reassess continuation of your stay in this hospital. Has there been some change about wanting to help yourself?" The difference in the latter approach is emphasis on the idea that the patient has responsibility for life situations; the control and the decisions are the patient's. It also communicates an attitude of respect, which could be a boost to the patient's self-esteem. The more the nurse is able to align with the nonregressed aspects of the patient's ego, the better are the chances for improved functioning.

Manipulative patients must also be held responsible for their behavior. They are skilled at placing responsibility on others. Staff members must communicate with each other so that consistent messages are given. These patients recognize any inconsistency and use it to focus attention on others. They usually resist rules. Staff and family members must collaborate in enforcing clear limits. Manipulative patients sometimes lie. It is important to confront the patient who consciously lies.

Masterson[20] describes guidelines for treating borderline patients that incorporate several of these principles. He emphasizes the need for availability of staff attention combined with structured discipline. There must be an expectation that the patient will meet standards of healthy behavior. Failure to meet the standard is identified, and acting-out is confronted. Loss of control may be dealt with by room restriction, with the patient in-

PATIENT EDUCATION PLAN
MODIFYING IMPULSIVE BEHAVIOR

Content	Instructional activities	Evaluation
Describe characteristics and consequences of impulsive behavior.	Select a situation in which impulsive behavior occurred. Ask the patient to describe what happened.	The patient will identify and describe an impulsive incident.
	Provide the patient with paper and a pen.	The patient will maintain a diary of impulsive behaviors.
	Instruct the patient to keep a diary of impulsive actions, including a description of events before and after the incident.	The patient will explore the causes and consequences of impulsive behavior.
Describe behaviors characteristic of interpersonal anxiety and relate anxiety to impulsive behavior.	Discuss the diary with the patient. Assist the patient to identify interpersonal anxiety related to impulsive behavior.	The patient will connect feelings of interpersonal anxiety with impulsive behavior.
Explain stress-reduction techniques.	Describe the stress response. Demonstrate relaxation exercises (see Chapter 28). Assist the patient to return the demonstration.	The patient will perform relaxation exercises when signs of anxiety appear.
Identify alternative responses to anxiety-producing situations.	Using situations from the diary and knowledge of relaxation exercises, assist the patient to list possible alternative responses.	The patient will identify at least two alternative responses to each anxiety-producing situation.
Practice using alternative responses to anxiety-producing situations.	Role-play each of the identified alternative behaviors. Discuss the feelings associated with impulsive behavior and the alternatives.	The patient will describe the relationship between behavior and feelings. The patient will select and perform anxiety-reducing behaviors.

A PATIENT SPEAKS

When I was hospitalized, the nurses were my link with the outside world. They were with me more than anyone else. They were also my link to the treatment that was prescribed by my psychiatrist. The doctor left prn orders because he thought I was a mature woman who could decide when I needed medication. I often felt a loss of dignity when the nurse questioned my need for the prn medication. Since the medicine decreased my anxiety, I think I was the best judge of when I needed it. Since the doctor made me responsible for requesting the medication, it was not the nurse's job to question my need for it unless I asked for more than was prescribed. Even if someone is in the hospital, they need to be treated with dignity and respect. They are sick, not children and not stupid. Nothing hurts more than being treated like a second-class citizen by people who are in a more powerful position. It is much easier to work with a nurse who is kind and supportive. ▼

structed to think about the episode so that it may be discussed in therapy. The length of the restriction should be based on the seriousness of the behavior. These approaches may lead to depression. The depressed feelings should be directed into formal psychotherapy sessions, but the staff can act as role models for appropriate behavior. A school program, occupational therapy, and the milieu may be used to teach age-appropriate social and achievement skills. Reality orientation may also be necessary.

You believe that a manipulative adolescent patient is exploiting another patient by "borrowing" money, clothing, and snacks. When confronted, the first patient claims that the items were gifts, "because we're friends." Do you think that limit setting is needed? If so, how would you set appropriate limits?

A FAMILY SPEAKS

It seems like my brother was always a problem. When we were growing up, he got us both into trouble all the time. Finally I learned to ignore his schemes and stay away from him. As he got older, the situation got worse. Our parents kicked him out of the house, but he would come back and promise to change and they would let him back in. Then it would start all over again. He began to get into trouble with the law. First there was vandalism for spray-painting graffiti on a building; then he was with a gang of kids who stole a car. He said he was just along for the ride, but I didn't really believe him.

The rest of the family was pretty embarrassed about his behavior. I thought about telling people I was adopted so they wouldn't think I was like him. I didn't do that because I knew it would hurt my parents and they had enough trouble already. I'll never forget the night when the phone rang at 4:00 AM and it was my brother saying he was in jail. He had been caught with drugs in a stolen car and had also resisted arrest. My parents refused to bail him out and he didn't have any money. The next day he called again to say that he was at the local psychiatric hospital. He had threatened to kill himself in jail, so they sent him to the hospital to see if he was really mentally ill.

My parents were really upset about this development. I think it was actually a good thing, though, because the doctors and nurses at the hospital explained to us that he has a personality disorder. It did help to know that there might be a reason for his behavior, although he hasn't really changed much. I think my parents are beginning to accept this, but I know it's really hard for them. ▼

Protection from Self-Harm

The deliberate self-destructive or self-mutilating behavior of the borderline patient is very difficult to treat (see Chapter 18). Often the nursing staff must observe the patient constantly to prevent serious physical harm. At the same time these patients have intense dependency needs related to an unresolved separation-individuation developmental phase. This makes it extremely difficult to wean them from constant staff attention, and contact must be decreased very gradually. Observation may need to be increased again if the patient seems out of control. Patient involvement in planning for decreased observation may be helpful. The patient must be reassured that less contact does not equal no contact. Consistent, scheduled time with a staff member is recommended. Primary nursing is particularly effective with a patient who needs to work through

CRITICAL THINKING ABOUT CONTEMPORARY ISSUES

Should Constant Close Observation Be the Primary Nursing Approach for Borderline Patients with Impulsive Self-Harming Behavior?

Patients with borderline personality disorder are most often hospitalized because of impulsive attempts at self-mutilation or suicide. The nursing intervention of constant close observation is usually initiated to protect the patient from impulsive behavior. This intervention activates the patient's conflicts about close relationships. Splitting may become evident as the patient establishes preferences for the staff assigned to observation. The patient is challenged to outwit the staff and find opportunities to act out. When efforts are made to decrease the level of observation, the patient's attachment conflicts become evident. There is often an effort to maintain the undivided attention of staff by renewed self-harming behavior.

Gallop[6] suggests that nurses can assist these patients to assume responsibility for their behavior and find ways to change it. The nurse should enlist the patient's assistance in defining and describing the harmful behavior. Identification of behavioral cues and triggers allows the patient to request assistance, thereby becoming an active participant in the therapeutic process. Nurses are less judgmental about the patient because they understand the source of the behavior and can be sensitive to the patient's feelings. The challenge to nurses is to maintain the patient's safety while facilitating behavioral change. ▼

these separation issues (see Critical Thinking about Contemporary Issues).

Focusing on Strengths

Patients with maladaptive social responses often are effective leaders within the patient group. A useful nursing approach is to encourage them to identify and use their strengths. They may be given responsibilities within the patient care unit and can be helpful to other patients. They are often intelligent and can participate actively in planning their own care. However, they are extremely resistant to recognizing or dealing with feelings and need consistent encouragement to verbalize these emotions.

Nurses become frustrated with these patients because they seem to be so aware of what is happening and in control of most situations, yet so unaware of others' needs. Nurses must remember that these patients have little tolerance for intimacy. Their maneuvering of others is a way to keep them at a safe distance. These patients are often charming, and it is easy to become involved with them. However, as soon as other people make demands or show signs of emotional closeness, the patients dilute the relationship by withdrawing, by frustrating others, or by distracting attention from themselves.

Journal writing is a nursing intervention that can be helpful to patients who have difficulty with close relationships. Keeping a diary of their thoughts and feelings helps them identify the various aspects of their interpersonal experiences and review them over time. Sebastian[29] has found that keeping a journal helps patients develop object constancy. It gives them an opportunity to see continuity of people and relationships. The nurse can review the journal with the patient to assist in making connections among experiences. Interpersonal strengths can be identified and reinforced. The nurse can also note behavioral strengths that the patient has not yet identified and assist the patient in recognizing these as well.

Behavioral Strategies

Various behavioral strategies can help decrease antisocial behavior (see Chapter 28). The patient is usually impatient with delays in gratification. Material rather than emotional rewards are preferred. Thus reinforcers used in a behavior modification program should be concrete and readily available. For example, points may be accumulated to qualify for privileges, such as a trip to the canteen. Other reinforcers might be a visit or a favorite food. Ignoring undesirable behavior is the least reinforcing but is not always possible. If behavior is disruptive and there must be a response, it should be matter of fact and one not desired by the patient. For instance, removal from contact with others for a specific period of time may discourage undesirable behavior, whereas a lecture that attracts attention may be a reinforcer.

Behavioral contracting has been tried with borderline patients. Miller[22] describes the contract as a mutually negotiated agreement that is explicit and that specifies the responsibilities of both parties. She describes the advantages of behavioral contracting as:

▼ Emphasizing the need for the patient's active collaboration in treatment
▼ Decreasing vulnerability to regression
▼ Reducing anxiety about medicolegal issues
▼ Assisting the treatment team in identifying countertransference feelings and splitting more quickly

▼ Countering an unrealistic sense of timeliness by establishing a prearranged discharge date

When a contract is negotiated, control is shared between the nurse and the patient. The nurse-patient contract is based on patient-identified strengths, learning needs, and goals. However, the patient must agree to basic expectations. These usually include agreement to refrain from harmful behavior, as well as defining the length of time that the contract will be in effect.

A Nursing Care Plan Summary for the patient with maladaptive social responses is presented on p. 536.

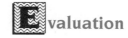 **valuation**

Evaluating the success of nursing intervention is difficult when the focus is on the quality of the therapeutic relationship. Since the relationship is central to effective delivery of nursing care, it is threatening for many nurses to examine their ability to relate to others. This type of evaluation must take place on two levels. One level focuses on the nurse and the nurse's participation in the relationship. Self-examination may be useful in accomplishing this, especially if the nurse reviews an interaction immediately. Blind spots about one's own feelings that may be present while involved with the patient may become clearer in retrospect. However, self-evaluation is colored by self-perceptions. Supervision from an experienced nurse therapist can be very helpful in identifying aspects of the relationship that may be less obvious to the nurse. Constructive supervision can help nurses identify the dynamics of the relationship. It can also help them deal with patients' resistance to change. No matter how experienced, nurses' perceptions of their participation in a relationship are affected by their self-concept. The need for supervision continues throughout their career.

The second level of evaluation focuses on the patient's behavior and the behavioral changes that the nurse works to facilitate. The patient is the primary source of input about these changes. Perceived changes in behavior should be validated with the patient to see if the patient is also aware of change. Sharing feelings and intimate thoughts denotes increased trust and a willingness to risk self-revelation. Nonverbally the patient also reveals responses to the therapeutic relationship. Accessibility to the nurse for scheduled meetings indicates trust and involvement in the relationship. Eye contact usually occurs more often when one person is comfortable with another. Initiation of activities with others indicates more openness to relatedness. Increased decision making and assumption of leadership roles imply improved self-esteem and increasing self-

NURSING CARE PLAN SUMMARY
Maladaptive Social Responses

Nursing Diagnosis: Impaired social interaction

Expected Outcome: The patient will obtain maximum interpersonal satisfaction by establishing and maintaining self-enhancing relationships with others.

Short-term Goals	Interventions	Rationale
The patient will participate in a therapeutic nurse-patient relationship.	Initiate a nurse-patient relationship contract mutually agreed on by patient and nurse Develop mutual behavioral goals Maintain consistent behavior by all nursing staff Communicate honest responses to the patient's behavior Provide honest, immediate feedback about behavioral change Maintain confidentiality Demonstrate accessibility	An atmosphere of trust facilitates open expression of thoughts and feelings A trusting relationship enables the patient to risk sharing feelings Honest responses reinforce openness Staff consistency creates a predictable environment that creates trust
The patient will describe interpersonal strengths and weaknesses	Provide opportunities to demonstrate strengths, e.g., helping other patients, assuming leadership roles Assist to analyze experiences that are perceived as failures Communicate acceptance of the patient as a person while not accepting maladaptive social behavior	Patients with maladaptive social responses are unable to identify accurately their interpersonal strengths and weaknesses, leading to fear of closeness and fear of failure. It is important to assist the patient to separate behavioral incidents from total self-worth and recognize that one can be liked even if imperfect.
The patient will establish or reestablish one interpersonal relationship that is mutually satisfying and adaptive.	Provide consistent feedback about adaptive and maladaptive social behavior Encourage patient to describe successful and unsuccessful relationship experiences orally or in a written journal Assist patient in initiating or resuming a relationship with one other person Review aspects of this relationship with the patient Reinforce the patient's adaptive social responses Evaluate with the patient alternatives to maladaptive social responses	Describing and evaluating one's behavior requires taking responsibility for the behavior and its consequences Patients need to go beyond understanding or insight to engaging in actual behavioral change It is important for the nurse to help the patient evaluate whether one's responses are adaptive or maladaptive Alternatives can then be identified to further the patient's goal achievement

Nursing Diagnosis: High risk for self-mutilation

Expected Outcome: The patient will select constructive rather than self-destructive ways of coping with interpersonal anxiety.

Short-term Goals	Interventions	Rationale
The patient will not engage in self-mutilation.	Develop a contract with the patient to notify staff when anxiety is increasing Provide close 1:1 observation of the patient when necessary to maintain safety Remove all potentially dangerous objects from the patient and the environment Provide prescribed medications	When the patient is not able to cope with anxiety, protection of safety is the nurse's highest priority A contract helps the patient assume responsibility and explore healthier coping responses

NURSING CARE PLAN SUMMARY—cont'd
Maladaptive Social Responses

Nursing Diagnosis: High risk for self-mutilation

Expected Outcome: The patient will select constructive rather than self-destructive ways of coping with interpersonal anxiety.

Short-term Goals	Interventions	Rationale
The patient will describe self-mutilating episodes.	Assist the patient in reviewing these events Identify cues and triggers that precede self-mutilating behavior Help the patient explore feelings related to these episodes	Self-mutilation is often a way of relieving extreme anxiety Structured interpersonal support can help the patient review these events
The patient will describe alternatives to self-mutilating behaviors.	Suggest alternative behaviors such as seeking interpersonal support or engaging in an adaptive anxiety-reducing activity	The nurse can help the patient review the full range of adaptive responses Supportive but critical evaluation is necessary for behavioral change
The patient will implement one new adaptive response when experiencing high interpersonal anxiety.	Assist the patient in selecting new adaptive responses Reinforce the patient's adaptive behavior Identify positive consequences of the adaptive responses Discuss ways these may be generalized to other situations	The nurses should taken an active role in setting limits, examining patient behaviors, and reinforcing adaptive actions These new learned responses can also be reviewed for their applicability to other life events

confidence. Such behaviors can be observed, documented, and validated with other staff members. Therefore these are useful evaluation criteria.

Significant others may also contribute to the evaluation. They have known the patient before the occurrence of any behavioral problem and can provide information about the patient's behavioral norms. They are particularly helpful in providing information about changes that continue when the patient is in the community. Some patients have difficulty transferring new behavior to their usual life settings. Involving families in this type of assessment helps to teach the family the behaviors learned by the patient. It gives them an idea of what is reasonable to expect from the patient.

Several questions may assist the nurse to evaluate the outcomes of intervention with the patient who has maladaptive social responses:

▼ Has the patient become less impulsive, manipulative, or narcissistic?

▼ Does the patient express satisfaction with the quality of interpersonal relationships?

▼ Can the patient participate in close interpersonal relationships?

▼ Does the patient verbalize recognition of positive behavioral change?

SUGGESTED CROSS-REFERENCES

Therapeutic Nurse-Patient Relationship	Chapter 2
A Stress Adaptation Model of Psychiatric Nursing Care	Chapter 4
Anxiety Responses and Anxiety Disorders	Chapter 14
Self-Concept Responses and Dissociative Disorders	Chapter 16
Self-Protective Responses and Suicidal Behavior	Chapter 18
Managing Aggressive Behavior	Chapter 27
Cognitive Behavioral Therapy	Chapter 28

SUMMARY

1. In a healthy interpersonal relationship, the individuals involved experience intimacy with each other while maintaining separate identities. Adaptive social responses include the capacity for solitude, autonomy, mutuality, and interdependence. Maladaptive responses include manipulation, narcissism, and impulsivity.

2. The behaviors associated with disruptions in relatedness include manipulation, impulsivity, and narcissism.

3. Predisposing factors for maladaptive social re-

sponses are described from developmental, biological, and sociocultural perspectives. Precipitating stressors that affect social responses include sociocultural values and norms and psychological pressures.

4. A wide array of relationships and interests provide coping resources. Coping mechanisms related to social responses may include idealization of others, devaluation of others, projection, acting-out, splitting, and projective identification.

5. Primary NANDA nursing diagnoses are personal identity disturbance, self-esteem disturbance, high risk for self-mutilation, social isolation, and high risk for violence—self-directed or directed at others.

6. Primary DSM-IV diagnoses are antisocial personality disorder, borderline personality disorder, and narcissistic personality disorder.

7. The expected outcome of nursing care is that the patient will obtain maximum interpersonal satisfaction by establishing and maintaining self-enhancing relationships with others.

8. The plan of nursing care must be realistic, considering the patient's ability to tolerate anxiety, and promote consistency of interventions.

9. Primary nursing interventions for patients with maladaptive social responses include establishing a therapeutic relationship, family involvement, milieu therapy, limit setting and structure, protection from self-harm, focusing on strengths, and behavior modification.

10. Evaluation is based on the patient's recognition of improvement of the quality and quantity of interpersonal relationships.

COMPETENT CARING
A CLINICAL EXEMPLAR OF A PSYCHIATRIC NURSE

Ernestine Cosby, BSN, RNC

I met Ms. X when she was admitted to my unit. She was 35 years of age with a diagnosis of borderline personality disorder and a history of five prior hospitalizations. Her previous hospitalizations were characterized by being in restraints for destructive behavior to herself and others, intense negative relationships with staff, and depression with a history of four suicide attempts. Ms. X had been a nun for 8 years until her self-destructive behavior became unmanageable at the convent, necessitating her first psychiatric admission. The order of nuns continued their involvement with her even when she was unable to return to the convent. They assisted with finding a teaching position for her in one of their schools.

Ms. X was the oldest of four siblings, all girls, with parents who provided "things" but not affection. She had hoped to find and fill the emptiness she felt all the time in the convent. She discovered that being a nun didn't make it "all better." On this admission she was depressed and had made a suicide attempt by overdosing on pills 2 days before admission. She was distrustful, unable to express anger, impulsive, and unable to relate to others unless angry or demanding. By the second week with us she was actively engaged in staff splitting, making requests that could not be met no matter how we tried, and cutting herself following conflict with staff. She refused to attend any groups, complaining of boredom. Predictably, the staff engaged in conflict with each other over how to deal with the patient. Since I frequently talked with her, my peers elected me to coordinate a plan to focus on the splitting, angry outbursts, and self-destructive behaviors. I was aware of two things I liked about Ms. X: one was her sense of humor and the other her ability to write. I spent the next 2 weeks meeting with her at planned times for a half hour. My goals were to establish rapport, attempt to engage her involvement, and establish some level of trust. I was anxious about the potential for creating dependency on me. But with her involvement I planned to help her branch out from me to others.

The initial plan we agreed on was an attempt to decrease the anxiety she felt related to abandonment feelings when she requested to talk with staff at the change of each shift. She denied that she requested to talk only at the change of shifts. This patient's strengths included an ability to express herself through writing. I offered several options of times when the staff had agreed that they could be with her one-on-one for 20 minutes. She selected her preferred times. We agreed that she would keep a journal of the issues, feelings, needs, or concerns to discuss with staff at the designated times. She would also write how she felt after each meeting with staff. Another nurse and I met with the patient to make a list of emergencies that would require an immediate response from the staff.

Ms. X and I met three times a week to review her contacts with the other staff. Initially this involved only complaints about the staff or how they talked to her. Eventually, she was able to explore her involvement in the interaction. Then she was able to listen to my feedback and later to ask other staff for their feedback. This process continued to provide stepping stones to engage her involvement in contracting to work on her self-destructive behavior, trying other coping skills to deal with anger, branching out to interact with patients, progressively attending groups, and recognizing her own manipulative behavior.

This process had peaks and valleys throughout. She would greet me in the morning (my worst time) at the door with a hostile and provoking interaction. She later explained the fear she experienced each day when it neared time for me to leave. She feared that I would not return, and at other times she would wish harm to me. This was reflected in her early morning behavior. The rewarding part of working with this patient was her continued attempt to carry out what she contracted to do, even though under protest most of the time. The staff and I were able to recognize her progress in the milieu, with staff and patients. This took longer for her to acknowledge, but one day she was able to write and share an interaction with staff that did not end in her losing control or cutting. She was ecstatic that she used options that she had worked out and that had resulted in a positive outcome. Since her discharge Ms. X has not required inpatient hospitalization. In outpatient therapy she has successfully continued to be actively involved in her treatment. ▼

REFERENCES

1. American Psychiatric Association: *Diagnostic and statistical manual of mental disorders*, ed 4, revised (DSM-IV), Washington, DC, 1994, The Association.
2. Cadoret RJ et al: Genetic and environmental factors in alcohol abuse and antisocial personality, *J Stud Alcohol* 48:1, 1987.
3. Caroline HA: Explorations of close friendship: a concept analysis, *Arch Psychiatr Nurs* 7:236, 1993.
4. Coccaro EF, Kavoussi RJ: Biological and pharmacological aspects of borderline personality disorder, *Hosp Community Psychiatr* 42:1029, 1991.
5. Danziger S: Major treatment issues and techniques in family therapy with the borderline adolescent, *J Psychosoc Nurs Ment Health Serv* 20:27, 1982.
6. Gallop R: Self-destructive and impulsive behavior in the patient with a borderline personality disorder: rethinking hospital treatment and management, *Arch Psychiatr Nurs* 6:178, 1992.
7. Gallop R, McCay E, Esplen MJ: The conceptualization of impulsivity for psychiatric nursing practice, *Arch Psychiatr Nurs* 6:366, 1992.
8. Gottschalk LA: Narcissism: its normal evolution and development and the treatment of its disorders, *Am J Psychotherapy* 42:4, 1988.
9. Grove WM et al: Heritability of substance abuse and antisocial behavior: a study of monozygotic twins reared apart, *Biol Psychiatry* 27:1293, 1990.
10. Gunderson JG: *Borderline personality disorder*, Washington, DC, 1984, American Psychiatric Press.
11. Hagerty BMK et al: Sense of belonging: a vital mental health concept, *Arch Psychiatr Nurs* 6:172, 1992.
12. Hagerty BMK, Lynch-Sauer J, Patusky KL, Bouwsema M: An emerging theory of human relatedness, *Image* 25:291, 1993.
13. Heath A, Martin NG: Psychoticism as a dimension of personality: a multivariate genetic test of Eysenck and Eysenck's psychoticism construct, *J Pers Soc Psychol* 58:111, 1990.
14. Hirschfeld RMA: Personality disorders: foreword. In

Frances AJ, Hales RE, eds: *Psychiatry update*, vol 5, Washington, DC, 1986, American Psychiatric Press.

15. Kaplan CA: The challenge of working with patients diagnosed as having a borderline personality disorder, *Nurs Clin North Am* 21:429, 1986.

16. Kernberg O, Haran C: Milieu treatment with borderline patients, *J Psychosoc Nurs Ment Health Serv* 22:29, 1984.

17. Lewis D et al: Biopsychosocial characteristics of children who later murder: a prospective study, *Am J Psychiatry* 142:1162, 1985.

18. Livesley WJ, Jang KL, Jackson DN, Vernon PA: Genetic and environmental contributions to dimensions of personality disorder, *Am J Psychiatr* 150:1826, 1993.

19. Livesley WJ, Schroeder ML: Dimensions of personality disorder, *J Nerv Ment Dis* 179:320, 1991.

20. Masterson JF: *Treatment of the borderline adolescent*, New York, 1985, Brunner/Mazel.

21. Meissner WW: *The borderline spectrum: differential diagnosis and developmental issues*, New York, 1984, Aronson.

22. Miller LJ: The formal treatment contract in the inpatient management of borderline personality disorder, *Hosp Community Psychiatry* 41:985, 1990.

23. Piccinino S: The nursing care challenge: borderline patients, *J Psychosoc Nurs Ment Health Serv* 28:22, 1990.

24. Pollock VE et al: Childhood antecedents of antisocial behavior: parental alcoholism and physical abusiveness, *Am J Psychiatry* 147:1290, 1990.

25. Reid WH: The antisocial personality: a review, *Hosp Community Psychiatry* 36:831, 1985.

26. Rinsley DB: A comparison of borderline and narcissistic personality disorders, *Bull Menninger Clin* 48:1, 1984.

27. Rinsley DB: Notes on the developmental pathogenesis of narcissistic personality disorder, *Psychiatr Clin North Am* 12:695, 1989.

28. Rogers C: *On becoming a person*, Boston, 1961, Houghton Mifflin.

29. Sebastian L: Promoting object constancy: writing as a nursing intervention, *J Psychosoc Nurs Ment Health Serv* 29:21, 1991.

30. Shostrom E: *Man, the manipulator*, Nashville, Tenn, 1967, Abingdon Press.

31. Simmons D: Gender issues and borderline personality disorder: why do females dominate the diagnosis? *Arch Psychiatr Nurs* 6:219, 1992.

32. Soloff P, Millward J: Developmental histories of borderline patients, *Compr Psychiatry* 22:574, 1983.

33. Spitz RA: *The first year of life: a psychoanalytic study of normal and deviant development of object relations*, New York, 1965, International Universities Press.

34. Sullivan H: *The interpersonal theory of psychiatry*, New York, 1953, WW Norton.

35. Surakic DM: Emotional features of narcissistic personality disorder, *Am J Psychiatry* 142:720, 1985.

36. Warren BJ: Explaining social isolation through concept analysis, *Arch Psychiatr Nurs* 7:270, 1993.

37. Widiger TA, Weissman MM: Epidemiology of borderline personality disorder, *Hosp Community Psychiatr* 42:1015, 1991.

ANNOTATED SUGGESTED READINGS

*Gallop R: The patient is splitting: everyone knows and nothing changes, *J Psychosoc Nurs Ment Health Serv* 23:6, 1985.

Uses a case study to illustrate the staff splitting caused by borderline patients and discusses approaches to dealing with countertransference.

Gorton G, Akhtar S: The literature on personality disorders, 1985-88: trends and controversies, *Hosp Community Psychiatry* 41:39, 1990.

Discusses problems differentiating disorders, research needs, and treatment issues. Recommended for advanced practitioners.

Gunderson JG: *Borderline personality disorder*, Washington, DC, 1984, American Psychiatric Press.

Written by a psychotherapist with extensive experience in providing therapy to borderline personality disorder patients. Invaluable description of the problem's etiology and suggestions regarding interventions.

*Kaplan CA: The challenge of working with patients diagnosed as having a borderline personality disorder, *Nurs Clin North Am* 21:429, 1986.

Explores the interplay of various treatment modalities during inpatient hospitalization of the borderline patient. Describes counterproductive staff responses and examines approaches aimed at maximizing treatment outcome.

Kernberg OF: The narcissistic personality disorder and the differential diagnosis of antisocial behavior, *Psychiatr Clin North Am* 12:553, 1989.

Describes in detail the intimate relationship between narcissistic personality disorder and antisocial personality disorder.

Miller LJ: The formal treatment contract in the inpatient management of borderline personality disorder, *Hosp Community Psychiatry* 41:985, 1990.

Examines advantages and disadvantages of behavioral contracts with borderline patients and points out several common contractual errors.

*Nehls N: Borderline personality disorder and group therapy, *Arch Psychiatr Nurs* 5:137, 1991.

Report of a nursing study in an outpatient setting of the effectiveness of group therapy for patients with borderline personality disorder.

*O'Brien P, Caldwell C, Transeau G: Destroyers: written treatment contracts can help cure self-destructive behaviors of the borderline patient, *J Psychosoc Nurs Ment Health Serv* 23:19, 1985.

Describes the application of treatment contracting to nursing intervention with borderline patients including the use of a case study.

Rinsley DB: Notes on the developmental pathogenesis of narcissistic personality disorder, *Psychiatr Clin North Am* 12:695, 1989.

Presents in-depth diagnostic and developmental considerations related to narcissistic character pathology.

*Runyon N, Allen CL, Ilnicki SH: The borderline patient on the med-surg unit, *Am J Nurs* 88:1644, 1988.

Provides a practical approach to the potentially disruptive behavior of the borderline patient in a medical-surgical setting. Includes sample interactions and a care plan.

Shea MT: Standardized approaches to individual psychotherapy of patients with borderline personality disorder, *Hosp Community Psychiatr* 42:1034, 1991.

Reviews the application of various psychotherapeutic approaches in the

*Nursing reference.

treatment of patients with borderline personality disorder, including psychoanalytic, expressive, interpersonal, behavioral, and cognitive.

*Simmons D: Gender issues and borderline personality disorder: why do females dominate the diagnosis? *Arch Psychiatr Nurs* 6:219, 1992.

Presents an interesting analysis of the interplay of gender role expectations and psychiatric diagnosis of borderline personality disorder.

*Valente SM: Deliberate self-injury: management in a psychiatric setting, *J Psychosoc Nurs Ment Health Serv* 29:19, 1991.

Applies theories of anxiety and behavior modification to develop guidelines for inpatient management of the patient who is self-injuring.

*Vogel CH et al: Exploring the concept of manipulation in psychiatric settings, *Arch Psych Nurs* 1:429, 1987.

Describes studies determining how nurses define manipulation.

---

*Nursing reference.

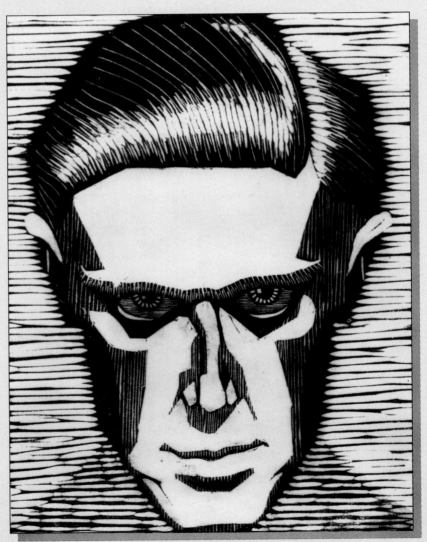

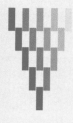

CHAPTER 21
Cognitive Responses and Organic Mental Disorders

SANDRA J. SUNDEEN

Cogito, ergo sum. I think, therefore I am.
Descartes

The ability to think and to reason is a distinguishing feature of the human being. This ability created civilization and allowed progress from the Stone Age to the Space Age. Knowledge is growing at such a rapid rate that there is an overwhelming demand for a person to assimilate new information. Society has moved from the time when power meant physical strength, to the use of money to acquire power, to an era in which power lies in information.

Intellectual functioning is highly valued. Most people fear the possibility of losing their cognitive abilities, which are reasoning, memory, judgment, orientation, perception, and attention. These functions allow the person to make sense of experience and interact productively with the environment. Maladaptive cognitive responses leave the affected person in a state of confusion, unable to understand experience and unable to relate current to past events. Memory is a key cognitive ability because to exercise judgment, make decisions, or even to be oriented to time and place, the person must remember past experiences. Therefore memory loss is a particularly frightening experience.

CONTINUUM OF COGNITIVE RESPONSES
Learning Model of Cognition

Psychology is the discipline that has historically been most involved in studying cognition as expressed through the learning process. Experimental psychologists have been interested in defining the process of learning and developing models that will explain learned behavior. Learning is a persistent change in the person's behavior related to a particular situation. It results from experience rather than instinct, reflex, or maturation. The behavioral model of learning relates behavioral change to reinforcement. When the individual experiences a **stimulus,** several behavioral **responses** are available. The person is most likely to select the response that has been **reinforced** in the past. In other words, the person has learned a particular response to a given stimulus or set of stimuli. If the response is not reinforced, an alternative behavior may be substituted. If the new behavior is reinforced, the person is more likely to continue to behave in that way. The following clinical example illustrates this process.

 CLINICAL EXAMPLE

Johnny M, age 3, asked his mother for a cookie. Ms. M told Johnny that he could have a cookie after he picked up his toys. Johnny began to kick and scream. Ms. M cuddled Johnny, gave him a cookie, and picked up the toys. When she discussed this experience with her neighbor, Ms. P, the mother of four children, Johnny's mother learned that he had a temper tantrum and that the behavior was likely to continue if she gave in to Johnny's demands. The next time Johnny demanded a cookie, Ms. M again requested that he pick up his toys first. Johnny began his temper tantrum. His mother placed him in another room and informed him again that when he picked up his toys, he could have a cookie. After a few minutes, Johnny quieted, then came out and put away his toys. His mother responded with cuddling and a cookie. Over time the temper tantrums disappeared.

By reinforcing Johnny's tantrums with cookies and cuddling, Ms. M had, in effect, taught him that his behavior was effective. When she stopped reinforcing Johnny's negative behavior, he learned that another be-

havior was more effective in meeting his needs. Gradually, with continued reinforcement, the potential for effective behavior increased. Learning theorists believe that this sequence is responsible for the development of many human behaviors. They also believe that behavior can be changed, or learning can take place, by altering the reinforcement.

This process is depicted in Fig. 21-1. Since response number 1 is not reinforced, it tends not to recur. Instead, the person tries response number 2. It is reinforced and thus will tend to recur the next time the stimulus is produced. Reinforcement need not be a reward, although rewards are certainly powerful reinforcers. Punishment can also be a reinforcer of behavior. In the preceding example, spanking Johnny would probably have been less effective than leaving him alone, since he would still be receiving his mother's attention. Also, a reinforcer need not be a material object. The cuddling may have been as effective in reinforcing Johnny's behavior as the cookie.

Social-Cognitive Model

Another major group of learning theorists proposes a social-cognitive model.[1,27] While recognizing that reinforcement of behavior is important, they believe that behavior is based on additional information about the environment. In this case, the stimulus is perceived as a **sign** that a desired resource may be available from the environment (e.g., a cookie). This perception creates a **demand** that, when combined with knowledge about the environment, leads the person to seek gratification. The person's perception of the environment is referred to as a **cognitive map.** Cognitive learning theorists would say that the change in Johnny's cookie-seeking behavior resulted from a change in his perception of his

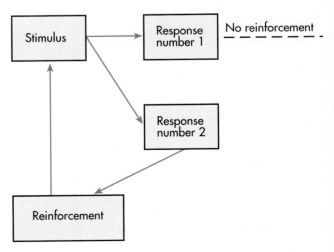

Fig. 21-1 The associationist, or behavioral, model of learning.

mother's behavior as a part of his environment. Her changed behavior blocked the pathway that had previously led him to a cookie, so he had to find a new route.

Observational learning is another example of the social-cognitive model.[1] It has been shown that people learn from watching others in similar situations. If Johnny had an older brother who stole cookies when his mother was not looking, he might have tried this as an alternative path to his reward. Role modeling is a form of observational learning that is often used by nurses to teach health-related behavior. Application of the behavioral and cognitive theories of learning in psychiatric nursing practice is presented in Chapter 28.

Piaget's Developmental Model of Cognition

Human cognitive development has been described by Piaget[18] and is summarized in Table 21-1. His research revealed three stages in the development of thought processes. The first developmental stage is "the period of sensorimotor intelligence." This phase lasts from birth until the development of language, usually about 2 years of age. This stage is action oriented, with the actions first directed toward the self and then gradually incorporating more space and the ability to locate the

self in space. Also, memory begins for objects that are out of sight. This is a necessary condition for the development of language using words to describe objects that are not present. The baby who plays "peekaboo" is practicing this ability.

The second stage is the "period of preparation and organization of concrete operations: of categories, relations, and numbers." This period lasts from 2 to 12 years of age and is divided into two substages.[12]

The first substage of preoperational behavior lasts from about 2 to 5 years of age. The child then enters the substage of concrete operations. At this point, the child is "capable of relatability, i.e., combinations, associations, negations and reversibility."[8] They learn to solve problems of conservation. For instance, if an object changes in shape, its weight remains the same.[12] During this period, children develop the capacity for syllogistic reasoning, which means that an action leads to a reaction or consequence. This enables them to make and follow rules. They also develop the ability to quantify experience.

The third stage is "the period of formal operations."[18] This develops between ages 12 and 14 years, resulting in the ability to conceptualize at an adult level. The period of formal operations enables people to explore idealistic concepts and to measure reality against possibilities. This pertains to observations of significant others, such as parents, and of cultural institutions, such as government and religions. The same process is applied to the self in the form of self-criticism. This developmental process provides the foundation for continued cognitive growth as life experiences enrich and modify the person's perceptions of the world.

In some people, cognitive responses do not develop fully or, once developed, deteriorate. When maladaptive cognitive responses occur during childhood, they are generally referred to as developmental disabilities or mental retardation. The reader is referred to a textbook of pediatric nursing for a discussion of these disorders. This chapter considers maladaptive cognitive responses in the adult. In most cases the person has developed to the level of formal operations. Although they may occur at any age, maladaptive cognitive responses are most common in the elderly. It is highly recommended that this chapter be read in conjunction with Chapter 36 because the content of the two chapters is complementary.

Maladaptive cognitive responses include impaired memory and judgment, disorientation, misperceptions, decreased attention span, and difficulties with logical reasoning. They may occur episodically or be present continuously. Depending on the stressor, the condition may be reversible or characterized by progressive deterioration in functioning. Fig. 21-2 illustrates the continuum of cognitive responses.

Table 21-1 Piaget's Levels of Cognitive Development

Stage	Age (years)	Characteristics
Sensorimotor	Birth to 2	Action oriented No language Develops awareness of body in space Develops memory for missing objects
Preparation and organization of concrete operations		
Preoperational phase	2 to 5	Symbolism appears Objects defined by function Magical thinking Imaginative play
Concrete operations	5 to 12	Capable of relatability Syllogistic reasoning Makes and follows rules Quantifies experience Understands conservation
Formal operations	12 to 14 and older	Abstraction Development of ideals Criticism of others Self-criticism

CONTINUUM OF COGNITIVE RESPONSES

Adaptive responses   **Maladaptive responses**

Decisiveness
Intact memory
Complete orientation
Accurate perception
Focused attention
Coherent, logical
thought

Periodic indecisiveness
Forgetfulness
Mild transient confusion
Occasional misperceptions
Distractability
Occasional unclear
thinking

Inability to make decisions
Impaired memory and judgment
Disorientation
Serious misperceptions
Inability to focus attention
Difficulties with logical reasoning

Fig. 21-2   Continuum of cognitive responses.

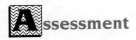 Cognitive functioning is affected by the individual's level of anxiety. Compare and contrast the cognitive functioning of a person experiencing a mild level of anxiety with one in a state of panic.

Assessment

Behaviors

Maladaptive cognitive responses are most apparent in people who have a medical diagnosis of delirium, dementia, and amnestic and other cognitive disorders (DSM-IV).[2] Discussions in this chapter focus primarily on delirium and dementia because these are the medical diagnostic categories that nurses encounter most frequently. Assessment relies heavily on both biological findings and results of the mental status examination described in Chapter 6.

Associated with Delirium. Delirium is characterized by clouded awareness involving sensory misperceptions and disordered thought. Disordered thought processes include disturbed attention, memory, thinking, and orientation. There are also disturbances of activity patterns and of the sleep-wake cycle. Generally there is a rapid onset and brief course of illness. The degree of impairment usually fluctuates. The delirious person may have occasional periods of mental clarity, but the condition is usually worse at night. This clinical example illustrates behavior that is typical of a patient who is delirious.

 ## CLINICAL EXAMPLE

Ms. S was brought to the emergency room of a general hospital by her parents. She was a 22-year-old single woman who was described as having been in good health until 2 days prior to admission, when she complained of malaise and a sore throat and stayed home from work. She was employed as a typist in a small office and had a stable employment record. According to her parents, she had an active social life and there were no significant conflicts at home.

On admission, Ms. S was extremely restless and had a frightened facial expression. Her speech was garbled and incoherent. When she was approached by an unfamiliar person, she would become agitated, trying to climb out of bed and striking out aimlessly. Occasionally she would slip into a restless sleep. Her temperature on admission was 104° F (40° C) rectally, pulse was 108 per minute, and respirations were 28 per minute. Her skin was hot, dry, and flushed. Her mother said she had had only a few sips of water in the last 24 hours and had not urinated at all, although she had had several episodes of profuse diaphoresis.

Her ability to cooperate with a mental status examination was limited. She would respond to her own name by turning her head. When her mother asked her where she was, she said "home," but could not say where her home was. She would give only the month when asked for the date and said it was January, when the actual date was February 19. She also refused to give the day of the week. A neurological examination was negative for signs of increased intracranial pressure or for localizing signs of CNS disease. The tentative medical diagnosis was that of delirium secondary to fever of unknown origin. Symptomatic treatment of the fever, including intravenous fluids, an aspirin suppository, and cool water mattress, was begun immediately while further diagnostic studies were carried out. Nurses caring for the patient noticed continued restlessness and disorientation. Her speech was still incoherent. In addition, they noticed that she was picking at the bedclothing. Suddenly she became extremely agitated, trying to get out of bed and crying out, "Bugs, get away, get bugs away." She was brushing and slapping at herself and the bed. As her mother and the nurse talked with her and held her, she gradually became calmer but periodically would continue to slap at "the bugs" and need reassurance and reorientation.

Later in the day additional laboratory results became available. A lumbar puncture was normal, as were skull x-ray films. Results of toxicological screening of blood were also negative. The electroencephalogram revealed diffuse slowing. There was an elevated white blood count and electrolyte imbalance consistent with severe dehydration. Cultures of her throat and blood were both positive for beta-hemolytic streptococci, so intravenous antibiotic therapy was begun at once while other supportive measures were continued.

As the infection gradually came under control and the fever decreased, Ms. S's mental state improved. A week later, when she was discharged from the hospital, her cognitive functioning was completely normal, with the exception of amnesia for the time during which she was delirious.

Selected Nursing Diagnoses:

▼ Hyperthermia related to infection as evidenced by elevated temperature; hot, dry, flushed skin; and diaphoresis

▼ Fluid volume deficit related to decreased fluid intake as evidenced by anuria for 24 hours and hot, dry, flushed skin

▼ High risk for injury related to fear and disorientation as evidenced by agitated behavior

▼ Impaired verbal communication related to altered brain chemistry as evidenced by garbled and incoherent speech

▼ Sensory/perceptual alteration (visual) related to altered brain chemistry as evidenced by hallucination of bugs

▼ Altered thought process related to altered brain chemistry as evidenced by disorientation

Ms. S demonstrates many behaviors often seen in patients who have delirium. The behaviors are related to alterations in neurochemical and electrical responses in the brain as a result of the stressor that causes the maladaptive response. Disorientation is generally present, sometimes in all three spheres of time, place, and person. Thought processes are usually disorganized. Judg-

ment is poor, and little decision-making ability exists. Stimuli may be misinterpreted, resulting in illusions or distortions of reality. An example of an illusion is the perception that a polka-dot drape is actually covered with cockroaches. Delirious patients may hallucinate. These hallucinations are usually visual and often take the form of animals, reptiles, or insects. They are real to the person and very frightening. Assaultive or destructive behavior may be the patient's attempt to strike back at a hallucinated image. At times, patients with delirium also exhibit a labile affect, changing abruptly from laughter to tearfulness, and vice versa, for no apparent reason. There may also be loss of usual social behavior, resulting in such acts as undressing, playing with food, and grabbing at others. Delirious patients tend to act on impulse.

Other behaviors may be specifically related to the cause of the behavioral syndrome. For example, the fever and dehydration experienced by Ms. S were a result of her systemic streptococcal infection, as was her brain syndrome. It is very important to describe observations of behavior carefully. This helps identify the stressor. Treatment is usually conservative until a specific stressor has been isolated. Although most patients recover, it is possible for the person to develop long-term disabilities or die as a result of the stressor's severity. If adequate intervention does not take place, delirium may become dementia.

Associated with Dementia. Dementia is a maladaptive cognitive response that features a loss of intellectual abilities and interferes with usual social or occupational activities. The loss of intellectual ability includes impairment of memory, judgment, and abstract thought. The patient with dementia does not have the clouding of awareness that is seen with delirium. Changes in personality frequently occur. The personality change may appear as either alteration or accentuation of the person's usual character traits. The onset of dementia is usually gradual. It may result in progressive deterioration or the condition may become stable. In some cases the process of dementia can be reversed, and the person's intellectual functioning improve if the underlying stressors are identified and treated.

Dementia may occur at any age but most often affects the elderly. According to Horvath et al.,[14] of the American population over 65 years old, 10% suffer from mild to moderate dementia, and slightly less than 5% have severe dementia. It is estimated that 4 million people in the United States suffer from Alzheimer's disease at an annual cost of $80 billion.[20,22] This is about 55% of those with dementia. After 75 years of age, Alzheimer's is the fourth leading cause of death. Dementia results from structural and neurochemical brain changes. These changes may be related to accidental or surgical trauma, a chronic infection such as tertiary syphilis, cerebrovascular disruptions such as arteriosclerosis or chronic hypertension, or the cause may be unknown. *Senility* is a nonspecific term and usually applies to those who have degenerative brain disease of unknown cause. Because of the negative connotation, use of the terms *senility* or *senile* is discouraged. This clinical example demonstrates behaviors associated with dementia.

 CLINICAL EXAMPLE

Mr. B is a 73-year-old widower who has resided in a nursing home for 3 years. He chose to move to the nursing home after the death of his wife, although his son encouraged him to live with him and his family. Mr. B stated that he did not want to burden his family and would be happier with others of the same age. He did well for the first 18 months. He was an active participant in social groups both in the home and in his church, where he continued to attend regularly. He also visited his son once a week and enjoyed seeing his grandchildren and puttering around his son's house.

About 18 months ago Mr. B began to seem forgetful. He would ask the same question several times and on occasion would prepare for church on a Friday or Saturday. He also became irritable and accused his son of not caring about him and abandoning him in "that place." Mr. B spent many hours taking papers from his desk and studying them. When asked what he was doing, he would say, "Attending to my business." He began to withdraw from activities and make flimsy excuses to avoid playing his favorite care game, gin rummy. When he was persuaded to play, he usually quit in frustration because he could not remember which cards had been played. At times Mr. B was quite anxious. He would periodically seem well oriented and expressed great concern about the changes he was experiencing, wondering if he was "going crazy."

Because of the concern of the nursing staff at the nursing home, Mr. B was scheduled for a complete physical examination by his family physician and for a psychiatric evaluation by the geriatric psychiatric nurse consultant who came to the nursing home weekly. The physical examination revealed generally good health for a man of Mr. B's age. He suffered from a mild hearing loss and slight prostatic hypertrophy. Hypertension had been diagnosed 10 years before this examination but was well controlled by diuretics. Neurological examination revealed normal reflexes, normal muscle strength, a slight intention tremor, normal response to sensation, normal cranial nerves, and no disturbance of gait. An electroencephalogram was normal, as were a skull x-ray film and the results of laboratory studies of blood and urine. Computed tomography studies of the brain revealed some atrophy of the cerebral cortex.

The mental status examination confirmed the deficits in cognitive functioning that had been observed by the nursing home staff and by Mr. B's son. He was oriented to person and place but stated that the date was April 6, 1958. The real date was March 11, 1994. He also thought the day of the week was Friday, whereas it was actually Tuesday. He correctly identified the season of the year as spring. Mr. B was able to give correctly his birth date, the date of his son's birth, and the year he began to work at his first job. He spoke at length and with great detail about his exploits as a young man. However, he could not repeat the names of three objects after 5 minutes and could not remember what he had eaten for lunch or the last name of the man who shared his room. He became distressed when he was trying to answer these questions. His vocabulary was excellent, as was his fund of general information. However, he was unable to remember the names of the two most recent presidents. He could, however, recite the names of the eight presidents preceding them.

Mr. B's judgment was somewhat impaired. When asked what he would do if he found a stamped, addressed, sealed envelope, he said he would "read it, then mail it." His ability for abstract thinking was slightly concretized. His attention span and ability to concentrate were normal. His eye-hand coordination was disrupted, as demonstrated by his difficulty in copying simple figures. He tremor was evident both when he was drawing and when he signed his name.

His affect was appropriate in quality and quantity to the content of the discussion. He appeared depressed when talking about his memory loss but cheerful and proud when describing his grandchildren. No abrupt mood swings were noted. The flow of speech was of a normal rate and volume. Content of speech was logical and coherent, except when Mr. B was trying to remember and describe recent events, when it became somewhat disjointed.

As a result of the data gathered in the physical and mental status examinations, he was diagnosed as having dementia not otherwise specified.

Over the next several months, Mr. B's condition continued to deteriorate gradually. He became increasingly forgetful and began to confabulate (fabricate stories). He was less conforming to social norms and needed reminding about hygiene and appropriate dress. He also became seductive with female residents and staff, making suggestive remarks and occasionally fondling someone. Visits to his son's home became impossible as his behavior deteriorated. His memory of the identity of family members sometimes was confused. He would misidentify his daughter-in-law as his wife and his grandson as his son. More and more, his conversation consisted of rambling reminiscences of his life in his youth. Because he is surrounded with caring people, Mr. B continues to live with dignity and respect despite his progressively limited ability to communicate.

Selected Nursing Diagnoses:

▼ Impaired verbal communication related to cognitive impairment as evidenced by recent memory loss and confabulation

▼ Impaired social interaction related to altered thought processes as evidenced by loss of conformity to social norms

▼ Bathing/hygiene self-care deficit related to cognitive impairment as evidenced by failure to perform personal hygiene activities without reminders

▼ Dressing/grooming self-care deficit related to cognitive impairment as evidenced by need for assistance in selecting appropriate clothing

▼ Altered thought processes related to cognitive impairment as evidenced by disorientation and memory loss

The behaviors associated with dementia reflect the brain tissue alterations that are taking place. In Alzheimer's disease behavioral change occurs slowly in the early and late stages and rapidly in the middle stage.[3] The cognitive changes are related to the actions of stressors that interfere with the functioning of the cerebral cortex. Other areas of the brain may be affected as well, which is one reason for ensuring that the patient has a complete medical and neurological examination. Another reason is that although the condition may be irreversible, progression may be stopped by identifying the stressor and treating the underlying dysfunction. For instance, treatment of hypertension may prevent further occurrence of small hemorrhages, which are a possible cause of dementia. Recent research has shown that many cases of dementia may be reversible. It has also been found that depression in the elderly is often misinterpreted as dementia and therefore not treated appropriately. This happens so often that the condition has been labeled **pseudodementia.** Behaviors related to delirium, dementia, and depression are compared in Table 21-2. One study found that individuals who have vascular dementia are more likely to have depression at any stage of their illness than are people with severe Alzheimer's disease.[10] Another study identified more severe behavioral retardation, depression, and anxiety in patients with vascular dementia as compared with those with Alzheimer's disease.[24]

Depressed elderly persons are often misdiagnosed as demented. What nursing observations will assist in determining whether a patient's mental disorder is primarily affective or cognitive?

A common behavior related to dementia is disorientation. Usually, time orientation is affected first, then place, and finally person. This behavior can be distressing to the patient, who may be aware of this difficulty and embarrassed or frightened by it. This is particularly true if the person's mental acuity is fluctuating. In these instances the person is aware, during periods of lucidity, of the confusion and disorientation experienced at other times.

Memory loss is another prominent characteristic of dementia. Immediate recall and recent memory are most seriously affected. Remote memory may be intact, although it will deteriorate as the condition progresses. In the last clinical example, Mr. B had trouble remembering what he had eaten for lunch but gave accurate dates for significant events earlier in his life. Most aging people dwell on the past, but people with recent memory loss have difficulty shifting to the present and at advanced stages may seem to live in the past. This is exemplified by Mr. B's misidentification of his grandson and his daughter-in-law. Another behavior related to memory loss is confabulation. This is a confused person's tendency to make up a response to a question when he cannot remember the answer. For instance, when Mr. B was asked if he knew one of the female residents of the home, he replied, "Of course I know her. I used to play gin with her husband." Actually, the woman's husband had been dead for many years and Mr. B had never met him. This behavior should not be viewed as lying or an attempt to deceive. Rather, it is the person's way of trying to save face in an embarrassing situation. He is aware that he should know the answer to the question and gives an answer that seems reasonable, not entirely disbelieving to himself. It is not unlike the situation in which a person meets an acquaintance and cannot recall the other's name or where they met. The person acts as if these facts are remembered, hoping that the other will offer clues about his identity. Denial of memory loss may also be related to the dementia's effect on the cognitive abilities needed for awareness of the problem.[21]

As Alzheimer's disease progresses, patients often develop **aphasia, apraxia,** and **agnosia.** Aphasia is difficulty finding the right word; apraxia is inability to perform familiar skilled activities; and agnosia is difficulty recognizing well-known objects.[28] These behaviors are related to the effect of the illness on the temporal-parietal-occipital association cortex.

Vocabulary and general information may be less affected by dementia, at least until its very late stages. This depends on when the information was learned. Facts learned early in life may be recalled well, whereas those learned recently may be quickly forgotten, as demonstrated by Mr. B's performance in listing the last 10 presidents.

These patients may have labile affective behavior,

Table 21-2 Comparison of Delirium, Depression, and Dementia

	Delirium	Depression	Dementia
Onset	Rapid (hours to days)	Rapid (weeks to months)	Gradual (years)
Course	Wide fluctuations; may continue for weeks if cause not found	May be self-limited or may become chronic without treatment	Chronic; slow but continuous decline
Level of consciousness	Fluctuates from hyperalert to difficult to arouse	Normal	Normal
Orientation	Patient is disoriented, confused	Patient may seem disoriented	Patient is disoriented, confused
Affect	Fluctuating	Sad, depressed, worried, guilty	Labile; apathy in later stages
Attention	Always impaired	Difficulty concentrating; patient may check and recheck all actions	May be intact; patient may focus on one thing for long periods
Sleep	Always disturbed	Disturbed; excess sleeping or insomnia, especially early-morning waking	Usually normal
Behavior	Agitated, restless	Patient may be fatigued, apathetic; may occasionally be agitated	Patient may be agitated or apathetic; may wander
Speech	Sparse or rapid; patient may be incoherent	Flat, sparse, may have outbursts; understandable	Sparse or rapid; repetitive; patient may be incoherent
Memory	Impaired, especially for recent events	Varies day to day; slow recall; often short-term deficit	Impaired, especially for recent events
Cognition	Disordered reasoning	May seem impaired	Disordered reasoning and calculation
Thought content	Incoherent, confused, delusions, stereotyped	Negative, hypochondriac, thoughts of death, paranoid	Disorganized, rich content, delusional, paranoid
Perception	Misinterpretations, illusions, hallucinations	Distorted; patient may have auditory hallucinations; negative interpretation of people and events	No change
Judgment	Poor	Poor	Poor; socially inappropriate behavior
Insight	May be present in lucid moments	May be impaired	Absent
Performance on mental status exams	Poor but variable; improves during lucid moments and with recovery	Memory impaired; calculation, drawing, following directions usually not impaired; frequent "I don't know" answers	Consistently poor; progressively worsens; patient attempts to answer all questions

From Holt J: Am J Nurs 93:32, 1993.

particularly if the limbic system has been affected by the disease process. There may also be some deterioration in social skills. Impulsive sexual advances may occur. These reflect decreased inhibition and impaired judgment. Frequently this behavior is also an attempt to establish interpersonal contact and is a way of asking for caring from others. It is also a way of reinforcing an important part of the person's identity, which is becoming less secure as mental functioning declines. Alteration in sexual functioning associated with Alzheimer's disease causes great concern for patients and their partners.

Loss of erection ability is a common problem among men who have Alzheimer's.[6] It is uncertain whether this is physiological or psychological in origin. However, both the patient and the sexual partner can benefit from continued sexual intimacy.

Restlessness and agitation are other behaviors that occur with dementia. Extreme agitation may occur at night; this is sometimes referred to as the **sundown syndrome.** It probably results from tiredness at the end of the day combined with fewer orienting stimuli, such as planned activities, meals, and contact with people.

Based on your understanding of "sundown syndrome," describe nursing interventions that would decrease the severity of this problem.

Disorientation can result in fear and agitation. When behavior becomes extremely agitated, it is referred to as a **catastrophic reaction.** Swanson and colleagues[25] have described the following precipitating factors related to catastrophic reactions:

1. A change in cognitive status, resulting in difficulty organizing and interpreting information; sensory or cognitive overload or misinterpretation of sensory stimuli may be contributing factors
2. Side effects of medications
3. Psychosocial factors resulting in increased demands to remember, such as "fatigue, changes in routines or caregivers, and disorienting stimuli"
4. Environmental factors, including changes in the environment, noise, and decreased light

The term **confusion** is frequently used when referring to the person with cognitive impairment. Although widely accepted as nursing and medical jargon, this term has not been specifically defined. It is better to use specific terms when describing a patient's behavior.

Some individuals who have maladaptive cognitive responses function at a level that is lower than would be expected based on objective measurements of their impairment. This type of functional deficit is called **excess disability.**[3] This problem adds to the frustration of the patient and to the burden that is placed on caregivers. Paradoxically, caregivers may contribute to the development of excess disability by performing activities for the person rather than coaching and assisting when needed. Functional abilities are then lost more rapidly.

Often patients who have a cognitive impairment are referred to a clinical psychologist for testing. This referral should be made for a specific purpose, since the testing is time consuming, expensive, and tiring for the patient. Some reasons for psychological testing include identification of the stressor(s) causing the disruption, understanding of the dynamics of the problem, developing guidelines for therapeutic intervention, and obtaining a prognosis for recovery. More information about psychological testing may be found in Chapter 6.

Predisposing Factors

Maladaptive cognitive responses are usually caused by a biological disruption in the functioning of the central nervous system (CNS). The CNS requires a continuous supply of nutrients to function. Any interference with the provision of supplies to the brain will cause functional disruptions. For instance, the difficulties in cognition experienced by some elderly people result from arteriosclerotic changes in cerebral blood vessels. These changes deprive the brain of needed oxygen, glucose, and other essential basic chemicals. Other vascular abnormalities, such as transient ischemic attacks (small strokes), cerebral hemorrhage, and multiple small infarcts in brain tissue caused by chronic hypertension, can also result in cognitive impairments.

Aging. Aging itself predisposes the individual to maladaptive cognitive responses. A cumulative degeneration of brain tissue is associated with aging, but it is not extensive enough to be particularly noticeable in most people. If other stressors are added, however, the person may experience difficulty. Some toxins collect in brain tissue, and a lifetime of exposure to a toxic chemical or a heavy metal may result in maladaptive cognitive responses.

Neurobiological. Alzheimer's disease is the most prevalent cause of maladaptive cognitive responses. It is now accepted that loss of mental abilities is not automatically associated with aging. Intensive research has focused on identifying the causes, characteristics, and treatment for Alzheimer's disease. Investigators have found that characteristic alterations occur in brain tissue. Selkoe[20] has summarized these as follows:

1. Plaques consisting of "altered axons and dendrites . . . surrounding an extracellular mass of thin filaments."[20] This central core is made up of amyloid beta- protein. Plaques also contain altered glial cells.
2. Neurofibrillary tangles which are "dense bundles of abnormal fibers in the cytoplasm of certain neurons."

These phenomena are found in the cortex, the amygdala, and the hippocampus, the center for short-term memory. This is consistent with the short-term memory loss characteristic of Alzheimer's disease. In addition, there is atrophy of the associational areas of the cortex. Alterations have also been noted in the neurotransmitter systems. In particular, there is a serious deficiency of acetylcholine.[14] Additional information regarding the biological aspects of Alzheimer's disease is included in Chapter 5. Other behaviors associated with this disease are found in most types of dementia.

Vascular dementia is much less common than dementia of the Alzheimer's type. This was previously called multi-infarct dementia because of the underlying cause. It results from disruptions in the cerebral blood supply.[14] Patients with hypertensive vascular disease may experience this type of dementia as the result of the sudden closure of the lumen of arterioles related to pressure changes. Atherosclerosis may lead to the formation of thrombi or emboli. In either case, the outcome is infarction of the brain tissue in the area supplied by the affected blood vessels. The resulting cognitive problems are related to the area of the brain that is involved. Another brain disorder that results in dementia is associated with HIV disease. AIDS dementia complex is discussed in Chapter 38.

Some metabolic disorders, such as chronic liver disease, chronic renal disease, and vitamin deficiencies, can result in maladaptive cognitive responses. Vitamin B—complex deficiency, particularly thiamine, is believed to cause the Wernicke-Korsakoff syndrome found in some chronic alcoholics. A prominent feature of this syndrome is a severe deficit in cognitive functioning. Malnutrition increases the person's risk of organic brain disease. This is often a problem in the elderly, who may lack the physical or financial resources needed for an adequate diet. However, young people with anorexia nervosa or bulimia nervosa are sometimes also at risk for cognitive impairment.

Genetic. Genetic abnormalities may also be a cause. An example of a hereditary degenerative brain disease is Huntington's chorea, which is inherited as an autosomal dominant trait. Although a specific genetic defect has not been identified, there is evidence that Alzheimer's disease occurs more often in first-degree relatives of some patients. However, in other families there is not a consistent pattern of occurrence.[4] It does occur more frequently in people with Down's syndrome, another hereditary brain disorder. For additional discussion of genetic factors related to Alzheimer's disease, see Chapter 5.

A degree of cognitive impairment may be found along with other maladaptive psychiatric responses. For instance, a delusional person may seem disoriented because he misidentifies his location. People who have affective disorders may have short attention spans. Depression may also result in memory disorders, although it is often difficult to determine whether the problem is related to memory loss or lack of motivation. The predisposing factors related to these maladaptive cognitive responses are also related to the primary problem.

Precipitating Stressors

Any major assault on the brain is likely to disrupt cognitive functioning. Wolanin[29] cites three major systemic problems that contribute to maladaptive cognitive responses: (1) hypoxia, (2) alterations in blood glucose content, and (3) toxicity. She further subdivides hypoxia into four types: (1) anemic; (2) histotoxic, or conditions that prevent cells from metabolizing oxygen; (3) hypoxemic, or problems with ventilation; and (4) ischemic.

Hypoxic. Anemic hypoxia may be insidious in onset. Possible stressors include aspirin ingestion, resulting in occult bleeding; other occult blood loss; or deficiencies of iron, folic acid, or vitamin B_{12}. Histotoxic hypoxia may be related to such stressors as dehydration, hyperthermia, or hypothermia. A possible stressor related to hypoxemic hypoxia is chronic obstructive lung disease. Others might include asthma or an acute respiratory tract infection. Ischemic hypoxia can result from congestive heart failure, atherosclerosis, hypotension, hypertension, or increased intracranial pressure resulting from a tumor, subdural hematoma, or normal pressure hydrocephalus.[29]

Metabolic. Metabolic disorders often affect mental functioning, especially when severe or of long duration. Endocrine malfunctioning, whether it involves underproduction or overproduction of hormones, can adversely affect cognition. For example, the thyroid hormone greatly influences mental alertness. People with hypothyroidism are sluggish and retarded in their thinking. Those with severe hypothyroidism (myxedema) may develop psychotic behavior characterized by delusional thinking. People with hyperthyroidism, on the other hand, are frequently hyperalert and agitated. Other endocrine disorders that may cause cognitive disruptions include hypoglycemia, hypopituitarism, and adrenal disease.

Based on a review of neurophysiology, compare and contrast the effects of hypoxia, hypothyroidism, and hypoglycemia on cerebral functioning.

Toxic and Infectious Agents. Toxic and infectious agents may also result in behavior typical of maladaptive cognitive responses. Toxins may originate within the individual or in the external environment. An example of an internally generated toxin is the elevated blood level of urea found in a patient with renal failure. Environmental toxins include various poisonous substances, e.g., toxic wastes and animal venoms. Increased levels of aluminum have been found in the brains of people with Alzheimer's disease. However, it is unclear how this is related to the illness. Acute viral and bacterial infections occur in the CNS, resulting in inflammation and impaired functioning. Infections in other body systems may also impair the CNS if temperature is extremely elevated. Chronic infections also affect the brain. One such condition is the neural manifestation of tertiary syphilis, general paresis. This is seldom seen because of the early treatment of syphilis. It has also been determined that people who are infected with human immunodeficiency virus type 1 (HIV-1) often develop an organic brain syndrome called AIDS dementia complex.

Prescription and over-the-counter drugs are also potential toxic stressors. Thorough assessment of drug use is critical with elderly patients because of their increased sensitivity to drugs and because confusion could lead to difficulty in following directions for taking drugs. Interactions between drugs or between drugs and other substances, particularly alcohol, may also lead to disruptions in cognitive functioning.

Structural Changes. Conditions that alter the structure of brain tissue are also reflected in impaired cognitive functioning. Tumors may cause proliferation or displacement of tissue, thus altering its function. Trauma, whether accidental or surgical, may result in a change in ability to process information. The specific effect depends on the location of the lesion.

Sensory Stimulation. Sensory underload or overload can result in cognitive dysfunction. Persons who are placed in environments with minimal stimuli seem to develop internally produced stimuli in the form of hallucinations. In contrast, the constant light and activity in intensive care units (ICUs) have led to confusion, delusions, and hallucinations, sometimes referred to as "ICU psychosis." However, it is difficult to determine how much of the cognitive impairment results from the sensory experience as opposed to other concurrent stressors, such as the introduction of multiple drugs into the system and the result of massive assaults on physical integrity.

 Either sensory overload or sensory deprivation may lead to maladaptive cognitive responses. In what way is this information significant in planning the nursing care of a patient who is confined to a seclusion room?

Nonspecific Stressors. Unfortunately, many times the specific stressor related to cognitive impairment cannot be identified. Understanding of the biochemical process of the brain and the response of brain and nervous tissue to stressors is still limited. As knowledge grows, specific biological components may be identified in the etiology of all psychiatric disorders. The fields of psychiatry and neurology may merge at some time as knowledge grows more sophisticated. For example, deficiency in the neurotransmitter acetylcholine has been observed in patients with Alzheimer's disease. It is not known whether this is a cause or effect of the illness.

In general when assessing maladaptive cognitive responses, physiological causes are ruled out first, then psychosocial stressors are considered. Even when physiological factors are present, psychosocial stress may further compromise the person's thought process. Each patient must receive a complete assessment so that nursing care can be planned in a holistic manner.

Coping Resources

Individual and interpersonal resources are important to the individual who is attempting to cope with maladaptive cognitive responses. The individual who has a varied repertoire of skills may be able to substitute for functional losses. For instance, it has been noted that people with Alzheimer's disease who have higher levels of educational attainment deteriorate less rapidly than those who have less education.[28]

Interpersonal resources are extremely important to the person with a cognitive impairment. Family members and friends often have a calming influence on the agitated person. They can provide the nurse with information about the person's usual life-style and can be sure that the environment contains familiar objects. Caregivers also need coping resources. These can often be found by attending self-help groups such as the Alzheimer's Disease and Related Disorders Association. The importance of family involvement is illustrated in A Family Speaks.

A FAMILY SPEAKS

My mother, Margaret, is 78 years' old and has been in a nursing home for the past 3 years. She is diagnosed with dementia. There are days when she does not recognize me and there are some days when she does, but her mood may not be very pleasant. Many days she only sits in her chair and responds to nothing. Frequently she cannot feed herself or express her needs. I visit her nearly everyday.

The nurses in the home are my only link to my mother. The doctor visits weekly but rarely communicates with me unless there is an emergency. The nurse gives me information about my mother's condition and *listens* to me when I have concerns about her. In the beginning the nurses were indifferent to me, and I worried that they were the same with my mother. I brought pictures of the family to the nursing home and shared them with the nurses. They began to see that her life had been very different. It allowed them to see a person instead of a patient. This helped them treat her with more respect and dignity. Now I really depend on the nurses to let me know how my mother is doing from day to day. ▼

Coping Mechanisms

How an individual copes with maladaptive cognitive responses is greatly influenced by past experience. A person who has developed a reservoir of effective coping mechanisms is better able to handle the onset of a cognitive problem than one who has not.

The person's response to the onset of dementia often mirrors that person's basic personality. For instance, a person who has usually reacted to stress with anger directed toward other people and the environment will probably react similarly when limitations in intellectual abilities occur. A person who is more apt to direct anger inward and become depressed will be more likely to respond with depressive behaviors. A person who has relied on a mechanism such as intellectualization will be more threatened by loss of intellectual ability than a person who has used a mechanism such as reaction formation.

Regression is often used to cope with advanced dementia. It may be caused in part by deterioration in mental function. It probably also results from the problem's behavioral manifestations, which cause the patient to become more dependent on others for the fulfillment of basic needs such as nutrition and hygiene. Encouraging patients to perform self-care also supports their use of healthier coping mechanisms.

Because the basic behavioral disruption in delirium is altered awareness, which reflects the severe biological disturbance in the brain, psychological coping mechanisms are not generally used. Therefore the nurse must protect the patient from harm and provide a substitute for the patient's coping mechanisms by constantly reorienting the patient and reinforcing reality.

A characteristic of early dementia is the mechanism of denial. Those with dementia attempt to pursue their usually daily routine and make light of memory lapses. They may be able to use some environmental resources to help them cope. For instance, a businessman who is experiencing difficulty with recent memory might ask his secretary to remind him of all his appointments and provide him with the names of the people with whom he is meeting and the meeting's purpose. As the impairment progresses, the person may become very resistant to any limitations on his independence. For instance, the family of a patient with Alzheimer's disease might become very concerned about his ability to continue to drive a car safely. The patient probably would be very reluctant to give up his driver's license and would deny that he was having any problem.

As cognitive ability decreases, efforts to cope become more obvious. For instance, a family member may complain that a relative has "always been irritable, but is now belligerent when he doesn't get his way." In other cases the patient's behavior may be perceived as a personality change. Some behaviors that are probably attempts to cope with loss of cognitive ability include suspiciousness, hostility, joking, depression, seductiveness, and withdrawal. Because it is threatening to admit that a close relative has dementia, family members may focus on the coping mechanism instead of the real problem, thus participating in the denial of the underlying cognitive impairment.

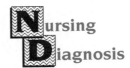

Nursing Diagnosis

The nursing diagnosis of the person with cognitive impairment must consider both the possible underlying stressors and the patient behaviors. Fig. 21-3 summarizes the stress adaptation model developed by Stuart related to maladaptive cognitive responses.

Most cognitive impairment disorders are physiological in origin. Therefore the nurse must consider the patient's physical needs, as well as the psychosocial behavioral problems. For instance, the delirious patient may be reacting to an infection or a drug overdose. The identified problem and all its effects must be reflected in a complete nursing diagnosis. Many people who are demented are also elderly. They experience many effects of the aging process in addition to impaired cognitive functioning. A thorough nursing diagnosis reflects all these influences on the patient's behavior. In addition, the nature of a cognitive impairment may inhibit the patient's ability to participate in the care planning process. The nurse must rely on observational skills and on the input of significant others to arrive at an accurate, relevant diagnosis. If the nursing diagnosis cannot be validated with the patient, a family member familiar with the person's behavioral patterns should be involved. The primary NANDA nursing diagnosis related to maladaptive cognitive response is altered thought processes. The range of frequently encountered NANDA nursing diagnoses and the DSM-IV medical diagnoses are included in the Medical and Nursing Diagnoses box on p. 556. The primary NANDA diagnoses and examples of complete nursing diagnoses are presented in the Detailed Diagnoses box on p. 557.

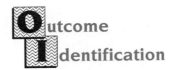

Outcome Identification

The expected outcome related to the patient who has maladaptive cognitive responses is:

The patient will achieve optimum cognitive functioning.

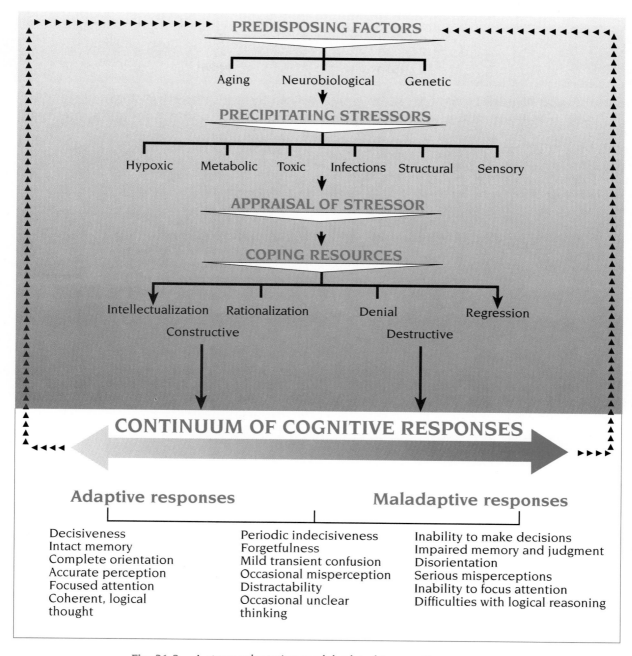

PREDISPOSING FACTORS

Aging   Neurobiological   Genetic

PRECIPITATING STRESSORS

Hypoxic   Metabolic   Toxic   Infections   Structural   Sensory

APPRAISAL OF STRESSOR

COPING RESOURCES

Intellectualization   Rationalization   Denial   Regression

Constructive   Destructive

CONTINUUM OF COGNITIVE RESPONSES

Adaptive responses   Maladaptive responses

Decisiveness	Periodic indecisiveness	Inability to make decisions
Intact memory	Forgetfulness	Impaired memory and judgment
Complete orientation	Mild transient confusion	Disorientation
Accurate perception	Occasional misperception	Serious misperceptions
Focused attention	Distractability	Inability to focus attention
Coherent, logical thought	Occasional unclear thinking	Difficulties with logical reasoning

Fig. 21-3   *A stress adaptation model related to cognitive responses.*

Goals may be directed toward an improved ability to process information, if this is realistic, or toward optimum use of the abilities the patient retains if the impairment is irreversible. For example, a goal for a patient who is disoriented because of drug withdrawal might be:

The patient will verbalize the complete date within 3 days.

In contrast, a goal for a patient who is disoriented because of chronic alcoholism and who is not in withdrawal might be:

Within 1 month the patient will find his own bed every night without assistance.

This patient may never be able to remember the exact date but may not need that information if he is to function in a protected setting. The first patient, however, will need that information. In addition, the nurse can use the assessment of the patient's orientation to time to assess the current status of mental functioning. Goals should be realistic to avoid discouragement. If the second patient had been required to learn the date, fre-

MEDICAL AND NURSING DIAGNOSES
RELATED TO MALADAPTIVE COGNITIVE RESPONSES

Related Medical Diagnoses (DSM-IV)*	Related Nursing Diagnoses (NANDA)†
Delirium due to a general medical condition	Anxiety
Substance-induced delirium	Bowel incontinence
Delirium due to multiple etiologies	Communication, impaired verbal
Dementia of the Alzheimer's type	Coping, ineffective family: compromised
Vascular dementia	Coping, ineffective individual
Substance-induced persisting dementia	Diversional activity deficit
Dementia due to multiple etiologies	Fear
Amnestic disorder due to a general medical condition	Fluid volume deficit, potential
Substance-induced persisting amnestic disorder	Health maintenance, altered
	Home maintenance management, impaired
	Injury, potential for
	Mobility, impaired physical
	Role performance, altered
	Self-care deficit (specify)
	Bathing/hygiene, feeding, dressing/grooming, toileting
	Sensory/perceptual alterations (specify)
	Visual, auditory, kinesthetic, gustatory, tactile, olfactory
	Skin integrity, potential impaired
	Sleep pattern disturbance
	Social interaction, impaired
	Social isolation
	‡**Thought processes, altered**
	Trauma, potential for

*American Psychiatric Association: *Diagnostic and statistical manual of mental disorders*, ed 4, Washington, DC, 1994, The Association.
†From North American Nursing Diagnosis Association: NANDA *nursing diagnoses: definitions and classifications* 1992-1993, Philadelphia, 1993, The Association.
‡Primary nursing diagnosis for maladaptive cognitive responses.

quent confrontation with deteriorated cognitive skills might result, leading to frustration, higher anxiety, and possibly less effective coping.

If an identified stressor is causing the patient's behavioral disruption, goals that focus on the stressor should also be developed. For instance, if a person is delirious because of a fever, a goal might state:

The patient's temperature will be maintained below 100° F (37.8° C).

When the cause of the elevated temperature is identified, appropriate goals will be written to address that problem. For example, dehydration may be a stressor contributing to an elevated temperature. A related nursing goal would then be:

The patient's fluid intake will be at least 3000 ml in each 24-hour period.

As the various elements of the person's behavior are explored and documented, nursing goals must be updated

and modified; new goals must be added and accomplished goals deleted.

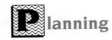 **Planning**

The nursing care plan for a patient with maladaptive cognitive responses must address all of the person's biopsychosocial needs. In most cases, the person either has or is at risk for physiological problems in addition to the psychosocial disruption. Life-threatening problems always receive the highest priority for nursing intervention. Protection of the person's safety is almost always a concern with these patients.

Mental health education related to patients with impaired cognition is often directed toward the family. They are frequently the caregivers for these patients. The

DETAILED DIAGNOSES
RELATED TO MALADAPTIVE COGNITIVE RESPONSES

NANDA Diagnosis Stem	**Examples of Complete Diagnoses**
Altered thought processes	Altered thought processes related to severe dehydration as evidenced by hypervigilance, distractibility, visual hallucinations, and disorientation to time, place, and person
	Altered thought processes related to barbiturate ingestion as evidenced by altered sleep patterns, delusions, disorientation to time and place, and decreased ability to grasp ideas
	Altered thought processes related to brain disorder as evidenced by inaccurate interpretation of environment, deficit in recent memory, impaired ability to reason, and confabulation

DSM-IV Diagnosis	**Essential Features***
Delirium (general criteria) (to be applied to all other categories of delirium)	Disturbed consciousness accompanied by a cognitive change that cannot be accounted for by a dementia.
	Impaired ability to focus, sustain or shift attention.
	Cognitive changes including impaired recent memory, disorientation to time or place, language disturbance or perceptual disturbance.
	Develops over a short time; tends to fluctuate during the course of a day.
Delirium due to a general medical condition	Evidence that the cognitive disturbance is the direct result of a general medical condition.
Substance-induced delirium	Evidence of substance intoxication or withdrawal, medication side effects, or toxin exposure judged to be related to the delirium.
Delirium with multiple etiologies	Evidence of multiple causes for the delirium.
Dementia (general criteria) (to be applied to all other categories of dementia)	Development of multiple cognitive deficits including memory impairment and at least one of the following: aphasia, apraxia, agnosia, or disturbed executive functioning (ability to think abstractly and plan, initiate, sequence, monitor, and stop complex behavior).
	Must cause severe impairment in social or occupational functioning.
Dementia of the Alzheimer's type	Gradual onset with continuing cognitive decline. All other causes of dementia must be ruled out.
Vascular dementia	Focal neurological signs and symptoms or laboratory evidence of cerebrovascular disease that are judged to be related to the dementia.
Dementia due to other general medical conditions	Evidence that the general medical condition (e.g., HIV disease, traumatic brain injury, Parkinson's disease, Huntington's disease, Pick's disease, Creutzfeldt-Jakob disease, normal-pressure hydrocephalus, hypothyroidism, brain tumor, vitamin B_{12} deficiency) is etiologically related to the dementia.

*Adapted from the American Psychiatric Association *Diagnostic and statistical manual of mental disorders*, ed 4, Washington, DC, 1994, The Association.

Continued.

DETAILED DIAGNOSES
RELATED TO MALADAPTIVE COGNITIVE RESPONSES—cont'd

DSM-IV Diagnosis—cont'd	Essential Features—cont'd
Substance-induced persisting dementia	Deficits do not occur exclusively during a delirium and persist beyond the usual duration of substance intoxication or withdrawal.
	Evidence that the deficits are related to persisting effects of substance use (e.g., drug of abuse, medication).
Dementia due to multiple etiologies	Evidence that the dementia has more than one etiology.
Amnestic disorder (general criteria)	Development of memory disorder as evidenced by impaired ability to learn new information or to recall previously learned information.
	Disturbance causes significant impairment in social or occupational functioning and represents a significant decline from a previous level of functioning.
	Does not occur exclusively during the course of delirium or dementia.
Amnestic disorder due to a general medical condition	Evidence that the disturbance is directly related to a general medical condition (including physical trauma).
Substance-induced persisting amnestic disorder	Evidence that the memory disturbance is etiologically related to the persisting effects of substance use (e.g., drug of abuse, medication)

---

nurse can help them cope with this difficult and demanding responsibility by providing them with information. Harvis and Rabins[13] found that educational approaches were helpful for caregivers or patients with dementia. One useful topic was information about problematic behaviors and problem-solving for the caregiver. Another was providing information on stress reduction, including individual ways to decrease stress, the use of respite care, and participation in a peer support group. A Family Education Plan for families of cognitively impaired persons is presented on p. 559.

Implementation

Intervening in Delirium

Physiological Needs. Highest priority is given to nursing interventions that will maintain life. If the individual is too disoriented or agitated to attend to basic physiological needs, nursing care must be planned to meet these needs. Nutrition and fluid balance may be maintained by intravenous therapy. If the patient is very agitated or restless, restraint may be necessary to keep

the intravenous line open. However, restraints can increase agitation and anxiety and thus should be applied only when absolutely necessary. A disoriented patient should never be restrained and left alone.

Sleep deprivation may be another problem. Intervention is important because lack of sleep can add to already existing cognitive dysfunction. Since sedative medication may complicate attempts to identify the original stressor, the physician may be reluctant to prescribe sedation. Nursing measures such as a back rub, a glass of warm milk, and soothing conversation may help a less agitated patient relax and fall asleep. The presence of a family member is also reassuring to the patient. Disoriented patients need to be in a lighted room. Shadows may be misinterpreted and add to the patient's fear. Also, environmental objects help the patient orient to place and person.

Do you think it is safer to use physical (mechanical) restraints than it is to use chemical restraints (medication) with an agitated delirious patient?

FAMILY EDUCATION PLAN
HELPING A FAMILY MEMBER WITH MALADAPTIVE COGNITIVE RESPONSES

Content	Instructional activities	Evaluation
Explain possible causes of maladaptive cognitive responses	Describe predisposing factors and precipitating stressors that may lead to impaired cognition; provide printed reference materials	The family identifies possible causes of the patient's disorder.
Define and describe orientation to time, place, and person	Define the three spheres of orientation; role play interpersonal responses to disorientation	The family identifies disorientation and provides reorientation.
Relationship of level of cognitive functioning to ability to communicate	Describe the impact of maladaptive cognitive responses on communication; demonstrate effective communication techniques; videotape and discuss return demonstration	The family adjusts communication approaches to the patient's ability to interact.
Effect of maladaptive cognitive responses on self-care behaviors	Describe the usual progression of gain or loss of self-care ability related to nature of disorder; encourage the family to assist in providing care to patient; provide written instructional materials	The family assists with activities of daily living as required by the patient's level of biopsychosocial functioning.
Referral to community resources	Provide a list of community resources; arrange to meet with staff members of selected community programs; visit meetings of selected programs and self-help groups	The family describes various programs that provide services relevant to the patient and family's needs; contacts appropriate programs or self-help groups when needed.

Hallucinations. Disoriented patients may need to be protected from hurting themselves or others, particularly during hallucinations. Visual hallucinations of delirium are often very frightening. Patients may try to run away or even jump out of a window. Patients' rooms must be safe, with security screens and a minimum of extra furniture or other objects placed where they might hurt themselves. Frequently these patients require one-to-one nursing observation and repetitive verbal reorientation.

It is tempting to help a frightened patient eliminate the hallucinated object. For instance, the patient might request help in brushing the bugs off the sheets. Agreeing to do this is not usually therapeutic. By participating in this activity, the nurse is nonverbally communicating to the patient that the hallucinated objects are real. This can make the patient even more frightened. In reality the hallucinations will continue until the underlying stressor is eliminated. A more appropriate response is to orient the patient continually to the reality of being sick and hospitalized. In addition, the patient can be assured that the nursing staff and physician are there to help and to keep the patient safe. Family members should also be helped to respond in a supportive way.

Communication. Patients with maladaptive cognitive responses need clear messages and instructions. Choices should be kept to a minimum. Independent decision making can be introduced into the plan of nursing care as the patient improves. Decisions related to orientation may be especially difficult for the patient. To respond appropriately to the question "What time would you like to take your bath?" requires knowledge of the present time and some idea of the usual routine.

Simple direct statements are reassuring and most likely to result in an appropriate response. Orienting phrases such as "here at the hospital" or "now that it's June" can be woven into a conversation. Patients who have difficulty dressing or feeding themselves need matter-of-fact, specific directions. Confused patients need to be fed or dressed in a manner that allows them to maintain their dignity. Families can often assist with this. Helping the patient can lessen the family's anxiety, and the patient may be reassured by the family's physical closeness and concern.

Patient Education. While recovering, patients may be concerned about what happened to them. The healthcare team needs to discuss this issue and arrive at a conclusion about the disruption in functioning that occurred. This should then be explained to patients and their families. The nurse should assess the patient's understanding of the nature of the problem, the stressors that were involved, any ongoing therapy that will be required, and preventive measures that will decrease the probability of a recurrence. Teaching may have to be repeated several times before the patient copes with personal feelings and then understands the information. Written materials can be helpful to patients who are having residual problems processing information. The teaching should include at least one responsible family member so that the information will be reinforced when the patient goes home.

If the patient is discharged from the hospital with a residual deficit in cognitive functioning, a community health nursing referral may be helpful. The community health nurse can then continue to implement the nursing care plan and can validate the patient's compliance with the treatment plan.

Intervening in Dementia

Nursing care of the patient with dementia is similar in some respects to that of the patient with delirium. Usually the stressors involved do not present an immediate threat to life; thus highest priority is given to nursing care that will help the patient maintain an optimum level of functioning. This will differ for each individual. Frequently an attitude of hopelessness evolves in those who work with chronically ill people. This can lead to stereotyping and decreased ability to see and appreciate the uniqueness of each person. It is challenging to search for this uniqueness and rewarding to find it. Individualized nursing care is probably most important for those who will be institutionalized for a long time.

Nursing approaches need to address the patient's need for social interaction. Some interventions that have been helpful include discussion groups with structured agendas; exercise groups to promote physical activity; reality orientation groups; sensory stimulation; and parties appropriate to the time of the year or to recognize important events such as birthdays. Arranging for visits from community volunteer groups provides stimulation as well as an opportunity to socialize. Referral to other members of the treatment team, especially the occupational, recreational, art, music, and dance therapists may be indicated.

Pharmacological Approaches. Pharmacological approaches to the treatment of dementia are related to theories about the cause of the disorder. Much of the research seeks a treatment for Alzheimer's disease. Tacrine (Cognex) is the only drug that has received approval as a specific treatment for this disorder. In doses up to 160 mg per day, it has been found to somewhat delay the progression of Alzheimer's. It maximizes the

function of cholinergic neurons by inhibiting the enzyme, anticholinesterase, preventing the degradation of acetylcholine.[17]

Medications must be used with care when treating persons with dementia. Elderly people are very sensitive to medications and combinations of medications. Drugs with anticholinergic effects and benzodiazepines (which interfere with learning) should be avoided.

Orientation. Disorientation is a common problem of people with cognitive impairment. Nursing interventions should help the patient function in the environment. In an institution it is helpful to mark patient rooms with large, clearly printed signs indicating the occupant's name. This also reminds forgetful people of others' names. Personal possessions can also be orienting devices. A favorite rocking chair, a hand-made afghan, or a family picture gives the person a sense of identity and helps to identify a personal area of the institution. Everyone needs a personal space. A light in the room at night helps the person remain oriented and decreases nighttime agitation. Some authorities recommend the use of small amounts of antipsychotic medications, such as phenothiazines and butyrophenones, to help patients rest, since barbiturate sedatives may cause paradoxical agitation in patients with organic brain syndromes.

Clocks with large faces aid in orientation to time. A digital clock is not recommended, since the confused person may not identify it as a clock. Calendars with a separate page for each day and large writing also help with time orientation. Newspapers provide other orienting stimuli and also help to stimulate interest in current events. An institutional newspaper provides a creative outlet that focuses on patient strengths and also helps patients maintain awareness of the environment.

Reality orientation is a nursing approach that is generally helpful to patients with cognitive impairments. Orientation includes the dimensions of time, place, and person. Systematic reality orientation includes attention to each of these dimensions. This approach often takes place in a group. It is most effective if the group meets daily, if possible, and at a standard time. A pattern of group activity should be established. For instance, the group might begin with each person introducing oneself, followed by informing the group of the date and time. A review of the schedule for the day is frequently helpful. A brief time is allowed for questions. In general, this type of group should only last for 15 to 20 minutes. If the members become fatigued, their cognitive ability will deteriorate.

Communication. Recent memory loss is another frequently encountered behavior. Patients may be frustrated when constantly confronted with evidence of failing memory. Conversational focus can be directed toward topics that the patient initiates. Most patients feel more comfortable talking about remote memories and may derive pleasure from discussing past experiences. Misperceptions of the present can be dealt with gently and diplomatically. For example, if an elderly woman who has been widowed for 10 years says that she expects her husband to come home soon, the nurse might reply, "You must have loved your husband very much. Sometimes it seems to you that he's still here." Explicitly or implicitly agreeing that her husband will "come home" is fostering false hope, perhaps leading to a disappointment. Abrupt confrontation with the reality of her husband's death is cruel and will increase her anxiety. Considerations about reality orientation are discussed in Critical Thinking about Contemporary Issues.

Farran and Keane-Hagerty[9] have recommended communication techniques for nurses who provide care for patients with dementia. The nurse should introduce

CRITICAL THINKING ABOUT CONTEMPORARY ISSUES

Is Reality Orientation Always the Best Nursing Intervention for Patients Who Are Experiencing Progressive Memory Loss?

Reality orientation is often recommended as a nursing intervention for patients who are disoriented. The rationale for this is that patients are reassured by being in touch with where they are in time and place. For the same reason, clocks and calendars are placed where patients can see them. Reality orientation is appropriate for patients who can process the information that is given to them. However, in the case of progressive memory loss related to dementia the question arises as to whether repeated efforts at reality orientation serve patients' needs.

Jones[15] describes a situation in which a patient was distressed at the nursing staff's attempts to convince him that he was in a hospital. When a nurse participated in his life situation as he was experiencing it and responded as if she were in his workplace with him, he was much happier. The nurse's rationale for this intervention was that she was assisting him to reminisce, which is an important developmental task for the elderly. Richards[19] refers to the "delicate balance" that nurses must maintain between providing the patient with needed information about the environment and denying the patient's inability to process that information in a meaningful way. This means that nurses must question the automatic use of reality orientation as the best intervention for every disoriented patient. ▼

oneself at each interaction with the patient. There should be an attitude of unconditional positive regard. Empathy, warmth, and caring are important. Verbal communication should be clear, concise, and unhurried. The voice should be modulated in relationship to the patient's ability to hear. Shouting may be interpreted as anger by a person who hears well. The use of pronouns should be avoided. Questions that require a "yes" and "no" answer are best. Behavior should be requested one step at a time and if repetition is required, it should be stated in exactly the same way as originally. Nonverbal communication skills are also important. A pleasant, calm, supportive tone of voice should be used. Verbal and nonverbal communication must be congruent. Sometimes nonverbal techniques, especially touch, may be reassuring to the patient. The nurse should try to understand who the patient was in the past. This can be accomplished by encouraging reminiscence and talking with family members. Pictures or music may assist the patient to remember past experiences.

Farran and Keane-Hagerty[9] further suggest providing an environment of "sheltered freedom." This includes a predictable, unhurried schedule, and the assignment of a primary nurse. Distraction or diversion along with decreased stimulation should be used if a patient appears to become agitated. Appropriate use of humor and flexibility on the part of the nurse assist the patient to function in the environment.

Reinforcement of Coping Mechanisms. Previously helpful coping mechanisms are often used by the patient with maladaptive cognitive responses. Sometimes these attempts to cope may be hard to understand unless placed in the appropriate context. An older man who pats and pinches nurses and makes lewd remarks may have had past success dealing with his anxiety by behaving seductively. An elderly woman who hoards food in her room may equate food with security. An aging person who has been suspicious of others in the past may become more suspicious over time. Because of the protective nature of these behaviors, they should not be actively confronted. Rather, the nurse should try to discover the source of the person's anxiety and attempt to alleviate it, thus allowing the person to behave less defensively.

Wandering. Wandering is a behavior that causes great concern to caregivers. In fact, it often leads to institutionalization or to the use of restraints. Fopma-Loy[11] recommends that nurses observe patients carefully to identify the situations that contribute to wandering behavior. She suggests that mapping of the behavior may be useful when attempting to understand it and plan appropriate interventions. In some cases, medications may cause agitation and restlessness. Some patients are extremely sensitive to stress and tension in the environ-

Table 21-3   Timetable of Discharge Planning Steps for Cognitively Impaired Patients

On admission	During hospitalization	Before discharge	Day of discharge
Assess	Monitor progress and continue to assess mental status	Monitor patient's physical and mental status	Evaluate health status
Baseline mini-mental state exam	Include family and significant others in plans	Review patient's and significant other's recall of health teaching	Administer mini-mental state exam
Existence and extent of cognitive impairment	Explore financial constraints and limitations	Reinforce teaching as needed	Review care with patient
Medications for possible impairment	Continue formulating discharge planning needs	Contact home nursing agency	Reinforce teaching
Patient's support systems	Schedule interdisciplinary conferences with all caregivers to evaluate progress and plan discharge	Confirm arrangements with community resources	Reconfirm home nursing or community agency visits schedule
How activities of daily living and related activities are usually managed (cooking, cleaning, medication administration, and personal care)		Complete referral forms	
	Locate community resources available for discharge assistance	Pack supplies	
Identify	Contact home nursing agencies		
Potential patient needs	Begin teaching patient and significant others care, including medication administration, activity, and diet restrictions		
Preliminary discharge needs			
Staff nurse responsible for discharge planning needs (use discharge planning nurse if available)			
Implement			
Interventions for cognitively impaired patients			

From Dellasega C, Shellenbarger T: *Nurs Health Care* 13:526, 1992.

ment. Their wandering may be an attempt to get away. Similarly, if patients are aware that an activity that they dislike is about to occur, such as bathing or medication administration, they may try to avoid it, If wandering meets needs for attention, efforts to control the behavior may actually reinforce it.

Fopma-Loy suggests decreasing stress in the environment, especially at night when many people have decreased stress tolerance. Eliminating distracting background noise or shadows may help. Safe areas should be provided where patients can move about freely. If possible, this should include an outside area with adequate staff supervision to ensure safety. Environmental design can be used to camouflage doorways or to incorporate distractions. Any method of increasing orientation can also decrease the need to wander. However, it is important to base nursing intervention on observation and analysis of the motivation for the patient's behavior.

Decreasing Agitation. Patients may also become agitated when pushed to do something unfamiliar or unclear. Expectations should be explained simply and completely. If the patient can make choices, they should be offered. An individual daily schedule of activities can help the person prepare for and plan his day. If a patient refuses to participate in an activity, continued in-

sistence usually leads to increased agitation and sometimes loss of behavioral control resulting in a catastrophic response. The best approach may be to wait a few minutes and then return to see if the patient will agree to the request. In the interim the approach to the patient can be examined to see if the nurse might have contributed to the problem. Perhaps the patient thought the nurse was too controlling and a power struggle developed, or perhaps the nurse initiated the request abruptly, not allowing the patient a time for transition.

Family and Community Interventions. Many individuals with dementia live in community settings with their families. It is important to support these caregivers because the patient usually derives great benefit from being with them. When hospitalization occurs, careful discharge planning is needed. Dellasega and Shellenbarger[7] have developed a timetable for discharge planning for cognitively impaired patients (Table 21-3).

Teusink and Mahler[26] have identified a family reaction process in relatives of patients with Alzheimer's disease. The same sequence of responses is probably characteristic of families of individuals with other dementing illnesses. This five-stage process closely parallels the grieving process identified in the significant others of dying persons. The stages are presented in Table 21-4.

Table 21-4 Pattern of Family Members' Responses to Alzheimer's Disease

Stage	Family behavior	Intervention
Denial	May ignore severe memory loss; may use relatively intact remote memory as evidence of no problem; may interfere with treatment planning	Education Confrontation
Overinvolvement	Sacrifice of usual family activities; reluctance to seek help, often related to ethnicity	Determine cultural norms; help to see problems related to overinvolvement
Anger	Reaction to burden of care and feeling of abandonment by patient; often projected or displaced onto care provider	Assist to recognize and express feelings; be aware of countertransference
Guilt	Reaction to recognition of anger and wish that patient would die; may also be caused by past interpersonal experiences with the patient	Educate about the illness and what the family can and cannot control; assist to make decisions about care, even if patient objects
Acceptance	Resolution of other stages; realistic understanding of what to expect and what can be done	Provide support and knowledge as required

Adapted from Teusink JP, Mahler S: *Hosp Community Psychiatry* 35:152, 1984.

Families may need assistance in providing 24-hour care for the patient. Home care agencies may provide nursing and homemaking services to enable patients to remain in their own homes. If family members are not available during the day, adult day-care centers are available in some communities. These programs provide help with activities of daily living, recreation, health supervision, rehabilitation, exercise, and nutrition. Families also receive support and assistance, particularly during the first few weeks of attendance, when the patient may be resistant because of difficulty adapting to a new experience. However, one study found that although caregivers recognized that supportive services were available, they tended not to use them.[5] A Nursing Care Plan Summary for patients who have maladaptive cognitive responses is presented on p. 564.

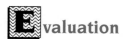 valuation

Expectations of the patient who has cognitive difficulty must be realistic but not pessimistic. One evaluation criterion is the appropriateness of the nursing goal to the individual. The nurse should assess whether the expectation is too high or too low. Levels of expectation can be increased until the patient is clearly unable to function and then lowered to the realistic level.

The evaluation of the nursing care of the patient who has maladaptive cognitive responses is based on achievement of the identified nursing care goals. If goals are not achieved, the nurse should ask the following questions:

▼ Was the assessment complete enough to correctly identify the problem?
▼ Were the goals individualized for this patient?
▼ Was enough time allowed for goal achievement?
▼ Did I have the skills that I needed to carry out the identified interventions?
▼ Were there environmental factors that affected goal achievement?
▼ Did additional stressors affect the patient's ability to cope?
▼ Was the goal achievable for this patient?
▼ What alternative approaches could be tried?

Colleagues are helpful in evaluating the nursing care plan. They may suggest alternate interventions or provide feedback about transference-countertransference issues. For instance, nurses who work with aging patients with dementia may respond to concerns about their own aging or that of their parents and have difficulty seeing patients as unique persons. Hallucinating patients frequently arouse anxiety in nurses, who may then respond with their own defense mechanisms. Regular supervision can help nurses to develop enhanced self-awareness and to determine when a particularly anxiety-provoking situation has bothered them and why.

SUGGESTED CROSS-REFERENCES

NURSING CARE PLAN SUMMARY
Maladaptive Cognitive Responses

Nursing Diagnosis: Altered thought processes

Expected Outcome: The patient will achieve optimum cognitive functioning.

Short-term goals	Interventions	Rationale
The patient will meet basic biological needs.	Maintain adequate nutrition; monitor fluid intake and output; monitor vital signs Provide opportunities for rest and stimulation Assist with ambulation if necessary Assist with hygiene activities as needed	Basic biological integrity is necessary for survival. Interventions that are related to survival are given high priority for nursing intervention.
The patient will be safe from injury.	Assess sensory and perceptual functioning Provide access to eyeglasses, hearing aids, canes, walkers, etc. if needed Observe and remove safety hazards (e.g., obstacles, slippery floors, open flames, inadequate lighting) Supervise medications if necessary Protect from injury during periods of agitation with one-to-one nursing care; restraints only if absolutely necessary	Maladaptive cognitive responses usually involve sensory and perceptual disorders that can endanger the patient's safety.
The patient will experience an optimum level of self-esteem.	Provide reality orientation Establish a trusting relationship Encourage independence Identify interests and skills; provide opportunities to use them Give honest praise for accomplishments Use therapeutic communication techniques to help patient communicate thoughts and feelings	Cognitive impairment is a threat to self-esteem. A positive nurse-patient relationship can assist the patient to express fears and feel secure in the environment. Recognition of accomplishments also raises self-esteem.
The patient will maintain positive interpersonal relationships.	Initiate contact with significant others Encourage patient to interact with others; involve in group activities Teach family and patient about the nature of the problem and the recommended health care plan Allow significant others to assist in patient care if they wish Meet with significant others regularly and provide them with an opportunity to talk Involve patient and family in discharge planning	Caring relationships with others promote a positive self-concept. Communication by significant others can often be understood more easily than that of strangers. Family and friends can provide help in knowing the patient's habits and preferences. Involvement of significant others in caregiving often helps them cope with the stress of the patient's health problem.

SUMMARY

1. The continuum of cognitive responses is related to the learning, social-cognitive, and developmental models.

2. Behaviors related to cognitive responses vary depending on whether the maladaptive response is acute and likely to resolve as in delirium, or progressive and chronic, as in dementia. Behaviors are re-

lated to disturbances in thought, memory, reasoning, judgment, orientation, perception, and attention.

3. Predisposing factors are described related to aging, neurobiological functioning, and genetic factors. Precipitating stressors are categorized as hypoxic, metabolic, toxic and infectious, structural, and those related to sensory stimulation.

4. Coping resources are based on individual and inter-

personal supports. Coping mechanisms that are used relative to cognitive responses include intellectualization, rationalization, denial and regression.

5. The primary NANDA nursing diagnosis is altered thought processes.

6. Primary DSM-IV diagnoses are categorized as dementia, delirium, and amnestic disorder.

7. The expected outcome of nursing care is that the patient will achieve the optimum level of cognitive functioning.

8. Interventions related to delirium include caring for physiological needs, responding to hallucinations, therapeutic communication, and patient education. Interventions related to dementia include pharmacological approaches, orientation, therapeutic communication, reinforcement of coping mechanisms, responding to wandering, decreasing agitation, and family and community approaches.

9. Evaluation of nursing care is based on goal accomplishment and involves feedback from the patient, significant others, peers, and supervisors.

COMPETENT CARING
A CLINICAL EXEMPLAR OF A PSYCHIATRIC NURSE

Royce Sampson, MSN, RN, CS

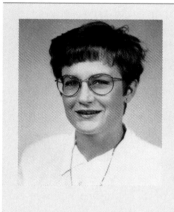

When I first saw this patient in his home, he was withdrawn and rarely spoke. He remained in his room all the time because he required total care and was incontinent of bowel and bladder. The medical history indicated that the patient had suffered a severe closed head injury several years before; that he was aphasic; and that he had a neurogenic bladder and bowel. His rehabilitation potential appeared poor. Through my multidimensional assessment of him and conversations with his family and home health aide, multiple needs and strengths were identified. By establishing a rapport with him and gaining his trust, I was able to identify what it was he thought he needed to feel better. He wanted adequate food, care, security, and safety. He wanted nursing home placement. I knew through my experience that many months would pass before nursing home placement could be obtained, if at all. After discussing all the alternatives with the patient and his family, we agreed on a few additional goals and selected a possible home. I would assist the family through the nursing home placement process, and in the meantime would coordinate additional services to meet his needs and maximize his ability to care for himself.

Through the assessment process, I identified that this patient was alert and oriented. He could communicate adequately and had through necessity (although unsafely) learned to transfer himself to his wheelchair. The home health aide also identified that the patient was capable of remaining continent if reminded. I talked to the patient about rehabilitation services in response to his remarks about his desire for increased independent mobility and function. He agreed that he would like to try these services. We decided that adult day-care services would be the best option to meet many of his needs with the limited community resources that were available.

Through negotiations with his physician and the other health-care providers, I arranged for the home health aide to get him ready for adult day care and for the adult day-care bus to pick him up and take him to the center where he would receive hot meals, group socialization, physical therapy, occupational therapy, and speech therapy. I also counseled his family about how they could better meet his needs at home. The patient had very limited social supports and financial resources and lived in a rural area, which complicated and sometimes thwarted the process of meeting his needs. Home-delivered meals were unavailable, and the adult day-care bus did not usually travel the distance to the patient's home.

Over the next few months the patient made tremendous progress. At day care, he met friends his own age from the boarding home that was attached to the center. These friends provided him with much needed socialization. An added advantage was the motivation for self-care and independence that the peer group invoked in the patient. When he was with his peer group, he wheeled his wheelchair independently and toileted himself. Periodically, he would stop going to the day-care center, and the day-care staff would call me to intervene. The expense of going to the patient's home when he would refuse to go to the center after the bus arrived at his home, combined with his loss in function when therapy was missed, threatened his termination of all services. Sometimes recoordination of services was needed, but many times it was psychological support and counseling that was really indicated.

Therapy was painful, frustrating, and difficult for the patient. At times he was afraid of what his increasing independence would mean for him. If he became too independent, he would not be eligible for nursing home placement, and he did not want to remain in his home environment. We discussed the possibility of placement in a less restrictive environment, such as the boarding home where the day-care center and his friends were located, but the patient was afraid that he would not be able to maintain the level of independence the facility required. By spending much time counseling and assisting him identify his abilities and the progress he had made, and negotiating with the boarding home for a trial placement, I was able to assist the patient to gain enough self-confidence to try the boarding home placement. I maintained contact with the patient and the facility for the next month to ensure that the patient was appropriately placed and happy. The placement was a huge success.

While I have always been an advocate for maintaining a patient in his or her own home if at all possible, in this instance the patient's physical and safety and security needs could not be adequately satisfied at home. Boarding home placement not only met those needs, but also helped him to meet higher needs of socialization through his peer group, increased self-esteem through the confidence he gained by being able to function in a less restricted environment, and self-actualization through reaching for his maximum potential.

I learned a great deal from my involvement with this patient as I constantly reevaluated my own values and goals for him. I wanted the patient to reach his maximum potential, and I had faith in his ability. But, as he taught me time and time again, it was *his* goals on which I had to focus, and *his* belief in himself that I had to foster. My skills in collaboration, advocacy, coordination of services, counseling, and clinical nursing enabled me to obtain a successful and satisfying outcome for my patient and a rewarding experience for myself. ▼

REFERENCES

1. Agras WS: Learning theory. In Kaplan HI, Sadock BJ, eds: *Comprehensive textbook of psychiatry*, ed 5, Baltimore, 1989, Williams & Wilkins.
2. American Psychiatric Association: *Diagnostic and statistical manual of mental disorders*, ed 4, Washington, DC, 1994, The Association.
3. Beck C et al: Dressing for success: promoting independence among cognitively impaired elderly, *J Psychosoc Nurs Ment Health Serv* 29:30, 1991.
4. Cohen GE: Alzheimer's disease: clinical update, *Hosp Community Psychiatry* 41:496, 1990.
5. Collins C, Stommel M, Given CW, King S: Knowledge and use of community services among family caregivers of Alzheimer's disease patients, *Arch Psychiatr Nurs* 5:84, 1991.
6. Davies HD, Zeiss A, Tinklenberg JR: 'Til death do us part: intimacy and sexuality in the marriages of Alzheimer's patients, *J Psychosoc Nurs Ment Health Serv* 30:5, 1992.
7. Dellasega C, Shellenbarger T: Discharge planning for cognitively impaired elderly adults, *Nurs Health Care*, 13:526, 1992.
8. Engelhardt K: Piaget: a prescriptive theory for parents, *Matern Child Nurs J* 3:1, 1974.
9. Farran CJ, Keane-Hagerty E: Communicating effectively with dementia patients, *J Psychosoc Nurs Ment Health Serv* 27:13, 1989.
10. Fischer P, Simanyi M, Danielczyk W: Depression in dementia of the Alzheimer type and in multiinfarct dementia, *Am J Psychiatry* 147:1484, 1990.
11. Fopma-Loy J: Wandering: causes, consequences, and care, *J Psychosoc Nurs Ment Health Serv* 26:8, 1988.
12. Greenspan SI, Curry JF: Piaget's approach to intellectual functioning. In Kaplan HI, Sadock BJ, eds: *Comprehensive textbook of psychiatry*, ed 5, Baltimore, 1989, Williams & Wilkins.

13. Harvis KA, Rabins PV: Dementia: helping family caregivers cope, *J Psychosoc Nurs Ment Health Serv* 27:7, 1989.

14. Horvath TB et al: Organic mental syndromes and disorders. In Kaplan HI, Sadock BJ, eds: *Comprehensive textbook of psychiatry*, ed 5, Baltimore, 1989, Williams & Wilkins.

15. Jones CP: In Sam's shop, *Am J Nurs* 94:51, 1994.

16. Jones PS, Martinson IM: The experience of bereavement in caregivers of family members with Alzheimer's disease, *Image J Nurs Sch* 24:172, 1992.

17. Knapp MJ et al: A 30-week randomized controlled trial of high-dose tacrine in patients with Alzheimer's disease, *JAMA* 271:985, 1994.

18. Piaget J: *The child and reality: problems of genetic psychology*, New York, 1973, Grossman Publishers.

19. Richards BS: Alzheimer's disease: a disabling neurophysiological disorder with complex nursing implications, *Arch Psychiatr Nurs* 4:39, 1990.

20. Selkoe DJ: Amyloid protein and Alzheimer's disease, *Sci Am* special issue, 1993.

21. Sevush S, Leve N: Denial of memory deficit in Alzheimer's disease, *Am J Psychiatry* 150:748, 1993.

22. Skelton WP, Skelton NK: Alzheimer's disease: recognizing and treating a frustrating condition, *Postgrad Med* 90:33, 1991.

23. Stern RG et al: A longitudinal study of Alzheimer's disease: measurement, rate, and predictors of cognitive deterioration, *Am J Psychiatry* 151:391, 1994.

24. Sultzer DL et al: A comparison of psychiatric symptoms in vascular dementia and Alzheimer's disease, *Am J Psychiatry* 150:1806, 1993.

25. Swanson EA, Maas ML, Buckwalter KC: Catastrophic reactions and other behaviors of Alzheimer's residents: special unit compared with traditional units, *Arch Psychiatr Nurs* 7:292, 1993.

26. Teusink JP, Mahler S: Helping families cope with Alzheimer's disease, *Hosp Community Psychiatry* 35:152, 1984.

27. Tolman EC: *Purposive behavior in animals and man*, New York, 1932, Century.

28. Ugarriza DN, Gray T: Alzheimer's disease: nursing interventions for clients and caretakers, *J Psychosoc Nurs Ment Health Serv* 31:7, 1993.

29. Wolanin MO: Physiologic aspects of confusion, *J Gerontol Nurs* 7:236, 1981.

ANNOTATED SUGGESTED READINGS

Baker FM: Screening tests for cognitive impairment, *Hosp Community Psychiatry* 40:339, 1989.

Comparison of the usefulness of five different screening tests for cognitive impairment with attention given to sociocultural and education factors.

*Batt LJ: Managing delirium: implications for geropsychiatric nurses, *J Psychosoc Nurs Ment Health Serv* 27:23, 1989.

Describes nursing interventions that are helpful in providing care to a patient with delirium.

Deptula D, Singh R, Pomara N: Aging, emotional states, and memory, *Am J Psychiatry* 150:429, 1993.

Report of a study that documented that negative affect states such as anxiety and depression adversely affect memory in elderly people.

Doernberg M: *Stolen mind: the slow disappearance of Ray Doernberg*, Chapel Hill, NC, 1989, Algonquin Books of Chapel Hill.

The wife of a man with progressive dementia describes her experiences and his reactions to his increasing dependence. Provides insight into the impact of this illness on the family.

*Fopma-Loy J, Austin JK: An attributional analysis of formal caregivers' perceptions of agitated behavior of a resident with Alzheimer's disease, *Arch Psychiatr Nurs* 7:217, 1993.

This nursing study applied attributional theory to the expectations of nursing home staff regarding the behavior of patients.

*Hall GR: This hospital patient has Alzheimer's, *Am J Nurs* 91:45, 1991.

This continuing education unit provides an excellent overview of the nursing care of a patient who has Alzheimer's disease.

*Hamdy RC, Turnbull JM, Clark W, Lancaster MM: *Alzheimer's disease: a handbook for caregivers*, ed 2, St Louis, 1994, Mosby.

This book provides a wealth of information about Alzheimer's disease. It is designed to be used by caregivers of people who have this illness but is very useful for nurses as well. Highly recommended.

*Liken MA, Collins CE: Grieving: facilitating the process for dementia caregivers, *J Psychosco Nurs Ment Health Serv* 31(1):21, 1993.

Addresses the nursing interventions that assist caregivers to cope with both predeath and postdeath when a loved one has a dementia.

Powell LS, Courtice K: *Alzheimer's disease: a guide for families*, Reading, Mass, 1993, Addison-Wesley.

Recommended as a reference for families with practical information that can be applied to everyday caregiving.

Rabins PV and Mace NL: *The 36-hour day*, Baltimore, 1981, The Johns Hopkins University Press.

Indispensable guide for families and other care providers for individuals with dementia. Provides practical information and explains behavioral changes in understandable terms. Excellent adjunct to health education.

*Rossby L, Beck C, Heacock P: Disruptive behaviors of a cognitively impaired nursing home resident, *Arch Psychiatr Nurs* 6:98, 1992.

Good example of the use of research to analyze a nursing care problem and identify interventions.

*Smith-Jones SM, Francis GM: Disruptive institutionalized elderly: a cost-effective intervention, *J Psychosooc Nurs Ment Health Serv* 30:17, 1992.

Describes nursing approaches to intervene in a difficult caregiving problem while maintaining the patient's dignity and staff satisfaction.

*Stolley JM, Buckwalter KC, Shannon MD: Caring for patients with Alzheimer's disease: recommendations for nursing education *J Geront Nurs* 17:34, 1991.

An excellent resource for nurse educators and in-service education instructors with recommended content for curricula.

*Taft LB: Conceptual analysis of agitation in the confused elderly, *Arch Psych Nurs* 3:102, 1989.

Identifies critical attributes of agitation using case studies.

*Nursing reference.

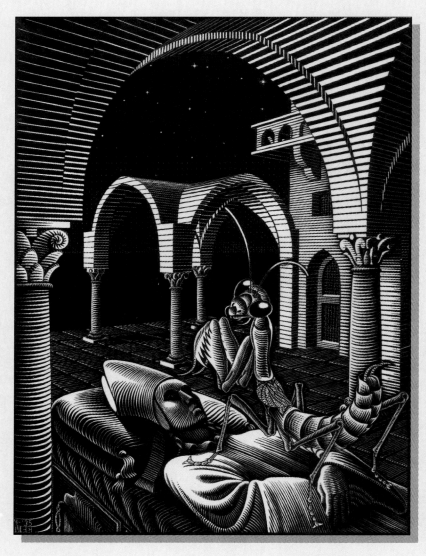

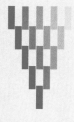

C H A P T E R 2 2

Chemically Mediated Responses and Substance-Related Disorders

LINDA V. JEFFERSON

Sleepmonger, deathmonger, with capsules in my palms each night, eight at a time from sweet pharmaceutical bottles I make arrangements for a pint-sized journey.
I'm the queen of this condition. I'm an expert on making the trip and now they say I'm an addict. Now they ask why. Why!

Anne Sexton: The Addict*

LEARNING OBJECTIVES

After studying this chapter the student should be able to:

▼ Describe the continuum of adaptive and maladaptive chemically mediated responses

▼ Discuss trends in the use of alcohol and drugs

▼ Identify behaviors associated with chemically mediated responses

▼ Analyze predisposing factors and precipitating stressors related to chemically mediated responses

▼ Describe coping resources and coping mechanisms related to chemically mediated responses

▼ Formulate nursing diagnoses for patients related to chemically mediated responses

▼ Assess the relationship between nursing diagnoses and medical diagnoses related to chemically mediated responses

▼ Identify expected outcomes and short-term nursing goals for patients related to chemically mediated responses

▼ Develop a patient education plan to promote patients' adaptive chemically mediated responses

▼ Analyze nursing interventions for patients related to chemically mediated responses

▼ Evaluate nursing care for patients related to chemically mediated responses

TOPICAL OUTLINE

Continuum of Chemically Mediated Responses
    Definition of Terms
    Attitudes Toward Substance Abuse
    Prevalence
Assessment
    Screening for Substance Abuse
    Behaviors of Abuse and Dependence
    Predisposing Factors
    Precipitating Stressors
    Coping Resources
    Coping Mechanisms
Nursing Diagnosis
Related Medical Diagnoses
Dual Diagnosis
Outcome Identification
Planning
Implementation
    Biological Interventions
    Psychological Interventions
    Social Interventions
    Intervening with Impaired Colleagues
    Preventive Interventions
Evaluation

---

*From Anne Sexton: *Live or die,* © 1966 by Anne Sexton.
Reprinted by permission of Houghton Mifflin Co.

Psychoactive substances have been used by humans in almost all cultures since prehistoric times. These substances have been seen as enhancers of individual and social functioning. People continue to use them for relief of negative emotional states, such as depression, fear, and anxiety; relief from fatigue or boredom; and as a break from daily routines through altered states of consciousness.[38] Alcohol and drugs also continue to be used in various religious ceremonies. Ethical and legal considerations aside, moderate use for any of these purposes would probably not result in major social or individual harm. However, history also shows that all cultures have recognized the negative effects of alcohol and drug use. Excessive use of these substances has contributed to profound individual and social problems.

Any drug that can produce pleasurable changes in mental or emotional states has potential for abuse. Drugs that cause the most marked and immediate desirable effects have the greatest abuse potential. Alcohol and cocaine are very popular because they produce effects on the brain within minutes. Drugs of abuse include legal drugs, such as alcohol and prescription drugs, and illegal drugs, such as heroin, cocaine, and marijuana. This chapter covers the main categories of abused drugs, including:

1. CNS depressants (alcohol, antianxiety agents, such as the benzodiazepines, and barbiturates)
2. Marijuana
3. Stimulants (amphetamines and cocaine)
4. Opiates
5. Hallucinogens (LSD)
6. PCP

CONTINUUM OF CHEMICALLY MEDIATED RESPONSES

Definition of Terms

A person may achieve a state of relaxation, euphoria, stimulation, or altered awareness in several ways. The range of these chemically mediated coping responses is illustrated in Fig. 22-1. Although there is a continuum from occasional drug use to frequent drug use to abuse and dependence, not everyone who uses drugs becomes an abuser, nor does every abuser become dependent. The definitions of the terms *use, abuse,* and *dependence* have changed through the years and vary greatly in the addiction literature. The nurse must realize that what one person or health-care professional means by addiction is not necessarily meant by another. Reading and discussion should start with agreement about meanings of terms.

Substance abuse, as described in the *Diagnostic and Statistical Manual of Mental Disorders*, fourth edition (DSM-IV),[2] refers to continued use despite the occurrence of related problems. The term **substance dependence,** related to either drugs or alcohol, indicates a severe condition, usually considered a disease. There may be physical problems as well as serious disruptions in the person's work, family, and social life. The psychosocial behaviors related to substance dependence are often called **addiction.** For most purposes, the terms *dependence* and *addiction* are used interchangeably.

Withdrawal symptoms and tolerance are signs that the person is **physically dependent** on the drug. **Withdrawal symptoms** result from a biological need that develops when the body becomes adapted to having the drug in the system. Characteristic symptoms occur when the level of the substance in the system decreases appreciably. **Tolerance** means that, with continued use, more of the substance is needed to produce the same effect. Physical dependence can occur independently from the symptoms of drug dependence. For example, a patient who receives narcotics for chronic pain may develop both tolerance and withdrawal, yet not have any of the other problems related to drug use such as preoccupation with getting the drug, loss of control, or use in spite of problems. This person would be described as physically dependent on the narcotic but would not be called a drug addict.

Whether people really progress from use to abuse to dependence is controversial. It is certain that a person cannot develop drug dependence and the related problems if drugs are never used. Once use has begun, the risk of becoming dependent is influenced by many biological, psychological, and sociocultural factors. Once dependent, the "disease" continues to progress and can be fatal.

Attitudes Toward Substance Abuse

Substance abuse is viewed differently, depending on the substance used, the person using it, and the setting in which it is used. Nurses should be aware of these social and cultural attitudes and recognize their impact on individual users and people close to them. For instance, a businessman who starts arguments after a few drinks with his associates would not usually be considered an alcohol abuser. If the same person was caught nipping from a bottle in his desk, he would probably be considered to have a drinking problem. Despite convincing evidence of medical problems related to smoking and the effects of secondary smoke inhalation, tobacco abuse is still widely accepted in the United States. On the other hand, a person who smokes opium would be considered deviant even if the behavior took place in private.

CONTINUUM OF CHEMICALLY MEDIATED COPING RESPONSES

Adaptive responses — **Maladaptive responses**

| "Natural high" Physical activity Meditation | Occasional use of tobacco, caffeine, alcohol, prescription drugs, illicit drugs | Frequent use of tobacco, caffeine, alcohol, prescription drugs, illicit drugs | Dependence Abuse Withdrawal Tolerance |

Fig. 22-1 Continuum of chemically mediated coping responses.

 Can you describe other examples of sociocultural mixed messages about the use of tobacco, alcohol, and marijuana? How would you as a health professional go about changing these attitudes?

Changing laws related to consumption, sale, and serving of alcohol and drugs may be a reflection of changing attitudes toward their use (see Critical Thinking about Contemporary Issues). Driving while intoxicated (DWI) laws are becoming tougher. When groups of friends go out, it is more common for one to be the "designated driver" and not drink. Places that serve alcoholic beverages can be held liable if a customer overindulges and then causes an accident. Mandatory sentencing for certain drug offenses is intended to show an unaccepting attitude toward drug abuse.

Many nurses have negative attitudes toward alcoholics and other drug abusers. Some have had negative experiences with family members or friends who have had substance-related problems. This may influence the nurse's ability to assess and care for these patients. Nurses often see substance abusers at their worst—during a medical or psychiatric crisis. They see these patients returning repeatedly for alcohol or drug-related health problems. Nurses rarely have contact with alcoholics and drug addicts who have recovered from their addiction because they are ill less often. When they do seek health care, these patients may try to hide their substance abuse history. The best way for nurses to change negative attitudes is to attend open meetings of self-help groups. There they will meet recovering alcoholics and addicts who have overcome tremendous odds to remain sober and lead healthy, productive lives.

 CRITICAL THINKING ABOUT CONTEMPORARY ISSUES

Should All Drugs Be Legalized?

In 1993 Joycelyn Elders, the Surgeon General of the United States, stated that she was in favor of legalization of drugs. Those who agree with her position argue that substance abuse is a public health problem and that criminalization of drug abusers creates a barrier to treatment. In addition, they point to the criminal activity that results from illegal sale of abused substances and the use of tax dollars to combat crime rather than support treatment programs.

Opponents say that they doubt legalization will decrease the crime associated with drug use. They worry about the enormous health-care costs that could be associated with providing treatment for chronic drug users. They believe that ready availability of drugs would encourage experimentation and result in increased rates of addiction. They are also strongly opposed to government sanction of what they view as an immoral behavior. ▼

Prevalence

Although reported use of all substances has decreased according to recent surveys,[3,14,24-26] the United States still has one of the highest levels of substance abuse in the industrialized world. Substance abuse is involved in numerous chronic illnesses, hospitalizations, emergency room visits, and deaths.

Prevalence is the proportion of persons who report enough symptoms at any point in their lives to meet the criteria for a medical diagnosis of a substance-

Table 22-1 Prevalence of Substance Abuse in Adults

Substance type	Prevalence (%)	Comments
Alcohol	Men: 23.8[14] Women: 4.6 Both: 13.8	>1.4 million treated for alcoholism (fiscal year 1987)[23] About 25% of all hospitalizations are alcohol related[22]
Illicit drugs[3]	Men: 7.7 Women: 4.8	Use seems to be decreasing
Prescription drugs[24]	All drugs: 12.5 Stimulants: 7.0 Analgesics: 6.1 Tranquilizers: 5.6 Sedatives: 4.3	Categories frequently abused include narcotics, barbiturates, amphetamines, benzodiazepines, meprobamate, and less often tricyclic antidepressants Diazepam is probably the most abused drug next to alcohol (5% of all prescriptions written in the United States)[38]

related disorder. Prevalence of substance abuse by adults is summarized in Table 22-1.

Adolescence is a critical time for the first experience with drugs. Although teenagers tend to progress from nicotine, alcohol, and marijuana (also known as the "gateway" drugs) to drugs that are perceived to be more dangerous, drug use patterns seem to be most related to availability. Information about substance abuse by adolescents is provided in Chapter 35.

Multiple Substance Use. The simultaneous or sequential use of more than one substance is a serious and increasing problem. For instance, barbiturates and amphetamines may be used alternately to achieve relaxation and then stimulation. Cocaine use is sometimes followed by heroin to moderate the stimulant effect or to ease the depression ("crash") that follows the high. This can be dangerous, particularly if synergistic drugs, such as barbiturates and alcohol, are used. It also complicates substance abuse assessment and intervention, since the patient may be demonstrating effects of or withdrawal from several drugs at the same time.

Substance-Related Disorders in Nurses. Despite claims that health-care professionals have a higher rate of substance abuse than the general public, there is little information to support this. In fact, at least one major epidemiological study contradicts these claims.[34] Trinkoff found that nurses were no more likely to have

used illicit drugs and were less likely to have had alcohol abuse problems than nonnurses. The Epidemiologic Catchment Area Study[14] surveyed the mental health status of 20,000 people in five locations across the United States. Based on prevalence figures from this study, about 10% of registered nurses probably have problems with alcohol or drug abuse/dependence. Since there are 2.2 million registered nurses in the United States, the number of RNs with drug- or alcohol-related problems would be estimated at 220,000.

State board of nursing disciplinary records provide additional information. According to statistics from the data bank of the National Council of State Boards of Nursing, 68.2% of all disciplinary actions taken against registered nurses in 1991 were drug related, down from 94.4% in 1987. It is well known that nurses are ignored, fired, or asked to resign rather than reported to state licensing boards. Therefore, these data probably reflect only a small segment of the problem.

Alcohol is the drug of choice for nurses, as in the general population. Also, as in the general population, the individual's choice of substance is influenced by availability and exposure. Of all health-care professionals, physicians and nurses use parenteral narcotics the most in their practices. Therefore, they are more likely to choose these drugs for their own use. The drug of choice for nurses is Demerol. Anesthesiologists and nurse anesthetists tend to favor fentanyl, a potent, short-acting narcotic. In general health-care professionals tend to abuse prescription drugs rather than "street" drugs, whether they acquire them by prescription or diversion.

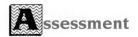

Assessment

Although accurate assessment of a patient's patterns of drug and alcohol use is important, it is sometimes very difficult to accomplish. Alcohol and drug addicts may use many defense mechanisms when discussing their chemical use. They tend to deny how much they use and its relationship to problems in their lives. They often rationalize their substance use. Patients should not be criticized for these unconscious mechanisms. They are often not aware of the extent or effects of their use. It is also true that some patients purposely distort the truth about drug use to avoid feared consequences. The nurse must be aware of these behaviors and take them into account.

Screening for Substance Abuse

Fortunately, there are ways to increase the accuracy of assessment. One is asking the right questions. People

Box 22-1

BRIEF DRUG ABUSE SCREENING TEST (B-DAST)

Instructions: The following questions concern information about your involvement and abuse of drugs. Drug abuse refers to (1) the use of prescribed or "over the counter" drugs in excess of the directions and (2) any nonmedical use of drugs. Carefully read each statement and decide whether your answer is yes or no. Then circle the appropriate response.

YES	NO	1.	Have you used drugs other than those required for medical reasons?
YES	NO	2.	Have you abused prescription drugs?
YES	NO	3.	Do you abuse more than one drug at a time?
YES	NO	4.	Can you get through the week without using drugs (other than those required for medical reasons?
YES	NO	5.	Are you always able to stop using drugs when you want to?
YES	NO	6.	Have you had "blackouts" or "flashbacks" as a result of drug use?
YES	NO	7.	Do you ever feel bad about your drug abuse?
YES	NO	8.	Does your spouse (or parents) ever complain about your involvement with drugs?
YES	NO	9.	Has drug abuse ever created problems between you and your spouse?
YES	NO	10.	Have you ever lost friends because of your use of drugs?
YES	NO	11.	Have you ever neglected your family or missed work because of your use of drugs?
YES	NO	12.	Have you ever been in trouble at work because of drug abuse?
YES	NO	13.	Have you ever lost a job because of drug abuse?
YES	NO	14.	Have you gotten into fights when under the influence of drugs?
YES	NO	15.	Have you engaged in illegal activities in order to obtain drugs?
YES	NO	16.	Have you ever been arrested for possession of illegal drugs?
YES	NO	17.	Have you ever experienced withdrawal symptoms as a result of heavy drug intake?
YES	NO	18.	Have you had medical problems as a result of your drug use (e.g., memory loss, hepatitis, convulsions, bleeding, etc.)?
YES	NO	19.	Have you ever gone to anyone for help for a drug problem?
YES	NO	20.	Have you ever been involved in a treatment program specifically related to drug use?

From Skinner HA: *Addict Behav* 7:363, 1982.
(Items 4 and 5 are scored in the "no," or false, direction.)

who drink, take drugs, or do both tend to be around others who drink and use drugs like they do. They do not have a good idea of what "normal" use patterns are. Therefore even people who deny drug and drinking problems are apt to answer certain questions truthfully. These questions have been included in screening tools, which are the first level of assessment for alcohol and drug dependence.

Simple screening tools are available that are very useful in identifying persons who are probably addicted to drugs. One of these, the Brief Drug Abuse Screening Test (B-DAST),[31] is presented in Box 22-1. It is a true/false self-administered questionnaire. Each item has a one-point value. Scores of 6 or above suggest significant drug abuse problems. Patients who score above established cutoff scores are considered to be addicted. Since the tools can be incorrect, all persons screened positive for addiction should be further assessed according to diagnostic criteria.

CAGE. The CAGE questionnaire is one of the simplest and most reliable screening tools for alcohol abuse.[11] CAGE is an acronym for the four questions it contains (Box 22-2). Answering "yes" to one or more questions

Box 22-2

THE CAGE QUESTIONNAIRE

▼ Have you ever felt you ought to **C**ut down on your drinking?
▼ Have people **A**nnoyed you by criticizing your drinking?
▼ Have you ever felt bad or **G**uilty about your drinking?
▼ Have you ever had a drink first thing in the morning to steady your nerves or get rid of a hangover (**E**ye-opener)?

Scoring: One "yes" answer calls for further inquiry.

From Ewing JA: *JAMA* 252:1905, 1984.

indicates that alcohol abuse is likely. Further assessment would be needed to make a diagnosis. The CAGE is recommended as an initial screening tool in a variety of settings because its questions and scoring can be remembered easily and included in any interview. The wording should be adapted to fit the general conversation, being sure to focus on **C**utting down, **A**nnoyance

Table 22-2 Comparison of Blood Alcohol Concentrations to Behavioral Manifestations of Intoxication

Blood alcohol level	Behaviors
Up to 0.1% (100 mg/100 ml)	Loud speech, decreased inhibitions, silliness
0.1% to 0.2%	Slurred speech, moodiness, unsteady gait, decreased coordination, shortened attention span, impaired memory
0.2% to 0.3%	Ataxia, tremor, irritability, stupor
0.3%	Unconsciousness

Modified from Butz RH: Intoxication and withdrawal. In Estes NJ, Heinemann ME: *Alcoholism: development, consequences, and interventions,* ed 2, St Louis, 1982, Mosby.

by criticism, **G**uilty feelings, and **E**ye-openers. Other tools for screening for substance abuse are found in Chapter 6.

Breathalyzer. The simplest biological measure to obtain is blood alcohol content (BAC) by use of a breathalyzer. Alcohol in any amount has an effect on the central nervous system.[7] The behaviors that can be expected from a nontolerant individual at different concentrations of alcohol in the blood are shown in Table 22-2. Remember that a person who has developed tolerance to alcohol would not demonstrate these behaviors and could have a high BAC without showing any signs of impairment. A level above 0.10% without associated behavioral symptoms indicates the presence of tolerance. The higher the level without symptoms, the more severe the tolerance. High tolerance is a sign of physical dependence.

Blood and Urine Screening. Blood and urine are the body fluids most often tested for drug content, although saliva, hair, breath, and sweat analysis methods have been developed and are being refined. Identification and measurement of drug levels in the blood is useful for treating drug overdoses or complications in emergency room and other medical settings. Otherwise, urine drug screening is the method of choice because it is noninvasive. Urine drug screening is sometimes used to test prospective employees and athletes for evidence of drug use. It is also used by drug treatment personnel to determine whether patients have used drugs while in treatment. Urine drug screening is frequently used in court to validate a person's drug use related to criminal activity.

The person being tested may try to alter the sample to hide drug use. The most common ways to do this are diluting the specimen with water from the toilet or substituting a "clean" specimen donated by a friend for the "dirty" specimen. To help prevent these practices, the specimen is frequently collected on random days under direct observation of a same-sex staff member. Another way is to have the person leave jackets, sweaters, purses, and so forth outside the stall, place drops of dye in the toilet water to alter its color, and test the specimen for temperature. Fresh, undiluted urine should feel warm through the cup and should be approximately 37° C.

The length of time that drugs can be found in blood and urine varies according to dosage and the metabolic properties of the drug. All traces of the drug may disappear within 24 hours or may still be detectable 30 days later.

Random urine testing for drugs is required for members of some occupations, including some nurses. This practice has been challenged as an invasion of privacy and an intrusion on professional integrity. What is your opinion about random urine testing for nurses?

Behaviors of Abuse and Dependence

There are many biopsychosocial consequences of using alcohol and drugs. Some are very serious and have led to great social concern. Life-styles associated with drug abuse carry risks. Accidents are frequent and violence is common. Self-neglect is the norm, contributing to physical, mental, and dental disease. The drugs and lifestyle also lead to complications of pregnancy and the risk of fetal abnormalities and fetal drug dependence.

Users of intravenous drugs and their sexual partners are at high risk for infection with bloodborne pathogens, particularly hepatitis B (HBV) and the human immunodeficiency virus (HIV), which causes the acquired immunodeficiency syndrome (AIDS). It is common for addicts to share needles when they are using drugs in a group. Since the needles are not cleaned, blood is transferred from one person to the others. This is an ideal situation for the transmission of HIV or HBV. Needle sharing and sexual relations with infected IV drug users are the primary routes of transmission of HIV to women. Their babies are often born with the dual problems of HIV and drug addiction.

Additional information regarding the consequences of substance abuse are included in Table 22-3.

CNS Depressants. This term is used for any drug that depresses excitable tissues at all levels of the brain. These drugs are also called sedative-hypnotics. Their primary effects are to reduce anxiety (the calming, anti-

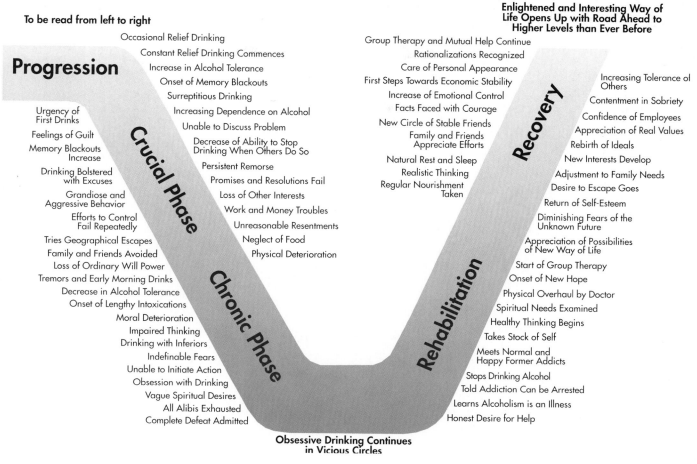

To be read from left to right

Enlightened and Interesting Way of Life Opens Up with Road Ahead to Higher Levels than Ever Before

Progression

Occasional Relief Drinking
Constant Relief Drinking Commences
Increase in Alcohol Tolerance
Onset of Memory Blackouts
Surreptitious Drinking
Increasing Dependence on Alcohol
Unable to Discuss Problem
Decrease of Ability to Stop Drinking When Others Do So
Persistent Remorse
Promises and Resolutions Fail
Loss of Other Interests
Work and Money Troubles
Unreasonable Resentments
Neglect of Food
Physical Deterioration

Urgency of First Drinks
Feelings of Guilt
Memory Blackouts Increase
Drinking Bolstered with Excuses
Grandiose and Aggressive Behavior
Efforts to Control Fail Repeatedly
Tries Geographical Escapes
Family and Friends Avoided
Loss of Ordinary Will Power
Tremors and Early Morning Drinks
Decrease in Alcohol Tolerance
Onset of Lengthy Intoxications
Moral Deterioration
Impaired Thinking
Drinking with Inferiors
Indefinable Fears
Unable to Initiate Action
Obsession with Drinking
Vague Spiritual Desires
All Alibis Exhausted
Complete Defeat Admitted

Crucial Phase

Chronic Phase

Group Therapy and Mutual Help Continue
Rationalizations Recognized
Care of Personal Appearance
First Steps Towards Economic Stability
Increase of Emotional Control
Facts Faced with Courage
New Circle of Stable Friends
Family and Friends Appreciate Efforts
Natural Rest and Sleep
Realistic Thinking
Regular Nourishment Taken

Recovery

Increasing Tolerance of Others
Contentment in Sobriety
Confidence of Employees
Appreciation of Real Values
Rebirth of Ideals
New Interests Develop
Adjustment to Family Needs
Desire to Escape Goes
Return of Self-Esteem
Diminishing Fears of the Unknown Future
Appreciation of Possibilities of New Way of Life
Start of Group Therapy
Onset of New Hope
Physical Overhaul by Doctor
Spiritual Needs Examined
Healthy Thinking Begins
Takes Stock of Self
Meets Normal and Happy Former Addicts
Stops Drinking Alcohol
Told Addiction Can be Arrested
Learns Alcoholism is an Illness
Honest Desire for Help

Rehabilitation

Obsessive Drinking Continues in Vicious Circles

Fig. 22-2 The progression and recovery of the alcoholic in the disease of alcoholism.
From Jellinek EM: *QJ Stud Alcohol* 13:672, 1952.

anxiety, or sedative effect), induce sleep (the hypnotic effect), or both. Included in this class are alcohol, barbiturates, and benzodiazepines. The signs and symptoms of the use of, overdose by, and withdrawal from CNS depressants are listed in Table 22-3. It should be noted that cross-tolerance develops among all drugs in this category. This means that as tolerance develops to one drug, it develops to all other drugs in this category as well. For example, a chronic alcoholic will need very high doses of benzodiazepines to control signs of withdrawal.

Alcohol. Although alcohol is a sedative, it creates an initial feeling of euphoria. This is probably related to decreased inhibitions. Symptoms of sedation of different central nervous system structures increase as the amount drunk increases.

Approximately 15% of drinkers progress to alcoholism. Figure 22-2 demonstrates characteristic elements of this process. The behaviors are categorized into phases according to severity.[16] A person's drinking may begin like everyone else's, or an individual may be able to drink more alcohol than others before feeling intoxi-

cated. In either case, the person likes the feeling, and continues to drink whenever possible. Gradually, drinking occurs more often and in larger quantities. As this happens, drinking begins to cause problems in the person's life, which are quickly explained away. The problems increase, the drinking increases, physical and psychological dependence develops, and the person begins to drink to avoid withdrawal symptoms. Or, the person drinks in binges. Not everyone progresses in the same way or displays all of these characteristics, and the time period over which the progression occurs varies widely. The following clinical example illustrates many of the behaviors described. Mr. H has the medical diagnoses of alcohol dependence and alcohol withdrawal delirium.

 CLINICAL EXAMPLE

Mr. H was admitted to the detoxification center of a large metropolitan hospital in acute alcohol withdrawal. He was delirious and having visual hallucinations of

Table 22-3 Characteristics of Substances of Abuse

Substance	Route (most common first)	Common street names	Dependence: physical / psychological	Use: signs and symptoms	Overdose: signs and symptoms	Withdrawal: signs and symptoms	Special considerations/ consequences of use
DEPRESSANTS							
Alcohol	Ingestion	Booze, brew, juice, spirits	Yes/Yes	Depression of major brain functions such as mood, cognition, attention, concentration, insight, judgment, memory, affect, and emotional rapport in interpersonal relationships. Extent of depression is dose dependent and ranges from slight lethargy through the various levels of anesthesia and death. Tranquilization, sedation, and sleep. Psychomotor impairment, increased reaction time, interruption of hand-eye coordination, motor ataxia, nystagmus. Decreased REM sleep leading to more dreams and sometimes nightmares. Benzodiazepines have minimal cardiovascular and respiratory effects.	Unconsciousness, coma, respiratory depression, death	*General depressant withdrawal syndrome:* Tremors, agitation, anxiety, diaphoresis, increased pulse and blood pressure, sleep disturbance, hallucinosis, seizures, delusions, DTs (severe tremors, delirium, disorientation, visual hallucinations, extremely elevated temperature, vomiting, and diarrhea). *Postacute Withdrawal:* Mood swings, difficulty sleeping, impaired cognitive functioning, increased emotionality, overreaction to stress. *Low-Dose Benzodiazepine Withdrawal:* Therapeutic doses for no more than 6 months; subtle symptoms, peak in about 12 days; wax and wane for 6-12 months; several symptom-free days, followed by acute anxiety, dilated pupils, elevated pulse, and blood pressure. *High-Dose Benzodiazepine Withdrawal:* Peaks in 2 to 3 days for short-acting drugs and 5 to 8 days for longer-acting; symptoms usually gone in 2 weeks.	Chronic alcohol use leads to serious disruptions in most organ systems: malnutrition and dehydration; vitamin deficiency leading to Wernicke's encephalopathy and alcoholic amnestic syndrome; impaired liver function, including hepatitis and cirrhosis; esophagitis, gastritis, pancreatitis; osteoporosis; anemia; peripheral neuropathy; impaired pulmonary function; cardiomyopathy; myopathy; disrupted immune system; and brain damage.[36] High susceptibility to other dependencies. Dependence on barbiturates and benzodiazepines may develop insidiously; users may underreport the actual amount taken because of guilt about multiple prescriptions and abuse.
Barbiturates	Ingestion Injection	Barbs, beans, black beauties, blue angels, candy, downers, goof balls, G.B., nebbies, reds, sleepers, yellow jackets, yellows	Yes/Yes				
Benzodiazepines	Ingestion Injection	Downers	Yes/Yes				
Marijuana	Smoking Ingestion	Acapulco gold, aunt mary, broccoli, dope, grass, grunt, hay, hemp, herb, J, joint, joy stick, killer weed, maryjane, pot, ragweed, reefer, smoke, weed	No/Yes	Altered state of awareness, relaxation, mild euphoria, reduced inhibition, red eyes, dry mouth, increased appetite, increased pulse, decreased reflexes, panic reaction.	Toxic psychosis	None	Pulmonary problems. Interference with reproductive hormones. May cause fetal abnormalities.
STIMULANTS							
Amphetamines	Ingestion Injection	A, AMT, bam, bennies, crystal, diet pills, dolls, eye-openers, lid poppers, pep pills, purple hearts, speed, uppers, wake-ups	Yes/Yes	Sudden rush of euphoria, abrupt awakening, increased energy, talkativeness, elation. Agitation, hyperactivity, irritability, grandiosity, pressured speech. Diaphoresis, anorexia, weight loss, insomnia. Increased temperature, blood pressure and pulse. Tachycardia, ectopic heartbeats, chest pain. Urinary retention, constipation, dry mouth. *High Dose:* Slurred, rapid, incoherent speech. Stereotypic movements, ataxic gait, teeth grinding, illogical thought processes, headache, nausea, vomiting. *Toxic Psychosis:* Paranoid delusions in clear sensorium; auditory, visual, or tactile hallucinations (may scratch at nonexistent bugs). Very labile mood. Unprovoked violence.	Seizures. Cardiac arrythmias, coronary artery spasms, myocardial infarctions. Increased increase in blood pressure and temperature that can lead to cardiovascular shock and death	*Crash:* Depression, agitation, anxiety, and intense drug craving followed by fatigue, depression, loss of drug desire, insomnia, desire for sleep followed by prolonged sleep then extreme hunger, renewed drug cravings, anergia, and anhedonia, which may increase for 1 to 4 days.[12] Pattern varies widely among patients; anxiety, depression, irritability, fatigue may last several weeks;[25] craving may return; relapse is a risk. Sometimes a user stops stimulants purposely to decrease tolerance, decreasing the amount needed to get high.	Certain amphetamines prescribed for attention deficit hyperactivity disorder in children because of a paradoxical depressant action. May be used alternately with depressants. Psychosis that does not clear may indicate preexisting vulnerability. Cocaine use may lead to multiple physical problems: destruction of the nasal septum related to snorting; coronary artery vasoconstriction; seizures; cerebrovascular accidents; transient ischemic episodes; sudden death related to respiratory arrest, myocardial infarction, or status epilepticus.[21] Intravenous use of stimulants may lead to the serious physical consequences described under Opiates.
Cocaine	Inhalation Smoking Injection Topical	Bernice, bernies, big C, blow, C, charlie, coke, dust, girl, heaven, jay, lady, nose candy, nose powder, snow, sugar, white lady. Crack = conan, freebase, rock, toke, white cloud, white tornado	Yes/Yes				

OPIATES

Drug	Route	Slang Names	Dependence (Physical/Psychological)	Possible Effects	Effects of Overdose	Withdrawal Syndrome	Comments
Heroin	Injection, Ingestion, Inhalation	H, horse, harry, boy, scag, shit, smack, stuff, white junk, white stuff	Yes/Yes	Euphoria, relaxation, relief from pain, "nodding out" (apathy, detachment from reality, impaired judgment, and drowsiness); constricted pupils, nausea, constipation, slurred speech, respiratory depression	Unconsciousness, coma, respiratory depression, circulatory depression, respiratory arrest, cardiac arrest, death. Anoxia can lead to brain abscess	*Initially:* Drug craving, lacrimation, rhinorrhea, yawning, diaphoresis. *In 12-72 hr:* Sleep disturbance, mydriasis, anorexia, piloerection, irritability, tremor, weakness, nausea, vomiting, diarrhea, chills, fever, muscle spasms (especially in legs), flushing, spontaneous ejaculation, abdominal pain, hypertension, increased rate and depth of respirations. *Protracted withdrawal:* Changes in respirations and temperature, decreased self-esteem, anxiety, depression, and abnormal responses to stressful situations. Lasts up to 6 months. [17]	Intravenous use leads to high risk for infection with bloodborne pathogens, such as HIV or hepatitis B. Other infections (e.g. skin abscesses, phlebitis, cellulitis, and septic emboli causing pneumonia, pulmonary abscess, or subacute bacterial endocarditis) may occur as a result of lack of asepsis or contaminated substances. Adulterants (e.g., talc, starch, strychnine) are deposited in the lungs, causing impaired function. Chronic use leads to lack of concern about physical well-being, resulting in malnutrition and dehydration. Criminal behavior may occur to acquire money for drugs. Multiple drug use is common.
Morphine	Injection						
Meperidine	Injection, Ingestion						
Codeine	Ingestion, Injection						
Opium	Smoking, Ingestion						
Methadone	Ingestion						
Hallucinogens	Ingestion, Smoking	Acid, big D, blotter, blue heaven, cap, D, deeda, flash, L, mellow yellows, microdots, paper acid, sugar, ticket, yello	No/No	Distorted perceptions and hallucinations in the presence of a clear sensorium. Distortions of time and space, illusions, depersonalization, mystical experiences, heightened sense of awareness. Extreme mood lability. Tremor, dizziness, piloerection, paresthesias, synesthesia, nausea and vomiting. Increased temperature, pulse, blood pressure, and salivation. Panic reaction, "bad trip."	Rare with LSD: convulsions, hyperthermia, death	None	Flashbacks may last for several months. Permanent psychosis may occur.
Phencyclidine (PCP)	Smoking, Ingestion	Angel dust, DOA, dust, elephant, hog, peace pill, supergrass, tic tac	No/No	Intensely psychotic experience characterized by bizarre perceptions, confusion, disorientation, euphoria, hallucinations (in clouded sensorium), paranoia, grandiosity, agitation. Anesthesia. Apparent enhancement of strength and endurance. Rage reactions. May be agitated and hyperactive with tendency toward violence and antisocial behavior or catatonic and withdrawn or vacillate between the two conditions. Red, dry skin; dilated pupils, nystagmus, ataxia, hypertension, rigidity, and seizures.	Seizures, coma, and death	None	If flashbacks occur, they are mild and usually not disturbing.

bugs in his bed. He was extremely frightened, thrashing around in bed and mumbling incoherently. Since he had a long and well-documented history of alcohol abuse, family members were contacted and confirmed that he had recently stopped drinking after a 2-week binge.

The patient had been a successful lawyer with a large practice. He specialized in corporate law and conducted much business over lunch or dinner. He also kept a well-stocked bar in his office to offer clients a drink. Without his really being aware of it, Mr. H's drinking gradually increased. After a few years he was drinking almost non-stop from lunchtime to bedtime. He then began to have a Bloody Mary with breakfast "just to get myself going."

His wife reported that he had become irritable, particularly if she questioned his drinking. On two occasions he had hit her during their arguments. She was seriously considering divorce. He had also become alienated from his children, who appeared frightened of him. Infrequently he would feel guilty about his neglect of his family and plan a special outing. Most of the time he was too drunk to carry out his plans. The family had also become less involved in activities with friends. Mrs. H and the children felt embarrassed about his behavior and so did not invite anyone to their home. On two occasions, Mr. H had tried to stop drinking. The first time he went to a private hospital, where he was detoxified. He abstained from drinking for about a month after discharge.

He then lost an important case and decided to have "just one drink" to carry him through the crisis. Soon his drinking was again out of control. His second hospitalization was at a general hospital with an active alcoholism rehabilitation program. He was introduced to Alcoholics Anonymous and started taking disulfiram (Antabuse). This program worked until he decided that he could manage without medication. A couple of weeks later his co-workers persuaded him to "help celebrate" at an office party. This was the start of a binge that ended when he had an automobile accident on the way home from a bar. A passenger in the other car was killed, and Mr. H was charged with vehicular homicide and driving under the influence of alcohol. He stopped drinking abruptly, which resulted in his current hospital admission 3 days later.

Selected Nursing Diagnoses:

▼ Sensory-perceptual alteration, visual, related to neurobiological changes induced by acute alcohol withdrawal as evidenced by hallucinations of bugs in the bed

▼ Ineffective individual coping related to repeated drinking as evidenced by work and family problems and denial of drinking problems

▼ High risk for injury related to drinking and driving as evidenced by recent automobile accident

▼ High risk for violence directed at others related to lack of control of behavior when drunk as evidenced by past pattern of self-destructive behavior

Barbiturates. Barbiturate drugs include barbital, amobarbital (Amytal), phenobarbital, pentobarbital (Nembutal), secobarbital (Seconal), and butabarbital. These drugs were once widely prescribed for their sedative and hypnotic effects. However, many problems were associated with their use, and they have been the major cause of overdose death from accidental poisonings and suicide. They produce excessive drowsiness, even at therapeutic doses. Also, tolerance to them develops rapidly. Like alcohol, barbiturates are depressants that cause an initial response of euphoria. Thus they are popular street drugs. Barbiturate use leads to both physical and psychological dependence. There is a synergistic effect between alcohol and barbiturates, meaning that either drug potentiates the effects of the other. For this reason, combinations of these drugs are particularly dangerous and can lead to accidental overdose and death. Despite these drawbacks, barbiturates are very useful for the treatment of epilepsy and general depressant withdrawal syndromes.

Benzodiazepines. In the 1960s benzodiazepines replaced barbiturates as the preferred treatment for anxiety and related disorders. This was based on three beliefs about these drugs:

1. They would relieve anxiety without drowsiness
2. They had a wide therapeutic index (the difference between the therapeutic dose and the lethal dose)
3. They were nonaddicting

It is now known that benzodiazepines do cause drowsiness, although less than barbiturates. They are also addicting, causing both physical and psychological dependence. They lead to the same withdrawal symptoms as alcohol. Because benzodiazepines are longer acting, the symptoms are less intense and continue over a longer period of time. They are safer in terms of overdoses. Despite their drawbacks, they are still widely prescribed in the United States. The clinical uses of benzodiazepines are described in Chapter 25.

Marijuana. Marijuana is sometimes classified as a hallucinogenic drug, but it rarely causes hallucinations. It causes sedation, but is not primarily a CNS depressant. The active ingredients in marijuana are the tetrahydrocannabinoids (THC). The marijuana cigarette can be smoked as it is, or through a water-pipe, or "bong," to cool the hot vapors. Marijuana generally produces an altered state of awareness accompanied by a feeling of relaxation and mild euphoria. Effects depend on the potency of the drug, as well as the setting and the experience of the user. Strength can vary widely from 1% to 14% THC. Prolonged use may lead to apathy, lack of energy, loss of desire to work or be productive, diminished concentration, poor personal hygiene, and preoccupation with marijuana. This cluster of symptoms is known as the **amotivational syndrome.** Although study findings are controversial, there seems to be general support for the existence of such a syndrome. Use of very large doses can lead to a toxic psychosis that clears as the substance is eliminated from the body. Marijuana may also precipitate psychosis when used by schizophrenics whose symptoms are otherwise controlled with antipsychotic drugs. It does not appear to lead to psychosis in nonschizophrenic individuals.[13]

The main physiological effects of marijuana are mild (see Table 22-3). Tolerance develops in heavy users, but there is no withdrawal pattern. Marijuana may have medicinal benefits in alleviating glaucoma as well as the nausea and vomiting associated with chemotherapy used in cancer treatment. However, its use in these ways has been limited legally in the United States.

> Supporters of legalization of marijuana say that the penalties are too severe for the behavior and that marijuana is no more harmful than legal substances such as alcohol and nicotine. What is your position on the legalization of marijuana?

Stimulants.

The stimulants have the ability to stimulate the central nervous system at many levels. The most common of these are the amphetamines and cocaine. People use these drugs for the feelings of euphoria, relief from fatigue, added energy, and alertness they provide. The signs and symptoms of use, overdose, and withdrawal are basically the same for all drugs in this class (see Table 22-3).

AMPHETAMINES. Amphetamine was first synthesized for use as a bronchodilator in the 1930s, and street abuse began shortly thereafter. The amphetamine drugs include amphetamine, methamphetamine, dextroamphetamine, and benzphetamine. Amphetamines are thought to act by crowding norepinephrine and dopamine out of storage vesicles and into the synapse. The increase of these catecholamines at the receptors causes increased stimulation. It was once believed that amphetamines did not cause physical dependence, but clear patterns of tolerance and withdrawal have been described. Tolerance develops to the euphoria and the "pleasant" effects of these drugs but not to the wakefulness effects. An amphetamine addict may reach a total daily intake of 30,000 mg intravenously.[21] Prolonged or excessive use of amphetamines can lead to psychosis, which is almost identical to paranoid schizophrenia.

In the 1950s and 1960s amphetamines were widely prescribed for weight loss (diet pills) and relief of fatigue and depression. Their effectiveness for both conditions was only temporary and often led to dependency. In 1970 the Food and Drug Administration (FDA) restricted the legal use of amphetamines to three types of conditions: narcolepsy, hyperkinetic behavior in children, and short-term weight reduction programs. Today, it is clear that the abuse potential of amphetamines outweighs the benefit of their medical use for almost any reason. Safer treatments for these conditions have been found and are generally preferred.

COCAINE. Cocaine may seem to be a drug of the 1990s, but it has been around for almost 2000 years. Its use in the United States grew when legal controls were placed on the production and sale of amphetamines. Cocaine is usually inhaled as a powder, injected intravenously, or smoked.

The smokable form of cocaine is produced by a process called free-basing. Early methods of free-basing required dangerous chemical reactions. More recently, the "crack" form of free-base cocaine has been produced by "cooking" street-grade cocaine in a baking soda solution. Its name is derived from the cracking sound it makes when it is smoked.

The euphoria caused by cocaine is relatively short acting, starting with a 10 to 20 second rush and followed by 15 to 20 minutes of less intense euphoria. A person who is "high" on cocaine feels euphoric, energetic, self-confident, and sociable. Although cocaine was not initially thought to produce physical dependence, a pattern of withdrawal symptoms very similar to that seen in amphetamine users has been observed, beginning with intense craving and drug-seeking behavior. The relapse rate for patients who try to discontinue cocaine use is very high. Cocaine use has been known to result in sudden death.

Biochemically, cocaine blocks the reuptake of norepinephrine and dopamine. Since more neurotransmitter is present at the synapse, the receptors are continuously activated. It is believed that this causes the euphoria. At the same time, presynaptic supplies of dopamine and norepinephrine are depleted. This causes the "crash" that happens when the effect of the drug wears off.

Cocaine use has been glamorized by the publicity given to it by movie stars, sports figures, and other well-known people. This makes it particularly inviting to adolescents who regard famous people as role models.

Addiction to barbiturates ("downers") and stimulants ("uppers"), particularly the amphetamines, often occurs simultaneously. Sometimes a patient who has been using downers develops a need for uppers to provide enough energy to function. The next clinical example illustrates this pattern. Ms. W's pattern is not uncommon. Aside from street use, many people slip into drug abuse without being aware of the consequences of their behavior.

 ## CLINICAL EXAMPLE

Ms. W was a 34-year-old woman who was moderately overweight. She had tried various diets on her own with little success. A friend told her about a "diet doctor" who had a reputation for helping his patients lose weight with minimum deprivation from eating their usual diet. Ms. W decided to see the physician and was accepted for treatment. She was given a diuretic and appetite depressant medication. The latter contained amphetamines. She began to lose weight as soon as she started the prescribed regimen and was delighted. She also liked the additional burst of energy she felt every time she took her medication. She completed projects that she had been planning to work on for months. However, her family began to complain because she was irritable and very restless. In addition, she developed insomnia and roamed about the house at night.

On the urging of her husband, she went to her family physician. She felt guilty about seeing another physician for her weight problem, so neglected to tell her regular physician about this. With the history of insomnia, irritability, and recent weight loss, her physician thought she might be depressed. He ordered an antidepressant medication and a barbiturate sedative. Ms. W soon found that she was able to sleep well with her sedative. However, she felt slightly hung over in the morning and still wanted to lose more weight, so she continued with her diet pills as well. For a while she was able to function well. Gradually, however, she found that she needed two sedatives and then she also began to use extra stimulants. Her husband questioned her drug use. Ms. W had read about drug abuse and with her husband's help identified that she had a problem. She decided to see her family physician again and this time told him the whole story. He then advised a brief hospitalization so she could be withdrawn from both drugs under medical supervision. Ms. W was very embarrassed by her addiction. While in the hospital, she needed a great deal of nursing support to integrate this experience.

Selected Nursing Diagnoses:
▼ Ineffective individual coping related to dependence on stimulants and depressants as evidenced by inability to function without the drugs and the development of tolerance

▼ Altered role performance related to drug dependence as evidenced by family concern over her behavior
▼ Altered nutrition, more than body requirements, related to repeated dieting failures as evidenced by seeking out a doctor who would help her lose weight with minimal deprivation

Opiates. The opiates include opium, heroin, meperidine, morphine, codeine, and methadone. The first two drugs were used for medical, and in the case of opium, religious and recreational purposes, but are no longer approved for this in the United States. Meperidine, morphine, and codeine are frequently used analgesics. Methadone is used to treat addiction to other opiates. It can be used either to aid withdrawal or to provide maintenance at a stable dose. It is useful because it does not interfere with the ability to function productively as other narcotics do. Patients taking a maintenance dose of methadone may work and live normally, although still addicted to narcotics.

Opiate use is less widespread than depressant or stimulant use but is still a serious social problem. Although some people use opiates for years with few problems, people with opiate addiction often deteriorate mentally and physically until they are unable to function productively. Illegal behavior such as stealing or prostitution to acquire money for drugs may result from addiction. Obtaining and using drugs becomes an all-consuming passion. The pattern of use is partially related to setting. For instance, the vast majority of soldiers who used heroin heavily while in Vietnam stopped using heroin completely when they returned to the United States.

One characteristic of narcotic addiction is the development of tolerance, which also increases the expense of the habit. Physiological effects of narcotics are included in Table 22-3.

The most important psychological response to opiate use is euphoria, or feeling "high." It is this powerful, pleasurable response that causes the person to use the drug repeatedly, leading to addiction. Other psychological effects of narcotics include apathy, detachment from reality, and impaired judgment. The phrase "nodding out" describes this group of behaviors combined with drowsiness. The next clinical example demonstrates the behaviors associated with opiate abuse.

 ## CLINICAL EXAMPLE

Mr. C was a 35-year-old man who had been jailed for auto theft. He was believed to be a member of a large ring of automobile thieves in a major metropolitan area. His previous arrest record included several episodes of armed robbery and breaking and entering. A few hours after he had been jailed, Mr. C complained of abdominal cramps and appeared very anxious. His nose and eyes were running, there were beads of perspiration on his brow, and he was rocking back and forth on his bunk. The guard called Ms. V, the correctional health nurse.

Ms. V observed Mr. C and performed a brief physical assessment. She noted that his pupils were dilated, his blood pressure was elevated, and he had "gooseflesh." In addition, there were multiple needle "tracks" on his arms. She asked him directly about drug use, and he admitted that he had been addicted to heroin. He stated that his addiction began in 1967 while he was stationed with the army in Vietnam. When he returned to the United States, he remained in the army for 18 months and was able to stop using drugs altogether. He planned to get a job and attend school after leaving the service. He related that he was disturbed by the attitude of people toward Vietnam veterans. While he was still in the service, he was able to use peer support to cope with his feelings. However, after his discharge, he was reluctant to talk about his military experience. Others seemed disinterested, embarrassed, or hostile when he talked about it.

Mr. C had difficulty finding a civilian job. He was an artillery specialist in the army and found that it was difficult to apply this experience. He began to have nightmares and "flashbacks" of his combat experiences. Because of the anxiety associated with this, he finally returned to drugs. Without a job, he used illegal means to finance his habit and therefore repeatedly went to jail.

Ms. V discussed Mr. C's problem with the physician in the prison health department. They decided to assess Mr. C's eligibility for a methadone drug treatment program and to request consultation from a counselor at the local Vietnam veterans counseling center.

Selected Nursing Diagnoses:

▼ Ineffective individual coping related to inability to obey the law as evidenced by repeated arrests

▼ Altered role performance related to difficulty adjusting to civilian life as evidenced by inability to find a job or seek out peer support

▼ Social isolation related to unresolved stressful military experiences as evidenced by reliance on drugs rather than people

▼ High risk for violence, directed at others, related to compelling need for drugs as evidenced by history of armed robbery

Withdrawal from narcotics is extremely uncomfortable but not usually life threatening. Overdosage of nar-

cotics, on the other hand, is very dangerous. It can lead rapidly to coma, respiratory depression, and death. Accidental overdoses among narcotic addicts sometimes occur, particularly when the user is uncertain of the drug's strength. Drugs are usually cut with inert (and sometimes toxic) substances before they are sold, resulting in the availability of varied strengths on the streets.

NATURAL OPIATES. In 1975 natural substances that acted very much like morphine were isolated in the brain. It was later learned that these biochemicals, known as endorphins or enkephalins, were neurotransmitters that bond with opiate receptors in the brain and pituitary gland. Release of these "natural opiates" results in a feeling of euphoria. This understanding has led to a theory of drug cravings: When large amounts of artificial opiates are taken over a long period of time, the brain responds by cutting off production of endorphins in an attempt to restore homeostasis. As the artificial opiates leave the system, there are no natural opiates to take their place. This deprivation is experienced as *craving*. Details of these mechanisms continue to be studied. It appears that what was thought of as a psychological response has a neurochemical basis. It is hoped that this knowledge will lead to effective biochemical treatments for drug dependence.

Hallucinogens. One behavior that represented the "drop-out" generation of the 1960s was the use of drugs that create experiences very similar to those typical of a psychotic state. These substances have been called *hallucinogens*, although they generally produce perceptual distortions, not true hallucinations. They have also been called *psychedelic* or "*mind-revealing*" drugs. LSD, peyote, mescaline, and psilocybin are commonly used hallucinogens, with LSD being the most commonly used.

LSD is generally swallowed. It is colorless and tasteless and is often added to a drink or food, such as a sugar cube. It may also be given to a person without that person knowing. Pleasurable effects of hallucinogen use include intensification of sensory experiences. Colors are described as more brilliant, and sounds, smells, and tastes are heightened. Sometimes users of these drugs report synesthesia, or a crossover of sensory experiences during which music may be seen or colors may be heard. Space and time are distorted.

The hallucinogens have not appeared to cause physical dependence. Tolerance does develop if they are used regularly. Hallucinogens also lead to self-destructive behavior because they cause impaired judgment. Vulnerable individuals who take these drugs may experience "bad trips," sometimes resulting in psychotic episodes. They may experience paranoid, grandiose, or somatic delusions, usually accompanied by vivid hallucinations.

The hallucinatory experience may be pleasant or frightening. Patients who are psychotic are not in contact with reality and frequently misinterpret environmental events. They may be unable to attend to any of their biological needs and also may inadvertently hurt themselves or others in response to hallucinations or while trying to escape from the frightening experience. Since there is no physical dependence, withdrawal symptoms do not occur. Usually there is a gradual decrease in psychotic behavior, although the patient may have "flashbacks" for several months. These brief recurrences of the hallucinogenic experience can be frightening. Patients often express the fear that they are crazy and will never be free of the after-effects of the drug.

A college classmate who is not a nursing major tells you that she overheard her 12-year-old brother talking with a friend about "doing microdots together." You suspect that he was talking about LSD. What would you advise her to do?

PCP. PCP use was very popular in the 1970s but today is less common than LSD in all age groups.[26,27] PCP was originally tested as an anesthetic-analgesic agent. It was withdrawn from testing on humans because of severe adverse reactions, sometimes including hallucinations, as the effects wore off. As a street drug it may be ingested, but it is frequently smoked in a mixture with another substance, such as marijuana. Severity of symptoms are dose dependent. At low doses (less than 5 mg) the user experiences a euphoric, floating feeling, along with heightened emotionality and incoordination. Distorted perceptions such as objects floating or growing in size, inability to judge distance, or feelings of being outside one's body are common. At higher doses PCP use may precipitate an intensely psychotic experience characterized by extreme agitation. Patients may become violent toward themselves or others. Because the drug is an anesthetic, PCP-intoxicated individuals feel little or no pain and may pound their head into a wall or strike out violently, causing serious injury to themselves or others. These persons may have other antisocial behaviors, such as insistence on removing their clothing or using profanity. Physical manifestations of PCP intoxication are noted in Table 22-3.

PCP use may cause the occurrence or exacerbation of a previously controlled psychosis. The unpredictability of the reaction to PCP makes it an extremely dangerous drug.

Co-dependence. When the term *co-dependence* was first coined in 1979, it referred to people who had become

dysfunctional as a result of living in a committed relationship with an alcoholic.[4] It was said that the alcoholic was addicted to the bottle, and the co-dependent was addicted to the alcoholic. The definition has expanded to include nonaddicted relationships, but the behaviors are the same. The co-dependent is obsessed with controlling other people's behavior. Other typical characteristics of co-dependents are listed in Box 22-3.

The co-dependent person has low self-esteem and tries to feel better by preoccupation with the lives, feelings, and problems of others. Although co-dependents want their loved ones to stop drinking or using drugs, their behavior may have the opposite effect and enable the person to continue drug or alcohol use.

The nurse may observe co-dependent behavior in family members of substance-dependent patients, in the patients themselves, or in nurses and other professionals. Simple questions to family members about efforts they have made to try to control the addict's use may uncover the pattern. Questions to the patient about relationships with others may indicate that co-dependence is at the root of the drug/alcohol problem. Listening to colleagues talk about their family and friends may reveal similar patterns in their relationships. Nurses tend to find great satisfaction in caring for others. When this behavior is the person's only source of self-esteem, it is done at the expense of personal health and welfare. It takes on a compulsive quality that is evidence of co-dependence.

Box 22-3

TYPICAL CHARACTERISTICS OF CO-DEPENDENCE

▼ Overcommit self
▼ Feel compelled to help others solve their problems
▼ Feel overly responsible for other people's feelings, thoughts, actions, needs, and well-being
▼ Feel worthless when not productive
▼ Feel trapped in relationships
▼ Feel "crazy" and wonder what is "normal"
▼ Afraid of own anger
▼ Tired and lack energy
▼ Feel uncomfortable when a compliment is given
▼ Always try to please others, not self
▼ Try to control events and how other people should behave
▼ Find it difficult to express emotions and make decisions
▼ Wish there was more time for exercise, hobbies, and sports
▼ Constantly seeking approval and affirmation

Adapted from Zerwekh J, Michaels B: *Nurs Clin North Am* 24:109, 1989.

Predisposing Factors

Several models or etiologies have been proposed for substance abuse. Belief in a particular model influences the assessment and intervention. Awareness of the differences between these models helps the nurse understand why patients, as well as other professionals, hold many different views about substance abuse treatment. Much research has been conducted concerning the factors that predispose a person to becoming chemically dependent. These factors may be biological, psychological, or sociocultural.

Biological.

A key biological factor is the tendency of substance abuse to run in families. Most genetic research has focused on alcoholism; very little is known about other drugs of abuse. There is much evidence from adoption, twin, and animal studies that heredity is significant in the development of alcoholism. Some research has identified subtypes of alcoholism that differ in inheritability. One type of alcoholism is associated with an early onset, inability to abstain, and an antisocial personality. This type appears to be primarily genetic in origin. Another type tends to be associated with onset after age 25, inability to stop drinking once started, and a passive-dependent personality. This type is influenced much more by the environment.[8]

Although still controversial, some researchers believe that they have identified a gene that is associated with transmission of alcoholism.[6] It is theorized that this genetic abnormality blocks feelings of well-being. This results in a tendency toward anxiety, anger, low self-esteem, or other negative feelings. There is a craving for a substance that will take the bad feelings away. Persons with such a disorder need alcohol or some other psychoactive drug just to feel "normal." Other researchers agree that there may be complex genetic factors involved in alcoholism, but they believe that a single gene is unlikely to be responsible for a large proportion of the illness.[12]

If genetic factors are clearly identified as major influences on the development of alcoholism in some people, what ethical issues are likely to be debated?

Biological differences in the response to alcohol may influence susceptibility. For example, many Asian people experience a physiological response to alcohol including flushing, tachycardia, and an intense feeling of discomfort. This appears to be related to the tendency for Asians to have a genetically inactive form of the enzyme aldehyde dehydrogenase. This leads to a buildup of the toxic substance acetaldehyde, an alcohol metabolite, which causes the symptoms.[32] This response may help explain why Asian-Americans have the lowest level of alcohol consumption and alcohol-related problems of the major racial and ethnic groups in the United States.

Psychological.

Many psychological theories have attempted to explain the factors that predispose people to developing substance abuse. *Psychoanalytic* theories see alcoholics as fixated at the oral stage of development, thus seeking need satisfaction through oral behaviors such as drinking. *Behavior* or *learning* theories view addictive behaviors as overlearned, maladaptive habits that can be examined and changed in the same way as other habits. *Family systems* theory emphasizes the pattern of relationships between family members through the generations as an explanation for substance abuse. It is easy to see how belief in any particular theory would influence assessment and treatment.

Clinicians have observed a link between substance abuse and several psychological traits such as depression, anxiety, antisocial personality, and dependent personality. There is no evidence that these psychological problems existed before or caused substance abuse. It is just as likely that they resulted from drug and alcohol use and dependence.

Many studies have tried to find common personality traits among persons addicted to alcohol or drugs. No addictive personality has been identified. Studies show a wide variety of personality types among alcoholics. Observed personality patterns result from the effects of the alcohol or drug on previously normal psychological functions, combined with ineffective responses to these effects.

Another theory of substance abuse focuses on the human tendency to seek pleasure and avoid pain or stress. Drugs create pleasure and reduce physical or psychological pain. Since pain returns when the effect of the drug wears off, the person is powerfully attracted to repeated drug use. It has been suggested that some people are more sensitive to the euphoric effects of drugs and are more likely to repeat their use. This repeated drug use leads to more problems and initiates the downhill spiral of substance use.

Some substance abusers have psychological problems related to childhood experiences. Many have histories of childhood physical or sexual abuse. Most have low self-esteem and difficulty expressing emotions. These problems may have influenced the initial use of drugs and progression into dependence. The nursing care of survivors of abuse is discussed in Chapter 37.

Sociocultural.

Several sociocultural factors influence a person's choice to use or not use drugs, which drugs to use, and how much to use them. Attitudes, values, norms, and sanctions differ according to nationality, religion, gender, family background, and social environment. Assessment of these factors is necessary to understand the whole person. Combinations of factors may make a person more susceptible to drug abuse and interfere with recovery.

Nationality and ethnicity influence alcohol use patterns. For example, it has been found that Northern Europeans have higher alcoholism rates than Southern Europeans. Values may influence the way in which addiction is viewed. Some believe that addiction results from moral weakness or lack of willpower. Unfortunately a moralistic approach may cause the person to feel guilty, often resulting in drinking to alleviate the guilt.

Formal religious belief can also affect drinking behavior. Members of religions that discourage the use of alcohol have much lower rates of alcohol use and alcoholism than members of those that accept or encourage its use. Of the major religious groups in the United States, Roman Catholics have the highest rate of alcoholism and Jews the lowest. During assessment, however, the nurse should not assume certain use or nonuse patterns related to ethnic or religious factors. For instance, a Jewish patient may be alcoholic even though that religion has the lowest rate of alcoholism.

Gender differences also have been noted in the prevalence of substance abuse. Research is needed to determine the influence of biological as opposed to sociocultural reasons for this. However, powerful gender-related cultural factors help to shape substance-using behaviors. There is much less acceptance of female alcoholism, which is often hidden. Women tend to deny having a drinking problem even longer than men do. In the United States more women than men abuse prescription drugs such as diazepam. This is more socially acceptable and sometimes even encouraged. In contrast, use of antianxiety drugs is viewed as weak and unmasculine, whereas the ability to drink large amounts of alcohol is considered manly.

Finally, broad, sociocultural factors have influenced drug use, abuse, and treatment since the 1960s. Multiple social crises have contributed to the risk for drug abuse in poor neighborhoods.[17] Affordable and decent housing and shelter are difficult to find. Job opportunities are limited, and many jobs are low paying. Social programs have often inadvertently fostered development of single-parent families. The drop-out rate in inner-city schools is high, and advanced education is difficult to obtain. Living in neighborhoods dominated by these problems plus poor health-care access, crime, and violence creates vulnerability to the escape some people find in drugs and alcohol. However, it is important to recognize that the majority of people living in these circumstances are not addicted to drugs, which

supports the belief that many factors influence the development of drug use patterns.

 What sociocultural factors have you observed that encourage the use of drugs and alcohol?

Precipitating Stressors

Withdrawal. Symptoms of withdrawal from particular drugs of abuse are listed in Table 22-3. Medically, withdrawal from CNS depressants is the most dangerous. It is important for the nurse to understand the expected symptoms of withdrawal and the associated medical dangers. With appropriate medical and nursing management, excessive discomfort and risk of serious complications can be minimized.

It is possible to predict the severity and duration of withdrawal symptoms by following three general guidelines:

1. The longer the period of time between last use and appearance of withdrawal symptoms and the longer these symptoms last, the less intense they will be.
2. The longer the half-life of the drug, the longer withdrawal symptoms will last.
3. The longer the half-life of the drug, the less intense the withdrawal symptoms will be.

For example, if a person has alcohol withdrawal symptoms within 2 hours after the last drink, the withdrawal syndrome will probably be more intense than if the symptoms appear after 18 hours. As another example, the withdrawal symptoms from methadone, which has a long half-life, are less severe than from heroin.

The pattern of withdrawal symptoms is so similar for all of the central nervous system depressant drugs that it has been called the "general depressant withdrawal syndrome."[15] Severe withdrawal symptoms can result when these drugs are taken at two or more times the maximum therapeutic range for more than a month.[37] Alcohol is the model for the withdrawal syndrome and is presented in more detail.

When a large amount of alcohol is ingested, unpleasant symptoms usually occur. If overindulgence is short-lived, symptoms are caused by the direct effect of alcohol on body cells. This results in headache and stomach and intestinal distress—the typical "hangover." However, if heavy drinking occurs over a long time, a decrease in blood alcohol level may cause symptoms of withdrawal.

Alcohol sedates the central nervous system. When alcohol is withdrawn, the symptoms resemble a "rebound reaction" in the CNS. The first symptoms usually occur

4 to 6 hours after the last drink and include agitation, anxiety, tremors, diaphoresis, insomnia, nausea, vomiting, mild tachycardia, and hypertension. The severity of symptoms depends on the quantity, frequency, and duration of consumption and how quickly the blood level drops. Symptoms usually disappear in hours or days but could last as long as 2 weeks. A person who drinks large amounts over long periods of time may develop more severe symptoms sometimes progressing to delirium tremens (DTs), which may be fatal.

Grand mal seizures, sometimes called "rum fits," may occur, usually between 6 and 48 hours after the last drink. A history of seizures or photophobia may predispose a person in withdrawal to seizures. Conditions such as hypomagnesemia, hypoglycemia, and respiratory alkalosis have also been associated with seizures.[5] Other causes of seizures should be explored, including trauma and use of other drugs. Seizures occurring after 10 to 14 days of abstinence generally indicate dependence on a long-acting CNS depressant.

Alcoholic hallucinosis is characterized by auditory, visual, or tactile hallucinations in the absence of other psychotic behavior. It usually occurs about 48 hours after the last drink. The person is usually oriented, rational, and may not even admit to hallucinations unless reassured that they are not due to mental illness. One way to obtain this information is to ask the patient about nightmares and vivid daydreams.[7] This condition generally lasts for a few hours or a day, although it may last 1 to 2 weeks and in rare instances becomes chronic.[5] The person experiencing alcoholic hallucinosis is not disoriented. Disorientation should be reported immediately because it may herald the onset of alcohol withdrawal delirium (delirium tremens, or DTs).

Alcohol withdrawal delirium is considered to be a medical emergency because it can be fatal even with appropriate medical intervention. It is characterized by an exaggeration of earlier symptoms plus paranoia, disorientation, delusions, visual hallucinations, elevated vital signs, vomiting, diarrhea, and diaphoresis. Alcohol withdrawal delirium usually occurs 3 to 5 days after the last drink and lasts 2 to 3 days.

The Clinical Institute Withdrawal Assessment–Alcohol (CIWA-AD)[30] is a tool that was developed for use in monitoring the symptoms of alcohol withdrawal to determine appropriate intervention. An opioid withdrawal assessment (CINA)[28] has also been developed. Nurses may find these tools helpful in monitoring patient responses to medication and other aspects of nursing care. Table 22-3 summarizes the important aspects of withdrawal from the opioids and other abused substances.

Pregnancy. Since most of the drugs that are abused cross the placental barrier, women should be counseled about the possible effects of substance use during pregnancy. Congenital abnormalities have occurred in infants of mothers who have taken drugs. A fetal alcohol syndrome has been identified, which involves a pattern of physical growth and mental deficiencies. In addition, use during pregnancy of drugs that cause physical dependence can result in the birth of an addicted baby who must be withdrawn from the drug. The safest pregnancy is one in which the mother is totally drug and alcohol free with one exception: for pregnant women addicted to heroin, methadone maintenance is safer for the fetus than acute opiate detoxification.

Some policymakers have proposed that pregnant women who abuse substances should be jailed, placed under house arrest, or committed to a mental hospital until the baby is born. Do you agree with this? Support your position. Do you have the same opinion related to all abused substances, including alcohol?

Coping Resources

Coping resources are those life skills that enable the person who abuses substances to survive. The nurse needs to identify these skills and assist the patient to redirect them toward overcoming addiction. Many persons develop very effective *communication* and *assertiveness skills* while trying to obtain drugs or convince others that they do not have a problem. Some have strong *social support systems* consisting of people who can be enlisted to help the person through recovery. This may be family and friends or members of a self-help group. *Pleasurable activities* that are not related to substance use should be identified, as should *stress reduction techniques* that may have been effective in the past. *Vocational skills* may be reinforced and offer a focus for future goals.

It is essential for the person who is facing recovery from substance abuse to have a strong *motivation* to change behavior. The nurse should identify the reasons that the patient has for seeking treatment and work to reinforce them. The person who has a low level of motivation is less likely to recover successfully.

Coping Mechanisms

People who abuse substances develop coping mechanisms to assist them to handle the painful emotions that are usually associated with the problem. These may include guilt, shame, depression, hopelessness, anger, and fear of discovery. Many attempt to cover up substance use. Small lies to hide the behavior may progress to *denial*, with the person involved believing the distortions in reality. *Rationalizations* are common. The alcoholic may claim that an alcohol-related automobile accident happened because the road was poorly lighted or may use *projection* and blame the other driver. *Minimization* of the amount of alcohol or drug used is frequent, except in some cultures that reward high intake of alcohol by men.

These ego defenses must be recognized for their anxiety-reducing function. During the intervention phase the nurse works with the patient to substitute effective coping resources for the ineffective coping mechanisms and the substance-abusing behavior.

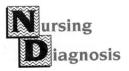

Nursing Diagnosis

After completion of the nursing assessment the nurse synthesizes the data regarding the patient's drinking or drug use behavior. Using the stress adaptation model (Fig. 22-3) and the NANDA classification system, appropriate nursing diagnoses are identified.

Addiction problems are very complex. They affect nearly every aspect of the patient's functioning. The nurse should be sure that the nursing diagnoses selected for an individual reflect the whole person. At least

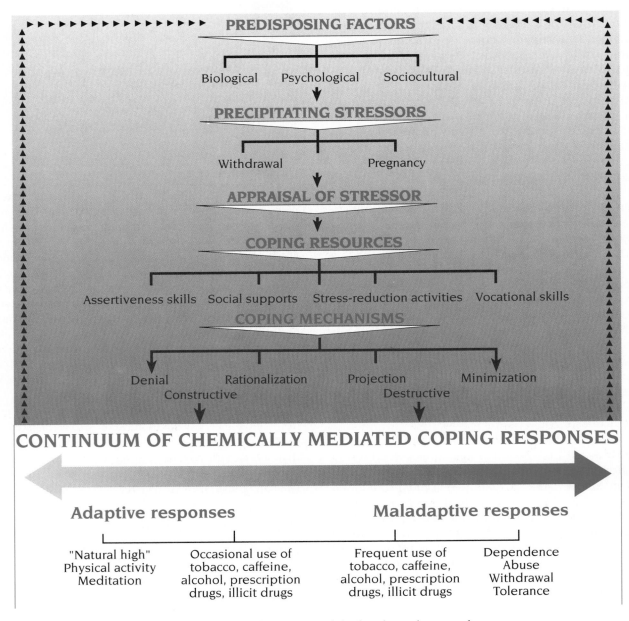

Fig. 22-3 A stress adaptation model related to substance abuse.

27 nursing diagnoses are common in addictions nursing practice,[1] which can be grouped into four categories: biological, cognitive, psychosocial, and spiritual. Nursing diagnoses related to chemically mediated responses and medical diagnoses for substance-related disorders are listed in the Medical and Nursing Diagnoses box. The primary NANDA diagnoses and examples of complete nursing diagnoses are presented in the Detailed Diagnoses box.

Related Medical Diagnoses

Disorders that are related to substance abuse are included in DSM-IV[2] in two ways. Diagnoses that are primarily related to alcohol or drug use are categorized as Substance-Related Disorders. The essential features of these are presented in the Detailed Diagnoses box.

However, if substance-induced intoxication or withdrawal is associated with another type of mental disorder, the diagnosis is located in that category. For example, if a person is depressed related to alcohol withdrawal, the medical diagnosis would be "substance-induced (withdrawal) mood disorder." The categories that include substance-induced diagnoses are delirium, dementia, amnestic, psychotic, mood, anxiety, sex, and sleep.

Dual Diagnosis

There are several ways to view the relationship between drug use and psychiatric illness. Psychiatric symptoms can be regarded as caused by or the cause of drug use. When psychiatric symptoms appear first, they are seen as the cause of drug use. Patients using drugs under these conditions are said to be "self-medicating" their psychiatric symptoms. This may be the case when the schizophrenic patient drinks or uses a drug to quiet auditory hallucinations; or when a person begins drinking after the death of a loved one. However, many addicts use dysphoric mood as a rationalization for drug use. In these situations the drugs cause the psychiatric problems. Examples are when alcoholism leads to depression or paranoia, or hallucinogen or amphetamine use leads to psychosis.

Drug intoxication or withdrawal can mimic any psychiatric symptom. In crisis situations or initial interviews it is often impossible to determine which condition came first. Information from other sources can be helpful. If the symptoms disappear after an extended period of abstinence, then most likely they were caused by, not the cause of, drug use.

It is also possible for the drug problem and psychiatric condition to coexist as separate illnesses. This is generally called *dual diagnosis*. In this case both conditions require treatment. Generally, abstinence is the first

goal so that other symptoms can be identified without the influence of the drug. However, the priority of treatment may shift to the psychiatric symptoms if these are creating a danger to the patient. For instance, if a patient is suicidal, then this problem takes priority over all others and psychiatric hospitalization may be required. The psychiatric symptoms may also need to be treated first if they interfere with the person's ability to abstain. Sometimes it is possible to treat both conditions at the same time.

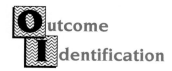 How would you respond to a patient who prefers street drugs over prescribed medication because of the side effects of the medication?

Outcome Identification

The expected outcome related to withdrawal is:
The patient will overcome addiction safely and with a minimum of discomfort.
Short-term goals related to this phase of recovery may include the following:
1. The patient will withdraw from dependence on the abused substance.
2. The patient will be oriented to time, place, person, and situation.
3. The patient will report symptoms of withdrawal.
4. The patient will correctly interpret environmental stimuli.
5. The patient will recognize and talk about hallucinations or delusions.

For persons dependent on drugs or alcohol, the expected outcome is:
The patient will abstain from all mood-altering chemicals.
Studies have shown that persons who are dependent on a drug or alcohol cannot safely return to any level of use of any addicting drug. If they do, eventually the vast majority return to their old addictive patterns. However, patients often become very anxious at the thought of never again using the substance to which they are addicted. Therefore it may be helpful to focus on short-term goals. Short-term goals related to abstinence may include the following:
1. The patient will agree to remain drug and alcohol free for 1 week, with the agreement to be renewed weekly.
2. The patient will make a daily commitment to be abstinent.

MEDICAL AND NURSING DIAGNOSES RELATED TO CHEMICALLY MEDIATED RESPONSES

Related Medical Diagnoses (DSM-IV)*

Alcohol dependence
Alcohol abuse
Alcohol intoxication
Alcohol withdrawal
Amphetamine (or related substance) dependence
Amphetamine (or related substance) abuse
Amphetamine (or related substance) intoxication
Amphetamine (or related substance) withdrawal
Caffeine intoxication
Cannabis dependence
Cannabis abuse
Cannabis intoxication
Cocaine dependence
Cocaine abuse
Cocaine intoxication
Cocaine withdrawal
Hallucinogen dependence
Hallucinogen abuse
Hallucinogen intoxication
Hallucinogen persisting perception disorder (flash-backs)
Inhalant dependence
Inhalant abuse
Inhalant intoxication
Nicotine dependence
Nicotine withdrawal
Opioid dependence
Opioid abuse
Opioid intoxication
Opioid withdrawal
Phencyclidine (or related substance) dependence
Phencyclidine (or related substance) abuse
Phencyclidine (or related substance) intoxication
Sedative, hypnotic, or anxiolytic dependence
Sedative, hypnotic, or anxiolytic abuse
Sedative, hypnotic, or anxiolytic intoxication
Sedative, hypnotic, or anxiolytic withdrawal
Polysubstance dependence
Other (or unknown) substance dependence
Other (or unknown) substance abuse
Other (or unknown) substance intoxication
Other (or unknown) substance withdrawal

Related Nursing Diagnoses (NANDA)†
Biological responses

Growth and development, altered
Infection, potential for
Injury, potential for
Nutrition, altered
Pain
Self-care deficit
‡Sensory-perceptual alteration
Sexual dysfunction
Sleep pattern disturbance

Cognitive responses

Knowledge deficit
Noncompliance
‡Thought processes, altered

Psychosocial responses

Anxiety
Communication, impaired verbal
‡Coping, ineffective individual
Family processes, altered
Fear
Growth and development, altered
Parenting, altered
Self-esteem disturbance
Social isolation
Violence, potential for

Spiritual responses

Grieving, dysfunctional
Hopelessness (also psychological)
Powerlessness
Spiritual distress

*From American Psychiatric Association: *Diagnostic and statistical manual of mental disorders*, ed 4, Washington, DC, 1994, The Association.
†From North American Nursing Diagnosis Association: NANDA *nursing diagnoses: definitions and classifications* 1992-1993, Philadelphia, 1992, The Association.
‡Primary nursing diagnosis for chemically mediated response.

DETAILED DIAGNOSES
RELATED TO CHEMICALLY MEDIATED RESPONSES

NANDA Diagnosis Stem	Examples of Complete Diagnosis
Sensory-perceptual alteration	Sensory-perceptual alteration related to hallucinogen ingestion as evidenced by visual hallucination of snakes in the bed
Altered thought processes	Altered thought processes related to alcohol withdrawal as evidenced by disorientation to time person and place
Ineffective individual coping	Ineffective individual coping related to cocaine abuse of 6 months' duration as evidenced by loss of job and lack of personal goals

DSM-IV Diagnosis	Essential Features*
Substance dependence	Maladaptive pattern of substance use characterized by any three of the following within 12 months: tolerance; withdrawal; using more of the substance or using for longer than planned; persistent desire or unsuccessful efforts to cut down or control use; much time spent in efforts to obtain, use, or recover from use; interference with social, occupational, or recreational activities; continued use despite knowledge of use-related recurrent physical or psychological problems
Substance abuse	Maladaptive pattern of substance use characterized by one or more of the following within 12 months: recurrent use resulting in failure to meet role obligations, recurrent use in physically hazardous situations, recurrent use-related legal problems, continued use despite persistent or recurrent use-related social or interpersonal problems, has never met the criteria for dependence for this class of substance

*Adapted from the American Psychiatric Association: *Diagnostic and statistical manual of mental disorders,* ed 4, Washington, DC, 1994, The Association. A single set of essential features has been developed for substance dependence and for substance abuse. The essential features of intoxication and withdrawal vary according to the substance and are listed in Table 22-3.

3. The patient will attend at least two support group meetings weekly.
4. The patient will contact a supportive person if he experiences an urge to use an addictive substance.

Development of some kind of support system is an essential expected outcome for drug-dependent patients. Once abstinence and support system goals are established, attention can turn to learning about dependence and recovery and development of alternate coping skills. Goals related to the person's job, relationships, or education should be deferred until later, unless any are a roadblock to recovery. For instance, a person is usually encouraged to focus on self and not on a relationship. However, if the person's spouse is an alcoholic and violence in the home is common, then the priority shifts to finding a safe place to live.

Goals should be worded so that it is clear that the patient is responsible for behavior. Addicted patients often want others to do the work for them. Nurses sometimes comply because they want to be helpful. However, such behavior does not help in the long run. Writing the goals and a specific plan of action into a contract and providing the patient with a copy of the contract will reinforce the patient's responsibility. The contract should be signed by both the nurse and the patient.

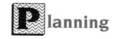 **lanning**

The nursing care plan should be developed by considering the expected long- and short-term outcomes of intervention. Priority must be given to the most immediate needs. For patients who are experiencing drug withdrawal, the highest priority is given to stabilization of the patient's physiological status until the crisis of withdrawal is over.

Once safety needs are met, abstinence and support system issues must be addressed. Plans related to these needs must be made in collaboration with the patient, considering the overall assessment and taking into account the patient's individual current life situation and desires. Family members and supportive friends may also be included in the planning process. This will assist them to understand the problems that the patient may encounter as recovery continues.

The nurse must be aware that it is rare for an addicted person suddenly to stop substance use forever. Most addicts try at least once and usually several times to use the substance in a controlled way. It is important for addicts to know that they should return to treatment after these relapses. Then they can learn from what they did and try to prevent further relapses. These issues should be addressed openly in the planning process.

Planning related to addictions often includes a major focus on education of the patient and support system members. Self-help groups such as Alcoholics Anonymous (AA) or Narcotics Anonymous (NA) are good sources of information related to substance abuse. Assisting patients to identify community educational programs sponsored by schools, hospitals, and other organizations is also helpful. In addition to receiving useful information, they may meet other people who are coping with similar problems.

Implementation

The nurse encounters patients with substance abuse problems in all health-care settings. The types of interventions recommended depend largely on the setting in which the nurse works. When encountering these patients outside of addiction treatment programs, the nurse may be able to refer the person to treatment. If a patient has a history of seizures or serious withdrawal symptoms or is at risk for developing symptoms because of a heavy, chronic use pattern, the first referral should be to a detoxification program. Otherwise, referral should be to the program that appears to match the patient's level of severity. Research is being conducted to determine the relationship between patient variables and treatment variables to ensure the best treatment outcome. This "treatment matching" approach holds promise for improving effectiveness and efficiency of care.

Biological Interventions

Substance abusers frequently come into contact with the health-care system because of a physiological crisis. It may be related to overdose, withdrawal, allergy, or toxicity. There may be physical deterioration caused by the damaging effects of drugs, including such conditions as malnutrition, dehydration, and various infections, including HIV. When an acute physical condition is present, it takes priority over the other health needs of the patient. It is particularly important to attend to the condition that the patient has identified as the problem. The nurse is then seen as potentially helpful and will have more credibility when other aspects of the addiction are addressed.

Only two drugs have been approved for the treatment of drug abuse:

1. Methadone, a partial agonist-antagonist that is taken in place of street heroin
2. Naltrexone, a narcotic antagonist that blocks the effects of opiates in the brain. Addicts who are motivated for abstinence may choose to take naltrexone to prevent a high if they should relapse and use heroin

Three other drugs are expected to be approved for use in drug abuse treatment in the near future. These are LAAM (1-acetyl-alpha-methadol), a long-acting substitute for heroin, and buprenorphine and clonidine, which are used for withdrawal symptoms.

Intervening in Withdrawal. If the patient is physically dependent on a drug, withdrawal symptoms may occur when the blood level of the drug drops suddenly. Since some of these symptoms are at best uncomfortable and at worst life threatening, medical and nursing interventions are planned to prevent severe withdrawal symptoms. The process of assisting an addict safely through withdrawal is called **detoxification.** Actually the liver detoxifies the substance. Medications and nursing actions only help to relieve the symptoms. Gradual weaning from the substance may be instituted, especially if the person is addicted to prescription drugs, such as barbiturates, amphetamines, or benzodiazepines. Another approach is the use of a longer-acting, cross-tolerant drug with a similar action to prevent the occurrence of withdrawal symptoms. For instance, chlordiazepoxide may be given to assist with alcohol withdrawal. The dose of the substituted drug is then tapered down and eventually discontinued. Such a process is best accomplished in an inpatient setting or in a closely monitored outpatient setting. Even with monitoring in place, it is possible for the patient to develop a dependence on the substitute drug or even continue to use the original substance.

A variation on this approach is used when daily

methadone is substituted for heroin. This is called **methadone maintenance.** The goal of the treatment program may be either gradual withdrawal from methadone or indefinite maintenance at a stable dose. The decision between these alternatives is based on assessment of the likelihood of recidivism (habitual relapsing) if the person becomes drug free. This treatment approach has been controversial because methadone is a narcotic. However, addiction to methadone does not cause impaired functioning; thus the person can be productive while addicted. Those in favor of methadone maintenance point out the benefits of avoiding the debilitating effects of heroin addiction and the life-style associated with obtaining illegal drugs on the streets.

Methadone maintenance is essentially substituting a legal narcotic for an illegal one. Do you believe that this is a responsible practice? State the reasons for your position.

Withdrawal symptoms may occur in spite of efforts to prevent them. Substance abusers do not always give accurate drug-use histories, although it is extremely important to obtain as specific an assessment as possible. If the amount of substance used has been understated or if multiple abuse is undetected, withdrawal symptoms may occur. The possibility of seizures should always be anticipated. Emergency equipment should be at hand. Drug abuse should always be considered possible when unexpected seizures occur. If drug abuse is suspected, the physician should be informed so that blood and urine specimens can be collected for laboratory analysis and an appropriate treatment plan initiated.

If withdrawal is appropriately managed, the patient should be slightly sedated, but not asleep. The nurse should be sure to look for objective signs of withdrawal, in addition to the patient's report. For example, a heroin patient may claim to have abdominal and muscle cramps because the nurse can't prove otherwise; the patient actually wants another dose of methadone. Alcoholic patients may claim to have vomited in the toilet; however, it is important that this be observed directly, since these patients may want a higher dose of the drug being used for withdrawal. The nurse should be alert for inconsistencies in the reported pattern of symptoms. It may mean that the patient is pretending more severe withdrawal or that another condition or type of withdrawal is superimposed on the first. Quick responses to any change in condition are necessary. Alcohol withdrawal is more easily controlled while in its mild form.

Once symptoms have progressed to DTs, little can be done except supportive care until the crisis is over.

A quiet, calm environment is helpful for patients experiencing the general depressant withdrawal syndrome. This helps the patient relax and decreases nervous system irritability. Reassurance in a calm, quiet tone of voice is also helpful. To help maintain the patient's orientation, the nurse should place a clock within sight and give frequent, low-key reminders about who they are, where they are, the nurse's name, and the day of the week. If possible, another patient who is further along in detoxification may be assigned as a buddy so that the patient is not left alone. A family member may also help.

The patient in withdrawal should be treated symptomatically. Fluids should be encouraged only if the person is dehydrated. Eating should be encouraged, and vitamins are usually ordered. Tylenol or Kaopectate, if ordered, may be given for discomfort or diarrhea. A small amount of milk may be offered frequently to help manage epigastric distress. Seizure precautions should be taken. A cool washcloth can be offered for use on the forehead if the patient is feeling warm or diaphoretic. Position changes, assistance with ambulation, and changing damp clothing are also indicated. Evidence suggests that offering this type of intense, supportive care can reduce withdrawal symptoms rapidly and often dramatically without medications.[30] If the patient is receiving large doses of benzodiazepines, the nurse should monitor for signs of toxicity, such as ataxia and nystagmus. Always, the patient should be treated with respect and dignity.

Intervening in Toxic Psychosis. Users of LSD, PCP, and stimulants often come to the emergency room in acute toxic psychosis. The behavior may be quite similar to that of the schizophrenic patient. However, there may be no history of abnormal behavior. Careful assessment of an acute psychotic reaction, particularly in an adolescent or young adult, should include exploration of drug use. It may be necessary to interview friends of the patient to obtain this information. An attempt should be made to identify the specific drug used, although LSD and PCP may be taken without the knowledge of the person involved.

There is an important difference in the nursing approach to users of PCP and amphetamine as opposed to those who have an adverse reaction to LSD. Unless the psychiatric symptomatology is severe, LSD users experiencing a "bad trip" frequently respond to reassurance and may be "talked down." Patient should be oriented frequently and discouraged from closing their eyes because this may make the symptoms worse. However, victims of PCP-induced psychosis do not respond well to attempts at interaction. Agitated PCP and amphetamine users are more likely to strike out in response to their misperceptions and panic. They are potentially more harmful to themselves and others.[35] This aggression may be totally unprovoked. In addition, since PCP is also an anesthetic, these patients feel minimal, if any, pain. For this reason, they seem to have enormous strength. They do not feel pain when they exceed the limits of their muscular capability and may continue pushing, pulling, or hitting until they seriously damage themselves or others.

Other elements of treatment are basically the same for acutely agitated LSD and PCP patients. Both require a safe environment that has minimum stimulation. Staff should not perform any procedures without a thorough explanation, should not touch the patient without permission, and should avoid rapid movements in the patient's presence. Adequate staff should be present to control impulsive behavior. Vital signs should be monitored and other physiological needs met. Although restraints may exacerbate muscle damage and agitation, they may be necessary, especially if a seclusion room is not available. Benzodiazepines are the treatment of choice, followed by high-potency antipsychotic medications if they are ineffective.[36] Excretion of PCP is aided by acidifying the urine by giving the patient cranberry juice or ascorbic acid.[35] Gastric lavage may be necessary for persistent symptoms or if an overdose has been taken, although this is not recommended for PCP patients because it increases agitation.

Disulfiram Therapy.

Another long-term biological approach to substance abuse is the prescription of disulfiram (Antabuse) for alcoholics. This drug interrupts the metabolism of alcohol, causing a buildup of a toxic substance in the body if the person uses alcohol in any form. The physiological response may include a severe headache, nausea and vomiting, flushing, hypotension, tachycardia, dyspnea, diaphoresis, chest pain, palpitations, dizziness and confusion. It can also lead to respiratory and cardiac collapse, unconsciousness, convulsions, and death. Antabuse should never be forced on a patient or given without the patient's stated willingness to comply. It is also important that the patient agree to take disulfiram only after careful instruction about the potential consequences of drinking while taking the drug. This instruction should include a written list of alcohol-containing preparations to be avoided, including cough medicines, rubbing compounds, vinegars, aftershave lotions, and some mouthwashes. Drinking must be avoided for 14 days after disulfiram has been discontinued. This medication cannot prevent someone who is determined to drink from drinking. This person can simply wait until the disulfiram has been excreted.

However, it helps to prevent impulsive drinking because the person does have to wait to be able to drink safely. This treatment should be used in conjunction with other supportive therapies, not by itself.

> Describe the information that should be provided to a patient who is to be treated with disulfiram (Antabuse). What issues related to informed consent should be considered in the use of this drug?

Psychological Interventions

Before initiating nursing intervention with a substance-abusing patient, the nurse must develop self-awareness of feelings and attitudes about the problem. It is recommended that a values clarification approach be used, as described in Chapter 2. Most people have had personal contact with substance abuse by family, friends, or colleagues. This problem creates many negative feelings. It is important that the nurse be able to differentiate feelings associated with past situations from those aroused by contacts with patients and their families. A supervisor, teacher, or senior clinical nurse can be of assistance when a nurse is having difficulty sorting out these feelings.

Group Therapy.

Group psychotherapy is the preferred method of treatment for persons with addiction. Chapter 29 provides detailed information about therapeutic groups. Addiction groups are somewhat different from other therapy groups. As mentioned earlier, addicts tend to deny their addiction and avoid emotional issues. Through their patterns of use, many have become very manipulative and "conning." They have learned to say what other people seem to want to hear or what will get them what they want. When uncomfortable, they may change the subject or give long, vague answers to questions. They tend to rationalize their behavior and minimize its effect on themselves and others. Addicts bring these same behaviors to the group. They need feedback to recognize and change these behavior patterns.[9]

Feedback is the honest reaction of group members to what the speaker says. It is based on the content of what the person says and on previous experiences with the speaker. Although feedback from one person, especially the therapist, may be discounted, it is difficult for the addict to ignore feedback from several group members. They are very sensitive to such behaviors because they have used them themselves. They are hard to fool.

When confronted in a focused way, the group pressure to examine and change negative behavior can be very intense.

 A group member says he has read a newspaper report saying that studies have found that some alcoholics can learn to drink in a controlled way. How would you respond?

Intervening in Denial. Denial must be confronted because it is a potential obstacle to recovery. Most patients deny their inability to control their substance-abusing behavior even when they have serious drug-related problems. For instance, an intoxicated person who has caused an automobile accident may claim to have drank "just a few beers." Barbiturate addicts may claim they can stop whenever they want to do so. The denial is partially related to the stigma of drug abuse.

It is difficult to apply the term *alcoholic* or *addict* to oneself. Denial also protects addicts or alcoholics from admitting that they are unable to control their behavior. Self-control is central to the self-concept of most people. Admitting a problem is also the first step toward behavioral change. Commitment to change frightens the substance-dependent person. It involves a decision to stop using a substance that has become the major focus of the person's life. Anyone who has tried to diet or stop smoking cigarettes can understand to some extent the anxiety aroused by this decision.

It is essential that denial be overcome and the patient make the commitment to behavioral change. Family members and co-workers too often enable the person to continue drinking, using drugs, and related inappropriate behavior by avoiding direct communication about these problems. To break through the denial, honest feedback with specific evidence of substance abuse problems must be given to the addict by people who care (see A Patient Speaks).

A specific method of intervention has been developed by the Johnson Institute.[18] In this method concerned persons meet in advance to plan the intervention. Each writes a list of specific instances that show how the patient's substance abuse has affected him or her personally. The group decides how to persuade the addict to come to a place where they will all be gathered. During the encounter each person takes a turn saying how important the person is and then reads items from the list aloud. This serves as a loving confrontation. Then they present the bottom line, which usually includes treatment options and consequences for choosing not to go into treatment. Arrangements have

A PATIENT SPEAKS

I have abused drugs and alcohol for many years. One thing that has been important is for nurses to spend time with me so I can learn to trust them. It helps when they make sure I schedule treatment appointments and keep them. Substance abuse education is very important, and it has to be repeated over and over.

I've been through detoxification many times. Some of the nurses in those programs have coddled me. This makes it easy for me to dance around issues of sobriety. I've had the best success with the nurse who will get in my face and cut me no slack. The nurses who confront me and have high expectations leave me enough room to help myself, but not enough to be dishonest. There needs to be a balance of empathy and toughness. It's not easy, but that's the role for the nurse to establish. ▼

been made to take the person directly to a treatment facility. Like group therapy, this technique serves as a very powerful incentive for behavioral change.

Intervening in Dependence. Some addicts are people-pleasers who are dependent on others for approval and self-esteem. This dependency is evident in all of the person's relationships. If the person is too dependent on others, this dependency may drive them away, thus increasing the person's need to depend on alcohol or drugs. Mr. B in the following clinical example illustrates this dependency.

CLINICAL EXAMPLE

Mr. B was a 45-year-old man who was admitted to the medical unit of a general hospital with a diagnosis of gastritis. He complained of abdominal pain, nausea, and vomiting. He had a slightly elevated temperature of 37.5° C (100° F). When the admitting nurse who was completing the nursing assessment asked Mr. B about alcohol use, he said he had "a couple of beers" after work everyday. He also reported that his wife had left him the day before admission. He said he was not sure why she left, but he was sure she would be back. Mrs. B did come to the hospital to visit her husband. His primary nurse met with them together and asked Mrs. B why she left. She said she was tired of putting Mr. B to bed every night after he passed out from drinking and did not want to continue to call his employer saying he was sick when he was really hung over. She had threatened to leave before, but Mr. B had always begged her to stay and she had relented. She had married him because she felt sorry for him. He had been living alone and was not taking good care of himself. She revealed that her first husband was also an alcoholic and her father had been one as well. She would agree to try again to make the marriage a success if he would agree to stop drinking and seek counseling. Mr. B said to the nurse, "I'll be good and do what she says. You tell her I'll be good."

Selected Nursing Diagnoses:

▼ Ineffective individual coping related to reluctance to be responsible for his behavior as evidenced by denial of why his wife left

▼ Ineffective family coping, disabling, related to repetitive dysfunctional behavior patterns of both spouses as evidenced by cycles of drinking, threats to leave, and promises to change

▼ Pain related to gastritis evidenced by verbal complaints

Mr. B used alcohol to avoid responsibility for his actions and his life. He used his wife in a similar way. When Mrs. B confronted him with her expectations, he responded in a childlike way and tried to place the nurse in the parental role. This avoidance of responsibility is a behavior that is very difficult to change. The nurse must be careful not to make decisions for the patient.

Mrs. B represents the co-dependence that may occur in spouses of substance-abusing patients. She is a woman who appears to be drawn to dependent men. She is probably a very maternal person who likes to take care of others. This increases the possibility that she will assume the role of enabler. The enabler perpetuates the substance abuse problem by not confronting the substance abuser and by helping to cover up the problem. When Mrs. B called Mr. B's employer to say he was sick, she was being an enabler. When significant others play an enabling role, family counseling or family support groups help the family accept and support the changing behavior of the patient.

Intervening in Low Self-Esteem. Assertiveness training can assist both the dependent substance abuser and significant others to accomplish a behavioral change. More information about assertiveness may be found in Chapter 27. An increase in assertiveness may also have a positive effect on self-esteem. Although some substance abusers appear self-confident, most have little basic regard for themselves. The relaxation, euphoria, or release of inhibitions given by the drug helps the person overcome this sense of inferiority. An

important goal of nursing care must be to find new ways of bolstering the person's self-esteem. This can be difficult because many of these patients have destroyed the relationships and activities that normally build self-esteem. One thing the patient can do without the help of anyone else is to use self-affirmations. Self-affirmations are positive self-statements meant to be repeated several times a day to oneself. The nurse also needs to help the person identify remaining strengths and build on them. Strengths may be related to overcoming the substance abuse problem itself. This is true of Bobby in the next clinical example.

 ## CLINICAL EXAMPLE

Bobby was a 17-year-old who was admitted to the hospital acutely psychotic with a history of recent use of PCP. The emergency room nurse noted scarring of the veins in Bobby's arm and surmised that he was also a user of heroin. Blood and urine testing confirmed this suspicion. Bobby recovered from his psychotic episode in 24 hours but was then extremely uncomfortable due to opiate withdrawal. The decision was made to use titrated doses of methadone to assist with the withdrawal. Mr. L, a young nurse, established a close relationship with Bobby during this time. Bobby requested the nurse's help in planning for his future, but doubted that he had the strength to stay away from drugs. He was advised to take a day at a time. Mr. L took Bobby on a visit to a drug treatment program, and he agreed to try membership in one of the groups at this center. Bobby did well in the group and was very helpful to new members, describing his experiences and encouraging them to "take 1 day at a time." Bobby expressed an interest in finishing school and said he would like to become a drug counselor. The staff of the drug treatment program agreed that Bobby seemed to have an aptitude for that role and encouraged him to pursue his goal.

Selected Nursing Diagnoses:

▼ Altered thought processes related to PCP use as evidenced by uncontrolled behavior in the emergency room

▼ Situational low self-esteem related to pessimism about ability to stop using drugs as evidenced by expressed self-doubt

Mr. L used his relationship with Bobby to communicate his belief that he could successfully give up drugs. This message has a core of positive regard for Bobby's potential strength. The staff of the drug treatment program added to this seed of self-esteem by encouraging Bobby to help others in the program and then to aim higher at becoming a counselor himself. This taught Bobby that there were rewards in life other than those attached to drug use. Gradually, he learned to value the interpersonal rewards more than the drug rewards while making positive use of his past difficulties.

Discuss the significance of the substance abuser's level of self-esteem to the recovery process. Describe nursing interventions designed to enhance self-esteem.

Intervening in Manipulation. Manipulative behavior is frequently displayed by alcoholics and addicts. Sometimes this is learned during the process of obtaining their supply and hiding their use and its consequences from others. The hospitalized person may promise to give up the substance in order to be discharged, then start using it again upon returning home. Drug abusers sometimes manipulate the health-care system by obtaining prescriptions from more than one physician or by forging prescriptions. This behavior must be confronted when it is discovered, and the patient should be helped to understand the self-defeating nature of this behavior. Although the behavior appears to be directed toward others, the real victim is always the patient.

Intervening in Anger. When substance abusers are confronted with their behavior and pressed to be responsible for it, they may become angry. The anger is usually related to the pain patients feel when deciding to give up a behavior that has been central to their existence. In addition, patients may be raging over the emerging understanding of the problems they have caused for themselves. For the recovering alcoholic, giving up alcohol is a loss, followed by grief. Anger is one stage of grief and can intensify as the alcoholic begins to realize the life experience lost during the drinking years.

Nurses must realize that the patient's anger may be directed toward them but usually is not related to their behavior. Nurses should not take the anger personally and should try to discover what triggered it. It is important to teach the patient that anger must be understood and controlled because it can be used as an excuse for returning to drugs or alcohol. The nurse can also demonstrate how human support can be helpful when confronting painful feelings.

There are several other ways the nurse can help the

patient cope with anger. One way of coping is by understanding the stressors and thought patterns that contribute to the angry response. The nurse can help the patient develop new coping behaviors such as exercise, recreation, music, crying, work, and humor. Talking with the patient about feeling angry is another useful nursing intervention. Drug users become so accustomed to avoiding feelings chemically that they have trouble even recognizing them. By interacting with others, they can be helped to label and eventually cope with their feelings.

The nurse also can teach how using "shoulds" and blaming others contribute to anger. Discussion can focus on how these thoughts are not helpful or rational and how to substitute more helpful, rational thoughts. All of this is aimed at helping the patient take personal responsibility for feelings and behaviors.

Intervening in Relapse. Although it is great when a person is able to quit drinking alcohol or using drugs forever on the first attempt, this does not usually happen. Most people in recovery have one or more slips in their attempt to stay clean and sober. Continued use leads to a full-scale relapse, and many addicts then return to their previous life-style. Without condoning substance use, it is important for the nurse to teach the patient ways of minimizing the possibility of slips and ways of preventing a slip from turning into a relapse.

The nurse should help the patient identify the environmental triggers that led to previous use or relapse. Some examples are driving down a street where the patient used to "cop" drugs, getting into an argument with a loved one, going to parties, or the sights and sounds associated with the drug using environment. The patient is asked to avoid these environmental triggers as much as possible, especially early in recovery. Eventually the patient is taught to cope with many of them. Sometimes it is helpful to bring triggers into the treatment setting and teach the patient how to cope with the support of the nurse. This behavioral technique is called *cue exposure*. Paraphernalia associated with use, substances simulating the appearance of the drug, or movie clips with use on the screen can all be used as "cues." Nurses teach patients to recognize their physical and psychological responses to cues and to cope with them when they occur. When cues are repeatedly not followed by drug use, they lose their potency. Avoidance of triggers (cues), coping with them, and development of new cognitive behavioral skills become part of the patient's relapse prevention plan (see Chapter 28).

Another key element of the relapse prevention plan includes what to do if the person actually uses drugs or alcohol. It must be taught that a slip does not make the patient a "failure" or a "bad" person. It must be learned that there are many decision points between first thinking of using drugs or alcohol, actual use, and relapse. It should be clear that the patient will be welcomed back into treatment if a slip occurs. Otherwise, guilt will cause a loss of perspective and feelings of hopelessness. There is a sense of failure in abstinence that gives a reason for continuing to use drugs. This kind of thinking is called the "abstinence violation effect."[20] It is one of the causes of a full-blown relapse.

Social Interventions

Family Counseling. Reliable support from caring people is crucial to the recovery of substance abusers. However, the family is often frustrated with the patient's behavior and finds it difficult to be supportive. The family seldom understands the nature of addiction and generally does all the wrong things in its attempt to help the substance abuser. The family frequently tries to protect the patient from consequences. Many times, family members cover up by making excuses to employers and other family members for the person's erratic behavior. They also tend to blame themselves for the behavior and go to great lengths to avoid confrontation with the user. All of these behaviors are called *enabling* behaviors. By shielding the person from the consequences of drug use, the family enables the person's continued use of the drug.

Addiction is a family problem (see A Family Speaks). Everyone in the family suffers, not just the alcoholic or drug addict. Some problems families experience include guilt, shame, resentment, insecurity, delinquency, financial troubles, isolation, fear, and violence. Families think their problems would be solved if their loved one simply stopped using drugs or alcohol. However, they can get help even if the user refuses. They should also realize that without help, many of the negative patterns of behavior developed over years of dysfunctional family life will continue after sobriety.

The nurse should encourage family members to seek counseling from a professional experienced in addictions treatment. Referral to AlAnon, a support group for friends and family of alcoholics, or NarAnon, for friends and family of narcotic addicts, is also helpful. These groups are based on the same twelve steps as AA and NA except that they are powerless over their alcoholic/addict instead of the substance itself. These families need to learn to pay attention to their own needs. They need to stop covering up for the addict. They need to be direct in their communication. They also need to know that they are not alone.

Self-Help Groups. The most common type of self-help group for substance abusers is the twelve-step

A FAMILY SPEAKS

When I met Jim in 1983, I knew he dabbled in drugs but I still married him. I had no idea how his growing drug abuse problem would impact on my life over the next decade. In 1986 Jim entered treatment for his heroin addiction for the first time. I was impressed with the nurses in that program. They were compassionate, understanding, and knowledgeable about addiction. They taught Jim the first steps in the recovery process and supported him through the difficult changes that he had to make to maintain a drug-free life-style.

One nurse was particularly helpful to me as a family member of a newly recovering addict. She stood out because she consistently showed genuine concern for Jim and me. She always asked about Jim by name. She talked like he was an individual, not just one of the patients in the program. This allowed me to open up to her. I was finally able to ask if some of the things he was going through were normal, and I was very relieved to find out that they were! In contrast, another nurse on the staff talked down to all the patients. Neither the patients nor the family members felt they could talk to her.

In spite of all the help he received, Jim relapsed after a few months of being clean. I was disappointed, but I had learned about relapse and I refused to give up on him. After 5 more years, Jim entered a methadone maintenance program. By then our marriage was falling apart. A nurse in the program had special training in working with families. We saw her together. With her help, Jim was able to recognize that he, not I, was responsible for his addiction. He became more responsible for himself. I learned about how I had enabled his addiction and how I would have to change for our drug-free marriage to succeed. It seemed like each of us could hear what the nurse said better than we could hear each other. Now, 4 years later, Jim is still taking methadone, and we are still together. I want nurses to know that little kindnesses as well as bigger interventions can make a positive difference in the lives of drug addicts and their families. ▼

group. AA (Alcoholics Anonymous) is the model for 12-step support groups. It is composed entirely of alcoholics who have a desire to stop drinking. They believe that mutual support can give the alcoholic strength to abstain. AA aims for total abstinence. The member must admit to alcoholism openly and publicly by introducing himself at meetings, saying, "My name is John and I am an alcoholic." At speaker meetings, one or more members share their life histories with the group. This shows that members are more alike than different, removing a common resistance to involvement. AA members also commit themselves to helping each other. Some AA members serve as sponsors, a role that involves availability and accessibility to another member whenever a member feels the need to drink. The sponsor also teaches the person how to "work" the twelve steps of the program. This reciprocal relationship gives the new member caring support and the sponsor improved self-esteem. AA also involves a strong spiritual orientation that is experienced as supportive by some alcoholics. The twelve steps of AA are listed in Box 22-4. They were conceived by recovering alcoholics in 1935. It is easy to see the therapeutic benefit of these steps. For example, admitting the problem, making amends for past behavior, and reaching out to others who need help are sound therapeutic processes.

There are aspects of twelve-step programs that do not appeal to everyone. One of these is the powerlessness that must be acknowledged. Many people believe that the power to change lies within oneself. Some people are upset by the need to "turn over one's will to a higher power." Members are told that this higher power can be the AA group, the sponsor, or anything else they want. Although the higher power does not have to be "God" in the religious sense, the meetings generally have a religious overtone and usually end with the Lord's prayer. Some members have formed AA groups especially for agnostics.

Other self-help groups have emerged. One of these is Women for Sobriety (WFS).[19] This program shows women how to change their way of life through a change of thinking. The program particularly fills women's needs by teaching them to overcome depression, guilt, and low self-esteem. WFS helps women overcome their drinking problems with the support of other group members who have the same problems and needs. The difference from AA is evident in the first statement of the WFS "acceptance program": "I have a drinking problem that once had me."[19] All of the 13 statements of WFS are worded positively.

Another very popular program is the Rational Recovery (RR) movement,[33] which is based on Albert Ellis' Rational Emotive Therapy. This program asserts that alcohol dependence is not biologically determined and beyond our control. Rather, it is seen as a way of thinking. Irrational thoughts keep the alcoholic drinking. Rational thoughts can get and keep the alcoholic sober. RR philosophy is one of personal power; there is no reference to a higher power. RR groups have professional advisors who provide occasional rational input and also observe members for problems that indicate a need for a higher level of care. Group meetings operate by discussion, also known as cross-talking. This is in contrast to AA, which strongly discourages interrupting or responding to others. Group members read rational literature, learn to think rationally, and become rational counselors to themselves and others.

It should be noted that total abstinence is the goal of each of the above programs. A program that allows controlled drinking for an individual who has experienced the loss of control characteristic of addiction has little support in the research literature.

Community Treatment Programs. A variety of community programs may be available for drug abusers. Some hospital programs are designed specifically for safe medical detoxification. They have been cut from 1 to 2 weeks in the 1980s to 2 to 3 days in the 1990s because of changes in insurance coverage and other economic forces. Intensive inpatient hospital rehabilitation programs were also drastically cut. Many have been forced to close, and others have reduced their length of stay from 28 days to 10 to 21 days. Some residential, free-standing rehabilitation programs provide services for 21 to 28 days. To cut costs, alternatives to expensive hospital and residential programs have developed. Outpatient detoxification programs are becoming more popular. Some offer methadone withdrawal or maintenance for opiate addicts. Methadone programs must have special licensure to operate and follow federal guidelines. Day or evening programs are also common. The patient spends most of the day in treatment and returns home at night or spends the day at work and several evenings per week in treatment. Regular outpatient programs that are attended once or twice per week are even less intensive. Most programs provide a mix of group, individual, and family therapy, vocational counseling, drug and health education, and involvement with 12-step self-help programs. 12-step programs such as Alcoholics Anonymous, may be an adjunct to or substitute for professionally run programs.

Employee Assistance Programs. Another potential resource for the substance-abusing patient is the employee assistance program that may be part of an employee health service. Many businesses have found that it is profitable for them to help substance-abusing employees. These programs generally offer counseling and health education. Employees with a substance abuse problem are usually required to participate in the program to retain their job. Nurses are often key staff members in employee assistance programs. The health-care system has been rather slow in developing these programs for health-care providers. Since nurses and physicians also have problems with drugs and alcohol, there is a need for programs that can focus on their problems.

A Nursing Care Plan Summary for patients who abuse substances is presented on pp. 599-600.

Intervening with Impaired Colleagues

It is usually difficult for nurses to respond to a colleague who is showing signs of a substance abuse problem. This is true of supervisors as well as peers. For the safety of the nurse, as well as the nurse's patients, it is necessary to identify the problem and take action. In addition, many states have laws requiring health-care professionals to report colleagues who show signs of working while impaired. In these states, reporting is both an ethical and a legal obligation.

It is not usually easy to be sure that a nurse's practice is impaired by drug or alcohol use. However, particular patterns of behavior and signs are characteristic of this problem (Box 22-5). The concerned nurse colleague should report incidents of this nature to the supervisor. It is also important that these incidents be documented in writing, with the time, date, place, description of the incident, and the names of others who were present. This documentation will make it easier to intervene.

Box 22-5
SIGNS OF IMPAIRED NURSING PRACTICE

JOB PERFORMANCE CHANGES

Controlled drug handling/records (potential drug diversion)

Drug counts incorrect
Excessive errors
Excessive wastage, often not countersigned
Medicine signed out to patient who has not been in pain
Two strengths of drug signed out to same patient, same time
Packaging appears to be tampered with
Patient complaints of ineffective pain control
Volunteers to give controlled drugs
Comes in early and/or stays late
Disappears into the bathroom after handling controlled drugs
Unexplained absences from the unit

General performance

Medication errors
Poor judgment
Euphoric recall for involvement in unpleasant situations, or confrontations on the job
Illogical or sloppy charting
Absenteeism, especially in conjunction with days off
Requesting leave time just before the assigned shift
Latenesses with elaborate excuses
Job shrinkage (does the minimum work required to get by)
Missed deadlines

BEHAVIOR/PERSONALITY CHANGES

Sudden changes in mood
Periods of irritability
Forgetfulness
Wears long sleeves even in hot weather
Socially isolates from co-workers
Inappropriate behavior
Has chronic pain condition
History of pain treatment with controlled substances

SIGNS OF USE

Alcohol on the breath
Constant use of perfumes, mouthwash, and breath mints
Flushed face, reddened eyes, unsteady gait, slurred speech
Hyperactivity, accelerated speech
Increasing family problems that interfere with work

SIGNS OF WITHDRAWAL

Tremors, restlessness, diaphoresis, pupil changes
Watery eyes, runny nose, stomach aches, joint pains, gooseflesh

NURSING CARE PLAN SUMMARY
Chemically Mediated Responses

Nursing Diagnosis: Ineffective individual coping

Expected Outcome: The patient will abstain from using all mood-altering chemicals.

Short-term Goals	Interventions	Rationale
The patient will substitute healthy coping responses for substance-abusing behavior	Confront the patient with the substance-abusing behavior and its consequences Assist the patient to identify the substance abuse problem Involve the patient in describing situations that lead to substance-abusing behavior Consistently offer support and the expectation that the patient does have the strength to overcome the problem	Motivation for change is related to recognition of a problem that is upsetting to the individual Identification of predisposing factors and precipitating stressors must precede planning for more adaptive behavioral responses
The patient will assume responsibility for behavior	Encourage the patient to agree to participate in a treatment program Develop with the patient a written contract for behavioral change that is signed by the patient and nurse Assist the patient to identify and adopt healthier coping responses	Denial and rationalization are dysfunctional coping mechanisms that can interfere with recovery Personal commitment will enhance the likelihood of successful abstinence
The patient will identify and use social support systems	Identify and assess social support systems that are available to the patient Provide support to significant others Educate the patient and significant others about the substance abuse problem and available resources Refer the patient to appropriate resources and provide support until the patient is involved in the program	Substance abusers are often dependent and socially isolated people who use drugs to gain confidence in social situations Substance-abusing behavior alienates significant others thus increasing the person's isolation It is difficult to manipulate people who have participated in the same behaviors Social support systems must be readily available over time and acceptable to the patient

Nursing Diagnosis: Sensory-perceptual alteration

Expected Outcome: The patient will overcome addiction safely and with a minimum of discomfort.

Short-term Goals	Interventions	Rationale
The patient will withdraw from dependence on the abused substance	Supportive physical care: vital signs, nutrition, hydration, seizure precautions Administer medication according to detoxification schedule	Detoxification of the physically dependent person can be dangerous and is always uncomfortable The patient's physical safety must receive high priority for nursing intervention
The patient will be oriented to time, place, person, and situation	Assess orientation frequently; orient the patient if needed; place a clock and calendar where they can be seen by the patient	Cognitive function is usually affected by addiction; disorientation is frightening

NURSING CARE PLAN SUMMARY—cont'd
Chemically Mediated Responses

Nursing Diagnosis: Sensory-perceptual alteration

Expected Outcome: The patient will overcome addiction safely and with a minimum of discomfort.

Short-term Goals	Interventions	Rationale
The patient will report symptoms of withdrawal	Observe carefully for withdrawal symptoms and report suspected withdrawal immediately	Withdrawal symptoms provide powerful motivation for continued substance abuse; judgment may be impaired by substance use
The patient will correctly interpret environmental stimuli	Explain all nursing interventions; assign consistent staff; keep soft light on in room; avoid loud noises; encourage trusted family and friends to stay with the patient	Sensory and perceptual alterations related to use of drugs or alcohol are frightening; consistency reduces the need to interpret stimuli
The patient will recognize and talk about hallucinations or delusions	Observe for response to internal stimuli; encourage patient to describe hallucinations or delusions; explain the relationship of these experiences to withdrawal from addictive substances	Assisting the patient to identify delusional or hallucinatory experiences and relate them to withdrawal is reassuring

An enabler is a person who supports someone in maintaining an addiction. Describe behaviors that would enable a colleague to continue drug or alcohol use that impairs performance of nursing roles. What alternative behaviors would be more helpful?

If the pattern of behavior indicates that impairment exists, an intervention should be planned. An advisor should be selected who has expertise in the area of impaired nursing practice. This advisor could be someone from the state nurse rehabilitation committee, if there is one. A team of people who have meaningful relationships with the nurse should be asked to prepare written statements demonstrating their observations of probable impaired practice. The team should consist of co-workers, the supervisor or other nurse administrator, and perhaps a family member. The team rehearses the statements in a meeting without the nurse present to work out any details and to ensure a nonmoralistic tone. They also anticipate various reactions the nurse may have and decide how to respond to these. Treatment options are discussed and plans made to escort the nurse directly from the meeting to a treatment facility.

After the above preparation, a meeting is called in which the team members read their statements to the nurse, who is informed of the bottom line that the team has decided on. The bottom line is usually that the nurse must enter treatment or resign from nursing and potentially lose the license to practice. The nurse is escorted to either an inpatient treatment program or an outpatient appointment. Since the suicide risk for nurses who have just gone through an intervention is great, the nurse should not be left alone after the intervention.

During treatment the supervisor should maintain contact with the treatment program to see how the nurse is progressing. It is strongly advised that a return-to-work contract be written that clearly describes the nurse's responsibilities upon return. If the state has a nurse rehabilitation committee, they can assume some responsibility for monitoring the nurse's progress and developing treatment and return-to-work contracts. This type of intervention makes it possible for the chemically dependent nurse to get the treatment needed, yet remain employed—a situation in which everyone benefits.

Preventive Interventions

Prevention of substance abuse is an important public health problem. Nurses must be aware of the need

PATIENT EDUCATION PLAN
PROMOTING ADAPTIVE CHEMICALLY MEDIATED RESPONSES

Content	Instructional activities	Evaluation
Elicit perceptions of substance use	Lead group discussion regarding knowledge about chemical use and experience with it; correct misperceptions	Patient will describe accurate information about substance use
Demonstrate negative effects of substance abuse	Show films of physical and psychological effects of substance abuse; provide written materials	Patient will identify and describe physical and psychological effects of substance abuse
Interaction with peer who has abused chemicals	Small group discussion with peer group member who has abused substances and quit because of negative experiences	Patient will compare and contrast advantages and disadvantages of using mind-altering substances
Obtain agreement to abstain from use of mind-altering substances	Discuss future plans for refusing abused chemicals if offered	Patient will verbally agree to abstain from using mind-altering substances

for primary prevention and incorporate this into their professional practice (see the Patient Education Plan above). Resnick[29] suggests the following components for drug abuse prevention programs:

1. Work to improve the social conditions that affect families
2. Focus on influencing the environment in which drug use occurs, including establishing drug education programs in schools
3. Strengthen individuals' interpersonal and social skills to increase self-esteem and resistance to peer pressure
4. Create a strong interagency network, encouraging resource sharing to increase the impact on the system
5. Share federal and state government resources

Nurses can play an important part in developing and initiating policies that support the development of good substance abuse prevention programs.

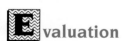valuation

The evaluation of substance abuse treatment is based on accomplishment of the expected outcomes and short-term goals. Estes, Smith-DiJulio, and Heinemann[10] have identified evaluation criteria for the treatment of alcoholics. These criteria apply to abusers of other drugs as well:

▼ Has the patient been able to progress significantly toward achieving the stated goals?
▼ Can the patient communicate without being defensive?

▼ Is the patient able to react appropriately, managing the demands of daily life without use of a drug?
▼ Is the patient actively involved in a variety of activities, using external social and activity resources?
▼ Does the patient use internal resources to be consistently productive at work and involved in meaningful interpersonal relationships?

The evaluation process should take place at regular intervals during the nurse-patient relationship.

SUGGESTED CROSS-REFERENCES

A Stress Adaptation Model of Psychiatric Nursing Care	Chapter 4
Biological Context of Psychiatric Nursing Care	Chapter 5
Psychological Context of Psychiatric Nursing Care	Chapter 6
Psychopharmacology	Chapter 25
Managing Aggressive Behavior	Chapter 27
Therapeutic Groups	Chapter 29
Adolescent Psychiatric Nursing	Chapter 35

SUMMARY

1. Adaptive chemically mediated responses include "natural highs," which may be related to physical activity or meditation. Maladaptive responses include substance dependence, substance abuse, and withdrawal from addiction.
2. Statistically the use of most illicit drugs has been declining, but deaths and drug-related emergency room visits have increased. Multiple substance abuse is a growing problem.

3. Patient behaviors related to chemically mediated responses are related to dependence, intoxication, or overdose and vary according to the abused substance(s). Abused substances may include CNS depressants, alcohol, barbiturates, benzodiazepines, marijuana, stimulants, opiates, hallucinogens, and PCP.

4. Predisposing factors that lead to maladaptive chemically mediated responses are described from the biological, psychological, and sociocultural perspectives. Precipitating stressors may include withdrawal from addiction and pregnancy.

5. Coping resources include communication and assertiveness skills, social support systems, pleasurable activities, stress-reduction techniques, vocational skills, and motivation to change. Maladaptive coping mechanisms often include denial, rationalization, projection, and minimization.

6. Primary NANDA nursing diagnoses related to maladaptive chemically mediated responses are sensory-perceptual alteration, altered thought processes, and ineffective individual coping.

7. Primary DSM-IV diagnoses are dependence, abuse, intoxication, or withdrawal related to a particular substance.

8. The expected outcome of nursing care is that the patient will abstain from using all mood-altering chemicals.

9. Planning is based on providing first for safe withdrawal, followed by developing ways to maintain abstinence. Support systems including family, friends, and self-help groups should be involved whenever possible.

10. Interventions include detoxification; treatment of toxic psychosis; disulfiram (Antabuse) therapy; group therapy; patient and family education; assisting the patient to manage behaviors related to denial, dependency, low self-esteem, manipulation, and anger; prevention of relapse; family counseling; and referral to self-help groups, community treatment programs, and employee assistance programs. Other interventions are related to prevention and impaired colleagues.

11. Evaluation criteria for nursing care related to chemically mediated responses include goal achievement, open communication, abstinence, adequacy of coping resources, and ability to participate in work and interpersonal relationships.

COMPETENT CARING
A CLINICAL EXEMPLAR OF A PSYCHIATRIC NURSE

Walter E. Roberson, Jr., RN, MA

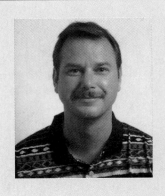

One of the most fulfilling experiences I have ever had with a chemically dependent patient occurred not long ago. This young woman came into the hospital after planning to throw herself into traffic. She had a history of cocaine and alcohol abuse and recently had to give up her son to the Department of Family Services because she had been unable to care for him.

When she first came into the hospital she demonstrated a lot of anger as well as extensive erratic behavior. I recognized this as part of her withdrawal symptoms and also the grief she was experiencing because of the loss of her son. She was unapproachable at first, and much of her conversation was confused and contradictory. Over and over again she refused to talk with me about how she was feeling and what she planned to do in her life. What I finally started to notice was a very subtle change in her affect. It was like very thin layers of an opaque material were being taken away as things inside her began to clear. I was persistent with making myself available for her while giving ongoing support. Finally she reached a point where she said she was ready to talk and she said many things were clear now that she did not understand before. Over the course of the next several weeks the rest of the treatment team and I began to offer her options. She ended up going into a halfway house for several months, and then she was able to move into an apartment and eventually regain custody of her little boy. She checks back in periodically to say hi and show us how well she is doing.

This has shown me that it is always important to keep trying and that the difference a person can make can be very significant in a patient's recovery. Don't ever give up. ▼

REFERENCES

1. American Nurses' Association and National Nurses Society on Addictions: *Standards of addictions nursing practice with selected diagnoses and criteria*, Kansas City, Mo, 1988, American Nurses' Association.
2. American Psychiatric Association: *Diagnostic and statistical manual of mental disorders*, ed 4, Washington, DC, 1994, The Association.
3. Anthony JC, Helzer JE: Syndromes of drug abuse and dependence. In Robins LN, Regier DA, eds: *Psychiatric disorders in America: the epidemiologic catchment area study*, New York, 1991, The Free Press.
4. Beattie M: *Codependent no more: how to stop controlling others and start caring for yourself*, New York, 1987, Harper/Hazelden.
5. Beeder AB, Millman RB: Treatment of patients with psychopathology and substance abuse. In Lowinson JH, Ruiz P, Millman RB: *Substance abuse: a comprehensive textbook*, ed 2, Baltimore, 1992, Williams & Wilkins.
6. Blum K et al: Allelic association of human dopamine D2 receptor gene in alcoholism, *JAMA* 263:2055, 1990.
7. Butz RH: Intoxication and withdrawal. In Estes NJ, Heinemann ME, eds: *Alcoholism: development, consequences, and interventions*, ed 3, St Louis, 1986, Mosby.
8. Cloninger CR: Neurogenetic adaptive mechanisms in alcoholism, *Science* 236:410, 1987.
9. Elder IR: *Conducting group therapy with addicts: a guidebook for professionals*, Blue Ridge Summit, Pa, 1990, Tab Books.
10. Estes NJ, Smith-DiJulio K, Heinemann ME: *Nursing diagnosis of the alcoholic person*, St Louis, 1982, Mosby.
11. Ewing JA: Detecting alcoholism, the CAGE questionnaire, *JAMA* 252:1905, 1984.
12. Gelernter J, Goldman D, Risch N: The A1 allele at the D2 dopamine receptor gene and alcoholism: a reappraisal, *JAMA* 239:1673, 1993.
13. Grinspoon L, Bakalar JB: Marihuana. In Lowinson JH, Ruiz P, Millman RB: *Substance abuse: a comprehensive textbook*, ed 2, Baltimore, 1992, Williams & Wilkins.
14. Helzer, JE, Burnam A, McEvoy LT: Alcohol abuse and dependence. In Robins LN, Regier DA, eds: *Psychiatric disorders in America: the epidemiologic catchment area study*, New York, 1991, The Free Press.
15. Jaffe JH: Drug addiction and drug abuse. In Gilman AG, Goodman LS, Rall TW, Murad F, eds: *Goodman and Gilman's pharmacological basis of therapeutics*, New York, 1985, Macmillan.
16. Jellinek EM: Phases of alcohol addiction, *QJ Stud Alcohol* 13:672, 1952.
17. Johnson BD, Muffler JM: Sociocultural aspects of drug use and abuse in the 1990s. In Lowinson JH, Ruiz P, Millman RB: *Substance abuse: a comprehensive textbook*, ed 2, Baltimore, 1992, Williams & Wilkins.
18. Johnson VE: *Intervention: how to help someone who doesn't want help*, Minneapolis, 1986, Johnson Institute Books.
19. Kirkpatrick J: *Turnabout: new help for the woman alcoholic*, ed 3, New York, 1990, Bantam Books.
20. Marlatt FA, Gordon JR, eds: *Relapse prevention*, New York, 1985, The Guilford Press.
21. Miller NS, Gold MS: Amphetamine and its derivatives. In Giannini AJ, Slaby AE, eds: *Drugs of abuse*, Oradell, NJ, 1989, Medical Economics Books.
22. Moore RD et al: Prevalence, detection, and treatment of alcoholism in hospitalized patients, *JAMA* 261:403, 1989.
23. National Institute on Drug Abuse: *National drug and alcoholism treatment unit survey (NDATUS): 1989 main findings report*, Rockville, Md, 1990, NIDA.
24. National Institute on Drug Abuse: *National household survey on drug abuse: highlights 1991*, Rockville, Md, 1993, NIDA.
25. National Institute on Drug Abuse: *Press release*, Rockville, Md, April 13, 1993, NIDA.
26. *National survey results from the monitoring the future study, 1975-1992*, vol I, NIH Pub No 93-3597, 1993.
27. National Institute on Drug Abuse: *Smoking, drinking, and illicit drug use among American secondary school students, college students, and young adults, 1975-1991*, vol II, Washington, DC, 1992, US Government Printing Office.
28. Peachey JE, Lei H: Assessment of opioid dependence with Naloxone, *Br J Addict* 83:193, 1988.
29. Resnick HS: *It starts with people: experience in drug abuse prevention*, Rockville, Md, 1978, Department of Health, Education, and Welfare.
30. Sellers EM, Sullivan JT, Somer G, Sykora K: Characterization of DSM-III-R criteria for uncomplicated alcohol withdrawal provides an empirical basis for DSM-IV, *Arch Gen Psychiatr* 48:442, 1991.

31. Skinner HA: The drug abuse screening test, *Addict Behav* 7:363, 1982.

32. Sue D: Use and abuse of alcohol by Asian Americans, *J Psychoactive Drugs* 19:57, 1987.

33. Trimpey J: *Rational recovery from alcoholism: the small book*, ed 3, Lotus, Calif, 1989, Lotus Press.

34. Trinkoff AM, Eaton WW, Anthony JC: The prevalence of substance abuse among registered nurses, *Nurs Res* 40:172, 1991.

35. Vourakis C, Bennett G: Angel dust: not heaven sent, *Am J Nurs* 79:649, 1979.

36. Weiss CJ, Millman RB: Hallucinogens, phencyclidine, marijuana, inhalants. In Frances RJ, Miller SI, eds: *Clinical textbook of addictive disorders*, New York, 1991, The Guilford Press.

37. Wesson DR, Smith DE, Seymour RB: Sedative-hypnotics and trycyclics. In Lowinson JH, Ruiz P, Millman RB, eds: *Substance abuse: a comprehensive textbook*, ed 2, Baltimore, 1992, Williams & Wilkins.

38. Westermeyer J: Historical and social context of psychoactive substance disorders. In Frances RJ, Miller SI, eds: *Clinical textbook of addictive disorders*, New York, 1991, The Guilford Press.

ANNOTATED SUGGESTED READINGS

Brower KJ, Blow FC, Beresford TP: Treatment implications of chemical dependency models: an integrative approach, *J Subst Abuse Treat* 6:147, 1989.

Describes five basic models of chemical dependency (moral, learning, disease, self-medication, and social) and their treatment implications.

Carroll KM, Rounsaville BJ, Keller DS: Relapse prevention strategies for the treatment of cocaine abuse, *Am J Drug Alcohol Abuse* 17:249, 1991.

Describes specific interventions and therapeutic strategies used in the treatment of cocaine abuse.

*Clement JA, Williams EB, Waters C: The client with substance abuse/mental illness: mandate for collaboration, *Arch Psychiatr Nurs* 7:189, 1993.

An excellent presentation of the special challenges posed by dual diagnosis, including information about neurophysiological changes related to drug use and the need for multidisciplinary training in service delivery.

Co-dependency, Deerfield Beach, Fla, 1988, Health Communications.

Short readings that present various viewpoints on co-dependency.

*Dodge VH: Relaxation training: a nursing intervention for substance abusers, *Arch Psychiatr Nurs* 5:99, 1991.

Presents a practical application of relaxation therapy as an intervention for this population, assisting them to resist the temptation to use drugs.

Elder IR: *Conducting group therapy with addicts: a guidebook for professionals*, Blue Ridge Summit, Pa, 1990, Tab Books.

Describes the nuts and bolts of the Friendly Forces model of conducting group therapy with addicts.

*Friedrich RM, Kus RJ: Cognitive impairments in early sobriety: nursing interventions, *Arch Psychiatr Nurs* 5:105, 1991.

Describes how cognitive impairment may manifest itself in alcoholic patients in early recovery and provides several nursing interventions designed to enhance the learning process in early alcoholic recovery.

*Hall JM: What really worked? A case analysis and discussion of confrontational intervention for substance abuse in marginalized women, *Arch Psychiatr Nurs* 7:322, 1993.

Thought-provoking article that challenges nurses to consider the ethical implications of using confrontation with substance-abusing women.

Hayes EN, ed: *Adult children of alcoholics remember*, New York, 1989, Harmony Books.

Collection of personal accounts of growing up in an alcoholic family. Provides an opportunity to understand the impact of parental alcoholism on the child.

*Nursing reference.

*Jefferson LV, Ensor BE: Confronting a chemically impaired colleague, Am J Nurs 82:574, 1982.

A classic but still current article about addicted nurses. Case studies illustrate the characteristics of drug- and alcohol-abusing nurses. Describes clues that should lead one to suspect substance abuse. Intervention section includes advice on confronting a nurse colleague who may be alcoholic or abusing drugs. Highly recommended for all nurses.

*Nursing interventions for addicted patients, Nursing Clinics of North America 24(1), 1989.

Entire volume deals with addictions nursing topics such as identifying the alcoholic client, the role of the psychiatric nurse in a community substance abuse prevention program, strategies for intervention, family recovery, cocaine addiction, and co-dependency. Excellent resource.

*Oswald LM: Cocaine addiction: the hidden dimension, Arch Psychiatr Nurs 3:134, 1989.

Describes neurochemical alterations in the brain thought to be responsible for cocaine addiction and the treatment implications for nurses.

Ray OS, Ksir C: Drugs, society, and human behavior, ed 6, St Louis, 1993, Mosby.

Highly recommended as a basic resource on all aspects of chemical dependence. Discusses both relevant psychosocial factors and pharmacological aspects.

*Sisney KF: Intervention: a strategy to help chemically dependent students, Nurse Educator 17:28, 1992.

Provides an example of an effective intervention with a student nurse.

*Sullivan EJ: Nursing care of clients with substance abuse, St Louis, 1995, Mosby.

Written specifically for nurses caring for clients with substance abuse. Provides numerous nursing care plans based on case studies.

Wing DM: Applying the "model of recovering alcoholics' behavior stages and goal setting" to nursing practice, Arch Psychiatr Nurs 7:197, 1993.

Presents a theoretical model of recovery that can assist the nurse in planning care for the alcoholic patient.

*Nursing reference.

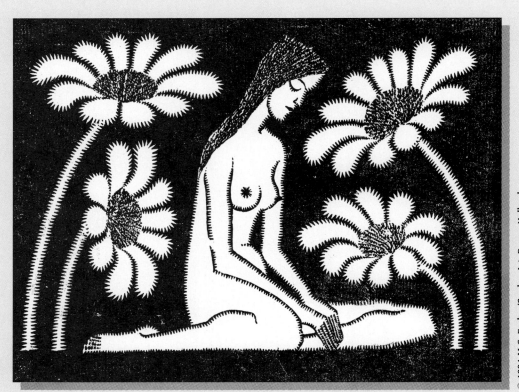

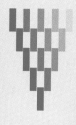

CHAPTER 23

Eating Regulation Responses and Eating Disorders

CAROLYN E. COCHRANE

Soon her eyes fell upon a little glass box that was lying under the table: she opened it, and found in it a very small cake, on which the words "EAT ME" were beautifully marked in currants. She ate a little bit, and said anxiously to herself, "Which way? Which way?," holding her hand on the top of her head to feel which way it was growing.

Lewis Carroll: *Alice's Adventures in Wonderland*

LEARNING OBJECTIVES

After studying this chapter the student should be able to:

▼ Describe the continuum of adaptive and maladaptive eating regulation responses
▼ Relate the prevalence of anorexia nervosa, bulimia nervosa, and binge eating disorder
▼ Identify behaviors associated with eating regulation responses
▼ Analyze predisposing factors and precipitating stressors related to eating regulation responses
▼ Describe coping resources and coping mechanisms related to eating regulation responses
▼ Formulate nursing diagnoses for patients related to eating regulation responses
▼ Assess the relationship between nursing diagnoses and medical diagnoses related to eating regulation responses
▼ Identify expected outcomes and short-term nursing goals for patients related to eating regulation responses
▼ Develop a family education plan to promote adaptive eating regulation responses
▼ Analyze nursing interventions for patients related to eating regulation responses
▼ Evaluate nursing care for patients related to eating regulation responses

TOPICAL OUTLINE

Continuum of Eating Regulation Responses
   Prevalence of Eating Disorders
Assessment
  Behaviors
  Predisposing Factors
  Precipitating Stressors
  Coping Resources
  Coping Mechanisms
Nursing Diagnosis
  Related Medical Diagnoses
Outcome Identification
Planning
  Choice of Treatment Setting
  Nursing Care Plan Contract
Implementation
  Nutritional Stabilization
  Exercise
  Cognitive Behavioral Interventions
  Body Image Interventions
  Family Involvement
  Group Therapies
  Medications
Evaluation

Food is essential to life because it supplies the individual with needed nutrients and sources of energy. As such, eating is a crucial self-regulatory activity. However, it can also assume importance and meaning beyond that of nutrition and become associated with biopsychosocial processes that promote or inhibit adaptive functioning.

CONTINUUM OF EATING REGULATION RESPONSES

As a pattern of self-regulation, properly controlled eating contributes to psychological, biological, and sociocultural health and well-being. Adaptive eating responses are characterized by balanced eating patterns, appropriate caloric intake, and body weight that conforms to the Metropolitan Standard Tables[33] for height and weight (Table 23-1). Although eating is a common occurrence, society appears to have difficulty understanding the idea of unregulated eating. For example, everyone has at times overeaten, skipped one or more meals, or seen adolescent boys consume large amounts of food at a single meal. Many women have premenstrual cravings for salty, sweet, or other types of foods. These eating behaviors are not viewed as problematic.

However, food can also be used in an attempt to satisfy unmet emotional needs, moderate stress, and provide rewards or punishments. People can also have unrealistic images of their ideal body size and desired body weight. Research has shown that most people think that they should weigh 10% less that they do, and this can result in a range of behaviors from fasting fads to severe dieting.[21] The inability to regulate eating habits and the frequent tendency to overuse or underuse food interferes with biological, psychological, and sociocultural integrity.

Illnesses associated with maladaptive eating regulation responses include anorexia nervosa, bulimia nervosa, and the newly named binge eating disorder (Fig. 23-1). About 90% of these disorders occur in adolescent and young adult women who are predominantly white and middle to upper class. Although not nearly as

Table 23-1   Metropolitan Standard Table for Height and Weight

How to Approximate Frame Size

$$r = \frac{\text{Height (cm)}}{\text{Wrist circumference (cm)}}$$

Frame size can be determined as follows:

Men	Women
r > 10.4, small	r > 11.0, small
r = 9.6 to 10.4, medium	r = 10.1 to 11.0, medium
r < 9.6, large	r < 10.1, large

Ideal weight*

	Men				Women		
Height	Small frame	Medium frame	Large frame	Height	Small frame	Medium frame	Large frame
5' 2"	128-134	131-141	138-150	4' 10"	102-111	109-121	118-131
5' 3"	130-136	133-143	140-153	4' 11"	103-113	111-123	120-134
5' 4"	132-138	135-145	142-156	5' 0"	104-115	113-126	122-137
5' 5"	134-140	137-148	144-160	5' 1"	106-118	115-129	125-140
5' 6"	136-142	139-151	146-164	5' 2"	108-121	118-132	128-143
5' 7"	138-145	142-154	149-168	5' 3"	111-124	121-135	131-147
5' 8"	140-148	145-157	152-172	5' 4"	114-127	124-138	134-151
5' 9"	142-151	148-160	155-176	5' 5"	117-130	127-141	137-155
5' 10"	144-154	151-163	158-180	5' 6"	120-133	130-144	140-159
5' 11"	146-157	154-166	161-184	5' 7"	123-136	133-147	143-163
6' 0"	149-160	157-170	164-188	5' 8"	126-139	136-150	146-167
6' 1"	152-164	160-174	168-192	5' 9"	129-142	139-153	149-170
6' 2"	155-168	164-178	172-197	5' 10"	132-145	142-156	152-173
6' 3"	158-172	167-182	176-202	5' 11"	135-148	145-159	155-176
6' 4"	162-176	171-187	181-207	6' 0"	138-151	148-162	158-179

Data from Metropolitan Insurance Company: 1979 *Build study*, New York, 1983, Society of Actuaries and Association of Life Insurance Medical Directors of America.
*Weights at ages 25-59 based on lowest mortality.

widespread, eating disorders are becoming more common among males, minorities, and women of all age groups. These disorders can cause biological changes including altered metabolic rates, profound malnutrition, and possibly death. Obsessions about eating can cause psychological problems including depression, isolation, and emotional lability. Sociocultural ideals concerning body size can cause eating disorders by influencing an individual to perceive body size as being larger or smaller than it actually is. This distorted body image may initiate an attempt to attain an unrealistic body size.

Before working with patients with maladaptive eating regulation responses, nurses must closely examine their own feelings and prejudices about weight and body size. Reflecting on the following questions may elicit answers requiring further examination:

1. What do I believe is the ideal body size and shape?
2. How do I feel about people who are overweight?
3. Can a person ever really be too thin?
4. Do I worry about my weight a lot?
5. Do I have biases about eating and weight that will interfere with my ability to take care of patients with eating disorders?

If a nurse suspects that she has an eating disorder, she may not be able to provide care for patients who cannot regulate their eating responses. She should seek out professional help for herself before attempting to care for others.

> Identify three sociocultural factors that influence the type and amount of food you eat and your perception of the ideal body size.

Prevalence of Eating Disorders

Anorexia Nervosa. Anorexia nervosa occurs in about 1% of the female population. Its onset is usually between the ages of 13 and 20, but the illness can occur in any age group, including the elderly and prepubertal children. Anorexia nervosa is also seen in males, although less frequently. The ratio of females to males with this disorder is thought to be about 20:1. Mortality from anorexia nervosa is estimated to be between 6% to 10%.[4,31,32]

Bulimia Nervosa. Bulimia nervosa occurs more frequently in the population than anorexia with estimates of between 2% and 4% and a prevalence of 4% to 15% in female high school and college students.[27] The age of onset is typically between 16 to 18 years of age, and the female to male ratio is 9:1. Bulimia and anorexia may be present in the same patient. As many as 50% of anorectic patients develop bulimic symptoms, and many bulimics can subsequently develop anorexia. Bulimia usually occurs in people of normal weight, but it may occur in obese and thin individuals.

Binge Eating Disorder. Binge eating disorder is a new diagnostic category in the fourth edition of the *Diagnostic and Statistical Manual of Mental Disorders*, in which individuals consume large amounts of calories but do not attempt to prevent weight gain.[3] Previous descriptions of this problem included obese bingers, compulsive overeaters, and pathological overeaters. Since the mid-1980s researchers sought to identify the differences between individuals who were obese but did not binge, those who were obese and binged, and those nonobese bulimics who both binged and purged. Many differences were found, and they are summarized in Table 23-2.

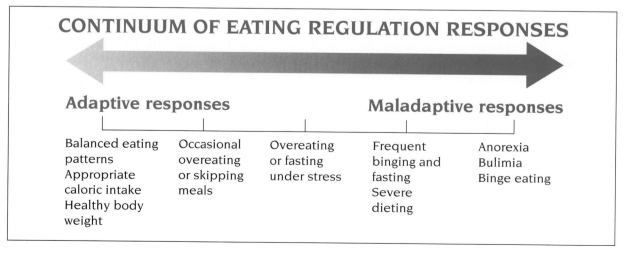

Fig. 23-1   Continuum of eating regulation responses.

Table 23-2 Differences in Obese Nonbingers, Obese Bingers, and Nonobese Bulimics

	Obese nonbingers	Obese bingers	Nonobese bulimics
Body image distortion	Low or none	Moderate to low	High level
Amount of binging	None or little	High amount but less than bulimics of normal weight	Very high level
Mood disturbance	Same as general population	One third chronic	One third to one half chronic and 75% to 80% lifetime
Purging	Rare	Infrequent	High level
Degree of control regarding binging	High	Medium to low	Low
Interest in food	Preoccupied at times	Obsessed	Obsessed
Problems with self-esteem	Same as general population	Low self-esteem	Low self-esteem
Substance abuse	Same as general population	Moderate to high	High

Not all patients with a diagnosis of binge eating disorder are obese. In one national study the incidence of binge eating disorder in females was determined to be 1.2% with the typical individual being of normal weight, any race, and any age.[7] In several multisite studies, participants in weight loss programs were surveyed. The incidence of binge eating disorder in this obese population was found to be between 29% to 30%.[14,39,40] These findings suggest that assessing for eating disorders should be an important part of weight management programs. Conclusions regarding the incidence of binge eating disorder in males have not yet been determined.

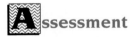ssessment

It is essential that patients with maladaptive eating regulation responses receive a comprehensive nursing assessment, including complete biological, psychological, and sociocultural evaluations.[31] A full physical examination should be performed with particular attention given to vital signs, weight for height, skin, the cardiovascular system, and evidence of laxative or diuretic abuse and vomiting. A dental examination may be indicated, and it is useful to assess growth, sexual development, and general physical development indicators. A psychiatric history, substance use history, and family assessment are also needed.

Specific attention should be focused on the assessment of eating regulation responses. Several questionnaires and rating scales have been developed to screen for the presence of eating disorders. Some of these are listed in Chapter 6. A recent study, however, found that asking just two questions may be as effective as more extensive questionnaires in identifying women with eating disorders.[18] They are:

1. Are you satisfied with your eating patterns?
2. Do you ever eat in secret?

These questions can be easily incorporated into the nursing assessment of all patients. If a patient is being evaluated for an eating disorder, additional information should be obtained including the following:

1. Actual and desired weight
2. Onset and pattern of menstruation
3. Food restrictions and avoidances
4. Frequency and extent of binge eating and vomiting
5. Use of laxatives, diuretics, diet pills, and ipecac
6. Body image disturbances
7. Food preferences and peculiarities
8. Ritualistic behavior regarding food and exercise

It is also helpful to explore the patient's understanding of how the illness developed and its impact on school, work, and social relationships so that a holistic view of the patient's world can be obtained.

Behaviors

Binge Eating. Binge eating is the rapid consumption of large quantities of food in a discrete period of time, although there is no agreement on exactly how many calories constitutes a binge. Anorectics who binge may describe a binge of several hundred calories. Bulimics who are not also anorectic may ingest several thousand calories at a sitting. Emphasis on the individual's perception of loss of control and perceived excessive caloric intake is more important to the nursing assessment than the total number of calories consumed during a binge.[38] Therefore it is important that the nurse carefully assess exactly what each individual patient means by a "binge." People usually binge secretively, and there is often considerable shame associated with their binging behavior. The bulimic typically is of average weight or slightly overweight and has a history of unsuccessful dieting. The severity of the binging can vary greatly, ranging from several times a week, to more than 10 times a day, to only occasional binges related to stressful situations.

Fasting or Restricting. Anorectics often do not consume more than 500 to 700 calories daily and may in gest as few as 200 calories a day, yet they see their intake as adequate for their energy needs. They may be vegetarians and eliminate even fish and chicken from their diets. Anorectics are also likely to exhibit obsessive-compulsive eating behaviors, such as eating the same foods at the same times every day or eating foods in a certain predetermined order. They may also have bizarre food preferences, avoid foods considered fattening, and have difficulty controlling any food intake. Some individuals with anorexia may not eat for days at a time. In spite of these restrictions, many anorectics are preoccupied or obsessed with food and may as a result do much of the family cooking or be employed in a food-related occupation. The following clinical example describes the fasting behavior seen in anorectics.

 ## CLINICAL EXAMPLE

Barbara is a 15-year-old white female who has been restricting her food intake for 6 months because she felt too fat. Her weight at the beginning of her food restriction was 128 pounds. This weight was appropriate for her age, her height of 5' 5", and her small body frame. Her current weight is 102 pounds, which is approximately 80% of what she should weigh. The patient denies having any eating problems and feels that her family is overreacting to her weight loss. She is willing to come for treatment only because her family wants her to do so.

Barbara was age 13 at menarche and had regular periods until they stopped 2 months ago. She says that she never tried or planned to lose weight but admits to becoming a vegetarian 6 months ago. Barbara, despite her low weight, thinks that she needs to lose another 10 pounds because she feels her thighs are too large. She is an avid ballet dancer and practices dancing 2 to 3 hours a day. Her family describes her as the perfect daughter.

Selected Nursing Diagnoses:
▼ Altered nutrition related to restricted food intake as evidenced by weight loss
▼ Body image disturbance related to eating disorder as evidenced by continued desire to lose weight
▼ Ineffective denial related to eating problems as evidenced by lack of acceptance of realistic weight parameters

Purging. A variety of purging behaviors may be used by individuals with maladaptive eating regulation responses to prevent weight gain. These include excessive exercise, over-the-counter and prescription diuretics, diet pills, laxatives, and steroids. Less well-known substances used to counteract weight gain include insulin, cocaine, heroin, thyroid replacements, nicotine, hallu-

cinogens, analgesics, benzodiazepines, antidepressants, ipecac, and sorbitol.[9] Many patients engage in more than one purging behavior. One study of 275 women with bulimia reported the following methods used by women to rid themselves of calories: vomiting (81.4%), exercise (76.1%), fasting (69.1%), and ingestion of laxatives (39.8%), diet pills (34.1%), and diuretics (20.2%).[35]

Exercising for these patients often becomes a grueling, time-consuming affair. Running or participating in high-impact aerobics for 2 to 3 hours each day is typical of the compulsive exerciser. Many patients with an eating disorder exercise so much that they sustain major skeletal injuries, but this still does not deter them from continuing this maladaptive behavior. This is seen in the clinical example that follows.

 ## CLINICAL EXAMPLE

Bill is a single, 30-year-old man with a 7-year history of anorexia nervosa and bulimia nervosa. Bill exercises compulsively at least 3 hours daily. He was exercising 6 to 7 hours a day from the age 23 until age 29. Examples of current and previous exercise rituals include running 25 miles followed by a 2- to 3-mile swim and bicycling 25 miles before allowing himself to eat a meal. His athletic abilities have been rewarded with numerous trophies. He is receiving fewer trophies lately because of damage to his knees from overuse.

In addition to exercising compulsively, Bill also vomits after binging and has periods of fasting lasting 2 to 3 days. When he does eat a regular meal he does so by eating only certain foods and eating these foods in a certain order. Bill also writes obsessively and is methodical about the order of his personal hygiene. He is depressed about the fact that his life revolves around his eating, hygiene, and exercise rituals and is eager to receive treatment.

Selected Nursing Diagnoses:
▼ Altered nutrition related to anxiety about body size as evidenced by binging and fasting
▼ Body image disturbance related to fears of gaining weight as evidenced by excessive exercise and food restrictions
▼ High risk for injury related to excessive exercise as evidenced by knee injuries

Laxative abuse often begins gradually. Initially the individual may use only one or two mild laxatives per week, and then increase the number in the subsequent weeks and months. Over time, more laxatives are needed to get the same effect as before. Individuals abusing laxatives commonly take 5 to 15 at a time, and it is not unusual for someone to take a total of 60 laxatives a week. Laxatives are one of the most inefficient ways to lose calories, since only 12% fewer calories are absorbed through the use of laxatives.[6]

Binging, fasting, and purging are sometimes described as addictive behaviors. Compare and contrast them to smoking, gambling, and substance abuse.

Medical Complications. Usually every individual with maladaptive eating regulation responses has some type of associated physical problem. For example, one study reported that 70% of the bulimic patients admitted for inpatient treatment required medical care, and 90% of the medical complications found on assessment were previously unrecognized.[22] The various complications associated with eating disorders are listed in Box 23-1.

Assessment of the individual's physical status can help reveal the magnitude of the eating problem. Patients below 20% or above 40% of their ideal body weight on the Metropolitan Standard Table (see Table 23-1) demonstrate more physical abnormalities than those who are between 20% and 40% of their ideal weight. Pa-

tients who are below 40% or above 100% of their ideal body weight will have clinical and laboratory findings that are often life threatening. Individuals who vomit and use laxatives or diuretics, regardless of their weight, usually have significant and sometimes life-threatening clinical findings and laboratory abnormalities.[5]

In anorexia nervosa, metabolic and endocrine abnormalities result from the body's reaction to malnutrition associated with starvation. All body systems are affected. Most commonly seen are amenorrhea, osteoporosis, and hypometabolic symptoms such as cold intolerance and bradycardia. Starvation may cause hypotension, constipation, and acid-base and fluid-electrolyte disturbances including pedal edema.[13]

In bulimia nervosa, potassium depletion and hypokalemia are often seen as a result of vomiting and laxative or diuretic abuse. Symptoms of potassium depletion include muscle weakness, cardiac arrhythmias, conduction abnormalities, hypotension, and other problems associated with electrolyte imbalance. Gastric, esophageal, and bowel abnormalities are common complaints in bulimics. Those who vomit are subject to erosion of the dental enamel and parotid enlargement.[23,29]

For those with binge eating disorder and concurrent morbid obesity, serious health problems caused by excess weight or prior health problems exacerbated by in-

---

Box 23-1
MEDICAL COMPLICATIONS OF EATING DISORDERS

CENTRAL NERVOUS SYSTEM

Decreased rapid eye movement and shortwave sleep
Cortical atrophy
Thermoregulatory abnormalities

RENAL

Hematuria
Proteinuria

HEMATOLOGIC

Leukopenia
Anemia
Thrombocytopenia

GASTROINTESTINAL

Dental erosion
Parotid swelling
Esophagitis, esophageal tears
Delayed gastric emptying
Gastric dilatation
Pancreatitis
Diarrhea (laxative abuse)
Hypercholesterolemia

METABOLIC

Dehydration
Acidosis
Hypokalemia
Hypochloremia
Hypochloremic alkalosis
Hypocalcemia
Hypophosphatemia
Hypomagnesemia
Osteoporosis
Hypercarotenemia

ENDOCRINE

Decreased luteinizing hormone and follicle-stimulating hormone
Decreased triiodothyronine, increased reverse triiodothyronine, rT3, normal thyroxin and thyroid-stimulating hormone
Irregular menses
Amenorrhea

CARDIOVASCULAR

Bradycardia
Postural hypotension
Dysrhythmia, sudden death

creased weight are common. Many have hypertension, cardiac problems, sleep apnea, difficulties in mobility, and diabetes mellitus. Some of the medical consequences of eating disorders are seen in the following clinical example.

 ## CLINICAL EXAMPLE

Audrey is a 25-year-old black woman with a 4-year history of restrictive intake and a 3-year history of binge eating and laxative abuse. Audrey has been concerned about her weight since high school, when she was a star basketball player, a competitive swimmer, and participant in track, volleyball, and tennis. She bypassed her senior year in high school. She began to diet at age 20, and her severe restriction of food at age 21 led to a 20-pound weight loss and amenorrhea. At age 22 she began to binge eat and use laxatives. Since that time she binges two to three times a week and uses an average of 30 to 60 stimulant-type laxatives each week.

She is constantly preoccupied with food and her weight and has periods of mood lability, sadness, lack of energy, social isolation, anxiety, irritability, and difficulty concentrating. Audrey also reports chronic constipation, bloating, edema of hands, feet, legs, and face, and lightheadedness. She has recently consulted a gastroenterologist for her severe constipation and was advised that her large intestine was grossly oversized. Audrey became very frightened by the report and immediately called a local eating disorder program for help.

Selected Nursing Diagnoses:

▼ Altered nutrition related to fear of gaining weight as evidenced by binging

▼ Body image disturbance related to anxiety about body size as evidenced by excessive use of laxatives

▼ Constipation related to maladaptive eating patterns as evidenced by pain, bloating, and enlarged intestine

Psychiatric Complications. Many patients seeking treatment for eating disorders have evidence of other psychiatric disorders. Comorbid major depression or dysthymia has been reported in 50% to 75% of anorectics. Obsessive-compulsive disorder may be found in 10% to 13% of anorectics with a lifetime prevalence of 25%. Among patients with bulimia, there have been reported increased rates of anxiety (43%), substance abuse disorders (49%), bipolar illness (12%), and personality disorders (50% to 75%). Disagreement exists regarding comorbidity rates for borderline personality disorder and eating disorder with reported estimates varying widely between 2% and 60%. In addition, many bulimics have dissociative symptoms, sexual conflicts, and a variety of impulsive behaviors that include overspending, shoplifting, promiscuity, and self-mutilation.[2] Fi-

nally, binge eating disorder has been found to be associated with higher rates of major depression, panic disorder, bulimia nervosa, borderline personality disorder, and avoidant personality disorder.[46]

Predisposing Factors

Biological, psychological, and sociocultural factors have been identified that may predispose an individual to the development of an eating disorder. These factors are involved in the regulation and control of food intake. It is generally agreed that the etiological factors are multidetermined and interactive, involving a combination of genetic, neurochemical, developmental, characterological, social, cultural, and familial factors (Fig. 23-2).

Biological. There is believed to be a genetic link involved in both anorexia nervosa and bulimia nervosa. Studies of twins have reported a higher incidence of anorexia and bulimia in monozygotic twins as compared with dizygotic twins. It has also been found that sisters and daughters of patients with anorexia have increased rates of the illness; data regarding sisters and daughters of bulimics are inconclusive.[27,43] Finally, there appears to be evidence for a familial association between bulimia and affective disorders, and a high prevalence of alcoholism among family members of these patients.

Biological models of the etiology of eating disorders focus on the appetite regulation center in the hypothalamus, which controls specific neurochemical mecha-

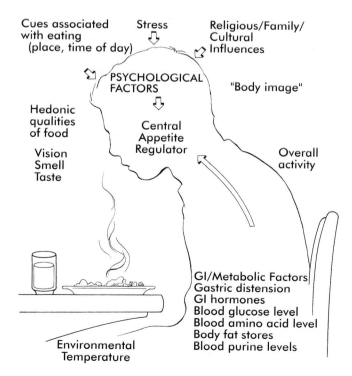

Fig. 23-2 Major peripheral inputs influencing appetite.

nisms for feeding and satiety. In patients with eating disorders it has been hypothesized that the neurotransmitters, neuromodulators, and hormones that control feeding and satiety are dysregulated. More specifically, the neurotransmitter, serotonin, is thought to be involved in the pathophysiology of eating disorders.[8] Serotonin primarily has been shown to inhibit food intake and is thought to be a satiety agent. It has also been reported that 3-methoxy-4-hydroxyphenylglycol (MHPG) in urine and cerebrospinal fluid is reduced, suggesting lessened norepinepherine turnover and activity.

Other hypotheses propose that eating disorders may be variants of mood disorders or may be caused by decreased endogenous opioid activity. This last theory is based on the clinical observations that carbohydrates, particularly sugar, play a role in binge eating and obesity, since many binge eaters preferentially eat sweets during a binge. Beta-endorphin has an appetite-stimulating mechanism, and if sugar stimulates beta-endorphin production, it can eventually lead to increased eating. Positron-emission tomography (PET) scans are also being conducted on anorectics,[16] and abnormal findings on computed tomography (CT) scans of the brain have been reported in more than half of patients with anorexia nervosa. All of these models are still in the developmental stage, however, and ongoing research in this area promises to shed more light on the biological factors that may predispose an individual to maladaptive eating regulation responses.

Analyze the hypothesized role serotonin plays in the development of both eating disorders and depressive disorders and the implications this has for the use of selective serotonin reuptake inhibitors as a medication strategy for both disorders.

Psychological. A variety of psychological factors have been suggested that may predispose an individual to the development of an eating disorder. Early histories of patients with eating disorders are often complicated by medical and surgical illnesses, separations, and family deaths. Women with bulimia also describe growing up in a conflicted family environment and experiencing more behavioral disturbances, such as drug abuse, suicide attempts, truancy, and other emotional problems.[44] Sexual abuse has been reported in 20% to 50% of patients with bulimia, but this rate may be similar to that found in other psychiatric populations.[26,36,44] Early separation and individuation conflicts, a pervasive sense of ineffectiveness and helplessness, difficulty interpreting feelings and tolerating intense emotional states, and fear of biological or psychological maturity may predispose an individual to

---

Box 23-2

PSYCHOLOGICAL CHARACTERISTICS ASSOCIATED WITH EATING DISORDERS

Anxiety
Compulsivity
Conflict avoidance
Depression
Difficulty expressing feelings, particularly anger
Exaggerated sense of guilt
Fear of sexuality and biological maturity
Feelings of alienation
Intolerance for frustration
Perfectionism
Poor impulse control
Self-consciousness
Sense of ineffectiveness

---

an eating disorder.[24] Additional personality and psychological characteristics of these patients are identified in Box 23-2.

Sociocultural. In the past 50 years there has been a steady increase in the incidence of diagnosed eating disorders, subclinical eating problems, and body image disturbances. In cultures where plumpness is either accepted or valued, eating disorders are rare. It has also been observed that the sociocultural milieu for adolescent and young women in this country has become progressively unstable, precipitating a range of problems in this age group, including eating disorders.[17,42] Shifting cultural norms for young women have forced them to face multiple, ambiguous, and often contradictory role expectations. Thus thinness is highly valued, culturally rewarded, and associated with achievement. Most women are imprinted with cultural ideals of body size and shape and find themselves struggling with body image concerns throughout their lives, as sociocultural norms become the yardsticks for their self-evaluation.

Cultural values regarding ideal body shape and size have varied throughout history. The contemporary American ideal woman is lean, strong, graceful, and feminine. One advantage to this profile is its emphasis on fitness and health. A disadvantage is the constant demand this norm places on women to focus on and control their bodies, often as a means for achieving desired goals. The result is intense social pressure on women for self-discipline, rigorous exercise, dieting, and often obsessive concern about weight and body image. The result is that at least 50% of American women are on a diet at any given time, and Americans spend over $5 billion on dieting products alone.

Children, teenagers, and young adults living in

FAMILY EDUCATION PLAN
PREVENTING CHILDHOOD EATING PROBLEMS

Content	Instructional activities	Evaluation
Describe self-demand feeding and its importance in healthy eating behaviors	Explore current feeding practices of parents and understanding of healthy eating Provide information to enhance knowledge of healthy eating behaviors	Parents will identify healthy eating behaviors and self-demand feeding and begin to explore how their relationship with food influences their children's eating
Describe physiological and psychological signs of hunger and satiety, as well as the meaning and difference of both types of signs Describe danger of psychological hunger	Explore parents' own signs of hunger and satiety and also have parents describe child's signs Explain the use of a hunger diary, which is a daily journal regarding signs of hunger	Parents will keep a hunger diary to record physical and psychological signs of hunger and satiety for themselves and their children Parents will be able to distinguish between psychological and physical hunger
Explore myths about feeding: e.g., "cleaning the plate" and "eating because other children are starving"	Describe the importance of allowing children to determine their feeding needs and the relationship of healthy eating to the children's ability to differentiate between physical and psychological signs of hunger and satiety Give homework assignment for each parent to interview three other adults about their current eating practices and memories of eating	Parents will complete homework assignment, discuss interview experiences, and describe how perpetuating myths about feeding can harm their child
Implement self-demand feeding at particular developmental stages of children	Review the stages that children experience with eating and the potential problems they may have at each stage	Parents will discuss the developmental stages of their children and plan for implementing self-demand feeding
Discuss parental experiences related to implementing self-demand feeding	Review parents' expectations and experiences with implementing self-demand feeding	Parents will relate any problem around self-demand feeding Nurse will evaluate family for further education and plan for follow-up if necessary

communities or going to schools where emphasis is placed on weight and size are often prone to developing eating disorders. Activities or occupations that emphasize beauty or fitness also promote preoccupation with weight and eating behaviors.[19] Ballet dancers, models, actors, athletes, fashion retailers, and flight attendants all have either tacit or explicit criteria dictated to them concerning body weight and size. These occupations and activities in and of themselves do not cause eating disorders but they do attract individuals who may measure their self-esteem, self-worth, and attractiveness by body parameters rather than accomplishments and personal satisfaction.

Parents who overemphasize athletics, reward slimness, or vocalize distaste of overweight individuals are placing their children at risk for eating disorders. Also, parents who continually skip meals, eat when distressed, and otherwise model poor nutritional habits are not teaching children about the appropriate value of food as nourishment. An important preventive nursing intervention is educating the parents of young children regarding healthy eating behaviors. The Family Education Plan for preventing childhood eating problems is presented above.

 Watch television for an evening and count the number of men and women who are overweight. Explain any sociocultural bias you observe.

Precipitating Stressors

Possessing or displaying one or more of the predisposing factors previously mentioned puts an individual at risk for an eating disorder. Individuals thus predisposed are especially vulnerable to environmental pressures and stress. Lacking an integrated self-concept and realistic body image, they rely on external feedback such as the reactions of others to their appearance and actions. They are unable to perceive or interpret stimuli from within the body, have difficulty describing their feelings and self-concepts, and lack an internal center of initiative and regulation. Thus they must rely on external cues to regulate themselves. Food becomes one of these cues and is used as an external replacement for a deficient internal regulator and inadequate integration of the body and mind.[28]

This individual is very susceptible to the impact of life stressors, such as the loss of a significant other, interpersonal rejection, and failure. Studies have shown a positive correlation between stress and the severity of binge eating, and other precipitating stressors may also play an important role.[25,45] For example, some studies report that bulimics reported their lowest mood status when at home alone, and the severity of bulimic symptoms was correlated with severity of mood, thus suggesting that daily solitude may be a precipitating stressor for these disorders.[30] Others have suggested that for individuals predisposed to eating disorders, exercise is not viewed as a way to lose weight but is actually an attempt to experience the reality of their bodies. Controlling their eating or vomiting is another effort at countering the anguish of emptiness, boredom, or tension. Although binge eating may momentarily release this tension, it sets in motion a cycle of binging and purging that, once begun, is very difficult to stop.[28] Some of the precipitating stressors related to eating disorders are evident in the following clinical example.

 ## CLINICAL EXAMPLE

Lydia is a 15-year-old female with a 6-year history of binging, a 9-month history of purging, and a 2-year history of restricting her food intake. She is the only child of parents who separated when she was 3 and divorced when she was 6. Her father has a history of frequent mood swings and was later diagnosed and treated for cyclothymic disorder. He had always been overly concerned not only about his bodily appearance but also about the appearance of his family. When Lydia was 9, her father moved to a city 500 miles away, and 2 years later he remarried. Lydia's mother remarried several months after her ex-husband did, but her marriage lasted less than a year. Her husband had concealed an alcohol problem, and Lydia and her mother were verbally abused by this man on numerous occasions.

After her second divorce, Lydia's mother socialized very little and became overprotective of Lydia. Lydia's mother has frequently criticized Lydia's father for his extramarital behavior while he was married to her. Lydia's mother had supported the father through college and dental school and was angry about her lowered standard of living since their divorce.

Lydia's parents continue to have a stormy relationship, and she feels caught between them at times. She avoids conflict by siding with her custodial parent, her mother, and avoiding any discussion about her mother with her father. Lydia tries to be the perfect daughter and strives not to displease either parent. She has become very overprotective of her mother and secretly despises her father. She feels that a number of people have hurt her mother and that she and her mother must protect each other. Lydia is afraid to grow up because her mother will be left alone. She states, "I'm the center of my mom's universe. If she's alone, her world will crumble. . . . I'm happiest when I'm worrying about my mom." Lydia does not think she has any eating problems and is very resistant to treatment. Her parents feel otherwise.

Selected Nursing Diagnoses:

▼ Altered nutrition related to unrealistic self-image as evidenced by binging, purging, and restricting food

▼ Ineffective denial related to family conflict as evidenced by overprotection of mother and ambivalence toward father

Coping Resources

One of the most important aspects of the assessment of patients with maladaptive eating regulation responses is their level of motivation to change behavior. This may be obtained by asking patients to rate their desire for treatment on a scale of 1 to 10, with 10 representing high motivation and 1 low motivation for change. Patients may also be asked to identify the advantages and disadvantages of giving up the behavior, and this information can be used to evaluate a patient's insight, identify coping resources, and stimulate therapeutic issues for future discussion.

The nurse might also inquire into how binging, fasting, and purging serve as a form of coping. Asking patients what precedes these episodes and how they feel afterward are important elements of the nurse's assessment. The patient should also be asked how stress and tension have been handled adaptively in the past and what supports in the environment that can be enlisted in the treatment process. These may include family members, friends, work, and leisure activities.

Coping Mechanisms

Anorectics are happiest when fasting, losing weight, or achieving their weight goals. Their use of **denial** is severely maladaptive, and they are unlikely to seek help on their own. Concerned family members, primary practitioners, nurses, or school counselors are usually the ones who identify a problem and attempt to obtain help. Anorectics are usually angry or impatient with the concern shown by others. Interestingly, as the family becomes more distraught about the loss of weight or signs of malnutrition, the anorectic's insistence of normalcy increases. For the patient, the issue is not about weight; it is about control of the anorectic's life and fears. Individuals with anorexia nervosa who fear maturity, independence, failure, sexuality, or parental demands believe they have found a solution to the problem by controlling their food intake and their bodies. With the increasing concerns of the family, the anorectic is now able to control the focus of significant others as well. For the anorectic this seems to be the perfect solution.

The defense mechanisms used by bulimics include **avoidance, denial, isolation of affect,** and **intellectualization.**[25] Bulimics, regardless of their weight, are usually very upset about their binging and purging behavior. They realize that their behavior is a sign that they are not in control or coping adaptively, but they do not know why. They are more likely to acknowledge that they have a problem than are patients with anorexia nervosa, although they may regard the symptoms as preferable to the prospect of weight gain, and it may be years before the bulimic accepts treatment.

Individuals with binge eating disorder share the bulimic's distress about binging, although it is unclear how motivated they are to seek treatment. Obese binge eaters are more likely to seek assistance on their own or be willing to be referred by their primary practitioner.

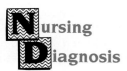

Nursing Diagnosis

In formulating the nursing diagnosis the nurse should review all aspects of the assessment phase as identified in the stress adaptation model (Fig. 23-3). Nursing diagnoses related to eating disorders encompass biological, psychological, and sociocultural concerns, and because of the complexity of these patients, many NANDA nursing diagnoses may be appropriate. Primary NANDA diagnoses for working with patients with maladaptive eating regulation responses include anxiety, body image disturbance, fluid volume deficit, high risk for self-mutilation, altered nutrition, powerlessness, and

self-esteem disturbance. The Medical and Nursing Diagnoses box on p. 619 presents nursing diagnoses associated with the range of possible maladaptive eating regulation responses and related medical diagnoses. Primary NANDA nursing diagnoses and examples of complete nursing diagnoses are presented in the Detailed Diagnoses box on p. 620.

For patients with moderate to extreme nutritional deficiencies, the nurse must exercise caution when determining nursing diagnoses. Patients with nutritional deficiencies exhibit symptoms of malnutrition that may be mistakenly related to other causes. Irritability, apathy, depression, obsessiveness, difficulty with concentration, anxiety, decreased interest in sex, and negativism are psychological symptoms that usually reverse with adequate nutrition.[11] The nurse may see a very different outward presentation in a patient who is no longer malnourished. Finally, family members may offer important insights into the patient's premorbid functioning and be able to give a clearer picture of the patient's personality before the eating disorder developed.

Related Medical Diagnoses. The medical diagnoses associated with maladaptive eating regulation responses include anorexia nervosa, bulimia nervosa, and binge eating disorder.[3] These medical diagnoses and their essential features are described in the Medical and Nursing Diagnoses box. The key features distinguishing anorexia nervosa from bulimia nervosa are listed in Box 23-3 on p. 621.

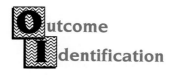

Outcome Identification

The expected outcome for the patient with maladaptive eating regulation responses is:

The patient will restore healthy eating patterns and normalize physiological parameters related to body weight and nutrition.

For anorectic and bulimic patients, this means that they will be able to eat 100% of all meals, without binging, purging, or engaging in other compensatory behavior. Obese patients with binge eating disorder should be encouraged to leave something (no more than 5% or less than 2%) on their plate at the end of the meal.

Short-term goals may further specify the steps the patient needs to take to demonstrate adaptive eating regulation responses. These might include the following:

1. The patient will identify cognitive distortions about food, weight, and body shape.
2. The patient will develop a week's menu of nutritionally balanced meals.

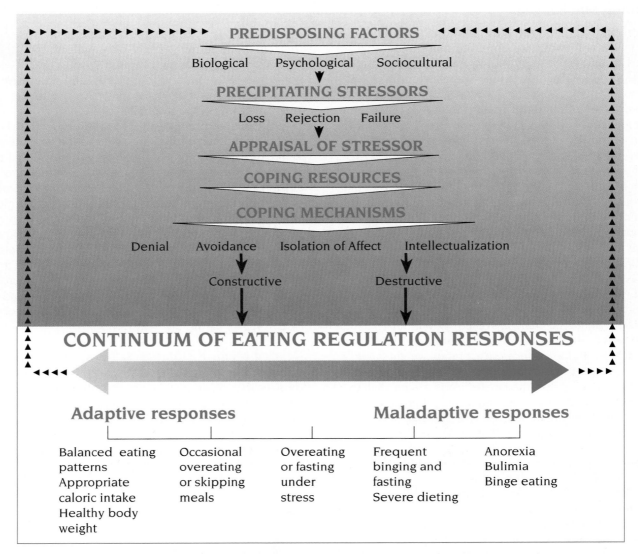

PREDISPOSING FACTORS

Biological   Psychological   Sociocultural

PRECIPITATING STRESSORS

Loss   Rejection   Failure

APPRAISAL OF STRESSOR

COPING RESOURCES

COPING MECHANISMS

Denial   Avoidance   Isolation of Affect   Intellectualization

Constructive   Destructive

CONTINUUM OF EATING REGULATION RESPONSES

Adaptive responses   **Maladaptive responses**

| Balanced eating patterns Appropriate caloric intake Healthy body weight | Occasional overeating or skipping meals | Overeating or fasting under stress | Frequent binging and fasting Severe dieting | Anorexia Bulimia Binge eating |

Fig. 23-3   A stress adaptation model related to eating regulation responses.

3. The patient will accurately describe body dimensions.
4. The patient will exercise in moderate amounts only when nutritionally and medically stable.
5. The patient will demonstrate positive family interactions and successful movement toward achievement of separation and individuation issues.

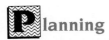**lanning**

Choice of Treatment Setting. Nursing care varies to some degree based on the treatment setting of the patient with maladaptive eating regulation responses. A number of factors affect the choice of treatment setting including the patient's physical and psychological con-

dition, financial resources, availability of treatment specialists, and patient preference. Clinical criteria for inpatient treatment of eating disorders are listed in Box 23-4.

Outpatient treatment may be considered the preferred setting because it allows the patient the greatest opportunity for self-control and autonomy. It requires a high level of patient motivation, the active support and involvement of family members, and ongoing physiological monitoring. Contingencies for outpatient treatment should be mutually agreed on expectations of behavioral change, including weight gain and decreased binging or purging, and the acceptance of inpatient or more intense day treatment programs if the patient is not making progress.

The important advantage of inpatient treatment is the availability of 24-hour nursing care to ensure patient safety, support needed behavioral change, and monitor

MEDICAL AND NURSING DIAGNOSES RELATED TO EATING REGULATION RESPONSES

Related Medical Diagnoses (DSM-IV)*

Binge eating disorder
Bulimia nervosa
Anorexia nervosa

Related Nursing Diagnoses (NANDA)†

Activity intolerance
‡**Anxiety**
‡**Body image disturbance**
Constipation
Decisional conflict
Denial, ineffective
Family process, altered
Fatigue
‡**Fluid volume deficit**
Growth and development, altered
High risk for injury
‡**High risk for self-mutilation**
Hopelessness
Individual coping, ineffective
‡**Nutrition, altered**
Personal identity disturbance
‡**Powerlessness**
Role performance altered
‡**Self-esteem disturbance**
Sexual dysfunction
Social interaction, impaired
Thought process, altered
Violence, potential

*From American Psychiatric Association: *Diagnostic and statistical manual of mental disorders*, ed 4, Washington, DC, 1994, The Association.
†From North American Nursing Diagnosis Association: NANDA *nursing diagnoses: definitions and classifications* 1992-1993, Philadelphia, 1992, The Association.
‡Primary nursing diagnosis for eating problems.

physiological responses. Patients with eating disorders can present a unique challenge to inpatient staff, and care requires a high level of interdisciplinary collaboration, coordination, and consistency. Team members must work closely together and maintain open communication and mutual respect to prevent some patients' tendencies for "splitting," or playing staff off against each other.

Nurse-Patient Contract. Nurse-patient contracts can be formulated for patients with eating disorders who are seen in either inpatient or outpatient settings. The terms of the contract may vary, but the goal is the same—to engage the patient in a therapeutic alliance and obtain commitment to the treatment process.

Eating can be better controlled in an inpatient rather than outpatient setting. Before a patient is admitted to an inpatient unit for treatment of an eating disorder, it is advisable to secure the patient's cooperation in treatment with a nurse-patient contract. By signing such a contract, patients will understand the treatment they will be receiving and be able to make informed decisions about their commitment to the treatment process and their ability to honor the contract. If a patient will not sign the contract and is not at risk for injury, the admission should be delayed and outpatient treatment should be recommended. Patients who are at risk for injury due to compromised physical status or suicidal behavior must be admitted, but their participation in an eating disorder program will be limited if they do not agree to the nursing care plan contract. They may, however, agree to sign the contract once admitted to the hospital.

How would you respond to a patient who wants to receive treatment for an eating disorder but does not want to sign the nurse-patient contract because it is "too restrictive"?

DETAILED DIAGNOSES RELATED TO EATING REGULATION RESPONSES

NANDA Diagnosis Stem	Examples of Complete Diagnosis
Anxiety	Anxiety related to fear of weight gain evidenced by rituals associated with food preparation and eating.
Body image disturbance	Body image disturbance related to fear of weight gain evidenced by verbalization of being "fat" while actually being 30% below ideal body weight.
Fluid volume deficit	Fluid volume deficit related to purging activities evidenced by weakness, poor skin turgor, hypokalemia, and hypotension.
High risk for self-mutilation	High risk for self-mutilation related to feelings of inadequacy evidenced by injuries due to excessive exercise and self-induced vomiting.
Nutrition, altered	Altered nutrition related to excessive intake of calories evidenced by being 40% above ideal body weight, sleep apnea, and difficulty with mobility.
Powerlessness	Powerlessness related to perceived lack of control over eating behaviors evidenced by inability to stop binge eating and avoidance of food-related settings.
Self-esteem disturbance	Self-esteem disturbance related to feelings of low self-worth evidenced by verbalization of sole standard of success being related to physical attractiveness.

DSM-IV Diagnosis	Essential Features*
Anorexia nervosa	An intense fear of gaining weight, even when underweight. There is a disturbance in the way the body is experienced and a refusal to maintain body weight above a minimal normal weight for age and height, leading to a body weight 15% below expected. In females there is also the absence of at least three consecutive menstrual cycles.
Bulimia nervosa	Recurrent episodes of binge eating with a feeling of lack of control over the eating behavior and persistent overconcern with body shape and weight. The individual also regularly engages in self-induced vomiting, use of laxatives, or rigorous dieting and fasting to counteract the effects of binge eating.
Binge eating disorder	Recurrent episodes of binging that are a cause of distress with a feeling of lack of control over the eating behavior but without behaviors used to prevent weight gain.

*Adapted from the American Psychiatric Association: *Diagnostic and statistical manual of mental disorders*, ed 4, Washington, DC, 1994, The Association.

mplementation

Nutritional Stabilization

Stabilizing the patient's nutritional status is a high priority for nursing intervention. Healthy target weights and expected rates of controlled weight gain or loss should be established. In life-threatening circumstances, patients who are malnourished may need refeeding interventions (see Critical Thinking about Contemporary Issues), but this option is exceptional.

In an inpatient setting, specific nursing interventions to promote weight stabilization and restore healthy eating patterns can be facilitated by program protocols that identify treatment goals, program components, and patient and staff responsibilities.[12] Some of these might include the following:

1. The time, frequency, and procedure for weighing the patient and if the patient may see the weight
2. The time when meals will be served and how many meals are to be eaten each day

---

Box 23-3
KEY FEATURES OF ANOREXIA NERVOSA AND BULIMIA NERVOSA

ANOREXIA NERVOSA

Rare vomiting or diuretic/laxative abuse
More severe weight loss
Slightly younger
More introverted
Hunger denied
Eating behavior may be considered normal and source of esteem
Sexually inactive
Obsessional features predominate
Death from starvation (or suicide, in chronically ill)
Amenorrhea
More favorable prognosis
Fewer behavioral abnormalities

BULIMIA NERVOSA

Vomiting or diuretic/laxative abuse
Less weight loss
Slightly older
More extroverted
Hunger experienced
Eating behavior considered foreign and source of distress
More sexually active
More hysterical or borderline features as well as obsessional features
Death from hypokalemia or suicide
Menses irregular or absent
Less favorable prognosis
Stealing, drug and alcohol abuse, self-mutilation, and other behavioral abnormalities

From Andersen AE: *Practical comprehensive treatment of anorexia nervosa and bulimia,* Baltimore, 1985, The Johns Hopkins University Press.

Box 23-4
CLINICAL CRITERIA FOR HOSPITALIZATION OF PATIENTS WITH AN EATING DISORDER

MEDICAL

Need for extensive diagnostic evaluation
Weight loss greater than 30% of body weight over 3 months
Heart rate less than 40 beats/min
Temperature less than 36° C or 96.8° F
Systolic blood pressure less than 70 mm Hg
Serum potassium less than 2.5 meq/L despite oral potassium replacement
Severe dehydration
Concurrent somatic illnesses (e.g., infection)

PSYCHIATRIC

Risk of suicide or self-mutilation
Severe depression
Psychosis
Family crisis
Failure to comply with treatment contract
Inadequate response to outpatient treatment

3. How the staff is to interact with the patient during mealtimes to maximize their therapeutic value
4. The amount of time the patient will be allowed to spend eating each meal, and the consequences if the meal is not completed
5. Whether diet foods, condiments, or food substitutions are allowed
6. The amount of water the patient may drink each day
7. The frequency of obtaining the patient's vital signs, intake and output, and required laboratory work
8. Times when visitors are allowed on the unit
9. Conditions regarding bathroom privileges
10. Indications for close observation by staff

Once inpatients have been able to master their meals, they can move toward more independence with eating and food selection. Selecting their own menus with assistance is next. The patient can then progress to selecting food from the hospital cafeteria, followed by shopping for and cooking food with supervision. By discharge the patient should have gained a high level of comfort with food and its preparation.

For anorectic outpatients, stabilizing their nutrition and promoting weight gain usually require a motivated patient and cooperative family. Obtaining the patient's agreement to stop trying to lose weight is the first obstacle the nurse must overcome, since patients are often very resistant to such an idea. Actually getting an anorectic to gain weight is an even more difficult task. Nurse-patient contracts can be effective tools with these patients because their need for control of food is so great. For example, the nurse and anorectic patient may set a realistic goal of gaining 1 pound per week. If the patient fails to gain 4 pounds in a month, the contract would stipulate that the patient would then agree to enter a hospital, day treatment program, or some other more intensive type of care.

Counseling about healthy eating patterns and behaviors is an essential aspect of nursing care for all patients, regardless of whether they may need to gain,

CRITICAL THINKING ABOUT CONTEMPORARY ISSUES

Should Tube Feeding Be a Component of an Eating Disorders Treatment Program?

The positive and negative consequences of nasogastric tube feeding or even total parenteral nutrition for patients with an eating disorder have been debated among clinicians and researchers in the field. Current guidelines recommend that refeeding interventions should be used only rarely and in life-threatening situations.[2] Specifically, there is recognition of the danger of rapid refeeding, which includes severe fluid retention and cardiac failure, and of forced nasogastric or parenteral feeding. Thus these procedures should not be used routinely. However, some severely malnourished anorectic patients may accept nasogastric feeding more willingly than eating, especially in the early stages of renourishment.

If forced feeding is to be considered, careful thought should be given to the patient's clinical condition, the patient's and family's opinion, and legal and ethical dimensions of the patient's treatment. Each one of these areas merits a full discussion by the interdisciplinary health-care team, and treatment decisions should include specific timelines, outcomes, and alternatives. ▼

lose, or maintain weight. The nurse should also clarify with patients the effect of poor nutrition on the body. Collaboration with a dietitian may be helpful in teaching patients about proper eating habits, as well as in planning menus with patients. Nurses should teach, clarify, and reinforce knowledge about proper nutrition and the importance of planning healthy meals using the recommended servings from each of the five food groups. Patients should be encouraged to make shopping lists, and the nurse may even accompany the patient to the grocery store. Nutritional assessment, education, and ongoing support are essential nursing care activities.

The patient who is struggling with major issues around food will not be ready for intensive psychological interventions. As the patient is feeling less need to be in control of food and eating, issues underlying the eating disorder may start to surface. This can be a difficult time for the patient who may actually begin to feel worse than when treatment began. If a patient is in the hospital there is someone available to talk with, but this is not always true for the outpatient. Thus the outpatient may need more frequent sessions with the nurse or more phone contacts between sessions. However,

when sufficient progress has been made toward nutritional rehabilitation, the patient will be better prepared both cognitively and emotionally to begin the next phase of treatment.

Exercise

As the patient's eating increases, the need to increase exercise or engage in a new purging or compensatory behavior will also be increased. On an inpatient unit the patient can be closely monitored to prevent such compensatory activity. However, as the patient stabilizes and responds to treatment it is often appropriate to begin a gradual exercise program. For some patients who exercise compulsively, this can be their most difficult period of treatment. The nurse should initially allow patients limited amounts of exercise with gradual increases over time. The focus of the exercise program should be on physical fitness as opposed to working off calories.[47] Consultation with a recreational therapist or exercise physiologist may be helpful to maximize the therapeutic value of the exercise regimen.

Cognitive Behavioral Interventions

It is important for the nurse to work with patients around their cognitive distortions and faulty thinking about body shape, weight, and food. Box 23-5 presents a list of cognitive distortions often used by patients with eating disorders and an example of each. Cognitive behavioral therapy is discussed in detail in Chapter 28.

Assisting the patient to become aware of these thoughts is the first step in changing them. The patient should be asked to monitor and record eating, binging, and purging behavior and thoughts and feelings regarding weight, shape, and food.[15] The goal of these exercises is for the patient to better understand the following:

1. The **cues** that trigger problematic eating responses
2. The **thoughts, feelings,** and **assumptions** associated with the specific cues
3. The connection between these thoughts, feelings, assumptions and **eating regulation responses**
4. The **consequences** resulting from the eating responses

Cues. Cues that can trigger maladaptive eating behavior can be social, situational, physiological, and psychological. Examples of social cues are loneliness, interpersonal conflict, social awkwardness, and holiday celebrations. Examples of situational cues include observation of diet advertisements, and walking by a store that sells

Box 23-5

COGNITIVE DISTORTIONS RELATED TO MALADAPTIVE EATING REGULATION RESPONSES

Magnification—Overestimation of the significance of undesirable events. Stimuli are embellished with meaning not supported by objective analysis. "I've gained 2 pounds, so I can't wear shorts any more."

Superstitious thinking—Believing in the cause-effect relationship of noncontingent events. "If I eat a sweet, it will instantly be turned into stomach fat."

Dichotomous or all-or-none thinking—Thinking in extreme or absolute terms such that events can only be black or white, right or wrong, good or bad. "If I gain 1 pound, I'll go on to gain 100 pounds."

Overgeneralization—Extracting a rule on the basis of one event and applying it to other dissimilar situations. "I used to be of normal weight and I wasn't happy. So I know gaining weight isn't going to make me feel better."

Selective abstraction—Basing a conclusion on isolated details while ignoring contradictory and more important evidence. "The only way I can be in control is through eating."

Personalization and self-reference—Egocentric interpretations of impersonal events or overinterpretation of events related to the self. "Two people laughed and whispered something to each other when I walked by. They were probably saying that I looked unattractive. I have gained 3 pounds."

From Garner D, Bemis K: Cognitive therapy for anorexia nervosa. In Garner D, Garfinkle P, eds: *Handbook of psychotherapy for anorexia and bulimia nervosa*, New York, 1985, The Guilford Press.

a food conducive to initiating a binge. Hunger and fatigue are the two most common physiological cues. Memory and mental images are two examples of psychological cues.

Specific cues such as these can trigger cognitive distortions and lead to maladaptive eating regulation responses. For example, when stepping on the scale a patient may see that she has gained a pound. She then may employ dichotomous thinking—"Since I've gained 1 pound, I will probably gain 20 pounds in the next week. I better take a package of laxatives so that I can lose the pound by tomorrow."

1. Stepping on the scale is the **cue.**
2. Believing she will gain 20 pounds is the related irrational **thought.**
3. Taking the laxatives is the maladaptive **eating regulation response** connected to the cognitive distortion.
4. Beginning another purge cycle is the **consequence** resulting from the maladaptive response.

Cues can be used as a strategy for change. Rearranging cues, avoiding a cue, and changing the response to a cue are ways of altering maladaptive responses. After continued recording about eating, binging, and purging behavior, and thoughts and feelings about food, shape, and weight, it is hoped that the patient will begin to see connections between thoughts and behaviors and recognize the consequences of the harmful activity.

Thoughts, Feelings, and Assumptions. The nurse helps patients challenge their faulty thoughts, feelings, and assumptions by questioning the evidence supporting or refuting the particular belief. In the previous example the nurse might ask the patient what specifically happened in the past when she gained a pound. Did she continue to gain 19 more pounds in the same week? If so, how often has it happened in the past? If not, why does the patient believe it will happen this time? It is also important for the nurse to ask the patient about the implications of this type of thinking. Do other people have the same problem if they gain a pound? If so, how do they deal with it? The nurse can then help the patient consider alternative explanations for her thoughts, and thereby gradually modify the irrational assumptions that underlie these beliefs. This is an example of the cognitive intervention of decentering.[15,20] These and other cognitive behavioral techniques may be successfully used in patients with maladaptive eating regulation responses (see A Patient Speaks).

Eating Regulation Responses. Patients with eating disorders need help in problem solving and making decisions. Rather than resorting to maladaptive responses, the patient must be helped to distinguish between adaptive and maladaptive coping responses and find alternative solutions.

One way of doing this is to encourage the patient to make a list of high-risk situations that cue them to exhibit maladaptive eating and purging behavior. The high-risk situation may be a certain day of the week, time of the day, season of the year, individual, group, event, or emotional response, such as anger or frustration. The nurse can then help the patient identify specific alternative ways of handling these high-risk situations that will be more adaptive.[15]

Decision-making strategies also may need to be reviewed and modified. Many patients with eating disorders know what they need to do in a given situation but may feel inadequate or shy about carrying out a certain plan of action. These individuals may benefit from assertiveness training and role modeling sessions with the nurse.

A PATIENT SPEAKS

Learning to separate my feelings from my eating has been the hardest part but the greatest benefit of treatment for my eating disorder. From early childhood, food had been my main outlet for almost every emotion. When I was sad, I comforted myself by eating. When I was happy, I celebrated by eating. Feelings of loneliness could be diminished by gathering up all my "food friends" and eating. Feeling angry at anyone beside myself was unacceptable, so I would eat and then I had a "good reason" to be angry and focus it all on myself.

Also discovering that everything in life is not black or white, good or bad, perfect or imperfect, hungry or full has enabled me to be kinder to myself and more accepting of my imperfections and humanity. I now realize that shades of gray do exist when making a decision, performing a task, feeling an emotion, and even experiencing hunger. Another benefit of this insight is a decrease in my level of anxiety along with feelings of worthlessness.

Each day is no longer a battle to control all aspects of my life, especially my food consumption. The struggle with food and my weight still remains, but now it doesn't completely overshadow everything else that happens in my life. Food is no longer the only friend and enemy life offers. I learned all this from a nurse who took the time to get to know me and in turn helped me to get to know myself. ▼

Consequences. It is particularly important for the nurse and patient to explore the positive and negative consequences that result from the cognitive distortion and maladaptive response. Consequences can be biological, psychological, and sociocultural, and there are positive and negative consequences resulting from each behavior. Some of these are presented in Table 23-3. A maladaptive behavior such as binging is maintained because positive consequences are more immediate or more valued than the negative consequences.

Strategies for change focusing on consequences involve the use of rewards that increase the likelihood of behavior change. In the above example in which the laxatives were taken in response to a 1 pound weight gain, rewards would be given if the individual was able to resist taking the laxative. The reward should be received immediately following the desired behavior change. It should be something pleasurable and can be either a material item or a psychological reinforcer, but it should not involve food.

 Should overweight nurses be assigned to care for patients with eating disorders? Why or why not?

Body Image Interventions

Body image distortions are one of the most difficult aspects of the eating disorder to treat. This is partly because researchers disagree on what exactly constitutes a body image distortion. The only agreement is that body image distortion in the eating disordered involves perceptual, attitudinal, and behavioral features[10] (Fig. 23-4). One also needs to distinguish between body image distortion and dissatisfaction.

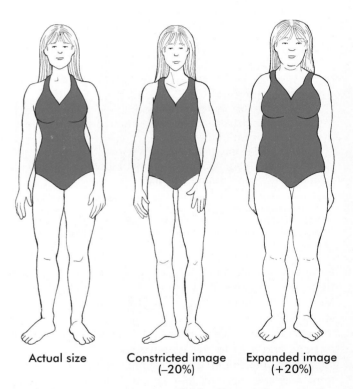

| Actual size | Constricted image (−20%) | Expanded image (+20%) |

Fig. 23-4 The perception of body shape and size can be evaluated through the use of special computer drawing programs that allow a subject to distort the width of an actual picture of a person's body by as much as 20% larger or smaller. Both anorectics and normal subjects adjusted the figures of other people's bodies to normal dimension. However, anorectics consistently adjusted their own body picture to a size 20% larger than its true form, suggesting that they have a major problem with the perception of self-image.

Adapted from Bloom F, Lazerson A: *Brain, mind, and behavior,* New York, 1988, WH Freeman.

Body image distortion is the discrepancy that exists between the patient's actual and perceived body size. Body dissatisfaction refers to the degree of unhappiness that a person feels in relation to body size.

While all individuals at sometime in their lives may express dissatisfaction with their bodies, the bulimic or anorectic's dissatisfaction is constant. Individuals with eating disorders place so much value on their appearance that it begins to exclusively define their self-worth. Behavioral features of body image disturbance are manifested in a life-style that revolves around a person's self-concern about the body. Examples of this range from constant weight measurement, wearing baggy clothes, and avoiding social situations in which the individual might be scrutinized about appearance. Overestimation of body size or of a body part is a common perceptual distortion in anorexia and bulimia.

A variety of interventions have been suggested for treating body image problems.[34] It is important for the nurse to first determine whether the patient has problems in perception, attitude, or behavior and then devise a treatment program targeting the specific problem area. Cognitive behavioral interventions are effective, as are dance and movement therapies, which create pleasant body experiences and can enhance the integration of mind and body, clarify body boundaries, and modulate negative feelings about the body.[37] Other therapeutic approaches include the use of imagery and relaxation, working with mirrors, and depicting self through art mediums. Researchers agree that body image interventions are crucial to the treatment of eating disorders, and much work remains to be done in this area.

Family Involvement

Families should be engaged from the beginning of treatment and included in family meetings and treatment planning sessions. The nurse should gather information about the family system and explore how the maladaptive eating response might serve a specific function within the family. Questions the nurse might ask include the following:

1. What part does the eating disorder serve in stabilizing the family system?
2. How has the family attempted to deal with the eating disorder?
3. What is the central theme surrounding the eating behavior?
4. What would be the consequences of change for each family member?
5. What is the underlying therapeutic issue from a family perspective?

Many young patients may need intensive family therapy after they have successfully completed the refeeding stage. The initial issue of such therapy is centered on the separation and individuation of the patient within the context of the family. This process requires much openness on the part of the family, and not every family may be able to complete it. However, the nurse should work with family strengths that have been identified and help involved family members work toward change (see A Family Speaks). Family therapy is described in more detail in Chapter 30.

Table 23-3 Consequences Resulting from Maladaptive Eating Regulation Responses

	Positive consequences	Negative consequences
Biological	▼ Reduced fear of fatness ▼ Reduced perception of hunger ▼ Avoidance of biological maturity	▼ Weakness, fatigue, dizziness ▼ Poor concentration ▼ Electrolyte disturbance ▼ Dental problems
Psychological	▼ Relief from tension, anger, and stress ▼ Relief from boredom ▼ Emotional anesthesia ▼ Feeling nurturance or pleasure ▼ Thoughts about avoiding weight gain	▼ Depression, guilt, shame ▼ Tendency to overact emotionally ▼ Increase in negative self-reference or guilt-related behavior
Sociocultural	▼ Avoidance of interpersonal conflict ▼ Social reinforcement for not gaining weight ▼ Distraction from adverse tasks ▼ Avoidance of responsibility and independence	▼ Social withdrawal ▼ Lying and lack of trust in relationships ▼ Occupational problems ▼ Financial problems ▼ Legal problems

Adapted from the University of Minnesota's Intensive Group Outpatient Treatment for Bulimia.

NURSING CARE PLAN SUMMARY
Eating Regulation Responses

I. Nursing Diagnosis: Altered nutrition

Expected Outcome: The patient will restore healthy patterns and normalize physiological parameters related to body weight and nutrition.

Short-term Goals	Interventions	Rationale
The patient will engage in treatment and acknowledge having an eating disorder.	Help patient identify maladaptive eating responses. Discuss positive and negative consequences of maladaptive eating responses. Contract with patient to engage in treatment.	The first step of treatment is for the patient to acknowledge the illness and see the need for help.
The patient will be able to describe a balanced diet based on the five food groups.	Complete a nutritional assessment including eating-related behaviors and preferences. Teach, clarify, and reinforce knowledge of proper nutrition.	Knowledge of healthy nutrition is essential to establishing and maintaining adaptive eating responses.
The patient's nutritional status will be stabilized by a specified targeted date.	Monitor physiological status for signs of compromised nutrition. Administer medications and somatic treatments for management of symptoms. Monitor and evaluate the patient's response to somatic treatments. Implement nursing activities as specified in the program contract and protocol.	Weight stabilization must be a central and early goal for the nutritionally compromised patient. Medications may assist the appetite regulation center and neurochemical responses to feeding and satiety.
The patient will participate in a balanced exercise program on a daily basis.	Review established exercise routines. Modify exercise patterns focusing on physical fitness rather than weight reduction. Reinforce new exercise and fitness behaviors.	The focus of a balanced exercise program should be on physical fitness rather than caloric reduction to lose weight.

II. Nursing Diagnosis: Body image disturbance

Expected Outcome: The patient will express clear and accurate descriptions of body size, body boundaries, and ideal weight.

Short-term Goals	Interventions	Rationale
The patient will correct body image distortions.	Modify body image misperceptions through cognitive strategies. Use dance and movement therapies to enhance the integration of mind and body. Employ imagery and relaxation interventions to decrease anxiety related to body perceptions.	Body image distortions involve perceptions, attitudes, and behaviors that place so much emphasis on appearance that they define self-worth.
The patient will modify cognitive distortions about body weight, shape, and eating responses.	Assist patient in identifying: 1. Cues that trigger problematic eating responses. 2. Thoughts, feelings, and assumptions associated with the specific cues. 3. Connections between these thoughts, feelings, assumptions and eating regulation responses. 4. The consequences resulting from the eating responses.	Cognitive distortions result in lowered self-esteem. Behavioral change occurs as a result of increased awareness of feelings and faulty cognitions.
The patient will identify social support systems that will reinforce accurate body perceptions and adaptive eating responses.	Include family members in the evaluation and treatment planning process. Assess the family as a system and the impact of the eating disorder on family functioning. Initiate group therapy to mobilize social support and reinforce adaptive responses.	Patients with eating disorders benefit from the involvement of family members and supportive group work.

A FAMILY SPEAKS

We have a 19-year-old daughter who has had an eating disorder for 8 years. The past 8 years have been most painful for our family as we went from doctor to doctor, counselor to counselor, and therapist to therapist—all with little or no results. What clinicians don't realize is how hard the day-to-day struggle is for families who want so much for their child to be healthy and happy, but who feel so helpless in how to make this happen.

Then we were referred to a nurse who we were told specialized in eating disorders, and slowly our lives began to change. Clearly, this nurse knew about our daughter's illness and together we went about treating it. Yes, we went through individual and family therapy, all in an attempt to help our daughter recover. Yes, at times it was painful and even frustrating. In the family sessions the nurse helped family members be aware of the part they had to play in our daughter's struggle and helped us realize that it would take a family team effort to help her get well. But the most important part is that all of the hard work of our daughter, each family member, and our nurse has been worth it. Our daughter now knows how to control her eating disorder, has had very few problems in the last 6 months, and our family has become even closer as we look back on the past with relief and into the future with hope. ▼

Group Therapies

Many models of group therapy are used for patients with eating disorders including cognitive behavioral, psychoeducational, psychodynamic, and interpersonal. Reality testing, supporting, and communicating with peers are essential therapeutic factors provided by group intervention. In addition, outpatient support groups may also be helpful if they serve to reinforce social alliances and encourage members to identify and express feelings.[41] Therapeutic groups are described in detail in Chapter 29.

Medications

Anorectics often resist medication, and no drugs have been found to be effective for this disorder. Medications that may be helpful for some patients include antidepressants for patients who are still depressed despite refeeding and antianxiety agents used before meals for anticipatory anxiety concerning eating. Unlike anorexia, some antidepressant medications, including imipramine, desipramine, trazadone, and fluoxetine, have been shown to be effective in reducing bulimic symptoms. The monoamine oxidase inhibitors phenelzine and isocarboxazid have also demonstrated efficacy.[2] Although antidepressants may make up one part of a

treatment plan for most bulimic patients, they should be used in conjunction with other therapeutic interventions. Finally, a single study has been conducted that supports the use of imipramine to reduce the frequency of binging in the treatment of binge eating disorder.[1] More research is needed regarding psychopharmacological treatments in this patient population.

The Nursing Care Plan Summary for patients with maladaptive eating regulation responses is presented on p. 626.

valuation

Patients with maladaptive eating regulation responses present special challenges to psychiatric nursing care. The evaluation of their care should begin with a focus on the therapeutic nurse-patient relationship. Nurses should determine if they provided effective role modeling, emotional support, biological monitoring, and reinforcement of the patient's attempts to explore and experiment with new cognitive and behavior patterns. Evaluation activities can then address three specific aspects of care:

1. Have normal eating patterns been restored?
2. Have the biological and psychological sequelae of malnutrition been corrected?
3. Have the associated sociocultural and behavioral problems been resolved so that relapse does not occur?

In answering these questions the nurse should review each aspect of the nursing process and modify care as needed to achieve the identified outcomes.

SUGGESTED CROSS-REFERENCES

SUMMARY

1. Adaptive eating regulation responses include balanced eating patterns, caloric intake, and weight.

Maladaptive responses include anorexia nervosa, bulimia nervosa, and binge eating disorder.

2. The majority of the maladaptive eating disorders occur in females and may range from 1% to 4% of adolescent and young adult women.

3. Patient behaviors related to eating regulation responses include binge eating, fasting or restricting, purging, and related medical and psychiatric complications.

4. Predisposing factors for eating regulation responses are described from biological, psychological, and sociocultural perspectives. Precipitating stressors that affect eating responses include peer pressure, interpersonal rejection, and daily solitude.

5. Level of motivation to change behavior is an important coping resource to assess. A variety of maladaptive coping mechanisms may be used including avoidance, intellectualization, isolation of affect, and denial.

6. Primary NANDA nursing diagnoses are anxiety, body image disturbance, fluid volume deficit, high risk for self-mutilation, altered nutrition, powerlessness, and self-esteem disturbance.

7. Primary DSM-IV diagnoses are anorexia nervosa, bulimia nervosa, and binge eating disorder.

8. The expected outcome of nursing care is that the patient will restore healthy eating patterns and normalize physiological parameters related to body weight and nutrition.

9. Planning activities involves decisions related to choice of treatment setting and the formulation of a nursing care plan contract.

10. Interventions include nutrition stabilization, exercise, cognitive behavioral interventions, body image interventions, family involvement, group therapies, and medications.

11. The nurse and patient should evaluate whether normal eating patterns have been restored and associated biopsychosocial problems have been resolved.

COMPETENT CARING
A CLINICAL EXEMPLAR OF A PSYCHIATRIC NURSE

Debra L. Davis, RN

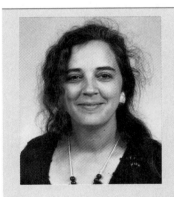

It seemed like a typically busy but uneventful day on our adult inpatient unit. After lunch, patients who had been participating in a group therapy session began returning to the unit. However, one patient was not in the company of the group. Upon inquiring I discovered that Miss G, a 22-year-old patient with an eating disorder, had failed to attend the group session. I told the charge nurse of her absence and, almost simultaneously, the phone rang informing us that someone had been spotted standing on top of our building. I went outside and encountered a security officer whom I followed to the site of the report. Sure enough, there on top of the three-story building was Miss G. who was saying she intended to jump.

As a staff nurse, I instantly assessed the situation as an emergency and knew that someone had to assume immediate crisis management. I also realized that this was a time when my considerable tenure as a mental health technician, licensed practical nurse, and now registered nurse, would lend itself to the task. Certainly, I faced many crises during my years in the mental health field, but none was more perilous than this one, and none had begged for quicker or more decisive action.

In horror, I fixed my gaze on the patient, her toes draped over the edge of the building some 60 feet above the ground. Her precariously positioned frame was teetering, and her state of mind seemed to be of similar disposition. Miss G again threatened to jump and continued to repeat her desire to "end it all."

I yelled up to her and asked what could I do to reduce her distress. She asked to see Shelley, a staff member who had established a therapeutic relationship with Miss G and was someone she obviously trusted. I successfully bargained with the patient to step back from the edge of the building and sit down while I ran inside to get Shelley.

I then directed the security officers to summon the mobile crisis unit to assist in managing this drama. In the interim, I knew we had to continue efforts to retrieve the distressed patient. "Someone's got to go in the building and try to reach that roof," I said to Drew, another staff member who was on the scene. He agreed and quickly hurried off to find a way up. Extremely anxious that Miss G would either jump or accidently fall. Shelley and I, along with some security personnel, dragged mattresses outside and placed them beneath where Miss G was standing.

Shelley began to communicate with the patient via a bullhorn, talking about the progress that Miss G had made and the plans she was looking forward to

as they had previously discussed. Suddenly, as we watched, a pair of arms wrapped around Miss G and pulled her back from the edge of the building. Drew had found access to the roof and had snatched the patient back to safety. Applause erupted on the ground, and with the help of the mobile crisis unit and the security officers, Miss G was lowered to the ground and escorted back to the unit.

Those of us involved in the crisis removed ourselves from the scene, and uninvolved staff began postcrisis management interventions on the unit. I breathed deeply and felt the muscles in my neck relax for the first time in hours. So much for a typically busy but eventful day in psychiatric nursing. ▼

REFERENCES

1. Alger S et al: Effect of a tricyclic antidepressant and opiate agonist on binge eating in normoweight bulimic and obese binge eating subjects, *Am J Clin Nutr* 53:865, 1991.
2. American Psychiatric Association: Practice guidelines for eating disorders, *Am J Psychiatry* 150:207, 1993.
3. American Psychiatric Association: *Diagnostic and statistical manual of mental disorders*, ed 4, Washington, DC, 1994, The Association.
4. Anderson AE, ed: *Males with eating disorders*, New York, 1990, Brunner/Mazel.
5. Blinder BJ, Chaitlin BF, Goldstein RS: *Medical and psychological basis of diagnosis and treatment*, New York, 1988, PMA Publishing.
6. Bo-Linn GW, Santa Ana CA, Morawski SG, Fortran HF: Purging and caloric absorption in bulimic patients and normal woman, *JAMA* 99:14, 1983.
7. Brewerton TD, Dansky BS, O'Neil PM, Kilpatrick DG: Prevalence of binge eating disorder in U.S. women. Paper presented at the American Psychiatric Association's Annual Meeting, San Francisco, May 1993.
8. Brewerton TD et al: Serotonin in the eating disorders. In Coccaro EF, Murphy DL, eds: *Serotonin in major psychiatric disorders*, Washington, DC, 1989, American Psychiatric Association Press.
9. Bulik CM: Abuse of drugs associated with eating disorders, *J Subst Abuse Treat* 4:69, 1992.
10. Cash T, Pruzinsky T: *Body images: development and deviance*, New York, 1990, The Guilford Press.
11. Casper R, Davis J: On the course of anorexia nervosa, *Am J Psychiatry* 134:974, 1977.
12. Conrad N, Sloan S, Jedwabny J: Resolving the control struggle on an eating disorders unit, *Perspect Psychiatr Care* 28:13, 1992.
13. Dardis PO, Hofland SL: Anorexia nervosa: fluid-electrolyte and acid-base manifestations, *J Child Adolesc Psychiatr Nurs* 3:85, 1990.
14. Devlin MJ, Walsh BT, Spitzer RL, Hasin D: Is there another binge eating disorder? A review of the literature on over-eating in the absence of bulimia nervosa, *Int J Eating Disorders* 11:333, 1991.
15. Fairburn C: Eating disorders. In Hawton K et al, eds: *Cognitive behavior therapy for psychiatric problems*, Oxford, 1989, Oxford University Press.
16. Fava M, Copeland PM, Schweiger U, Herzog DB: Neurochemical abnormalities in anorexia nervosa and bulimia nervosa, *Am J Psychiatry* 146:963, 1989.
17. Fontaine KL: The conspiracy of culture: women's issues in body size, *Nurs Clin North Am* 26:669, 1991.
18. Freund KM, Graham SM, Lesky LG, Moskowitz MA: Detection of bulimia in a primary care setting, *J Gen Intern Med* 8:236, 1993.
19. Garfinkle PE, Garner DM: *Anorexia nervosa: a multidimensional perspective*, New York, 1982, Brunner/Mazel.
20. Garner D, Bemis K: Cognitive therapy for anorexia nervosa. In Garner D, Garfinkle P, eds: *Handbook of psychotherapy for anorexia and bulimia nervosa*, New York, 1985, The Guilford Press.
21. Garner PE, Garfinkle DM, eds: *Handbook of psychotherapy for anorexia nervosa and bulimia nervosa*, New York, 1985, The Guilford Press.
22. Hall CW, Beresford TP: Medical complications of anorexia and bulimia nervosa, *Psychiatr Med* 7:165, 1989.
23. Hofland SL, Dardis PO: Bulimia nervosa: associated physical problems, *J Psychosoc Nurs Ment Health Serv* 30:23, 1992.
24. Johnson C: The initial consultation for patients with bulimia nervosa and anorexia nervosa. In Garner DM, Garfinkle PE, eds: *Handbook of psychotherapy for anorexia nervosa and bulimia nervosa*, New York, 1985, The Guilford Press.
25. Johnson C, Connors ME: *The etiology and treatment of bulimia nervosa: a biopsychosocial perspective*, New York, 1987, Basic Books.
26. Kanter RA, Williams BE, Cummings C: Personal and parental alcohol abuse and victimization in obese bingers and the nonbinging obese, *Addict Behav* 17:439, 1992.
27. Kendler KS et al: The genetic epidemiology of bulimia nervosa, *Am J Psychiatry* 148:1627, 1991.

28. Krueger DW: Eating disorders: A model developmental arrest of body self and psychological self. In *Body self and psychological self: a developmental and clinical integration of the disorders of the self*, New York, 1992, Brunner/Mazel.

29. Laraia MT, Stuart GW: Bulimia: a review of nutritional and health behaviors, *J Child Adolesc Psychiatr Nurs* 3:91, 1990.

30. Larson R, Johnson C: Bulimia: disturbed patterns of solitude, *Addict Behav* 10:281, 1985.

31. Love CC, Seaton H: Eating disorders: highlights of nursing assessment and therapeutics, *Nurs Clin North Am* 26:677, 1991.

32. Lucas AR, Beard CM, O'Fallon WM, Curlan LT: 50-year trends in the incidence of anorexia nervosa in Rochester, Minn.: a population-based study, *Am J Psychiatry* 148:917, 1991.

33. Metropolitan Insurance Company: 1979 *Build study*, New York, 1983, Society of Actuaries and Association of Life Insurance Medical Directors.

34. Miller KD: Body-image therapy, *Nurs Clin North Am* 26:727, 1991.

35. Mitchell JE, Hatsukami D, Eckert ED, Pyle RL: Characteristics of 275 patients with bulimia nervosa, *Am J Psychiatry* 142:482, 1985.

36. Pope HG, Hudson JI: Is childhood sexual abuse a risk for bulimia nervosa? *Am J Psychiatry* 17:455, 1991.

37. Rice J, Hardenbergh M, Hornyak L: Disturbed body image in anorexia nervosa: dance/movement therapy interventions. In Hornyak L, Baker E, eds: *Experiential therapies for the eating disorders*, New York, 1989, The Guilford Press.

38. Rositer EM, Agras WS: An empirical test of the DSM III-r definition of a binge, *Int J Eating Disorders* 9:513, 1990.

39. Spitzer RL et al: Binge eating disorder: a multisite field trial of the diagnostic criteria, *Int J Eating Disorders* 11:191, 1991.

40. Spitzer RL et al: Binge eating disorder: its further validation in a multisite study, *Int J Eating Disorders* 13:137, 1993.

41. Staples NR, Schwartz M: Anorexia nervosa support group: providing transitional support, *J Psychosoc Nurs Ment Health Serv* 28:6, 1990.

42. Steiner-Adair KS: The body politic: normal female adolescent development and the development of eating disorders. In Gilligan C, Lyons NP, Hammer TJ, eds: *Making connections: the relational worlds of adolescent girls at Emma Willard School*, Cambridge, 1990, Harvard University Press.

43. Strober M et al: A controlled family study of anorexia nervosa: evidence of familial aggregation and lack of shared transmission with affective disorders, *Int J Eating Disorders* 9:239, 1990.

44. Stuart G, Laraia M, Lydiard R, Ballenger J: Early family experiences of women with bulimia and depression, *Arch Psychiatr Nurs* 4:43, 1990.

45. Wolfe EM, Crowther JH: Personality and eating habit variables as predictors of severity of binge eating and weight, *Addict Behav* 8:335, 1983.

46. Yanovski S et al: Association of binge eating disorder and psychiatric comorbidity in obese subjects, *Am J Psychiatry* 150:1472, 1993.

47. Yates A: *Compulsive exercise and the eating disorders: toward an integrated theory of activity*, New York, 1991, Brunner/Mazel.

ANNOTATED SUGGESTED READINGS

*Conrad N, Sloan S, Jedwabny J: Resolving the control struggle on an eating disorders unit, *Perspect Psychiatr Care* 28:13, 1992.

Describes the process by which the nursing staff of an eating disorder program identified an ineffective treatment model and implemented the therapeutic/administrative split model to improve patient care.

*Fontaine K: The conspiracy of culture: women's issues in body size, *Nurs Clin North Am* 26:669, 1991.

Reviews the influence of culture and weight prejudices that are socially based.

*Forisha B, Grothaus K, Luscombe R: Dinner conversation: meal therapy to differentiate eating behavior from family process, *J Psychosoc Nurs Ment Health Serv* 28:13, 1990.

Meal therapy was developed by the authors as a family therapy approach to treating families within the psychosocial context of a family meal.

Freeman R: *Body love: learning to like our looks and ourselves*, Cambridge, 1989, Harper & Row.

Self-help manual for common problems about appearance that concern all women.

Garner D, Garfinkel P, eds: *Handbook of psychotherapy for anorexia nervosa and bulimia*, New York, 1985, The Guilford Press.

Presents various theoretical foundations for the treatment of anorectics and bulimics, including psychodynamic, behavioral, cognitive, family, and group therapy approaches. Classic in the area.

Harper-Giuffre H, MacKenzie K: *Group psychotherapy for eating disorders*, Washington, DC, 1992, American Psychiatric Press.

Excellent resource describing almost every type of group currently used in eating disorders.

Hirschmann J, Zaphiropoulos L: *Preventing childhood eating problems: a practical positive approach to raising children free of food and weight conflicts*, Carlsbad, Calif, 1993, Gurze Books.

Comprehensive guide for parents in understanding eating behaviors from infancy through adolescence. Practical, valuable, and clearly written.

*Irwin E: A focused overview of anorexia nervosa and bulimia: Part I. Etiological issues; Part II. Challenges to the practice of psychiatric nursing, *Arch Psychiatr Nurs* 7:342, 1993.

Excellent two-part overview of these eating disorders with detailed implications for nursing care.

Kaplan A, Garfinkel P, eds: *Medical issues and the eating disorders*, New York, 1993, Brunner/Mazel.

Thorough review of the medical problems of eating disorder patients.

*Laraia M, Stuart G: Bulimia: a review of nutritional and health behaviors, *J Child Adolesc Psychiatr Nurs* 3:91, 1990.

The epidemiology, early precipitants, physiology, and biochemistry of bulimia are reviewed with implications for holistic nursing care.

*Love C, Seaton H: Eating disorders: highlights of nursing assessment and therapeutics, *Nurs Clin North Am* 26:677, 1991.

Highly recommended article describing nursing assessment and treatment strategies for eating disorder patients. Includes sample care plans.

*Miller K: Body image therapy, *Nurs Clin North Am* 26:727, 1991.

Explores characteristic disturbances, assessment issues, and specific strategies of body image therapy. Good reference article.

*Staples N, Schwartz M: Anorexia nervosa support group: providing transitional support, *J Psychosoc Nurs Ment Health Serv* 28:6, 1990.

---

*Nursing reference.

Describes the goals, structure, process, and themes of an anorexia support group.

Vandereycken W, Koge E, Vanderlinden J, eds: *Family approach to eating disorders*, Great Neck, NY, 1989, PMA Publishers.

Questions assumptions and knowledge about families of eating disorder patients. Offers innovative research results as well as treatment principles for families.

Working Group on Eating Disorders: American Psychiatric Association Practice Guidelines: practice guidelines for eating disorders, Am J Psychiatry 150:207, 1993.

Consensus report for current standards of care by eating disorder clinicians and researchers based on existing research in the field.

Zerbe K: *The body betrayed: women, eating disorders, and treatment*, Washington, DC, 1993, American Psychiatric Association Press.

Authoritative and comprehensive book on eating disorders and their treatment, written in an accessible and compassionate manner.

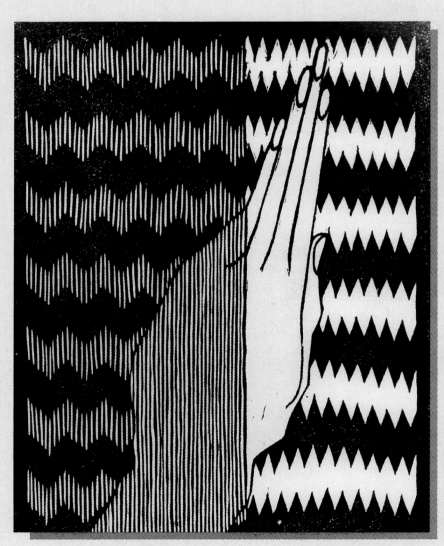

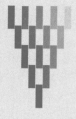

CHAPTER 24

Sexual Responses and Sexual Disorders

SUSAN G. POORMAN

I locked myself away from you
Too long,
Tossing aside my feelings
For you.
Looking for a way out, an excuse
Not to touch you;
Because I want to,

Inciting a riot within me.
To reach out for you
Is difficult,
But less difficult
Than turning away.

Leslie Bertel

LEARNING OBJECTIVES

After studying this chapter the student should be able to:

▼ Describe the continuum of adaptive and maladaptive sexual responses and the four phases of the nurse's growth in developing self-awareness of human sexuality
▼ Identify behaviors associated with sexual responses
▼ Analyze predisposing factors and precipitating stressors related to sexual responses
▼ Describe coping resources and coping mechanisms related to sexual responses
▼ Formulate nursing diagnoses for patients related to their sexual responses
▼ Assess the relationship between nursing diagnoses and medical diagnoses related to sexual responses
▼ Identify expected outcomes and short-term nursing goals for patients related to sexual responses
▼ Develop a patient education plan to promote patients' adaptive sexual responses
▼ Analyze nursing interventions for patients related to their sexual responses
▼ Evaluate nursing care for patients related to their sexual responses

TOPICAL OUTLINE

Continuum of Sexual Responses
    Adaptive and Maladaptive Sexual Responses
    Self-Awareness of the Nurse
Assessment
    Behaviors
    Predisposing Factors
    Precipitating Stressors
    Coping Resources
    Coping Mechanisms
Nursing Diagnosis
    Related Medical Diagnoses
Outcome Identification
Planning
Implementation
    Health Education
    Sexual Responses within the Nurse-Patient Relationship
    Maladaptive Sexual Responses due to Illness
    Maladaptive Homosexual and Bisexual Responses
    Maladaptive Transsexual Responses
    Dyfunctions of the Sexual Response Cycle
Evaluation

Sexuality broadly refers to all aspects of being sexual and is one dimension of the personality. It includes more than the act of intercourse and is an integral part of life. It is evident in the individual's appearance and in beliefs, behaviors, and relationships with others and includes gender identity. Accepting a broad concept of sexuality allows nurses to explore ways in which people are sexual beings and understand more fully their feelings, beliefs, and actions. Nurses are often called on to intervene in the sexual concerns of patients when providing holistic patient care. Therefore it is important that nurses develop skills and competence in addressing sexual issues by increasing awareness through education.

As nurses become educated in the basic principles of sexuality, they will better understand sexual needs and problems. If nurses are comfortable with sexual issues, they will convey this to the patient, who will also feel more comfortable in discussing such issues. Patients are often experiencing pain and change as a result of threats to health or even as a part of normal growth and development. Thus it is important that the nurse-patient relationship allow for honest discussions about sexuality.

In answering the question, "What do nurses need to know about sexuality?," several factors emerge. First, nurses need to know themselves and be aware of their feelings and values regarding sexuality. If nurses are not aware of their feelings, they cannot help patients meet their needs. Second, nurses need to understand that other people's feelings and values about sexuality will be different from their own. Third, all nurses can become educated about sexual health and use sound counseling methods with patients. Specifically, nurses can do the following:

1. Develop confidence in their ability to discuss sexual issues with patients
2. Learn interviewing skills for sexual assessment and history taking
3. Counsel or refer patients for counseling

Education can be gained through nursing courses and continuing education programs. Some nurses pursue additional education and may become sex educators in schools, outpatient clinics, and planned parenthood agencies. Nurses prepared at the graduate level may become sex therapists through postgraduate work in human sexuality and extensive clinical supervision.

CONTINUUM OF SEXUAL RESPONSES
Adaptive and Maladaptive Sexual Responses

It is difficult to define "normal" sexual behavior without making value judgments. *Normal* is frequently defined as what we ourselves do and feel comfortable about, and *abnormal* is what others do that seems different or odd to us. Parents, relatives, friends, and society are all likely to have different views on normal sexuality. Goldstein[12] defines normal sexual behavior as any sexual act between adults that is consensual, lacks force, and is performed in private, away from unwilling observers. If Goldstein's definition is accepted, then homosexuality, sexual pleasure between members of the same sex, would be considered normal. Conversely, pedophilia, obtaining sexual pleasure through child molestation, would not meet Goldstein's requirements.

Experts in sexuality do not agree on what is normal. For years many people believed that only sexual relations between married heterosexual partners for procreation was normal. Today people view sexual behavior with a wider range of attitudes. Sexuality, on a continuum, ranges from adaptive to maladaptive (Fig. 24-1). The most adaptive responses meet the following cri-

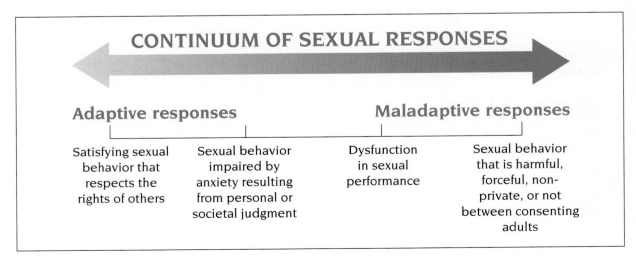

Fig. 24-1   Continuum of sexual responses.

teria: between two consenting adults, mutually satisfying to both, not psychologically or physically harmful to either party, lacking in force or coercion, and conducted in private.

Sometimes, however, sexual behavior can meet the criteria for adaptive responses but may be altered by what society deems acceptable and unacceptable. Unfortunately, society often decides this based on fear, prejudice, and lack of information rather than on data and facts (see Critical Thinking About Contemporary Issues). For example, the homosexual person may have the potential for healthy responses but be impaired by anxiety about societal disapproval.

Maladaptive sexual responses include behaviors that do not meet one of more of the criteria for adaptive responses. The degree to which these behaviors are maladaptive will vary. Some sexual behaviors may not meet any of the criteria mentioned. For example, incest may include force and be psychologically harmful. However, other sexual responses may meet four of the five criteria for adaptive responses but still be maladaptive. For example, a couple with a sexual dysfunction, such as premature ejaculation, may meet Goldstein's criteria for normal behavior, but their sexual behavior may be un-

satisfactory or even psychologically harmful to one or both members.

Caution must be used when attempting to label sexual behaviors as adaptive or maladaptive. There will never be total agreement, and there will always be exceptions to the rule. The continuum shown in Fig. 24-1 is free of moral judgment and was developed to aid the nurse in developing self-awareness and understanding the range of sexual responses.

 How do you define "normal" sexuality? Compare your views with those of a friend, a family member, and a health-care provider.

Self-Awareness of the Nurse

The nurse's level of self-awareness is critically important in discussing sexual issues with patients. The first step in developing self-awareness involves clarification of values regarding human sexuality. Foley and Davies[9] identified growth experiences developed around the nursing care of rape victims. Their model is also applicable to sexual counseling and consists of four phases of the nurse's growth: cognitive dissonance, anxiety, anger, and action (Fig. 24-2).

Cognitive Dissonance. The first phase of growth in developing sexual self-awareness is cognitive dissonance, which arises when two opposing beliefs exist at the same time. For example, nurses grow up learning what society, family, and friends believe about sexual issues. If a nurse is raised in an environment that teaches that "it is impolite to talk about sex; it's too personal a subject," the nurse will carry that belief into nursing practice. When a patient wants to discuss a sexual concern, the nurse may feel two opposing reactions simultaneously: (1) "I should not ask questions about such a personal subject as sex"; and (2) "As a professional, I should be able to discuss any problem, including sexual problems, with my patient."

The nurse has opposing thoughts based on the different role expectations that make the nurse uncomfortable. However, the discomfort can be positive because it forces the nurse to examine feelings about the issue. The nurse resolves the cognitive dissonance in one of two ways: (1) continues to believe that sexual concerns are too personal to discuss with patients or (2) examines the fact that sexuality is an integral part of being human.

Both of these beliefs have consequences for how the nurse relates to patients who voice sexual concerns. If the nurse continues to believe that sex is too personal to discuss with the patient, the nurse may become un-

CRITICAL THINKING ABOUT CONTEMPORARY ISSUES

Does Sex Education in Schools Promote Teenage Promiscuity?

Some people in this country believe that teenagers are sexually active because they are taught sex education in their schools. The issue of sex education for youth in this country has raised a storm of questions and controversy. Unfortunately, much of it is based on values, beliefs, and personal opinion instead of facts. People who oppose sex education fight against comprehensive sex education programs in public education. In contrast, many parents believe that their children are receiving sex education in school when, in fact, they often are not.

Research provides some answers to this controversial question. Studies have demonstrated that comprehensive sex education programs can delay the initiation of first intercourse, reduce unprotected intercourse, and decrease unwanted teen pregnancy.[22,37] Based on these findings, along with the rising incidence of teen pregnancy and sexually transmitted diseases, the more important question this country faces is whether we can afford not to provide comprehensive sex education in our schools. ▼

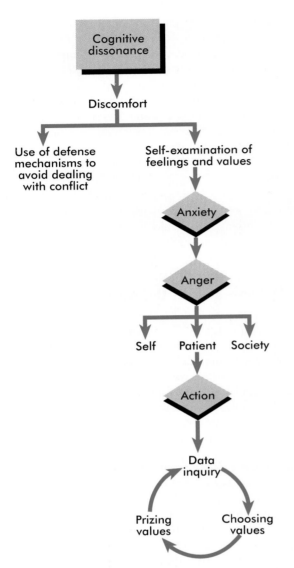

Fig. 24-2 Phases of the nurse's growth in developing self-awareness of human sexuality.

comfortable and choose not to follow-up on sexual issues. This discomfort may be projected onto the patient, with the nurse stating, "The patient seemed too upset to talk about that right now." In this case the nurse should explore personal values and beliefs about sexuality and ask, "Do I believe these ideas about discussing sexual concerns because I have researched the facts and have accurate, current information?" Only when the nurse has examined the available information and made an informed choice on values will clarification of those values occur. If the nurse examines personal and professional values and believes that sexuality is an integral part of being human, a second phase of growth occurs.

Anxiety. Most people think that anxiety is a negative emotion. However, a mild level of anxiety can be posi-

tive because it can promote an awareness of danger, give extra energy, or stimulate professional growth by creating enough discomfort to initiate some type of action. In this second phase the nurse realizes that uncertainty, insecurity, questions, and problems regarding sexuality are normal. The nurse begins to understand that everyone is capable of a variety of sexual feelings and behaviors and that anyone can have a sexual dysfunction or question sexual identity. The nurse experiencing anxiety may exhibit behaviors that hinder discussion of sexual issues such as talking too much (not allowing patients to verbalize their feelings), failing to listen (not picking up on patients' cues and messages), and diagnosing and analyzing (becoming preoccupied with facts rather than feelings). As the anxiety level rises, the nurse becomes more uncomfortable and tries to reduce it. Learning about sexuality and facing conflicting values bring the nurse to the third phase of growth.

Anger. Anger generally arises after anxiety, fear, and shock subside. It is generally self-directed or directed to the patient or society. The nurse begins to recognize that issues associated with sex or sexuality are emotional and sometimes highly volatile. Rape, abortion, birth control, equal rights, child abuse, pornography, and religious issues all are related to sexuality and give rise to controversy and debate. This realization often breeds anger and contempt in the nurse. For example, the nurse may become angry at a colleague or a friend who makes judgmental remarks about pro-life or pro-choice activists.

During this phase of anger, the nurse tends to choose words and actions that may be as judgmental as the attitudes the nurse is fighting against. The nurse may lecture other nurses about the need for sex education or critically judge a teenager who does not fear the consequences of having unprotected sex with someone known to be HIV positive. The nurse may also be angry with society for perpetuating ignorance about sexuality. Some nurses may spend time and energy at school-based clinics discussing issues such as date rape and not understand when others do not share their enthusiasm for changing society's beliefs. Toward the end of this phase the nurse begins to understand that blaming self or society for lack of proper awareness does not help patients with sexual concerns. This realization helps defuse the anger, and the nurse is ready for the final phase.

Action. The final step in the growth experience is the action phase. Several behaviors emerge during this final phase of the growth experience: data inquiry, choosing values, and prizing values. Data inquiry occurs when the nurse seeks out additional information about sexual issues. Once the information is obtained, the nurse may wish to discuss and debate the issues. These are healthy ways of exploring and deciding what to believe, and the nurse will eventually make some choices about a value position.

After choosing a value position, the final behavior is one of prizing the value position, which consists of an awareness and cherishing of feelings and values and being willing to share them publicly. Although prizing values is considered the final step in a positive growth experience, it does not mean that what is valued now will not change. Values are never static; they evolve and shift as a person changes, grows, and acquires new experiences. Thus a person who once ascribed to pro-life values may later become understanding and empathetic toward women who have abortions. The following clinical example illustrates the phases of growth health professionals experience while increasing their awareness about sexuality. Chapter 5 has additional content on developing self-awareness and the nurse's therapeutic use of self.

CLINICAL EXAMPLE

Ms. G worked as a staff nurse at an outpatient psychiatric clinic. One day at an interdisciplinary team meeting, Ms. G presented a new case to the treatment team for review. Her case was a 29-year-old female patient who came to the clinic because she thought she was transsexual. Ms. G began to explain the patient's history to the treatment team when one of the team members interrupted, stating "If this isn't the sickest thing I've ever heard of . . . . I hope you don't expect us to treat this woman, or should I say man!" The other members of the treatment team began to snicker and continued to make jokes about the transsexual patient.

After the team meeting, Ms. G felt very confused. She usually respected her co-workers' clinical judgment and considered them to be good clinicians. However, her new patient was obviously experiencing problems with her sexuality and was serious about wanting treatment for sexual reassignment. Ms. G was also anxious because of her lack of facts and knowledge about transsexuality. She decided to research the nature of transsexualism to help her patient. She found a psychologist in the city who worked with transsexual patients and made an appointment to talk about transsexuality.

Ms. G explained her co-workers' reaction to the psychologist, her anger at their ignorance, and her own difficulties in understanding transsexuality and in finding an appropriate referral for the patient. "This isn't the first time this has happened at our clinic," Ms. G told the psychologist. "Anytime we get a patient with sexual\ problems, everybody makes jokes and nothing is ever really done for them." The psychologist offered to do an in-service program on sexuality for the staff.

The next day Ms. G told the staff at the team meeting of the psychologist's offer to talk with them about providing care to patients expressing sexual preferences that differ from their own. One of the team members responded by laughing, "We don't need anyone to teach us about sex—I think we know everything we need to know." Everyone laughed and agreed. Ms. G, although anxious, spoke up stating, "If we all know so much, why all this nervous laughter? Look, I know it's hard to talk about sex and sexual issues, but we have to admit that we don't do a very good job addressing some of the sexual issues or problems that patients present us with here."

After Ms. G spoke up, there was a long silence in the room until another nurse spoke. "You know, I think Ms. G is right. There are lots of times I just don't know what to say or do for people who come in here with sexual concerns. What could it hurt to have an in-service?" After some discussion, the staff agreed to set up the in-service program.

 Which phase of growth are you in related to the development of self-awareness of human sexuality?

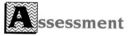 **ssessment**

Some people who feel stress regarding their sexual identity may be reluctant to accept help. Others may seek help indirectly by describing a vague symptom that masks an underlying sexual problem. The nurse is often the first health professional to come in contact with these patients. Any basic health history needs to include questions regarding sexual history.

A nurse who is comfortable in discussing sexuality conveys the message that it is normal to talk about sexual health in a health assessment interview. If nurses are able to eliminate the attitude that "sex should not be discussed" by being calm and professional, questions about patients' sexual health can be asked naturally. The patient can discuss sexual matters without embarrassment. At times, it may be helpful to assess an individual's sexual health in more detail. A sexual health assessment form such as the one in Box 24-1 may be useful.

Behaviors

There are many modes of sexual expression. In 1948, Kinsey used a seven-point rating scale to examine sexual preference (Fig. 24-3); 0 represented exclusively heterosexual experiences, 6 represented exclusively ho-

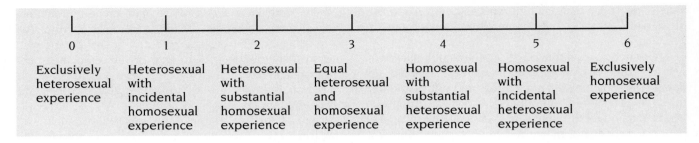

Fig. 24-3   Kinsey's rating scale of sexual preference.
From Kinsey AC, Pomeroy WB, Martin EC: *Sexual behavior in the human female*, Philadelphia, 1953, WB Saunders.

Box 24-1
SEXUAL HEALTH ASSESSMENT FORM

1. How were your questions about sex answered when you were a child? Where did your sexual information come from? (Appropriate for adolescents.) When you were a teenager, how were your questions about sex answered? (Appropriate for adults.)
2. How did you first find out about sexual intercourse (how babies are made)? (Appropriate for adolescents and young adults.)
3. How would you describe your current sexual activity?
4. What, if anything, would you change about your current sexual activity?
5. How important is a sexual relationship to you at this time in your life?
6. Do you have any concerns about birth control?
7. Do you have any health problems that, in your opinion, affect your sexual health or happiness?
8. Are you taking any medicines that, in your opinion, affect your sexual health or happiness?
9. Is there anything about these questions that you would like clarified or explained?

From Mims FH, Swenson M: *Sexuality: a nursing perspective*, New York, 1980, McGraw-Hill.

---

as sexual preference or sexual orientation. Some prefer the term *sexual orientation* over *sexual preference* in that preference infers that homosexuals choose to be homosexual. Although sexual behaviors do involve choice, sexual orientation includes emotion and erotic attraction and may be genetically determined rather than a matter of free will.[4] The actual incidence of homosexual behavior is unknown. Conservative estimates range from 3% to 5% in adult females and 5% to 10% in adult males. This estimate does not include bisexual behavior.[24]

For many years the medical profession, including psychiatry, has searched for causes of homosexuality. Although many psychological and biological theories have been suggested, there is no compelling evidence to support any one specific theory.[6] Some experts suggest that there should be less emphasis on determining the cause of homosexuality and more focus placed on learning more about modes of sexual expression. Research findings indicate that gays and lesbians function as well psychologically, emotionally, and sexually as heterosexual persons.[2] If current estimates of homosexuality are accurate, nurses come into contact with homosexuals daily but often know little about homosexuality and frequently assume that all patients are heterosexual.

 How are health-care providers' views of homosexuality influenced by social norms and cultural values?

mosexual experiences, and 2, 3, and 4 indicated a bisexual orientation. He suggested that most individuals are not exclusively heterosexual or homosexual. His studies indicated that a substantial percentage of men and women had experienced both heterosexual and homosexual activity. Specifically, the Kinsey study reported that 25% of U.S. males and 6% to 14% of females have had more than incidental homosexual experience.[21]

Homosexuality. Homosexuality can be defined as sexual attraction to members of the same sex. The term *gay* is used to refer to both male and female homosexuals; however some use the term to refer only to male homosexuals and the term *lesbian* to refer to female homosexuals. An individual's attraction to individuals of the same sex, opposite sex, or both sexes is referred to

Bisexuality. Bisexuality has been misunderstood in American society, and little interest in bisexuality research has been generated. There has also been inconsistency in the literature in defining the term *bisexuality*. Bisexuality, sometimes called *ambisexuality*, can be defined as a sexual attraction to persons of both sexes and the engagement in both homosexual and heterosexual activity.[35] Zinik[41] defines bisexuality as eroticizing or being sexually aroused by both females and males, engaging in (or desiring) sexual activity with both, and adopting bisexuality as a sexual identity label (rather than labeling oneself as heterosexual or homosexual). The prefix *bi-* implies equal (50/50) relations and eroticizing of both sexes; however, this is not the norm. Bisexuals do eroticize both sexes, but not necessarily to the same degree. For example, a bisexual individual may lean toward one sex or the other in more of a 60/40 or 70/30 ratio. Bisexuals may also have a preference for one sex or another but eroticize both sexes.

There has also been a long-standing debate regarding the nature of bisexuality. One theory, the conflict model, sees bisexuality as characterized by conflict and ambivalence, since it is based on the idea that sexual orientation is a dichotomy (one is either heterosexual or homosexual) and the bisexual cannot decide on sexual preference. Another view of bisexuality is the flexibility model in which bisexuality is seen as the coexistence of same and opposite sex erotic feelings and behaviors and an integration of homosexual and heterosexual identities. The flexibility model proposes that homosexual and heterosexual interests coexist without conflict and may, in fact, more fully reflect the integration of human experiences.

The incidence of bisexuality is difficult to determine because of the inconsistencies in the definition of bisexuality and the fact that there is no way of knowing how many people would actually identify themselves as being bisexual. It has been estimated that approximately 25 million Americans exhibit some combination of heterosexual and homosexual behavior. Although there has been limited research on bisexuality, the research that does exist indicates that bisexuals are as well adjusted as heterosexuals and homosexuals.[41]

Transvestism. Transvestism is defined as cross-dressing, or dressing in the clothes of the opposite sex. Clinically defined, "transvestism is a condition in which a male has a sexual obsession for or addiction to women's clothes, such that he periodically experiences intolerable psychic stress if he does not dress up as a female."[29] Most often the transvestite who seeks treatment is a male; very little is known about female transvestism. No reliable statistics concerning the incidence of transvestism are available; however, many professionals believe it is more common than generally assumed.

Transvestites tend to be married men who report heterosexual behavior. Although they occasionally or frequently dress in female clothes, they do not wish hormonal or surgical sex change. Many transvestites try to find willing partners, and typically their activities of cross-dressing do not prevent sexual relationships with others.[24]

Transsexualism. The word *transsexual* simply implies going from one sex to another. More specifically, a transsexual is a person who is anatomically a male or female but who expresses, with strong conviction, that he or she (1) has the mind of the opposite sex, (2) lives as a member of the opposite sex part-time or full-time, and (3) seeks to change his or her original sex legally and through hormonal and surgical sex reassignment.[29] Many times the transsexual patient will describe himself as "feeling trapped in the wrong body." Transsexuals genuinely believe they belong to the other sex. Many experience intense emotional turmoil because of stigma from society. There are no accurate estimates of the incidence of transsexualism; however postoperative transsexuals in the United States now number in the thousands.

Transsexuality is different from homosexuality in that homosexuals are comfortable with their anatomical identity and do not want to change their sex. Many transsexuals are heterosexual and express distaste for homosexual activity. Transsexuals are essentially heterosexual, not homosexual, but are often mistaken by others or themselves as homosexual as seen in this clinical example.

 ## CLINICAL EXAMPLE

Mr. L is a 21-year-old biological male who was admitted to the psychiatric unit for evaluation after a serious suicide attempt. Mr. L told his nurse that he tried to kill himself because he has been "sexually mixed up for years" and is tired of feeling like a freak of nature. He said that his friends make fun of him and tell him he is a homosexual. Although he does feel sexually attracted to other men, he does not believe he is a homosexual. "I guess I don't feel like a man, I feel like a woman inside a man's body, and as a woman I am attracted to men."

Selected Nursing Diagnoses:

▼ Altered sexuality patterns related to conflicting sexual feelings as evidenced by verbalizations of confusion and happiness

▼ Potential for self-directed violence related to sexual identity confusion as evidenced by suicide attempt

> Think of a patient you took care of last week. How would your care have been different if you knew this patient was a homosexual, bisexual, transvestite, or transsexual?

The Sexual Response Cycle. In addition to modes of sexual expression or sexual orientation, the physiological and psychological responses to sexual stimulation can also be described. Masters and Johnson[27] were the first to report the physiological changes that occur in men and women during sexual activity. They described the sexual response cycle as consisting of four phases: excitement, plateau, orgasmic, and resolution. Kaplan[18] also identified three stages of the sexual response cycle: desire, excitement, and orgasm. Currently the accepted stages of the sexual response cycle are a combination of those previously defined by Masters and Johnson and Kaplan and are listed in Box 24-2.

Impairment in sexual response may occur in any one of the phases of the sexual response cycle. For example, when the orgasm stage of the sexual response cycle is disrupted, premature or retarded ejaculation in males or orgasmic inhibition in females may result. If the excitement phase is inhibited, it may produce erectile dysfunction in males and a general sexual dysfunction in females. If the appetitive phase is absent, it may be evidenced by hypoactive sexual desire disorder or sexual arousal disorders. Although sexual dysfunction can occur when any phase is disrupted, resolution phase inhibition is rarely responsible for specific sexual dysfunctions.

The etiology of sexual dysfunctions is varied and complex. Sex therapists agree that many sexual dysfunctions are caused by psychological factors ranging from unresolved childhood conflicts to adult problems such as performance anxiety, lack of knowledge, or failure to communicate with a partner. Sexual dysfunction can also be caused by physiological factors such as vascular and endocrine disorders and medication side effects and is often the result of the interaction of psychological and physiological factors.[36]

Predisposing Factors

No one theory can adequately explain sexual development or predisposing factors of maladaptive sexual responses. Several theories have been proposed, however, and are now briefly described.

Biological. Biological factors are initially responsible for the development of gender, that is, whether a person is genetically male or female. Somatotype includes chromosomes, hormones, internal and external genitalia, and gonads. Sex differentiation is determined by the Y chromosome. Research in humans confirms the general rule that maleness and masculinity depend on fetal and perinatal androgens.

A biological female typically has XX chromosomes, with estrogen as the predominant hormone, appropriate internal and external genitalia, and ovaries. A biological male typically has XY chromosomes, with androgen as the predominant hormone, appropriate internal and external genitalia, and testicles. However, each of these typical configurations may vary. A person may have triple chromosomes, such as XXX, XXY, or XYY, or a single chromosome, XO. There is no YO chromosomal pattern. The triple pattern XXX and the single pattern XO (Turner's syndrome) will result in a female body, whereas the triple patterns XXY (Klinefelter's syndrome) and XYY will result in male bodies. Assuming no variation occurs, the biological factors result in a single, fully developed gender, either male or female.

Based on family studies and DNA samples of homosexual brothers it has been suggested a gene may be related to homosexuality. Early work in the field suggested that homosexuality may be inherited from the maternal side of the family through the X chromosome. Before such research is accepted as definitive, however, it will have to be validated by replication, and similar studies of lesbians have not yet been completed. In addition, such findings cannot account for all cases of homosexuality, but they do support a possible biological basis.

Psychoanalytical. Freud saw sexuality as one of the key forces of human life. In *Three Essays of the Theory of Sexuality*,[10] he theorized about the nature of sexuality and sexual development and proposed that sexuality was established before the onset of puberty. He also believed that a person's choice of sexual expression depended on a mix of heredity, biology, and social factors. He wrote extensively about childhood sexuality and believed sexuality during infancy was central to personality development.

Box 24-2

STAGES OF THE SEXUAL RESPONSE CYCLE

Stage 1
Appetitive
Sexual fantasies and the desire for sexual activity

Stage 2
Excitement
Subjective sense of sexual pleasure along with physiological changes, including penile erection in the male and vaginal lubrication in the female

Stage 3
Orgasm
Peaking of sexual pleasure and the release of sexual tension accompanied by rhythmic contractions of the perineal muscles and pelvic reproductive organs

Stage 4
Resolution
Sense of general relaxation, muscular relaxation, and well-being. Females may be able to respond to additional stimulation almost immediately during this stage; however, most males need some time before they can be restimulated to orgasm

The child, according to Freud, passes through a series of developmental stages in which a different erogenous zone is dominant. The first is the oral stage (birth to 12 or 18 months), in which the infant's chief sense of pleasure is derived from stimulation of the lips and mouth, that is, sucking. In the second, or anal, stage (ages 1 to 3 years), the child's attention is focused on elimination functions and control over body sphincters. The phallic stage follows (ages 3 to 5 years), in which the child's focus is on the genitals. An important occurrence in this stage is the development of the Oedipus complex in boys and the Electra complex in girls.

In the Oedipus/Electra complex the child experiences sexual feelings for the parent of the opposite sex and resents the parent of the same sex. According to Freud, the boy fears retaliation from his father for desiring the mother and fantasizes that the father will cut off his penis (castration anxiety). This fear is the impetus for the young boy's eventually giving up the resentment of the father and identifying with him and the male gender role. The girl, on the other hand, has no penis to fear losing. She believes that at one time she had a penis but it was cut off, and she blames her mother for this.

After the resolution of the Oedipus or Electra complex, the child enters a prolonged stage where sexual impulses are repressed (latency stage). This stage lasts until adolescence, when the child enters the genital stage and sexual urges reawaken. The reemergence of Oedipal/Electra feelings and the need to assert themselves with parents also occur during this phase of development. The adolescent then makes the final transition into mature genital sexuality.

In recent years there has been much criticism of Freud's theory of psychosexual development. Feminists argue that psychoanalytical theory is male centered and views women as anatomically inferior to men (because they have no penis). Lack of scientific evidence is one of the major problems with Freud's theory. Most of Freud's concepts have not been verified by any of the usual scientific methods. Other criticisms include that Freud was a victim of the Victorian era, a time of sexual repression, and that his thoughts and writings were bound by the period in which he lived. Finally, Freud's data were collected from observations of his patients, who were probably not representative of the total population and were to some degree emotionally ill.

 What impact has Freud's theory of psychosexual development had on society's view of women?

Behavioral. From a behaviorist's perspective, the most legitimate basis for understanding sexual reactions is the observable response to overt, measurable stimuli. Behaviorists are not concerned with the complex intrapsychic process of early childhood and adolescence; rather, they view sexual behavior as a measurable response, with both physiological and psychological components, to a learned stimulus or reinforcement event.

Behaviorists consider the sexual behavior of adults who care for children as important in the children's later sexual development. They are thus interested in sexual difficulties that result from sexual abuse in childhood. Although the research is limited, it does appear that adults who were sexually abused as children may have significant adjustment problems. In one study, women with sexual abuse histories were more likely than their nonabuse counterparts to have sexual problems as well as suicidal ideation, suicide attempts, histories of drug abuse, and self-mutilation.[5] Another study found that young adult women who had experienced childhood incest reported less satisfaction with their sexual functioning than did a control group.[16] In this study, 65% of the victims met the DSM-III criteria for one or more of the sexual dysfunctions such as inhibited sexual desire, inhibited orgasm, inhibited sexual excitement, dyspareunia, or vaginismus.[1] Finally, an examination of the aftermath of child sexual abuse in black and white American women found that one of the lasting effects of child sexual abuse included sexual problems for women of both ethnic groups.[40] The care of individuals who have been victims of abuse and violence is described in detail in Chapter 37.

Precipitating Stressors

Feelings about oneself as a sexual being change throughout the life cycle. Sexual identity cannot be separated from self-concept or body image. Therefore when bodily or emotional changes occur, sexual responses change as well.

Illness and Injury. Physical and emotional illness may alter sexuality. The patient may find that hospitalization alone changes sexual feelings and behavior. Nurses frequently care for patients with sexual dysfunctions or altered sexuality patterns; they need to discuss and therapeutically intervene in patients' responses to these changes. A person with rheumatoid arthritis may have body disfiguration and a change in body image caused by swollen areas around joints. The same patient may have decreased sexual interest because of joint pain during intercourse. People who have had a myocardial infarction may have decreased sexual interest because they fear sexual arousal may cause a heart attack.

Psychiatric illness also affects an individual's sexuality as well as the sexual behavior and satisfaction of the individual's partner (see A Family Speaks). Depression can be either the result or cause of sexual dysfunction. As many as 70% of depressed patients have decreased sexual desire and decreased frequency of intercourse. Most often, depressed men engage in intercourse less frequently; depressed women may participate in sex but with less enjoyment. In contrast, hypersexuality may be the first symptom of a manic episode. Individuals with bipolar illness have decreased sexual inhibitions, often impulsively choose sexual partners or begin extramarital affairs, display inappropriate sexual behavior, or act seductively or flirtatiously. Finally, individuals with schizophrenia may become preoccupied with sex and have sexual delusions about being a member of the opposite sex, being homosexual, being pregnant, having lovers, or having misperceptions about their sexual organs.

Some medications contribute to sexual dysfunction, such as a woman's failure to reach orgasm and a man's impotence or failure to ejaculate. Nurses should be knowledgeable about the medications they administer. Sexual side effects of antipsychotic medications, including problems with erection, ejaculation, libido, and menstrual difficulties, are estimated to occur in 30% to 60% of persons taking medication.[34] Side effects are also associated with some antidepressants. Psychotropic medications and their side effects are described in Chapter 25.

Nurses should be familiar with the sexual side effects of medications, educate their patients about them, and encourage patients to notify a health professional when these effects occur. For example, a patient may not be aware that his medication can cause impotence, yet he may be embarrassed and hesitant to talk with the physician or nurse about the problem. Often the medication itself or the dosage can be changed to correct the problem. Abuse of alcohol or nontherapeutic drugs may also have a debilitating effect on sexuality. Although many people believe alcohol is a sexual stimulant, prolonged use can cause erectile difficulty and other dysfunctions.

Fear of contracting a sexually transmitted disease (STD) may be a stressor that creates change in sexual behavior. The most frightening STD is acquired immune deficiency syndrome (AIDS), which is caused by the human immunodeficiency virus (HIV). More than a decade ago the first cases of AIDS were discovered in homosexual men. Since that time AIDS/HIV infection has become a leading worldwide health problem that is spreading rapidly. Over the years there have been many changes in the incidence of this disease. First, there is a decreasing incidence in the number of cases in homosexual men because of the significant increase in safer sexual practices among gay men.[11,32] Widely

A FAMILY SPEAKS

Our daughter was diagnosed with schizophrenia 5 years ago when she was 17 years of age. Since that time we have been fortunate to have received very good care for her. While we understand that she may never be completely well, she has her illness under control and has even started taking some courses at the local community college. She has also met some people her age and seems to enjoy their company.

But ever since she began doing better, we have had the added concern about her sexual needs and activities. As involved parents, we raised this issue with the different health-care providers who were managing her care over the years. In each case, almost without exception, we were told "don't worry about such things; be grateful your daughter is as healthy as she is." While their intentions may have been good, they didn't help resolve our questions or fears. But then our daughter was assigned a nurse who we were told would be her case manager. The first time they met, the nurse took a detailed history and asked our daughter the unthinkable—what sexual feelings did our daughter have and how was she managing her sexual needs. It was as if the floodgate had opened for all of us, and that session marked the beginning of an ongoing discussion we would all have about the very topic we had worried so much about. For the question of that nurse we will always be grateful, and if we could share one thought with future nurses in training, it would be to remember that patients are whole people and that sexuality is as important to those with psychiatric illness as it is to people everywhere. ▼

used strategies to promote safe sex include the following:

1. Using condoms
2. Reducing the number of sexual partners
3. Promoting sexual behaviors that decrease the exchange of body fluids

Second, HIV infection is now spreading most rapidly among heterosexuals and children. The greatest proportion of this increase includes women who have been using intravenous (IV) drugs, had sexual relations with partners using IV drugs, or had sexual contact with bisexual men.[15] Third, the number of young people in the United States today who have AIDS and the number who are infected with HIV continue to increase. Today, individuals in their twenties account for over 20% of all AIDS cases, the majority of whom were probably infected as adolescents, and the number of teenagers who have AIDS has increased more than 70% in the past 2 years.[14] Clearly, this illness has a significant impact on all aspects of an individual, and it is discussed in more detail in Chapter 38.

Patients who become disfigured because of injury or surgery may also experience alterations in sexuality due to changes in body image. Sudden injury leaves little or no time to prepare for the loss. People with spinal cord injuries may lose sexual functioning because of full or partial paralysis, but they continue to be sexual beings with feelings, needs, and desires. The most common surgical procedures that may cause difficulty with sexual responses include the following:

1. Loss of an external body part, such as mastectomy or penectomy
2. Loss of internal organs, such as prostatectomy or hysterectomy
3. Loss of body function, such as surgery that would result in impotence
4. Relocation of a body orifice, such as colostomy or ileostomy

Maladaptive self-concept and body image responses are discussed in detail in Chapter 16.

 Consider two medications that you commonly administer to patients. Do you know if they have sexual side effects, and have you talked about this possibility with your patients?

The Aging Process. In the past, researchers suggested that sexual activity decreased with aging. More recent studies indicate that patterns of sexual activity actually remain stable over middle and late adulthood years with only a small decline in later life. In reviewing the studies on sexuality and older adults, Kaplan[19] found that most elders who are in good health remain sexually active on a regular basis until the end of their lives.

There is nothing in the biology of aging that automatically shuts down sexual functioning; however, specific physiological changes do occur. In postmenopausal women there is little to no increase in breast size, and less muscle tension occurs during sexual arousal. Vaginal functioning changes in two ways; there is reduced elasticity in the walls of the vagina and decreased vaginal lubrication. The decrease in vaginal lubrication is the result of decreased blood flow to the vagina, which is caused by low estrogen levels. In men over the age of 55, several physiological changes occur in sexual response. Greater time and more direct stimulation are often needed for the penis to become erect, and erections tend to be less firm. The amount of semen is reduced, ejaculation is less intense, and the physical need to ejaculate is diminished. The refractory period also becomes greater with age.[27]

In Western culture the myth of the older adult as asexual still prevails. Many personality theorists have encouraged the myth of the older adult as an asexual or childlike being, and people have been taught that it is normal for older adults to have little or no interest in sex. Therefore when health professionals care for older individuals who express an interest in sex or who are sexually active, the professional often judges the older adult to be an exception to the rule. Older adults themselves may accept society's false beliefs about sexuality and aging. Many deny sexual attractions and feelings because they also have been socialized to believe that sexual behavior in older people is abnormal or perverted. Older adults are influenced by cultural values of Western society that currently prize youth and vitality and often disapprove of an elderly person doing anything other than sitting in a rocking chair.

One extremely important variable affecting altered sexuality because of aging is attrition by disuse: "use it or lose it." Prolonged abstinence from sexual activity causes more physiological problems in the older adult. For example, the older female who abstains from sexual activity will have greater shrinkage in vaginal size than a sexually active female of the same age. The older male who abstains from sexual activity may experience difficulty having erections when attempting to return to sexual activity.

Psychological factors, such as self-esteem, can also influence sexual activity in older adults. Older adults may be less inclined to be sexually active if they believe the physical changes that occur with aging make them unattractive. Marital status can also influence sexuality. Because men die at younger ages than women, women are more likely to be widowed and live the last part of their lives alone. Since there are fewer men in the population, it is more difficult for older women to find partners than it is for men.[7]

Organic factors similarly affect sexual functioning. From clinical observation, Kaplan[19] found that half of her patients over the age of 50 had some degree of interference with sexual functioning caused by disease states or medication side effects. For example, beta blockers and diabetes can contribute to impotence in men. Testosterone deficiency can create anorgasmy in women. She further reports that although these disorders cause some degree of physical impairment, the patient may regard them as quite serious. Frequently these impairments can be treated.

Finally, about 5% of individuals over the age of 65 reside in nursing homes and other long-term care facilities.[7] Many nursing homes restrict physical activity, so residents lack privacy from staff, who tend to care for older adults in a parental way. Physical contact between nursing home residents is often discouraged by nursing home staff, and many residents may feel restricted in their sexual expression. However, nurses are becoming more sensitive about the sexual needs and feelings of nursing home residents. By seeing them as individuals with sexual needs, nurses can act as advocates and help residents with sexual expression by encouraging discussion of sexual concerns, closing doors to ensure privacy, and allowing socialization with sexual partners.

> While working in a long-term care facility you walk into a patient's room and see two patients engaged in sexual relations. How would you respond?

Coping Resources

It is important for the nurse to assess the patient's coping resources because these can have a significant impact on sexual health. Resources may include the individual's knowledge about sexuality, positive sexual experiences the patient has had in the past, supportive individuals in the patient's environment, and social or cultural norms that encourage healthy sexual expression. It is also helpful to include the individual's sexual partner whenever possible; this allows the nurse to evaluate the quality of this relationship and to frame all nursing interventions within the context of a supportive, loving partnership.

Coping Mechanisms

Coping mechanisms related to sexual response may be adaptive or maladaptive, depending on how and why they are being employed. **Fantasy** is a coping mechanism used by individuals who wish to enhance their sexual experiences. Men and women may escape to erotic fantasies with unknown lovers during sex with their spouse. Although many people fear that fantasies about individuals other than their sexual partner indicate they are unsatisfied or unattracted to their partner, this is typically not the case. Fantasies are often a creative way to increase sexual excitement and enjoyment and are not usually indicative of dissatisfaction with a current partner. However, excessive fantasy can be maladaptive when used as replacement for actual sexual expression or the development of intimate relationships with others.

Maladaptive coping mechanisms may result from problems with self-concept. Often one member of a sexually dysfunctional couple may use **projection** in blaming his partner for the total problem, absolving himself from any responsibility: "I never had a sex problem with any of my previous lovers; I think you are the problem." Projection is also the coping mechanism used when a person's thoughts and feelings are unacceptable and anxiety producing. For example, a wife constantly accuses her husband of wanting to have an affair when actually the wife is contemplating an affair. Because her feelings are unacceptable to her, she projects them onto her husband and accuses him.

Denial and **rationalization** are also common coping mechanisms. Both allow the individual to avoid dealing with sexual issues. The following are maladaptive examples:

Denial: "I don't have a problem with sex", or "I never feel sexual."

Rationalization: "I don't need sex; I'm fine without it. Besides, a good marriage is a lot more than just sex."

To cope with unacceptable feelings about becoming vulnerable and the resulting ambivalent feelings about intimacy, some individuals withdraw from any form of sexual behavior. Others may engage in increased sexual behavior with multiple partners to protect themselves from one intimate relationship.

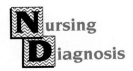 **Nursing Diagnosis**

When developing nursing diagnoses for variations in sexual response, the nurse should consider all the information gathered in the assessment phase and the components of the stress adaptation model (Fig. 24-4). The identified nursing diagnoses serve as a foundation for future problem solving. There are two primary NANDA nursing diagnoses concerned with sexual response. The first is altered sexuality patterns, which includes difficulties, limitations, or changes in sexual behaviors or activities. The second is sexual dysfunction, which includes lack of sexual satisfaction, alterations in perceived sex role, and conflicts involving values.

Other related nursing diagnoses that address additional behavioral problems may also need to be included. For example, a patient may be sexually functional but sexual identity may be unclear. Nursing diagnoses related to the range of possible maladaptive responses and related medical diagnoses are identified in the Medical and Nursing Diagnoses box on p. 646. The primary NANDA diagnoses and examples of complete nursing diagnoses are presented in the Detailed Diagnoses box on p. 647.

Related Medical Diagnoses

Many people who have transient variations in sexual response do not have a medically diagnosed health problem. Those with more severe or persistent problems are classified into one of three categories of variations in

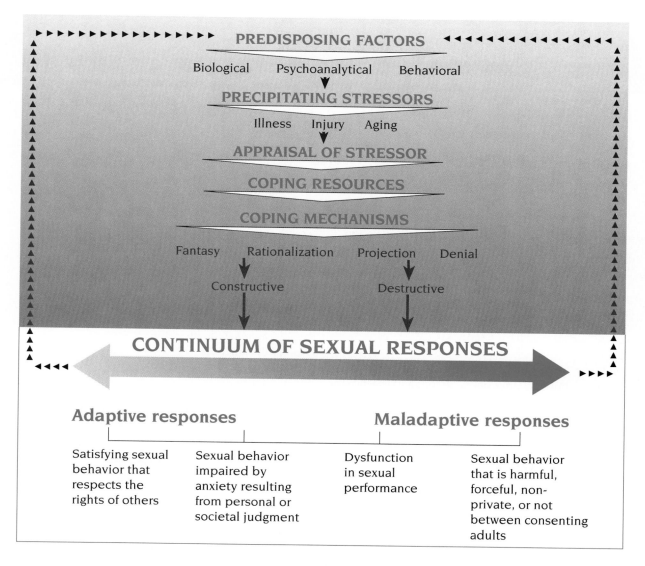

Fig. 24-4   A stress adaptation model related to sexual responses.

sexual response according to DSM-IV: sexual dysfunctions, paraphilias (sexual perversions or deviations), or gender identity disorders.[1] The medical diagnoses and their essential features that fall under each of these diagnostic classes according to the DSM-IV are described in the Detailed Diagnoses box.

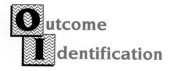

Outcome Identification

Goals must be formulated realistically, remembering the uniqueness of each person. The expected outcome for patients with maladaptive sexual responses is:

The patient will obtain the maximum level of adaptive sexual responses to enhance or maintain health.

This outcome can be made more specific through the use of short-term goals. These goals must be mutually identified with the patient, priorities established, and criteria used to measure progress toward the goals must also be defined. Examples of short-term goals include the following:

1. The patient will describe personal values and beliefs regarding sexuality and sexual expression.
2. The patient will identify sexual questions and problems.
3. The patient will relate accurate information about sexual concerns.
4. The patient will implement one new behavior to enhance sexual functioning.

MEDICAL AND NURSING DIAGNOSES RELATED TO VARIATIONS IN SEXUAL RESPONSE

Related Medical Diagnoses (DSM-IV)*

Hypoactive sexual desire disorder
Sexual aversion disorder
Sexual arousal disorder
Orgasmic disorder
Premature ejaculation
Dyspareunia
Vaginismus
Sexual dysfunction due to a general medical condition
Substance-induced sexual dysfunction
Exhibitionism
Fetishism
Frotteurism
Pedophilia
Sexual masochism
Sexual sadism
Voyeurism
Tranvestic fetishism
Gender identity disorder of childhood, adolescence, or adulthood

Related Nursing Diagnoses (NANDA)†

Anxiety
Body image disturbance
Decisional conflict
Fear
Grieving, dysfunctional
Health maintenance, altered
Health-seeking behaviors
Mobility, impaired physical
Pain
Personal identity disturbance
Powerlessness
Role performance, altered
Self-care deficit
Self-esteem disturbance
Sensory/perceptual alterations
‡Sexual dysfunction
‡Sexuality patterns, altered
Sleep pattern disturbance
Social interactions, impaired
Spiritual distress (distress of the human spirit)
Violence, potential for: self-directed or directed at others

*From American Psychiatric Association: *Diagnostic and statistical manual*, ed 4, Washington, DC, 1994, The Association.
†From North American Nursing Diagnosis Association: *Nursing diagnosis: definitions and classifications*, 1992-1993, Philadelphia, 1992, The Association.
‡Primary nursing diagnosis for variations in sexual response.

5. The patient will report decreased anxiety and greater satisfaction with sexual health.

After identifying goals in partnership with the patient, the nurse begins to implement the appropriate nursing interventions.

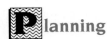

Planning

The nurse's level of expertise determines the degree of planning. The planning phase can simply involve reviewing assessment data, exploring options, and making referral sources known and available. This phase can also include sexual instruction for the patient or the patient and partner together. The nurse and patient can discuss a specific sexual issue and approaches that will provide the needed information. A Patient Education Plan for patients recovering from an organic illness is presented on p. 649.

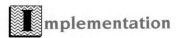

Implementation

Health Education

Primary prevention strives to promote health and prevent problems through specific methods such as teaching and planning, described in Chapter 11. Before engaging in health education or counseling, however, nurses must examine their values and beliefs about sexual behavior. This can be facilitated by exploring commonly held myths regarding human sexuality.[26] Table 24-1 lists some common sexual myths, the results of believing them, and the facts related to each one.

Education is the most frequent method of primary prevention of sexual problems. The content and methods of sex education have changed little over the past several decades.[8] Many people continue to receive most of their sex education from friends who may not provide accurate information. Too few parents discuss sexual issues with their children, and school sex educa-

DETAILED DIAGNOSES RELATED TO SEXUAL RESPONSES

NANDA Diagnosis Stem	Examples of Complete Diagnosis
Sexual dysfunction	Sexual dysfunction related to prenatal weight gain as evidenced by verbal statements of physical discomfort with intercourse.
	Sexual dysfunction related to joint pain as evidenced by decreased sexual desire.
Sexuality patterns, altered	Altered sexuality patterns related to financial worries as evidenced by inability to reach orgasm.
	Altered sexuality patterns related to mastectomy as evidenced by statements such as "My husband won't want to touch me," and "I don't feel like a woman."
	Altered sexuality patterns related to fear of pregnancy as evidenced by stopping before penetration.

DSM-IV Diagnosis	Essential Features*
Hypoactive sexual desire disorder	Persistent or recurrent deficit or absence of sexual fantasies and desire for sexual activity is present.
Sexual aversion disorder	Persistent or recurrent extreme aversion to and avoidance of all or almost all genital sexual contact with a sexual partner occurs.
Sexual arousal disorder	Persistent or recurrent partial or complete failure to attain or maintain the physiological response of sexual activity or persistent or recurrent lack of a subjective sense of sexual excitement and pleasure during sexual activity occurs.
Orgasmic disorder	Persistent or recurrent delay in or absence of orgasm occurs following a normal sexual excitement phase during sexual activity that is judged by the clinician to be adequate in focus, intensity, and duration, taking into account the individual's age.
Premature ejaculation	Ejaculation persistently or recurrently occurs with minimal sexual stimulation, before, on, or shortly after penetration, before the individual wishes it.
Dyspareunia	Recurrent or persistent genital pain occurs before, during, or after sexual intercourse.
Vaginismus	Recurrent or persistent involuntary spasm of the musculature of the outer third of the vagina occurs and interferes with coitus.
Sexual dysfunction due to a general medical condition	Clinically significant sexual dysfunction etiologically related to a general medical condition.
Substance-induced sexual dysfunction	Clinically significant sexual dysfunction that developed during significant substance intoxication or withdrawal.
Exhibitionism	A persistent association occurs, lasting at least 6 months, between intense sexual arousal, desire, acts, or fantasies, and exposing one's genitals to an unsuspecting stranger.
Fetishism	A persistent association occurs, lasting at least 6 months, between intense sexual arousal, desire, acts, or fantasies, and nonliving objects (e.g., female undergarments).

Adapted from the American Psychiatric Association: *Diagnostic and statistical manual of mental disorders*, ed 4, American Psychiatric Association, Washington, DC, 1994, The Association.

DETAILED DIAGNOSES
RELATED TO SEXUAL RESPONSES—cont'd

DSM-IV Diagnosis—cont'd	Essential Features—cont'd
Frotteurism	A persistent association occurs, lasting at least 6 months, between intense sexual arousal, desire, acts, or fantasies, and rubbing against a nonconsenting person.
Pedophilia	A persistent association occurs, lasting at least 6 months, between intense sexual arousal, desire, acts, or fantasies, and one or more children, aged 13 years or younger.
Sexual masochism	A persistent association occurs, lasting for at least 6 months, between intense sexual arousal, desire, acts, or fantasies, and being humiliated, beaten, bound, or otherwise being made to suffer (real or imagined).
Sexual sadism	A persistent association occurs, lasting at least 6 months, between intense sexual arousal, desire, acts, or fantasies, and the affliction of real or simulated psychological or physical suffering (including humiliation).
Voyeurism	A persistent association occurs, lasting at least 6 months, between intense sexual arousal, desire, acts, or fantasies, and observing unsuspecting people who are either naked, in the act of disrobing, or engaging in sexual activity.
Transvestic fetishism	A persistent association occurs, lasting at least 6 months, between intense sexual arousal, desire, acts, or fantasies, and cross-dressing.
Gender identity disorder of childhood, adolescence, or adulthood	Persistent and intense distress about being a male or a female is present, with an intense desire to be the opposite sex, a preoccupation with the activities of the opposite sex, and a repudiation of one's own anatomical structures.

tion programs, to avoid discussion of controversial subjects, often focus only on biological factors, which is insufficient for the needs of today's youth. Opponents of sex education propose that the less children and adolescents know about sex, the less likely they are to become sexually active. However, studies on this topic do not support this belief. Well-designed evaluations of sex education programs have demonstrated that programs can markedly reduce unprotected intercourse and delay initiation of first intercourse.[22,37]

Recently, because of the epidemic rates of teenage pregnancies and abortion and the advent of the AIDS crisis, many experts are suggesting more comprehensive sex education programs, and some are suggesting that these programs begin as early as preschool and kindergarten. Sex education is a lifelong process with the primary goal of promoting sexual health. This includes helping people develop positive views of sexuality, gain information and skills about taking care of their sexual health, and acquire decision-making abilities regarding sexual issues. A comprehensive sex education program has the following four primary goals[31]:

1. Communicating accurate information about sexuality
2. Providing an opportunity to develop values, beliefs, and attitudes about sexuality
3. Helping individuals develop relationships and interpersonal skills
4. Encouraging the exercise of responsibility in sexual relationships

It is also clear that teaching information about sex and sexuality is not enough. For a sex education program to be effective it must promote behavioral change. The most effective sex education programs are compre-

PATIENT EDUCATION PLAN
SEXUAL RESPONSE AFTER AN ORGANIC ILLNESS

Content	Instructional activities	Evaluation
Describe the variety of human sexual response patterns	Discuss the range of sexual desires, modes of expression, and techniques	Patient identifies personal sexual orientation and typical level of sexual functioning
Define the patient's primary organic problem	Provide accurate information regarding the disruption caused by the organic impairment	Patient understands the specific organic illness
Clarify relationship between the organic problem and patient's level of sexual functioning	Reframe distorted or confused perceptions regarding the impact of the illness on patient's sexual functioning	Patient accurately describes the impact of the illness on sexual functioning
Identify ways to enhance patient's sexual functioning and improve interpersonal communication	Describe additional experiences that would add to the sexual satisfaction and the relationship between the patient and patient's partner	Patient and partner report reduced anxiety and greater satisfaction with their sexual responses

hensive and skill based. More specifically, it is not enough to teach students to say no to sex, but they must be taught how to say no. This could be done by teaching decision-making skills, assertiveness training, and role playing potentially difficult sexual situations.

Sexual Responses Within the Nurse-Patient Relationship

Sexual Responses of Nurses to Patients. A clinical situation in which a nurse feels sexual attraction to a patient can be a problem. Although this occurs, it has received little attention in the nursing literature. One major reason is that nurses often deny sexual feelings for their patients. However, sexual attraction and sexual fantasies are part of the human experience. If these feelings are not examined, they can interfere with the quality of care by shifting the focus from the patient's needs to those of the nurse.

First, nurses must acknowledge their feelings without judging them. Often nurses try to ignore or deny these feelings because they are uncomfortable and frightening. They make judgments about themselves, such as, "What's wrong with me? I shouldn't feel this way about my patients. I must be really weird" and "I'm sure I'm the only nurse who ever had these feelings." The nurse who admits these feelings without judging them is able to deal with them. Edelwich and Brodsky[8] offer the following suggestions:

1. Do not share personal information with patients.
2. Do not become overly involved in patients' problems.
3. Do not discuss with the patient feelings of sexual attraction to him or her.
4. Seek consultation.

Asking for consultation from a more experienced nurse or a supervisor often helps the nurse sort out feelings and, most important, maintain a professional therapeutic relationship with the patient. It is never acceptable for a nurse to engage in sexual behavior of any kind with a patient. Such activity can lead to litigation and loss of the nurse's license to practice.

Sexual Responses of Patients to Nurses. One of the most common sexual behaviors of hospitalized patients is acting out or displaying seductive behaviors toward the nurse; this includes making passes and sexual comments, inappropriate touching, asking for their phone numbers, and requesting a date. Nurses are often extremely uncomfortable when they are the recipients of such behavior. One recent survey of nursing and occupational therapy students revealed that 40% had been victims of sexual harassment from patients. Of these students, 16% were victims of a forceful physical sexual assault by a patient.[20]

Which sexual myth from Table 24-1 did you believe before reading this chapter? How will knowing the "fact" affect your nursing practice?

The first step in intervening is to let the patient know that such behavior is unacceptable. The nurse needs to respond in a firm, matter-of-fact manner that clearly states what limits are being set. For example, "Mr. Moore, I am uncomfortable when you suggest that I get

Table 24-1   Ten Common Myths and Facts about Human Sexuality

Myth	Result of myth	Fact
Patients become embarrassed when nurses bring up the subject of sexuality and would prefer that nurses not ask questions about sex.	If nurses believe this, they deny the patient the opportunity to ask questions and clarify concerns related to sexual issues.	Research indicates that patients would prefer that nurses initiate discussions of sexuality with them.[23,39]
Excessive masturbation is harmful.	Individuals often feel guilty or ashamed about masturbating; some individuals deny themselves this experience because of uncomfortable feelings perpetuated by society.	There is no evidence that masturbation causes physical problems. Masturbation seems to be a self-limiting practice. If masturbation leads to satisfaction and pleasure, it is unlikely to be a problem.[27]
Sexual fantasies about having sex with a partner other than lover or spouse indicate relationship difficulties.	Individuals may become uncomfortable about having a fantasy with a different partner. They may experience guilt feelings and view the fantasy as a sign of infidelity.	Imagining sex with a different partner is one of the most common sexual fantasies and does not necessarily indicate any desire on the part of the individual to act out the fantasized behavior.[27]
Sex during menstruation is unclean and harmful.	Women often view their bodies as unclean and even unfit or inferior during menstruation. Women use menstruation as an excuse to avoid intercourse rather than simply saying no without a "good reason."	Medically, menstrual flow is in no way harmful or dirty. If women desire, there is no reason to abstain from intercourse during menstrual flow.[26]
Oral and anal intercourse are perverted and dangerous.	Many individuals refrain from these behaviors or indulge in them only to feel ashamed and guilty afterward.	According to Masters and Johnson, "nothing could be further from the truth"; they suggest certain precautions when performing anal intercourse, such as avoiding contamination of the vaginal tract and wearing a condom to prevent the transmission of disease.[26]
Most homosexuals molest children.	Known homosexuals are often fired from teaching jobs, and many parents will not allow their children to spend any time with anyone who is homosexual.	Research shows that the adult heterosexual male poses a far greater risk to the underage child than does the adult homosexual male.[13]
Homosexuals are sick and cannot control their sexual behavior.	Homosexuals are denied jobs and are sometimes jailed for their homosexuality. Homosexual partners may have their children taken away by courts.	According to Bell and Weinberg,[2] most homosexuals' social and psychological adjustment is the same as the heterosexual majority, and objectionable sexual advances are far more likely to be made by a heterosexual (usually male to female) than by a homosexual.[2]
Because of sex education programs, most adolescent and young adults are aware of the risks of getting sexually transmitted diseases and practice safe sex.	When health educators believe that young adults have adequate knowledge about sexually transmitted diseases, they may not take the time to further assess, add to this knowledge, and correct any misperceptions.	A study of over 500 freshmen at a large university reported that of those who had multiple partners, fewer than 50% used condoms to lower the risk of disease.[30]
Advancing age means the end of sex.	Many older adults become victims of this myth not because their bodies have lost the ability to perform, but because they believe that they have lost the ability to perform.	Sexually, men and women in good health can function effectively throughout their lives.[19]
Alcohol ingestion reduces inhibitions and therefore enhances sexual enjoyment.	Many individuals use alcohol in the hope that it will increase their sexual pleasure and performance. Alcohol ingestion can also provide an excuse for engaging in sexual behaviors—"I would never have gone to bed with him if I hadn't had all that wine."	Data do not support the belief that alcohol ingestion reduces inhibitions and enhances sexual enjoyment.[38]

into bed with you. Please stop saying that"; or "Mr. Dean, take your hand off my breast."

Nurses are sometimes embarrassed or afraid to confront patients and attempt to laugh it off or ignore it with a "boys will be boys" attitude. Providing health care to patients does not give them permission to be verbally offensive or to touch nurses' bodies without permission. Nurses are taught to be accepting of patients' behavior, and this principle is difficult to dispute. However, when the behavior violates nurses' rights, limits need to be set.

Nurses have a responsibility as professionals to attempt to understand sexual behaviors and to analyze their possible meanings. Patients may show seductive behaviors for various reasons, which may or may not include a serious desire for sex with the nurse. Seductive behavior is often a way of getting the nurse's attention. Hospitalized patients can also feel unattractive or inse-

cure about themselves sexually; thus seductive behaviors may be a request for reassurance. Sometimes patients confuse their gratitude for and appreciation of the nurse with sexual attraction. These feelings may in turn generate thoughts such as, "Wouldn't my nurse make a wonderful wife. She's so giving and understanding all the time." In this case the patient views professional behavior and concern as self-sacrificing and altruistic.

Finally, patients may have difficulty understanding the difference between a professional and a social relationship. In many ways the nurse-patient relationship is idealized for the patient. The patient receives all the attention and caring and is not expected to give anything in return. It is easy to see how the patient could be confused about his relationship with the nurse. The clinical example that follows illustrates this point. Table 24-2 summarizes nursing considerations in sexual responses of patients to nurses.

Table 24-2   Summary of Nursing Considerations in Sexual Responses of Patients to Nurses

Goal—Maintain a professional nurse-patient relationship that will enable the nurse to provide therapeutic nursing care

Principle	Rationale	Nursing considerations
Establish a trusting relationship	An atmosphere of trust allows for open, honest communication between patient and nurse; when this occurs, the nurse can aid the patient in discovering the underlying issues related to sexual feelings and behavior.	Express nonsexual caring and concern for the patient. Be a responsive listener, especially to feelings and needs that the patient may not be able to directly express. Reinforce the purpose of the professional therapeutic nurse-patient relationship.
Awareness of nurse's own feelings and thoughts	When the nurse is aware of her feelings and thoughts, she will begin to understand how they influence her behavior; with increased self-awareness the nurse will be able to increase the effectiveness of her interactions with patients.	Recognize own feelings and thoughts. Identify any specific patient interaction or behavior that influences the nurse's feelings and thoughts. Identify the influence of the nurse's feelings and thoughts on one's behavior in an attempt to increase the effectiveness of nursing interventions.
Decrease patient's expressions of sexual feelings and behavior	If the nurse is able to help the patient see that his sexual interactions and behavior are being expressed to an inappropriate partner (the nurse), the sexual acting out will usually decrease; this allows the nurse to help the patient begin to identify the reasons for his behavior.	Set limits on patient's sexual behavior. Use a calm, matter-of-fact approach without implying judgment. Reaffirm nonsexual caring for the patient. Explore the meaning of the patient's feelings and behaviors.
Expand patient's insight into sexual feelings and behavior	Once the patient begins to identify the reasons for his sexual feelings and behaviors, he is able to see that the nurse is not an appropriate outlet for these feelings and behaviors and can move toward a more appropriate and therapeutic relationship with the nurse.	Clarify misconceptions regarding any feeling patient may have about the nurse as a possible sexual partner. Point out the futile nature of his romantic or sexual interest in the nurse. Redirect patient's energies toward appropriate health-care issues.

CLINICAL EXAMPLE

Mr. P has been hospitalized for an exacerbation of a chronic illness for the past 3 weeks. Ms. S has been his primary nurse during this hospitalization. The following is a conversation between the nurse and patient the day before his discharge.

MR. P: I wish my wife were more like you, Ms. S.

MS. S: Mr. P, I'm not sure I understand what you are saying.

MR. P: Well, it's just that you are always so concerned about me. You always try to make me feel good and want to help me all the time. Sometimes my wife's a grouch; she's so wrapped up in her job and the kids she doesn't always pay as much attention to me as you do.

MS. S: I'm glad you feel taken care of, Mr. P, but I think it's impossible to compare my role as your nurse with your wife's role.

MR. P: I'm not sure I follow you. . . .

MS. S: They are very different types of relationships. It's nice to have someone take care of us when we can't take care of ourselves, but when we are healthy, we don't need someone to take care of us all the time. Your relationship with your wife is more of a sharing one with mutual benefits. You take care of her needs, and she takes care of your needs in return. If you feel that your relationship with your wife is not a satisfying one, perhaps you need to talk this over with her.

Maladaptive Sexual Responses Due To Illness

Stress, physical and emotional illness, injury, and aging can lead to changes in sexuality and sexual functioning. These changes and related nursing interventions differ based on whether the illness is acute or chronic. It is important for the nurse to obtain complete information on the nature and course of the illness, the types of medications used in its treatment, the patient's appraisal of the impact of the illness, and any physical limitation imposed by the illness that affects the patient's sexual health.

Several major nursing interventions can then be implemented to facilitate the patient's adaptive sexual responses. The first is for the nurse to act in a facilitative and supportive way and to help the patient express feelings, fears, and problems. Open communication between the patient and partner should also be encouraged. The nurse can reinforce the positive attributes of the patient, prevent social isolation, mobilize available coping resources, and support adaptive coping mechanisms that have helped the patient deal with stressors in the past.

The nurse can also offer anticipatory guidance and give accurate information about the illness or injury including what the patient may expect from medical or psychiatric treatment and its impact on sexual health (see A Patient Speaks). The nurse can also initiate counseling about sexuality and alternative means of sexual expression. Relaxation techniques, autoerotic activities, and variations in movement and positions may be suggested. The nurse should emphasize that pleasure can be obtained in a variety of ways and stress the importance of a loving relationship. Finally, if the problem is complex and of a long duration, the patient should be referred for psychotherapy or sex therapy from a qualified professional.

 Should sexual behavior be permitted among patients who are residents of a long-term psychiatric facility? If so, what issues need to be addressed by staff? If not, how will the sexual needs of these patients be met?

A PATIENT SPEAKS

It's bad enough to be depressed, but how's a person supposed to feel when the people taking care of them don't give them all the information they need? From what I can see from talking to other patients in my group, my story is not that unusual.

For about 6 months I felt myself slipping deeper and deeper into the black hole of depression. I saw some ads on television and decided that maybe I needed some outside help, since I clearly wasn't getting better by myself. So off I go to a nearby clinic where I see someone who diagnoses me with depression and gives me some pills to take. In the beginning, the drugs made me kind of jittery, but gradually I got over it. In a couple of months I actually almost felt like my old self again—all except for sex, that is. In that one area of my life I simply couldn't experience the satisfaction I used to have and didn't know what was going on. Well, it turns out that the pills I'm on limit my sexual performance, but nobody every bothered to mention this to me. I guess they thought it wasn't important or something, but they were really wrong.

Now that I understand what's going on I can work around it, since the drugs have helped me in almost every other way. But still, it would have been nice if the people that you turn to for help could give you all the information you need and not just talk about the parts that they think are important or limit themselves to the topics they're comfortable talking about. ▼

Maladaptive Homosexual and Bisexual Responses

Most homosexual and bisexual people accept their orientations, although some have difficulties and seek professional help. Because of the homosexual element of bisexuality, bisexuals often encounter many of the same difficulties stemming from societal attitudes as homosexuals. Another factor that may present a problem for the bisexual is isolation from a support group. Because bisexuals are frequently accused of fence-sitting, they can be rejected by heterosexuals and homosexuals. Bisexuals may complain about lack of support; friends and family may pressure them to decide on one sexual orientation (usually heterosexual) so that they will be accepted by society.

The first step in counseling the homosexual or bisexual who views his or her sexual responses as maladaptive is the nurse's acceptance. Most patients are extremely perceptive of their caregiver's values and attitudes toward them. Nurses who believe they are hiding their prejudices are only fooling themselves. Because nurses have grown up in a homophobic society, it is often difficult to examine the myths and search for facts. **Homophobia** is a persistent and irrational fear of homosexuals, as well as a negative attitude and hostility toward homosexuals.[7] It may also include the individual's fear of having an actual or potential homosexual orientation.[28] The homosexual patient has grown up in the same society where negative attitudes regarding homosexuality still exist and therefore often experiences the same homophobia as anyone else.

An important step in working with homosexual patients is to avoid focusing on the causal factors of homosexuality ("Why did this happen to me?") and to encourage patients to explore their beliefs and values about homosexuality.[33] The patient may have internalized some of society's prejudices, such as "Homosexuality is a sick and abnormal behavior and therefore, because I am a homosexual, I am sick and abnormal and should not act on my sexual feelings because they are wrong." Responses can be varied and include denial, confusion, and sexual promiscuity, especially among those trying to prove to themselves that they are not gay. It is helpful to have patients list their beliefs about homosexuality and bisexuality and to discuss each one. However, a review of beliefs about homosexuality may not be sufficient. Encouraging the person to read about homosexuality and bisexuality is also helpful. Throughout this process, the patient will be extremely sensitive to the nurse's acceptance or rejection.

Confidentiality is also a central issue. It is helpful for the nurse to demonstrate an appreciation for patients' concerns about unwanted exposure of their homosexuality to family members, friends, or co-workers. The nurse should not encourage nor discourage the patient's disclosure of homosexual concerns but rather assist the homosexual patient in exploring and processing the choice of disclosure or lack of disclosure with others, as in this clinical example.

 ## CLINICAL EXAMPLE

Ms. A, a 25-year-old single female, came to the mental health clinic with the complaint of a "sexual problem." Her history revealed that she had been sexually inactive for the past 5 years. At the age of 20, Ms. A had a brief sexual encounter with a man she had been dating for 2 years. She ended the relationship shortly afterward because she had no interest in maintaining a sexual relationship with the man. Recently, she became involved in a relationship with a woman that was very satisfying to her. She felt she had to end the relationship because she would not tolerate thinking of herself as a homosexual. During one of the initial counseling sessions, Ms. A told the nurse that she must end the relationship before "it" happens again.

NURSE: What are you afraid will happen?

MS. A: I'm afraid I'll feel attracted to her again.

NURSE: What about that frightens you?

MS. A: (becoming upset) That will mean I'm homosexual!

NURSE: What does being homosexual mean for you?

MS. A: It means I'm sick. It's a sin, I couldn't go to church anymore.

NURSE: Are all homosexuals sick?

MS. A: Yes.

NURSE: How do you know this?

MS. A: Everybody knows that homosexuality is morally wrong. Homosexuals have a lot of emotional problems.

NURSE: Do you know any homosexual people?

MS. A: Well, not exactly. . . .

NURSE: What have you read about homosexuality?

MS. A: Nothing.

NURSE: Then it looks to me like you are basing all of your conclusions on hearsay and not real knowledge. I think that you and I need to explore your beliefs in more detail, then you can do some reading to find out the facts.

Selected Nursing Diagnoses:

▼ Altered sexuality patterns related to questions about sexual preference related to recent interpersonal relationship

▼ Spiritual distress related to conflicting values as evidenced by questions about religous beliefs

In the preceding clinical example, the nurse and Ms. A developed a plan often used in sexual counseling to explore homosexuality. Some of the interventions included the following:

1. Ms. A described her beliefs about homosexuality and homosexuals.
2. The nurse encouraged Ms. A to explore the literature on homosexuality and suggested readings to help dispel the myths.
3. The nurse then discussed these with Ms. A and suggested that she attend a social gathering for gay people to test out her new knowledge. The nurse suggested the social gathering because many people struggling with a homosexual identity are frightened to test out situations that would dispel the myths.
4. Finally, the nurse helped Ms. A. explore her responses to these activities and integrate them into a positive view of self.

Maladaptive Transsexual Responses

Treatment of the transsexual person has been a controversial topic in recent years. Recommendations range from long-term psychotherapy to surgical reassignment. Standards of care developed by the Harry Benjamin International Gender Dysphoria Association set guidelines for those who are to receive psychotherapy, hormonal therapy, or surgical reassignment, since not all transsexuals choose surgical reassignment.[3] The standards help trained professionals who treat transsexual patients give quality care. Criteria include the following:

1. The person must demonstrate discomfort with self and express the wish to live in the genetically opposite sex role.
2. Along with criterion no. 1, the person must be known to a professional therapist (who is an expert in sexuality) for 3 to 6 months.

If the person meets these criteria, the therapist then endorses hormonal therapy. A male changing to a female receives estrogen; a female changing to a male receives testosterone. Before starting hormonal therapy, the patient receives a complete physical examination with specific blood work serum glutamic pyruvic transaminase (SGPT) levels in females changing to males, SGPT, bilirubin, triglyceride, and fasting glucose levels in males changing to females. If surgical reassignment is desired (penectomy, castration, or vaginoplasty for a male changing to a female; hysterectomy, vaginectomy, or phalloplasty for a female changing to a male), the patient must be known to the professional therapist for at least 6 months. The individual must have been successful in living as the genetically opposite sex role for at least 1 year and up to 2 years. Before the transsexual receives surgical alteration, the original therapist's endorsement must be agreed on by a second therapist who has evaluated the person.

Professionals who care for transsexual patients must be educated in sexuality. The assessment phase of treatment is especially important. The patient and therapist must be certain that implementing the treatment plan is the best approach because the surgery is not reversible.

A Nursing Care Plan Summary for maladaptive sexual responses is presented on p. 655.

Dysfunctions of the Sexual Response Cycle

Treating sexual dysfunctions is beyond the scope of the nurse generalist. However, the nurse should be aware of the principles involved and should also know of creditable sex therapists in the community for referral of patients. Two common models of sex therapy are briefly discussed here: the Masters and Johnson and the Helen Singer Kaplan models.

Masters and Johnson Model. Masters and Johnson began pioneering research in sexuality in the 1950s. Their book, *Human Sexual Inadequacy*,[25] describes their research and counseling methods. Before the work of William Masters and Virginia Johnson, patients with problems in sexuality were generally referred to a psychiatrist for psychotherapy or psychoanalysis. Health professionals assumed that anyone who had a problem with sexuality was emotionally disturbed. Problems with dysfunction of sexual response are usually not psychiatric problems but are the result of sociocultural deprivation and ignorance of sexual physiology. Masters and Johnson's treatment includes short-term education with step-by-step instructions regarding the physical aspects of sexual activity and supportive psychotherapy. The researchers believe that attitudes and ignorance are responsible for most sexual dysfunctions.

Their approach to patients begins with obtaining a detailed sexual and background history. They recommend a male-female therapeutic team. On day one of the treatment, the therapists meet with the couple in a roundtable discussion to review and clarify their histories taken the previous day. Then the couple is instructed to carry out a sensate focus exercise in which each partner instructs the other in specific ways of caressing for sensual pleasure without involving the breasts or genitals. The activity is done first by one partner and then the other. The next day the exercise is repeated, including breasts and genital areas, but without performing coitus. The exercise's purpose is to alleviate performance anxiety and to enhance warm, comfortable feelings between partners. After the sensate focus exercises are completed, the therapy is directed to the sexual dysfunction. The Masters and Johnson model emphasizes education, communication, and cooperation between partners.

NURSING CARE PLAN SUMMARY
Maladaptive Sexual Responses

Nursing Diagnosis: Altered sexuality patterns

Expected Outcome: The patient will obtain the maximum level of adaptive sexual responses to enhance or maintain health.

Short-term Goals	Interventions	Rationale
The patient will describe values, beliefs, questions, and problems regarding sexuality.	Listen to sexual concerns implied and expressed. Help the patient explore sexual beliefs, values, and questions. Encourage open communication between the patient and partner.	An accepting therapeutic relationship will allow patients to be free to question, grow, and seek help with sexual concerns. Communicate respect, acceptance, and openness to sexual concerns.
The patient will relate accurate information about sexual concerns.	Clarify sexual misinformation. Dispel myths. Provide specific education about sexual health practices, behaviors, and problems. Give professional "permission" to continue sexual behavior that is not physically or emotionally harmful. Reinforce positive attitudes of the patient.	Accurate information is helpful in changing negative thoughts and attitudes about particular aspects of sexuality. It can also prevent or limit dysfunctional behavior. Giving permission allows the person to continue the behavior and alleviate anxiety about normalcy. It allows patients to incorporate sexual behavior in a positive and accepting self-concept.
The patient will implement one new behavior to enhance sexual response.	Set clear goals with the patient. Identify specific behaviors that can be carried out focusing on enhancing self-concept, role functioning, and sexuality. Encourage relaxation techniques, redirection of attention, positional changes, and alternative ways of sexual expression as appropriate. Become familiar with the sex therapy resources available in the community. Refer the patient to a qualified sex therapist as needed.	Giving a patient direct behavioral suggestions can help relieve a sexual problem or difficulty and is a useful intervention when the problem is of recent onset and short duration. While all nurses need to screen for maladaptive sexual responses and provide basic nursing care, complex problems should be referred to qualified sex therapists for further treatment.

Helen Singer Kaplan Model. Kaplan's[17] method of treating sexual dysfunctions combines specific tasks with psychodynamic insights, dream interpretations, and gestalt and transactional techniques. She differs from Masters and Johnson in that she believes the single therapist is as effective as cotherapists of opposite sexes. According to Kaplan, the primary objective of sex therapy is symptomatic relief, achievable by treating the patient without a partner in some cases.

Kaplan's treatment begins with an extensive evaluation, including marital, psychiatric, sexual, medical, and family history from both partners. If serious intrapsychic or interpersonal difficulties are found, the couple may

be referred to individual or conjoint therapy and is not accepted for sex therapy at that time. According to Kaplan, sex therapy is usually not advised for couples who are severely emotionally disturbed.

As with Masters and Johnson, Kaplan employs sensate focus exercises and variations, such as showering together, to begin sex therapy or to further evaluate a client's suitability for sex therapy. Therapy itself consists of erotic tasks performed at home plus weekly or semi-weekly meetings with the therapist. Clients and the therapist explore feelings experienced during the erotic exercises. The exercises take into account the motivations and dynamics of the relationship. The integration of experiential and dynamic modes is a major feature of Kaplan's approach. The role of the therapist includes education, clarification, and support.

Both Kaplan and Masters and Johnson emphasize communication between partners and exploration of the relationship and emotional concerns. The reader is referred to original works of these therapists for more information.[17,18,25,27]

Evaluation

In the evaluation phase the nurse works with the patient to evaluate the effectiveness of the sexual counseling or intervention. Factors to consider include the following:

1. *Sense of well-being.* How does the person feel about himself or herself? Have these feelings improved during the treatment?
2. *Functioning ability.* If the individual was dysfunctional, is functional ability restored? Somewhat improved? What about the person's ability to function within primary relations at work? With friends?
3. *Satisfaction with treatment.* Does the patient believe that the treatment was helpful? Were the patient's goals adequately met?

Evaluation of any form of sexual counseling or intervention should be ongoing. The nurse and patient should work together on goals, problems, and alternatives.

SUGGESTED CROSS-REFERENCES

SUMMARY

1. Sexuality is defined as a desire for contact, warmth, tenderness, and love. Criteria for adaptive sexual behavior are identified as consensual, free of force, performed in private, neither physically nor psychologically harmful, and mutually satisfying.
2. Patient behaviors related to sexual responses include homosexuality, bisexuality, transvestism, transsexualism, and physiological and psychological responses to sexual stimulation.
3. Predisposing factors for variations in sexual response are described from biological, psychoanalytical, and behavioral perspectives. Precipitating stressors that may change sexuality include physical and emotional illness, therapeutic and nontherapeutic drugs, surgical intervention, hospitalization, and aging.
4. A variety of coping mechanisms are used with expressions of sexuality: fantasy, projection, denial, and rationalization.
5. Primary NANDA diagnoses are sexual dysfunction and altered sexuality patterns.
6. Primary DSM-IV diagnoses are categorized as sexual dysfunctions, paraphilias, and gender identity disorders.
7. The expected outcome of nursing care is that the patient will obtain the maximum level of adaptive sexual responses to enhance or maintain health.
8. Interventions include sex education and preventive counseling and intervening in sexual feelings and behaviors within the nurse-patient relationship, maladaptive modes of sexual expression, and dysfunctions of the sexual response cycle.
9. The nurse and patient should consider the following factors in evaluating nursing care: the patient's sense of well-being, functioning ability, and satisfaction with treatment.

COMPETENT CARING
A CLINICAL EXEMPLAR OF A PSYCHIATRIC NURSE

Donald Ribelin, RN, C

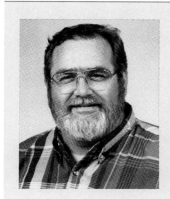

Having worked in nursing for over 20 years, I tend to have certain defined responses to almost any given situation. This works well until something comes along that doesn't fit into those preconceived notions of how things should be. I was working as evening charge nurse on an adult acute care psychiatric unit when one of the mental health assistants came to the desk to report that he had seen Mr. B and Mrs. G sneaking into the solarium and that they appeared to be "getting it on." Almost every psychiatric, or med-surg nurse for that matter, has had to confront patients, visitors, or both in a sexual situation of one type or another. We'd had our share of such encounters in the past, but the staff reacted very differently this time.

To begin with, Mr. B was a 72-year-old "street" person who had been admitted with a diagnosis of rule-out dementia, and Mrs. G was a lovely 70-year-old widow with a diagnosis of situational depression. Mr. B's apparent dementia had proven to be secondary to malnutrition and vitamin B_{12} deficiency. Once he had received treatment for these, we had found him to be a remarkable person whose ready sense of humor lightened many an evening group. Mrs. G had been admitted with one of the flattest affects I had ever seen. Her family reported that she had been increasingly depressed ever since her husband's death 3 years ago. This depression increased dramatically around the anniversary of Mr. G's death, which was right around this time of the year.

Over the past week, Mrs. G's depression had lifted noticeably. She could be seen talking, laughing, and joking with Mr. B during any free moment. They seemed to always be together, sitting next to each other during groups or meals or walking side by side on outings. We had all commented on how much they had helped each other and what a nice couple they made. Suddenly Mr. B and Mrs. G had stopped being a nice "old" couple and had become two psychiatric patients sneaking off to have "sex."

I found myself torn between several reactions to this news. The empathic nurse in me responded, "this is great—two lonely people in their twilight years of their lives have found love and companionship." The analytical nurse in me wondered if this relationship would really be therapeutic for Mrs. G given Mr. B's background. The cautious nurse in me wondered if Mr. B could simply be trying to ensure he had somewhere to stay after discharge. But the administrative nurse in me won out thinking that I don't let other patients behave in this manner; therefore I have to intercede.

Somewhat loudly I walked down the hall and into the solarium, taking a very long time fumbling for the light switch. The lights revealed Mrs. G and Mr. B sitting side by side, holding hands and red faced. Mrs. G's blouse was only partially buttoned, and she was obviously upset. I apologized to them, explaining that I had planned to spend my break in the solarium and hadn't meant to startle them. As they quickly stood up and headed toward their rooms, I could see a look of sadness and possibly shame replacing the happy smile that we had been seeing the past few days on Mrs. G's face. Mr. B also looked sad, and for a moment I thought I saw the return of the shuffling gait he had at admission. By doing the "right" thing, I now felt like I had done the very worst thing possible.

During my shift report, I gave the incident only brief comment. Talking more about the possible therapeutic benefits of the relationship, I didn't mention the sexual aspects at all. Guilt can be a great censor and rewriter of history, and I was obviously really feeling guilty.

Well, time may heal all wounds, but it only gives rumors time to grow. I was very surprised when, upon returning to work the next evening, my nurse manager asked where was the incident report on Mr. B and Mrs. G having sex in the solarium. She also wanted to know why I hadn't documented the incident in my nursing notes. By the time I had explained the previous evening's happenings, what had started out as two people wanting to be together had become a major event.

Damage control began with a meeting of all unit staff, where we discussed what had and had not happened. It didn't stop there. A psychiatric unit is often like a small town where there are no secrets. That evening, in group, the patients brought up our hapless couple's "making out." Again I found myself in a position where I felt anything I said could and probably would be wrong. After careful thought I responded by first reminding them that this was a hospital and there were certain rules of conduct that had to be adhered to, even when we might personally disagree with them. Members of the group were asked to share their feelings about these rules and why they were or were not necessary. As the group proceeded, I kept a careful eye on Mrs. G and Mr. B. They were sitting about as far from each other as possible and both were very quiet.

As the patients talked, I kept trying to think of something to say or do to alleviate the obvious pain and embarrassment of our elderly who were now the center of attention. Suddenly Mr. B stood up, smiled at the group, and said, "You know, I've been feeling real bad today. I felt like I had done something wrong and that I was just waiting for my punishment to come." Then he stated, "Yeah! I was feeling real bad until just a moment ago, when I remembered a button I saw once. It said, 'Old people need love too,' and you know that's right because everyone needs to know that someone cares about them, needs them, and loves them. So it really doesn't matter what any of you think because I've found someone to love me and for me to love."

I'll always remember that moment as a time that patients and staff clapped, cried, and laughed together. ▼

REFERENCES

1. American Psychiatric Association: *Diagnostic and statistical manual of mental disorders*, ed 4, Washington, DC, 1994, The Association.

2. Bell AP, Weinberg MS: *Homosexualities: a study of diversity among men and women*, New York, 1978, Simon & Schuster.

3. Berger L et al: *Standard of care*, 1981, The Harry Benjamin International Gender Dysphoria Association.

4. Biery RE: *Understanding homosexuality: The pride and the prejudice*, Austin, Tex, 1990, Edward-William Publishing.

5. Briere J, Zaidi L: Sexual abuse histories and sequelae in female psychiatric emergency room patients. *Am J Psychiatry* 146:1602, 1989.

6. Byne W, Parsons B: Human sexual orientation: the biological theories reappraised, *Arch Gen Psychiatry* 50:228, 1993.

7. Denney NW, Quadango B: *Human sexuality*, ed 2, St Louis, 1992, Mosby.

8. Edelwich J, Brodsky A: *Sexual dilemmas for the helping professional*, New York, 1991, Brunner/Mazel.

9. Foley T, Davies M: *Rape: nursing care of victims*, St Louis, 1983, Mosby.

10. Freud S: *Three essays of the theory of sexuality*, ed 3, London, 1962, Hogarth Press (originally published 1905).

11. Gallagher D: HIV/AIDS: The epidemic continues. *Imprint* 39:62, 1992.

12. Goldstein B: *Human sexuality*, New York, 1976, McGraw-Hill.

13. Groth AN, Birnbaum NJ: Adult sexual orientation and attraction to underage persons, *Arch Sex Behav* 7:3, 1978.

14. Haffner D: Yough still at risk, yet barriers to education remain: SIECUS testimony for the National AIDS Commission, *SIECUS Report* 21:10, 1992.

15. Haynes YL: A woman's issue: HIV/AIDS. *Perspect Psychiatr Care* 29:23, 1993.

16. Jackson JL, Calhoun KS, Amick AE, Maddever HM, Habif VL: Young adult women who report childhood intrafamilial sexual abuse: subsequent adjustment, *Arch Sexual Behav* 19:211, 1990.

17. Kaplan HS: *The illustrated manual of sex therapy*, New York, 1975, New York Times Book Co.

18. Kaplan HS: *Disorders of sexual desire and other new concepts and techniques in sex therapy*, New York, 1979, Brunner/Mazel.

19. Kaplan HS: Sex, intimacy, and the aging process. *J Am Acad Psychoanal* 18:185, 1990.

20. Kettl P et al: Sexual harassment of health care students by patients, *J Psychosoc Nurs Ment Health Serv* 31:11, 1993.

21. Kinsey AC, Pomeroy WB, Martin EC: *Sexual behavior in the human female*, Philadelphia, 1953, WB Saunders.

22. Kirby D: Sexuality education: it can reduce unprotected intercourse, *SIECUS Report* 21:19, 1992.

23. Krueger JC, Hassell J, Goggins DB, Ishimatsu T, Pablico MR, Tuttle EJ: Relationship between nurse counseling and

sexual adjustment after hysterectomy, *Nurs Res* 28:145, 1979.

24. Marmor J, ed: *Homosexual behavior: a modern reappraisal*, New York, 1980, Basic Books.

25. Masters WH, Johnson VE: *Human sexual inadequacy*, Boston, 1970, Little, Brown.

26. Masters WH, Johnson VE: Ten sex myths exploded. In Barbour JR, ed: *Human sexuality 79/80*, Guilford, Conn, 1979, Dushkin Publishing.

27. Masters WH, Johnson VE, Kolodny RC: *Masters and Johnson on sex and human loving*, Boston, 1986, Little, Brown.

28. McDonald HB, Steinhorn AL: *Homosexuality: a practical guide to counseling lesbians, gay men, and their families*, New York, 1990, Continuum Publishing.

29. Money J, Wiedeking C: Gender identity role: normal differentiation and its transpositions. In Wolman BB, Money J, eds: *Handbook of human sexuality*, Englewood Cliffs, NJ, 1980, Prentice-Hall.

30. Pepe MV, Sanders DW, Symons CW: Sexual behaviors of university freshmen and the implications for sexuality educators, *J Sex Educ Ther* 19:20, 1993.

31. SIECUS fact sheet #3, on comprehensive sexuality education: sexuality education and the schools: issues and answers, *SIECUS Report* 20:13, 1992.

32. Siegel K, Glassman M: Individual and aggregate level changes in sexual behavior among gay men at risk for AIDS, *Arch Sex Behav* 18:335, 1989.

33. Smith GB: Nursing care challenges: homosexual psychiatric patients, *J Psychosoc Nurs Ment Health Serv* 30:16, 1992.

34. Sullivan G, Lukoff D: Sexual side effects of antipsychotic medication: evaluation and interventions, *Hosp Community Psychiatry* 41:1238, 1990.

35. Thomas SP: Bisexuality: a sexual orientation of great diversity, *J Psychosoc Nurs Ment Health Serv* 18:19, 1980.

36. Trudel G, Boulos L, Matte B: Dyadic adjustment in couples with hypoactive sexual desire, *J Sex Educ Ther* 19:31, 1993.

37. Vincent M, Clearie AF, Schluchter MD: Reducing adolescent pregnancy through school and community-based education, *JAMA* 257:3382, 1987.

38. Wilsnack SC: Alcohol abuse and alcoholism in women. In Pattison EM, Kaufman E, eds: *Encyclopedia handbook of alcoholism*, New York, 1982, Gardner Press.

39. Wilson ME, Williams HA: Oncology nurses' attitudes and behaviors related to sexuality of patients with cancer, *Oncol Nurs Forum* 15:49, 1988.

40. Wyatt GE: The aftermath of child sexual abuse of African-American and white American women: the victims' experience, *J Fam Violence* 5:61, 1990.

41. Zinik G: Identity conflict or adaptive flexibility? bisexuality reconsidered, *J Homosexuality* 11:7, 1985.

ANNOTATED SUGGESTED READINGS

Bancroft J: *Human sexuality and its problems*, New York, 1989, Churchill Livingstone.

Written for health professionals who are interested in working with people with sexual problems. Excellent review of the field including sexual development, behavior, problems, and treatments.

Civic D, Walsh G, McBride D: Staff perspectives on sexual behavior of patients in a state psychiatric hospital, *Hosp Community Psychiatry* 44:887, 1993.

Reports the results of a study that assessed staff experiences with and attitudes toward patients' sexuality. Thought-provoking reading for nurses working in inpatient settings.

*Deevey S: Lesbian self-disclosure, *J Psychosoc Nurs Ment Health Serv* 31:21, 1993.

Challenges nurses who are lesbians to share information about lesbian culture with their colleagues and provide healthy role models for their patients and peers.

Denney N, Quadrango B: *Human sexuality*, ed 2, St Louis, 1992, Mosby.

Comprehensive sexuality textbook that provides good information on a wide variety of sexuality topics.

Edelwich J, Brodsky A: *Sexual dilemmas for the helping professional* ed 2, New York, 1991, Brunner/Mazel.

Provides nurses with many helpful suggestions for intervening in sexual situations. Covers such rarely discussed topics as client seduction of therapist and vice versa; referring clients who arouse sexual feelings in the therapist; and ethical responses to feelings of attraction and seductive behavior.

*Fogel C, Lauver D: *Sexual health promotion*, Philadelphia, 1990, WB Saunders.

Provides nurses with an excellent biopsychosocial approach for promoting the sexual health of patients. Particularly good discussion of illness, chronic disease, and sexuality.

*Fontaine K: Unlocking sexual issues: counseling strategies for nurses, *Nurs Clin North Am* 26:737, 1991.

Good overview of sexual issues including assessment and counseling strategies.

*Hacker S: Students' questions about sexuality: implications for nurse educators, *Nurse Educ* 10:28, 1984.

Identifies major areas of concern for graduate and student nurses in regard to human sexuality.

*Kettl P et al: Sexual harassment of health care students by patients, *J Psychosoc Nurs Ment Health Serv* 31:11, 1993.

Reports on a survey of sexual harassment by patients and a training program to deal with this problem.

Martin H: The coming-out process for homosexuals, *Hosp Community Psychiatry* 42:158, 1991.

Describes the stages of the coming-out process and the clinical implications for therapy with homosexual patients.

Masters W, Johnson V, Kolodny R: *Masters and Johnson on sex and human loving,* Boston, 1986, Little, Brown.

The authors present the biological, psychological, and social aspects of sexuality in a highly readable fashion. This book is an excellent resource for the health professional and also the general public.

Poorman S: Human sexuality and the nursing process, Norwalk, Conn, 1988, Appleton & Lange.

Explores concepts of human sexuality from a nursing process perspective. Sample nursing care plans demonstrate the transfer of theoretical knowledge to actual clinical experience. Sexual acting out behavior and the sexual components of the nurse-patient relationship are also explored.

*Skeen P, Walters L, Robinson B: How parents of gays react to their children's homosexuality and to the threat of AIDS, J Psychosoc Nurs Ment Health Serv 26:7, 1988.

Describes the five-stage mourning process experienced by parents who learn of their child's homosexuality and the supports available to them.

*Smith G: Nursing care challenges: homosexual psychiatric patients, J Psychosoc Nurs Ment Health Serv 30:15, 1992.

Helps nurses examine their attitudes toward homosexuals and provide an atmosphere of acceptance. Includes specific recommendations for nursing care of the homosexual psychiatric patient.

Sullivan G, Lukoff D: Sexual side effects of antipsychotic medication: evaluation and interventions, *Hosp Community Psychiatry* 41:1238, 1990.

Reports on sexual dysfunctions due to psychotropic medication side effects and interventions that may be helpful.

---

*Nursing reference.

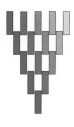

Treatment Modalities

Maybe there have been times when you've felt that the problems people experience are truly overwhelming and you've wondered how you, as an individual, can ever really help. Sure you're a nurse, but how can one person impact on the enormity of stress, illness, and social injustice? Although it's true that societal problems are great, it's also true that the contribution of each person is like a ripple in a pool that can eventually turn the tide of life. But to be effective you need to have the right tools for the task, tools that will allow you to help people think about their life situation and change their behavior, tools that will help you work therapeutically with individuals, families, and groups.

In this unit you will be exposed to a wide range of treatment tools, but don't think that these strategies will pertain only to patients with psychiatric illnesses. The fact is that many people take psychotropic medications, and nurses deal with individuals who struggle with issues of control, aggression, and violence in almost all clinical settings. So too, strategies to change negative thinking patterns and problematic behavior can apply to children and adults throughout their experiences with health and illness. And finally, aren't groups an essential part of every health-care delivery system, and don't all patients have families? As you can see, the skills you will learn in this unit will enhance your nursing practice regardless of setting. So grab your highlighters and get ready to add to your growing repertoire of nursing skills and competencies, because the fact is, you can and will make a difference.

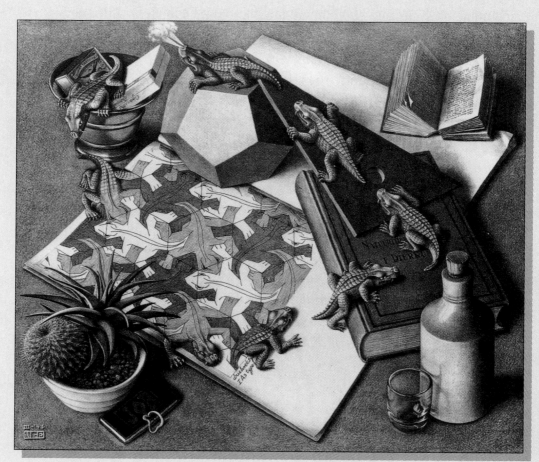

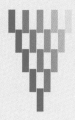

C H A P T E R 2 5
Psychopharmacology

MICHELE T. LARAIA

Medicines are nothing in themselves, if not properly used, but the very hands of the gods, if employed with reason and prudence.

Herophilus

LEARNING OBJECTIVES

After studying this chapter the student should be able to:

▼ Identify the role of the nurse in psychopharmacological treatments

▼ Describe pharmacokinetics and problems of polypharmacy and drug interactions

▼ Discuss the mechanism of action, clinical use, and adverse reactions related to antianxiety and sedative-hypnotic drugs

▼ Discuss the mechanism of action, clinical use, and adverse reactions related to antidepressant drugs

▼ Discuss the mechanism of action, clinical use, and adverse reactions related to mood stabilizing drugs

▼ Discuss the mechanism of action, clinical use, and adverse reactions related to antipsychotic drugs

▼ Evaluate the emergence of new psychopharmacological agents

▼ Describe psychiatric nursing practice issues including psychopharmacology guidelines, documentation, patient education, and promoting patient adherence

TOPICAL OUTLINE

Role of the Nurse
  Patient Assessment
  Coordination of Treatment Modalities
  Psychopharmacological Drug Administration
  Monitoring Drug Effects
  Medication Education
  Drug Maintenance Programs
  Interdisciplinary Clinical Research Drug Trials
  Prescriptive Authority
Pharmacokinetics
  Drug Interactions
  Biological Basis for Psychopharmacology
Antianxiety and Sedative-Hypnotic Drugs
  Benzodiazepines
  Nonbenzodiazepines
Antidepressant Drugs
  Tricyclic Antidepressants
  Selective Serotonin Reuptake Inhibitors
  Monoamine Oxidase Inhibitors
Mood Stabilizing Drugs
  Lithium
  Anticonvulsants
Antipsychotic Drugs
  Mechanism of Action
  Clinical Use
  Adverse Reactions
Future Psychopharmacological Agents
Psychiatric Nursing Practice
  Psychopharmacology Guidelines
  Documentation
  Patient Education
  Promoting Patient Adherence

The past 40 years have produced a revolution in the treatment of psychiatric disorders and in the theories about the etiologies of these disorders. This revolution was sparked by the introduction of neuropsychopharmacology: drugs that treat the symptoms of mental illness and whose actions in the brain provide models to understand better the mechanisms of mental disorders. This sense of "revolution" continues as new theories are debated by experts in drug research and as more centers around the world are funded for clinical research drug studies.

Amid the growth and controversy involving new scientific information, the nurse frequently is the one professional to integrate these drug treatments with the wide range of nonpharmacological treatments in a manner that is knowledgeable, safe, effective, and acceptable to the patient. Regardless of the nurse's theoretical framework, the reality of drug treatment of psychiatric illness must be recognized. Nurses should continue to incorporate psychopharmacology into the knowledge base of nursing theory, the arena of nursing research, and the art and science of nursing care. Nurses should also continue to do what nurses do best—lead the patient through the maze of health-care possibilities in a holistic manner, incorporating them into an individualized and effective treatment plan.

This chapter is designed to introduce the nurse to psychopharmacology and to describe some of the important principles of drug treatment in psychiatry. The theoretical framework suggested here is one of integration: drug therapy can complement problem-solving procedures and the wide range of psychodynamic, psychosocial, and interpersonal interventions. Drug therapy should never be viewed as "an easy way out," "a quick fix," or "a miracle pill." Currently, drug therapy treats symptoms of mental illness with some success, but drugs do not treat the patient's personal, social, or environmental responses to the mental illness. In addition, side effects and adverse reactions of drug therapy add another level of concern and need for expertise and judgment in the care of people receiving these treatments. Thus this is a very exciting time in psychiatric treatment, and nurses are in an excellent position to add new dimensions to their role from this expanding aspect of patient care.

ROLE OF THE NURSE

Psychopharmacological treatment is intended to be integrated with the principles of psychiatric nursing practice presented throughout this text. The psychiatric nurse has a wealth of knowledge and techniques that make nursing unique in the care of people with psychiatric disorders. Following are some examples of the nurse's role in psychopharmacological treatment regimens.

Patient Assessment

Psychoactive drugs treat symptoms of mental disorders. However, not all behaviors are treated by drug therapy, and not every identified personality trait is a symptom of illness targeted for treatment with drugs. It thus is essential to obtain baseline information about each patient before drug treatment. This information helps describe aspects of the patient's psychiatric illness as compared with the patient's personality before the illness. As a result, a list of psychiatric symptoms can be identified as appropriate targets for drug treatment. Residual symptoms of the illness and personality characteristics not related to the illness then can be addressed by nonpharmacological treatments. In addition, drug side effects can be identified and appropriately treated as they appear. Symptoms of organ system dysfunction caused by drug treatment can also be identified and treated. Finally, careful assessment of each patient can help identify medical illnesses that are concurrent with psychiatric illness or that possibly cause psychiatric symptoms. Box 25-1 provides a medication assessment tool for the nurse to use in taking a drug history.

Coordination of Treatment Modalities

The nurse has an important role in designing a viable treatment program for the patient. The most appropriate treatment choices, integrated in a holistic manner and individualized for each patient, should be reflected in the care plan designed by the nurse. The coordination of treatment modalities is often the primary responsibility of the nurse who works with the patient in an ongoing therapeutic alliance.

Psychopharmacological Drug Administration

No one on the health-care team has a greater daily impact on the patient's experience with psychopharmacological agents than the nurse. The nurse administers each medication dose, works out a dosing schedule based on drug requirements and the patient's preferences, and is continually alert for drug effects. This role defines the nurse as a key professional in working to maximize therapeutic effects of drug treatment and to minimize drug side effects in such a way that the patient is included as a true collaborator in the medication regimen.

Monitoring Drug Effects

The nurse is the most available professional to the patient and has the important role of consistently monitoring the effects of psychopharmacological drugs, including their effects on target symptoms of illness, side effects, and adverse reactions and the

---

Box 25-1

MEDICATION ASSESSMENT TOOL

1. **Psychiatric medications** (for each medication ever taken by the patient obtain the following information):
   a. Name of drug
   b. Why prescribed
   c. Date started
   d. Length of time taken
   e. Highest daily dose
   f. Who prescribed it
   g. Whether it was effective
   h. Side effects or adverse reactions
   i. If it was taken as prescribed; if not, explain
   j. If anyone else in family has been prescribed this drug; if so, for what reason and if it was effective

2. **Prescription (nonpsychiatric) medications** (for each medication taken by the patient in the past 6 months and for major medical illnesses if more than 6 months ago, obtain the following information):
   a. Name of drug
   b. Why prescribed
   c. Date started

   d. Highest daily dose
   e. Who prescribed it
   f. Whether it was effective
   g. Side effects or adverse reactions
   h. If drug was taken as prescribed; if not, explain

3. **Over-the-counter (nonprescribed) medications** (for each medication taken by the patient in the past 6 months, obtain the following information):
   a. Name of drug
   b. Reason taken
   c. Date started
   d. Frequency of use
   e. Whether it was effective
   f. Side effects or adverse reactions

4. **Alcohol, caffeine, nicotine, and street drugs**
   a. Name of substance
   b. Date of first use
   c. Frequency of use
   d. Summarize effects
   e. Adverse reactions
   f. Withdrawal symptoms

---

overall yet often subtle effects on the patient's self-concept and sense of trust.

Medication Education

The nurse is in a pivotal position to educate the patient and the family about medications. This includes conveying complex information to the patient so that it is understandable, acceptable, achievable, and often critical for the patient's health and safety.

Drug Maintenance Programs

For some patients the medication maintenance program could last many years. The nurse can assume the important role of continuing a therapeutic alliance with a patient on drug maintenance in the aftercare setting.

Interdisciplinary Clinical Research Drug Trials

As a member of the interdisciplinary research team, the nurse can contribute to the body of scientific knowledge, often adding a nursing perspective to team research efforts. The nurse can be included on several levels, from data collector to coinvestigator to principal investigator. The nurse's roles in interdisciplinary clinical research drug trials in the clinical setting are just beginning to be appreciated and defined.

Prescriptive Authority

Within the last 5 years legislation has been passed in most states in this country authorizing clinical nurse specialists to prescribe medications. Psychiatric nurses who are qualified by education and experience in accordance with their state practice act are thus able to prescribe pharmacological agents to treat the symptoms and improve the functional status of patients with psychiatric illness.[41] Specific pharmacological agents can be prescribed by psychiatric clinical nurse specialists based on clinical indicators of the patient's status, and the role of nurses in psychopharmacological treatments has been expanded once again to increase patients' access to quality and cost-effective health care.

 Does your state grant prescriptive authority to psychiatric clinical nurse specialists? If so, what are the requirements for practice?

PHARMACOKINETICS

Drugs are chemicals with specific properties that affect treatment. For example, it is important to know a drug's **half-life**. The half-life determines how long it takes to achieve a steady state of concentration. **Steady state** means that the amount of drug excreted equals the amount ingested, and it occurs in approximately four to six half-lives. Until steady state is reached, the drug level continues to build, and it changes after each dosing. This accounts for some acute side effects in some patients. It also means that until steady state is reached, the optimum dose for a particular patient cannot be determined nor is a blood level accurate in determining a proper dose range. It may take longer to reach steady state in the elderly because of slower gastrointestinal activity and liver metabolism.

Another significance of half-life is in the frequency of dosing. Usually a drug with a half-life of 24 hours or more can be administered once a day when steady state is reached; a drug with a shorter half-life should be administered more often to achieve constant clinical effects. Termination of drug treatment is also affected by half-life. In general, the effects of drugs with a long half-life can last a long time (sometimes weeks) after the last dose. Drugs with a short half-life usually must be tapered (discontinued gradually over several days or weeks). In general, all psychoactive drugs should be discontinued by a tapering period.

This chapter focuses on the adult patient, although children and the elderly are frequently given psychoactive drugs. Generally, adults and children metabolize drugs similarly, although children exhibit a variable response to these drugs. Children must receive lower drug

doses because of their lower body weight. The elderly and newborns are particularly sensitive to psychotropic drugs. For the elderly, drug distribution, hepatic metabolism, and renal clearance are all affected by age. If a pregnant woman takes psychoactive drugs before delivery, the infant may experience withdrawal symptoms unless the baby is detoxified from the drug. The infant whose mother takes psychoactive drugs generally should not be breast-fed.[10] Patients with liver disease are extremely sensitive to most psychoactive drugs, and patients with renal impairment are particularly sensitive to lithium.

Drug Interactions

Drugs can interact with each other on two levels:
1. **Pharmacokinetic**—one drug interferes with the absorption, metabolism, distribution, and excretion of another drug, thus raising or lowering the levels of the drug in the blood and tissue
2. **Pharmacodynamic**—one drug combines with another to increase or decrease the drugs' effects in an organ system

Concurrent use of drugs, or polypharmacy, can enhance a specific therapeutic action, may be necessary to treat concurrent illnesses, and can counteract unwanted effects of one of the drugs. Unfortunately, a number of problems have been associated with concurrent drug use; confusion over therapeutic efficacy and side effects and development of drug interactions are just two.[42] In general, polypharmacy in psychiatry should be used only when necessary and with caution. Box 25-2 lists guidelines for polypharmacy, and Box 25-3 alerts the nurse to patients at a higher risk for drug interactions. Table 25-1 is a reference list for the more common drug interactions of psychotropic drugs.

This chapter refers to drugs by their generic names. There is a strong movement in practice to use generic

---

Box 25-2

GUIDELINES FOR POLYPHARMACY

1. Identify specific target symptoms for each drug.
2. If possible, start with one drug and evaluate effectiveness and side effects before adding a second drug.
3. Be alert for adverse drug interactions.
4. Consider the effects of a second drug on the absorption and metabolism of the first drug.
5. Consider the possibility of additive side effects.
6. Change the dose of only one drug at a time and evaluate results.
7. Be aware of increased risk of medication errors.
8. Be aware of increased cost of treatment.
9. Be aware of decreased patient compliance in the aftercare setting when medication regimen is complex.
10. In follow-up treatment, eliminate as many drugs as possible and establish the minimum effective dose of the drugs utilized.
11. Patient education programs regarding concomitant drug regimens must be particularly clear, organized, and effective.
12. Patient follow-up contacts should be more frequent.

Box 25-3

INCREASED RISK FACTORS FOR DEVELOPMENT OF DRUG INTERACTIONS

Polypharmacy
High doses
Geriatric patients
Debilitated/dehydrated patients
Concurrent illness
Compromised organ system function
Inadequate patient education
History of noncompliance
Failure to include patient in treatment planning

TABLE 25-1

INTERACTIONS OF PSYCHOTROPIC DRUGS AND OTHER SUBSTANCES

Drug/category	Interacting drug/class	Possible consequences
ANTIPSYCHOTIC AGENTS		
	Oral antacids	Antacids may inhibit absorption of orally administered phenothiazines
	Central nervous system depressants: alcohol, barbiturates, antianxiety agents, antihistamines, narcotic analgesics	Additive central nervous system depression, increasing the risk of mental or physical impairment of performance
	Anticholinergic agents: levodopa* (Bendopa, Larodopa, Levopa)	Additive atropine-like side effects; antiparkinson effects of levodopa may be antagonized by antipsychotic agents
Clozapine	Carbamazepine*	Additive bone marrow suppression; increased incidence of agranulocytosis and aplastic anemia
ANTIANXIETY AGENTS		
Benzodiazepines	Central nervous system depressants: alcohol, barbiturates, antipsychotics, antihistamines, cimetidine	Potential additive central nervous system effects, especially sedation and decreased daytime performance
		Interferes with metabolism of long-acting benzodiazepines
ANTIDEPRESSANT AGENTS		
Tricyclics	MAO inhibitors*	May cause hypertensive crisis if tricyclic is added to MAO inhibitors
	Alcohol, other central nervous system depressants	*Acute*: additive CNS depression; *Chronic*: may increase tricyclic metabolism
	Antihypertensives*: guanethidine (Ismelin), methyldopa (Aldomet), clonidine (Catapres)	Antagonism of antihypertensive effects with loss of control of blood pressure
	Antipsychotics	Additive atropine-like effects
	Anticholinergics	
	Antiarrhythmics: quinidine, procainamide	Additive antiarrhythmic effects, prolongation of QRS complex
MOOD STABILIZER		
Lithium	Diuretics*: hydrochlorothiazide	Diuretic-induced sodium depletion can increase lithium levels; may cause toxicity
	Nonsteroidal antiinflammatory agents*: ibuprofen, indomethacin, phenylbutazone	Increases lithium blood levels; may cause toxicity
SEDATIVE-HYPNOTIC AGENTS		
	Alcohol—acutely Analgesics—narcotics Antihistamines Antidepressants Antipsychotics	Combined use of sedative-hypnotics with other central nervous system depressants may impair mental and physical performance (e.g., motor vehicle operation) and result in lethargy, respiratory depression, coma, or death. These drugs may enhance the sedative effects of barbiturates and nonbarbiturates.
	Anticoagulants*—oral	Increased rate of coumarin anticoagulant metabolism, decreasing plasma levels of coumarin and reducing its ability to prevent blood coagulations; higher dose of coumarin required; when barbiturate withdrawn and dose of coumarin not reduced, bleeding episode may occur.

*Potentially clinically significant.

names instead of trade names to be more accurate, to take advantage of price differences, and to prevent confusion when a drug becomes generic (when the patent runs out and the drug can be made by any company, thus reducing cost). Once a drug becomes generic, the patient should be taught to use the same brand of a drug because the bioavailability of psychoactive drugs may vary significantly from one brand to another, thus affecting drug dose and steady state. The patient can use one pharmacy regularly and can ask the pharmacist to use the same company when filling generic prescriptions of a particular drug.

Why do you think patients often fail to report over-the-counter medications when asked about current medications? How can you, as a nurse, be sure to obtain this information?

Biological Basis for Psychopharmacology

All communication in the brain involves neurons "talking" to each other at synapses. These nerve cells are the basic functional unit of the nervous system, and the study of this communication process forms the basis of much of the neurosciences. The following description is simplified to present a very basic frame of reference from which to view the rather overwhelming complexity of neuropharmacological mechanisms.

The synapse is a narrow gap separating two neurons (the presynaptic cell and the postsynaptic cell) at a transmission site (Fig. 25-1). During neurotransmission the chemical neurotransmitter is released from a storage vesicle in the presynaptic cell, crosses the synapse, and is recognized by the receptor on the postsynaptic cell membrane (this recognition is called *binding*). Receptors are the cellular recognition sites for specific molecular structures such as neurotransmitters, hormones, and many drugs. Thus their action is selective for specific chemicals. Neurotransmitters, the "chemical messengers" that travel from one brain cell to another, are synthesized by enzymes from certain dietary amino acids, or precursors. At the synapse, neurotransmitters act as receptor activators (agonists) or inhibitors (antagonists) and trigger complex biological responses within the cell. The chemical remaining in the synapse is either reabsorbed and stored by the presynaptic cell or is

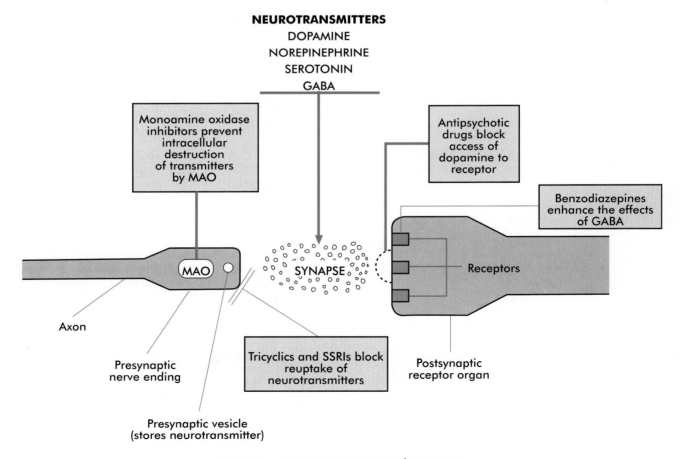

NEUROTRANSMITTERS
DOPAMINE
NOREPINEPHRINE
SEROTONIN
GABA

Monoamine oxidase inhibitors prevent intracellular destruction of transmitters by MAO

Antipsychotic drugs block access of dopamine to receptor

Benzodiazepines enhance the effects of GABA

MAO

SYNAPSE

Receptors

Axon

Presynaptic nerve ending

Tricyclics and SSRIs block reuptake of neurotransmitters

Postsynaptic receptor organ

Presynaptic vesicle (stores neurotransmitter)

Fig. 25-1   Neurotransmission at the synapse.

metabolized (inactivated) by enzymes, one of which is monoamine oxidase.

Many of the psychiatric disorders are thought to be caused by an overresponse or an underresponse somewhere along the complex process of neurotransmission. For instance, psychosis is thought to involve excessive dopamine neurotransmission. Depression and mania are thought to result from disruption of normal patterns of neurotransmission of norepinephrine, serotonin, and other neurotransmitters. Anxiety is thought to be a dysregulation of gamma-aminobutyric acid (GABA) and endogenous antianxiety chemicals.

If a particular psychiatric illness is known to result from "too much" or "too little" neurotransmission in a particular neurotransmitter system and if the mechanism of action of the psychiatric drugs is understood, then some order in the various pharmacological strategies used in psychiatry can be recognized. This process of cell-to-cell communication at the synapse can be affected by drugs in several important ways:

1. *Release:* More neurotransmitter is released into the synapse from the storage vesicles in the presynaptic cell.
2. *Blockade:* The neurotransmitter is prevented from binding to the postsynaptic receptor.
3. *Receptor sensitivity changes:* The receptor becomes more or less responsive to the neurotransmitter.
4. *Blocked reuptake:* The presynaptic cell does not reabsorb the neurotransmitter well, leaving more neurotransmitter in the synapse and therefore enhancing or prolonging its action.
5. *Interference with storage vesicles:* The neurotransmitter is either released again into the synapse (more neurotransmitter) or is released to metabolizing enzymes (less neurotransmitter).
6. *Precursor chain interference:* The process that "makes" the neurotransmitter is either facilitated (more neurotransmitter is synthesized) or disrupted (less neurotransmitter is synthesized).
7. *Synaptic enzyme interference:* Less neurotransmitter is metabolized, so more remains available in the synapse.

Not all of the above strategies have yielded clinically relevant treatments. Several have, however, and these are emphasized in this chapter (see Fig. 25-1): antipsychotic drugs block dopamine from the receptor site; tricyclic antidepressants and selective serotonin reuptake inhibitors (SSRIs) block the reuptake of norepinephrine and serotonin and regulate the areas of the brain that manufacture these chemicals; monoamine oxidase inhibitors (MAO inhibitors or MAOIs) prevent enzymatic metabolism of norepinephrine and serotonin; and benzodiazepines potentiate GABA.

Understanding this process has led to the variety of treatment approaches in pharmacotherapy that attempt to change or modify one or more of the steps in neuro-

transmission. Unfortunately, to date the actions of psychopharmacological drugs are not confined to the specific brain areas that are thought to be associated with psychiatric symptoms. These drugs spread throughout the body, causing unwanted drug reactions or side effects and undesirable drug interactions during concomitant drug therapy. Current psychopharmacological research attempts to better understand the cause of psychiatric illness at the neurotransmission level and the increased specificity of psychopharmacological drugs.

ANTIANXIETY AND SEDATIVE-HYPNOTIC DRUGS

The diagnosis of anxiety is based on the patient's description, the nurse's observation of behaviors, and the elimination of alternative diagnoses. The possibility of a medical cause must be considered. Hyperthyroidism, hypoglycemia, cardiovascular illness, and severe pulmonary disease are characteristic illnesses associated with high levels of anxiety. In addition to a careful physical assessment and a review of laboratory tests, the patient should be asked about use of over-the-counter drugs, "recreational" substances, alcohol, and caffeine. Anxiety also accompanies many psychiatric disorders. In general, the primary disorder should be treated with the appropriate medication. Anxiety may be associated with psychosis or an affective disorder and often goes away when the target symptoms for the primary disorder subside with appropriate treatment.

This section divides antianxiety and sedative-hypnotic drugs into two categories: the benzodiazepines and nonbenzodiazepines; the latter group includes several classes of drugs. The benzodiazepines are the most widely prescribed drugs in the world, and within the last two decades they have almost entirely replaced the barbiturates in the treatment of anxiety and sleep disorders. Their popularity is related to their effectiveness and wide margin of safety, and they are the principal drugs used in the treatment of anxiety and insomnia.

Benzodiazepines

Mechanism of Action. The benzodiazepines are thought to reduce anxiety because they are powerful potentiators of the inhibitory neurotransmitter GABA, although the role of GABA in anxiety is not yet clear. A postsynaptic receptor site specific for the exogenous benzodiazepine molecule has been discovered. The search for a naturally occurring "antianxiety" chemical has recently resulted in the discovery of an endogenous benzodiazepine-binding inhibitor (DBI). The benzodiazepine molecule and GABA do not compete for the same receptor site. However, the benzodiazepines do compete with DBI for a role in neurotransmission, indicating that DBI may be the antianxiety neurotransmitter. Research in this field promises to provide a great deal of information in the future.

 What sociocultural factors may help to explain why benzodiazepines are the most commonly prescribed medications in the United States?

Clinical Use. The benzodiazepines are the drug treatment of choice in the management of anxiety, insomnia, and stress-related conditions. The target symptoms for use of these drugs are listed in Box 25-4. The major indications for their use are generalized anxiety disorder, anxiety associated with other psychiatric diagnoses, sleep disorders, anxiety associated with phobic disorders, posttraumatic stress disorder, alcohol and drug withdrawal, anxiety associated with medical disease, skeletal muscle relaxation, seizure disorders, and the anxiety and apprehension experienced before surgery.[35] Major studies are beginning to show that higher-dose benzodiazepines, particularly alprazolam, a triazolobenzodiazepine, appear to have specific antipanic effects in the treatment of panic disorder.

The specific types of benzodiazepines have no significant clinical advantages over each other. Some of the differences suggested for the use of these drugs can be attributed more to marketing strategies than clinical efficacy. Prescribing decisions can be made based on whether or not the drug breaks down into active metabolites that extend drug half-life (Table 25-2). Duration of action after a single dose can be relatively brief, depending on how rapidly the drug is metabolized and how extensively it is distributed to body tissues (in turn, this is based on lipid solubility). Duration of action at steady state can be much longer. Differences in half-life can be clinically useful. For example, patients with persistent high levels of anxiety should take a drug with a long half-life. Patients with fluctuating anxiety might be better off with short-acting drugs. When used as hypnotics the benzodiazepines ideally should induce sleep rapidly, and their effect should be gone by morning. The rate of absorption of the different benzodiazepines from the gastrointestinal tract varies considerably, thus affecting the rapidity and intensity of onset of their acute effects. Diazepam and clorazepate are absorbed fastest, whereas prazepam and oxazepam are slowest. Antacids or food in the stomach slows down this process.

Because the benzodiazepines are in the same pharmacological class as alcohol, they can be used to suppress the alcohol withdrawal syndrome. The concomitant use of these two substances can be dangerous because it produces extreme sedation. Any of the benzo-

---

Box 25-4

TARGET SYMPTOMS FOR ANTIANXIETY AND SEDATIVE-HYPNOTIC BENZODIAZEPINES

PSYCHOLOGICAL

Vague sense of irritability and uneasiness
Sense of impending doom or panic
Insomnia

PHYSICAL

Flushed skin
Hot or cold flashes
Sweating
Dilated pupils
Dry mouth
Nausea or vomiting
Diarrhea
Tachycardia, palpitations
Dizziness, light-headedness
Shortness of breath
Hyperventilation, with paresthesias
Tremor
Restlessness
Headache
Urinary frequency

---

diazepines can be an effective sedative-hypnotic when administered at bedtime.

Although some patients may need to take antianxiety drugs for extended periods, the drugs have their drawbacks and should always be used with nonpharmacological treatments for the patient with chronic anxiety. Psychotherapy, behavioral techniques, environmental changes, stress management, and an ongoing therapeutic relationship continue to be important in the treatment of anxiety disorders.

Most experts believe that treatment with benzodiazepines should be brief, used during a time of specific stress. Those drugs with a long half-life (longer than 18 to 24 hours) can be given once a day. Drugs with a short half-life (8 to 15 hours) need to be given more frequently; they can be taken as needed for increased symptoms of anxiety as such symptoms occur. The patient should be observed frequently during the early days of treatment to assess target symptom response and to monitor side effects so that the dose can be adjusted. Some patients require long-term antianxiety medication treatment.

Concentrations of benzodiazepine drugs in the blood have not yet been firmly correlated to clinical effects. All benzodiazepines are rapidly absorbed by mouth. The injectable benzodiazepines have been proven reliable when administered in the deltoid muscle and lead to

TABLE 25-2

ANTIANXIETY AND SEDATIVE-HYPNOTIC DRUGS: BENZODIAZEPINES

Drug family				Drug dosage		
Chemical class generic name (trade name)	Active metabolites	Half-life (hr)	Days to steady state	Equivalence (mg)	Usual adult dosage range (mg/day)	Available forms (mg)
ANTIANXIETY DRUGS						
Benzodiazepines						
Alprazolam (Xanax)	Yes (not significant)	6-20	3	0.5	0.5-4	tabs: 0.25, 0.5, 1.0
Chlordiazepoxide (Librium)	Yes	5-200	1-3	10	20-100	tabs: 5, 10, 25 inj: 100
Clorazepate (Tranxene)	Yes	30-200	5-16	7.5	7.5-60	tabs: 3.75, 7.50, 15
Clonazepam (Klonopin)	No	18-50	3-8	—	1.5-2	tabs: 0.5, 1, 2
Diazepam (Valium)	Yes	20-200	4-8	5	10-40	tabs: 2, 5, 10, sustained release 15 inj: 5/ml
Halazepam (Paxipam)	Yes	20-100	4	20	80-160	tabs: 20, 40
Lorazepam (Ativan)	No	10-20	2-3	1	2-6	tabs: 0.5, 1, 2 inj: 2/ml, 4/ml
Oxazepam (Serax)	No	5-15	1-2	15	15-90	tabs: 10, 15, 30
Prazepam (Centrax)	Yes	30-200	5-32	10	10-60	tabs: 5, 10, 20
SEDATIVE-HYPNOTIC DRUGS						
Benzodiazepines						
Estazolam (ProSom)	No	10-24	1-2	1	1-2	tabs: 1, 2
Flurazepam (Dalmane)	Yes	30-250	4-8	15	15-60	caps: 15, 30
Temazepam (Restoril)	No	10-20	2-3	15	15-30	caps: 15, 30
Triazolam (Halcion)	No	1.5-4	1	0.25	0.25-0.5	tabs: 0.25, 0.50

rapid and predictable rises in the blood level when used intravenously. When given intravenously, administration should be slow (over 1 minute) and direct, not mixed in an IV infusion, because plastic tubing absorbs the drug and the drug can precipitate when mixed with saline or dextrose.

Another clinical indication for the use of benzodiazepines is as a sedative-hypnotic to improve sleep. Insomnia (poor sleep) includes difficulty falling asleep, difficulty staying asleep, or awakening too early. It is a symptom with many causes and often responds to nonpharmacological strategies such as talking about problems, increased daytime exercise, and physical comfort measures at night. Drugs to induce sleep have their place but should be used with discretion and are never a substitute for good nursing care.

Adverse Reactions. Because the benzodiazepines have a very high therapeutic index, overdoses of benzodiazepines alone almost never cause fatalities. Side effects are common, dose related, and almost always harmless. Table 25-3 summarizes these reactions and nursing considerations. The benzodiazepines generally do not live up to their reputation of being strongly addictive if they are discontinued gradually, if they have been used for appropriate purposes, and if their use has not been complicated by other factors such as chronic use of barbiturates or alcohol.

Tolerance does develop to the sedative effects of benzodiazepines, but it is unclear whether induced sleep or antianxiety effects develop tolerance. These drugs should be discontinued relatively slowly to minimize withdrawal symptoms and rebound symptoms of insom-

Table 25-3   Benzodiazepine Side Effects and Nursing Considerations

Side effects	Nursing considerations
ACUTE/COMMON	
Drowsiness, sedation	Activity helps; caution when using machinery
Ataxia, dizziness	Caution with activity, prevent falls
Feelings of detachment	Discourage social isolation
Increased irritability or hostility	Observe carefully, offer support, be alert for disinhibition of control over socially unacceptable impulses
Anterograde amnesia	Inability to recall events that occur while the drug is active; desirable in preoperative use
LONG-TERM/COMMON	
Minor tolerance to some effects	Short-term use if possible; discontinue, using a slow taper; not recommended for use
Dependency	with people with history of drug or alcohol abuse
Rebound insomnia/anxiety	
RARE (CAUSAL RELATIONSHIP UNCERTAIN)	
Increased appetite and weight gain	Weight control measures
Cutaneous reactions	Usually not clinically significant
Nausea	Dose with meals, decrease dose
Headache	Usually responds to mild analgesic
Confusion	Decrease dose
Gross psychomotor impairment	Dose related, decrease dose
Depression	Decrease dose; may require antidepressant treatment
Paradoxical rage reaction	Discontinue drug

nia or anxiety. The general rule is a decrease by 5% of the dose each 1 to 3 days, although this varies. All benzodiazepines, regardless of half-life, should be discontinued by tapering. When these drugs are discontinued too rapidly or are stopped precipitously, especially with prolonged use of high doses, a benzodiazepine withdrawal syndrome can occur as described in Box 25-5. If this occurs, the dose must be raised until symptoms are gone and then tapering is resumed at a slower rate.[38]

An elderly patient is more vulnerable to side effects because the aging brain is more sensitive to sedatives. Dosing ranges from ½ to ⅓ of the actual daily dose.[43] The benzodiazepines with no active metabolites (see Table 25-2) are less affected by liver disease, the age of the patient, or drug interactions. Use of benzodiazepines during pregnancy has been associated with infant cleft lip/cleft palate, multiple congenital deformities, and intrauterine growth retardation, especially when used during the first trimester. When used late in pregnancy or during breast-feeding, these drugs have been associated with floppy infant syndrome, neonatal withdrawal symptoms, poor sucking, and hypotonia.

Nonbenzodiazepines

The advantages of the benzodiazepines compared with most other antianxiety and sedative-hypnotic agents have led to greatly decreased use of some of the older,

---

Box 25-5

BENZODIAZEPINE WITHDRAWAL SYNDROME

Usually worsens several days after taper begins, increases over several weeks, then subsides. Minimize by slowing taper.

MILD SYMPTOMS	SEVERE SYMPTOMS
Tremulousness	Diarrhea
Insomnia	Hypotension
Dizziness	Hyperthermia
Headaches	Neuromuscular irritability
Tinnitus	Psychosis
Anorexia	Seizures
Vertigo	
Blurred vision	
Agitation	
Anxiety	

---

more dangerous nonbenzodiazepines. Nonbenzodiazepine anxiolytics and sedative-hypnotics, listed in Table 25-4, are used when alternatives to benzodiazepines are sought or when preferred by clinicians or patients. An exception to this is zolpidem, the first of a new class of compounds for short-term (up to 10 days) treatment of insomnia. Structurally unrelated to benzodiazepines,

TABLE 25-4

ANTIANXIETY, SEDATIVE-HYPNOTIC DRUGS:
NONBENZODIAZEPINES

Chemical class generic name (trade name)	Dose (mg)	Half-life (hr)
Barbiturates		
Secobarbital (Seconal)	100-200	19-34
Pentobarbital (Nembutal)	100-200	15-48
Amobarbital (Amytal)	100-200	8-42
Butabarbital (Butisol)	100-200	34-42
Phenobarbital (Luminal)	100-200	24-140
Propanediols		
Meprobamate (Equanil, Miltown)	800	10
Acetylenic alcohols		
Ethchlorvynol (Placidyl)	500-1000	10-25
Piperidinediones		
Glutethimide (Doriden)	250-500	5-22
Methyprylon (Noludar)	200-400	4
Chloral derivative		
Chloral hydrate (Noctec)	500-2000	4-10
Antihistamines		
Diphenhydramine (Benadryl)	50	unknown
Hydroxyzine (Atarax)	100 tid	unknown
Beta-adrenergic blocker		
Propranolol (Inderal)	10 qid	3
Anxiolytic		
Buspirone (BuSpar)	10-40	2-5
Imidazopyridine		
Zolpidem (Ambien)	10	2.5

zolpidem binds more selectively to neuronal receptors involved in inducing sleep. It is well tolerated and appears to have little antianxiety, anticonvulsant, or muscle-relaxant properties. Side effects include daytime drowsiness, dizziness, and diarrhea. Zolpidem is a schedule IV controlled substance.[32]

The barbiturates have been largely replaced by the benzodiazepines, although the former are used occasionally. Barbiturates have numerous disadvantages: tolerance develops to their antianxiety effects; they are more addictive; they cause serious, even lethal withdrawal reactions; they are dangerous in overdose and cause central nervous system (CNS) depression; and they can cause a variety of dangerous drug interactions.

The propanediol drug, meprobamate, has also dropped in popularity. Its adverse effects, drug interactions, potential for abuse, and withdrawal syndromes are similar to those observed with barbiturates. Also, many studies show meprobamate to be no more effective than a placebo.

Ethchlorvynol, an acetylenic alcohol, has a variety of side effects: confusion, hangover, ataxia, hypotension,

and gastrointestinal distress. Physical dependence occurs, tolerance develops, abuse is possible, and discontinuation can cause withdrawal reactions.

The piperidinedione derivatives have all the drawbacks of the barbiturates without any added advantages. They have remained in use despite their low therapeutic index, high lethality, and addiction potential because they produce relatively few unwanted effects at therapeutic doses.

Chloral hydrate can cause gastrointestinal irritation and causes a variety of drug interactions. Tolerance, physical dependence, addiction, and a withdrawal syndrome are all problems.

Antihistamines, especially hydroxyzine, are usually not as effective as the benzodiazepines; they cause sedation but do not cause physical dependence or abuse. A disadvantage of the antihistamines is that they lower the seizure threshold.

Propranolol blocks beta-noradrenergic receptors centrally and in the peripheral cardiac and pulmonary systems. This drug probably decreases certain physiological symptoms of anxiety, especially tachycardia, rather than centrally acting on anxiety. More research is needed to define a proper role for propranolol in the treatment of anxiety.

Buspirone, a nonbenzodiazepine anxiolytic drug, has been the subject of much discussion. It appears to be a potent antianxiety agent with no addictive potential. Buspirone is effective in the treatment of anxiety and does not exhibit muscle-relaxant or anticonvulsant activity, interaction with CNS depressants, or sedative-hypnotic properties. It is not effective in the management of drug or alcohol abuse.[37]

ANTIDEPRESSANT DRUGS

The 1950s were an important time in the history of psychopharmacology with the discovery of drugs that were effective in treating depression. Early in the 1950s dramatic improvements in mood and well-being were noted in tuberculosis patients being treated with iproniazid before improvement in the tuberculosis lesion was noted. This led to the use of MAOIs as primary drug treatments for depression. At this same time, the first tricyclic antidepressant (TCA), imipramine, was tested for potential antipsychotic activity. It was found to be an ineffective antipsychotic, but depression improved. Imipramine was marketed in 1958 for its significant antidepressant properties.

Research on the biology of depression has led to many new discoveries and even more questions. It has been proposed that either serotonin or norepinephrine or both are reduced in depression and that an excess of norepinephrine is produced in mania. The biological understanding of antidepressant drugs supports this theory: MAO inhibitors "inhibit" the metabolism of these neurotransmitters, and tricyclic antidepressants, and even more specifically, the SSRIs, block their re-uptake at the presynaptic neuron. Both these mechanisms allow more neurotransmitter to remain in the synapse, thereby solving the functional "deficit" in depression. Several problems challenge the simplicity of this theory: 25% to 30% of people who are depressed do not respond to antidepressant drugs, and several new drugs that seem to be effective antidepressants do not appear to affect norepinephrine or serotonin levels. There is also evidence that antidepressants regulate the locus ceruleus, the part of the brain that makes most of the norepinephrine.

The primary clinical indication for use of antidepressant drugs is major depressive illness. These drugs are also useful in the treatment of panic disorder and enuresis in children. A variety of preliminary research studies suggest that they are useful in attention deficit disorders in children and in narcolepsy. The SSRIs are receiving attention for their effectiveness in treating bulimia and their low side effect profile. Clomipramine (Anafranil) and fluoxetine (Prozac) have been shown to be effective in obsessive-compulsive disorder. Table 25-5 presents a side effect profile of these medications.

> Your patient who has been taking antidepressant medication for 3 months tells you that he feels better and wants to stop taking it. How would you respond?

Patients who respond to the initial course of treatment with antidepressants should continue taking the drugs at the same dosage for 4 to 9 months afterward. This is known as *continuation treatment*. If they are symptom free during this time, they can then be tapered off the medication. Patients who have relapses after the continuation treatment is ended may require long-term maintenance medication to prevent recurring depression.[15] Patients who have had three or more episodes of major depression have a 90% chance of having another and are therefore potential candidates for long-term maintenance antidepressant medication. The maintenance medication given is generally the same type and dosage found to be effective in the acute phase of treatment.[18]

Tricyclic Antidepressants

Mechanism of Action. Although the class of tricyclic antidepressants includes some drugs that are structur-

Table 25-5 Side-Effect Profiles of Antidepressant Medications

Drug	Side effect*						
		Central nervous system		Cardiovascular			Other
	Anticholinergic†	Drowsiness	Insomnia/ agitation	Orthostatic hypotension	Cardiac arrhythmia	Gastrointestinal distress	Weight gain (over 6 kg)
Amitriptyline	4+	4+	0	4+	3+	0	4+
Desipramine	1+	1+	1+	2+	2+	0	1+
Doxepin	3+	4+	0	2+	2+	0	3+
Imipramine	3+	3+	1+	4+	3+	1+	3+
Nortriptyline	1+	1+	0	2+	2+	0	1+
Protriptyline	2+	1+	1+	2+	2+	0	0
Trimipramine	1+	4+	0	2+	2+	0	3+
Amoxapine	2+	2+	2+	2+	3+	0	1+
Maprotiline	2+	4+	0	0	1+	0	2+
Trazodone	0	4+	0	1+	1+	1+	1+
Bupropion	0	0	2+	0	1+	1+	0
Fluoxetine	0	0	2+	0	0	3+	0
Paroxetine	0	0	2+	0	0	3+	0
Sertraline	0	0	2+	0	0	3+	0
Monoamine oxidase inhibitors (MAOIs)	1	1+	2+	2+	0	1+	2+

From Depression Guideline Panel: *Depression in primary care*, vol 2, *Treatment of major depression. Clinical practice guideline*, Number 5 (AHCPR publication no. 93-0551), Rockville, Md, 1993, US Department of Health and Human Services, Public Health Service, Agency for Health Care Policy and Research.
*0, Absent or rare; 1+; 2+, in between; 3+; 4+, relatively common.
†Dry mouth, blurred vision, urinary hesitancy, constipation.

ally dissimilar, the drugs in this class are quite similar in their clinical effects and adverse reactions. They are divided into several categories: tertiary tricyclics (or parent drugs), secondary tricyclics (or metabolites), and a newer nontricyclic (or heterocyclic) group of drugs.

Clinical Use. The antidepressant drugs are listed in Table 25-6. Elderly patients and patients with a concomitant medical illness may require lower doses of these drugs than healthy adults and careful assessments for side effects while they are taking the drugs. For patients with an acceptable cardiac history and an ECG within normal limits, particularly for patients over 40 years of age, tricyclic antidepressants are safe and ef-

fective in the treatment of acute and long-term depressive illness.

Unfortunately, all antidepressants must be taken for 3 to 4 weeks or longer before a therapeutic response is evident. Table 25-7 describes the target symptoms for these drugs in the approximate order of the time it takes for each symptom to begin to improve. When caring for suicidally depressed patients, it is important to remember that they become more motivated and begin to look better long before their subjective depressive feelings and suicidal thoughts are relieved. The nursing care plan must include suicide assessments and suicide precautions for weeks after these patients begin to look less depressed.

TABLE 25-6
ANTIDEPRESSANT DRUGS

Chemical class generic name (trade name)	Usual dosage range (mg/day)	Available forms (mg)
TRICYCLIC DRUGS		
Tertiary (parent drug)		
Amitriptyline (Elavil, Endep)	50-300	tabs: 10, 25, 50, 75, 100, 150
		inj: 10/ml
Doxepin (Adapin, Sinequan)	50-300	caps: 10, 25, 50, 75, 100, 125, 150
		oral conc: 10/ml
Imipramine (SK-Pramine, Tofranil)	50-300	tabs: 10, 25, 50
		caps: 75, 100, 125, 150
		inj. 25/2 ml
Trimipramine (Surmontil)	50-300	caps: 25, 50, 100
Clomipramine (Anafranil)	50-250	tabs: 25, 50, 75
Secondary (metabolite)		
Desipramine (Norpramin, Pertofrane)	50-300	tabs: 25, 50, 75, 100, 150
Nortriptyline (Aventyl, Pamelor)	50-150	caps: 10, 25, 75
		solution: 10/5 ml
Protriptyline (Vivactil)	15-60	tabs: 5, 10
NONTRICYCLIC DRUGS		
Amoxapine (Asendin)	50-600	tabs: 25, 50, 100, 150
Maprotiline (Ludiomil)	50-225*	tabs: 25, 50, 75
Trazodone (Desyrel)	50-600	tabs: 50, 100, 150
Bupropion (Wellbutrin)	50-600*	tabs: 50
SELECTIVE SEROTONIN REUPTAKE INHIBITORS		
Fluoxetine (Prozac)	20-80	caps: 10, 20
Sertraline (Zoloft)	50-200	tabs: 50, 100
Paroxetine (Paxil)	20-50	tabs: 20, 30
NONSELECTIVE UPTAKE INHIBITOR		
Venlafaxine (effexor)	150-375	tabs: 25, 37.5, 50, 75, 100
MONOAMINE OXIDASE INHIBITORS		
Isocarboxazid (Marplan)	30-70	tabs: 10
Phenelzine (Nardil)	45-90	tabs: 15
Tranylcypromine (Parnate)	20-60	tabs: 10

*Antidepressants with a ceiling dose due to dose-related seizures.

Table 25-7 Antidepressant Drug Target Symptoms

Onset of drug effect	Symptom
Week 1	Middle and terminal insomnia
	Appetite disturbances
	Anxiety
Week 2	Fatigue
	Poor motivation
	Somatic complaints
	Agitation
	Retardation
Week 3	Dysphoric mood
	Subjective depressive feelings (anhedonia, poor self-esteem, pessimism, hopelessness, self-reproach, guilt, helplessness, sadness)
	Suicidal thoughts

TABLE 25-8

THERAPEUTIC PLASMA LEVELS FOR ANTIDEPRESSANT DRUGS

Drug	Therapeutic range (ng/l)
Imipramine and desipramine	150-250
Desipramine	125-300
Amitriptyline and nortriptyline	80-250
Nortriptyline	50-150
Protriptyline	70-260
Doxepin and desmethyldoxepin	150-250
Maprotiline	200-600
Amoxapine and 8-hydroxyamoxapine	200-600
Trazodone	800-1600

Two of the tricyclic antidepressants, imipramine and nortriptyline, have rigorously studied blood plasma levels that have been correlated with clinical response. Plasma levels for most other antidepressants, although less extensively researched, are also widely used.[34] Plasma level guidelines are helpful, since each patient metabolizes drugs at a different rate. A plasma level can help keep the dose within the therapeutic range (listed in Table 25-8). It also ensures that enough drug is in the patient's system to be effective. Some drugs, particularly nortriptyline, have a "therapeutic window" (the range within which the drug is considered to be therapeutic), and a plasma level below or above the range limits results in a decrease in antidepressant effectiveness. Blood for a plasma level should be drawn 8 to 12 hours after a single (usually bedtime) dose. Measuring the level soon after drug ingestion results in an artificially high level, representing the peak of the drug metabolism rather than the steady-state level.

It is estimated that about 25% of patients with depressive illness have chronic or recurrent symptoms. These patients may benefit from a maintenance regimen of antidepressant drugs. A tricyclic that has been successful in the past for a particular patient may be continued indefinitely.

Adverse Reactions. The nurse should know the common side effects of the antidepressants and their nursing treatments, as described in Table 25-9. Most of these side effects cause minor discomfort, but some can produce serious illness.[29] These drugs have no known long-term adverse effects, tolerance to therapeutic effects does not develop, and persistent side effects often can be minimized by a small decrease in dose. Because antidepressants do not cause physical addiction, psychological dependence, or euphoria, they have no abuse potential. Their long half-life (24 hours or longer) allows

them to be conveniently administered once a day, at night for most people. If the bedtime dose interferes with sleeping or causes nightmares, the dose should be given in the morning or divided into several doses throughout the day. Patients with bipolar illness may be switched into mania by these drugs; they should be watched closely for increased activity, greater difficulty concentrating and eating, and decreased sleeping patterns.

Because these drugs are among the most toxic substances available when taken in excessive amounts, overdoses and suicide attempts using tricyclic antidepressants are extremely serious and require emergency medical attention. Ingestion of 1000 to 3000 mg can be lethal. This may represent barely a 1-week supply of medication. For inpatients, mouth checks may be necessary. Even for outpatients who are not suicidal, antidepressants should be prescribed in small amounts, and frequent assessments should be made. Accidental overdoses in children whose parents are taking an antidepressant are unfortunately common and often lethal. The health teaching and care of these patients should include an assessment of household members, and patients should be cautioned to keep these drugs in the childproof bottles received from the pharmacy, to keep the drugs out of the reach of children, and to discard leftover drugs when pharmacotherapy is completed.

Most patients develop tolerance to side effects, and most side effects are dose related; thus they can be minimized by increasing the dose gradually when the drug is first prescribed. This gives the patient time to physiologically adjust to the drug. This is especially true when these drugs are used to treat panic disorder. Patients with panic disorder are particularly sensitized to any drug side effects that remind them of symptoms of anxiety or panic attacks (e.g., rapid heartbeat, dizziness, nausea, blurred vision). In the case of severely depressed patients or those who are suicidal, doses are

Table 25-9 Tricyclic Antidepressant Side Effects and Nursing Considerations

Side effects	Nursing considerations
GASTROINTESTINAL	
Heartburn, nausea, vomiting	Administer drug with meals or at bedtime
Decrease in intestinal motility, paralytic ileus	Occurs in half of all patients; elderly are particularly susceptible; promote bran, bulk laxatives, high-fiber foods, stool softeners; decrease dose; change to a less anticholinergic drug
Dry mouth	Common; tolerance can develop; encourage adequate hydration, sugar-free products, mouth lubricants; try bethanecol (cholinergic agent—25 mg tid); lower dose; change to a less anticholinergic drug
HEMATOLOGICAL	
Leukopenia and thrombocytopenia	Monitor; rarely clinically significant
Agranulocytosis: Allergic response of sudden onset; appears 40 to 70 days after initiation of drug (low white blood cell count, normal red blood cell count, infection of the pharynx, fatigue, malaise)	Very rare; discontinue drug and place patient in reverse isolation immediately; never administer drug again; try antidepressant with a different chemical structure and follow patient closely
HEPATIC	
Liver toxicity within first 8 weeks of treatment: abdominal pain, anorexia, fever, mild transient jaundice, abnormal liver function tests	Rare hypersensitivity response; discontinue drug; switch to another type of antidepressant
ENDOCRINE	
Amenorrhea, galactorrhea	Due to increased prolactin caused by amoxapine; rare with other tricyclics
Menstrual irregularities	Rare and reversible; decrease dose; change to a different tricyclic
OPHTHALMOLOGICAL	
Blurred vision caused by ciliary muscle relaxation	Tolerance can develop over the first few weeks of treatment; distant vision is usually intact; do not use with patients with narrow-angle glaucoma
CARDIOVASCULAR	
Postural hypotension: lightheadedness or dizziness on rising due to decrease in blood pressure on rising	Occurs frequently; take vital signs with patient sitting and then standing ½ hour after dose; have patient rise slowly and dangle feet; tolerance can develop in first few weeks; not dose related; can continue to raise dose
Tachycardia: rapid heartbeat	Occurs frequently; tolerance usually develops; can increase symptoms of angina in patients with coronary artery disease; very frightening to panic disorder patients; in other patients, not clinically significant
ECG changes	QRS and QT interval prolongation; worsening of intraventricular conduction problems; take a careful cardiac history and do a pretreatment ECG, especially with patients over 40 years of age
Sudden death	Rare; patients at risk for cardiac heart block: over 50 years of age, family history of heart disease, preexisting cardiac disease or recent myocardial infarction, or bundle-branch block

Continued.

Table 25-9—cont'd   Tricyclic Antidepressant Side Effects and Nursing Considerations

Side effects	Nursing considerations
NEUROLOGICAL	
Sedation, psychomotor slowing, difficulty concentrating and planning	Inform patients, especially if they operate machinery or must perform mental tasks; tolerance can develop
Muscle weakness, fatigue, nervousness, headaches, vertigo, neuropathies, tremors, ataxia, paresthesias, twitching	Not common; tolerance can develop; lower dose
Lowered seizure threshold	Start drugs at lower dose and increase more gradually with seizure disorder patients
Extrapyramidal side effects (EPS): acute dystonic reactions, akathisia, Parkinson's syndrome, tardive dyskinesia	Rare, since they do not block dopamine; *amoxapine*, the exception, can cause all the common EPS reactions, possibly tardive dyskinesia with long-term use
Psychiatric symptoms: increased anxiety, depression, insomnia, nightmares, psychotic reactions, or confusional states with delusions, hallucinations, and disorientation; mania	Uncommon, may have to discontinue drug; mania may be precipitated if patient has prior history of mania in self or family (avoid tricyclics if possible in patients predisposed to mania)
CUTANEOUS	
Maculopapular rashes, petechiae, photosensitivity	Rare; can give an antihistamine; may have to discontinue antidepressant
GENITOURINARY	
Increased or decreased sexual desire, delayed ejaculation	Decrease dose, change to a less anticholinergic drug; take daily dose after sexual intercourse, not immediately before, for delayed ejaculation
Urinary retention	Lower dose, change to a less anticholinergic drug, try bethanecol; rare: acute renal failure following an atonic bladder
MISCELLANEOUS	
Tinnitus, weight loss, increased appetite and weight gain, psychomotor stimulation, parotid swelling, alopecia, allergic response: edema, generalized on face, tongue, and orbits	Very rare; weight control; decrease dose; may have to discontinue drug and try an antidepressant that is structurally different
Pathological sweating	Occurs in 25% of patients; head, neck, and upper extremities; episodic, or occurs only at night
WITHDRAWAL SYNDROME	
Mild withdrawal after sudden discontinuation: malaise, muscle aches, coryzia, chills, nausea, dizziness, anxiety	Taper patient off drug gradually (one to several weeks)
INTOXICATION SYNDROMES	
Poisoning: usually seen in overdose with CNS depression and/or cardiotoxicity: hallucinations, delirium, agitation, sensitivity to sounds, dilated pupils, hypothermia, hyperpyrexia, seizures, coma, arrhythmias, respiratory arrest	Treat aggressively; recovery can be slow; induce emesis, gastric lavage; cardiac monitoring; respiratory support; blood chemistry, arterial blood gases, tricyclic plasma levels monitored; carefully administer physostigmine, valium, mannitol, lidocaine, and other symptomatic treatments
ANTICHOLINERGIC SYNDROMES	
Confusion, delirium, disorientation, agitation, hallucinations, anxiety, motor restlessness, seizures, delusions, constipation, urinary retention, decreased sweating, increased pupillary size, dry mouth, increased temperature, motor incoordination, flushing, tachycardia	Usually occurs with high doses of several psychoactive drugs with anticholinergic effects; physostigmine, cardiac monitoring, respiratory support; in sensitive or aged patients, may occur at normal, therapeutic levels

generally increased more rapidly to minimize the time it takes to reach steady state and therapeutic effectiveness.

Tricyclic antidepressants, like all psychiatric drugs, should be avoided if possible during pregnancy, especially in the first trimester. However, these drugs have been given throughout pregnancy without harmful effects on the fetus and should be considered if a pregnant woman is severely depressed, especially if suicide is a risk.

Selective Serotonin Reuptake Inhibitors

SSRIs not only represent a new approach to the treatment of depression and perhaps other disorders, but also may provide a safer treatment option. The SSRIs inhibit the reuptake of serotonin at the presynaptic membrane. This results in an increase of available serotonin in the synapse, and therefore at the postsynaptic membrane. Thus these drugs promote the neurotransmission of serotonin in the brain. Their selectivity for serotonin means they do not have significant effects at the transmission sites of other neurotransmitters and thus have fewer side effects.[8] The newest antidepressant, venlafaxine (Effexor), raises the levels of serotonin and norepinephrine. Thus it has a broader spectrum of activity and is therefore called a nonselective uptake inhibitor. Early studies show that between 35% to 40% of patients previously resistant to antidepressant treatment responded to Effexor.

The SSRIs have antidepressant effects comparable to the other classes of antidepressant drugs, yet without significant anticholinergic, cardiovascular, and sedative side effects. They also do not cause weight gain, thus making them more acceptable to patients with bulimia and other individuals who are concerned about gaining weight. In addition, they are relatively safe in overdose. These properties have made them very popular in the short period of time that they have been available, even though they are more expensive than many of the older tricyclic compounds. Table 25-10 lists the side effects and nursing interventions of the four SSRIs currently available. The next few years will undoubtedly see several new SSRIs approved by the Food and Drug Administration (FDA).

Monoamine Oxidase Inhibitors

MAOIs are very effective antidepressant/antipanic drugs that have been underused and overly feared. The MAOIs currently used in psychiatry are listed in Table 25-6. Because of the potential for a hypertensive crisis when tyramine-containing foods and certain medicines are taken along with these drugs, careful health teaching of a reliable patient is quite important. The patient must

Table 25-10   Selective Serotonin Reuptake Inhibitor Side Effects and Nursing Considerations

Side effect	Nursing consideration
Nausea	Administer drugs with meals or at bedtime; tolerance can develop; treat with antinausea medication
Diarrhea	Bland diet; adequate hydration; lower dose temporarily; treat with antidiarrheal medication
Insomnia	Dose as early in the day as possible; good sleep regimen: decrease activities, relaxation techniques, omit caffeine from diet; lower dose
Dry mouth	Encourage adequate hydration; sugarfree lozenges and gum
Nervousness (fluoxetine)	Relaxation techniques; lower dose; change to another SSRI or a different class of antidepressants
Headache (fluoxetine)	Medicate with mild analgesics; lower dose; change to another SSRI or a different class of antidepressants
Male sexual dysfunction (sertraline and paroxetine)	Take daily dose after sexual intercourse not immediately before
Drowsiness (paroxetine)	Dose at bedtime; encourage daytime activity; avoid using machinery
Dizziness (paroxetine and venlafaxine)	Inform the patient; protect against falls; lower dose
Sweating (paroxetine)	Good hygiene, good hydration, cotton clothing

avoid certain foods, drinks, and medicines (Box 25-6), must know the warning signs, symptoms, and even treatment of a hypertensive crisis (Box 25-7), and must be taught the more common side effects of MAOIs (Table 25-11). For various indications these drugs are effective and are safe when used as prescribed. They generally cause fewer anticholinergic, sedative, and cardiovascular effects than tricyclics. They are nonaddicting, and tolerance does not develop toward therapeutic effects; however, safety in pregnancy has not been established. The patient should be on the restricted diet several days before beginning the medication, while on the medication, and for 2 weeks after stopping the medication. No more than one MAOI should be given at a time. Neither should these drugs be used along with other antidepressants except in limited cases and under expert supervision.

Tyramine is an amino acid released from proteins in food when they undergo hydrolysis by fermenting, aging, pickling, smoking, and spoiling. It is deactivated by monoamine oxidase in the gut wall and liver. When monoamine oxidase is inhibited, tyramine may reach

Box 25-6

DIETARY RESTRICTIONS 1 DAY BEFORE, DURING, AND 2 WEEKS AFTER TAKING MAOIS

FOOD AND BEVERAGES TO AVOID

Cheese, especially aged or matured
Fermented or aged protein
Pickled or smoked fish
Beer, red wine, sherry, liqueurs, cognac
Yeast or protein extracts
Fava or broad bean pods
Beef or chicken liver
Spoiled or overripe fruit
Banana peel
Yogurt

FOOD AND BEVERAGES TO BE CONSUMED IN MODERATION

Chocolate
Yogurt and sour cream
Clear spirits and white wine
Avocado
New Zealand spinach
Soy sauce
Caffeine drinks

MEDICATIONS TO AVOID

Cold medications
Nasal and sinus decongestants
Allergy and hay fever remedies
Narcotics, especially meperidine
Inhalants for asthma
Local anesthetics with epinephrine
Weight-reducing pills, pep pills, stimulants
Other MAO inhibitors
Other medications without first checking
    with a clinician

SAFE FOOD AND BEVERAGES

Fresh cottage cheese
Cream cheese
Fresh fruits
Bread products raised with yeast (bread)

SAFE MEDICATIONS

Aspirin, Tylenol
Pure steroid asthma inhalants
Codeine
Plain Robitusin or terpin-hydrate with codeine
Local anesthetics without epinephrine
All laxatives
All antibiotics
Antihistamines

MEDICATIONS THAT MAY NEED DOSE DECREASED

Insulin and oral hypoglycemics
Oral anticoagulants
Thiazide diuretics
Anticholinergic agents
Muscle relaxants

ILLICIT DRUGS TO AVOID

Cocaine
Amphetamine

Modified from Zisook S: *Psychosomatics* 26:240, 1985; and Moreines R, Gold MS: In Gold MS, Lydiard RB, Carman JS, eds: *Advances in psychopharmacology: predicting and improving treatment response*, Boca Raton, Fla, 1984, CRC Press.

adrenergic nerve endings, causing the release of large amounts of norepinephrine and producing a hypertensive reaction. Also, sympathomimetic drugs act on the neurotransmission process by releasing norepinephrine from the storage vesicles in the presynaptic nerve ends. Because monoamine oxidase has been inhibited when MAOIs are used, large amounts of norepinephrine are released and a severe hypertensive reaction can occur. Thorazine, an antipsychotic drug, and the alpha-adrenergic blocking agent phentolamine bind to the norepinephrine receptor sites, preventing norepinephrine stimulation and resolving the hypertensive crisis.

A new MAOI, moclobemide, although not yet approved for use, is novel because it is a reversible MAOI; thus there are no dietary restrictions. It also seems to have a lower side effect profile than the current MAOIs.[17]

It remains to be seen if the current MAO inhibitors will continue to be used for certain patient populations or if they will be used less frequently for depression and other disorders when reversible MAOIs become available.

MOOD STABILIZING DRUGS
Lithium

Lithium, a naturally occurring salt, was noted to have medicinal properties during the nineteenth century, when it was found to be present in the waters of some European mineral springs. It was described as having antimanic properties in 1949 but was not accepted for use in the United States until 1970 because of reports

Table 25-11 MAOI Side Effects and Nursing Considerations

Side effects	Nursing considerations
Postural lightheadedness	Get up slowly, dangle feet; wear elastic hose; increase salt intake; reduce dose
Constipation	Bran, bulk laxatives, stool softeners, fiber; exercise; reduce dose
Delay in ejaculation or orgasm	Separate last dose and sexual intercourse by as many hours as possible (e.g., 8 AM and noon dose, evening sexual intercourse); reduce dose
Muscle twitching	300 mg/day vitamin B_6 often helps; reduce dose
Drowsiness	Encourage activity; avoid using machinery; take short daytime naps
Dry mouth	Lemon/glycerin swabs, sugarless gum and candies, fluids
Fluid retention	Low-dose thiazide diuretics
Insomnia	Last dose should be as early in the day as possible; encourage patient not to remain physically active all evening but to start relaxing several hours before bedtime; reduce dose
Urinary hesitancy	Urecholine may help; reduce dose

Box 25-7

SIGNS AND TREATMENT OF HYPERTENSIVE CRISIS ON MAOI

WARNING SIGNS

Increased blood pressure, palpitations, frequent headaches

SYMPTOMS OF HYPERTENSIVE CRISIS

Sudden elevation of blood pressure
Explosive headache, occipital that may radiate frontally
Head and face are flushed and feel "full"
Palpitations, chest pain
Sweating, fever
Nausea, vomiting
Dilated pupils
Photophobia
Intracranial bleeding

TREATMENT

Hold next MAOI dose
Do not lie patient down (elevates blood pressure in head)
IM chlorpromazine 100 mg, repeat if necessary (*Mechanism of action*: blocks norepinephrine)
IV phentolamine, administered slowly in doses of 5 mg (*Mechanism of action*: binds with norepinephrine receptor sites, blocking norepinephrine)
Fever: Manage by external cooling techniques

---

of its toxic effects. Today it is readily and safely administered under careful clinical guidelines and has an important clinical role as a mood stabilizer in the treatment of cyclical affective disorders.

Mechanism of Action. The exact mechanism of action of lithium is not fully understood, but many neurotransmitter functions are altered by the drug. It has been suggested that lithium corrects an ion exchange abnormality; alters sodium transport in nerves and muscle cells; normalizes synaptic neurotransmission of norepinephrine, serotonin, and dopamine; increases the reuptake and metabolism of norepinephrine; and changes receptor sensitivity for serotonin. Its clinical effectiveness is likely the result of several of these complex actions.

Clinical Use. Acute episodes of mania and hypomania and recurrent bipolar illness are the most frequent indications for lithium treatment. Other disorders with an affective component, such as recurrent unipolar depressions, schizoaffective disorder, catatonia, and alcoholism, are sometimes effectively treated with lithium, especially when they are periodic or cyclical. In addition, lithium has been reported to be effective in treating nonaffective disorders such as aggressive conduct disorder, borderline personality disorder, and eating disorders. In general, lithium is not as helpful in the initial treatment of an acute depressive episode but can be given with antidepressant drug treatment. Box 25-8 lists the target symptoms of mania and depression for lithium therapy.

Before treatment with lithium, a complete history and physical examination are required, with special attention to the kidneys (lithium is excreted by the kidneys) and the thyroid. Regular medical checkups (Box 25-9) are essential while the patient is on maintenance lithium treatment.

In acute episodes lithium is effective in 1 to 2 weeks, but it may take up to 4 weeks or even a few months to treat the symptoms fully. Sometimes an antipsychotic agent is used during the first few days or weeks of an acute episode to manage severe behavioral excitement and acute psychotic symptoms. In a maintenance regimen lithium decreases the number of affective episodes, their severity, and the frequency of occurrence. However, mild mood swings or the recurrence of affective symptoms are not uncommon while on lithium maintenance.

Box 25-8

TARGET SYMPTOMS FOR LITHIUM THERAPY

MANIA	DEPRESSION
Irritable	Irritable
Expansive	Sadness
Euphoric	Pessimistic
Manipulative	Anhedonia
Labile with depression	Self-reproach
Sleep disturbance (decreased sleep)	Guilt
Pressured speech	Hopelessness
Flight of ideas	Somatic complaints
Motor hyperactivity	Suicidal ideation
Assaultive/threatening	Motor retardation
Distractibility	Slowed thinking
Hypergraphia	Poor concentration and memory
Hypersexual	Fatigue
Persecutory and religious delusions	Constipation
Grandiose	Decreased libido
Hallucinations	Anorexia or increased appetite
Ideas of reference	Weight change
Catatonia	Helplessness
	Sleep disturbance (insomnia or hypersomia)

Box 25-9

PRELITHIUM WORKUP

Renal: Urinalysis, BUN, creatinine, electrolytes, 24-hour creatinine clearance; history of renal disease in self or family; diabetes mellitus, hypertension, diuretic use, analgesic abuse
Thyroid: TSH (thyroid-stimulating hormone), T_4 (thyroxine), T_3 RU (resin uptake), T_4 I (free thyroxine index); history of thyroid disease in self or family
Other: Complete physical, history; ECG, fasting blood sugar, CBC

MAINTENANCE LITHIUM CONSIDERATIONS

Every 3 months: Lithium level (for the first 6 months)
Every 6 months: reassess renal status, lithium level, TSH
Every 12 months: reassess thyroid function, ECG
Assess more often if patient is symptomatic

Box 25-10

FACTORS PREDICTING LITHIUM RESPONSIVENESS

POSITIVE RESPONSE

Family history of mania or bipolar illness
Positive response of family member to lithium
Prior manic episode
Onset of illness with mania
Alcohol abuse
Cyclothymic personality features (numerous periods of mood disturbances but lack symptom severity and duration to meet DMS-IV bipolar diagnostic criteria)
Euphoria and grandiosity
Diagnosis of primary affective disorder
History of treatment compliance with pharmacotherapy

NEGATIVE RESPONSE

Rapid cycling (more than two episodes a year)
Thought disorder with depression and paranoia
Anxiety
Obsessive features
Onset after age 40

---

until steady state is reached, usually in 7 days. Then a blood level is drawn in the morning, 12 hours after the last dose. Even though the half-life of lithium is 18 to 36 hours, it cannot be given in a single daily dose because of toxic effects of high doses at its peak (3 hours after dosing). Thus b.i.d. or t.i.d. dosing is necessary. Lithium maintenance can be switched to sustained-release capsules for once daily dosing. Table 25-12 lists lithium preparations. Because of the low therapeutic index of lithium, toxic blood levels can be reached quickly. Also, because lithium is a salt, the sodium and fluid balance of the body affects lithium regulation. It is essential clinical practice to monitor serum blood levels regularly (every week for the first month, then every 3 to 6 months) to regulate the dose based on these levels and to teach the patient about lithium toxicity symptoms and issues regarding salt and fluid intake.

The dose is increased until bipolar symptoms are reduced, until side effects are too great, or until the upper limit of the therapeutic blood level is reached. The therapeutic range is considered between 0.6 and 1.4 mEq/l for adults. After the patient has had a good response to lithium, the maintenance lithium dose usually is set much lower to maintain a therapeutic blood level. Raising a daily dose by 300 mg usually increases the level by 0.2 mEq/l.

In geriatric patients or those with medical illness, a serum lithium level of 0.6 to 0.8 mEq/l is recommended.

These problems usually respond to a temporary increase in lithium dose or short-term psychotherapeutic support. The maintenance dose for each patient must be individualized and may vary from time to time. Box 25-10 lists factors predictive of a lithium response.

Lithium therapy usually is started with 300 mg t.i.d.

TABLE 25-12
LITHIUM PREPARATIONS

Lithium salts (trade name)	Available forms (mg)
Lithium carbonate (generic)	150, 300
Lithium carbonate (Eskalith) (Lithotabs) (Lithane) (Lithonate)	300
Lithium carbonate sustained release (Eskalith C-R) (Lithobid)	450 300
Lithium citrate concentrate (Cibalith-S)	5 ml/300

Use of lithium in pregnancy is not recommended. Various congenital abnormalities have been reported in babies exposed to lithium in utero, particularly during the first trimester.

> Your patient's wife calls you and is upset. Her husband says he enjoys his manic "highs" and does not want to take his medication, which "dulls" his enjoyment of life. How would you go about helping this family?

Adverse Reactions. Although lithium is used often, it is a challenge to patient education for nurses and other clinicians. Usually patients are treated with lithium for several years, and various physiological and environmental factors can rapidly raise their blood levels of lithium above the therapeutic limit. Patients must be taught the difference between acute and long-term side effects and signs of lithium toxicity (Box 25-11). Patients must also be taught the common causes for an increase in the lithium level and ways to stabilize a therapeutic level as described in Box 25-12. Lithium toxicity is an emergency. Management of serious toxic states is outlined in Box 25-13.

A lithium treatment failure can occur, even at therapeutic blood levels of lithium. Several alternatives to lithium alone include the addition of some anticonvulsants for manic breakthroughs or the addition of antidepressant drugs for depression breakthroughs. Electroconvulsive therapy (ECT) for either mania or depression is also effective and should be considered, particularly when the suicide risk seems high. Most importantly, there is no psychopharmacological substitute for a strong therapeutic relationship, patient education, psy-

---

Box 25-11
LITHIUM SIDE EFFECTS

ACUTE/COMMON/USUALLY HARMLESS

CNS: Fine hand tremor (50% of patients), fatigue, headache, mental dullness, lethargy
Renal: Polyuria (60% of patients), polydipsia, edema
Gastrointestinal: Gastric irritation, anorexia, abdominal cramps, mild nausea, vomiting, diarrhea (dose with food or milk; further divide dose)
Dermatological: Acne, pruritic maculopapular rash
Cardiac: ECG changes, usually not clinically significant, may be persistent
Body image: Weight gain (60% of patients); can be persistent

LONG-TERM/ADVERSE/USUALLY NOT DOSE RELATED (PATIENT USUALLY CAN CONTINUE TO TAKE LITHIUM)

Endocrine: (1) Thyroid dysfunction—hypothyroidism (5% of patients); replacement hormone may be necessary
(2) Mild diabetes mellitus—may need diet control or insulin therapy
Renal: (1) Nephrogenic diabetes insipidus—decreasing dose can help; patient must drink plenty of fluids; thiazide diuretics paradoxically reduce polyuria and may be helpful
(2) Microscopic structural kidney changes: (10% to 20% of patients on lithium for 1 year); usually does not cause significant clinical morbidity

LITHIUM TOXICITY/USUALLY DOSE RELATED

Prodrome of intoxication (lithium level ≥2.0 mEq/l)
Anorexia, nausea, vomiting, diarrhea, coarse hand tremor, muscle fasciculations, twitching, lethargy, dysarthria, hyperactive deep tendon reflexes, ataxia, tinnitus, vertigo, weakness, drowsiness
Lithium intoxication (lithium level ≥2.5 mEq/l)
Fever, decreased urine output, decreased blood pressure, irregular pulse, ECG changes, impaired consciousness, seizures, coma, death

---

chodynamic intervention, and regular maintenance evaluations.

Anticonvulsants

Carbamazepine (Tegretol), marketed since the 1950s as an anticonvulsant, was also seen to have mood stabilizing effects on patients with temporal lobe epilepsy. Research has demonstrated that carbamazepine is helpful in the treatment of acute mania and in the long-term prevention of manic episodes when lithium is ineffective or contraindicated.[20] Carbamazepine has its peak ef-

---

Box 25-12

STABILIZING LITHIUM LEVELS

COMMON CAUSES FOR AN INCREASE IN LITHIUM LEVELS

1. Decreased sodium intake
2. Diuretic therapy
3. Decreased renal functioning
4. Fluid and electrolyte loss: sweating, diarrhea, dehydration, fever, vomiting
5. Medical illness
6. Overdose
7. Nonsteroidal antiinflamatory drug therapy

WAYS TO MAINTAIN A STABLE LITHIUM LEVEL

1. Stable dosing schedule by dividing doses or use of sustained-release capsules
2. Adequate dietary sodium and fluid intake (2 to 3 liters/day)
3. Replace fluid and electrolytes during exercise or gastrointestinal illness
4. Monitor signs and symptoms of lithium side effects and toxicity
5. If patient forgets a dose, a dose may be taken if less than 2 hours have elapsed; if longer than 2 hours, the dose should be skipped and the next dose taken; never double up on doses

---

Box 25-13

MANAGEMENT OF SERIOUS LITHIUM TOXICITY

1. Rapid assessment of clinical signs and symptoms of lithium toxicity; if possible, obtain rapid history of incident, especially dosing, from patient; explain procedures to patient and offer support throughout
2. Hold all lithium doses
3. Check blood pressure, pulse, rectal temperature, respirations, level of consciousness. Be prepared to initiate stabilization procedures, protect airway, provide supplemental oxygen
4. Obtain lithium blood level immediately; obtain electrolytes, BUN, creatinine, urinalysis, CBC when possible
5. Electrocardiogram; monitor cardiac status
6. Limit lithium absorption; if acute overdose, provide an emetic; nasogastric suctioning may help because lithium levels in gastric fluid may remain high for days
7. Vigorously hydrate: 5 to 6 liters/day; keep electrolytes balanced; IV line and indwelling urinary catheter
8. Patient will be bedridden: range of motion, frequent turning, pulmonary toilet
9. In moderately severe cases:
   a. Implement osmotic diuresis with urea, 20 g IV two to five times per day, or mannitol, 50 to 100 g IV per day
   b. Increase lithium clearance with aminophylline, 0.5 g up to every 6 hr and alkalinize the urine with IV sodium lactate
   c. Ensure adequate intake of sodium chloride to promote excretion of lithium
   d. Implement peritoneal or hemodialysis in the most severe cases. These are characterized by serum levels between 2.0 and 4.0 mEq/l with severe clinical signs and symptoms (particularly decreasing urinary output and deepening CNS depression)
10. When appropriate: interview patient; ascertain reasons for lithium toxicity; increase health teaching efforts; mobilize postdischarge support system; arrange for more frequent clinical visits and blood levels; assess for depression and/or suicidal intent; consider concomitant antidepressant drug treatment and supportive nonpharmacological therapy

---

fects within 10 days of administration. Other psychiatric applications of carbamazepine, although still experimental, include the treatment of borderline personality disorder, schizophrenia, and schizoaffective disorder. Side effects include skin rash, sore throat, mucosal ulceration, low-grade fever, drowsiness, vertigo, ataxia, diplopia, blurred vision, nausea, vomiting, hepatotoxicity, and a temporary and benign 25% decrease in the white blood cell count. A rare but serious problem is carbamazepine-induced agranulocytosis, a significant decrease in the white blood cell count that does not return to normal. Thus blood levels and complete blood counts are monitored regularly.

Carbamazepine is administered initially at 200 mg/day and can be gradually increased to as much as 1600 mg/day. In some rare cases patients may even receive higher doses. Maintenance doses range from 200 to 1600 mg/day. Therapeutic serum levels range from 6 to 12 μg/l with neurotoxic side effects more common above 10 μg/l. Caution is advised when carbamazepine is used along with haloperidol for the control of excited psychosis (since plasma levels of haloperidol may be reduced) and with lithium (since neurotoxicity may be potentiated).

Another anticonvulsant medicine used in psychiatry is valproate. This drug has been shown to be effective in the manic phase of bipolar disorder and schizoaffective disorder, even in patients who failed to respond to or were unable to tolerate conventional drug therapy.[18,28] This drug is well tolerated in general. The most common side effects include gastrointestinal complaints such as anorexia, nausea, vomiting, and diarrhea; neurological symptoms of tremor, sedation, and ataxia; increased appetite; and weight gain. Very rare but serious side effects include pancreatitis and severe hepatic dysfunction. Liver function and hematology levels are checked monthly during the first 6 months of therapy, and then every 3 to 6 months.

Valproate is begun at 500 to 1000 mg/day in two to four divided doses until a serum level of 50 to 125 μg/l is achieved. Response usually occurs in 1 to 2 weeks. Valproate is not safe for use during pregnancy. It can be used in long-term maintenance alone or with other drugs such as lithium, antipsychotics, or antidepressants.

ANTIPSYCHOTIC DRUGS

The antipsychotic pharmacological family has become a mainstay in the treatment of psychotic disorders and some nonpsychotic conditions. Although they do not offer a cure for psychosis, these drugs are effective in reducing psychotic symptoms. The discovery in 1952 that chlorpromazine produced significant behavioral changes in psychiatric patients revolutionized psychiatric care. Despite the potential for severe side effects, antipsychotic drugs are widely prescribed and offer an alternative for some patients who might otherwise face a lifetime of institutionalization.

Mechanism of Action

The antipsychotic drugs are dopamine antagonists and block dopamine receptors in various pathways in the brain. Their effectiveness is thought to be the result of their ability to block dopamine receptors in the limbic system, which is the emotional part of the brain. Unfortunately, they also block dopamine receptors in other parts of the brain. This explains their side effects and the differences in tolerance to desired and undesired drug effects.[40] Most recently two atypical antipsychotic drugs, clozapine and risperidone, offer an alternative to the traditional antipsychotic drugs for the treatment of refractory schizophrenia.

Clinical Use

The most frequently prescribed antipsychotic drugs are listed in Table 25-13. With the exception of clozapine,[30] these drugs are not different from each other in terms of overall clinical response at equivalent doses; they all have an equal chance of treating the target of psychosis. What distinguishes the chemical classes of the antipsychotic drugs is the extent, type, and severity of side effects produced. Thus an understanding of the side effects of each class of drug becomes a major nursing fo-

cus when caring for patients receiving antipsychotic medications.[14]

Past success with a psychiatric drug in a patient or in a patient's first-degree relative may be the first reason to select a particular antipsychotic drug. The most common cause of treatment failure in acute psychosis is an inadequate dose. The most common cause of relapse seems to be patient noncompliance with maintenance drug therapy.

The major uses for antipsychotic drugs are in the management of schizophrenia, organic brain syndrome with psychosis, and the manic phase of manic-depressive illness. Their occasional use may be indicated in severe depression with psychotic features or in severe anxiety, particularly when the patient may have a tendency toward drug or alcohol dependency. Nonpsychiatric uses for antipsychotic drugs include treatment of vomiting, vertigo, and the increased effects of analgesics for pain relief.

The clinical symptoms of psychosis that are considered the major target symptoms for pharmacotherapy with the antipsychotic drugs are listed in Box 25-14. The initial nursing care plan should address drug dose, target symptom response, and observed side effects and their treatment, along with patient safety, education, and reassurance. Although the relationship the nurse establishes with the patient who is very psychotic forms the basis for an ongoing therapeutic alliance, active nonpharmacological treatment of the residual symptoms of psychosis is more successful when the patient's behavior, mood, and thought processes begin to show improvement with pharmacotherapy.

Clozapine (Clozaril) differs markedly from standard antipsychotic drugs in that it more selectively blocks specific types of dopamine neurotransmitter receptors. Clinical effects of Clozaril that are superior to other classes of antipsychotic drugs include improvement in symptoms of disorganization and social dysfunction and in negative and positive symptoms of schizophrenia.[4] It also has minimal acute extrapyramidal side effects and no reported cases of tardive dyskinesia to date. Thus it has been shown to be more effective for many patients who are nonresponders to adequate trials of standard antipsychotic drugs. It is also indicated for patients who are responders to standard antipsychotics but have developed intolerable side effects. Clozapine does not worsen preexisting tardive dyskinesia, and in some cases, symptoms of tardive dyskinesia improved after the standard antipsychotic had been discontinued and clozapine therapy had been initiated.[24] Unfortunately, clozapine does cause orthostatic hypotension, tachycardia, sedation, anticholinergic effects, weight gain, and a paradoxical hypersalivation, especially during sleep. There is a seizure risk that increases with dosage, and

TABLE 25-13
ANTIPSYCHOTIC DRUGS

Chemical class subtype generic name (trade name)	Drug dosage: equivalence (mg)	Usual maintenance dosage range (mg/day)	Available forms (mg)
PHENOTHIAZINES			
Aliphatic type Chlorpromazine (Thorazine)	100	300-1400	tabs: 10, 25, 50, 100, 200 time released: 30, 75, 150, 200 caps: 300 syrup: 10/5 ml conc: 30/ml; 100/ml supp: 25, 100 inj: 25/ml
Piperidine type Thioridazine (Mellaril)	100	300-800*	tabs: 10, 15, 25, 50, 100, 150, 200 conc: 30/ml, 100/ml susp: 25/5 ml, 100/5 ml
Mesoridazine (Serentil)	50	100-500	tabs: 10, 25, 50, 100 conc: 25/ml inj: 25/ml
Piperazine type Perphenazine (Trilafon)	10	8-64	tabs: 2, 4, 8, 16 conc: 16/5 ml inj: 5/ml
Trifluoperazine (Stelazine)	5	10-80	tabs: 1, 2, 5, 10 conc: 10/ml inj: 2/ml
Fluphenazine (Prolixin)	2	5-40	tabs: 0.25, 1, 2.5, 5, 10 conc: 5/ml elix: 0.5/5 ml
THIOXANTHENE			
Thiothixene (Navane)	4-5	10-60	caps: 1, 2, 5, 10, 20 conc: 5/ml inj: 2/ml, powder 5/ml
BUTYROPHENONE			
Haloperidol (Haldol)	2	5-100	tabs: 0.5, 1, 2, 5, 10, 20 conc: 2/ml inj: 50/ml
DIBENZOXAZEPINE			
Loxapine (Loxitane)	15	50-250	caps: 5, 10, 25, 50 conc: 25/ml inj: 50/ml
DIHYDROINDOLONE			
Molindone (Moban)	10-15	25-250	tabs: 5, 10, 25, 50, 100 conc: 20/ml
ATYPICAL			
Clozapine (Clozaril)	100	300-600	tabs: 25, 100, 7-day pack
Risperidone (Risperdal)	—	4-6	tabs: 1, 2, 3, 4

*Upper limit to avoid retinopathy.

Box 25-14

ANTIPSYCHOTIC DRUG TARGET SYMPTOMS

APPEARANCE

Bizarre or disheveled
Poor hygiene, poor nutrition

BEHAVIOR

Hyperactivity
Bizarre actions
Hostility, assaultiveness
Insomnia
*Motivation—poor
*Social functioning—poor

MOOD AND AFFECT

Flat affect
Agitation
Anxiety and tension

INTELLECTUAL FUNCTIONING—POOR

*Unrealistic planning
*Lack of insight
*Poor judgment

THOUGHT PROCESSES

Loose associations
Delusional ideas
Hallucinations
Suspiciousness
Negativism

---

*Residual symptoms: not highly responsive to traditional antipsychotics.

---

often a rapid return of psychotic symptoms when the drug is discontinued.

The most serious adverse effect of clozapine is agranulocytosis, which occurs in approximately 1% to 2% of patients (this is 10 to 20 times greater than that for standard antipsychotic drugs). This risk continues to increase during the first 6 months of treatment, then declines gradually, but it never entirely disappears. Weekly CBCs to monitor for declines in white cell count and Clozaril prescriptions 1 week at a time are mandated aspects of good clinical care. White cell count recovers if the drug is stopped in time.[22] Once a patient has this problem with Clozaril, reinstatement of the drug is contraindicated.[36] Obviously, this adds a significant cost to the treatment of patients taking clozapine. For the schizophrenic patient who needs this drug and can be monitored weekly for agranulocytosis, can afford the additional burden of cost, and does not need concomitant drugs that also lower white blood cell count, such as

carbamazepine, Clozaril may make a significant difference in treatment outcome.

Finally, while clozapine does reduce the negative symptoms of schizophrenia, patients taking this medication still need help with other aspects of their psychosocial functioning. Psychoeducation, social skills training, group support, and other rehabilitative interventions are beneficial in improving their overall level of functioning and their resulting quality of life.

Risperidone (Risperdal), another new atypical antipsychotic, is similar to clozapine but does not require frequent blood monitoring. It also has a low incidence of extrapyramidal symptoms.

 How would you help a family evaluate the risk/benefit ratio for clozapine treatment of their relative?

General Pharmacological Principles. Dosage requirements for individual patients vary considerably and must be adjusted as the target symptom changes and side effects are monitored. Initially the patient is dosed several times a day, and the daily dose can be raised every 1 to 4 days until symptoms improve. Some patients respond in 2 to 3 days, some take as long as 2 weeks. Response to clozapine may take several months. Full benefits may take 6 weeks or more. Parenteral high doses can be used initially to control a highly excited or dangerous patient.

When the patient has been stabilized for several weeks, the daily dose can be lowered to the lowest effective dose. The half-life of antipsychotic drugs is greater than 24 hours, so the patient can be dosed once a day after steady state is reached (approximately 4 days). Bedtime dosing allows the patient to sleep through side effects when they are at their peak. After approximately 6 to 12 months of stable maintenance drug therapy, the patient can be slowly tapered from medication to assess the need for continued drug treatment. Some schizophrenic patients require a lifetime of continuous medication management. A patient who is unresponsive to an adequate trial (6 weeks at a proper dose) frequently responds to another chemical class of antipsychotic drug, so a second drug trial usually is given.

Most antipsychotic drugs can be administered by oral and intramuscular routes. Fluphenazine comes in two depot injectable forms that can be given every 7 to 28 days. Haloperidol decanote is an injectable form of haloperidol that has a 4-week duration of action. It is not appropriate to treat an acute psychotic episode with haloperidol decanote alone because it takes 3 months to reach steady state drug levels. Thus this drug is more of a long-term maintenance medication. Acute psychotic episodes require a shorter-acting drug. The patient's ability to take these drugs should be tested by first administering the oral form for several days. Long-acting injectables have been important in treating the outpatient who requires supervision of medication intake because of noncompliance. With the exception of thioridazine, antipsychotic drugs also have antinausea effects.

Contrary to package inserts, there are no ceiling doses for these medicines with the exception of thioridazine, which can cause pigmentary retinopathy when given in amounts over 800 mg/day. Abruptly stopping antipsychotic drugs can cause dyskinetic reactions and some rebound side effects. The drugs should be tapered slowly over several days to weeks.

Antipsychotic drugs do not cause chemical dependency, nor is there tolerance to their antipsychotic effects over time. Because of their wide therapeutic index, overdoses of these drugs ordinarily do not result in death; thus they have a very low suicide potential. Because they do not produce euphoria, they also have a very low abuse potential. Antipsychotic drugs are not respiratory depressants but produce an added depressant effect when combined with drugs that produce respiratory depression. Therefore patients who also may be taking drugs such as benzodiazepines must be carefully observed. The effects of antipsychotics on the fetus are inconclusive. It is always best to avoid any drug during the first trimester, although what is best for a psychotic pregnant mother must be carefully considered.

Adverse Reactions

The side effects of antipsychotic drugs are many and varied and demand a great deal of attention from the nurse. Table 25-14 is a comprehensive list of side effects that includes risk factors and treatment considerations. Some side effects are merely uncomfortable for the patient; most are easily treated, but some are life threatening. The nurse should refer to this list frequently but should pay particular attention to the extrapyramidal symptoms (EPS), both short term and long term. It is important to minimize the patient's fears, increased sense of stigmatization, and possible noncompliance with drug treatment through effective patient education and support (see Critical Thinking about Contemporary Issues).

Acute EPS side effects are common, effectively treated, and not dangerous consequences of drug treatment. Drug strategies to treat EPS include lowering the dose of the antipsychotic drug, changing to an antipsychotic drug with a lower profile for that side effect (Table 25-15), or administering one of the drugs listed in Table 25-16. These drugs are administered with antipsychotic drugs if acute extrapyramidal symptoms occur. Since tolerance to these symptoms usually occurs in the first 3 months of antipsychotic drug treatment, drugs to treat EPS are used only during the first 3 months and then discontinued. Long-term use usually is not necessary.

Unfortunately the common long-term extrapyramidal symptom, tardive dyskinesia, has no effective treatment to date, although research continues in this area.[1] Thus primary preventive measures are important[6,16,25] (Fig. 25-2). The abnormal involuntary movement scale (AIMS) should be a part of every patient's treatment (Box 25-15). A serious and potentially fatal (14% to 30% mortality) EPS of dopamine-blocking agents is neuroleptic malignant syndrome. It is described in Table 25-14.

Because of their importance in managing patients treated with psychotropic medications and the problems they present the clinician in making the appropriate diagnosis, medication-induced movement disorders are now to be coded on Axis I of the DSM-IV.[3] Although they are labeled "medication-induced," it is often difficult to establish the causal link between medication exposure and the development of the movement disorder because some of these disorders occur in the absence of medication exposure. Nonetheless, the following disorders are to be listed on Axis I:

▼ Neuroleptic-induced parkinsonism
▼ Neuroleptic malignant syndrome
▼ Neuroleptic-induced acute dystonia
▼ Neuroleptic-induced acute akathisia
▼ Neuroleptic-induced tardive dyskinesia
▼ Medication-induced postural tremor
▼ Medication-induced movement disorder not otherwise specified
▼ Adverse effects of medication not otherwise specified

Currently the correlation between plasma blood levels of antipsychotic drugs or serum dopamine receptor binding and clinical response has yet to be determined, but these tests hold promise for refining drug selection and dosing regimens. Psychopharmacological research has just begun to discover chemical classes of antipsychotic drugs that have mechanisms of action highly specific for the target symptoms of psychosis and yet that do not produce a variety of unwanted side effects.

Text continued on p. 694.

Table 25-14 Side Effects and Adverse Reactions of Antipsychotic Drugs

Side effects/adverse reactions	Mechanism of action	Risk factors	Treatment and nursing considerations
ACUTE/COMMON/SIDE EFFECTS			
Neurological	Dopamine blockade: Acetylcholine/dopamine balance is disturbed	Extrapyramidal symptoms (EPS): 40% of all patients get EPS; differs between neuroleptics, highest with high-potency drugs	*General EPS treatment principles* 1. Tolerance usually develops by the third month 2. Decrease dose of antipsychotic drug if possible 3. Add an anticholinergic drug for 3 months then taper 4. Change to an antipsychotic with lower EPS profile 5. Patient education and supportive care
Extrapyramidal symptoms *1. Acute dystonic reactions: occur suddenly and are very frightening to the patient; spasms of major muscle groups of the neck, back, and eyes; catatonia; respiratory compromise		1. 10% of all EPS; occurs within the first 5 days; non-geriatric patients, especially children; males twice as often as females; high potency antipsychotics	*Acute dystonic reactions* Administer a drug from Table 25-15; parenteral routes work more rapidly than PO; have respiratory support equipment available
*2. Akathisia Patient cannot remain still; pacing, inner restlessness; leg aches that are relieved by movement		2. 50% of all EPS; high-potency antipsychotic drugs	*Akathisia* Rule out anxiety or agitation (difficult but important distinction)
*3. Parkinson's syndrome a. Akinesia—absence or slowness of motion; patient turns like one solid block of wood; gait is inclined forward with small, rapid steps; masklike facies b. Cogwheel rigidity and muscle stiffness on physical examination c. Bilateral fine tremor, anywhere in body; "pill-rolling" motion of the fingers		3. 40% of all EPS; females twice as often as males; geriatric patients; occurs within weeks to several months or longer after drug treatment begins	*Parkinson's syndrome* Tolerance does not develop in all patients; the dopamine agonist, amantadine, is sometimes effective (patient must have good renal function to avoid amantadine toxicity); use step 3 (above) early and vigorously
Behavioral *Sedation* Sleepy, groggy, fatigued		Peaks 2 to 3 hours after dosing	Tolerance occurs within days to several weeks; rule out overmedication; dose once daily at h.s.; change to an antipsychotic drug with a lower sedation profile; titrate dose more slowly
Autonomic *Anticholinergic side effects* Blurred vision, constipation, tachycardia, urinary retention, decreased gastric secretion, decreased sweating and salivation (dry mouth), heat stroke, nasal congestion, decreased pulmonary secretion; *"atropine psychosis"* in geriatric patients: hyperactivity, agitation, confusion, flushed skin, dilated pupils that are slow to react, bowel hypomotility, dysarthria, tachycardia	Cholinergic receptor blockade at some central and peripheral sites	Concurrent use of anticholinergic drugs; geriatric patients; patients with tachycardia; low-potency antipsychotic drugs; can return as rebound symptoms during antipsychotic drug withdrawal; men with prostatic hypertrophy may have particular difficulty with urinary retention	Tolerance develops in days to weeks; change to drug with a lower anticholinergic profile; treat symptomatically: frequently moisten dry mouth, use sugarless candy and gum; bulk diets, stool softeners, fluids, and exercise for constipation; avoid operating machinery if vision is blurred; cholinergic agonist (bethanecol) for urinary retention; IM physostigmine for severe atropine psychosis; avoid polypharmacy if possible; avoid getting overheated

Continued.

Table 25-14—cont'd Side Effects and Adverse Reactions of Antipsychotic Drugs

Side effects/adverse reactions	Mechanism of action	Risk factors	Treatment and nursing considerations
Cardiac (autonomic) *Orthostatic hypotension* Dizziness, tachycardia, drop in diastolic blood pressure by >40 mm Hg with a change of position from lying to sitting or sitting to standing	Alpha-adrenergic blockade producing vascular dilation and pooling of blood	Concurrent administration of antihypertensives, diuretics, antidepressants; geriatric patients; worse with injectable low-potency drugs	Tolerance develops in several weeks; lower dose; change to an antipsychotic with a lower hypotension profile, monitor blood pressure; increase fluid intake to expand vascular volume; have patient rise slowly and dangle feet while sitting; have patient wear support hose; use a pure alpha-adrenergic pressor agent (metaraminol) for hypotensive crisis
ACUTE/RARE ADVERSE REACTIONS **Allergic reactions**	Hypersensitivity reaction		
Hematological Agranulocytosis: develops abruptly; fever, malaise, ulcerative sore throat, leukopenia (WBC below 500)		Occurs within 3 to 8 weeks of treatment; very rare; twenty times more common with clozapine; phenothiazines, especially chlorpromazine; thiothixene; geriatric women; 30% mortality rate	This is an *extreme emergency*; be alert for high fever and ulcerative sore throat with patients taking these drugs, particularly geriatric women; monitor WBC with this risk group; if this occurs, discontinue drug immediately and initiate reverse isolation; antibiotics when appropriate
Dermatological 1. Systemic dermatosis: maculopapular, erythematous, itchy rash on face, neck, chest, extremities; contact dermatitis when touching drug		Occurs 2 to 8 weeks after treatment; chlorpromazine	Not dose related; discontinue drug and start again cautiously when rash disappears; change to a drug in another chemical class; topical steroids if necessary
2. Photosensitivity: severe sunburn		Low-potency drugs; brief exposure to direct sunlight	Lower dose; change to a high-potency drug; use sunscreen and wear clothing over exposed areas; topical relief of sunburn
Hepatic Jaundice: fever, nausea, abdominal pain, malaise, pruritus; abnormal liver function tests		Rare; was more common in the 1950s and 1960s due to impurities in the drugs; phenothiazines, especially chlorpromazine; occurs in first month of treatment	Discontinue drug, reversible and self-limiting; bedrest; high protein/carbohydrate diet
Cardiovascular ECG *abnormalities*	Effects in the hypothalamus and the heart	Preexisting cardiac conditions; geriatric patients; low-potency drugs, especially when combined with tricyclic antidepressants (thioridazine and amitriptyline are worst)	Baseline and follow-up ECG and vital sign monitoring for patients with pre-existing cardiac disease; change to high-potency drug
Neurological *Seizures* Usually grand mal, no warning aura	These drugs lower the seizure threshold	Patients with preexisting seizure disorder; patients who are poorly controlled psychiatrically; low-potency drugs; during sedative-hypnotic or alcohol withdrawal	Decrease dose; change to a high-potency drug; anticonvulsants do not protect non–seizure disorder patients.

Table 25-14—cont'd Side Effects and Adverse Reactions of Antipsychotic Drugs

Side effects/adverse reactions	Mechanism of action	Risk factors	Treatment and nursing considerations
LONG-TERM/COMMON ADVERSE REACTIONS			
Neurological	After prolonged blockade from dopamine, postsynaptic receptor site becomes overactive, supersensitive	Estimated that between 15% and 50% of all people receiving antipsychotics, particularly high doses for long-term use (occurs usually after years, but can occur as early as 4 months); geriatric patients, especially women; brain-damaged patients; anticholinergic drugs given for EPS may increase risk	These are stereotyped, involuntary movements that may be mild or become severely crippling; employ primary preventive measures (see Fig. 25-2); patients with severe tardive dyskinesia can become very distressed; may need soft foods, and soft shoes for feet movements; there is no treatment for tardive dyskinesia, although several drugs are in the experimental stages; may be irreversible, especially if not discovered early and if antipsychotic drugs cannot be stopped
Extrapyramidal symptoms *Tardive dyskinesia: tongue protrusion, lip smacking, puckering, sucking, chewing, blinking, lateral jaw movements, grimacing; choreiform movements of the limbs and trunk, shoulder shrugging, pelvic thrusting, wrist and ankle flexion or rotation, foot tapping, toe movements			
Endocrine Galactorrhea, amenorrhea, breast enlargement and engorgement, decreased libido, ejaculatory incompetence, appetite increase and weight gain, hypothermia or hyperthermia, false-positive pregnancy test	Effects on the hypothalamus and pituitary causing an increase in prolactin and luteotropic hormone secretion	Low-potency drugs, especially thioridazine	Partial tolerance over many months or years may develop; decrease dose or change to high-potency drug, especially with persistent symptoms; be sure that female patients are not actually pregnant; for weight gain: diet and exercise regimen (molindone has fewer appetite-stimulant effects); women should have periodic breast examinations especially with a personal or family history of breast cancer, although there is no clear evidence that the risk of breast cancer is increased
LONG-TERM/RARE/ADVERSE REACTIONS			
Ophthalmologic problems *Toxic pigmentary retinopathy* Patient notices brownish discoloration of vision, loss of visual accuity, possible blindness	Doses of thioridazine above 800 mg/day, even for brief periods of time	Degenerative and irreversible; completely avoidable; never **give** thioridazine above 800 mg/day; change to another drug if 800 mg/day of thioridazine does not treat target symptoms of psychosis	
Skin/eye syndrome Sunlight-exposed skin turns slate gray to metallic blue or purple; color changes are also noted in eyes, without vision impairment	Deposits of drug substance and pigment in the cornea, lens, and the skin	Prolonged use of chlorpromazine or thiothixene and exposure to sunlight	Change to another drug class; deposits disappear over many months after drug is discontinued

Continued.

Table 25-14—cont'd   Side Effects and Adverse Reactions of Antipsychotic Drugs

Side effects/adverse reactions	Mechanism of action	Risk factors	Treatment and nursing considerations
SHORT-TERM OR LONG-TERM/RARE/LIFE THREATENING			
Neuroleptic malignant syndrome High fever, tachycardia, muscle rigidity, stupor, tremor, incontinence, leukocytosis, elevated serum CPK, hyperkalemia, renal failure, increased pulse, respirations, and sweating	Presumably extreme dopamine receptor blockade is at least part of mechanism	This develops explosively over 1 to 3 days, from hours to many months after drug treatment begins; high-potency drugs are worse, but other psychiatric drugs have been implicated also; patients with marked dehydration; patients with organic brain disease; 20% mortality *Speculative:* young adult men, frail elderly; polypharmacy; haloperidol, fluphenazine; parenteral; depot preparations; long-term drug use	This is an *extreme emergency*—early recognition is critical; avoid marked dehydration in all patients; discontinue all drugs immediately; supportive symptomatic care: nutrition, hydration, renal dialysis for renal failure, ventilation for acute respiratory failure, reduction of fever *Speculative:* dantrolene, bromocriptine; antipsychotic drugs can be cautiously reintroduced

*Medication–induced movement disorder to be coded on Axis I, DSM-IV (1994).

Table 25-15   Acute Side Effects Profile: Antipsychotic Drugs

Drugs	Sedation	Extrapyramidal symptoms	Anticholinergic	Postural hypotension
LOW POTENCY				
Chlorpromazine	4	2	3	4
Thioridazine	4	1	4	4
HIGH POTENCY				
Trifluoperazine	2	3	2	2
Thiothixene	2	3	2	1
Loxapine	2	3	2	2
Molindone	2	3	2	2
Mesoridazine	3	2	3	3
Perphenazine	2	3	2	2
Fluphenazine	1	4	2	1
Haloperidol	1	4	1	1

1 = lowest incidence; 4 = highest incidence.

TABLE 25-16
DRUGS TO TREAT EXTRAPYRAMIDAL SIDE EFFECTS: NEUROTRANSMITTER SPECIFICITY

Chemical class generic name (trade name)	Equivalence (mg)	Usual dosage range (mg/day)	Available forms (mg)
ANTICHOLINERGIC			
Benztropine (Cogentin)	2	1-6	tabs: 0.5, 1, 2; inj: 1/ml
Trihexyphenidyl (Artane)	5	1-10	tabs: 2, 5; 5 sustained release; elix: 2/5 ml
Biperiden (Akineton)	4	2-6	tabs: 2; inj: 5/ml
Procyclidine (Kemadrin)	5	6-20	tabs: 5
Diphenhydramine (Benadryl)	50	25-300	tabs: 50; caps: 25, 50; elix: 12.5/5 ml; inj: 10/ml, 50/ml
DOPAMINERGIC			
Amantadine (Symmetrel)	100	100-300	caps: 100 mg; syrup: 50/5ml
GABAMINERGIC			
Diazepam (Valium)	10	(see Table 25-2)	
Lorazepam (Ativan)	2		

TREATMENT CONSIDERATIONS OF ANTICHOLINERGIC DRUG THERAPY

1. Geriatric patients are particularly sensitive to these drugs.
2. They can produce euphoria and have abuse potential.

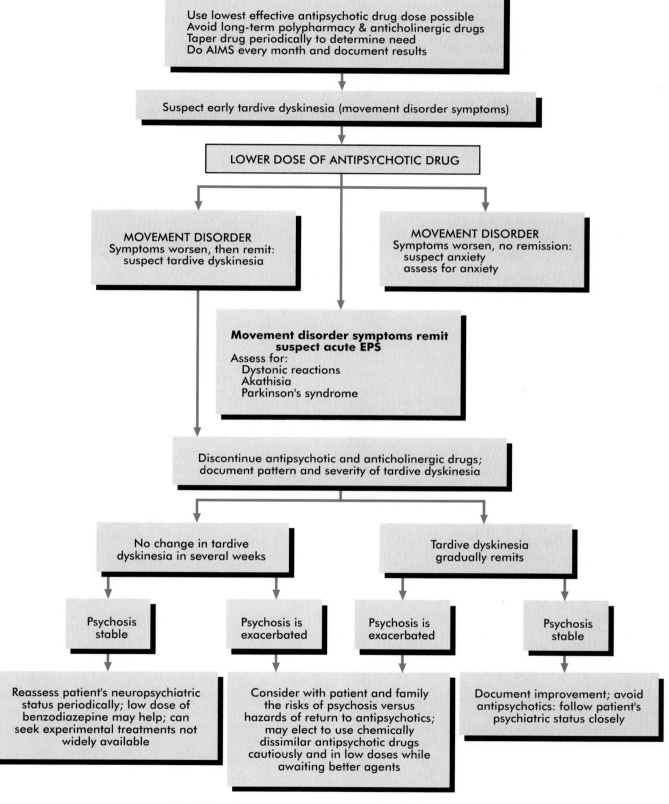

Fig. 25-2   Preventive measure for tardive dyskinesia (TD).

Box 25-15

ABNORMAL INVOLUNTARY MOVEMENT SCALE: AIMS

A Simple Method to Determine Tardive Dyskinesia Symptoms—Total Score Equals the Sum of the Items

Patient Identification: _____ Date: _____

Rated by: _____ Treatment period: _____

Either before or after completing the examination procedure, observe the patient unobtrusively at rest (e.g., in waiting room).

The chair to be used in this examination should be a hard, firm one without arms.

After the patient is observed, he may be rated on a scale of 0 (none), 1 (minimal), 2 (mild), 3 (moderate), and 4 (severe) according to the severity of symptoms at time of interview.

Ask the patient whether there is anything in his mouth (e.g., gum, candy) and if there is, ask him to remove it.

Ask the patient about the *current* condition of his teeth. Ask if he wears dentures. Do his teeth or dentures bother him *now*?

Ask the patient whether he notices any movement in mouth, face, hands, or feet. If yes, ask him to describe such movement and to what extent it *currently* bothers him or interferes with his activities.

0 1 2 3 4   Have the patient sit in a chair with hands on knees, legs slightly apart, and feet flat on floor. (Look at entire body for movements while in this position.)

0 1 2 3 4   Ask the patient to sit with hands hanging unsupported. If male, between legs; if female and wearing a dress, hanging over knees. (Observe hands and other body areas.)

0 1 2 3 4   Ask the patient to open mouth. (Observe tongue at rest within mouth.) Have him do this twice.

0 1 2 3 4   Ask the patient to protrude tongue. (Observe abnormalities of tongue movement.) Have him do this twice.

0 1 2 3 4   Ask the patient to tap thumb with each finger as rapidly as possible for 10 to 15 seconds separately with right hand then with left hand. (Observe facial and leg movements.)

0 1 2 3 4   Flex and extend patient's left and right arms (one at a time).

0 1 2 3 4   Ask the patient to stand up. (Observe in profile. Observe all body areas again, hips included.)

0 1 2 3 4   *Ask the patient to extend both arms outstretched in front with palms down. (Observe trunk, legs, and mouth.)

0 1 2 3 4   *Have the patient walk a few paces, turn, and walk back to chair. (Observe hands and gait.) Do this twice.

*Activated movements.

FUTURE PSYCHOPHARMACOLOGICAL AGENTS

Based on current trends in psychoactive drug research, the nurse can expect to see new drugs approved for use in mental disorders on a regular basis (Box 25-16). It is important to evaluate new drugs with a great deal of scrutiny as they come into clinical use.[19] The nurse should determine the advantages and disadvantages of a new drug as compared to the standard drugs in that class and in relationship to the patient's reactions and preferences. The following list is a partial guide to help evaluate a new drug and separate the pertinent facts from a drug company's merchandising descriptions. The nurse should be able to answer questions concerning whether each new drug has:

1. A different mechanism of action more specific to desired biological actions
2. Quicker onset of action
3. Fewer drug interactions
4. A lower side effect profile
5. No addictive or abuse potential
6. No long-term adverse effects

Box 25-16
A NEW TREATMENT FOR ALZHEIMER'S DISEASE

TACRINE (COGNEX)

Tacrine is the first drug to treat mild to moderate dementia related to Alzheimer's disease. Tacrine prevents or slows the breakdown of acetylcholine by inhibiting the action of the metabolizing enzyme, acetylcholinesterase. An excessive loss of the neurotransmitter acetylcholine is thought to cause the memory problems associated with Alzheimer's disease.

Dosing

10 mg qid po for the first 6 weeks with weekly transaminase levels. Titrate by 10-mg increments to 40 mg qid, at 6-week intervals for each dose, given stable or slightly elevated transaminase levels and patient tolerability. If levels become extreme, stop tacrine until they return to normal and then carefully rechallenge. Transaminase levels every 3 months at maintenance doses.

Side effects

Nausea, vomiting, diarrhea, dyspepsia, anorexia, muscle aches and ataxia. Monitor patients for elevated transaminase levels and abnormal liver function, tacrine-induced bradycardia in patients with sick sinus syndrome, and symptoms of occult or active GI bleeding.

Drug interactions

Can increase theophylline's half-life and plasma concentration. Cimetidine (Tagamet) increases and prolongs blood levels of tacrine. Synergistic effects are expected when given with succinylcholine and other cholinesterase inhibitors or cholinergic agonists.

Drug limitation

Tacrine's beneficial effects diminsh over time as Alzheimer's disease progresses.

Box 25-17
DRUGS OF CURRENT INTEREST IN CLINICAL TRIALS

ANTIPSYCHOTIC COMPOUNDS

	Manufacturer
Olanzapine	Eli Lilly
Amperozide	Kabi-Pharmacia/Sandoz
Brofaramine	Ciba
Ondansetron	Glaxo
Terguride	Sandoz
Tiospirone	Bristol-Myers Squibb

ANTIDEPRESSANT COMPOUNDS

	Manufacturer
Reboxetine	Kabi-Pharmacia
Duloxetine	Eli Lilly
Amesergide	Eli Lilly
Nefazodone	Bristol-Myers Squibb
Fluvoxamine	Upjohn

PSYCHIATRIC NURSING PRACTICE
Psychopharmacology Guidelines

Psychotropic medications are commonly used in the treatment of psychiatric disorders. It is therefore essential for psychiatric nurses to possess the knowledge and skills related to psychopharmacology. In response to recent developments in the field, the American Nurses' Association and the National Institutes of Mental Health established a task force in 1992 to identify the psychopharmacology guidelines for psychiatric–mental health nursing. The result of their work is a document published in 1994 that describes the skills and knowledge, modified by the specific setting, psychiatric nurses need to meet the standards of practice for the discipline.[2] The document identifies specific areas that nurses can review to evaluate their ability to deliver competent nursing care. The complete document on psychopharmacology guidelines can be obtained from the American Nurses' Association; Box 25-18 outlines the major areas.

Documentation

In addition to routine documentation of pharmacological activities, the nurse may have special documentation considerations in the pharmacological treatment of mental illness. The following issues are particularly important to document when working with psychiatric patients:

1. Drugs administered outside daily recommended levels
2. Rationale for medication changes

7. No suicide potential
8. Permanent or curative effects on neurotransmitter regulation
9. Several routes of administration, at least by mouth and intramuscularly
10. A wide therapeutic index
11. Fewer discontinuation problems
12. Advantage in cost effectiveness

Box 25-17 lists new drugs currently under review by the FDA. There are, in fact, over 300 drugs for mental disorders currently in development in the United States. Nurses can expect to see many of these medications approved for use with psychiatric patients at some time in the future.

Box 25-18

PSYCHOPHARMACOLOGY GUIDELINES FOR PSYCHIATRIC–MENTAL HEALTH NURSING

NEUROSCIENCES

Commensurate with level of practice, the psychiatric–mental health nurse integrates current knowledge from the neurosciences to understand etiological models, diagnostic issues, and treatment strategies for psychiatric illness.

PSYCHOPHARMACOLOGY

The psychiatric–mental health nurse involved in the care of patients taking psychopharmacological agents demonstrates knowledge of psychopharmacological principles, including pharmacokinetics, pharmacodynamics, drug classification, intended and unintended effects, and related nursing implications.

CLINICAL MANAGEMENT

The psychiatric–mental health nurse applies principles from the neurosciences and psychopharmacology to provide safe and effective management of patients being treated with psychopharmacological agents. Clinical management includes assessment, diagnosis, and treatment considerations.

Assessment

The psychiatric–mental health nurse has the knowledge, skills, and ability to conduct and interpret patient assessments of psychopharmacological agents. Assessments include physical, neuropsychiatric, psychosocial, and psychopharmacological parameters.

Diagnosis

The psychiatric–mental health nurse has the knowledge, skills, and ability to utilize appropriate nursing, psychiatric, and medical diagnostic classification systems to guide the psychopharmacological management of patients with mental illness.

Treatment

The psychiatric–mental health nurse takes an active role in the treatment of patients with mental illness and integrates prescribed psychopharmacological interventions in a cohesive, multidimensional plan of care.

Adapted from American Nurses' Association: *Psychiatric mental health nursing psychopharmacology project: ANA task force on psychopharmacology*, Washington, DC, 1994, The Association.

CRITICAL THINKING ABOUT CONTEMPORARY ISSUES

Is Noncompliance a Patient Problem or a Nursing Problem?

Every nurse and many patients and their families have had the difficult experience of facing relapse in psychopharmacologically treated psychiatric illness. An obvious problem-solving approach includes an assessment of compliance—is the patient taking the drug as prescribed? In the absence of concomitant medical illness, differences in bioavailability between generic brands of a drug, and increases in life stressors, the nurse and family return to the issue of compliance and wonder why the patient deviated from a previously effective drug regimen. Even if patients deny noncompliance, they usually carry the burden of blame for relapse, and their future relationships with mental health care providers may be jeopardized.

The interactions of cultural belief systems and psychotropic drug effects are poorly understood. A relatively unacknowledged but well-documented fact is that the effects of pharmacoactive agents are not solely determined by their pharmacological properties.[23] In the cultural context of care it must be recognized that psychotropic drugs affect diverse populations in diverse ways. Thus cultural differences must be considered in the patient and family medication education plan and in interactions with patients throughout the course of treatment.

The potential incompatibility between lay and professional values and between belief systems and explanatory models of illness often determines patients' satisfaction with treatment, medication compliance, clinical outcome, and most important, self-disclosure in the treatment setting.[21,39] The understanding, acceptance, and communication necessary to create a culturally competent and effective plan of care for the patient with mental illness rest with the nurse and the mental health team. If treatment planning is individualized and is a mutual and shared responsibility between the nurse and patient, then patient compliance or noncompliance must be viewed as a shared outcome of that responsibility. ▼

Box 25-19

TEACHING: PRESCRIBED MEDICATION

DEFINITION

Preparing a patient to safely take prescribed medications and monitor for their effects

ACTIVITIES

Instruct the patient to recognize distinctive characteristics of the medication(s) as appropriate
Inform the patient of both the generic and brand names of each medication
Instruct the patient on the purpose and action of each medication
Instruct the patient on the dosage, route, and duration of each medication
Instruct the patient on the proper administration/application of each medication
Evaluate the patient's ability to self-administer medications
Instruct the patient to perform needed procedures before taking a medication (e.g., check pulse, glucose) as appropriate
Inform the patient what to do if a dose of medication is missed
Instruct the patient on which criteria to use when deciding to alter the medication dosage/schedule as appropriate
Inform the patient of consequences of not taking or abruptly discontinuing medication(s) as appropriate
Instruct the patient on specific precautions to observe when taking medication(s) (e.g., no driving/using power tools) as appropriate
Instruct the patient on possible adverse side effects of each medication
Instruct the patient how to relieve and/or prevent certain side effects as appropriate
Instruct the patient on appropriate actions to take if side effects occur
Instruct the patient on the signs and symptoms of overdosage and underdosage
Inform the patient of possible drug/food interactions as appropriate
Instruct the patient how to properly store the medication(s)
Instruct the patient on the proper care of devices used for administration
Provide the patient with written information about the action, purpose, side effects, and so forth of medications
Assist the patient to develop a written medication schedule
Instruct the patient to carry documentation of his/her prescribed medication regimen
Instruct the patient how to fill his/her prescription(s) as appropriate
Inform the patient of possible changes in appearance and/or dosage when filling generic medication prescription(s)
Warn the patient of the risks associated with taking expired medication
Caution the patient against giving prescribed medication to others
Determine the patient's ability to obtain required medications
Provide information on medication reimbursement as appropriate
Provide information on cost-savings programs/organizations to obtain medications and devices as appropriate
Provide information on medication alert devices and how to obtain them
Reinforce information provided by other health-care team members as appropriate
Include the family/significant others as appropriate

From McCloskey J, Bulachek G: *Nursing interventions classification*, St Louis, 1992, Mosby.

---

3. Drugs used for other than the indications approved by the FDA
4. Continued use of a drug that is causing clinically significant side effects
5. Polypharmacy rationale

Patient Education

Patients taking psychotropic drugs must be knowledgeable about them. Serious consequences can result from what appears to be minor changes in some of the instructions for drug use, such as skipping medication one day, eating cheese, or failing to recognize certain side effects. A recent survey of 253 psychiatric patients discharged from a short-stay hospitalization reported that more than half did not know the name and dosage of the psychiatric medications prescribed for them and why they were taking them, even though they had received both group and individual medication instruction during hospitalization.[9] Results suggest the need for more active forms of medication education, such as supervised self-administration in the final days of hospitalization.[13]

Patients and their families need thorough and ongoing instruction on psychotropic drug treatment. Nursing programs focused on patient education need to address essential elements, such as missed medication dosages,[44] focus on self-management,[11] and document their effectiveness. Box 25-19 identifies specific nursing activities from the nursing interventions classification (NIC)[27] related to teaching a patient to take prescribed medications safely.

Many chronic mentally ill persons have social workers as their case managers. What skills and knowledge would psychiatric nurses bring to this patient population that differs from that of social workers?

Promoting Patient Adherence

Patients who do not take their medications as prescribed or who do not recognize warning signs of drug problems are at risk for unsuccessful results and adverse reactions. Yet it has been estimated that 30% to 55% of Americans do not follow their drug regimens properly.[31] The threats to patient adherence are many. Some of them reside primarily with the mental health team, others with the patient, and still others reflect a shared failure of the therapeutic alliance (see Critical Thinking about Contemporary Issues).

The administration of psychotherapeutic drugs places the nurse in a position of power and control over the patient.[7] The nurse should be aware of this issue and not use the administration of medications to punish or manipulate the patient. The nurse should never withhold a drug that the patient needs and is clinically indicated. It is also the nurse's obligation to be aware of countertransference issues and personal attitudes toward the patient, the prescribing clinician, the patient's diagnosis, and the drug treatment regimen that may negatively affect the patient's care.

Nurses and patients should work together to minimize misunderstandings and unnecessarily complex medication regimens. Too often, however, clinicians blame patients for noncompliance without fully evaluating the treatment plan from the patient's perspective. For example, a consumer of mental health services identified the following common mistakes clinicians make in prescribing medication for psychiatric patients[5]:

1. Incorrect prescribing as a result of misdiagnosis
2. Excessive dosages of medications
3. Too many drugs
4. Downplaying side effects
5. Overlooking the consumer's expertise
6. Discouraging consumer education
7. Inability of the prescriber to see the consumer from a holistic perspective

In addition, a number of studies have explored reasons given by patients for noncompliance with their medication regimen.[12,26,33] Risk factors for potential patient noncompliance are listed in Box 25-20. Understanding this issue from the patient's perspective will allow the nurse to anticipate problems and design nursing interventions that can target areas of potential difficulty.

For example, many patients decrease or completely stop taking their medications as soon as they start feeling better. If they have a bad day, they may take medication again for a day to two. Explaining to these patients how the medication works in the body and the need for therapeutic levels of the medicine in the bloodstream may help patients better understand their illness and adhere to the treatment plan. Still other patients may fear that the medications are addicting, that they will become dependent on them, or are embarrassed about the stigma of being on a psychiatric medication. Clarifying the use of the medication and the positive impact it can have on all aspects of the patient's life may help to reframe the issue of taking medication in a way that promotes adherence. Most important, patients should be encouraged by the nurse to discuss their questions, fears, problems, and concerns about medication before treatment is altered. Finally, the nurse

---

Box 25-20

RISK FACTORS FOR PATIENT MEDICATION NONCOMPLIANCE

Failure to form a therapeutic alliance with the patient
Devaluation of pharmacotherapy by treatment staff
Inadequate patient and family education regarding treatment
Poorly controlled side effects
Insensitivity to patient beliefs, wishes, or complaints about medication
Multiple daily dosing schedule
Polypharmacy
History of noncompliance
Social isolation
Expense of drugs
Failure to appreciate patient's role in drug treatment plan
Lack of continuity of care
Increased restrictions on patient's life-style
Unsupportive significant others
Remission of target symptoms
Increased suicidal ideation
Increased suspiciousness
Unrealistic expectations of drug effects
Concurrent substance use
Failure to target residual symptoms for nonpharmacological therapies
Relapse or exacerbation of clinical syndrome
Failure to alleviate intrafamilial and environmental stressors that precipitate symptoms
Potential for stigmatization

should realize that the quality of the nurse-patient relationship and the strength of the therapeutic alliance play an extremely important role in whether a patient will adhere to the pharmacological treatment plan and successfully recover from psychiatric illness.

SUGGESTED CROSS-REFERENCES

SUMMARY

1. Psychopharmacology is the fastest growing treatment in the current practice of psychiatry, and the psychiatric nurse makes a unique contribution to the implementation of this treatment strategy.

2. Various aspects of pharmacokinetics include half-life, steady state, polypharmacy, drug interactions, and the role of neurotransmitters in the development of psychiatric disorders.

3. Benzodiazepines, the most widely prescribed class of drugs, have almost completely replaced other classes of antianxiety and sedative-hypnotic agents. They are therapeutic and have a wide margin of safety when taken alone. They can be mildly addictive, especially when taken in high doses over long periods of time or when used with alcohol or barbiturates. Common side effects include drowsiness, dizziness, slurred speech, and blurred vision.

4. Antidepressant drugs are effective, nonaddicting, and can be lethal in overdose. Tricyclics, heterocyclics, and selective serotonin reuptake inhibitors are more commonly used than monamine oxidase inhibitors because they are safer in combination with other substances. Side effects of antidepressants are usually mild.

5. The mood stabilizer, lithium, is effective in the treatment of bipolar illness in short- and long-term treatment regimens. Lithium is not addictive but can be toxic. The therapeutic dose range is narrow and must be monitored by regularly assessing serum lithium levels. Some anticonvulsants also have mood stabilizing effects.

6. The various classes of antipsychotic drugs have similar therapeutic effects but are dissimilar in side effect profiles. Side effects are varied and can be disabling and life threatening. Clozapine and risperidone are new antipsychotic agents with positive clinical effects. Patients taking clozapine need to be closely monitored for agranulocytosis, which is its most serious side effect.

7. New psychopharmacological agents are currently being tested in clinical drug trials throughout the country. Many of them will be beneficial to patients with psychiatric illness.

8. Important issues related to psychopharmacology and psychiatric nursing practice include following ANA psychopharmacology guidelines, documentation, patient education, and promoting patients' adherence to their pharmacological treatment plan.

COMPETENT CARING
A CLINICAL EXEMPLAR OF A PSYCHIATRIC NURSE

Diana Laikam, MS, RN, CS

Even after 25 years in practice as a psychiatric nurse I continue to be surprised at the profound effect nursing interventions can have on patients. I was reminded of that again when I recently conducted a medication education group for inpatients on an acute care inpatient psychiatric unit. The group met for six sessions with approximately eight patients in attendance. One older man, Mr. F, paid particularly close attention to the content related to obtaining information about medication, knowing correct self-administration, identifying side effects of medication, and negotiating medication issues with health-care providers. Mr. F did not read very well but followed along as the content of the simple handouts was presented. He was early for each class, asked questions, and did homework with the assistance of the nursing staff.

At the last meeting, the patients were given certificates with their name on it acknowledging their successful completion of the medication education group. I will always remember that Mr. F had a broad smile on his face as I handed him his certificate and read it to him. Upon leaving the room he turned to me and said with great pride and joy, "When I leave the hospital I'm going to frame this certificate and hang it over my sofa in the living room."

Before that moment I had really not thought of the emotional impact the medication education group may be having on patients. My goal for the group was that members have increased medication compliance through education. What Mr. F taught me, however, was that completing the class in itself was an accomplishment of which he was extremely proud. It is patients like Mr. F who inspire me to put renewed energy into the practice of my profession each and every day. ▼

REFERENCES

1. Adler LA, Peselow E, Rotrosen J, Duncan E, Lee M, Rosenthal M, Angrist B: Vitamin E treatment of tardive dyskinesia, *Am J Psychiatry* 150:1405, 1993.
2. American Nurses' Association:*Psychiatric mental health nursing psychopharmacology project*: ANA *task force on psychopharmacology*, Washington, DC, 1994, The Association.
3. American Psychiatric Association: *Diagnostic and statistical manual*, ed 4, Washington, DC, 1994, The Association.
4. Barrett N, Ormiston S, Lolyneux V: Clozapine: a new drug for schizophrenia, *J Psychosoc Nurs Ment Health Serv* 29:24, 1990.
5. Blaska B: The myriad medication mistakes in psychiatry: a consumer's view, *Hosp Community Psychiatry* 41:993, 1990.
6. Bostrom AC: Assessment scales for tardive dyskinesia, *J Psychosoc Nurs Ment Health Serv* 26:9, 1988.
7. Carey N, Jones SL, O'Toole AW: Do you feel powerless when a patient refuses medication? *J Psychosoc Nurs Ment Health Serv* 28:19, 1990.
8. Charney DS, Krystal JH, Delgado PL, Heninger GR: Serotonin-specific drugs for anxiety and depressive disorders, *Annu Rev Med* 41:437, 1990.
9. Clary C, Dever A, Schweizer E: Psychiatric inpatients' knowledge of medication at hospital discharge, *Hosp Community Psychiatry* 43:140, 1992.
10. Cohen LS: Psychotropic drug use in pregnancy, *Hosp Community Psychiatry* 40:566, 1989.
11. Collins-Colon T: Do it yourself: medication management for community-based clients, *J Psychosoc Nurs Ment Health Serv* 28:25, 1990.
12. Conn V, Taylor SG: Medication management by recently hospitalized older adults, *J Community Health Nurs* 9:1, 1992.
13. Coudreaut-Quinn EA, Emmons MA, McMorrow MJ: Self-medication during inpatient psychiatric treatment, *J Psychosoc Nurs Ment Health Serv* 30:32, 1992.
14. Dauner A, Blair DT: Akathisia: when treatment creates a problem, *J Psychosoc Nurs Ment Health Serv* 28:13, 1990.
15. Depression Guideline Panel: *Depression in primary care*, vol 2, *Treatment of major depression. Clinical practice guidelines, no. 5*, (AHCPR publication no. 93-0551), Rockville, Md, 1993, US Department of Health and Human Services, Public Health Service, Agency for Health Care Policy and Research.
16. Dillon NB: Screening system for tardive dyskinesia: development and implementation, *J Psychosoc Nurs Ment Health Serv* 30:3, 1992.
17. Fitton A, Faulds D, Goa KL: Moclobemide: a review of its pharmacological properties and therapeutic use in depressive illness, *Drugs* 43:561, 1992.
18. Frank E, Kupfer D, Perel J, et al: Three-year outcomes for maintenance therapies in recurrent depression, *Arch Gen Psychiatry* 47:1093, 1990.
19. Glod C: Prozac: pros and cons, *J Psychosoc Nurs Ment Health Serv* 28:33, 1990.
20. Glod CA, Mathieu J: Expanding uses of anticonvulsants in the treatment of bipolar disorder, *J Psychosoc Nurs Ment Health Serv* 31:37, 1993.
21. Jacobsen FM: Ethnocultural assessment. In Comas-Diaz L, Griffith EE, eds: *Clinical guidelines in cross-cultural mental health*, New York, 1988, John Wiley & Sons.
22. Jaretz N, Flowers E, Millsap L: Clozapine: nursing care considerations, *Perspect Psychiatr Care* 28:19, 1992.
23. Lin KM, Poland RE, Nakasaki G: *Psychopharmacology and psychobiology of ethnicity*, Washington, DC, 1993, American Psychiatric Press.
24. Littrell K, Magill AM: The effect of clozapine on preexisting tardive dyskinesia, *J Psychosoc Nurs Ment Health Serv* 31:14, 1993.
25. Lohr JB, Caligiuri MP: Quantitative instrumental measurement of tardive dyskinesia: a review, *Neuropsychopharmacology* 6:231, 1992.
26. Lund VE, Frank DI: Helping the medicine go down: nurses' and patients' perceptions about medication compliance, *J Psychosoc Nurs Ment Health Serv* 29:6, 1991.
27. McCloskey J, Bulechek G: *Nursing interventions classification*, St Louis, 1992, Mosby.
28. McElroy SL, Keck PE, Pope HG, Hudson JI: Valproate in psychiatric disorders: literature review and clinical guidelines, *J Clin Psychiatry* 50:23, 1989.
29. Meador-Woodruff JH: Psychiatric side effects of tricyclic antidepressants, *Hosp Community Psychiatry* 41:84, 1990.
30. Meltzer HY: New drugs for the treatment of schizophrenia, *Psychiatr Clin North Am* 16:365, 1993.
31. Merkatz R, Couig MP: Helping America take its medicine, *Am J Nurs* 1992:56, 1992.
32. Meyer C: In the realm of the brain, *Am J Nurs* 1993:58, 1993.
33. Mulaik JS: Noncompliance with medication regimens in severely and persistently mentally ill schizophrenic patients, *Issues Ment Health Nurs* 13:219, 1992.
34. Orsulak PJ: Therapeutic monitoring of antidepressant

drugs: diagnostic update, *Ment Illness Neurol Disorders* 3:1, 1989.

34. Peden JG: Benzodiazepine use at the medicine/psychiatry interface, *Psychiatr Ann* 23:301, 1993.

35. Rifkin A: Pharmacologic strategies in the treatment of schizophrenia, *Psychiatr Clin North Am* 16:351, 1993.

36. Robinson DS: Buspirone in the treatment of anxiety. In Tunnicliff G, Eison AS, Taylor DD, eds: *Buspirone: mechanisms and clinical aspects*, New York, 1991, Academic Press.

37. Roy-Byrne PP, Cowley DS, eds: *Benzodiazepines in clinical practice: risks and benefits*, Washington, DC, 1991, American Psychiatric Press.

38. Smith M, Lin KM, Mendoza R: Nonbiological issues affecting psychopharmacotherapy: cultural considerations. In Lin KM, Poland RE, Nakasaki G, eds: *Psychopharmacology and psychobiology of ethnicity*, Washington, DC, 1993, American Psychiatric Press.

39. Stern RG, Kahn RS, Davidson M: Predictors of response to neuroleptic treatment in schizophrenia, *Psychiatr Clin North Am* 16:313, 1993.

40. Talley S, Brooke P: Prescriptive authority for psychiatric clinical nurse specialists: framing the issues, *Arch Psychiatr Nurs* 6:71, 1992.

41. Watsky EJ, Salzman C: Psychotropic drug interactions, *Hosp Community Psychiatry* 42:247, 1991.

42. Wengel SP, Burke WJ, Ranno AE, Roccaforte WH: Use of benzodiazepines in the elderly, *Psychiatr Ann* 23:325, 1993.

43. Zind R, Furlong C, Stebbins M: Educating patients about missed medication doses, *J Psychosoc Nurs Ment Health Serv* 30:10, 1992.

ANNOTATED SUGGESTED READINGS

Arana GW, Hyman SE: *Handbook of psychiatric drug therapy*, Boston, 1991, Little, Brown.

Practical and succinct pocket guide that includes relevant and up-to-date information on psychobiological issues, assessment techniques, and drug administration considerations.

Biederman J, Steingard R: Pediatric psychopharmacology. In Gelenberg AJ, Bassuk EL, Schoonover SC, eds: *The practitioner's guide to psychoactive drugs*, New York, 1991, Plenum.

Thorough coverage of medications used with children and adolescents with clear and helpful tables and examples, practical information, and a careful review of the sometimes scant research in pediatric psychopharmacology.

*Blair T, Dauner A: Neuroleptic malignant syndrome: liability in nursing practice, *J Psychosoc Nurs Ment Health Serv* 31:5, 1993.

Thought-provoking nursing review of NMS from a medicolegal point of view that should be essential reading for all psychiatric nurses.

Cadieux RJ: Geriatric psychopharmacology, *Postgrad Med* 93:281, 1993.

Provides the basis for understanding the effects of psychotropic agents in the elderly in a comprehensive and easy to understand format.

Cardoni AA: Pharmacotherapy of schizophrenia in the 1990s: current status and future outlook, *Am J Pharm Educ* 57:165, 1993.

Excellent overview of the use of antipsychotic medications and future pharmacological treatment strategies for schizophrenia.

*Carey N, Jones SL, O'Toole AW: Do you feel powerless when a patient refuses medication? *J Psychosoc Nurs Ment Health Nurs* 28:19, 1990.

Reports on research of nurses' responses to a common clinical problem—medication refusal by patients. Thought provoking and relevant to current practice.

*Collins-Colon T: Do it yourself: medication management for community-based clients, *J Psychosoc Nurs Ment Health Serv* 28:25, 1990.

Thorough description of a nursing education program to increase the knowledge and skill of patients living in the community regarding medication management.

*Coudreaut-Quinn EA, Emmons MA, McMorrow MJ: Self-medication during inpatient psychiatric treatment, *J Psychosoc Nurs Ment Health Nurs* 30:32, 1992.

Describes an interesting and innovative nursing program of patient self-medication in an inpatient setting as a way of addressing the issue of future medication adherence.

*Glod C: Prozac: Pros and cons, *J Psychosoc Nurs Ment Health Serv* 28:33, 1990.

Helps nurses sift through the confusing media coverage of this first-of-a-kind drug and get to the essential information necessary to actually make rational decisions regarding the use of Prozac for depressed patients.

*Jaretz N, Flowers E, Millsap L: Clozapine: nursing care considerations, *Perspect Psychiatr Care* 28:19, 1992.

Discusses assessment, planning, implementation, and evaluation issues of nurses working with patients who were taking clozapine.

*Keltner NL, Folks DG: *Psychotropic drugs*, St Louis, 1993, Mosby.

Includes an overview of psychobiology, review of drug uses in psychiatric and related illnesses, chapters on substance abuse, ECT, and treatments of EPS, and sections specific to different developmental stages.

Lin KM, Poland RE, Nakasaki G, eds: *Psychopharmacology and psychobiology of ethnicity*, Washington, DC, 1993, American Psychiatric Press.

Brief and compelling review of research in pharmacology and ethnicity that enhances understanding of cross-cultural issues in the care of psychiatric patients.

*Norris AE, Dilsaver SC, Del Medico VJ: Carbamazepine treatment of psychosis, *J Psychosoc Nurs Ment Health Serv* 28:13, 1990.

Uses a case study, tables, and descriptions of rating scales to help understand this complex and potentially dangerous treatment for patients with psychosis.

*Schwertz DW: Basic principles of pharmacologic action, *Nurs Clin North Am* 26:245, 1991.

Excellent and in-depth review of basic principles of pharmacokinetics and pharmacodynamics.

*Talley S, Brooke P: Prescriptive authority for clinical specialists: framing the issues, *Arch Psychiatr Nurs* 6:71, 1992.

Overview of prescriptive authority legislation, legal issues associated with prescribing psychotropic drugs, and prescriptive activities common to psychiatry with implications for psychiatric clinical nurse specialists.

---

*Nursing reference.

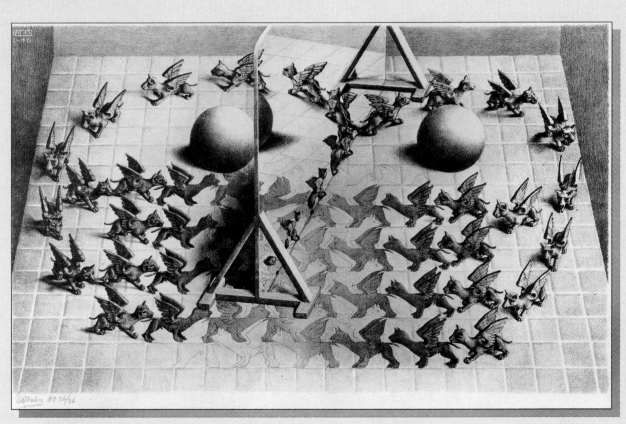

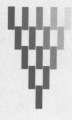

CHAPTER 26
Somatic Therapies

GAIL W. STUART

Canst thou not minister to a mind diseas'd,
Pluck from the memory rooted sorrow,
Raze out the written troubles of the brain,
And with some sweet oblivious antidote
Cleanse the stuff'd bosom of the perilous stuff
Which weights upon the heart?

William Shakespeare: *Macbeth*, Act V

LEARNING OBJECTIVES

After studying this chapter the student should be able to:

▼ Describe the use, indications, mechanism of action, and adverse effects of electroconvulsive therapy (ECT) as a treatment strategy for psychiatric illness
▼ Discuss the nursing care needs of the patient receiving ECT
▼ Describe the use, indications, mechanism of action, and adverse effects of phototherapy as a treatment strategy for psychiatric illness
▼ Describe the use, indications, mechanism of action, and adverse effects of sleep deprivation therapy as a treatment strategy for psychiatric illness

TOPICAL OUTLINE

Electroconvulsive Therapy
  Indications
  Mechanism of Action
  Adverse Effects
Nursing Care in Electroconvulsive Therapy
  Education and Emotional Support
  Informed Consent for Electroconvulsive Therapy
  Pretreatment Nursing Care
  Nursing Care during the Procedure
  Posttreatment Nursing Care
  Interdisciplinary Collaboration
  Nursing Staff Education
Phototherapy
  Indications
  Mechanism of Action
  Adverse Effects
Sleep Deprivation Therapy
  Indications
  Mechanism of Action
  Adverse Effects

With the emergence of biological psychiatry and the growing knowledge bases in the neurosciences, interest has increased in somatic therapies for psychiatric illness. The limitations of psychotropic medications, increase in treatment-resistant psychiatric disorders, refinement in treatment techniques, and growing research support for a biochemical basis of psychiatric illness have placed greater emphasis on evaluating the indications for and efficacy of somatic therapeutic interventions.

Psychiatric nurses are usually involved in caring for patients who are receiving somatic therapy. Thus it is essential that all nurses understand the way in which these treatment modalities work and the nursing care that enhances their effectiveness. This chapter discusses three contemporary somatic therapies—electroconvulsive therapy, phototherapy, and sleep deprivation therapy.

ELECTROCONVULSIVE THERAPY

Electroconvulsive therapy (ECT) was first described by Cerletti and Bini in 1938 as a treatment for schizophrenia. At that time it was believed that epileptics were rarely schizophrenic. It was therefore hypothesized that convulsions would cure schizophrenia. Later research did not support this hypothesis. Further experience with ECT demonstrated that it is much more effective as a treatment for affective disturbances than it is for schizophrenia. It has also been noted that epilepsy and schizophrenia do sometimes occur concurrently. ECT is now most frequently used as a treatment for severe depression.

ECT is a treatment in which a grand mal seizure is artificially induced in an anesthetized patient by passing an electrical current through electrodes applied to the patient's temples. Traditionally the electrodes have been applied bilaterally. More recently, unilateral electrodes have been used. It has been reported that patients have fewer cognitive side effects with unilateral placement, including less disorientation, fewer disturbances of verbal and nonverbal memory, and few pathological electroencephalogram (EEG) changes.[7] However, some data also suggest that unilateral ECT may not always be as effective.[3] Unilateral ECT is therefore most strongly recommended when it is particularly important to minimize cognitive impairment, whereas bilateral ECT should be considered for more severely ill patients.

For the treatment to be effective, a grand mal seizure must occur. The voltage is generally adjusted to the minimum level that will produce the therapeutic effect. The number of treatments in a series varies according to the patient's presenting problem and therapeutic response. For affective disorders, 6 to 12 treatments are normally administered. As many as 20 to 30 may be given for schizophrenia. ECT is most commonly given three times a week on alternate days, although it can be given daily or more than once a day.[3]

In some cases, after a successful initial treatment episode, continuation therapy with outpatient ECT may be recommended. The precise timing of continuation ECT varies, but weekly treatments for the first month after remission, followed by a gradual tapering to monthly treatments, appears to be effective.[7] Successful treatment with ECT may also be followed by antidepressant medication to prevent relapse.

Indications

The primary indication for ECT is major depression, which probably accounts for about 90% of referrals for

---

Box 26-1

CRITERIA FOR THE USE OF ELECTROCONVULSIVE THERAPY (ECT)

PRIMARY USE

Situations in which ECT may be used before a trial of psychotropic agents include, but are not necessarily limited to, the following:
1. When a need for rapid, definitive response exists on either medical or psychiatric grounds
2. When the risks of other treatments outweigh the risk of ECT
3. When a history of poor drug response and/or good ECT response exists for previous episodes of the illness
4. Patient preference

SECONDARY USE

In other situations, a trial of an alternative therapy should be considered before referral for ECT. Subsequent referral for ECT should be based on at least one of the following:
1. Treatment failure (taking into account issues such as choice of agent, dosage, and duration of trial)
2. Adverse effects that are unavoidable and that are deemed less likely and/or less severe with ECT
3. Deterioration of the patients' condition to the degree that criterion no. 1 is met

From American Psychiatric Association: *The practice of electroconvulsive therapy: recommendations for treatment, training, and privileging*, Washington, DC, 1990, The Association.

ECT in the United States. ECT's response rate of 80% or more is equal to or better than response rates to antidepressant medications. It is particularly useful for people who cannot tolerate or fail to respond to treatment with medication. Box 26-1 lists the primary and secondary criteria for the use of ECT as determined by the American Psychiatric Association (APA) Task Force on Electroconvulsive Therapy.[3]

The primary conditions are ones in which ECT may play a lifesaving role, for example, for the patient who is extremely suicidal or one who is so hyperactive that there is grave danger of self-harm. On occasion, ECT may be used for conditions other than affective disorders. ECT is believed to be quite effective in treating acute mania, and although controversy surrounds its usefulness for treating schizophrenia, some schizophrenic patients with catatonic stupor or catatonic excitement may respond well to ECT. Finally, ECT should be considered as an initial intervention when its anticipated side effects are less than those associated with drug therapy, such as with the elderly, for patients with heart block, and during pregnancy. Box 26-2 summarizes behaviors for which ECT is and is not effective.[11]

Box 26-2

TARGET BEHAVIORS FOR ELECTROCONVULSIVE THERAPY

ECT EFFECTIVE

Hyperemotionality
Hypermotility
Catatonia
Severe psychosis with acute onset
Life-threatening psychiatric conditions
Rigidity of parkinsonism or neuroleptic malignant syndrome

ECT INEFFECTIVE

Severe character pathology
Substance abuse and dependence
Sexual identification disorders
Psychoneuroses
Chronic illness without obvious psychopathology

 Why would ECT be particularly indicated for depressed patients with heart block?

Mechanism of Action

The specific way in which ECT works has been the subject of extensive research, but the precise mechanism of action is still not known. It is believed that the electric current passing through the brain causes a biochemical response. Most theories about the mode of action of ECT focus on its efficacy with depressed patients. The following theories have been proposed[17]:

1. *Neurotransmitter theory*—suggests that ECT acts like tricyclic antidepressants by enhancing deficient neurotransmission in monoaminergic systems. Specifically it is thought to improve dopaminergic, serotonergic, and adrenergic neurotransmission.
2. *Neuroendocrine therapy*—suggests that ECT releases hypothalamic or pituitary hormones or both, which results in its antidepressant effects. ECT releases prolacting, thyroid-stimulating hormone, adrenocorticotropic hormone, and endorphins, but the specific hormones responsible for the therapeutic effect is not known.
3. *Anticonvulsant theory*—suggests that ECT treatment exerts a profound anticonvulsant effect on the brain that results in an antidepressant effect. Some support for this theory is based on the fact that a person's seizure threshold rises and the seizure duration decreases over the course of ECT and that some patients with epilepsy have fewer seizures after receiving ECT.

In spite of unanswered questions regarding its mechanism of action, ECT is an effective treatment for many psychiatric disorders and is safe when properly administered.

Adverse Effects

The mortality rate associated with ECT is estimated to be the same as that with general anesthesia in minor surgery (approximately one death per 10,000 patients). Mortality and morbidity are believed to be lower with ECT than with the administration of antidepressant medications despite the frequent use of ECT in patients with medical complications and in the elderly.[3,7]

Medical adverse effects can to some extent be anticipated and prevented. Patients with preexisting cardiac illness, compromised pulmonary status, a history of central nervous system problems, or medical complications following anesthesia are likely to be at increased risk. Thus a complete medical workup should precede ECT and include a complete blood count, urinalysis, serum chemistry profile, chest and spinal x rays, electrocardiography, and optional computed tomography (CT) scan of the head. Adverse effects can potentially occur in the following categories:

1. *Cardiovascular effects.* Cardiovascular complications are the major cause of morbidity and mortality associated with ECT; therefore a cardiovascular evaluation before ECT is essential.
2. *Systemic effects.* Headaches, nausea, muscle aches and soreness, weakness, drowsiness, anorexia, and amenorrhea occasionally occur after ECT, but they usually respond to supportive management and nursing intervention.
3. *Cognitive effects.* ECT is associated with a range of cognitive side effects including a period of confusion immediately after the seizure and memory disturbance during the treatment course. These side effects subside after the treatment course, although a few patients report persistent deficits. The onset of cognitive side effects varies considerably among patients. It is believed that patients with preexisting cognitive impairment, neuropathological conditions, and those receiving psychotropic medications during ECT may be at increased risk for more profound side effects.[1]

NURSING CARE IN ELECTROCONVULSIVE THERAPY*

The effectiveness and limitations of ECT have been the subject of considerable debate within the field of psychiatry (see Critical Thinking about Contemporary Issues). Since it is a somatic therapy for psychiatric illness, nurses have participated in both the debate and the implementation of ECT as a treatment option for

---

*Adapted from Burns C, Stuart G: Nursing care in electroconvulsive therapy, P*sychiatr Clin North Am* 14:971, 1991.

CRITICAL THINKING ABOUT CONTEMPORARY ISSUES

Is ECT a Therapeutic Treatment or a Primitive Form of Punishment?

ECT remains a controversial treatment in health care. The controversy is not about its efficacy or safety, since these have been well established in numerous studies.[3] Rather, the controversy is about its presumed effects on the brain, public fears, and health-care professionals' lack of education related to its beneficial effects. Some people regard ECT as a punishment, believing that administering it is inhumane. Still others are concerned that permanent brain damage could result.

The opposing view holds that it is more inhumane to allow a person to suffer a severe emotional disorder when ECT provides prompt relief. They believe that the stigmatization related to ECT does considerably more harm than the treatment. Part of the stigma associated with ECT stems from the fact that mental illness is seen as social deviance rather than as a medical disorder. As a result, the treatment of mental illness is seen as a stigmatizing punishment.[12] The second major reason for the stigmatization of ECT is that few people have knowledge of the current administration of the procedure. Properly administered, ECT induces far less discomfort and medical complications than most surgical and many psychopharmacological treatments. The third reason rests in the language used to describe the treatment. The fact that it used to be called "shock therapy" conjures up the image of pain and discomfort that further stigmatizes this treatment option.

It is up to each professional to reach a personal resolution on this issue. This decision, however, should be based on objective data, observation of the treatment, and personal experiences in working with patients who have and have not received ECT. ▼

their patients. Although sometimes thought to be an infrequently used form of therapy, the increasing number of ECT devices, as well as the volume of recently published articles and books on the subject, suggests that ECT usage may be rising.[10]

Although psychiatric nurses have always had a role in assisting with the ECT procedure, the nursing functions have historically been limited to supportive and adjunctive care. With the growing sophistication of nursing science and clinical practice, this role is evolving to include independent and collaborative nursing actions.[2]

Education and Emotional Support

Nursing care begins as soon as the patient and family are presented with ECT as a possible treatment option. Initially an important role of the nurse is to allow the patient an opportunity to express feelings, including any myths or fantasies about ECT. Patients may describe fear of pain, dying of electrocution, suffering permanent memory loss, or experiencing impaired intellectual functioning. As the patient reveals these fears and concerns, the nurse can clarify misconceptions and emphasize the therapeutic value of the procedure. Supporting the patient and family in their need to discuss, question, and explore their feelings and concerns about ECT should be an essential component of nursing care before, during, and after the course of treatment.

Once the patient has had an opportunity to express feelings, the nurse can begin ECT teaching, which should take into consideration the patient's anxiety, readiness to learn, and ability to comprehend. Optimally, family teaching should occur at the same time as patient teaching, and the amount of information to be shared should be individualized for each patient and family. The nurse should review with the family and patient the information they have received from the physician regarding the procedure and attempt to respond to any questions they might have about this information.

During this assessment process, the nurse should also attempt to define specific patient behaviors the family associates with the patient's illness and determine whether the patient or family member has received ECT in the past. Any information about the family's previous experiences with ECT helps the nurse to identify familial beliefs about the patient's illness, the ECT treatment, and the expected prognosis. Both patient and family should also be asked what else they may know about ECT, such as through friends who have received it or by reading about it or seeing ECT portrayed in movies. Open-ended questions may give the nurse the opportunity to identify and correct misinformation and address specific concerns the patient or family has about the procedure. These nursing actions may facilitate the family's ability to provide support to the patient during the treatment course and thus further alleviate the patient's anxiety.

Various media may also be used to supplement the teaching of the patient and family about ECT, including written materials and videotape presentations.[5] A tour of the treatment suite itself may help familiarize the patient with the area, procedure, and equipment. Encouraging the patient to talk with another patient who has benefited from ECT may be worthwhile. Finally the nurse should facilitate flexibility in family arrangements, particularly during the patient's first few treatments, allowing for family presence before and after ECT if the patient and family desire. This serves to allay the family's anxieties and concerns about the patient's treatment, while encouraging the family to support the patient.

If the family is unable or does not wish to be present during these times, the nurse should contact the family after the treatments to provide information and describe the patient's response. The nurse should also encourage the family throughout the course of treatment to discuss changes they observe or questions that arise. Providing emotional support and responding to the educational needs of both patient and family are essential components of the nursing role throughout the patient's treatment.

> There are many misconceptions regarding ECT. Many of these are perpetuated by movies. Observe ECT in person, then watch the movies *One Flew Over the Cuckoo's Nest*, *Frances*, and *Ordinary People* and critique the way in which ECT is presented.

Informed Consent for Electroconvulsive Therapy

Before ECT treatment is begun, the patient should sign an informed consent form (see Chapter 8). If the patient does not have the capacity to consent, it can be signed by another legally designated person. This consent acknowledges the patient's rights to obtain or refuse treatment. Although it is the physician's ultimate responsibility to provide an explanation of the procedure when obtaining consent, then nurse plays an important part in the consent process.

Informed consent is a dynamic process that is not completed with the signing of a formal document; it implies a process that continues throughout the course of treatment. As such, it suggests a number of nursing activities.[4,22] First, it is helpful if a nurse is present at the time when the information for consent is discussed with the patient. The most appropriate nurse is one who has

established a trusting and therapeutic relationship with the patient and who is best able to assess whether the patient comprehends the explanation. The presence of a nurse at this time may facilitate the patient's confidence in asking questions, and the nurse may help to simplify the language if necessary. The nurse can also ensure that the patient has been provided with a full explanation, understands the nature, purpose, and implications of the treatment, including the option to withdraw consent at any time, and has had all questions answered before signing the consent form. After signing the informed consent, but before the beginning of treatment, the nurse should again thoroughly review this information and discuss the treatment in an open and direct manner, thus communicating that this is an accepted and beneficial form of treatment.

Certain patients pose particular challenges to the nurse in obtaining informed consent. If a patient is unable to make independent judgments and meaningful decisions about care and treatment, the nurse is responsible for acting as a patient advocate. For example, concentration is frequently impaired in depressed patients, and therefore they are less likely to comprehend and retain new information. For these patients it is essential that the nurse repeat the information at regular intervals, since new knowledge is seldom fully absorbed after only one explanation. Then, throughout the patient's treatment course, the nurse should reinforce what the patient already understands, provide reminders of anything that has been forgotten, and be there to answer new questions.

Pretreatment Nursing Care

Providing optimal nursing care for the ECT patient includes evaluating the pretreatment protocol to ensure that it has been followed according to hospital policy. This involves completing appropriate consultations, noting that any abnormalities in laboratory tests have been addressed, and checking that equipment and supplies are adequate and functional. The treatment nurse is responsible for ensuring that the treatment suite is properly prepared for the ECT procedure. Box 26-3 provides a list of standard equipment needed to provide optimal ECT patient care as designated by the APA Task Force on ECT.[3] Although not required to be in the treatment room itself, a crash cart with defibrillator should be readily available for emergency use.

Since ECT is not unlike a brief surgical procedure, patient preparation is similar. Because general anesthesia is required, fluids should be withheld from the patient for 6 to 8 hours before treatment to prevent the potential for aspiration. The exception to this NPO status is in the case of patients who routinely receive cardiac medications, antihypertensive agents, or H2 blockers.

Box 26-3

EQUIPMENT FOR ELECTROCONVULSIVE THERAPY

Treatment device and supplies, including electrode paste and gel, gauze pads, alcohol preps, saline, EEG electrodes, and chart paper

Monitoring equipment, including ECG and EEG electrodes

Blood pressure cuffs (2), peripheral nerve stimulator, and pulse oximeter

Stethoscope

Reflex hammer

Intravenous and venipuncture supplies

Bite blocks with individual containers

Stretchers with firm mattress and siderails with the capability to elevate the head and feet

Suction device

Ventilation equipment, including tubing, masks, Ambu bags, oral airways, and intubation equipment with an oxygen delivery system capable of providing positive-pressure oxygen

Emergency and other medications as recommended by anesthesia staff

Miscellaneous medications not supplied by the anesthesia staff for medical management during ECT such as labetalol, emolol, glycopyrrolate, caffeine, curare, midazolam, diazepam, thiopental sodium (Pentothal), methohexital sodium (Brevital), and succinylcholine

---

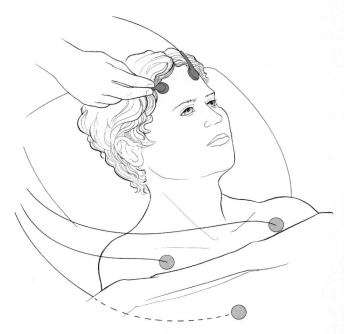

Fig. 26-1 EEG and ECG monitoring during electroconvulsive therapy.

These drugs should be administered several hours before treatment with a small sip of water. The patient should be encouraged to wear comfortable clothing, including street clothes, pajamas, or a hospital gown, provided that it can be opened in the front to facilitate the placement of monitoring equipment. The patient should also be reminded to remove prostheses before coming to the treatment area to prevent loss or damage. This includes dentures, glasses, contact lenses, and hearing aids. The patient's hair should be clean and dry for optimal electrode contact. Hairpins, barrettes, hair nets, and other hair ornaments should also be removed for placement of electrodes.

The patient should void immediately before receiving ECT to help prevent incontinence during the procedure and to minimize the potential for bladder distention and damage during treatment. An intramuscular injection of glycopyrrolate (usual dose 0.2 to 0.4 mg) is administered at least 30 minutes before each ECT. Atropine (usual dose 0.3 to 0.6 mg) may be given as an alternative.[25] These medications are administered both to prevent the potential for aspiration by decreasing the amount of oral secretions during the treatment and to help minimize cardiac bradyarrhythmias in response to the electrical stimulation.[3]

Nursing Care during the Procedure

The patient should be brought to the treatment suite either ambulatory or by wheelchair, depending on individual need, accompanied by a nurse with whom the patient feels at ease. If possible, the nurse should remain with the patient throughout the treatment to provide support. Since there will be a number of people in the room, including a psychiatrist, the treatment nurse, and the anesthesia staff, the patient should be introduced to each member of the treatment team and given a brief explanation of everyone's role in the ECT procedure.

The patient should then be assisted onto a stretcher and asked to remove shoes and socks. This allows for the placement of a blood pressure cuff on an ankle and clear observation of the patient's extremities during the treatment. Once the patient is positioned comfortably on the stretcher, a member of the anesthesia staff inserts a peripheral intravenous line while the treatment nurse and other members of the treatment team place leads for various monitors. One member of the treatment team should explain the procedure while it is occurring.

EEG monitoring consists of two electrodes, one on the forehead and one on the left mastoid. Two sets of 3-lead ECGs, one connected to the ECT machine and the other to the oscilloscope, are placed on the patient's chest (Fig. 26-1). A pulse oximeter is clipped to the patient's finger to monitor oxygen saturation. Blood pressure monitoring throughout the treatment is accomplished by a manual or automatic cuff. A peripheral

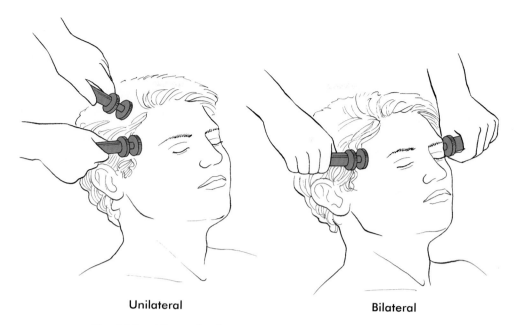

Unilateral   **Bilateral**

Fig. 26-2   Electrode placement in electroconvulsive therapy.

nerve stimulator, placed on the wrist over the ulnar nerve, serves to determine muscle relaxation.

The treating psychiatrist or nurse cleans areas of the patient's head with alcohol and gel at the sites of electrode contact. The area may be wetted with saline as well. This cleansing process facilitates optimal stimulus electrode contact during treatment, thus eliminating the potential for skin burns and minimizing the amount of electrical stimulus needed for the treatment. The areas being cleaned will be either both temples, if bilateral electrode placement is to be used, or the right temple and top of the head 1 inch to the right of the midline, if unilateral placement is used (Fig. 26-2).

Once the preparation is completed, an anesthetic is administered intravenously at a dosage titrated to the patient's weight, age, and physical status. Methohexital, an ultra short-acting agent, is frequently used for this purpose at a dose of approximately 1.0 mg/kg. When the patient is asleep, the blood pressure cuff on the ankle is inflated, allowing it to serve as a tourniquet. A muscle relaxant, succinylcholine (usual dose approximately 0.75 mg/kg), is then administered to minimize the patient's motor response to the ECT treatment. Since the tourniquet is in place on one ankle, the succinylcholine is not effective in that extremity. This is a desired effect, since it is used to assist in determining the presence of a motor response to the seizure. Progressive muscle relaxation is monitored by the nerve stimulator, as well as by observing the patient for the cessation of fasciculations. As the muscle relaxant takes effect, anesthesia provides oxygen by mask to the patient through positive-pressure ventilation.

Although most muscles become completely relaxed,

the patient's jaw muscles are stimulated directly by the ECT, causing the patient's teeth to clench. This creates the need for a protective device, or bite block, to be inserted in the patient's mouth by the treatment nurse before the electrical stimulus. This disposable or autoclavable device prevents the potential for tooth damage and tongue or gum laceration during the stimulus. The bite block should be placed with the thick rubber portion between the upper and lower teeth with the front rim separating the lips and teeth. The nurse should then support the patient's chin firmly against the bite block during delivery of the brief electrical stimulus. After delivery of the stimulus, the bite block may be removed.

The electrical stimulus causes a brief generalized seizure, the motor manifestations of which, due to muscle relaxation, can be observed only in the cuffed foot. Characteristic EEG changes may also be observed. One member of the treatment team records the time elapsed during the seizure. A seizure lasting 30 to 60 seconds is generally considered adequate to produce therapeutic effect, and seizures lasting longer than 2 minutes should be terminated using a benzodiazepine, such as diazepam or thiopental sodium (Pentothal), to prevent the potential for a prolonged postictal state. Anesthesia staff continuously ventilate the patient with pure oxygen throughout the procedure until the effects of the anesthetic and muscle relaxant subside and the patient is able to breathe spontaneously. Vital signs should be monitored by the nurse both before and after the ECT treatment. Once stabilized, the anesthesiologist clears the patient for transfer to the recovery area.

Posttreatment Nursing Care

The recovery area should be adjacent to the treatment area to provide accessibility for anesthesia staff in case of an emergency. The area should contain oxygen, suction, pulse oximeter, vital sign monitoring, and emergency equipment.[18] The area should be appropriately staffed and provide a minimal amount of sensory stimulation. Once in the recovery area with pulse oximeter in place, the patient should be unobtrusively observed by a staff member in close proximity until the patient awakens. At this time the staff should be aware of the potential for falls from the stretcher caused by patient restlessness and be prepared to engage assistance to maintain patient safety.

When the patient awakens, a nurse should discuss the treatment and check vital signs. Most patients do not remember receiving the treatment and may be confused and disoriented, similar to patients recovering from anesthesia. The nurse therefore should provide frequent reassurance and reorientation and repeat this information at regular intervals until the patient retains it. Being postictal, the patient's thinking may also be somewhat concrete. Providing brief, distinct direction is most beneficial in interacting with patients at this time.

When the patient indicates being awake and ready to return to the hospital room, has maintained a continuous oxygen saturation level of 90% or above, and when vital signs and mental status have returned to an acceptable level, the nurse should assist moving the patient from the stretcher to a wheelchair for transport from the recovery area.[8] When a wheelchair is used, the seatbelt should be securely fastened. The patient may be allowed to ambulate if so desired.

At this time the ECT treatment nurse should convey as much information as possible about the patient's condition to the unit nursing staff. The most beneficial information includes medications given to the patient that may be evidenced in the patient's behavior or vital signs and any change in the procedure or the patient's response to treatment that may affect the patient's behavior upon return to the unit. Table 26-1 identifies some common problems patients have at this time and related nursing interventions.

The patient's condition should be assessed by the nurse in the patient's room to determine the level of observation that is required of the nursing staff. If desired, the patient may return to bed and sleep, but the nurse should encourage eating breakfast and resuming normal activities as soon as possible. If the patient chooses to return to bed, the siderails should be in an upright position.

The patient should be observed a minimum of once every 15 minutes, and, if agitated, confused, or restless, one-to-one observation may be required until the patient's condition has stabilized. Level of orientation should be assessed every 30 minutes if the patient is

Table 26-1 Common Patient Problems and Nursing Interventions Related to Electroconvulsive Therapy

Patient problem	Nursing interventions
Pretreatment with beta-blockers may cause a decrease in blood pressure, pulse, or both.	Vital signs should be monitored frequently until they return to baseline.
Lengthy seizures (i.e., greater than 2 minutes) may increase the duration of disorientation or confusion.	Reorientation may need to be repeated frequently for longer period than usual.
If given a barbiturate or benzodiazepine to terminate the seizure, the patient may be more drowsy than usual.	Patient may need more time to rest after treatment.
Restlessness may increase potential for injury.	Intensity of observation may need to be increased to prevent falls.
Nuasea/vomiting creates potential for aspiration.	Increase intensity of observation. Extended stay in the recovery area may be necessary to provide access to suctioning equipment.
Headache creates alteration in comfort.	After assessment for gag reflex return, an analgesic may be administered. If headache is a recurrent problem, a standing order for analgesia to be given as soon as possible after each treatment may be obtained. Change in activity schedule and environment to provide for a darkened room or quiet area may be necessary.

awake until mental status returns to baseline. If sleeping, the patient should remain undisturbed unless additional nursing intervention is warranted. Sleeping may help the patient return to baseline values more quickly.

The return of the gag reflex should be assessed before administering medication or offering breakfast to the patient. When fully awake, the patient should be observed when getting out of bed for the first time to ensure full muscle functioning after administration of muscle relaxants. Throughout the posttreatment inter-

Table 26-2 Nursing Interventions for the Patient Receiving Electroconvulsive Therapy

Principle	Rationale	Nursing intervention
Informed participation in the procedure	A patient who understands the treatment plan will be more cooperative and have less stress than one who does not; an informed family is able to provide the patient with emotional support	Educate regarding ECT, including the procedure and expected effects; teach family about the treatment; encourage expression of feelings by patient and family; reinforce teaching after each treatment
Maintain biological integrity	General anesthesia and an electrically induced seizure are physiological stressors and require supportive nursing care	Check emergency equipment before procedure; maintain NPO status several hours before treatment; remove potentially harmful objects, such as jewelry and dentures; check vital signs; maintain patent airway; assist to ambulate; offer analgesia or antiemetic as needed
Maintain dignity and self-esteem	Patients are usually fearful before ECT treatment; amnesia and confusion may lead to anxiety and distress; patient will need assistance to function appropriately in the milieu	Remain with the patient and offer support before and during treatment; maintain the patient's privacy during and following the treatment; reorient the patient; assist family members to understand behavior related to amnesia and confusion

val, provision of support and reminders to the patient of having received ECT eliminate patient distress from posttreatment amnesia.

Potential side effects the patient may experience immediately after treatment that may be treated symptomatically include headache, muscle soreness, and nausea. Any confusion or disorientation is likely to be of short duration and may respond well to restricted environmental stimulation and frequent nursing contacts reminding the patient of ECT treatment and providing reorientation.[24] Memory loss primarily affects material that has been recently learned, as well as information acquired during the time of the ECT treatments themselves.

Although memory loss may be distressing for the patient, the nurse should reinforce that such difficulty will pass within several weeks, with a minimal amount lasting up to 6 months. Some information, however, will not return, including the experience of the treatment itself and events just before the procedure, such as IV placement. In addition, events occurring throughout the course of treatment may be unclear. A summary of nursing interventions for patients receiving ECT is presented in Table 26-2.

What kind of post-ECT environment do you think would be most conducive to the patient's recovery? How would you go about answering this nursing question?

Interdisciplinary Collaboration

The nurse is part of a interdisciplinary treatment team that not only administers the treatments but also collaborates to evaluate the effectiveness of ECT and recommend changes in the patient's treatment plan as appropriate.[2] Within the team the nurse identifies patterns of patient behavior and evaluates their implications for treatment. These include behaviors indicative of a positive treatment response, such as improvement in activities of daily living, adaptive changes in social interactions with others, increases in energy, appetite, and weight, or other positive changes in target symptoms. The nurse might also report any adverse behaviors associated with ECT, including prolonged periods of confusion or disorientation, recurrent nausea or headaches, elevation in blood pressure that does not resolve within several hours after treatment, or an increase in the intensity or occurrence of target symptoms. In addition, the nurse's work with the patient's family provides information important for planning treatment.

With these clinical observations and judgments made during the nursing assessment before and after treatment, the nurse becomes an active participant in the decision-making process of the treatment team regarding the patient's illness and proposed plan of care. Together the team evaluates such issues as the length of ECT treatment course, the need for alternative management strategies and adjustments in the frequency of treatments, considerations for maintenance ECT, indications for additional consultations, and other possible modifications in the patient's treatment plan.

Give specific examples of ways in which the psychiatric nurse's role in ECT has evolved from the dependent function of implementing physicians' orders to more independent and interdependent areas of psychiatric nursing practice. How have patients benefited from this change?

Nursing Staff Education

In spite of recent increases in the use of ECT and its effectiveness in the treatment of certain psychiatric illnesses, the procedure continues to elicit emotional responses from the general public and from within the medical and nursing communities.[9,23] Some of these responses may be positive, as indicated by a survey that explored the attitudes of a group of patients, professionals, and members of the general public concerning their perceptions of ECT.[16] In this study there was general agreement that ECT is an appropriate treatment for certain conditions and that it does result in clinical improvement.

The literature also suggests, however, that many react negatively to ECT based on outdated ideas and procedures. Also, some patients develop a pathological fear of ECT over the course of treatment.[13] It is critically important therefore that when a patient is referred for ECT, the patient and family be presented with information regarding treatment options in a balanced and unbiased manner. If a nurse has ambivalent or negative feelings about ECT, these feelings will likely be communicated to the patient and render the treatment course less effective. To function as patient advocates nurses need to examine their attitudes and have as much information about the procedure as possible.[26]

Educational efforts should be directed particularly toward nurses who work on units where ECT is implemented as a treatment strategy. Programs should be developed that address both cognitive and attitudinal content, since it has been shown that the more knowledge and clinical experience mental health professionals have with ECT, the more positive their attitude will be toward it as an effective treatment modality.[15]

Such programs should be offered on a regular basis and might be initiated by asking staff to discuss their present beliefs and feelings about ECT, including its potential therapeutic value, perceived risks, the nature of the procedure itself, and ethical and legal issues concerning its use. An open and forthright exchange should be encouraged for the staff to become aware of their existing beliefs and preconceptions before attending to new information about ECT.

The content can then progress to a discussion of factual material about ECT including the rationale for the treatment, possible mechanisms of action, its efficacy relative to other treatment options, risks and side effects resulting from ECT, and current research on its indications and benefits. Time should be spent discussing the way in which the procedure itself has changed over the years, and all nurses should be encouraged to observe the ECT procedure as performed in their institution.

The members of the ECT treatment team could be introduced to the nursing staff, and one of them be identified as the resource person for additional questions or information. These discussions might also be supplemented with written handouts, reference articles, and teaching videotapes about ECT. Finally, this information can be formalized and incorporated into the unit's daily nursing care by the establishment of nursing standards of care for patients receiving ECT[6] and the development of a standardized nursing care plan that identifies appropriate nursing diagnoses, goals, and interventions. These documents will provide the staff with specific references they can use in providing nursing care to ECT patients.

In addition to informing nurses who care for ECT patients, there is a need for teaching the larger nursing community about ECT. Psychiatric nurses who work with ECT can offer to provide in-services to nurses in other clinical settings, such as geriatrics, neurology, or medicine, to dispel myths, clarify misconceptions, and provide current, accurate information about ECT. Finally, nursing students need to be taught about ECT and other somatic therapies in their basic educational programs and have the opportunity to observe the procedure and learn about it. Given the increasing incidence of psychiatric illness and the growing number of elderly persons in this country, knowledge about ECT as a psychotherapeutic treatment option would appear to be essential knowledge for the contemporary nurse clinician.

What stereotypes did you have about ECT before reading this chapter? How have they changed, and how might this experience help you educate patients and colleagues about this treatment procedure?

PHOTOTHERAPY

Phototherapy, or light therapy, is a relatively new somatic treatment option. It consists of exposing patients to artificial therapeutic lighting about 5 to 20 times brighter than indoor lighting. Patients usually sit, with eyes open, about 3 feet away from and at eye level with a set of broad-spectrum fluorescent bulbs designed to produce the intensity and color composition of outdoor daylight. They then can engage in their usual activities

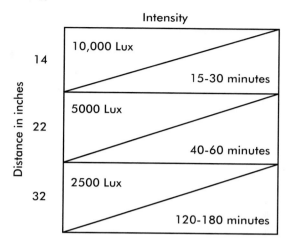

Fig. 26-4   Timing, dosage, and exposure to light. All times are average durations and may vary with each individual. *Lux*, Luminous flux density (unit of illuminance).

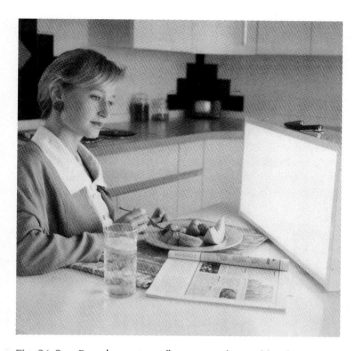

Fig. 26-3   Broad-spectrum fluorescent lamps like this one are used in daily therapy sessions from autumn into spring for people with SAD (seasonal affective disorder), who report feeling less depressed within 3 to 7 days.
Courtesy Medlight.

such as reading, writing, or eating (Fig. 26-3). Light boxes currently cost between $350 and $500.

The most recently developed light therapy devices are "light visors," a device shaped like a baseball cap and worn on the head, with the light contained in a visor portion suspended above and in front of the eyes. The obvious advantage to such a device is that it allows the person to move about while receiving treatment. However, the results of studies testing the device show great variability in effectiveness.

The timing and the dosage of the light vary from person to person. Some patients respond best to treatment given in the morning, whereas others prefer treatment in the evening. The amount of light to which a person is exposed depends not only on the person but also on the intensity of the light source and the duration of the exposure.[20] The brighter the light, the more effective the treatment per unit of time. For example, 2 hours of treatment with 2500 lux per day appears to have an antidepressant effect equal to that of 30 minutes per day at 10,000 lux (Fig. 26-4).

Light therapy appears to have important positive effects. Treatment is rapid and can be repeated. Most patients feel relief after 3 to 5 days and they relapse equally rapidly after light treatment is stopped. Patients do not appear to develop tolerance to phototherapy, and many have used the treatment for years.[28] Treatment can be received at home, and it need not disrupt daily routine. Light therapy also allows a person to actively participate in the treatment process, which enhances the patient's sense of control in recovering from illness.[14,19] However, the long-term efficacy of light therapy has not been fully evaluated.

Indications

Phototherapy relieves up to 75% of the symptoms of patients with well-documented, nonpsychotic winter depression or seasonal affective disorder (SAD).[20] SAD is a cyclical illness characterized by periods of depression that begin in October and subside in April (see Chapter 17). Although people in all latitudes can suffer from SAD, the prevalence of the disorder increases in the northernmost parts of the country. About 6% of the adult population in the United States, or 15 million people, suffer from the symptoms of SAD, which include sadness, irritability, increased appetite, carbohydrate craving, weight gain, hypersomnia, and decreased energy. In addition, 14% of Americans experience a more mild condition called "winter blues."

Light therapy should be administered by a professional with experience and training. It is a less-conventional treatment that may be of value to patients who do not respond to drug therapy, who prefer nonpharmacological treatments, or as an adjunct to drug treatments.

Mechanism of Action

Phototherapy is based on biological rhythms, particularly those related to light and darkness (see Chapter 5). However, scientists are not sure exactly how phototherapy works. An early theory suggested that melatonin secreted by the pineal gland of the brain played a critical role, but it has not been supported by recent research.[21] The therapeutic effect appears to be mediated primarily by the eyes, not the skin. Ongoing studies of the mechanism of phototherapy are exploring the eye itself, the way in which the eyes send messages to the brain, and the role of brain neurotransmitter systems such as serotonin and dopamine.[21] It also appears that certain individuals may have a neurochemical vulnerability, possibly inherited, that causes them to develop SAD in the absence of adequate exposure to environmental light.

Do you think that people who experience common disturbances in body rhythms such as jet lag and shift work can be helped by phototherapy?

Adverse Effects

Side effects, when they occur, are generally mild. However, light therapy, like any other psychiatric treatment, should be carefully monitored. The most common adverse effects of phototherapy are reported to be eyestrain, headache, irritability, insomnia, fatigue, nausea, and dryness of the eyes, nasal passages, and sinuses. These can usually be managed by decreasing the duration of therapy or increasing the patient's distance from the light. The long-term effects of phototherapy, if any, are currently unknown. Light therapy should be used with caution with specific ophthalmic conditions.

SLEEP DEPRIVATION THERAPY

It has been reported that as many as 60% of depressed patients improve immediately after one night of total sleep deprivation.[29] Unipolar and bipolar patients appear to do equally well. In addition, partial sleep deprivation that allows for as much as 3½ hours of sleep may also be effective. Although these findings have been reported in the literature, few randomized controlled clinical studies have been conducted on sleep deprivation. Furthermore, in the existing studies it is difficult to know the effect of the patient's expectations on the treatment outcome. Thus these findings should be considered with caution.

Unfortunately, many patients who respond to this therapy become depressed again when they resume sleeping even as little as 2 hours a night. This disadvantage has tended to discourage the use of sleep deprivation in clinical practice. There is some suggestion,

however, that improvement can be maintained if the sleep manipulation can be used repeatedly over time, such as by shifting the timing of sleep to earlier in the night. For example, the patient can go to sleep at 5:00 PM and arise at 2:00 AM.

In addition, medications may help prevent relapse after sleep deprivation therapy. It is interesting to note that some antidepressants, especially the monoamine oxidase inhibitors, often interfere with sleep (see Chapter 25). This has led some researchers to wonder if part of the efficacy of these drugs is due to their ability to induce partial sleep deprivation.

How can a patient's expectations of a treatment influence its effectiveness? Can you think of a placebo treatment for sleep deprivation therapy that would control this problem?

Indications

Evidence suggests that depressed patients with symptoms of marked diurnal variation are those most likely to improve after sleep deprivation. Patients who respond favorably to sleep deprivation also appear to have abnormally elevated nighttime body temperatures.

Mechanism of Action

The biological mechanisms of the antidepressant effects of sleep deprivation have not been identified. It has been hypothesized that sleep deprivation works by interrupting REM sleep (see Chapter 5). Another theory proposes that neuroendocrine changes accompanying sleep deprivation account for its antidepressant effects. Yet another hypothesis focuses on the body's thermoregulatory mechanisms and suggests that cold exposure and sleep deprivation may work together to produce antidepressant effects.[28]

Adverse Effects

Unfortunately, sleep deprivation appears to induce mania in some bipolar patients. Thus sleep deprivation, like some antidepressant medications, should be used with caution with patients who are susceptible to mania or have a family history of bipolar illness.

On the other hand, the knowledge that sleep deprivation may induce mania can have important preventive applications.[27] For example, individuals who are biologically vulnerable to bipolar illness might monitor disruptions to their sleep caused by work schedules, travel, drugs, or other life events. Thus for vulnerable individuals prevention of sleep loss at times of stress might help prevent mania.

SUMMARY

1. Electroconvulsive therapy (ECT) is an effective treatment for major depression with an efficacy rate of 80% or more, which is equal to or better than response rates to antidepressant medications. It is particularly useful for people who cannot tolerate or fail to respond to treatment with medication.

2. Nursing care in ECT involves providing emotional and education support to the patient and family; assessing the pretreatment protocol and the patient's behavior, memory, and functional ability before ECT; preparing and monitoring the patient during the actual ECT procedure; and observing and interpreting patient responses to ECT with recommendations for changes in the treatment plan as appropriate.

3. Phototherapy, or light therapy, consists of exposing patients to bright, artificial therapeutic lighting for a specified period of time each day. It is a relatively new treatment option for patients with nonpsychotic winter depression or seasonal affective disorder (SAD).

4. Sleep deprivation therapy has been reported to be effective with depressed patients; however, many become depressed again when they resume sleeping even as little as 2 hours a night. More research is needed to determine the efficacy and mechanism of action for this treatment strategy.

COMPETENT CARING
A CLINICAL EXEMPLAR OF A PSYCHIATRIC NURSE

Dean Olivet, RN, C

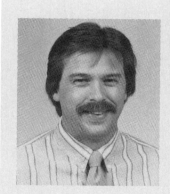

On this particular morning, I arrived at work as usual and performed all the morning rituals that a nurse does before venturing out on the clinical floor. After having several days off, it was apparent from reports and from listening to my co-workers that the acuity on the unit was high. Not only was the unit psychiatrically tense, but several geriatric patients had been admitted for evaluation and electroconvulsive therapy (ECT). On a general psychiatric unit, these patients often elicit a variety of feelings from the staff, ranging from mild anxiety to downright fear. Therefore I opted to take a few of the older, acute patients, including Mr. J., who was 80 years of age. This patient was newly admitted for evaluation of medications and a possible course of ECT. The staff who had contact with him described him as needy, confused, and wanting constant reassurance.

My first contact with Mr. J. found him asleep in his bed. He was disheveled, as was the condition of his room. I introduced myself to him and found out immediately why he seemed to have caused the staff to be anxious. He grabbed my arm and spoke to me in a high-pitched whine that anyone would want to avoid. My initial reaction was a flight response. To resist this, I began to assess his level of independence, and it became clear in a short period of time that he was unable to make any choices with regard to planning his morning. In organizing my care, the approach I decided on was to outline the morning routine for him in small time increments and assess his ability to make decisions with regard to his basic needs.

We began with his activities of daily living. Mr. J. needed assistance to meet these physiological needs, and his anxiety level made it necessary for me to maximize his safety and security. He told me that his daughter and son had helped him the night before. He assured me that I was too busy and they would help him the next time they visited as well. My nursing pride was somewhat injured, and I was puzzled about the necessity for his family to perform what seemed to be a nursing responsibility. Nonetheless, I carried on with my care and convinced him to bathe while I cleaned up his room and made his bed. Implementing this minor intervention made me feel more comfortable in his room, and he didn't seem quite as overwhelmed.

Since his anxiety was still moderately high, I consulted with the nurse giving his medications and also reviewed his chart. Here I learned that this was his second hospitalization, with many years free of symptoms of depression. During his first hospital stay he received a course of ECT that was very successful in helping him get well. I also learned that he was being cared for by his wife and daughter. Their treatment of choice was to medicate him until he slept. Learning this, I sensed the need to evaluate the quality of his experience with his last course of ECT, as well as the need for possible ECT and medication education for the family. These two educational needs became an ongoing process dependent on his and his family's readiness to learn.

My plan of care was quite simple. I would make sure that his activities of daily living were completed each morning, his environment kept orderly, and his introduction to the milieu would be made in short intervals. This was necessary to keep him safe from patients with less impulse control, thereby not overwhelming him or the other patients. The man needed some peer contact as well, and I introduced him to other patients as appropriate.

That afternoon his family came in to visit, and I met with them to assess their need for information and their readiness to learn. I outlined Mr. J.'s day and apologized for his insistence that they perform his activities of daily living. I thought that perhaps they may be annoyed about this issue and was relieved when they expressed their appreciation for my interest in their husband and father. They explained to me that I was the first person they had substantial contact with since he was admitted. In fact, they were quite upset with their husband/dad's condition the night before, and were considering raising the issue to staff. After listening to their concerns, I outlined my plan of care for Mr. J. and explained that in my absence the rest of the nursing staff would use the care plan to meet his daily needs. At this point, the family became an ally to the total hospital experience, and I became a resource to the patient and the family. This brought comfort to the family, which in turn allowed Mr. J. to meet his basic needs and have the security to meet the challenge of recovering from his illness.

The family members were satisfied with my interventions, and a possible problematic hospital experience was diverted by my nursing actions. As nurses, we all can relate to experiences when we care for patients only to have family members complain about the care or lack of care their significant other received. We can also describe occasions when it was very rewarding to have a patient respond to our care and to have the family recognize this nursing effort. Given this dichotomy, which do you prefer? The answer really reflects the crux of good psychiatric nursing practice. ▼

REFERENCES

1. Abrams R: *Electroconvulsive therapy*, ed 2, New York, 1992, Oxford University Press.
2. American Nurses' Association: *Standards of psychiatric and mental health clinical nursing practice*, Washington, DC, 1994, The Association.
3. American Psychiatric Association: *The practice of electroconvulsive therapy: recommendations for treatment, training, and privileging*, Washington, DC, 1990, The Association.
4. Barker P, Baldwin S: Shock story, *Nurs Times* 86:52, 1990.
5. Baxter LRJ, Roy-Byrne P, Liston EH, Fairbanks L: Informing patients about electroconvulsive therapy: effects of a videotape presentation, *Convulsive Therapy* 2:25, 1986
6. Burns C, Stuart G: Nursing care in electroconvulsive therapy, *Psychiatr Clin North Am* 14:971, 1991.
7. Coffey CE, Weiner RD: Electroconvulsive therapy: an update, *Hosp Community Psychiatry* 41:515, 1990.
8. Duffy WF, Conradt H: Electroconvulsivei therapy: the perioperative process, *AORN J* 50:806, 1989.
9. Fine M, Jenike MA: Electroshock: exploding the myth, *RN* 48:58, 1985.
10. Fink M: Is ECT use decreasing? *Convulsive Therapy* 3:171, 1987.
11. Fink M: Who should get ECT? In Coffey C, ed: *The clinical science of electroconvulsive therapy*, Washington, DC, 1993, American Psychiatric Press.
12. Fink P, Tasman A, eds: *Stigma and mental illness*, Washington, DC, 1992, American Psychiatric Press.
13. Fox H: Patients' fear of and objection to electroconvulsive therapy, *Hosp Community Psychiatry* 44:357, 1993.

14. Hyman J: *The light book*, Los Angeles, 1990, Jeremy P. Tarcher.
15. Janicak P, Mask J, Trimakas K, Gibbons R: ECT: an assessment of mental health professionals' knowledge and attitudes, *J Clin Psychiatry* 46:262, 1985.
16. Kalayam B, Steinhart M: A survey of attitudes on the use of electroconvulsive therapy, *Hosp Community Psychiatry* 32:185, 1981.
17. Kellner C, Pritchett J, Coffey C: *Handbook of ECT*, Washington, DC (in press).
18. Litwack K, Jones EE: Practical points in the care of the postelectroconvulsive therapy patient, *J Post Anesth Nurs* 3:182, 1988.
19. Rosenthal N: *Winter blues: SAD—what it is and how to overcome it*, New York, 1993, The Guilford Press.
20. Rosenthal N, Sack D, Skewrer R, Jacobson F, Wehr T: Phototherapy for seasonal affective disorder. In Rosenthal N, Blehar M, eds: *Seasonal affective disorders and phototherapy*, New York, 1989, The Guilford Press.
21. Rosenthal N, Wehr T: Towards understanding the mechanism of action of light in seasonal affective disorders, *Pharmacopsychiatry*, 25:56, 1992.
22. Royal College of Nursing: RCN nursing guidelines for ECT, *Convulsive Therapy* 3:158, 1987.
23. Sands D, McCary RC, Bigler ED, Becker HA, Waller PR: Understanding ECT, *J Psychosoc Nurse Ment Health Serv* 25:27, 1987.
24. Suedfeld P et al: Reduction of post-ECT memory complains through brief, partial restricted environmental stimulation (REST), *Prog Neuropsychopharmacol Biol Psychiatry* 13:693, 1989.
25. Swartz C, Saheba N: Comparison of atropine with glycopyrrolate for use in ECT, *Convulsive Therapy* 5:56, 1989.
26. Talbott K: ECT: exploring myths, examining attitudes. *J Psychosoc Nurs Ment Health Serv* 24:6, 1986.
27. Wehr T: Sleep loss: a preventable cause of mania and other excited states, *J Clin Psychiatry* 50(Suppl):8, 1989.
28. Wehr T: Manipulations of sleep and phototherapy: non-pharmacological alternatives in the treatment of depression, *Clin Neuropharmacol* 13(suppl):S54, 1990.
29. Wehr T: Effects of wakefulness and sleep on deprivation and mania. In Montplaisir J, Godbout R, eds: *Sleep and biological rhythms*, New York, 1990, Oxford University Press.

ANNOTATED SUGGESTED READINGS

Abrams R: *Electroconvulsive therapy*, ed 2, New York, 1992, Oxford University Press.
Comprehensive textbook on the clinical practice of ECT.

American Psychiatric Association: *The practice of electroconvulsive therapy: recommendations for treatment, training, and privileging*, Washington, DC, 1990, The Association.
Presents APA guidelines for the safe and effective use of ECT. Includes recommendations, rationale, bibliography, and appendices. The definitive document on the topic.

Coffey CE, Weiner RD: Electroconvulsive therapy: an update, *Hosp Community Psychiatry* 4:515, 1990.
Clear, concise, and easy-to-read review article on ECT.

*Glod C: Circadian dysregulation in abused individuals: a proposed theoretical model for practice and research, *Arch Psychiatr Nurs* 6:347, 1992.
Thought-provoking article that explores a possible link between the sleep disruptions seen in abused children with circadian and rhythmic theories from a nursing perspective.

Hyman J: *The light book*, Los Angeles, 1990, Jeremy P. Tarcher.
Easy-to-read text on how natural and artificial light affect our health, mood, and behavior. Well documented and interesting.

Kellner C, ed: *The Psychiatric Clinics of North America* vol 14, 1991.
The entire volume of this journal is dedicated to ECT, focusing on areas of clinical and scientific importance.

Kellner C, Pritchett J, Coffey C: *Handbook of ECT*, Washington DC (in press).
Excellent guide to contemporary ECT practice by experts in the field.

*Loving R, Kripke D: Daily light exposure among psychiatric patients, *J Psychosoc Nurs Ment Health Serv* 30:15, 1992.
Describes a study examining the 24-hour light exposure of psychiatric patients and identifies nursing interventions to increase light exposure in therapeutic environments.

Rosethal N: *Winter blues: SAD—what it is and how to overcome it*, New York, 1993, The Guilford Press.
Best book on the market to describe in layperson terms the illness of SAD and its treatment with phototherapy. Excellent for patient education.

*Valente S: Electroconvulsive therapy, *Arch Psychiatr Nurs* 4:223, 1991.
Overview article on ECT written from a nursing perspective.

*Nursing reference.

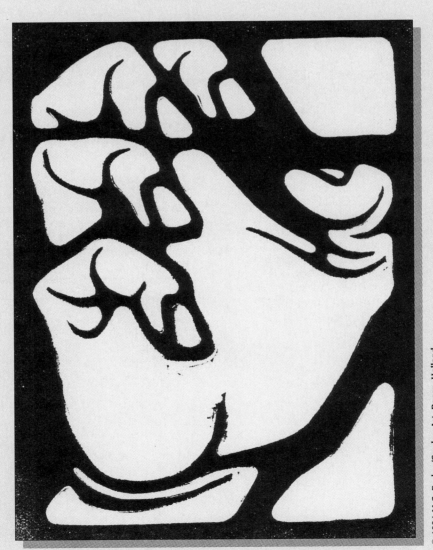

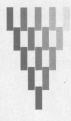

CHAPTER 27

Managing Aggressive Behavior

CHRISTINE C. HAMOLIA

Healthy children raised in decent conditions among loving people in a gentle and just society where freedom and equality are valued will rarely commit violent acts toward others.

Ramsay Clark: A Few Modest Proposals to Reduce Individual Violence in America

LEARNING OBJECTIVES

After studying this chapter the student should be able to:

▼ Discuss the prevalence of aggressive behavior among psychiatric patients and reasons for its increase

▼ Compare and contrast passive, assertive, and aggressive behavioral responses

▼ Describe five theories on the development of aggressive behavior

▼ Identify factors useful in predicting aggressive behavior among psychiatric patients

▼ Assess patients for aggressive behavioral responses

▼ Analyze nursing interventions for patients related to their aggressive behavior

▼ Describe the implementation of crisis management techniques

▼ Evaluate the need for staff development related to educating staff, working with staff who have been assaulted, and understanding legal implications

▼ Develop a patient education plan to promote patients' appropriate expression of anger

TOPICAL OUTLINE

Nurses provide care for patients with many types of problems. People who enter the health-care delivery system are often in great distress and may exhibit maladaptive coping responses. Nurses who work in certain settings, such as emergency rooms, critical care areas, and trauma centers, often care for individuals who respond to events with angry and aggressive behavior that can pose a significant risk to themselves, other patients, and their health-care providers. Thus managing aggressive behavior is an important skill for all nurses to master.

Psychiatric nurses in particular work with patients whose coping mechanisms for dealing with stress have proven to be inadequate. Patients admitted to an inpatient psychiatric unit are usually in crisis, and therefore their coping skills are even less effective. It is during these times of stress that acts of physical aggression or violence frequently occur. It is also true that nursing staff spend more time with patients on an inpatient unit than any other mental health discipline. As such they are more likely to be involved in managing aggressive behavior and are more at risk for being victims of physical acts of violence by patients. For these reasons, it is critical that psychiatric nurses be able to assess patients at risk for violence and intervene effectively with patients before, during, and after an aggressive episode.

DIMENSIONS OF THE PROBLEM

High rates of assaultive behavior have been reported in a variety of health-care settings including outpatient clinics, nursing homes, and emergency departments. By far the highest rates of assaults occur in psychiatric settings. Furthermore, injury to staff working on inpatient units has been identified as a major occupational risk, particularly for nursing staff.

Much has been written about violence in psychiatric populations in an attempt to describe and predict episodes of violence. Despite the common public misconception, most mentally ill persons do not commit violent acts. In fact, a minority of patients are responsible for a majority of the violent incidents. Differences in research methodology have made it difficult to identify the exact degree of violence in psychiatric facilities. The reported prevalence of both threatened and actual violence on inpatient units ranges from about 6% to 46%, although serious incidents are rare.[8,20] There is also some evidence that the rates of violence may be increasing over time and that rates are higher in the United States than in other countries.[8]

Many reasons help to explain the increasing incidence of violent behavior in psychiatric settings. First, as more emphasis is placed on outpatient and partial hospital treatment programs in the community, an increasing number of patients referred for inpatient care are hospitalized because they display aggressive or dangerous behavior. Before patients can be committed to the hospital, most states require evidence that patients are dangerous to themselves or others (see Chapter 8). This results in a larger proportion of aggressive and violent patients on inpatient units.

Second, the nature of the inpatient milieu has changed because of increasing patient acuity and shortened lengths of stay (see Chapter 31). In addition, economic constraints have resulted in fewer nursing staff assigned to inpatient units and limited availability and accessibility of medical staff to assist in managing patients.

Finally, evolving legal directives and perplexing ethical issues challenge the use of chemical and mechanical restraints and raise questions regarding patients' rights to refuse treatment and the nature of the "least restrictive" environment (see Chapter 8). This often results in conflict and confusion for inpatient staff, who try to manage patients effectively at a time of distress and dyscontrol.

Members of different disciplines sometimes have different views on how to manage aggressive behavior. Talk with nurses and physicians who care for psychiatric patients about their personal experiences and clinical judgments regarding this problem.

BEHAVIORAL RESPONSES

Within each person lies the capacity for passive, assertive, and aggressive behavior. In a threatening situation the choices are to be passive, fearful, and to flee; to be aggressive, angry, and to fight; or to be assertive, self-confident, and to confront the situation directly. The situation and the characteristics of the individuals involved define the appropriate response.

Passive Behavior

Passive individuals consistently subordinate their own rights to their perception of the rights of others. When passive individuals become angry, they try to camouflage it, thereby creating increased tension in themselves. In addition, if other people become aware of the anger by observing nonverbal cues, passive individuals are unable to confront the issue. This can also increase their tension. This pattern of interaction can seriously impair interpersonal growth. The following clinical example illustrates passive behavior.

 ## CLINICAL EXAMPLE

Ms. J was a staff nurse on a busy surgical unit. She enjoyed her work and liked the patients. She also placed a high value on getting along with her co-workers. Other staff members always spoke positively of her. Ms. C, the head nurse, valued Ms. J as an employee, stating particularly, "She's not like the rest of them. She never complains."

Ms. J made it a practice never to refuse a request made by a patient or another staff member. If a patient who was assigned to another nurse asked her to explain his diet or straighten his bed, she would do so, even if she was then behind in her own work. She never asked for help from others, since she felt that her assignment was her responsibility. If a co-worker asked to change days off with her, Ms. J always agreed, even if she had plans, rationalizing that the other person probably had more important plans.

Ms. C began to sense a tenseness when she was around Ms. J. Since she could not think of any problem at work, she assumed that Ms. J must have been having a problem at home. She was concerned and asked Ms. J if she could help. To her amazement, Ms. J recited a long list of angry feelings related to the work situation. Ms. C then felt guilty when she realized that she and the other staff members had been taking advantage of Ms. J.

Although Ms. J had thought that she was acting in a healthy way, she was actually negating her own needs and diminishing her self-respect. Her co-workers, who superficially liked her, in reality felt uncomfortable with her because they were never allowed to reciprocate when she had been helpful. Ms. C's guilty response quickly changed to anger when she realized that she had been a victim of Ms. J's passivity. If Ms. J had informed Ms. C of her feelings, she would have treated her more equitably.

Passivity is also expressed nonverbally. The person may speak softly, frequently in a childlike manner. There is little eye contact. Body language communicates diffidence and self-denial. The person may be slouched in posture and generally arms are held close to his body. Fidgeting also communicates passivity. Gestures are seldom used, although the head may be nodded in agreement (even when the person really disagrees).

Sarcasm is another indirect expression of anger. This usually provokes anger in the person who is the target. It is differentiated from assertive behavior because it usually infringes on the rights of the other. A sarcastic remark generally conveys the message "You are not worthy of my respect." Sarcasm may be disguised as humor. Confrontation may then be responded to with a disclaimer such as "Can't you take a joke?" Humor that derogates another person is hostile and is indulged in for the purpose of self-enhancement. It tends to backfire because the joker is revealed as insecure.

Assertive Behavior

Assertiveness is at the midpoint of a continuum that runs from passive to aggressive behavior. Assertive behavior conveys a sense of self-assurance but also communicates respect for the other person. Assertive individuals speak clearly and distinctly. They observe the norms of personal space appropriate to the situation. Eye contact is direct but not intrusive. Gestures emphasize speech but are not distracting or threatening. Posture is erect and relaxed. The body language may be symmetrical with that of the other party. The overall impression is one of strength, but not threatening.

Assertive persons feel free to refuse an unreasonable request. They will, however, share their rationale with the other person. They will also base the judgment about the reasonableness of the request on their own priorities. On the other hand, assertive individuals do not hesitate to make a request of others, assuming that they will inform them if their request is unreasonable. If the other person is unable to refuse, assertive individuals will not feel guilty about making the request.

Assertiveness also implies communicating feelings directly to others. As a result, anger is not allowed to build up, and the expression of feeling is more likely to be in proportion to the situation. If dissatisfaction is verbalized, the reason for the feeling is included. Assertive people also remember to express love to those to whom they are close. Compliments are given when deserved. Assertion also involves acceptance of positive input from others.

Aggressive Behavior

At the opposite end of the continuum from passivity is aggression. Aggressive people ignore the rights of others. They assume that all persons must fight for their own interests, and they expect the same behavior from others. Life is a battle. An aggressive approach to life may lead to physical or verbal violence. The aggressive behavior frequently covers a basic lack of self-confidence. Aggressive people enhance their self-esteem by overpowering others and thereby proving their superiority. The next clinical example describes aggressive behavior.

CLINICAL EXAMPLE

Suzy was a 9-year-old girl brought to the child psychiatric clinic by her mother on referral from the school nurse. She was described as a tomboy who loved active play and hated school. She was the first girl to make the neighborhood Little League baseball team and had proved her right to be there by beating up several male team members. Suzy was sent to the clinic after the teacher caught her forcing younger children to give her their lunch money.

When Suzy came to the clinic, she presented a facade of toughness. She did not deny her behavior and explained it by saying that the "little kids don't need much to eat anyway. I let them keep some of the money." Suzy was saving money for a new baseball glove. When she was asked about school, she said angrily, "I'm not dumb. I could learn that junk, but who needs it. I just want to play ball."

Psychological testing revealed that Suzy's IQ was slightly below average. She attended school with a group of upper middle class college-bound children. Even in the fourth grade she was feeling insecure and unable to compete. She masked her insecurity with her bullying behavior, striving for acceptance in sports, where she did have ability. The medical diagnosis was conduct disorder, undersocialized, aggressive. When Suzy's problem was explained to her parents and the school, some of the pressure for academic achievement was alleviated. Her parents spent extra time helping her with her homework. Also, she was given genuine recognition for her athletic ability, demonstrated by the gift of a new baseball glove. Suzy gradually responded to the positive input from others by developing a sense of positive regard for herself. As she did so, she no longer needed to bully other children and began to grow into some real friendships.

Aggressive adults are not unlike Suzy. They try to cover up their insecurities and vulnerabilities by acting aggressive. The behavior is self-defeating because it drives people away, thus reinforcing the low self-esteem and vulnerability to rejection. Aggressive behavior is also communicated nonverbally. Aggressive individuals may invade personal space. They speak loudly and with great emphasis. They usually maintain eye contact over a prolonged period of time so that the other person experiences it as intrusive. Gestures may be emphatic and often seem threatening (e.g., they may shake their fists, stamp their feet, or make slashing motions with their hands). Posture is erect, and often aggressive people lean forward slightly toward the other person. The overall impression is one of power and dominance. Table 27-1 summarizes the major characteristics of passive, assertive, and aggressive behaviors.

> Do you use passive, assertive, or aggressive behaviors most often in your personal life? How does this compare with your professional life as a nursing student?

THEORIES ON AGGRESSION

It is useful for nurses to view aggressive and violent behavior along a continuum with verbal aggression at one end and physical violence at another.[25] As such, violence represents the result of extreme anger (rage) or fear (panic). Specific reasons for aggressive behavior vary from person to person. Nurses need to communicate with patients to understand the events that they perceive as anger provoking. In general, anger occurs in response to a perceived threat. This may be a threat of physical injury, or more common, a threat to the self-concept. When the self is threatened, individuals may

Table 27-1 Comparison of Passive, Assertive, and Aggressive Behaviors

	Passive	Assertive	Aggressive
Content of speech	Negative Self-derogatory "Can I?" "Will you?"	Positive Self-enhancing "I can" "I will"	Exaggerated Other derogatory "You always" "You never"
Tone of voice	Quiet, weak, whining	Modulated	Loud, demanding
Posture	Drooping, bowed head	Erect, relaxed	Tense, leaning forward
Personal space	Allows invasion of space by others	Maintains a comfortable distance; claims right to own space	Invades space of others
Gestures	Minimal, weak gesturing, fidgeting	Demonstrative gestures	Threatening, expansive gestures
Eye contact	Little or none	Intermittent, appropriate to relationship	Constant stare

not be entirely aware of the source of their anger. In this case, the nurse and patient need to work together to identify the nature of the threat.

A threat may be external or internal. Examples of external stressors are physical attack, loss of a significant relationship, and criticism from others. Internal stressors might include a sense of failure at work, perceived loss of love, and fear of physical illness. Anger is only one of the possible emotional responses to these stressors. Some individuals might respond with depression or withdrawal. However, those reactions are usually accompanied by anger, which may be difficult for the person to express directly. Depression is sometimes viewed as anger directed toward the self, and withdrawal may also be a passive expression of anger (see Chapter 17).

Frequently anger seems out of proportion to the event that seemed to cause it. A relatively insignificant stressor may be "the last straw" and result in the release of a flood of feelings that have been stored up over time. Nurses need to be aware of this and not personalize anger expressed by a patient. The nurse may seem to be a safer target than significant others with whom the patient may also be angry.

A number of theories on the development of aggressive behavior have influenced the treatment of violent patients. They can be categorized as psychoanalytical psychological, behavioral, sociocultural, and neurobiological. Current thinking in the field suggests that aggressive behavior is the result of the interaction of a person's biological, psychological, and sociocultural characteristics and that each of these factors must be considered when determining nursing care.

Psychoanalytical Basis

Psychoanalytical theory suggests that aggressive behavior is the result of instinctual drives. Freud proposed that two primary drives influence human behavior, the life force expressed through sexuality and the death force expressed through aggression. He believed that life was a struggle to maintain a balance between the two drives and that the behavior exhibited by humans was simply the result of the more powerful drive. This theory had a great impact on early thinking in the field. However, little research has supported this theory. It has also been criticized as having limited clinical usefulness, since it suggests that humans are innately aggressive and that they do not have a choice in this disposition. Furthermore, it discourages individual responsibility and accountability for behavioral response.

Psychological Basis

According to the frustration-aggression theory, aggression occurs as the result of a buildup of frustration.[9]

Frustration results when a person's attempt to achieve a desired goal is blocked. These feelings are then reduced through aggressive behavior. This theory has been criticized for simplifying the complexity of the human spirit and not considering other stressors that might also lead to aggression. In addition, it implies that the absence of aggression is simply caused by the absence of frustration. Thus there is no allowance for choosing alternative ways of handling frustration.

Another psychological view of aggressive behavior suggests the importance of predisposing developmental or life experiences that limit the person's capacity to select nonviolent coping mechanisms.[20] Some of these experiences are listed in Box 27-1. They may restrict a person's ability to use supportive relationships, leave the person very self-centered, or make the individual particularly vulnerable to a sense of injury that can easily be provoked into retaliatory rage. Box 27-2 presents background information about the patient that may also be associated with violence.

Behavioral Basis

Social learning theory proposes that aggressive behavior is learned through the socialization process as a result of internal and external learning. Internal learning occurs through the personal reinforcement received when enacting aggressive behavior. This may be the result of achieving a desired goal or experiencing feelings of importance, power, and control. For example, 4-year-old Johnny wants a cookie just before dinner. When his mother refuses, Johnny has a temper tantrum. If his mother then gives him a cookie, Johnny has learned that an aggressive outburst will be rewarded and he will obtain what he wants. If similar situations occur, Johnny

---

Box 27-1

DEVELOPMENTAL FACTORS LIMITING USE OF NONVIOLENT COPING TECHNIQUES

▼ Organic brain damage, mental retardation, or learning disability, which may impair capacity to deal effectively with frustration

▼ Severe emotional deprivation or overt rejection in childhood, or parental seduction, which may contribute to defects in trust and self-esteem

▼ Exposure to violence in formative years, either as a victim of child abuse or as an observer of family violence, which may instill a pattern of using violence as a way to cope

From Menninger W: *Bull Menninger Clin* 57:208, 1993.

Box 27-2

BACKGROUND INFORMATION
ASSOCIATED WITH VIOLENT BEHAVIOR

▼ Childhood cruelty to animals or other children
▼ Fire setting or similar dangerous actions
▼ Recent violent behavior toward self or others
▼ Recent accidents, threats, or poor judgment in potentially dangerous situations
▼ Altered states of consciousness
▼ Escalating irritability, sensitivity, or hostility
▼ Fear of losing control
▼ Efforts to obtain help
▼ Bothering family, neighbors, police
▼ History of abuse of alcohol or other disinhibiting substances

From Menninger W: *Bull Menninger Clin* 57:208, 1993.

will continue to use an aggressive approach to need satisfaction.

External learning occurs through the observation of role models such as parents, peers, siblings, sports heroes, and entertainment figures. Sociocultural patterns that lead to the imitation of aggressive behavior suggest that violence is an acceptable way of solving problems and achieving status in society. According to this view, activities such as violent crime, aggressive sports, and war depicted through the media or witnessed in person reinforce aggressive behavior in individuals (see Critical Thinking about Contemporary Issues).

A recent addition to the social learning perspective suggests that violence is a functional behavior that is designed to control others purely for self-gain.[22] There is some evidence that this coercive interactional style may be a strong predictor of violent behavior.[23] It was discovered from direct interviews with patients who were asked the question "Why are you violent?" and responded "Because I'm tired of these people and I want to get them off my back." This theory thus proposes that some patients use violence to get what they want.

Sociocultural Basis

Social and cultural factors may also influence aggressive behavior. Cultural norms help to define acceptable and unacceptable means of expressing aggressive feelings. Sanctions are applied to violators of the norms through the legal system. By this means, society controls violent behavior and attempts to maintain a safe existence for its members. Unfortunately, this prohibition against violent behavior may also be extended to include any expression of anger. This can inhibit people from the healthy expression of angry feelings and lead to other maladaptive responses. A cultural norm that

CRITICAL THINKING ABOUT CONTEMPORARY ISSUES

Does Television, Movie, and Video Violence Lead to Greater Acts of Aggression in Society?

Some people believe that graphic scenes of violence in television, movies, and video games is directly linked to human aggression. Proponents of this view support measures to decrease video violence and restrict types of video programming. Others think that the relationship has not been clearly established. These individuals believe that violence is multidetermined by socioeconomic, biological, psychological, cultural, and familial factors.

Research suggests that although many instances of children and adults imitating video violence have been documented, no court has ruled that video violence actually causes harm. It has been suggested, however, that while the typical viewer may be mentally resilient and invulnerable to any ill effects, a small group of vulnerable viewers may be more impressionable and therefore more likely to suffer negative effects from violent programming.[13] More research is needed to identify characteristics of such a vulnerable population. It is also important to remember that the public must accept responsibility for the escalation of video violence. If the product were unappealing it would fail. Instead, the entertainment industry appears to exploit a public already fascinated with violence. ▼

supports verbally assertive expressions of anger will help people deal with anger in a healthy manner. A norm that reinforces violent behavior will result in physical expression of anger in destructive ways.

Neurobiological Basis

Current neurobiological research has focused on three areas of the brain believed to be involved in aggression: the limbic system, the frontal lobe, and the temporal lobe.[11,12] Neurotransmitters have also been suggested as having a role in the expression or suppression of aggressive behavior. Each of these areas is described in detail in Chapter 5.

The limbic system is associated with the expression of human emotions and behaviors such as eating, aggression, and sexual response. It is also involved in the processing of information. Structures commonly included in discussion of the limbic system are the hippocampus, amygdala, cingulate gyrus, and hypothala-

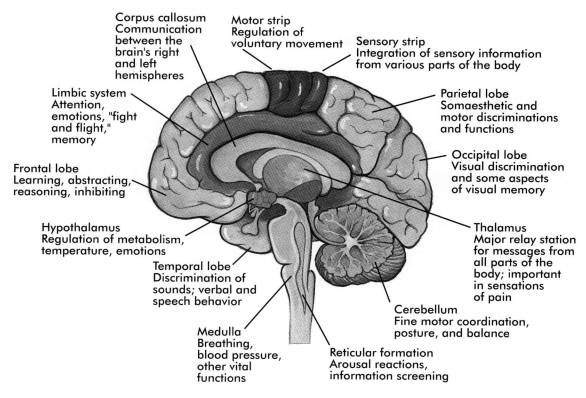

Fig. 27-1   Structures of the limbic system.

mus (Fig. 27-1). Damage to the limbic system may result in an increase or decrease in the potential for aggressive behavior.

The frontal lobes play an important role in mediating purposeful behavior and rational thinking. They are the part of the brain where reason and emotion interact. Damage to the frontal lobes can result in impaired judgment, personality changes, problems in decision making, inappropriate conduct, and aggressive outbursts.

The temporal lobes play a role in memory and the interpretation of auditory stimuli. The temporal lobe problem most often linked to aggressive behavior is epilepsy, particularly in those individuals with partial complex seizures. Aggressive behavior may occur during or after seizure activity.

Neurotransmitters are brain chemicals that are transmitted to and from neurons through synapses. An increase or decrease in these substances can influence behavior. The neurotransmitters most often associated with aggressive behaviors are the monoamines serotonin (5-hydroxytryptamine) and dopamine (3-hydroxytyramine) and the amino acid gamma-aminobutyric acid (GABA).

PREDICTING AGGRESSIVE BEHAVIOR

Researchers have tried to determine which patients are more likely to become violent. Demographic variables such as age, sex, race, marital status, education, and socioeconomic level have not been found to be useful in predicting violent behavior. In contrast, psychiatric diagnosis has frequently been correlated with assaultiveness. However, the ability of this variable to predict violence is complicated by the fact that many patients have more than one diagnosis. In addition, patients may have different clinical symptoms depending on the severity and acuity of their illness. Thus a patient's diagnosis is suggestive at best.

In general, psychotic inpatients probably have the greatest potential to commit violence during the acute phase of their illness, which typically occurs relatively early in the hospital stay. Temporary states of violence are also exacerbated by drug abuse. In the fourth edition of *Diagnostic and Statistical Manual of Mental Disorders* (DSM-IV), aggressive behavior is associated with a number of other psychiatric illnesses.[1] For some of these disorders the diagnosis of aggressive behavior requires prior aggressive activity; for others the behavior is an essential feature; whereas for other disorders, aggres-

---

Box 27-3

MENTAL ILLNESSES CHARACTERIZED BY AGGRESSIVE BEHAVIOR

REQUIRED FOR THE DIAGNOSIS

▼ Intermittent explosive disorder
▼ Organic personality syndrome, explosive type
▼ Conduct disorder
▼ Sexual sadism

ESSENTIAL FOR THE DIAGNOSIS

▼ Antisocial personality disorder
▼ Borderline personality disorder
▼ Alcohol idiosyncratic intoxication

ASSOCIATED BUT NOT INVARIABLY PRESENT

▼ Attention-deficit hyperactivity disorder
▼ Other psychoactive substance intoxication (especially PCP)
▼ Certain organic mental disorders
▼ Mental retardation
▼ Schizophrenia
▼ Brief reactive psychosis
▼ Schizoaffective disorder
▼ Manic episode
▼ Bipolar disorder
▼ Posttraumatic stress disorder
▼ Adjustment disorder

From Menninger W: *Bull Menninger Clin* 57:208, 1993.

sive behavior is often encountered but is not necessary for the diagnosis (Box 27-3).[20]

In recent years research efforts have focused on identifying clinical variables that have been shown to be predictors of violence. The best single predictor of violence appears to be a history of violence.[4,30] Another significant clinical variable is the length of time spent on an inpatient unit, with more assaultive patients being found to have spent significantly more time than non-assaultive patients on inpatient units since their first admission.[21]

Although knowledge about a patient's history is important in evaluating the risk for violence, it is also important to assess the patient's current clinical condition and situation. High levels of aggression before admission and absence of signs of anxiety at admission are believed to be good predictors of violence.[4] In addition, increased motor activity and an indication of poor impulse control or strong aggressive drives in psychological testing may also be significant in predicting patient assaultiveness.[17] Other studies report that correlates of violent behavior include a variety of behavioral and cognitive cues such as conceptual disorganization, loud ver-

balizations, tension, mannerisms and posturing, hostility, suspiciousness, uncooperativeness, hallucinatory behavior, unusual thought content, excitement, and disorientation.[8,18]

Finally, situational and environmental factors are also believed to play a role in escalating patient behavior from dangerousness to violence. This includes aspects of the physical facilities and the presence of staff and other patients. For example, several studies have found that the number of violent incidents is greater when patients move or gather in groups, are overcrowded, lack privacy, or are inactive.[8] Clinicians may also intentionally or inadvertently contribute to or precipitate an outbreak of violence, since staff attitudes and behavior have a powerful impact on modulating patient behavior. Staff provocation and inexperience, poor milieu management, close physical encounters, inconsistent limit setting, and a "norm of violence" may all negatively affect the inpatient environment.

Issues of Provocation

Research suggests that many assaultive patients view their victim as provoking the attack.[22,30] This is an important issue for nurses to consider. A primary factor of provocation is that of limit setting.[16] Failing to set effective limits may lead to provocation and assault. There is also increased risk of assault when limits are set inconsistently. Taking things away from patients such as food, beverages or cigarettes also appears to increase the likelihood of an attack.

Staff attitude is another important issue related to aggressive patient behavior.[3] Aggressive verbal and nonverbal behavior on the part of the staff frequently escalates the patient's distress and violent behavior. When the nursing staff act in a controlling manner, patients are more likely to use aggression and violence to get control. Staff who are authoritarian and inflexible in their approach to patients and who have not been trained in crisis management techniques are also more likely to provoke aggressive behavior. Finally, violent behavior may be a way of getting the staff's attention or may lead to a tangible reward.

Finally, locked units, inflexible unit structures, and nontherapeutic milieus can increase the risk for assaultive behavior by suggesting that aggressive behavior is acceptable or even expected (see Chapter 31). Overly strict unit structure may render staff unable to respond to patients empathically. In turn, patients may perceive the unit as coercive, controlling, and threatening and feel their behavioral options are limited to disruptive, desperate, or violent acts. Such settings often provoke the very behavior they are attempting to control.

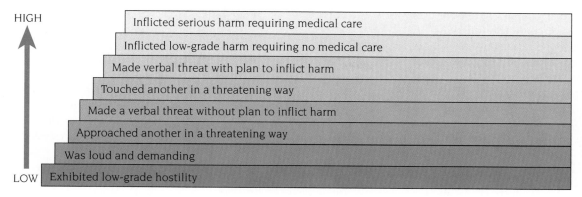

HIGH

Inflicted serious harm requiring medical care

Inflicted low-grade harm requiring no medical care

Made verbal threat with plan to inflict harm

Touched another in a threatening way

Made a verbal threat without plan to inflict harm

Approached another in a threatening way

Was loud and demanding

LOW   Exhibited low-grade hostility

Fig. 27-2   Hierarchy of aggressive and violent patient behaviors.

Discuss the fine line that exists between talking about ways staff can provoke patients and blaming the staff who are the victims of the aggressive behavior.

NURSING ASSESSMENT

Although researchers have made progress in determining reliable predictors of violence, a completely accurate prediction of patient violence is not possible. For this reason it is important for psychiatric nurses to be alert for symptoms of increasing agitation that could lead to violent behavior. For example, a correspondence has been shown between nurses' clinical estimates of patients' chances of becoming violent and the number of patients who later displayed some type of inpatient aggression.[19]

Some evidence also shows that a hierarchy of aggressive behaviors exists and that lower levels of aggression may lead to more violent behavior (Fig. 27-2).[24] Some of these early behaviors include motor agitation such as pacing, inability to sit still, clenching or pounding fists, and tightening of jaw or facial muscles. There also may be verbal clues such as threats to real or imagined objects or intrusive demands for attention. Speech may be loud and pressured, and posture may become threatening.

Another critical factor in the assessment of a potentially violent patient is the affect associated with escalating behaviors. Anger frequently is seen in patients who are imminently violent. Inappropriate euphoria, irritability, and lability in affect may indicate that a patient is having difficulty in maintaining control. Changes in level of consciousness may also be an indication of future violent behavior (Box 27-4).

Finally, in addition to evaluating possible precipi-

Box 27-4

BEHAVIORS ASSOCIATED WITH AGGRESSION

MOTOR AGITATION

Pacing
Inability to sit still
Clenching or pounding fists
Jaw tightening
Increased respirations
Sudden cessation of motor activity (catatonia)

VERBALIZATIONS

Verbal threats toward real or imagined objects
Intrusive demands for attention
Loud, pressured speech
Evidence of delusional or paranoid thought content

AFFECT

Anger
Hostility
Extreme anxiety
Irritability
Inappropriate or excessive euphoria
Affect lability

LEVEL OF CONSCIOUSNESS

Confusion
Sudden change in mental status
Disorientation
Memory impairment
Inability to be redirected

---

tants of violent behavior and issues related to provocation, nurses need to be aware of biological factors as well. This will help the nurse to better predict aggressive behavior, anticipate how it will be expressed, and plan the most appropriate nursing intervention. Five criteria that distinguish aggressive behavior with biological etiology include the following[7]:

1. Neuropsychological test scores or results of neurological examinations will likely show evidence of central nervous system lesions or dysfunctions.
2. Organically based incidents are typically sudden and relatively unprovoked.
3. Violent outbursts of patients with biologically based aggression are relatively less controlled.
4. Organically based incidents have clear changes from calm to rage and back to calm relatively quickly.
5. Patients with biologically based rage typically show remorse.

In summary, psychiatric nurses should carefully assess all patients for their potential for violence. A screening or assessment tool such as the one presented in Fig. 27-3 may be useful in this process. Such a tool

Directions:
a. Assess each key factor.
b. Circle one (of three) descriptor for each factor which BEST describes the patient.
c. Add the points for each circled item to obtain the Total Score

Key Factors	High Risk	Moderate Risk	No Precautions
History of Violence	Any single episode of violence with injury to others while hospitalized. -OR- Multiple assaults with injury while outside hospital. 2	Destruction of property without injury to others while in hospital. -OR- A single assault outside the hospital resulting in injury. -OR- Multiple assaults outside the hospital not resulting in injury. 1	Violence only when using drugs or alcohol. -OR- Destruction of property outside hospital. -OR- No history of violence. 0
History of Recent Aggression	Physically threatening at time of referral/admission. 2	Verbally threatening at time of referral/admission. 1	Nonthreatening at time of referral/admission. 0
History of Aggression in Family of Origin	Victim or perpetrator of physical and/or sexual abuse. 2	Witness of physical and/or sexual abuse 1	Witness or victim of verbal aggression. -OR- No history of aggression in family. 0
Substance Abuse Status	Recent alcohol/substance abuse actively detoxing. -OR- Currently under the influence of alcohol or drugs. 2	Recent substance/alcohol abuse with absence of withdrawal symptoms. 1	Rehabilitated abuser. -OR- No history of alcohol/substance abuse. -OR- Past history (>3 months ago) alcohol/substance abuse with no rehab. 0
Paranoia/Hostility	Paranoia and/or hostility generalized to people in the immediate environment. 2	Paranoia and/or hostility generalized towards inaccessible people. 1	No apparent paranoia. No apparent hostility. 0
Impulsivity	Physically impulsive. 2	Verbally impulsive. -OR- History of physical impulsivity. 1	No apparent impulsivity. 0
Agitation	Psychomotor agitation with constant pressured physical activity. 2	Psychomotor agitation with intermittent bursts of hyperactivity. 1	No apparent psychomotor agitation. 0
Sensorium	Disoriented with impaired memory. 2	Oriented with impaired memory. 1	Oriented with intact memory. 0

Scoring Key:
9 or more = High-Risk Precautions
3-8 = Moderate Risk Precautions
0-2 = No Precautions

Total Score: _____

Assessed by (RN): _____

Date: _____

Time: _____

Fig. 27-3 Assault/violence assessment form.
Courtesy of the Division of Psychiatric Nursing, Medical University of South Carolina.

not only should identify individuals at risk for aggressive behavior, but also should alert the nurse to the need for specific nursing interventions.

NURSING INTERVENTIONS

The nurse can implement a variety of interventions to manage aggressive behavior. These interventions can be thought of as existing on a continuum (Fig. 27-4). They range from preventive strategies such as self-awareness, patient education, and assertiveness training to anticipatory strategies such as verbal and nonverbal communication, environmental changes, behavioral interventions, and the use of psychopharmacological agents. If the patient's aggressive behavior continues to escalate in spite of these actions, the nurse must then implement crisis management techniques including seclusion and restraints.

Self-Awareness

The most valuable resource of a nurse is the ability to use the self to help others.[31] To ensure the most effective use of self, it is important to be aware of personal stress that can interfere with the ability to communicate therapeutically with patients. If the nurse is tired, anxious, angry, or apathetic, it will be difficult to convey an interest in the concerns and fears of the patient. Furthermore, if the nurse is overwhelmed with personal problems, the energy available for patients is greatly diminished.

When dealing with potentially aggressive patients, it is important to be able to assess the situation objectively despite the positive or negative countertransference that might be present. Countertransference is an emotional reaction to some aspect or behavior of the patient (see Chapter 2). Negative countertransference reactions have been found to be a significant factor in the occurrence of violence in hospitals.[8] To prevent this situation the nurse must demonstrate ongoing self-

---

Assault/Violence Assessment Instructions

The following potential for violence assessment tool is used on admission if:
    1. The patient has a history of violence.
    2. The patient is currently threatening violence.
    3. The patient was threatening violence at the time of referral.

The assessment tool is also utilized during hospitalization if:
    1. A physician orders violence precautions.
    2. The patient becomes threatening.
    3. A violent incident has occurred and the attached care plan is used as a treatment plan.

The purpose of this guide is to assist the nurse in:
    1. Developing a therapeutic alliance with the patient.
    2. Assessing his/her potential for violence.
    3. Developing a plan of care.
    4. Implementing the plan of care.
    5. Preventing violence/aggression in the milieu.

Following the assessment, if the patient is believed to be potentially violent:
    1. Identify level of precaution and notify co-workers.
    2. Assess environment and make necessary changes.
    3. Notify M.D. and inquire for PRN medication changes.
    4. Assess need to notify security.
    5. Implement appropriate care plan.
    6. Organize milieu plan for management of anxiety throughout shift.

Fig. 27-3, cont'd.   For legend see opposite page.

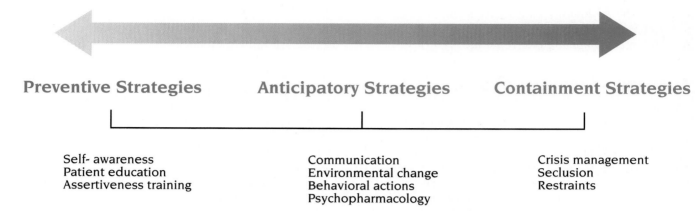

Fig. 27-4   Continuum of nursing interventions in managing aggressive behavior.

awareness and supervision with the goal of separating personal needs from those of the patient.

Patient Education

Teaching patients about communication and the appropriate way to express anger can be one of the most successful interventions in preventing aggressive behavior (see the Patient Education Plan on p. 731). Many patients have difficulty identifying their feelings, needs, and desires and even more difficulty communicating these to others. Teaching patients that feelings are not right or wrong or good or bad can allow them to explore feelings that may have been bottled up, ignored, or repressed. The nurse can then work with patients on ways to express their feelings and evaluate whether the responses they select are adaptive or maladaptive.

Assertiveness Training

Teaching assertive communication skills is an important nursing intervention (see Chapter 28). Interpersonal frustrations often escalate to aggressive behavior because patients have not mastered the assertive behaviors previously discussed in this chapter. Assertive behavior is a basic interpersonal skill that includes the following:

▼ Communicating directly with another person
▼ Saying no to unreasonable requests
▼ Being able to state complaints
▼ Expressing appreciation as appropriate

For example, the nurse might discuss with the patient how, if the patient talks about angry feelings toward a co-worker with another noninvolved co-worker, it does nothing to solve the problem and may even generate more negative emotions. So, too, if the patient pretends to not be angry, the anger is allowed to build up inside.

It is likely that the anger will be misdirected at a later time or expressed out of proportion in another unrelated situation.

Patients with few assertive skills can learn them by participating in structured groups and programs. In these settings patients can watch staff demonstrate specific skills and then role play the skills themselves. Staff can provide feedback to patients on the appropriateness and effectiveness of their responses. Homework can also be assigned to patients to help them generalize these skills outside the group milieu. It is expected that aggressive behaviors will diminish as the patient learns new and more effective social skills.

Do you think that a nurse who has difficulty being assertive with peers and interdisciplinary colleagues can effectively teach assertiveness skills to patients?

Communication Strategies

The psychiatric nurse can often prevent a crisis situation through the use of early verbal and nonverbal intervention. This is sometimes referred to as "talking the patient down." Since it is much less dangerous to prevent a crisis than it is to respond to one, every effort should be made to carefully monitor patients who are at risk for violent behavior and then to intervene at the first possible sign of increasing agitation.

Speaking to the patient in a calm, low voice can help to decrease a patient's agitation. Agitated patients often speak loudly and frequently use profanity. It is important that nurses not respond by raising their voice or by using profanity, since this will likely be

PATIENT EDUCATION PLAN
APPROPRIATE EXPRESSION OF ANGER

Content	Instructional activities	Evaluation
Help the patient identify anger	Focus on nonverbal behavior Role play nonverbal expression of anger Label the feeling using the patient's preferred words	The patient can demonstrate an angry body posture and facial expression
Give permission for angry feelings	Describe situations in which it is normal to feel angry	The patient describes a situation in which anger would be an appropriate response
Practice the expression of anger	Role play fantasized situations in which anger is an appropriate response	The patient participates in role play and identifies behaviors associated with expression of anger
Apply the expression of anger to a real situation	Help identify a real situation that makes the patient angry Role play a confrontation with the object of the anger Provide positive feedback for successful expression of anger	The patient identifies a real situation that results in anger The patient is able to role play expression of anger
Identify alternative ways to express anger	List several ways to express anger, with and without direct confrontation Role play alternative behaviors Discuss situations in which alternatives would be appropriate	The patient participates in identifying alternatives and plans when each might be useful
Confrontation with a person who is a source of anger	Provide support during confrontation if needed Discuss experience after confrontation takes place	The patient identifies the feeling of anger and appropriately confronts the object of the anger

Adapted from the model of intervention developed by Maynard CK, Chitty KK: J Psychiatr Nurs 17:36, 1979.

perceived as competition and will only further escalate the volatile situation. The nurse should use short, simple sentences and avoid laughing or smiling inappropriately.

The nurse can also help reduce a rising level of agitation in a patient by acknowledging the patient's feelings and reassuring the patient that the staff are there to help. It may be useful to allow the patient to ventilate without interruption. It is important that the nurse communicate expected behavior in a way that encourages the patient to maintain control of any violent impulses. At this early stage, some patients with encouragement may be willing to remove themselves from an overstimulating environment, thus facilitating their self-control.

The specific nonverbal communication used by the nurse can also greatly affect the outcome of the intervention. A calm and relaxed posture that does not tower over the patient is much less intimidating than a posture in which hands are placed on the hips and the nurse looms over the patient. Crossing the arms across the chest is another nonhelpful posture that communicates emotional distance and an unwillingness to help. The nurse's hands should be kept open and out of pockets. Threatening, nervous, and sudden gestures should be avoided. Altering position so that the nurse's eyes are at the same level as those of the patient allows the patient to communicate from an equal rather than inferior position.[31]

The nurse should assume a supportive stance that is at least one leg length or 3 feet from the patient. It is helpful if the nurse remains at an angle to the patient and that the patient's need for personal space is respected. It has been noted that violence-prone people need four times greater personal space than nonviolence-prone people. Thus intrusion into a patient's personal space can be perceived as a threat and provoke aggression. Finally, when approaching potentially violent patients, nurses should carefully observe their behavior. Clenched fists, tightening of the facial muscles, and movement away from the nurse may suggest that the patient is feeling threatened. The nurse should respond by giving the patient as much distance as possible.

Why do you think that standing at an angle to the patient is less threatening than facing the patient full face? Try the two stances with a friend and describe your feelings about each one.

Environmental Strategies

Violent behavior is more likely to occur in a poorly structured milieu with undefined program rules and a great deal of unscheduled time for patients.[7] Units that are overly stimulating, either visually or aurally, may also increase aggressive behavior. Thus treatment settings should be structured by unit rules so that levels of sensory stimulation are low to moderate. Televisions, stereos, lighting, temperature, wall colors, and air quality should not be overstimulating.

Inpatient units that provide many productive activities such as games, reading, and group programs reduce the chance of inappropriate patient behavior and increase adaptive social and leisure functioning. Both the unit norms and the rewards associated with such activities may reduce the amount of disorganized patient behavior and the number of aggressive acts. The impact of the environment is seen in the following clinical example.

 CLINICAL EXAMPLE

Mr. T was a 36-year-old man who was admitted for the third time to an acute care unit at a state psychiatric hospital. His medical diagnosis was bipolar disorder, manic. The nursing staff was apprehensive because the patient had a history of assaultive behavior on earlier admissions. At the time of this admission, the unit atmosphere was tense because one of the other patients had made a suicide attempt requiring emergency room treatment.

Mr. I was Mr. T's primary nurse from his previous admission. He was working when the patient arrived on the unit. During the nursing assessment, Mr. I discussed the nursing interventions that had seemed to be helpful in the past. He validated with Mr. T that he had usually been able to maintain control of his behavior by participating in a structured physical activity when he was feeling upset. In addition, he recalled that the patient would begin to pace rapidly and sing when he was losing control. Mr. T agreed with these observations.

Mr. T responded very quickly to the tension on the unit. He began to pace up and down the hall and sing in a moderately loud tone of voice. Other patients also began to show signs of increased agitation. The nursing staff held a brief consultation. They decided that the charge nurse would gather the patients for a community meeting to discuss their feelings about the suicide attempt. Meanwhile, Mr. I would take Mr. T to the nearby gym with one of the nurse's aides. They would perform structured calisthenic exercises. The interventions were successful. None of the patients needed to be restrained.

Room Program. In an inpatient setting, the use of a structured room program is another effective tool for the management of agitated patients whose self-control is tenuous and who have not yet decompensated to the point where seclusion or restraints is necessary. A **room program** is the titration of the amount of time patients are allowed in the unit milieu. For example, patients initially may be asked to stay in their rooms for a certain length of time, or conversely be allowed out of their rooms for a specified amount of time every hour. The amount of time in the milieu may then be increased by increments of 15 minutes as patients tolerate the environment. Another way of implementing a room program is to allow patients to come out of their rooms during certain designated hours, such as when the ward is quiet or when other patients are off the unit.

Such a structured program allows patients time away from situations that may increase agitation and provides a way to regulate the amount of stimulation patients receive. Its purpose is the prevention of a crisis that could result in more serious patient complications. A sample room program is presented in Box 27-5.

Behavioral Strategies

Other interventions include applying principles of behavior management with the aggressive patient (see Chapter 28). Effective limit setting is perhaps one of the most basic interventions in this area.

Limit Setting. Limit setting is a nonpunitive, nonmanipulative act in which the patient is told what behavior is acceptable, what is not acceptable, and the consequences of behaving unacceptably. The nurse does not assume responsibility for the patient's behavior, adaptive or maladaptive. It is recognized that the patient has the right to choose a behavior and knows the consequences of it. Limits should be clarified before negative consequences are applied.

Once a limit has been identified, the consequences must take place if the behavior occurs. Every staff member must be aware of the plan and carry it out consistently. If staff do not do so, the patient is likely to manipulate staff by acting out and then point out areas of inconsistent limit setting. Clear, firm, and nonpunitive enforcement of limits is the goal. It is also important for nurses to understand that when limit setting is implemented, the maladaptive behavior will not immediately decrease. In fact, it may briefly increase. This is consistent with behavioral principles and testing behavior. If staff understand the dynamics of this intervention they will be able to implement this strategy effectively and understand that patient behavior will eventually change.

Box 27-5
ROOM PROGRAMS

PURPOSE

Patients admitted and receiving on-going treatment for mental and emotional problems are often difficult to control. Their behavioral disorders can create problems that adversely affect their own safety, their peers' safety and the milieu of the unit. Therefore room programs that decrease stimulation, as well as reinforce self-control, are instituted. Room programs are initiated for patients who are having difficulty maintaining safety (of self, others, or both) on a unit or for patients who are advancing from seclusion or restraints. (A room program would *not* be instituted for patients who require periodic behavior modification time-outs for inappropriate behaviors.)

PROCEDURE

1. Patients will be informed about the proposed room program, the rationale for the program, and the responsibilities of the patient for progression to the status leading to return to milieu.
2. Patients will be given a copy of the program with indication as to the status being implemented.
3. Patients will be advanced in status as their behavior and level of stimuli tolerance indicate.
4. Patients may regress in status or remain at same status if this is indicated by patients' behavior or noncompliance with the protocol.
5. Discussions for status changes will be initiated by the shift coordinator, nurse team leaders, and primary caregiver for that shift.
6. Length of stay for each status change will be established at the beginning of the protocol. This information will be listed on patients' care plans and information given to patients. Time is calculated as *time awake, actively participating in program,* and *demonstrating control.*
7. Although there are established minimum time frames for change in status, the primary caregiver can make a decision based on patient behavior that more time at a particular status is required.
8. Any change in protocol, that is, lag times for status changes, will be communicated to patients and staff, as well as corrected on care plans.
9. Patients may begin room program at any level status, according to patients' behavior and discretion of the patients' primary caregivers for that shift.

Status I

Time in room: 55 minutes
Time out of room: 5 minutes
Patient will be restricted to unit and will not attend groups. Meals will be eaten on the unit in patient's room. Visitors are not allowed. Phone calls are not allowed.
Minimum time required for compliance and behavior control: *two cycles*

Status II

Time in room: 45 minutes
Time out of room: 15 minutes
Patient will be restricted to unit and will not attend groups. Meals will be eaten on the unit in patient's room. Visitors are not allowed. One 10-minute phone call is allowed during time out of room.
Minimum time required for compliance and for behavior control: *two cycles*

Status III

Time in room: 30 minutes
Time in milieu: 30 minutes
Patient will be restricted to unit and will not attend groups. Meals will be eaten on the unit in milieu. Visitors are not allowed. Two 10-minute phone calls are allowed during time out of room.
Minimum time required for compliance and behavior control: *two cycles*

Status IV

Time in room: 15 minutes
Time out of room: 45 minutes
Patient will be restricted to unit and will not attend groups. Meals will be eaten on the unit. Visitors are not allowed. Two 10-minute phone calls are allowed.
Minimum time required for compliance and behavior control: *two cycles*

Status V

Patient will be restricted to unit for a minimum of 24 hours and will not attend groups. Meals will be eaten on the unit. Visitors are allowed. Patient may have unlimited access to phone privilege.

Courtesy of the Division of Psychiatric Nursing, Medical University of South Carolina.

Behavioral Contracts. If a patient uses violence to gain control and make personal gains, the nursing care must be planned to eliminate the rewards the patient receives while allowing the patient to assume as much control as possible. Once the rewards are understood, nursing care can be planned that does not reinforce aggressive and violent behavior. Behavioral contracts with the patient can be very helpful in this regard. For example, head-injured patients with low impulse control can be told that staff will take them for a walk if they can refrain from using profanity for 4 hours.

To be effective, contracts require detailed information about the following:

▼ Unacceptable behaviors
▼ Acceptable behaviors
▼ Consequences for breaking the contract
▼ The nurse's contribution to care

Patients should also have input into the development of the contract to increase their sense of self-control. This negotiated process increases the mutuality of the therapeutic alliance and reduces the possibility of aggressive behavior.

Time-outs. Time-out from reinforcement is a behavioral technique in which socially inappropriate behaviors can be decreased by short-term removal of the patient from overstimulating and sometimes reinforcing situations. Time-outs are most effective with patients who feel loss of social contact as a negative consequence. With time-out, patients have more control over the process, and thus this intervention offers an alternative that involves less humiliation and less risk of injury.

With implementation of this intervention, patients who appear to be escalating are prompted to enter time-out, which is usually a quiet, low-traffic area of the unit. They remain there until they have been nonaggressive for a couple of minutes. Patients who do not comply with time-out instructions are told to enter the seclusion room for further protection of themselves and others.

Token Economy. Another effective behavioral strategy is the implementation of a token economy. In this intervention identified interpersonal skills and self-care behaviors are rewarded with tokens that can be used by the patient to purchase specific items. Behaviors to be targeted are specific to each patient. Guidelines should clearly specify desired behaviors required to receive tokens, the number of tokens to be received for each behavior, and the length of time a desired behavior must be exhibited to receive tokens. Furthermore, in a token economy undesired behaviors can result in the loss of tokens.

Research has shown that inpatient units that have implemented token economies have significantly fewer aggressive episodes than more traditional settings. This strategy for managing aggressive behavior is particularly useful with chronic lower functioning patient populations. This clinical example describes the use of this intervention.

 CLINICAL EXAMPLE

A regressed patient, Mrs. S, refused to get out of bed in the morning. She would not shower, dress, or wash her clothes. When encouraged to do these things, Mrs. S became agitated, swore, and threatened to hit anyone who attempted to assist her.

A token store was set up with the number of tokens required to purchase each item. The following contract was then written for Mrs. S:

Mrs. S will receive two tokens for each of the following behaviors:

▼ Getting out of bed by 7:30 AM
▼ Showering before 8:00 AM
▼ Dressing before 8:00 AM
▼ Being at breakfast table by 8:15 AM
▼ Eating 100% of breakfast tray by 8:45 AM
▼ Arriving to community meeting by 9:00 AM

Penalties
An episode of swearing will result in the loss of 4 tokens.

Psychopharmacology

Pharmacological interventions have proven to be effective in the management of aggressive behavior.[7] They include a variety of therapeutic agents, all of which are discussed in greater detail in Chapter 25.

Antianxiety and Sedative-Hypnotics. These drugs are effective in the management of acute agitation. Benzodiazepines such as lorezapam and clonopin are frequently used during psychiatric emergencies to sedate combative patients. They are not recommended for long-term use because they can result in confusion and dependency and may worsen depressive symptoms. Furthermore, some patients have experienced a disinhibiting effect from benzodiazepines that can result in increased aggressive behavior.

Researchers have also begun to study buspirone, an antianxiety drug that may be effective in the management of aggressive behavior associated with anxiety and depression. In preliminary reports buspirone has also been shown to decrease aggression and agitation in patients with head injuries, dementia, and developmental disabilities.

Antidepressants. Antidepressants have been shown to be effective in controlling impulsive and aggressive behavior associated with mood changes. Amitriptyline and trazodone have been reportedly effective in treating aggression associated with head injuries and organic mental disorders.

Mood Stabilizers. Studies have shown lithium to be effective in the treatment of aggression resulting from mania. Some evidence also shows that lithium may be useful in decreasing aggression resulting from other disorders such as mental retardation, head injuries, schizophrenia, and personality disorders. In patients with temporal lobe epilepsy, lithium may actually increase the frequency of aggressive acts. More research is needed to study the effects of this drug on aggressive behavior.

Carbamazepine has been shown to be effective in managing aggressive behavior in patients with abnormal electroencephalograms (EEGs). In one study eight patients with schizophrenia with abnormal EEGs demonstrated a decrease in aggressive behavior after being treated with carbamazepine despite a previously negative response to neuroleptics. There is also some evidence that carbamazepine may be effective in managing agitated behavior associated with dementia. Although very effective for many patients, carbamazepine is not without its risks. It can have adverse side effects such as aplastic anemia and hepatotoxicity.

Antipsychotics. Neuroleptics have been commonly used for the treatment of aggression. They cause sedation, and it is this sedation rather than the antipsychotic properties that are often effective for treating acute aggressive behavior. If the agitation is the result of delusions, hallucinations, or other psychotic behavior, the antipsychotic properties may be helpful but may take 2 to 3 weeks before their effects may be evident. Long-term management of aggressive behavior with antipsychotic medications is not recommended because of the potentially debilitating side effects of tardive dyskinesia.

Other Medications. Several case reports have suggested that naltrexone, an opiate antagonist, may reduce self-injurious behavior. This effect has been particularly notable in patients with developmental disabilities.

Beta-blockers such as propranolol have also been shown to decrease aggressive behavior in children, adults, and particularly in patients with organic mental disorder. Nurses should be aware of the side effects of beta-blockers including hypotension, bradycardia, and in some cases, depression.

How do the strategies for managing aggressive behavior relate to the theories of aggression described earlier in this chapter?

CRISIS MANAGEMENT TECHNIQUES

There are times when attempts at early intervention are unsuccessful and more active intervention is necessary. If the patient is exhibiting behavior that is dangerous either to self or others it may be unwise and unsafe to attempt a verbal intervention. This is evident in the following clinical example.

CLINICAL EXAMPLE

Mr. B was a 32-year-old man with a medical diagnosis of paranoid personality disorder. He was admitted to the locked ward of a psychiatric hospital because he had been arrested after his neighbors complained that he was letting the air out of their tires. He said that he did this because the neighbors laughed at him and talked about him when he was out walking his dog. He was angry about being arrested and wanted to leave the hospital, but he was held under commitment because he also threatened to burn down the house of the neighbor who had called the police.

Mr. B resisted the admission procedure. He belligerently demanded to be released, threatening to call the governor and "sue everybody in the place." When he was asked to undress for a physical examination, he ran down the hall and barricaded himself in the dining room. As staff forcibly entered the room, he began to lash out. Several staff members removed him to a seclusion room, where he was given intramuscular medication and isolated until he regained control of his behavior. He paced the floor and pounded on the door for 30 minutes before he began to appear calmer.

Several days later, when Mr. B was used to the staff and felt more comfortable in the hospital, he related to a nurse, "I hope I didn't hurt you the other night, but I didn't know what you wanted to do to me. A man has to protect himself, you know."

Experience and wisdom are needed to determine when the time for talking is over and when physical intervention is necessary. Nonviolent physical control and restraint should be used only as a last resort. Like medical emergencies, psychiatric emergencies require immediate action.

Team Response

Effective crisis management must be organized and should be directed by one clearly identified crisis leader (Box 27-6).[5] Since psychiatric nurses are responsible for the management of patient care 24 hours a day, it is most appropriate that the crisis leader be a nurse. The leader may be the charge nurse, the primary nurse, nurse manager, or a staff nurse; however, the individual should be decided in advance. Other staff members, including physicians, nurses, and counselors, can be used for support. The crisis leader must decide the intervention necessary to ensure the safety of both patients and staff. This decision can be a difficult one to make, especially when the acuity of the situation does not always allow adequate time to discuss all possible strategies with the entire treatment team.

Box 27-6

PROCEDURE FOR MANAGING PSYCHIATRIC EMERGENCIES

1. Identify crisis leader
2. Assemble crisis team
3. Notify security officers if necessary
4. Remove all other patients from area
5. Obtain restraints if appropriate
6. Devise a plan to manage crisis and inform team
7. Assign securing of patient limbs to crisis team members
8. Explain necessity of intervention to patient and attempt to enlist cooperation
9. Restrain patient when directed by crisis leader
10. Administer medication if ordered
11. Maintain calm, consistent approach to patient
12. Review crisis management interventions with crisis team
13. Process events with other patients and staff as appropriate
14. Gradually reintegrate patient into milieu

Once the decision to intervene has been made, the crisis leader must organize and assemble assistance to manage the crisis. All members of the crisis team should be trained in team crisis management and have experience working as a cohesive group. The staff should be prepared to intervene under the direction of the crisis leader. In many inpatient facilities, hospital security personnel also are notified when assistance is needed. It is the responsibility of the crisis leader to be acquainted with the security officers, give them a brief description of the situation, describe the intervention, and identify the role of security personnel in managing the crisis. Since security officers are not mental health professionals, their assistance should be used only when the patient cannot be physically managed by the nursing staff. Often, there is little time for planning, and the leader must balance the need to act quickly with the need to be organized so that the safety of the patients and the staff is not jeopardized.

The leader is also responsible for ensuring the safety of the other patients during a crisis. This can be accomplished by assigning a staff member to remove the other patients from the area. Quite often the other patients become more acutely distressed in response to a psychiatric emergency on the unit and require extra nursing attention both during and after the crisis. After the crisis has passed, allowing patients to verbalize their anxiety and concern about the crisis and processing it with them can be helpful. It is not appropriate to encourage this activity during a crisis intervention.

A room without furniture should always be readily available for an emergency. If restraints are necessary, they need to be obtained from an easily accessible place. To protect the patient and the staff, the leader must assess the situation quickly and devise a plan. This should include a brief explanation to the staff of the patient's behavior and the intervention necessary. Those staff members who will be directly involved in the intervention should each be assigned to secure one of the patient's limbs when directed to do so. The leader must also explain to the team what will be said to the patient and on what signal the staff should secure the patient's limbs. As they approach within 6 to 8 feet from the patient, the leader should express concern for the patient's safety and the behavior demonstrated that has caused such concern. The patient should then be escorted to the appropriate room and informed of the necessary intervention. It should be emphasized that the intervention is not a punishment but is being provided to help ensure the safety of the patient and the rest of the unit.

If restraints are to be used, the patient should be asked to lie on the bed with arms at one's side. Quite often, the presence of several staff is enough to enlist the patient's cooperation. If the patient is unable to cooperate, the patient should be told that the staff will be assisting. Patients often hesitate at this point in their attempt to remain in control. If patients cannot cooperate within several seconds, they may be unable to cooperate at all, and the leader must then direct the staff to restrain the patient as planned. This can be very frightening for patients and they may need several reminders that they will not be hurt but that the staff will protect them from their impulses.

During this time it is critically important that the leader relate to the patient in a calm, steady voice and manner. Any anxiety or ambivalence will be conveyed to the patient and contribute to a feeling of insecurity. A leader who is anxious will be unable to think clearly about the situation. Many patients are afraid of losing control, and they become assaultive not because they want to frighten people but because they, themselves, are frightened. If the staff shows control of the situation, the patient's escalation is often defused. When the crisis team is overwhelmed by their own fears of the patient, they cannot be effective in reducing the patient's fear. Consistency is also important so that the patient cannot bargain with or manipulate staff members. If the leader is indecisive, inconsistent, or easily manipulated, the patient will not be assured that the staff can guarantee safety by controlling the situation.

After the crisis is over, it is recommended that the team discuss any concerns they may have had during the crisis, since this type of intervention can be stressful for both staff and patients. The patient's behavior may have evoked feelings of guilt, anger, or aggression in the staff. These issues should be discussed as a team so that care is consistent, interventions are therapeutic, and staff do not become discouraged, negative, or burned out. The final intervention is a reevaluation of the patient's status and the gradual reintegration of the patient into the milieu.

Seclusion

There are times when secluding or separating the patient from others in a safe, contained environment is the most appropriate nursing intervention. It is a useful nursing intervention when the goal is to protect a patient, other patients, and staff from potential harm. As such, seclusion is a therapeutic intervention with specific indications for how it is implemented and anticipated outcomes.

Often staff members may have negative or conflicting views about using restrictive interventions such as seclusion and restraints. They may believe that they will betray the patient's trust and could jeopardize the relationships between the staff and patient. Some staff may believe that it is unethical or nontherapeutic to restrict a patient's freedom.[32] However, used appropriately, seclusion and restraints are legal, ethical, and therapeutic nursing interventions.

Degrees of seclusion vary. They include confining a patient in a room with a closed but unlocked door to placing a patient in a locked room with a mattress but no linens and with limited opportunity for communication. Patients may be dressed in their clothes or in hospital clothing. A mattress and sheet or blanket are the minimally acceptable conditions for seclusion.

The theoretical and clinical rationale for the use of seclusion is typically based on three principles:

1. Containment
2. Isolation
3. Decrease in sensory input

Using the principle of containment, the patient is restricted to a place where he is safe from harming himself, and the rest of the unit is also safe from the patient's impulsive behavior. Isolation addresses the need for the patient to distance oneself from relationships, which because of the illness, are pathologically intense. Some patients, particularly those with paranoia, distort the meaning of the interactions around them. Their distortions create such psychic pain that seclusion may provide some relief and may be the only place they feel safe from their "persecutors". Seclusion also provides a smaller area for these patients to master, allowing for a gradual increase in their interactions with others. The third principle is that seclusion provides a decrease in sensory input for those patients whose illness results in a heightened sensitivity to external stimulation. The quiet atmosphere and monotony of a seclusion room may provide some relief from the sensory overload. Nursing interventions related to seclusion are presented in Box 27-7.

Legal requirements for the care of the secluded patient vary from state to state. Good nursing care includes optimum fulfillment of basic human needs and concern for personal dignity. The nurse must assist the patient to meet biological needs by providing food and fluids, a comfortable environment, and opportunity for use of the bathroom. Frequent observation is essential. The room must be constructed so the patient can be observed without being unnecessarily exposed to those who are not involved in his care. Staff should be able to communicate with the patient. Careful records should include all nursing care and observation of the isolated patient. The need for continued isolation should be assessed on a regular basis. It may be necessary for the nurse to initiate this review of the patient's condition with other health team members.

There appears to be a gap between the understanding of staff and patients regarding each others' feelings and intentions related to seclusion.[27,33] Therefore it is recommended that staff spend more time talking with patients about the issues that led to seclusion and alternative methods of coping that might help the patient avoid seclusion in the future.

The nursing staff should always review the events that led up to the decision to isolate a patient. In particular, staff should be encouraged to give each other feedback about interpersonal relationships involving the secluded patient. Preventive measures that may assist the patient to gain control in the future without requiring seclusion should be identified. It is also useful for staff to ventilate their own feelings following an episode of seclusion. Management of violent behavior is physically and emotionally stressful.

One of the best ways to understand the patients' point of view is to "walk in their shoes." Arrange to spend 15 minutes alone in the seclusion room on a psychiatric unit. Dare you try on the restraints? Describe your thoughts and feelings during this time.

Restraints

Restraints involve the use of mechanical or manual devices to limit the physical mobility of the patient. Such an intervention may be indicated to protect the patient or others from injury, particularly if less restrictive interventions, such as environmental change and behavioral strategies, have failed.

Box 27-7

NURSING INTERVENTIONS RELATED TO SECLUSION

DEFINITION

Solitary containment in a fully protective environment with close surveillance by nursing staff for purposes of safety or behavior management

ACTIVITIES

Obtain a physician's order, if required by institutional policy, to use a physically restrictive intervention

Designate one nursing staff member to communicate with the patient and to direct other staff

Identify for patient and significant others those behaviors that necessitated the intervention

Explain procedure, purpose, and time period of the intervention to patient and significant others in understandable and nonpunitive terms

Explain to patient and significant others the behaviors necessary for termination of the intervention

Contract with patient (as patient is able) to maintain control of behavior

Instruct on self-control methods as appropriate

Assist in dressing in clothing that is safe and in removing jewelry and eyeglasses

Remove all items from seclusion area that patient might use to harm self or nursing staff

Assist with needs related to nutrition, elimination, hydration, and personal hygiene

Provide food and fluids in nonbreakable containers

Provide appropriate level of supervision/surveillance to monitor patient and to allow for therapeutic actions as needed

Acknowledge your presence to patient periodically

Administer PRN medications for anxiety or agitation

Provide for patient's psychological comfort as needed

Monitor seclusion area for temperature, cleanliness, safety

Arrange for routine cleaning of seclusion area

Evaluate at regular intervals patient's need for continued restrictive intervention

Involve patient, when appropriate, in making decisions to move to a more/less restrictive form of intervention

Determine patient's need for continued seclusion

Document the rationale for use of restrictive intervention, patient's response to the intervention, patient's physical condition and nursing care provided throughout the intervention, and rationale for terminating the intervention

Process with the patient and staff, upon termination of the restrictive intervention, the circumstances that led to the use of the intervention as well as any patient concerns about the intervention itself

Provide the next appropriate level of restrictive intervention (e.g., physical restraint, area restriction) as needed

From McCloskey JC, Bulechek GM: *Nursing interventions classification*, St Louis, 1992, Mosby.

The American Psychiatric Association[2] has outlined the following five criteria for the appropriate use of physical intervention, seclusion and restraint:

1. To prevent imminent harm to the patient or other persons when other means of control are ineffective or inappropriate
2. To preclude serious disruption of the treatment program or significant damage to the physical environment
3. To maintain treatment as part of an ongoing plan of behavioral therapy
4. To decrease the amount of stimulation a patient receives
5. To comply with a patient's own request

The primary indication for restraints is the control of violent behavior, either self-directed or directed toward others, that cannot be controlled by medication or psychosocial techniques. Patients who benefit from the use of this technique include those whose physical condition prevents or limits the use of medication. For example, a patient who may have developed a toxic reaction to anticholinergic medication may require restraints to control problematic behaviors until the toxicity has resolved. For these patients the use of restraints may be less harmful than the use of additional medications. Other indications for the use of restraints include hyperactivity, insomnia, decreased food and fluid intake, and grossly impaired judgment. Restraints may also be used to reduce disruptive effects of excessive stimulation that have resulted in increased agitation and confusion. Finally, patients sometimes request the use of restraints. Their request for external control should be acknowledged but should be differentiated from attempts to gain excessive attention, ensure dependency gratification, or legitimize regression. Each situation should be assessed carefully for the most appropriate and least restrictive intervention. Nursing interventions related to the use of restraints are presented in Box 27-8.

The patient in mechanical restraint may be confused or delirious and will probably be frightened at the limitation of movement. The nurse should not assume that the patient understands the need for restraint. Support and reassurance are essential. Restraints should be applied efficiently and with care not to injure a combative patient. Adequate personnel need to be assembled before the patient is approached. Each staff member should be assigned responsibility for controlling specific body parts. Restraints should be available and in working order. Padding of cuff restraints helps to prevent skin breakdown. For the same reason, the patient should be positioned in anatomical alignment. Provision of privacy is important. If visitors are allowed, the nurse should explain the treatment and the reason for it before they see the patient; this may help them accept the situa-

---

Box 27-8

NURSING INTERVENTIONS RELATED TO PHYSICAL RESTRAINT

DEFINITION

Application and monitoring of mechanical restraining devices or manual restraints to limit physical mobility of patient

ACTIVITIES

Obtain a physician's order, if required by institutional policy, to use a physically restrictive intervention

Provide patient with a private yet adequately supervised environment in situations where a patient's sense of dignity may be diminished by the use of physical restraints

Provide sufficient staff to assist with safe application of physical restraining devices or manual restraints

Designate one nursing staff member to direct staff and communicate with the patient during the application of physical restraints

Use appropriate hold when manually restraining patient in emergency situations or during transport

Identify for patient and significant others those behaviors that necessitated the intervention

Explain procedure, purpose, and time period of the intervention to patient and significant others in understandable and nonpunitive terms

Explain to patient and significant others the behaviors necessary for termination of the intervention

Monitor the patient's response to procedure

Avoid tying restraints to siderails of bed

Secure restraints out of patient's reach

Provide appropriate level of supervision/surveillance to monitor patient and to allow for therapeutic actions as needed

Provide for patient's psychological comfort as needed

Provide diversional activities, when appropriate (e.g., television, read to patient, visitors, mobiles) to facilitate patient cooperation with the intervention

Administer PRN medications for anxiety or agitation

Monitor skin condition of restraint site(s)

Monitor color, temperature, and sensation frequently in restrained extremities

Provide for limited movement according to patient's level of self-control

Position patient to facilitate comfort and to prevent aspiration and skin breakdown

Provide for movement of extremities in patient with multiple restraints by rotating the removal/reapplication of one restraint at a time (as safety permits)

Assist with periodic changes in body position

Provide the dependent patient with a means of summoning help (e.g., bell, call light) when caregiver is not present

Assist with needs related to nutrition, elimination, hydration, and personal hygiene

Evaluate, at regular intervals, patient's need for continued restrictive intervention

Involve patient, when appropriate, in making decisions to move to a more/less restrictive form of intervention

Remove restraints gradually (i.e., one at a time if in four point restraints) as self-control increases

Monitor patient's response to removal of restraints

Process with the patient and staff, upon termination of the restrictive intervention, the circumstances that led to the use of the intervention as well as any patient concerns about the intervention itself

Provide the next appropriate level of restrictive intervention (e.g., area restriction, seclusion) as needed

Document the rationale for use of restrictive intervention, patient's response to the intervention, patient's physical condition and nursing care provided throughout the intervention, and rationale for terminating the intervention

---

From McCloskey JC, Bulechek GM: *Nursing interventions classification*, St Louis, 1992, Mosby.

tion. Physical needs must be included in the nursing care plan. Vital signs should be checked, and regular observation of circulation in the extremities is necessary. Fluids should be offered regularly and opportunities for elimination provided. Skin care is also essential. Restraints must be released at least every 2 hours to allow exercise of the extremities.

Despite explanations of the therapeutic purpose of the intervention, it is not uncommon for patients to perceive the use of restraints as a punishment. This may result in further discomfort in the staff. Designating an authority figure, such as the charge nurse, as the crisis leader may help to preserve the therapeutic alliance between the patient and the staff members working more closely with the patient.

Terminating the Intervention

The decision to terminate the use of seclusion or restraints should be well planned. Reviewing the behavior that precipitated the intervention and patient's current capacity to exercise control over their behavior are key factors. Patients should be told which behaviors they need to exhibit and which behaviors or impulses they need to control before the intervention can be discontinued. Communication and careful documentation are critical in making an accurate assessment of a patient's level of control. The difficulty arises when patients appear to be in control for brief periods of time but then quickly decompensate. Their behavior may be subject to diurnal variation and changes in response to different staff members.

Patients should be gradually reintegrated into the milieu. This allows them to test out their control without feeling overwhelmed. Patients are initially reintegrated by reducing restraints from four points to three points and then to two points as soon as they begin to regain control. However, a patient should not be left in just a one point restraint because the risk of injury is potentially high. Once restraints have been discontinued altogether, or once a patient no longer requires locked seclusion, the patient may be given a specified amount of time out of the room. This amount of time will be gradually increased as the patient is successfully able to maintain control in the milieu. The primary nurse, in collaboration with the treatment team, can coordinate this into the interdisciplinary plan of care.

The success of the patient's reintegration into the milieu depends largely on the consistency of the staff. Some staff members may question the need to follow the time-structured outline if the patient appears to be in control. However, if the staff do not see the importance of the plan, neither will the patient, and cooperation will be more difficult to enlist. Some staff may wish to adhere to a structured room program only if the patient decompensates, but patients who are thrust back into a busy unit can be quickly overwhelmed with the sudden increase in stimulation. Sending them to their room after they have lost control again only reinforces their inability to stay in control and is more likely to be viewed by the patient as punishment. Thus gradual reintegration into the milieu is more likely to ensure the success of these patients to maintain control and increase their feelings of achievement.

Finally, debriefing is an important part of terminating the use of seclusion or restraints. **Debriefing** is a therapeutic intervention that includes reviewing the facts related to an event and processing the response to them. It provides staff and patients with an opportunity to clarify the rationale for the seclusion, offer mutual feedback, and promote more adaptive functioning. When staff engage in this activity it is sometimes referred to as a **postmortem.**

STAFF DEVELOPMENT

Effective management of potentially dangerous patients requires highly skilled staff. Nurses, physicians, and other support staff, including security personnel, all need to be trained in emergency psychiatric care and crisis management techniques. It has been found that the rate of staff injury from patient violence can be reduced significantly if staff are trained in crisis management techniques.[6] Education should focus on assessment of the patient, particularly mental status, motor behavior, affect, and speech. Verbal intervention should be stressed as a way of defusing agitation, and helpful and nonhelpful responses should be reviewed.

Education

All nursing interventions should be grounded in theory, and crisis intervention in psychiatric emergencies is no exception. The theoretical basis for various intervention strategies should be discussed as part of the training. Pharmacological interventions should be reviewed with particular attention given to the choice medication, its purpose, and its potential adverse effects. Ongoing practice sessions in crisis management should be required of all staff. These sessions should include basic self-protection maneuvers and strategies for restraining assaultive patients. Each member of the staff should be able to function as a leader in the event of a crisis, and the staff as a whole must be able to function smoothly as a cohesive emergency team. The nursing and medical care of these patients should be reviewed as well as the impact of countertransference issues. Finally, it is strongly recommended that the current state laws regarding the civil rights of patients be discussed in staff meetings to ensure that care given to patients is both proper and respectful of their rights.

Staff Assault

Unfortunately, nurses are sometimes assaulted by patients. It is impossible to succeed in predicting and preventing all episodes of violent behavior in a psychiatric setting. If a staff member is assaulted, the support and assistance of colleagues are needed. Lanza[14,15] has studied the reactions of nursing staff to physical assault by a patient. The response is similar to that experienced during the posttraumatic stress syndrome. Surprisingly, she found that many staff members were reluctant to identify any response to the assault. She thought that this might be related to a sense of guilt for not having prevented the episode and concern that others would not understand.

Ryan and Poster[29] studied the responses of 61 nurses who had been assaulted by patients. Their responses included "anger, anxiety, helplessness, irritability, soreness, hyperalertness, sadness, depression, shock, disbelief that the assault occurred, feeling sorry for the patient who committed the assault, and a feeling that they should have done something to prevent the assault." Eighty-two percent of the nurses had resolved their crisis state by the sixth week after the assault.

Nursing staff members who have been assaulted can be helped in a number of ways. One idea is the peer support group, which legitimizes staff responses and allows for the expression of feelings in a supportive setting. Another approach is to develop a staff action program made up of volunteers who work with staff in critical incident debriefing, running support groups and offering specialized services such as family and community meetings.[10] A final suggestion is the implementation of a nursing consultation support service that responds to the needs of assault victims and sets the tone for institutional attitudes of nonblaming concern.[26] All of these programs have merit and each organization should select the best way to deal with the problem of staff assault based on their environment, group process, and institutional resources.

Legal Action

Finally, there has been debate about whether staff should be encouraged to file legal charges against a patient who has intentionally assaulted them. Phelan and associates[28] presented several points in support of filing charges. They included the creation of a public record of assaultive behavior, allowing a judge and jury to fulfill their duty of determining responsibility, possible deterrence of future attacks, and the potential for harsher penalties for repeat offenders. Phelan and associates attributed much of the difficulty that staff have in pursuing this course of action to the ethical dilemma of deciding whether assaultive patients were actually responsible for their behavior. In addition, if care providers feel guilty for allowing the incident to occur, they are unlikely to take legal action against the patient.

This is an issue that must be resolved by the nurse based on the situation. In doing so, it would be very helpful to seek the advice of a trusted professional mentor.

SUMMARY

1. High rates of assaultive behavior have been reported in a variety of health-care settings including outpatient clinics, nursing homes, and emergency departments. By far the highest rates of assault occur in psychiatric settings.

2. Within each person lies the capacity for passive, assertive, or aggressive behavior. The situation and the characteristics of the individual define the most appropriate response.

3. Theories on the development of aggressive behavior include psychoanalytical, psychological, behavioral, sociocultural, and neurobiological.

4. The best single predictor of violence is a history of violence. It is also important to assess the patient's current clinical condition and situation.

5. Nurses need to assess possible precipitants of violent behavior, issues related to provocation, and biological factors. A screening tool may be useful in this process.

6. Many nursing interventions may be helpful in dealing with aggressive behavior including self-awareness, patient education, assertiveness training, communication strategies, environmental strategies, behavioral strategies, and psychopharmacology.

7. Effective crisis management must be organized and clearly directed by one team leader. Seclusion and restraint should be used only as a last resort.

8. Staff development issues include educating staff in crisis management techniques, working with staff who have been assaulted, and understanding the implications of possible legal action.

COMPETENT CARING
A CLINICAL EXEMPLAR OF A PSYCHIATRIC NURSE

Mary Brown, RN

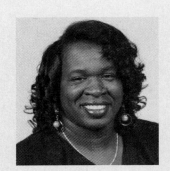

When I think about aggressive behavior, I think back to an incident that could have ended badly, but instead the people involved received the help needed. I was working as a case manager for an agency that provided intensive case management for chronically mentally ill individuals. The event took place on a weekend. Office hours were 9 AM until 5PM during the week, and there was someone on call after working hours and on all weekends.

I was on call this particular weekend. One of the agency's patients had been hospitalized and was now ready for discharge. This particular patient was deaf, and I was to pick him up from the hospital and see that he was settled in his home. After leaving the hospital with the patient, my beeper went off and I needed to call the answering service. I was close to the office, so I stopped there to use the phone. The building has two stories, and I had access to only the top floor. I climbed the stairs, the discharged deaf patient behind me, unlocked the door, and turned around to shut the door, but a large hand kept me from doing so.

The owner of this big hand was over 6 feet tall, weighed approximately 250 pounds, and appeared to be psychotic. He forced his way into the building with the patient and myself. I was now terrified. He stated, "I came to get my money," in an angry and loud tone of voice.

I then recognized him as a patient I had worked with before and could see the changes in him, which made me feel unsafe to be alone with him. I tried very hard not to let him know how frightened I was of him. I told him the office was closed and he needed to come back Monday, when the appropriate people could help him. He shouted, "I want my money now!" I became increasingly frightened. There was no panic button to push for help. There were no other staff to distract him to allow me to get my deaf patient and myself to safety. I was the one who needed to protect the patient and myself.

In a calm tone of voice, I told him I couldn't help him with getting his money. I told him I would need to go to the staff room, (he was aware that patients were not allowed in this room) and call someone to help him. He followed me into the room. I firmly told him that he was not allowed to be in the room and to please leave. He sat down anyway. I told him I was only at the office to return an emergency call. I called the service and the doctor who paged me was checking to see if everything went okay with the discharged patient. I told him about the intrusion from the angry and irrational man who was insisting on not leaving before he got his money. The doctor said he would call the police. While waiting for the police, I kept trying to get the patient to leave the room. He repeatedly refused. He sat at one end of the table and I sat at the other end. The deaf patient was watching our interaction intensely.

The angry patient appeared to be responding to internal stimuli. He was looking at me and began to laugh. He stopped laughing and said, "Why won't you go out with me," as he proceeded to my end of the table. I told him firmly that this behavior was not appropriate. I reinforced that I was his nurse and again I asked him to leave the room. He stopped, looked at me unexpectedly, and said, "I'll be back on Monday to get my money."

When I heard the door slam, I quickly locked the door. The doctor called back to say that the police were on their way and asked if everything was okay. While shivering, I said yes. The police picked the angry patient up downstairs and found a screwdriver on him. He told them that he was at the office before I arrived and intended to break into the office to take his money. The deaf patient who was watching all this communicated with me by writing on a piece of paper—"Are you alright? I can tell you were afraid of him." I was amazed. Nonverbal communication works both ways.

As a nurse, I am trained to look at what is not being said and make a determination. I realized that the deaf patient could look at my nonverbal communication and also make a determination. I also realized the value of setting firm limits and at all times giving clear, consistent and nonthreatening messages when managing aggressive behavior. ▼

REFERENCES

1. American Psychiatric Association: *Diagnostic and statistical manual of mental disorders*, ed 4, Washington, DC, 1994, The Association.
2. American Psychiatric Association: *Report of the task force on psychiatric uses of seclusion and restraint*, Washington, DC, 1985, The Association.
3. Blair D, New S: Assaultive: know the risk behavior, *J Psychosoc Nurs Ment Health Serv* 29:11, 1991.
4. Blomhoff S, Seim S, Friis S: Can prediction of violence among psychiatric inpatients be improved? *Hosp Community Psychiatry* 41:771, 1990.
5. Cahill C, Stuart G, Laraia M, Arana G: Inpatient management of violent behavior: nursing prevention and intervention, *Issues Ment Health Nurs* 12:239, 1991.
6. Carmel H, Hunter M: Compliance with training in managing assaultive behavior and injuries from inpatient violence, *Hosp Community Psychiatry* 41:558, 1990.
7. Corrigan P, Yudofsky S, Silver J: Pharmacological and behavioral treatments for aggressive psychiatric inpatients, *Hosp Community Psychiatry* 44:125, 1993.
8. Davis S: Violence by psychiatric inpatients: a review, *Hosp Community Psychiatry* 42:585, 1991.
9. Dollard J: *Frustration and aggression*, New Haven, Conn, 1939, Yale University Press.
10. Flannery R, Fulton P, Tausch J, DeLoffi A: A program to help staff cope with psychological sequelae of assaults by patients, *Hosp Community Psychiatry* 42:935, 1991.
11. Harper-Jacques S, Reimer M: Aggressive behavior and the brain: a different perspective for the mental health nurse, *Arch Psychiatr Nurs* 6:312, 1992.
12. Jaques S, Reimer M: Aggressive behavior and the brain: a different perspective for the mental health nurse, *Arch Psychiatr Nurs* 6:312, 1992.
13. Lande R: The video violence debate, *Hosp Community Psychiatry* 44:347, 1993.
14. Lanza M: The reactions of nursing staff to physical assault by a patient, *Hosp Community Psychiatry* 34:44, 1983.
15. Lanza M: A follow-up study of nurses' reactions to physical assault, *Hosp Community Psychiatry* 35:492, 1984.
16. Lanza M: Factors relevant to patient assault, *Issues Ment Health Nurs* 9:239, 1988.

17. Lanza M: Predictors of patient assault on acute inpatient psychiatric units: a pilot study, *Issues Ment Health Nurs* 9:259, 1988.

18. Lowenstein M, Binder R, McNiel D: The relationship between admission symptoms and hospital assaults, *Hosp Community Psychiatry* 41:311, 1990.

19. McNiel D, Binder R: Clinical assessment of the risk of violence among psychiatric inpatients, *Am J Psychiatry* 148:1317, 1991.

20. Menninger W: Management of the aggressive and dangerous patient, *Bull Menninger Clin* 57:208, 1993.

21. Miller R, Zadolinnyj K, Hafner R, Phil M: Profiles and predictors of assaultiveness for different psychiatric ward populations, *Am J Psychiatry* 150:9, 1993.

22. Morrison E: Violent psychiatric patients in a public hospital, *Scholar Inq Nurs Pract* 4:65, 1990.

23. Morrison E: A coercive interactive style as an antecedent to aggression and violence in psychiatric patients, *Res Nurs Health* 15:421, 1992.

24. Morrison E: A hierarchy of aggressive and violent behaviors among psychiatric inpatients, *Hosp Community Psychiatry* 43:505, 1992.

25. Morrison E: Toward a better understanding of violence in psychiatric settings: debunking the myths, *Arch Psychiatr Nurs* 7:328, 1993.

26. Murray M, Snyder J: When staff are assaulted, *J Psychosoc Nurs Ment Health Serv* 29:24, 1991.

27. Norris M, Kennedy C: How patients perceive the seclusion process, *J Psychosoc Nurs Ment Health Serv* 30:7, 1992.

28. Phelan L, Mills M, Ryan J: Prosecuting psychiatric patients for assault, *Hosp Community Psychiatry* 36:581, 1985.

29. Ryan J, Poster E: The assaulted nurse: short-term and long-term responses, *Arch Psychiatr Nurs* 3:323, 1989.

30. Sheridan M, Henrion R, Robinson L, Baxter V: Precipitants of violence in a psychiatric inpatient setting, *Hosp Community Psychiatry* 41:776, 1990.

31. Stevenson S: Heading off violence with verbal de-escalation, *J Psychosoc Nurs Ment Health Serv* 29:6, 1991.

32. Stilling L: The pros and cons of physical restraints and behavior controls, *J Psychosoc Nurs Ment Health Serv* 30:18, 1992.

33. Tooke S, Brown J: Perceptions of seclusion, *J Psychosoc Nurs* 30:23, 1992.

ANNOTATED SUGGESTED READINGS

American Psychiatric Association Task Force on Clinician Safety: *Clinician safety (task force report 33)*, Washington, DC, 1993, American Psychiatric Association.

Small booklet containing tips for clinicians, two case reports, and a bibliography.

*Blair D, New S: Assaultive: know the risk behavior, *J Psychosoc Nurs Ment Health Serv* 29:11, 1991.

Excellent overview from a nursing perspective of the risk factors and interventions related to assaultive behavior.

*Chenevert M: STAT: *special techniques in assertiveness training for women in the health professions*, St Louis, 1993, Mosby.

Applies the principles of assertiveness theory to the experience of women, especially nurses, in health-care settings. Good practical suggestions.

Corrigan P, Yudofsky S, Silver J: Pharmacological and behavioral treatments for aggressive psychiatric inpatients, *Hosp Community Psychiatry* 44:125, 1993.

Excellent and sophisticated overview of current behavioral and pharmacologic treatments for aggressive behavior.

---

*Nursing reference.

*Craig C, Ray F, Hix C: Seclusion and restraint: decreasing the discomfort, J Psychosoc Nurs Ment Health Serv 27:16, 1989.

Analyzes the many variables related to restrictive treatment including structural change, staffing, education, and interdisciplinary involvement.

Davis S: Violence by psychiatric inpatients: a review. Hosp Community Psychiatry 42:585, 1991.

Perhaps the best summary of factors related to violence in the inpatient psychiatric setting, including incidence and prevalence and individual, situational, and structural factors.

*Harper-Jacques S, Reimer M: Aggressive behavior and the brain: a different perspective for the mental health nurse, Arch Psychiatr Nurs 6:312, 1992.

Describes the biological basis for aggressive behavior with suggestions for proactive nursing interventions.

*Lanza M: Factors relevant to patient assault, Issues Ment Health Nurs 9:239, 1988.

Good example of nursing research related to patient assault. More research like this is needed in the field.

*Morrison E: Toward a better understanding of violence in psychiatric settings: debunking the myths, Arch Psychiatr Nurs 7:328, 1993.

Explores five myths about violence and offers alternatives to nurses interested in changing their approach to dealing with violent behavior.

*Norris M, Kennedy C: How patients perceive the seclusion process, J Psychosoc Nurs Ment Health Serv 30:7, 1992.

Reports in detail patients' perceptions of seclusion and the need for debriefing with the patient at the end of the intervention.

*Stevenson S: Heading off violence with verbal deescalation, J Psychosoc Nurs Ment Health Serv 29:6, 1991.

Nice review of verbal deescalation techniques for nurses.

Tesar G: The agitated patient: Part I. Evaluation and behavioral management, Hosp Community Psychiatry 44:329, 1993.

Discusses the evaluation, differential diagnosis, and behavioral treatment of agitated patients in the emergency room setting.

*Tooke S, Brown J: Perceptions of seclusion, J Psychosoc Nurs Ment Health Serv 30:23, 1992.

Compares and contrasts the perceptions of patients and nurses regarding seclusion. Interesting and important differences are described.

*Turnball J, Aiken I, Black L, Patterson B: Turn it around: short-term management for aggression and anger, J Psychosoc Nurs Ment Health Serv 28:7, 1990.

Describes in detail a training course that was developed to give nursing staff crisis management skills. Useful for inservices.

---

*Nursing reference.

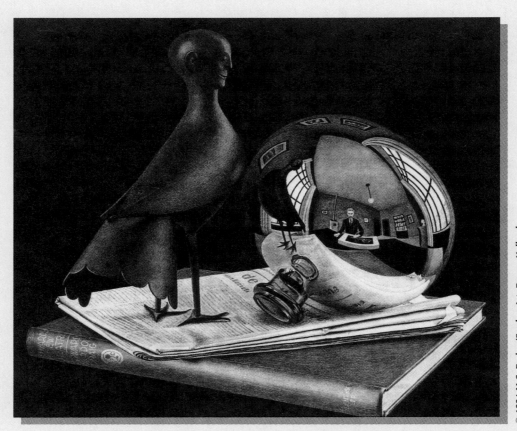

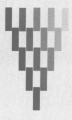

C H A P T E R   2 8
Cognitive Behavioral Therapy

GAIL W. STUART

But humanism stands for the whole person, the whole individual striving to become as conscious and responsible as possible about everything in the universe. But now you sit there quite calmly and as a humanist you say that due to the complexity of scientific achievement the human being must never expect to be whole, he must always be frightened.

Doris Lessing: The Golden Notebook

LEARNING OBJECTIVES

After studying this chapter the student should be able to:

▼ Define behavior
▼ Distinguish between classical and operant conditioning
▼ Describe operant conditioning procedures that increase and decrease behavior
▼ Relate the role of cognitions in adaptive and maladaptive coping responses
▼ Compare cognitive behavioral therapy and the nursing process
▼ Identify elements of a cognitive behavioral assessment
▼ Apply cognitive behavioral treatment strategies to nursing practice
▼ Discuss the role of the nurse in cognitive behavioral therapy

TOPICAL OUTLINE

Definition of Behavior
Classical Conditioning
Operant Conditioning
   Increasing Behavior
   Decreasing Behavior
Role of Cognition
Cognitive Behavioral Therapy and the Nursing Process
Cognitive Behavioral Assessment
Treatment Strategies
   Anxiety Reduction
   Cognitive Restructuring
   Learning New Behavior
Role of the Nurse

Cognitive behavioral therapy is the application of various learning theories to problems of living. The aim is to help people overcome difficulties in any area of human activity and experience. Frequently, these problems occur within the context of a clinical disorder. However, the techniques of cognitive behavioral therapy can be applied to education, the workplace, consumer activities, and sports. In these situations, cognitive behavioral therapy can help individuals achieve personal growth by expanding their coping skills. It can be used by nurses with any background and in any health-care setting to promote healthy coping responses and change maladaptive behavior. As such, it represents an important area of knowledge for nursing intervention across the health-illness continuum.

Historically, behavioral therapy was based on the principles of classical conditioning and operant learning. Over time, the social learning theory of Bandura[2] added to the field the importance of cognitions and information processing in influencing behavior. Most recently, this approach has been expanded to include cognitive therapy, which focuses on modifying thoughts, attitudes, and beliefs as well as behaviors.

Cognitive behavioral therapy is problem focused,

goal oriented, and deals with here-and-now issues. It views the individual as the important decision-maker about goals and issues to be dealt with in treatment. This chapter reviews the key concepts of cognitive behavioral therapy, the treatment process, and specific strategies that can be used in nursing practice.

DEFINITION OF BEHAVIOR

Behavior is any observable, recordable, and measurable act, movement, or response of the individual. Before a behavior can be measured it must be accurately described, which is done in different ways. For example, the behavior of eating can be broken down into parts such as selecting the food items, preparing the meal, setting the table, eating the meal, and cleaning the dishes when the food is eaten. In contrast, it can be more globally described as eating dinner. This shows that there can be several different and accurate definitions of what appears to be a single, simple behavior. It also points to the need to begin by describing what is seen or heard and then clarifying this information until the participants agree with the description.

A behavior is what is observed—not the conclusion, inferences, or interpretations drawn from observation. For example, hyperactivity is not a behavior; it is a conclusion drawn from a set of behaviors. Hyperactivity cannot be measured. What can be measured is the number of times a child gets out of his seat, interrupts a conversation, drops a book, or completes required homework assignments. Thus treatment for the child should focus not on hyperactivity but on the specific behaviors that interfere with the child's adjustment to school, home, or the community.

Other examples of inferences rather than behaviors are psychiatric diagnoses and the labeling of patients as uncooperative, aggressive, difficult, noncompliant, or hostile. These adjectives globally describe an individual but do not reflect the specific behavior that led to such conclusions. Similarly, when formulating a nursing diagnosis it is essential that the nurse identify those specific defining characteristics of the nursing diagnosis that apply to the patient. In this way treatment can address the patient's specific behaviors and problems at that particular point in time. In addition, the nurse will have recorded specific behaviors that can be measured over time. These can then be used to evaluate the patient's progress toward expected outcomes.

A clear definition of a behavior minimizes subjective interpretations. A clear definition of a behavior is measurable, is not subject to interpretation, and states what the person does.

CLASSICAL CONDITIONING

Classical conditioning focuses on the process by which **involuntary behavior** is learned. It is derived from Pavlov's[19] famous work in which he taught dogs to salivate at the sound of a bell by associating the bell with meat presented at the same time as the bell. The explanation is that an event occurs when one stimulus, by being paired with another stimulus, comes to produce the same response as the other stimulus. Other examples of classical conditioning include the following:

▼ Blinking in response to directing a puff of air to someone's eye
▼ Salivating at the aroma of fresh cookies baking
▼ Automatically raising the leg when the patellar tendon is struck

A clinical example is when a person becomes conditioned to feel fear in neutral situations that have come to be associated with anxiety, such as fear of heights or travelling in public places. Inconsistent pairings of the two stimuli, however, leads to less reliable learning, and the response gradually disappears if the pairings are discontinued.

OPERANT CONDITIONING

Operant conditioning has been credited to the work of B.F. Skinner and his co-workers.[21] It is concerned with the relationship between **voluntary behavior** and the environment. Operant behaviors are those behaviors that are influenced by the consequences of the action and are regarded as a more complex form of learning. Examples include correcting a spelling mistake when writing a letter or studying class notes before an examination. The basic idea is that behaviors are influenced by their consequences and that operant behaviors are cued by environmental stimuli. Behaviors that have a positive consequence will be stronger and are likely to be repeated. In contrast, behaviors that result in negative consequences will be weakened and are less likely to occur.

For example, if a person tells a joke and everyone who is listening to it laughs heartily, the person will probably repeat that joke in another social setting. If, however, the person tells the joke and everyone stares blankly or appears quiet and embarrassed, it is probable that the person will not repeat the joke in the future.

Unlike classical conditioning, operant conditioning is strengthened rather than weakened by inconsistent pairings of the behaviors and consequences. That is, when a certain behavior is followed unpredictably by positive or negative consequences, it is more likely to recur (Fig. 28-1).

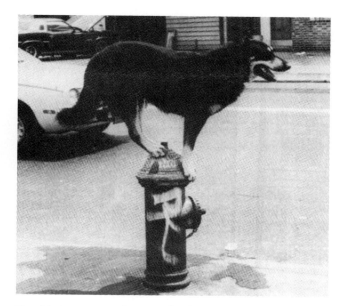

Fig. 28-1   No one knows why, but Joey jumps on the fire hydrant every time he passes it and stays there as long as he is allowed to. Joey's behavior has somehow been operantly conditioned by the promise of a reward that only Joey knows about.

From Barbara Phillips.

Many of the techniques used in operant conditioning fall under the heading of behavior modification. They are based on the assumption that high-frequency, preferred activity can be used to reinforce lower-frequency, nonpreferred activity. For example, if a boy enjoys playing with toy racing cars, this high-frequency preferred activity can be used to reinforce the lower-frequency, nonpreferred activity of tidying his room. However, the terms *reinforcement* and *punishment* when used in operant conditioning do not have the same meaning as when used by most laypeople.

> Give an example of classical and operant conditioning from your work in a psychiatric setting related to either patient or staff behavior.

Increasing Behavior

Reinforcers are literally anything that increase the frequency of a behavior. By far the most commonly applied form of reinforcement to be used is **positive reinforcement,** or rewarding stimuli, for example, when teachers praise students for remaining in their assigned seats. Because of the praise, the students are likely to remain seated more often. However, what is regarded as a posi-

tive reward can be quite subjective, and many times people intending to decrease a behavior actually wind up reinforcing it. For example, when a father yells at his son for fighting with his sibling, the yelling may represent to the son a form of desired parental attention and thus may be interpreted as positive reinforcement. As a consequence the son is likely to continue fighting with his sibling.

Negative reinforcement also increases the frequency of a behavior by reinforcing the behavior's power to control an aversive, rather than rewarding, stimuli. An example is putting on sunglasses in glaring sunlight. The sunlight is an aversive stimulus; putting on the sunglasses is the behavior; escaping the sun's glare is the negative reinforcer. It is negative because it removes or subtracts something from the environment (sunlight) resulting in an increase in the desired behavior (wearing sunglasses). Other examples of negative reinforcement include the following:

1. A child, who is being scolded by his mother, goes up to her and kisses her, and her scolding stops.
2. An adolescent who is having trouble in school runs away from home, thus avoiding his parents' displeasure.
3. Drivers maintain the speed limit to avoid receiving a traffic ticket.

Decreasing Behavior

Three techniques are used to reduce the frequency of behavior—punishment, response cost, and extinction. **Punishment** is an aversive stimuli that occurs after the behavior and serves to decrease its future occurrence. An example is a child who has to stay in from recess because of disrupting the class.

Response cost decreases behavior through the experience of a loss or penalty following a behavior. Examples include paying a fine for overdue library books, losing allowance for not keeping a clean room, or not being able to attend the next school dance because of coming home after curfew.

Extinction is the process of eliminating a behavior by ignoring it or not rewarding it. For example, a child who has frequent temper tantrums is sent to summer camp. On the first day at camp, the child had a tantrum because of not being allowed to sleep in a specific bunk. The counselor ignored the child and continued to interact with the other campers. In the next 2 days the child had three more tantrums, and the counselor continued to ignore the outbursts. After the fourth day the child had no more temper tantrums.

The procedures of operant conditioning are summarized in Box 28-1. They are incorporated in many of the cognitive behavioral treatment strategies, and they can

---

Box 28-1

OPERANT CONDITIONING PROCEDURES

INCREASING BEHAVIOR

Procedure: **Positive reinforcement**
Definition: Adding a rewarding stimulus as a consequence of a behavior, thus increasing the probability that it will occur again

Example: Behavior → Rewarding stimulus → Behavior ↑

Procedure: **Negative reinforcement**
Definition: Removing an aversive stimulus as a consequence of a behavior, thus increasing the probability that it will occur again.

Example: Aversive stimulus → Behavior → Aversive stimulus removed → Behavior ↑

DECREASING BEHAVIOR

Procedure: **Punishment**
Definition: Presentation of an aversive stimulus as a consequence of a behavior, thus decreasing the probability that it will occur again.

Example: Behavior → Aversive stimulus → Behavior ↓

Procedure: **Response cost**
Definition: Loss or withdrawal of a reinforcer as a consequence of a behavior, thus decreasing the probability that it will occur again.

Example: Behavior → Loss of reinforcer → Behavior ↓

Procedure: **Extinction**
Definition: Withholding of a reinforcer as a consequence of a behavior, thus decreasing the probability that it will occur again.

Example: Behavior → Reinforcement → Behavior → No reinforcement → Behavior ↓

---

be used by nurses in all areas of practice to help patients overcome a wide range of problems and resume productive lives.

> Do you think the procedures of operant conditioning can be used by nurses working in medical-surgical settings? Give an example from your experience.

ROLE OF COGNITION

Cognition means the act or process of knowing. In developing the framework for cognitive therapy, Beck[5] and Ellis[9,10] built on previous work in the field, proposing that it is not the events themselves but people's expectations and interpretations of events that cause anxiety and maladaptive responses. Thus they suggested that maladaptive behaviors can be altered by dealing directly with a person's thoughts and beliefs.

Specifically, cognitive therapists believe that maladaptive responses arise from cognitive distortions. These might include errors of logic, mistakes in reasoning, or individualized views of the world that do not reflect reality. Such distortions may be either positive or negative. For example, someone may consistently view

life in an unrealistically positive way and thus take dangerous chances, such as denying health problems and claiming to be "too young and healthy for a heart attack." Cognitive distortions also may be negative, as expressed by a person who interprets all unfortunate life situations as further proof of a complete lack of self-worth. Common cognitive distortions are listed in Box 28-2.

The goal of cognitive therapy is to alter irrational beliefs, faulty reasoning, and negative self-statements. Research has shown that cognitive therapy is an effective intervention for a wide range of clinical problems, particularly depression, anxiety, and eating disorders. It is also true that psychiatric nurses spend a good deal of time assessing and analyzing patients' cognitions, including how patients view themselves and how they see themselves in relation to their world. Thus interventions that include principles of cognitive therapy have much to contribute to psychiatric nursing practice.[4]

> Give an example from your personal experiences of each cognitive distortion listed in Box 28-2. What was the consequence of each distortion, if any?

Box 28-2
COGNITIVE DISTORTIONS

Distortion: **Overgeneralization**
Definition: Draws conclusions about a wide variety of things on the basis of a single event
Example: A student who has failed an examination thinks "I'll never pass any of my other exams this term and I'll flunk out of school."

Distortion: **Personalization**
Definition: Relates external events to oneself when it is not justified
Example: "My boss said our company's productivity was down this year, but I know he was really talking about me."

Distortion: **Dichotomous thinking**
Definition: Thinking in extremes—that things are either always good or all bad
Example: "If my husband leaves me I might as well be dead."

Distortion: **Catastrophizing**
Definition: Thinking the worst about people and events
Example: "I better not apply for that promotion at work because I won't get it and I'll feel terrible."

Distortion: **Selective abstraction**
Definition: Focusing on details but not on other relevant information
Example: A wife believes her husband doesn't love her because he works late, but she ignores his affection for her, the gifts he brings her, and the special vacation they are planning together.

Distortion: **Arbitrary inference**
Definition: Drawing a negative conclusion without supporting evidence
Example: A young woman concludes "my friend no longer likes me" because she did not receive a birthday card

Distortion: **Mind reading**
Definition: Believing that one knows the thoughts of another without validation
Example: "They probably think I'm fat and lazy."

Distortion: **Magnification/minimization**
Definition: Exaggerating or trivializing the importance of events
Example: "I've burned the dinner, which goes to show just how incompetent I am."

Distortion: **Perfectionism**
Definition: Needing to do everything perfectly to feel good about oneself
Example: "I'll be a failure if I don't get an A on all my exams."

Distortion: **Externalization of self-worth**
Definition: Determining one's value based on the approval of others
Example: "I have to look nice all the time or my friends won't want to have me around."

COGNITIVE BEHAVIORAL THERAPY AND THE NURSING PROCESS

There are many misperceptions about cognitive behavioral therapy. One misperception is that it is controlling of the patient. Another misperception is that relationship factors are neglected in the treatment process. Neither of these perceptions is true.[15] The major characteristics of cognitive behavioral therapy are listed in Box 28-3.

Cognitive behavioral therapy is totally patient centered. It views the person as a unique individual who has a problem of living rather than a psychopathological condition. Cognitive behavioral therapists may seem more accepting of patients because patients' problems are not viewed with suspicion about subconscious motivation or irrational underlying dynamics.[23] Maladaptive behaviors, as well as adaptive coping responses, are believed to be acquired through the process of learning. Thus much emphasis is placed on behavioral monitoring and the completion of homework by the patient. Rather than trying to remove problems by changing subconscious dynamics, the cognitive behavioral therapist works with the patient to plan experiences that encourage the development of new skills.

Another important characteristic is the high degree of mutuality that exists in the treatment process. Cognitive behavioral therapists do not control the patient. Rather, they collaborate with the patient in defining the problem, identifying goals, formulating treatment strat-

---

BOX 28-3

CHARACTERISTICS OF COGNITIVE BEHAVIORAL THERAPY

▼ The patient and therapist focus on defining and solving current problems of living. They discuss the here and now and not the history of the patient.

▼ Dysfunctional behavior is attributed to maladaptive learning. Relearning more adaptive responses is the goal of the treatment.

▼ Collaboration with the patient and active participation by the patient in the treatment process is the norm. Cognitive behavioral therapy helps people to change. The patient does the changing, not the therapist.

▼ The theraputic process is open and explicit. The patient and the therapist share a common understanding of what is going on in treatment.

▼ It is a scientific and patient-centered approach that uses a rigorous assessment process to define the problems and environmental factors that influence the problems.

▼ Explicit treatment goals are identified by the patient and therapist. They are then used to evaluate the patient's progress and treatment outcome.

▼ Treatment strategies are derived from clinical and experimental research. Emphasis is placed on validating the appropriateness of treatment strategies implemented.

▼ The patient is often given homework assignments for data collecting, skill practice, and reinforcement of new responses.

▼ Baseline measurements of the problem behavior are made during the assessment process. These measurements are repeated at regular intervals during and at the completion of treatment. Thus the treatment process is rigorously monitored.

▼ Change and progress in treatment must be meaningful to the patient and have a positive impact on the quality of the patient's life.

---

egies, and evaluating progress. Because the focus is on the patient's self-control, cognitive behavioral therapy is seen as educational and skill building rather than curative, with the therapist taking a facilitative role. Genuineness, warmth, empathy, and the therapeutic relationship are important, and full recognition is given to their significance in influencing the effectiveness of treatment.

From this overview it is evident that cognitive behavioral therapy has many things in common with the nursing process. The steps of the nursing process closely resemble the steps involved in cognitive behavioral therapy. Similarly, both approaches are patient centered

and strongly emphasize mutuality in the treatment process. Finally, cognitive behavioral therapy places a strong emphasis on an objective assessment process. Specifically, it uses standardized measurement tools, bases treatment strategies on research evidence, and values ongoing evaluation of patient progress.

These characteristics suggest that cognitive behavioral therapy can make a significant contribution to the therapeutic effectiveness of nursing care. Thus it has relevance for psychiatric nurses practicing in any setting and with any patient population.

COGNITIVE BEHAVIORAL ASSESSMENT

Cognitive behavioral therapy places great importance on assessment.[20,22] In this process there is little interest in personality traits, defensive styles, personality dynamics, or dispositions. Instead, cognitive behavioral therapist assess the patient's actions, thoughts, and feelings in particular situations. Assessment includes collecting information, identifying problems from the data, defining the problem behavior, deciding how to measure the problem behavior, and identifying environmental variables that influence the problem behavior. It also includes a review of the patient's strengths and deficits and minimizes the use of assumptions and unvalidated inferences.

It is noteworthy that nurses most often form conclusions about the physiological problems of patients only after using a variety of tools and tests to collect objective evidence. Nurses dealing with psychosocial problems, however, often forget to use the scientific approach and base their care on unsubstantiated inferences. The cognitive behavioral assessment, in contrast, is based on validation and supporting evidence through the use of observation, interviewing, and measurement.

It is important that the problem be defined as clearly as possible. Initially the nurse addresses the following questions:

1. What is the problem?
2. Where does the problem occur?
3. When does the problem occur?
4. Who or what makes the problem occur?
5. What is the feared consequence related to the problem?

The nurse can them proceed to assess the problem's frequency, intensity, and duration.

The next step is to find out more about the patient's experience with the problem. This is determined by using a behavioral analysis (Fig. 28-2), which consists of the following three parts (**the ABCs of behavior**):

1. **Antecedent**—the stimulus or cue that occurs before behavior that leads to its occurrence

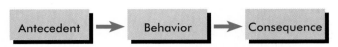

Fig. 28-2 Phases of behavior.

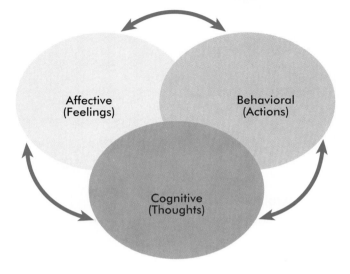

Fig. 28-3 Interacting systems in human behavior.

2. **Behavior**—what the person does or does not say or do
3. **Consequence**—what kind of effect (positive, negative, or neutral) the person thinks the behavior has

Antecedents can include the physical environment, social environment, or the person's behavior, feelings, or thoughts. Behaviors can also be broken down into discrete actions or series of steps. Finally, consequences can be viewed as powerful rewards or punishments of a person's actions. Thus they are critical elements of the assessment. An example of a behavioral analysis is as follows:

▼ Problem = anxiety
▼ Feared consequence = fear of losing control or dying
▼ Antecedent = leaving the house
▼ Behavior = avoiding stores, restaurants, and public places
▼ Consequence = restriction of daily activities

Another way of assessing an individual's experiences is to consider the three systems **(the ABCs of treatment)** that are interrelated in this treatment framework:

1. **Affective**—emotional or feeling responses
2. **Behavioral**—outward manifestations and actions
3. **Cognitive**—thoughts about the situation

Fig. 28-3 shows that these three elements are interrelated in explaining human behavior because:

▼ Feelings influence thinking
▼ Thinking influences actions
▼ Actions influence feelings

An assessment of each one of these areas has important implications for understanding the problem and effectively treating it.

Another aspect to be considered in the assessment process is whether the problem is expressed as observable behavior and if it is current and predictable. Mutually agreed on treatment goals and strategies can then be determined. Finally, throughout the treatment process, cognitive behavioral therapists use various methods to measure problem severity. These may include case-specific measures, as well as standardized rating scales. Chapter 6 discusses psychological evaluation and measurement issues in greater detail.

Are standardized rating scales used by staff working with patients in your psychiatric setting? If so, how are they used? If not, how would they influence patient care?

TREATMENT STRATEGIES

Cognitive behavioral therapy has been shown to be effective for treating a variety of clinical problems across all age groups. These include anxiety, affective, eating, schizophrenic, substance abuse, and personality disorders.[7,8] It is useful in working with children, adolescents, adults, elderly, and families and may be implemented both individually and in groups. In general, cognitive behavioral treatments include techniques aimed at the following:

1. Increasing activity
2. Reducing unwanted behavior
3. Increasing pleasure
4. Enhancing social skills

The three groups of cognitive behavioral treatment strategies are listed in Box 28-4. These techniques may be used alone or in combination. They also require practical skills and efforts from both the nurse and patient. This may include activities outside the office setting such as taking a bus ride, riding an elevator, or going to a supermarket.

Anxiety Reduction

Relaxation Training. As a therapeutic tool, relaxation training effectively decreases tension and anxiety. It can be used alone, in combination with other cognitive behavioral techniques, or in addition to supportive or insight therapy. The basic premise is that muscle ten-

---

Box 28-4

COGNITIVE BEHAVIORAL TREATMENT STRATEGIES

ANXIETY REDUCTION

Relaxation training
Biofeedback
Systematic desensitization
Flooding
Response prevention

COGNITIVE RESTRUCTURING

Monitoring thoughts and feelings
Questioning the evidence
Examining alternatives
Decatastrophizing
Reframing
Thought stopping

LEARNING NEW BEHAVIOR

Modeling
Shaping
Token economy
Role plating
Social skills training
Aversive therapy
Contingency contracting

Box 28-5

MANIFESTATIONS OF RELAXATION

PHYSIOLOGICAL

Decreased pulse
Decreased blood pressure
Decreased respirations
Decreased oxygen consumption
Decreased metabolic rate
Pupil constriction
Peripheral vasodilation
Increased peripheral temperature

COGNITIVE

Altered state of consciousness
Heightened concentration on single mental image
Receptivity to positive suggestion

BEHAVIORAL

Lack of attention to and concern for environmental stimuli
No verbal interaction
No voluntary change of position
Passive movement easy

---

sion is related to anxiety. If tense muscles can be made to relax, anxiety will be reduced.

The various relaxation procedures all involve rhythmic breathing, reduced muscle tension, and an altered state of consciousness. Clinical experience suggests that there are individual differences in the experience of relaxation. Not everyone demonstrates all of the characteristics of a relaxed physiological state. The physiological, cognitive, and behavioral manifestations of relaxation are listed in Box 28-5.

Relaxation training involves the tensing and relaxing of voluntary muscles in an orderly sequence until the body, as a whole, is helped. The patient should be seated in a comfortable chair. Soft music or pleasant visual cues may be present. Before beginning the exercises, a brief explanation should be given about how anxiety is related to muscle tension. The relaxation procedure should also be described.

The patient begins by taking a deep breath and exhaling slowly. A sequence of tension-relaxation exercises is then begun. The patient is instructed to tense each muscle group for about 10 seconds while the nurse describes how tense and uncomfortable this body part feels. The nurse then asks the patient to relax this muscle group, as the nurse comments, "Notice how all the hardness and tension is draining from your hands.

Now notice how they feel—warm, soft, and calm. Compare this feeling to when they were tense and see how much better they feel now." The patient should be reminded to tense only the muscle group named. The patient then proceeds to the next muscle group in the sequence listed in Box 28-6.

The final exercise asks the patient to become *completely* relaxed, beginning with the toes and moving up through the body to the eyes and forehead. When the patient learns the procedure, exercises can be performed only for the muscles that usually become tense. This is different for each person and may include the shoulders, forehead, back, or neck. Patients may also eliminate the tensing exercises and perform only the relaxation ones.

Systematic relaxation may be followed or replaced by another approach to evoke the relaxation response *meditation*. The basic components for meditation include the following:

1. A quiet environment
2. A passive attitude
3. A comfortable position
4. A word or scene to focus on

The first three components are necessary for any relaxation procedure. The fourth component refers to the process in which the patient selects a cue word or scene with pleasant connotations. The nurse then instructs the patient to close both eyes, relax each of the major

Box 28-6
SEQUENCE OF PROGRESSIVE MUSCLE RELAXATION

1. **Hands.** First the fists are tensed and relaxed, then the fingers are extended and relaxed.
2. **Biceps and triceps.** These are tensed and relaxed.
3. **Shoulders.** They are pulled back and relaxed and then pushed forward and relaxed.
4. **Neck.** The head is turned slowly as far to the right as possible and relaxed, then turned to the left and relaxed. It is then brought forward until the chin touches the chest and relaxed.
5. **Mouth.** The mouth is opened as wide as possible and then relaxed. The lips form a pout and then relax. The tongue is extended out as far as possible and then relaxed, then retracted into the throat and then relaxed. It is pressed hard into the roof of the mouth and relaxed, then pressed hard into the floor of the mouth and relaxed.
6. **Eyes.** They are opened as wide as possible and relaxed, the closed as hard as possible and relaxed.
7. **Breathing.** The patient inhales as deeply as possible and relaxes, then exhales as much as possible and relaxes.
8. **Back.** The trunk of the body is pushed forward so that the entire back is arched, then relaxed.
9. **Midsection.** The buttocks muscles are tensed and then relaxed.
10. **Thighs.** The legs are extended and raised about 6 inches off the floor and then relaxed. The backs of the feet are pressed into the floor and relaxed.
11. **Stomach.** It is pulled in as much as possible and relaxed, then extended and relaxed.
12. **Calves and feet.** With legs supported, the feet are bent with the toes pointing toward the head and then relaxed. Feet are then bent in the opposite direction and relaxed.
13. **Toes.** The toes are pressed into the bottom of the shoes and relaxed. They are then bent to touch the top inside of the shoes and relaxed.

muscle groups, and then begin repeating the word silently at each exhalation.

Name four clinical settings in which nurses can use relaxation training with patients. Identify whether it would be a primary, secondary, or tertiary prevention activity in each setting.

Biofeedback. Biofeedback uses a machine to reduce anxiety and modify behavioral responses. Small elec-

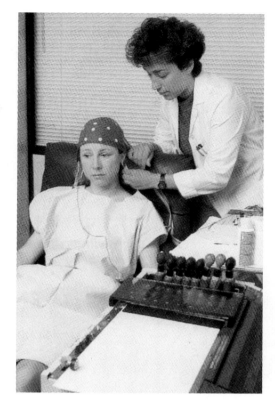

Fig. 28-4 This woman, using biofeedback, can reduce the pain of a migraine headache by learning to lower the temperature of her forehead.
From Melanie Brown/Photo Edit.

trodes connected to the biofeedback equipment are attached to the patient's forehead (Fig. 28-4). Brain waves, muscle tension, body temperature, heart rate, and blood pressure can then all be monitored for small changes. These changes are communicated to the patient by auditory and visual means. The more relaxed the patient becomes, the more pleasant sounds or sights are presented. These stop when the patient stops relaxing and resumes when the patient reachieves the relaxed state. After developing the ability to relax, the patient is encouraged to apply the technique in stressful situations.

Systematic Desensitization. Systematic desensitization was designed to decrease avoidance behavior linked to a specific stimulus such as heights or airplane travel. The goal of systematic desensitization is to help the patient change the response to a threatening stimulus. It involves combining deep muscle relaxation with imagined scenes of situations that cause anxiety. The assumption is that relaxation is incompatible with anxiety. So if the person is taught to relax while imagining such scenes, the real life situation that the scene depicted will cause much less anxiety.

With systematic desensitization the patient must first be able to relax the muscles. Additional steps are then taken. Next, a hierarchy of the anxiety-provoking or feared situations is constructed. These are ranked from 1 to 10 in order of difficulty, with 1 evoking little or no anxiety and 10 evoking intense or severe anxiety. Box 28-7 presents a sample hierarchy of a patient with agoraphobia.

With in vitro, or imaginal, desensitization, the patient proceeds with the imagined pairing of the hierarchy items with the relaxed state, progressing from the least to the most anxiety provoking. In vivo desensitization exposes the patient to real rather than imagined life situations. In vivo exposure is widely considered to be the treatment of choice for simple and social phobias, as well as for obsessive-compulsive disorders.

This technique works through a combination of positive reinforcement for confronting anxiety-provoking stimuli and the extinction of maladaptive behavior by realizing that the feared negative consequences never occurred. It is helpful for the nurse to share the following thoughts with the patient during exposure therapy:

1. Anxiety is unpleasant but is not dangerous, that is, the patient will not die or lose control.
2. Anxiety does eventually decrease and does not continue indefinitely.
3. Practice makes perfect, and the more the patient repeats a particular exposure exercise the easier it becomes.

For example, a boy may have a fear of spiders. His daily schedule may then include a series of planned activities involving reading about spiders. He may then begin gradual exposure to pictures and photographs of spiders, followed by looking at real spiders in his yard. Thus the exposure gradually leads to his anxiety reduction and more adaptive behaviors.

Flooding. Flooding is another form of exposure therapy in which the patient is immediately exposed to the most anxiety-provoking stimuli instead of being exposed gradually or systematically to a hierarchy of feared stimuli. If this technique uses an imaginary as opposed to real life event, it is called *implosion*.

Response Prevention. In response prevention the patient is encouraged to face a particular fear or situation without engaging in the accompanying behavior. It is based on the concept that repeated exposure to the anxiety-producing stimulus without the presence of the anxiety-reducing response will lead to a reduction in the anxiety because the feared consequence does not occur.

For example, a patient may fear using a public restroom and engage in hand washing up to 20 times a day. With response prevention treatment, the patient's daily schedule would include using a public restroom, turning on the water faucets, and washing hands for only 30 seconds. Over time, the maladaptive behaviors would be reduced, since the feared consequence of germs and illness did not occur.

Box 28-7
SAMPLE PATIENT HIERARCHY FOR PHOBIAS

A hierarchy of phobias is a list of your fears and avoidances in order of severity. Your greatest phobia should be at the top of the list and your smallest fear at the bottom. In between rank your other fears and phobias in order of severity. Try to list 10 but not more than 20 phobias. These activities should be convenient to do, as you will be doing them from several times a day to at least several times per week.

For example, think of yourself standing at the end of a football field marked off in 10 yard lines. Closest to you at the nearest end of the field at the 0 yard line is something you are mildly fearful of or avoid doing sometimes but not always; the farthest end of the field is your biggest fear; at the 50 yard line is a medium fear; and on the 10 yard line is a minor fear but one that is stronger than at the 0 yard line.

Remember everyone's hierarchy will be different. There are no "right" or "wrong" hierarchies. Your hierarchy is a tool to help you approach feared situations in a systematic and controlled way.

SAMPLE HIERARCHY

100	Driving alone across a high bridge in the rain
90	Driving alone on the interstate far from home
80	Driving alone on side streets that are unfamiliar
70	Speaking in front of groups of people
60	Using elevators alone
50	Eating in restaurants alone
40	Going to large public gatherings with safe people
30	Eating with friends or family in familiar restaurants
20	Driving more than several miles from home with a passenger in the car
10	Going shopping with a safe person in big stores and malls
0	Going shopping with a safe person in small stores near home

---

Do you think a highly anxious nurse can effectively implement anxiety-reduction strategies with patients? Why or why not?

Cognitive Restructuring

Monitoring Thoughts and Feelings. Changing cognitions begins with the identification of what is reinforcing and maintaining the patient's dysfunctional thinking and maladaptive behavior. An important first step is for patients to heighten their self-awareness and monitor their own thinking and feeling. Patients can be helped to do this through the use of the "Daily Record of Dysfunctional Thoughts Form" developed by Beck.[6] This consists of five columns (Fig. 28-5): the situation, feelings, automatic thoughts in response to the situation, the more rational response, and the outcome or consequence. Through the use of such a form patients are taught to distinguish between thoughts and feelings and to identify adaptive responses that would be alternatives to the situation. They also begin to recognize the connection between certain thoughts and maladaptive emotions and behaviors.

Questioning the Evidence. The next step is for the patient and therapist to examine the evidence that is used to support a certain belief. Questioning the evidence also involves examining the source of the data. Patients with distorted thinking often give equal weight to all sources or ignore all data except those that support their distorted thinking. Having patients question their evidence with staff, family, and other members of their social support network can clarify misinformation and result in more realistic and appropriate interpretations of the evidence.

Examining Alternatives. Many patients see themselves as having lost all options. This is particularly evident in suicidal patients. Examining alternatives involves working with patients to generate additional options based on patients' strengths and coping resources.

Decatastrophizing. Decatastrophizing is also called the *What if* technique. It involves helping patients to evaluate if they are overestimating the catastrophic nature of a situation. Questions that the nurse can ask include, "What is the worst thing that can happen?" "Would it be so terrible if that really took place?" "How would other people cope with such an event?" The goal of this intervention is to help the patient see that the consequences of life's actions are generally not "all or nothing" and thus are less catastrophic.

Reframing. Reframing is a strategy that modifies or changes a patient's perception of a situation or behavior. It involves focusing on other aspects of the problem or encouraging a patient to see the issue from a different perspective. Patients who dichotomize events may see only one side of a situation. Weighing the ad-

Date	Situation Describe: 1. Actual event leading to unpleasant emotion, or 2. Stream of thoughts, daydream, or recollection, leading to unpleasant emotion	Emotion(s) 1. Specify sad/anxious/angry etc. 2. Rate degree of emotion, 1-100	Automatic Thought(s) 1. Write automatic thought(s) that preceded emotion(s) 2. Rate belief in automatic thought(s) 0-100%	Rational Response 1. Write rational response to automatic thought(s) 2. Rate belief in rational response, 0-100%	Outcome 1. Re-rate belief in automatic thought(s), 0-100% 2. Specify and rate subsequent emotions, 0-100

Explanation: When you experience an unpleasant emotion, note the situation that seemed to stimulate the emotion. (If the emotion occurred while you were thinking, daydreaming, etc., please note this.) Then note the automatic thought associated with the emotion. Record the degree to which you believe this thought: 0%, not at all: 100%, completely. In rating degree of emotion: 1, a trace; 100, the most intense possible.

Fig. 28-5 Daily record of dysfunctional thoughts.
From Beck A, Rush A, Shaw B, Emery G: *Cognitive therapy of depression*, New York, 1979, The Guilford Press.

vantages and disadvantages of maintaining a particular belief or behavior can help patients gain balance and develop a new perspective. By understanding both the positive and negative consequences of an issue, the patient can attain a broader perspective of it. For example, suggesting that a mother's overinvolvement with her son is actually a sign of her loving concern may help a family see the situation in a new light.

This strategy also creates an opportunity to help challenge the meaning of a problem or behavior in the belief that once the meaning of a behavior changes, the person's response will also change. For example, it might involve helping a patient see an adversity as a potentially positive event. Thus the loss of a job may be perceived as a stressor, but it can also be viewed as an opportunity for pursuing a new job or career.

> Think of a problem you encountered in the past year. How might you have used the technique of cognitive reframing to see the situation in a more positive way?

Thought Stopping. Dysfunctional thinking can often have a snowball effect on patients. What may begin as a small or insignificant problem can, over time, gather importance and momentum that can be difficult to stop. The technique of thought stopping is best used when the dysfunctional thought first begins. The patient can picture a stop sign, imagine a bell going off, or envision a brick wall to stop the progression of the dysfunctional thought.

To begin, the patient identifies the problematic thought and talks about it as the problem scene is imagined. The nurse interrupts the patient's thoughts by shouting "STOP." Thereafter the patient learns to interrupt thoughts in a similar way. Finally, the patient converts the "stop" into an inaudible phrase or image and thus learns to use the technique quietly in everyday situations.

Learning New Behavior

Modeling. Modeling is a strategy used to form new behavior patterns, increase existing skills, or reduce avoidance behavior. The target behavior is broken down into a series of separate stages that are ranked in order of difficulty or distress with the first stage being the least anxiety provoking. The patient then observes an individual modeling the behavior that the patient finds difficult in a controlled environment. After this the patient imitates the model's behavior. In participant modeling the model and patient perform the behavior together before the patient does so alone. It is particularly important that the model selected for this treatment be credible to the patient for the treatment to be most effective.

Shaping. Shaping induces new behaviors by reinforcing behaviors that approximate the desired behavior. Each successive approximation of the behavior is reinforced until the desired behavior is attained. Skillful use of the technique requires that the nurse carefully look, wait, and reinforce. The nurse needs to look for the desired behavior, wait until it occurs, and then reinforce it when it does occur. An example of this strategy is when the nurse notices that an aggressive child is playing cooperatively with a peer and then praises the child for this behavior.

Token Economy. Token economy is a form of positive reinforcement used most often on a group basis with children or psychiatric hospital inpatients. It consists of rewarding the patient in various ways, such as with tokens, passes, or points for performing desired target behaviors. Behaviors might include hygienic grooming, attending classes, or verbally expressing frustration rather than striking out at others. Tokens also may be lost for inappropriate behaviors. If tokens or points are used, they may periodically be cashed in for rewards such as free time, off-unit outings, games, or sugarless candy.

Role Playing. Role playing allows patients to rehearse problematic issues and obtain feedback about their behavior. It can provide practice for decision making and exploring consequences. A related practice is that of role reversal in which the patient switches roles with someone else and thus experiences the difficult situation from another point of view.

Social Skills Training. Smooth social functioning is central to most human activity, and social skill problems exist in many psychiatrically ill patients. This technique is based on the belief that skills are learned and therefore can be taught to those who do not have them. The principles of skill acquisition include:
▼ Guidance
▼ Demonstration
▼ Practice
▼ Feedback

These principles must be included in implementing an effective social skills training program, which is often a component of psychiatric rehabilitation programs (see Chapter 13). Guidance and demonstration are usually used early in the treatment, followed by practice and feedback. Treatment typically follows four stages:
1. Description of the new behavior to be learned

2. Learning of new behavior through the use of guidance and demonstration
3. Practice of the new behavior with feedback
4. Transfer of the new behavior to the natural environment

The types of behaviors that are often taught in these programs include asking questions, giving compliments, making positive changes, maintaining eye contact, asking others for specific behavior change, speaking in a clear tone of voice, and avoiding fidgeting and self-criticism. This treatment strategy is most often used with patients who lack social skills, assertiveness (assertiveness training), or impulse control (anger management) and those with antisocial behavior.

Aversion Therapy. Aversion therapy helps to reduce unwanted but persistent maladaptive behaviors. Aversive conditioning applies an aversive or noxious stimulus when a maladaptive behavior occurs. An example is for a patient to snap a rubber band on the wrist when being bothered by an intrusive thought. Covert sensitization is an aversive technique in which patients imagine scenes that pair the undesired behavior with an unpleasant consequence. By imagining aversive consequences for a behavior such as overeating, the patient gains control by providing a form of punishment for one's own behavior.

Aversive therapy has sometimes been criticized as unethical and detrimental to patients' well-being. Do you agree? If not, what conditions should be present before implementing aversive therapy to patients?

Contingency Contracting. Contingency contracting involves a formal contract between the patient and the therapist defining what behaviors are to be changed and what consequences follow the performance of these behaviors. Included are positive consequences for desirable behaviors and negative consequences for undesirable behaviors.

ROLE OF THE NURSE

Much of the history of behavioral therapy started in the United States. The first report of nurses functioning as behavioral therapists came in 1959 when Ayllon and Michael[1] taught nurses to use operant skills to modify the behavior of patients in long-term psychiatric institutions. It was believed that nurses were a natural choice because they made up the majority of the staff caring for the patients. Since that time, however, the practice of behavioral therapy nursing has been more dominant in Britain than in the United States.

In 1975 Isaac Marks, a psychiatrist and researcher in London, established the first program to prepare nurses to be behavioral therapists working under little or no supervision. The clinical outcomes these nurses achieved were at least as good as those obtained by other professionals. Thus it was established that nurses could be prepared to be effective therapists.[17] Marks also calculated the cost-benefit of employing nurses as behavioral therapists. He found that people treated by nurses used fewer health-care resources after treatment than before, resulting in a significant savings of resources.[13] These were impressive findings, and behavioral therapy became an increasingly important component of the nurse's role in England and Scotland in the years that followed.

In contrast, cognitive behavioral therapy needs to be more aggressively integrated into the role of the psychiatric nurse in the United States. It is true, for example, that nurses are the frontline providers of care. They are the group most often called on to carry out selective reinforcement, modeling, extinction, skills training, shaping, and role playing. Because of their direct care contact, nurses are also best able to observe patients, assess problem areas, and recommend targets for cognitive behavioral intervention. Yet few nurses are skilled in the principles and techniques of cognitive behavioral therapy.

Several explanations have been suggested for this[7,15] (see Critical Thinking about Contemporary Issues). First, nurses may have little formal exposure to cognitive behavioral treatment strategies in the course of their education. Second, nurses have been traditionally reinforced for their unconditional nurturance of patients and their compliance with physicians' orders. In contrast, cognitive behavioral therapy requires the use of independent judgment, limit setting, reframing, and selective use of rewards that may not be encouraged for nurses in clinical settings. Third, American nurses have placed great emphasis on the therapeutic use of self, whereas British nurses have assumed a more pragmatic approach to nursing care. The American approach to nursing has sometimes created confusion between the concepts of caring and treatment. It incorrectly suggests that these are different events, with nurses responsible for caring and physicians responsible for treating.

Current changes in the scope and functions of contemporary psychiatric nursing practice, however, underscore the need for cognitive behavioral therapy skills by all nurses. Contemporary psychiatric nursing practice includes both caring and treating activities. The reality is that nurses have always been involved with helping patients reduce anxiety, change cognitions, and learn new behaviors. As influential agents of behavioral change,

CRITICAL THINKING ABOUT CONTEMPORARY ISSUES

Does Humanistic Nursing Care Result in the Promotion of Maladaptive Patient Behaviors?

Many assume that humanistic nursing care is always therapeutic and health promoting. However, some research in the field that examined the traditional caring orientation of nursing suggests that this notion be reconsidered. One study reported that psychiatric patients who demonstrated desirable or nonproblematic behavior were largely ignored by the nursing staff.[12] Conversely, nurses gave a great deal of attention to those who were perceived as sicker or who exhibited disturbed behavior. A more recent study of the interactional dimensions of the inpatient milieu found that nursing practice in the psychiatric inpatient setting did not regularly promote confirming or open patient-staff interactions.[11] The authors suggest that this interpretation of humanistic care results in the unintentional reinforcement of maladaptive behaviors and the promotion of the sick role.

Two other studies shed further light on this issue. The first examined unit structure on a therapeutic milieu and found that the highest rates of nurse-patient interaction occurred on highly structured units that were based on a behavioral treatment program.[14] The second study compared the effectiveness of the treatment programs of three units—a traditional program, a milieu therapy program, and a social learning program.[18] The social learning program was particularly effective in reducing dangerous and aggressive acts. It also increased the cognitive, social, and instrumental functioning of the patients, prevented rehospitalization in 97% of discharged patients, and was the most cost effective. Although there are relatively few studies in this area, they do suggest the need for psychiatric nurses to reevaluate the basis of their caregiving and treatment activities and to frame their interventions from a more cognitive behavioral and social learning perspective. ▼

nurses need to be aware of their ability to promote adaptive or maladaptive responses and increase their skills and knowledge in effective treatment strategies.

Three basic roles have been identified for nurses involved in cognitive behavioral therapy.[16] Each of these roles can be performed by all nurses at various levels of expertise, ranging from novice through generalist and specialist. They include:

1. Direct patient care
2. Planning treatment programs
3. Teaching others the use of cognitive behavioral techniques

Psychiatric nurses provide direct patient care in both inpatient and community settings, and the value of cognitive behavioral therapy is evident throughout the continuum of care. Most treatments are ideally suited to community settings, and they can include interventions across the continuum of coping responses from promoting health, to intervening in acute illness, to fostering rehabilitation. Nurses also may function as planners and coordinators of complex treatment programs, consultants, and teachers of other nurses, professionals, patients, and their families.[3] It is clear that with the current emphasis on cost-effective treatment and documented outcomes of care, cognitive behavioral therapy will be a growing area of expertise for all psychiatric nurses in the next decade.

SUGGESTED CROSS-REFERENCES

A Stress Adaptation Model of Psychiatric Nursing	Chapter 4
Psychological Context of Psychiatric Nursing Care	Chapter 6
Legal Context of Psychiatric Nursing Care	Chapter 8
Primary Mental Health Prevention	Chapter 11
Crisis Intervention	Chapter 12
Psychiatric Rehabilitation	Chapter 13
Anxiety Responses and Anxiety Disorders	Chapter 14
Emotional Responses and Mood Disorders	Chapter 17

SUMMARY

1. Cognitive behavioral therapy is aimed at helping people overcome difficulties in any area of human activity and experience. Behavior is any observable, recordable, and measurable act, movement, or response of the individual. It is what is observed, not the conclusions drawn from the observation.
2. Classical conditioning focuses on the processes by which involuntary behavior is learned.
3. Operant conditioning focuses on the processes by which voluntary behavior is learned, including increasing and decreasing behavior.
4. Cognitive therapists believe that maladaptive responses arise from cognitive distortions, and the goal of therapy is to correct faulty thinking that underlies behavioral problems.
5. Cognitive behavioral therapy is similar to the nursing process in that both are patient centered, emphasize mutuality, and place a strong emphasis on measurement of progress and evaluation.
6. Cognitive behavioral assessment includes collecting information, identifying problems, defining the problem, deciding how to measure the problem, and

identifying environmental variables that influence the problem behavior.

7. A variety of cognitive behavioral treatment strategies may be used alone or in combination. They focus on anxiety reduction, cognitive restructuring, and learning new behavior.

8. Three basic roles for nurses involved in cognitive behavioral therapy include direct patient care, planning treatment programs, and teaching others the use of behavioral techniques. These roles may be enacted by all nurses in various practice settings.

COMPETENT CARING
A CLINICAL EXEMPLAR OF A PSYCHIATRIC NURSE

Darcy O'Neill, RN

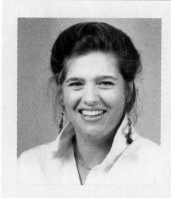

I first met A, a 13-year-old black girl, when she was admitted to our combined child and adolescent psychiatric unit by her mother. Her mother reported that A was becoming increasingly oppositional, refusing to attend school, having sexual relations with multiple partners, running away from home for long periods, and exhibiting destructive outbursts when confronted. A was admitted to our unit following a 3-day runaway. She appeared tired and disheveled, somewhat older than her chronological age, and was extremely angry about hospitalization. However, despite her angry demeanor, it was rapidly apparent that A was a very bright and charming young girl. I was intrigued.

During this hospitalization A continued to have unpredictable violent outbursts. At times the most benign redirection would result in verbal threats, screaming, and cursing, which would frequently escalate into physical attacks on staff. At other times, a similar or more emphatic directive would be calmly accepted and performed. I was puzzled and rather frustrated by trying to balance this child's need to express some deeply felt anger while maintaining the safety of the milieu.

Our unit utilizes a token economy as part of a patient's treatment. Patients earn points, or stickers, depending on age and cognitive abilities, for attending activities and participating in treatment. Points are earned as rewards and they may then be exchanged for special privileges. Although we specialize in short-term assessment and evaluation, many children quickly engage in this token economy, or point system, and are able to address behavioral issues in a direct and timely fashion. Unfortunately, A was not one of these children. Her participation in the point system was as unpredictable and sporadic as her behavior.

The team began to discuss the therapeutic effectiveness of an individually designed behavioral program for A. As a new graduate nurse who knew little about the utilization of behavioral therapies, I balked. I felt that what A needed was more one-to-one time to process the strong emotions underlying her behavior. A and I were beginning to have regular but brief interactions in which she began to share some of her feelings. I feared that by making a more concrete program, obviously different from the program her peers experienced, we risked alienating a child who already had great difficulties with trust. I also feared that from a position of frustration we were falling into a punitive stance. Unfortunately, A was discharged to an outpatient program before the formulation of a new behavioral program. It seemed that many of my questions concerning the therapeutic value of special behavioral programs would remain unanswered.

After I had been on the unit for 6 months A was readmitted. At this admission her mother reported an increase in the severity and frequency of the behaviors that had precipitated A's first admission. In the time that passed since her first admission, I had had quite a few opportunities to work with individually designed behavioral programs. I had begun to appreciate this therapeutic approach and understand that for many children these programs provided a sense of security and an opportunity to address their problem behaviors more concretely. What I had not understood at the time of A's first admission was that these programs increase the amount of one-to-one while assisting children in taking more control of their behavior. I had discovered that behavioral programs provided the framework for increased teaching and learning.

From the outset of her second admission, A was increasingly difficult to reach. She had become more physically and verbally threatening. I continued to try to engage her in the point system, with moderate success. In addition, early in her hospitalization A eloped. She reluctantly returned in 3 days. After establishing her immediate physical well-being, staff were faced with a new set of problems. One of the privileges earned in our program is increased freedom off the unit. This increase in privileges was often the motivation for patients to engage in the point system. Since A was at great risk for repeat elopement and her safety was a primary therapeutic concern, she would need to remain on unit supervision. It was quickly apparent that we would need a new motivator.

After her elopement A was even more unpredictable. At one minute she was willing to discuss her emotions and open to nurturance and support, while at the next she was isolated and violent, with no tolerance of any perceived frustration. I was quickly exasperated. I truly liked this charming, bright young girl who showed me through her behavior that she was in a great deal of pain. Many times after a violent or threatening outburst she would cry inconsolably, curled in the fetal position, appearing much younger than her 13 years. I agonized along with the team members on how to help this child out of a self-destructive downward spiral.

Quickly, the team returned to the discussion of a special behavioral program. Almost as quickly staff became divided on how to best design and imple-

ment this program. Individual philosophies, differing levels of appreciation for behavioral therapies, as well as personal limits and tolerances, were shared in numerous discussions. With A's full participation and albeit tenuous acceptance, a preliminary program was designed and implemented. Within 3 days some minor improvements were noted. However, they were buried in continually violent and impulsive behavior. It took a great deal of painstaking discussion for staff to identify the positive behavior changes and suggest appropriate modifications in the behavior plan in an effort to increase these positive behaviors. Unfortunately, this was not effective for A, and within the next few days she needed seclusion to remain safe.

Again, the team reassessed the program and decided to adopt a more concrete contract with A. By either exhibiting new positive behaviors or refraining from old negative behavior A could earn immediate rewards. The hope was to extinguish the dangerous, self-destructive behaviors while replacing them with new coping strategies. Again, the changes were subtle and erratic, surrounded by what appeared to be setbacks. This program necessitated hypervigilance on the part of staff to be aware of any positive change, no matter how slight.

I recall one time I was attempting to process with A after she was placed in open seclusion secondary to threatening staff. I found myself desperately searching for positive feedback to offer her. All I could immediately identify was total frustration with her behavior and the program, in addition to my own feelings of inadequacy. Yet, as I reviewed her behavioral contract I was able to see a number of significant changes. She had walked to seclusion independently, she only needed one directive to go to the seclusion room, and she was able to sit there without swearing at or threatening me. As soon as I realized all the changes I was witnessing I became elated. Although she was still unable to talk with me, I continued to state how impressed I was by her ability to eliminate these behaviors. I made a point of sharing this information with passing staff, loud enough for A to hear. With time she was able to process what had happened and reintegrate into the milieu.

Through this trying, challenging experience I feel I was able to grow professionally and personally. I learned in a very deep way the therapeutic necessity of a fully functioning interdisciplinary team, and my integral role on that team. But more important, I gained a new respect for behavioral programs and the opportunities they offer not only patients but nurses. A well-designed behavioral program provides numerous opportunities for teaching, one-to-one relationship building, and a framework for continual assessment, planning, and evaluation. Although the desired outcomes may be slow in coming and the process difficult, I readily look forward to the next opportunity to creatively use my skills in designing and implementing a behavioral treatment program. ▼

REFERENCES

1. Ayllon T, Michael J: The psychiatric nurse as a behavioral engineer, J Exp Anal Behav 2:323, 1959.
2. Bandura A: Social learning theory, Englewood Cliffs, NJ, 1977, Prentice Hall.
3. Barker P: Behavior therapy nursing, London, 1982, Croom Helm.
4. Barker P: Cognitive therapy model: principles and general application. In Reynolds W, Cormack D, eds: Psychiatric and mental health nursing, London, 1990, Chapman & Hall.
5. Beck A: Cognitive therapy and the emotional disorders, Philadelphia, 1976, Center for Cognitive Therapy.
6. Beck A, Rush A, Shaw B, Emery G: Cognitive therapy of depression, New York, 1979, The Guilford Press.
7. Bellack A, Hersen M: Handbook of behavior therapy in the psychiatric setting, New York, 1993, Plenum Press.
8. Dryden W, Rentoul R: Adult clinical problems: a cognitive-behavioral approach, London, 1991, Routledge.
9. Ellis A: Reason and emotion in psychotherapy, New York, 1962, Lyle Stuart.
10. Ellis A: Rational-emotive therapy and cognitive behavioral therapy, New York, 1984, Springer.
11. Emrich K: Helping or hurting: interacting in the psychiatric nursing milieu, J Psychosoc Nurs Ment Health Serv 27:12, 1989.
12. Gelfand D, Gelfand S, Dobson W: Unprogrammed reinforcement of patients' behavior in a mental hospital, Behav Res Ther 5:201, 1967.
13. Ginsberg G, Marks I: Costs and benefits of behavioral psychotherapy: a pilot study of neurotics treated by nurse therapists, Psychol Med 7:685, 1977.
14. Hodges V, Sandford D, Elzinga R: The role of ward structure on nursing staff behaviors, Acta Psychiatr Scand 73:6, 1986.
15. Hume A: Behavior therapy model: principles and general application. In Reynolds W, Cormack D, eds: Psychiatric and mental health nursing, London, 1990, Chapman & Hall.
16. LeBow M: Applications of behavior modification in nursing practice. In Hersen M, Eisler, R, Miller P, eds: Progress in behavior modification, vol 2, New York, 1976, Academic Press.
17. Marks I, Hallam R, Connolly J, Philpott R: Nursing in behavioral psychotherapy, London, 1977, Royal College of Nursing.
18. Paul G: Residential treatment programs and aftercare for the chronically institutionalized. In Mirabi M, ed: The chronically mentally ill: research and services, New York, 1984, Luce.
19. Pavlov I: Conditioned reflexes, London, 1927, Oxford University Press.
20. Richards D, McDonald B: Behavior psychotherapy: a handbook for nurses, Oxford, 1990, Heinemann Nursing.
21. Skinner B: Science and human behavior, New York, 1953, The Free Press.
22. Stern R, Drummond L: The practice of behavioral and cognitive psychotherapy, Cambridge, 1991, Cambridge University Press.
23. Thorpe G, Olson S: Behavior therapy: concepts, procedures, and applications, Boston, 1990, Allyn & Bacon.

ANNOTATED SUGGESTED READINGS

*Barker P: *Behavior therapy nursing*, London, 1982, Croom Helm.

   One of two nursing texts to explain behavior therapy and apply it to nursing practice. Published in London but relevant for American psychiatric nursing practice.

*Barker P: Cognitive therapy model: clinical applications. In Reynolds W, Cormack D, eds: *Psychiatric and mental health nursing*, London, 1990, Chapman & Hall.

   Excellent chapter with a case example of a nurse using cognitive therapy with a patient.

Bellack A, Hersen M: *Handbook of behavior therapy in the psychiatric setting*, New York, 1993, Plenum Press.

   All-inclusive manual for practicing behavioral therapy in psychiatric settings. It includes general principles and applies them to adults, children, and families.

*Dodge V: Relaxation training: a nursing intervention for substance abusers, *Arch Psychiatr Nurs* 5:99, 1991.

   Good article describing nursing's use of relaxation training for substance abusers. Includes a case example.

Dryden W, Rentoul R: *Adult clinical problems: a cognitive-behavioral approach*, London, 1991, Routledge.

   Provides a systematic and in-depth coverage of adult clinical problems and their treatment from a cognitive-behavioral perspective.

*Hume A: Behavior therapy model: principles and general application. In Reynolds W, Cormack D, eds: *Psychiatric and mental health nursing*, London, 1990, Chapman & Hall.

   This chapter reviews behavioral therapy from a nursing perspective and provides historical information on its development and use.

*Laraia M, Stuart G, Best C: Behavioral treatment of panic-related disorders: a review, *Arch Psychiatr Nurs* 3:125, 1989.

   Behavioral techniques for panic-related disorders are reviewed. One of the few articles describing behavioral treatments in the nursing literature.

*Pizzello L, Breitmayer B: Evaluation of treatment integrity on a child psychiatric unit: an illustration, *J Child Psychiatr Nurs* 6:15, 1993.

---

*Nursing reference.

Described the evaluation of a token economy on a child inpatient unit. Results indicate staff inconsistencies and need for greater monitoring of behavioral nursing treatments.

*Reeder D: Cognitive therapy of anger management: theoretical and practical considerations, *Arch Psychiatr Nurs* 5:147, 1991.

Presents premises of cognitive therapy and applies them to working with patients in the control of anger.

*Richards D, McDonald B: *Behavior psychotherapy: a handbook for nurses,* Oxford, 1990, Heinemann Nursing.

The one book nurses should purchase for added knowledge in this field. Clear, clinically focused and very applicable to all types of nursing practice.

*Scahill L et al: Inpatient treatment of obsessive-compulsive disorder in childhood: a case study, *J Child Psychiatr Nurs* 6:5, 1993.

Excellent article describing the use of behavior therapy techniques by nurses working on a child inpatient unit. Clear discussion of theory with case study.

Stern R, Drummond L: *The practice of behavioral and cognitive psychotherapy,* Cambridge, 1991, Cambridge University Press.

Clear and simple text for the clinician who wants to learn therapeutic skills in this area. Filled with clinical examples.

*Whitley G: Ritualistic behavior: breaking the cycle, *J Psychosoc Nurs Ment Health Serv* 29:31, 1991.

Case report of interventions for a patient with OCD, including behavioral therapy integrated into the nursing care.

Wright J, Thase M, Beck A, Ludgate J: *Cognitive therapy with inpatients: developing a cognitive milieu,* New York, 1993, The Guilford Press.

Explains the use of cognitive therapy with inpatients and their families, adolescents, depressed elderly, alcoholics, and patients with eating disorders. Good chapter on the role of psychiatric nurses in implementing a cognitive milieu.

*Nursing reference.

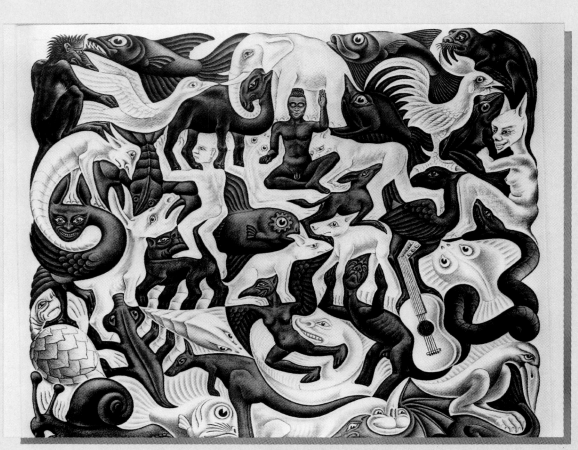

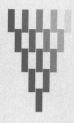

CHAPTER 29
Therapeutic Groups

PAULA C. LASALLE
ARTHUR J. LASALLE

Self and world are correlated, and so are individualization and participation. . . Participation means: being a part of something from which one is, at the same time, separated.

Paul Tillich: *The Courage To Be*

LEARNING OBJECTIVES

After studying this chapter the student should be able to:
▼ Define a group
▼ Identify and describe the components of a small group
▼ Compare and contrast the stages of group development
▼ Describe small group evaluation factors
▼ Discuss the responsibilities and qualities of nurses as group leaders
▼ Compare and contrast types of nurse-led groups

Agroup provides nurses with a potentially more therapeutic modality than the two-person, nurse-patient encounter. It offers its members a variety of relationships as they interact with each other and with the group leader. Group members come from many backgrounds and must "deal with their likes, dislikes, similarities, dissimilarities, envy, timidity, aggression, fear, attraction, and competitiveness."[17] All of this takes place in the context of the dynamics of the group process in which, with careful leadership, members give and receive feedback about the meaning and effect of their various interactions with each other.

Groups can be conducted in a variety of settings including inpatient units, community and university health centers, and places of employment. Families of individuals with serious illness may join a group for instruction, assistance with coping, mutual support, and crisis intervention. School nurses may lead groups for children who share developmental milestones or life problems, such as parental divorce or death. In each of these situations the format, setting, and goal of the group would vary. Thus leading a group requires the nurse to understand its structure and process.

Nurses are well prepared to use groups as a therapeutic treatment strategy. Throughout the nursing education program the nurse learns about the person both as an individual and as a part of a family group, a work group, a social group, and a cultural group. Understanding the individual as part of a larger system allows the nurse to better identify ways in which a person may benefit from a group experience. The flexibility of nurses enables them to assume different roles when working with a group, adapt to the group process, and utilize the therapeutic potential inherent in groups. Nurses who have learned therapeutic communication and relationship skills will have a sound basis for group leadership and the implementation of group programs. Thus group work is an important skill for all nurses to master, regardless of their practice setting or specialty area.

> Think of some specific patient situations in which a group approach would be more useful than an individual nurse-patient encounter. Discuss the reasons for this. Describe other situations in which a group format would be less helpful.

DEFINITION

A group is a collection of individuals who have a relationship with one another, are interdependent, and may

have common norms. Therapeutic groups have a shared purpose. For example, a group's purpose might be to help members who consistently enter destructive relationships identify and change maladaptive behaviors. Each group has its own structure and identity. The power of the group lies in the contributions of each member and the leader to the shared purpose of the group. These contributions are content and process oriented.

Content functions of the group are met when members share their experiences to help another member. When members share the methods they used to solve a common problem, they are addressing the group's content functions.

Process functions allow the individual to receive feedback from other members and the leader about how the member interacts and is perceived within the group. The group is used as a laboratory or arena to see, experiment, and define relationships and behaviors. For example, a member who complains that his wife is always accusing him of being domineering may receive feedback from the group as to whether others see him acting similarly in the group. Then he has the opportunity to work on changing his behavior in the group and risking the change in the outside world.

The group has primary and secondary tasks. The primary task is necessary for the group's survival or existence; secondary tasks may enhance the group but are not basic to its survival. An example of a primary task for a group of mothers might be to improve mothering skills; a secondary task might be to add to the mother's social network. Relationships in the group may either limit or enhance their willingness to share concerns about mothering.

COMPONENTS OF SMALL GROUPS

To be effective in therapeutic group work, it is necessary to understand the complex processes that occur and be able to use various approaches to increase the therapeutic potential of the group for its members. The components of small groups are summarized in Table 29-1. This chapter focuses on these processes and approaches only as they relate to small groups. The study of large groups, such as community meetings, is beyond the scope of this chapter.

Group Structure

Group structure refers to the group's underlying order. It describes the boundaries, communication and decision-making processes, and authority relationships within the group. The structure offers the group stability and helps to regulate behavioral and interactional patterns.

Table 29-1 Components of Small Groups

Components	Characteristics
Group structure	The group's underlying order; includes boundaries, communication, and decision-making processes, as well as authority relationships; offers stability and helps regulate behavior and interactional patterns
Group size	Preferred size is seven to ten members
Length of sessions	Optimum length of a session is 20 to 40 minutes for lower-functioning groups and 60-120 minutes for higher-functioning groups (divided into time for a brief warm-up, work time, and a brief wrap-up)
Communication	Feedback is used to help members identify group dynamics and communication patterns
Roles	Determined by behavior and responsibilities assumed by the members of the group
Power	Ability to influence the group and other members
Norms	Standards of behavior in the group; influence communication and behavior; communicated overtly or covertly
Cohesion	The strength of the members' desire to work together toward common goals; related to group's attraction and member satisfaction

Group Size

The preferred size of an interpersonally oriented group is seven to ten members. The group must have enough people to give members the opportunity for consensual validation, as well as the expression of different viewpoints. If the group has too many people, not all members will be given enough time to speak and some will feel excluded. There will also be insufficient time to analyze and discuss interactions. If the group has too few members, not enough sharing and interaction may occur.

Length of Sessions

The optimum length of a session is 20 to 40 minutes for lower-functioning groups and 60 to 120 minutes for higher-functioning ones. For the latter groups a few minutes are spent warming to the task of working, then most of the session is spent on group work, and finally the group summarizes and takes care of "unfinished business" from that session.

Communication

One of the group leader's primary tasks is to observe and analyze the communication patterns within the

group. Using feedback, the leader helps members become aware of the group dynamics and communication patterns so that they may realize the significance of these patterns for the group and for themselves. The group or individual members may then experiment and change these patterns if they choose.

Observable verbal and nonverbal elements of the group's communication include:

▼ Individual member communications
▼ Spatial and seating arrangements
▼ Common themes expressed by the group
▼ How frequently and to whom members communicate
▼ How members are listened to in the group
▼ What problem-solving processes occur in the group

These behaviors help the leader assess resistance within the group, interpersonal conflict, the roles assumed by some of the members, the level of competition, and how well the members understand and are working on the task.

Group Roles

In studying groups it is important to observe the roles that members assume in the group. Each role has certain expected behaviors and responsibilities.

The role a member takes can be determined by observing communication and behavioral patterns. The following factors influence role selection: the member's personality, the interaction in the group, and the individual's position in the group. Benne and Sheats[2] described three major types of roles individuals can play in groups:

1. **Building or maintenance roles,** which involve group processes and functions
2. **Task roles,** which deal with completing the group's task
3. **Individual roles,** which are not related to the group's tasks or maintenance; they may be self-centered and distracting for the group

These roles are summarized in Table 29-2. A person who acts as a harmonizer and peacemaker would be taking a maintenance role. A person in a task role might clarify and seek new information. The importance of group maintenance and task roles has been observed by Bales and Slater,[1] whose studies demonstrate evidence that groups encourage members to specialize in one of these two role functions.

Members may experience a conflict when there is a difference between the role they seek or assume and the role given to them by the group. For example, a member may be expected to be a peacemaker because of having performed that role previously. Now, however, this member may be under additional stress or angry with

Table 29-2   Group Roles and Functions

Role	Function
Maintenance roles	Function in group
Encourager	To be positive influence on the group
Harmonizer	To make/keep peace
Compromiser	To minimize conflict by seeking alternatives
Gatekeeper	To determine level of group acceptance of individual members
Follower	To serve as interested audience
Rule maker	To set standards for group behaviors (e.g., time, dress)
Problem solver	To solve problems to allow group to continue its work
Task roles	**Function in group**
Leader	To set direction
Questioner	To clarify issues and information
Facilitator	To keep group focused
Summarizer	To state current position of the group
Evaluator	To assess performance of the group
Initiator	To begin group discussion
Individual roles	**Function for individual**
Victim	To deflect responsibility from self
Monopolizer	To actively seek control by incessant talking
Seducer	To maintain distance and gain personal attention
Mute	To seek control passively through silence
Complainer	To discourage positive work and ventilate anger
Truant/late comer	To invalidate significance of the group
Moralist	To serve as judge of right and wrong

Modified from Benne KD, Sheats P: J *Soc Issues* 4:41, 1948.

someone in the group and may choose to start rather than resolve conflict. The group will often be confused and upset by this new role.

> Consider the last task-oriented group of which you were a member. Identify the roles that were taken by each group member. Which helped and which interfered with task accomplishment? Give an example of the behavior that was associated with each role.

Power

Power is the member's ability to influence the group and its other members. The power structure in the group is usually resolved in its initial stages. To determine the power of various members, it is helpful to assess which member(s) receive the most attention, which are listened to most, and which make decisions for the group.

Resolution of the power struggle does not necessarily mean that everyone will be satisfied with the arrangement. Sometimes a continual struggle for power occurs within the group. This may be functional if the members are trying to gain new leadership that contributes to their therapeutic goals. It can also be dysfunctional when it takes the group's energy and attention away from other tasks.

Norms

Norms are standards of behavior. They are expectations of how the group will act in the future based on its past and present experiences. It is important to understand norms because they influence the quality of communication and interaction within the group. The observance of norms results in conforming. The member who does not follow the norms may be considered rebellious or resistant by the other group members. Conforming to group norms is essential to being a fully accepted member. A member who is always late to meetings that the group has decided will start on time is not conforming to group norms. The group will decide to what extent it will tolerate this behavior.

Norms are created to:

1. Facilitate accomplishment of the group's goal(s) or tasks
2. Control interpersonal conflict
3. Interpret social reality
4. Foster group interdependence

Norms may be communicated overtly or covertly. Overt expression of norms may be written or clearly stated. For example, members may tell a new member that smoking is not allowed in the group. Covert expression of norms may be implied through members' behavior. For example, a member who uses foul language may be ignored by the other members. It must be noted that a highly cohesive group may have appropriate or inappropriate norms. For example, a group of patients may unite to help a patient sneak a cigarette when such behavior is contraindicated because of that patient's health problems. The group may also unite to do what it can to prevent that patient from smoking.

> Identify and describe norms that have been observed in a selected clinical setting and in the classroom. Did anyone deviate from a norm? How did the group respond? How did the leader respond?

Cohesion

Cohesion is the strength of the members' desire to work together toward common goals. It influences members

Table 29-3   Developmental Phases in Small Groups

Tuckman phases	Yalom phases	Definition	Task activity	Interpersonal activity
Forming	Initial orientation	Group members concerned with orientation	To identify task and boundaries regarding it	Relationships tested; interpersonal boundaries identified; dependent relationship with leaders, other group members or preexisting standards established
Storming	Initial conflict	Group members resistive to task and group influence	To respond emotionally to task	Intragroup conflict
Norming	Initial cohesion	Resistance to group overcome by members	To express intimate personal opinions around task	New roles adopted; new standards evolved in group feelings; cohesiveness developed
Performing	Working	Creative problem solving done; solutions emerge	To direct group energy toward completion of task	Interpersonal structure of group becomes tool to achieve its task; roles become flexible and functional

Modified from Tuckman B: *Psychol Bull* 63:384, 1965.

to remain in the group. It is related to each member's attraction to and satisfaction received from the group. Cohesion is a basic fiber of any group because it affects its life span and success. Many factors contribute to the level of cohesion, including agreement of members on group goals, interpersonal attractiveness between the members, degree to which the group satisfies individual needs, similarities among members, and satisfaction of members with the leadership style. Since cohesion is such an important dimension, some group leader interventions are aimed toward promoting it. These may include encouraging members to talk directly with each other, discussing the group in "we" terms, and encouraging all members to sit within the space reserved for the group. A leader can also promote cohesion by pointing out similarities among group members, helping members listen to each other, and encouraging cooperation among the members.

The group leader continually monitors the level of cohesion in the group. Group leaders might observe how much members express interest in each other and recognize each other for their individuality. Another way to measure cohesion is to find out if members identify with the group as a whole and whether they want to remain in the group.

GROUP DEVELOPMENT

Groups, like individuals, have capacity for growth and development. Likewise, they have the ability to regress and resist working effectively. Stages of development have been described for small groups. Bennis and Sheppard[3] theorized that the central concepts of group development are dependency and interdependency.

Schutz[14] stated that every group develops according to a series of three interpersonal stages: inclusion, or being "in or out"; control, or being "top or bottom"; and affection, or being "near or far." Each stage is characterized by members expressing various aspects of the same interpersonal issue or conflict.

Tuckman[15] believed that any group is concerned with the completion of its task. He referred to the group structure as the interpersonal relationships among the members and task activity as the interactions directly related to the task. Tuckman summarized the various phases of group development as forming, storming, norming, and performing. Table 29-3 summarizes Tuckman's categories and model.

Group development does not occur in distinct phases. Phases may overlap, and a group may regress to a previous phase. For example, group regression can occur when a new member is added. Phases of group development can be thought of as a path that a group takes to form and accomplish its objectives. The leader's task is to understand and assist the group as it moves along its growth path.

Pregroup Phase

An important factor to consider in starting a group is its goal or goals. The group's purpose will greatly influence many of the leader's behaviors. There may be more than one group goal; if so, the primary goal should be clear. To guarantee success, the group's goals must be understood by all persons involved, including the members and sponsoring agencies. It is the leader's role to clarify the task and assist the group in achieving it. An example of a group goal for survivors of spouse abuse would be to provide support for each member.

Once the purpose is established, the leader must be sure that the group has administrative permission. A written group proposal is one effective way to request this. Box 29-1 lists information to include in a group proposal. To avoid possible problems, the leader should explore any administrative limitations. For example, an agency may not permit a group to meet beyond its physical facilities or may prefer that the leader not use certain techniques in the group. Also, any potential cost to the agency should be clearly identified.

The leader is also responsible for finding physical space for the group. The leader identifies the room requirements of the group. For example, in a patient education group resources such as a blackboard or movie projector may be needed. A psychotherapy group may need space for comfortable chairs to be placed in a circle without a table. In a group that plans to use human relations exercises, a more spacious room will probably be needed. In all cases the group room should be comfortable, private, and quiet. The same room should be used for each meeting. Leaders often have to adapt inadequate space to fit the needs of the group. The session itself is more important than where it is conducted.

The next responsibility of the group leader is to select members. The selection is based on the purposes of the group, referrals to the group, and interviews with potential members. The leader and/or the agencies must provide information about the group to potential sources of referrals. All information should clearly identify the group's purpose and state the criteria for membership eligibility and the time, place, and duration. The leaders' names and professional credentials should be provided.

Membership will greatly influence the group's outcome. In selecting members, the leader should consider group cohesion and therapeutic problem solving. Selection criteria include problem areas, motivation, age, sex, cultural factors, educational level, socioeconomic level, ability to communicate, intelligence, and coping and defensive styles. Homogeneous groups will share preselected criteria; for example, all members will be women who suffered incest as a child. Heterogeneous groups will include a mixture of individuals, such as a group for men and women who want to build their self-esteem.

In a mixed (homogeneous and heterogeneous) group, members share an essential characteristic (e.g., depression), but their age, sex, and educational and family backgrounds vary. Yalom and Vinogradov[17] advocated that cohesion should serve as a primary guide for selection of patients for therapy groups and that heterogeneous factors be chosen to provide demographic variation.

If possible, the leader should decide whether the membership of the group will be closed or open before screening members. A group is closed if no new members are added once the group is started. In an open group, members leave and new members are added throughout the duration of the group. Open groups may maintain the same purpose, with both members and leaders changing. They usually continue indefinitely with no termination date. The closed group offers the advantage of consistency of leadership, norms, and expectations. The open group, on the other hand, continually brings fresh ideas and opportunities for learning to its members.

The screening interview's primary purpose is to determine the appropriateness of the potential member to the group. Secondary purposes accomplished during the screening interview include:

1. Beginning to develop a relationship between the leader and the member
2. Determining the motivation of the possible member

Box 29-1

GROUP PROPOSAL GUIDELINE

1. List the group goal(s)
   a. Primary goal
   b. Secondary goal
2. List group leader(s) and their related expertise
3. List theoretical framework(s) utilized by the leader(s) to meet the group goals
4. List criteria for membership
5. Describe the referral and screening process
6. Describe the structure of the group
   a. Meeting place_____
   b. Meeting time_____
   c. Length of each meeting_____
   d. Number of members_____
   e. Length of group_____
   f. Expected member behaviors_____
   g. Expected leader behaviors_____
7. Describe the evaluation process for members and the group
8. Describe resources needed for the group, such as coffee, a movie projector, or audiovisual equipment
9. If pertinent, describe the expected cost and financial benefits incurred by the group.

3. Determining if the candidate's goals are in agreement with the group goals
4. Educating the candidate about the nature of the group
5. Determining the type of group experience the individual has had
6. If appropriate, beginning to review the group contract

In addition to or instead of the screening interview, some clinicians use a "group intake." Several new members meet in a group for one to three sessions to learn about the group process and identify some possible treatment goals. This approach is less costly and has the same objectives as the screening interview.

As soon as possible a decision should be made about group membership. Candidates not selected should be referred to other treatment options. The reasons for not being selected should be explained to the individual, and if appropriate, to the person who made the referral.

Initial Phase

The initial phase includes meetings in which the group's members begin to "settle down" to work. This phase is characterized by anxiety regarding being accepted by the group, the setting of norms, and the casting of various roles. Curative factors such as catharsis and universality begin to operate. This phase has been subdivided into three stages by Yalom[17]: the orientation, conflict, and cohesive stages. The stages correspond to Tuckman's[15] first three stages of group development (see Table 29-3).

Orientation Stage. During this stage the leader is more directive and active than in other stages. The leader orients the group to its primary task and helps the group arrive at a group contract. Some common factors that may be included in the group contract are goals, confidentiality, meeting times, honesty, structure, and communication rules (e.g., only one person may talk at a time). Since an important part of this phase is norm setting, the leader should ensure that the norms will help the group achieve its primary and secondary goals. Another task of the leader in this stage is to foster a sense of belonging or cohesion among the members. To accomplish this, the leader encourages interaction among members and maintains the group at a working level of anxiety. For example, the leader could refer to the group as "our" group and suggest how members can help each other. Members could be encouraged to state what they hope to learn from the group. The leader would then reinforce realistic expectations and give examples of how the group might meet them.

During the first stage the members are evaluating each other, the group, and the leader. They are deciding if they are going to be a part of the group and how much they will participate. Some common conscious or unconscious concerns of members during this stage are fear of being rejected, fear of self-disclosure, and fear of not being seen as an individual. Social behaviors are important, and the members are attempting to develop their social roles. The roles members assume during this stage are often renegotiated during other stages. The group is dependent, and members will often test out their dependency needs and wishes on the leader. They look to the leader for structure, approval, and acceptance, and may try to please the leader with reward-seeking behaviors. The leader must not meet all the dependency wishes of the members but must encourage members to interact more with one another. This supports members in becoming more interdependent and less dependent on the leader. The dependency issue between the leader and the members may lead the group into conflict and thus into the second stage.

Conflict Stage. This stage of the group corresponds to Tuckman's[15] storming stage of group development. Issues related to control, power, and authority become primary. Members are concerned about the "pecking order" or deciding who is "top or bottom" in regard to control and decision making. The dependency conflict may be openly or covertly expressed, with members polarized between independent and dependent issues. Bennis and Sheppard[3] describe this stage as a struggle between the counterdependent and dependent members, with the counterdependent members wanting to assume the leader's role. For example, a group may be divided over the issue of whether members can telephone each other. Some members may want the leader to decide, whereas others may think that the leader's statements are irrelevant. During this phase the counterdependent members might sit in the leader's chair and let the leader know the directions have been unsuccessful or unheard. The dependent members might ask the leader for more directions. Other members who are neutral (neither dependent nor counterdependent) eventually may assist the group in resolving this conflict.

Subgroups usually form within the group, and hostility may be expressed. Often the hostility is directed toward the leader, but it may also be expressed toward other members. The leader's tasks are to allow expression of both negative and positive feelings, to help the group understand the underlying conflict, and to prevent and/or examine nonproductive behaviors such as scapegoating. This phase is usually the most difficult for the new leader because some members may lead the leader to believe he or she has failed the group by not living up to its unrealistic expectations.

The leader must be careful not to avoid or suppress the group members' anxiety and, at times, should encourage the expression of hostility. If hostility toward the leader is expressed indirectly, such as anger toward other authority figures (e.g., staff members, teachers, parents), the leader should assist the group in expressing its anger more directly. A useful technique is for the leader to give the group permission to discuss its anger by acknowledging that the group may be disappointed or angry at the leader.

By the end of the conflict stage the leader may be dethroned, and his or her omnipotent role, with its "magical" solutions, may be discarded. Slowly the leader becomes humanized. Members learn that responsibilities for the group are shared. Members may also learn that expressions of anger and disappointment do not destroy the leader and may help the group assess its resources and limitations more accurately. The group's resources can then be used to achieve its primary and secondary tasks. Members may realize that conflicts need not be avoided; instead, through discussion, conflicts may increase the group's maturity and usefulness.

Cohesive Stage. Tuckman's norming phase[15] is closely related to the cohesive stage. Group members, after resolving the second stage, feel a strong attraction toward one another and a strong attachment to the group. Positive feelings toward one another and the group are frequently expressed, and negative feelings are usually not shared.

At this stage, members feel free to give self-disclosing information and share more intimate concerns. However, the group's problem-solving ability is restricted because negative communication is usually avoided in order to maintain the high group morale. The leader's task is to make a connection between the members' disclosures and the group's primary task. The leader should not interfere with the group's basic cohesion but should encourage the group to use its problem-solving ability. The leader shows how a group member can have individual concerns and values and still be productive within the group. In other words the leader demonstrates that differing and opposite opinions may not destroy the group identity.

At the resolution of this stage, members may learn that self-discoveries and differences should not be feared. They also learn that similarities and differences between the members may help the group achieve its tasks. At the end of the cohesive stage the group begins to see task achievement as a reality. The members gain a more realistic and honest view of their ability to work together and accomplish their primary and secondary tasks.

 Compare and contrast behaviors that would indicate that a group is in the orientation stage, the conflict stage, and the cohesive stage. Give specific examples. What leader interventions would be appropriate at each stage?

Working Phase

The working phase of a group can be compared with Tuckman's performing stage of group development. During this stage the group becomes a team. It directs its energy mainly toward completing its tasks. Although they are hard at work, this phase is an enjoyable one for both the leader and the members. Responsibility for the group is more equally shared, anxiety is usually decreased and tolerated better, and the group is more stable and realistic.

Yalom and Vinogradov[17] have described some of the positive forces that occur in group therapy. They listed 11 curative factors that may occur (Table 29-4). Although these factors were identified in relationship to therapy groups, they are relevant to experiences in all types of groups. The new reality in inpatient psychiatric settings involves greater acuity of illness and shorter stays. Hoge and McLoughlin[6] identified seven therapeutic factors that are important in promoting positive change in short-term groups. They include self-responsibility, self-understanding, instillation of hope, group cohesiveness, catharsis, altruism, and universality. The last five are also included in Yalom's factors.

In a psychotherapy group, members begin seriously to work through their concerns related to their therapeutic goals. They begin a more in-depth exploration of the various goals related to their group's tasks. For example, in a psychotherapeutic group for mothers with chronically ill children, the members may discuss their various reactions to the children, their ambivalent feelings, some of their thoughts regarding the reason for their feelings, and alternative ways to cope with their daily realities.

The leader's major role is to help the group complete its task or tasks by maximizing effective use of its curative properties. Because the members are fully participating in the group's work, the leader's activity level decreases. The leader now acts more as a consultant to the group. The leader helps to keep the group goal-directed and tries to decrease the impact of anything that may regress or retard the group.

Because this phase is the group's creative problem-solving and resolution phase, there are few, if any, specific guidelines for the leader. The leader's interventions

Table 29-4 Yalom's Curative Factors

Factor	Definition
Imparting information	Receiving didactic information and advice
Instillation of hope	Increasing hopefulness of group members
Universality	Realization that others experience same thoughts, feelings, and problems
Altruism	Experience of sharing part of oneself to help another
Corrective reenactment of primary family group	Ability of members to alter learning experience previously obtained in their families
Development of social interaction techniques	Opportunity to increase awareness of social interactions and develop social skills
Imitative behaviors	Opportunities to increase skills by imitating behaviors of others in group
Interpersonal learning	Ability to engage in wider range of interpersonal exchanges, thereby increasing each member's understanding of responsibility and complexity of interpersonal relationships and decreasing member's interpersonal distortions
Existential factors	Ability of group to help members deal with meaning of their own existence
Catharsis	Opportunity to express feelings previously unexpressed
Group cohesion	Attraction of member for group and other members

Modified from Yalom ID, Vinogradov S: *Group psychotherapy*, Washington, DC, 1989, American Psychiatric Press.

are primarily based on theoretical frameworks, experiences, personality, and intuition, as well as the needs of the group and its members. In addition to fostering group cohesion, maintaining its boundaries, and encouraging the group to work on its tasks, the leader may help the group solve specific problems. Because these problems are unique to the group, many are not predictable. Some of the more common problems are the formation of subgroups, the management of conflict, and determining the optimum level of self-disclosure.[17]

Subgroups that conflict with the group's goals and are not acknowledged by the group can restrict its work. Other members may feel excluded, and loyalties will be divided between the subgroup and the whole group. For example, in a women's group, two of the members may become close friends, keeping secrets from the group and engaging in private conversations during the session. Other members may feel excluded from this pair and be ineffective in working with them. To decrease the negative impact of a subgroup, its consequences and the group's reactions should be openly discussed.

Conflict is unavoidable and can be used to foster growth. However, expression of conflict may need to be controlled so that the intensity does not exceed the group's tolerance. Examples of conflict are competition among members for the leader's attention and a disagreement between two members. A leader may manage conflicts by identifying the conflict, explaining that conflicts are natural and can lead to growth, and encouraging members to discuss the reasons for the conflict. Successful conflict resolution is related to the amount of group cohesion, trust, and acceptance among the members.

The amount of *self-disclosure* is usually related to the amount of acceptance and trust the member feels. Self-disclosure is always risky. If persons give private information too quickly, they will feel vulnerable. On the other hand, if persons disclose too little during the working phase they may not be able to form supportive interpersonal relationships. Their growth potential in the group may be decreased.

Resistance, or holding back the therapeutic process, can be expected in therapy groups. Resistance to working on the therapeutic goal can occur at both an individual and a group level. It is one matter to agree on goals and another to work on obtaining the actual therapeutic outcomes. Resistance by individual members may take many forms, such as avoiding discussion of a conflict, frequent or prolonged silences, attempting to become an assistant leader, absence from the group, pairing between two members, and prolonged or unusually intense expression of hostility. Resistance by the group or a majority of its members may be expressed in ways similar to those used by individuals. Other examples of group resistance include shared silence among the members, unusual amounts of dependency on the leader, scapegoating, subgroup formations, and the wish for magical solutions to resolve group conflict.

Resistance may occur because of increased anxiety related to conflict or change. The management of resistance depends on the type of group, the group contract, and the therapist's theoretical framework. Some methods of decreasing resistance are to make observations regarding the group process or individual behaviors, offer interpretations, counteract the resistant behavior, and demonstrate more adaptive behavioral patterns.

By the end of the second phase, members have made significant progress toward goal achievement. They have a sense of their own productiveness and accomplishments. The need for the group or their involvement in the group is less apparent. The group must begin to deal more actively with its final task—separation.

Termination Phase

The work of termination begins during the first phase of the group. However, as the group or individual members approach termination, certain processes are more likely to occur. The termination phase is not always discussed as a definite phase in the literature. It is discussed as a separate phase here because of the significance that it may have for the members.

There are two types of termination: termination of the group as a whole and termination of individual members. A closed group usually terminates as an entire group; in an open group, members (and perhaps the leader) terminate separately. Members and groups may terminate prematurely, unsuccessfully, or successfully.

Termination is a highly individual process. Members and groups will terminate in unique ways. If the group has been successful, termination is painful and involves grieving or a sense of loss. It may cause the group to experience increased anxiety, regression, and a feeling of accomplishment. Permitting members to avoid discussing termination would prevent them from having a possible successful growth experience. Leadership behaviors include encouraging an evaluation of the group or its terminating members, reminiscing about important events that occurred in the group, and encouraging members to give each other feedback. Evaluation usually focuses on the amount of achievement of the group's or individual's goals. Leaders must be careful not to collude with members in denying termination; rather, they must encourage full discussion. Termination should be talked about several sessions before the final session to allow members time to work through issues that surface. Termination may lead to discussion of many related topics, such as other separations, death, aging, and the use and passage of time. If terminated successfully, members may feel a sense of resolution about the group experience and use these experiences in many other life situations.

Premature termination means that the group ends before its tasks are completed or a member leaves the group before his or her work is finished. Premature termination may occur for appropriate and inappropriate reasons. Appropriate reasons include moving to another city before the group is terminated. Inappropriate reasons might include a member's unwillingness to discuss an issue central to the group but painful to that person.

As a staff nurse you are given the responsibility for developing a transition group for hospitalized schizophrenic patients who are soon to be discharged. Outline the points you will need to consider and the steps you would take to establish the group.

EVALUATION OF THE GROUP

Evaluation of the group and the group members' progress is an ongoing process that begins in the selection interview. Notes describing group sessions should be descriptive to assist in identifying goal achievement. To make record keeping easy, it is usually helpful to have a "group notebook." In this notebook leaders can write pertinent data on individual members, such as their goals, their telephone numbers, their addresses, the screening note, any individual comments, and a termination summary note. In another section of the group notebook the leaders can describe each group meeting. One format for quickly recording each group meeting is provided in Box 29-2. In most agencies summary notes are also included in individual members' clinical records.

In addition, it is helpful to determine each member's goal attainment periodically during the course of the group. This can be done using subjective ratings by the group leaders and by obtaining individual members' perceptions on how they are meeting their goals. For a slightly more objective evaluation, members are asked to rate their goal achievement on a Likert scale (one that allows members to rate their response along a con-

---

Box 29-2

GROUP SESSION NOTE OUTLINE

Date _____ Group Meeting No. _____
1. Membership:
   a. List members attending (state if new member)
   b. List members who were late
   c. List absent members
2. List individual members' pertinent issues or behaviors discussed in the group
3. List group themes
4. Identify important group process issues (e.g., developmental stage, roles, norms)
5. Identify any critical leadership strategy used
6. List proposed future leadership strategies
7. Predict member and group responses for the next session

tinuum, for example, 1 being low, 5 being high). Members' goal achievement should always be evaluated at termination.

Along with the descriptive evaluation the clinician may decide to administer a before- and after-group written test(s). The tests selected should be related to the expected changes in the group. For example, an anxiety scale could be administered to members attending a group whose major goal is to reduce anxiety. If this type of evaluation is used, it is critical that the clinician use the most appropriate standardized scale available and that the agency's and the members' permissions are obtained. Commonly used rating scales are described in Chapter 6. It is very important that all parties involved know the intent of using such tests and the disposition of test results.

It is also essential to identify outcomes so that the impact and validity of nursing group interventions can be communicated to consumers and health-care organizations. For example, vanServellen et al.[16] identified possible short-term outcome measures for nurse-led groups including increased knowledge of coping skills and increased insight into the members' own effective and ineffective coping behaviors. These were measured by a pre- and postgroup coping test. Longer term outcomes included a decrease in hopelessness measured by the Beck Hopelessness Scale; decreased depression measured by the Beck Depression Scale; and decreased manic behavior measured by the Young Manic Scale.

Guillory and Riggin[5] developed a nursing staff support group model. They listed the following measurable outcomes:

1. Use of a problem-solving approach
2. Development of a communication tool
3. Assertive handling of conflict
4. Seeking assistance from each other when stressed
5. Decreased patient complaints
6. Decreased staff turnover

NURSES AS GROUP LEADERS
Nurse Leadership Qualities

Nurses who are group leaders must be concerned about the many previously discussed factors regarding the group. The group leader must be able to study the group and participate in it at the same time. The leader must constantly monitor the group and, whenever necessary, help the group achieve its goals.

The qualities of an effective nurse leader are the same qualities that are important in the therapeutic relationship (see Chapter 2). In particular, these include the responsive and active dimensions of empathy, genuineness, and confrontation. In addition, creativity and opportunism are helpful qualities for leaders to possess.

While they are listening to members' words, leaders also need to be aware of the group process. They must be alert to opportunities for the group to use themes and behaviors and see how these are related to individual issues. Leaders may be likened to an orchestra conductor who seeks to focus on the sound of a particular instrument for the appreciation and reaction of the total orchestra. The leader may encourage examination of the music from different perspectives and look for possible variations that would create a new piece of music. Opportunities for creativity may also lead to the development of innovative group techniques (see Critical Thinking about Contemporary Issues).

CRITICAL THINKING ABOUT CONTEMPORARY ISSUES

Do Computer Networks Provide a New Way for Nurses To Intervene with Groups of Patients?

Interaction through on-line computer networks is growing in popularity. Nurses have begun to identify opportunities to establish patient groups using this technology. Nurses have reported on the effectiveness of facilitating computer network groups for people with AIDS and for caregivers of people with Alzheimer's disease.[13] They found that all of Yalom's curative factors could be identified during the course of these groups. Advantages to the members included convenience, ability to relate to a variety of people in similar situations, and ready access to peer support. This approach also offers the option of anonymity to group members.

Psychiatric nurses need to consider the implications of this new way of conducting groups. The inability to perceive nonverbal communication removes an important dimension from the communication process. Since interaction among members is not simultaneous, time gaps occur between interventions and the responses of various members. Spontaneity may also be lost. The development of trust among group members could proceed differently than in traditional groups. Confidentiality may be even more of a concern to members than it is in face-to-face groups.

Identifying and exploring the dimensions of computer network groups offer a challenge to psychiatric nurses. Nurses who lead groups need to adapt their skills to enhance the advantages of the technology and minimize the disadvantages. As more people become computer-literate and accustomed to on-line relationships, the potential for this new form of group support will evolve. ▼

Group leaders must make it safe for members to challenge their authority. In examining this interplay between the leader and the members, there are opportunities to practice conflict management, confrontation, and assertive communication. The leader needs to accept confrontation without taking it personally.

Leaders also need to have assertive communication skills so that they can foster independence in the group but also help the group focus to reach its goals. Achieving this balance requires a blend of skills and judgment that can be gained with practice in group leadership, supervision by an experienced group facilitator, and study of group process.

It is also critical for leaders to be able to organize a great deal of information and to identify themes for the session. Novice leaders usually need to review the group experience with a supervisor after the session so that they can identify and analyze the important events.

Finally, a nurse leader also needs a sense of humor. Laughter helps reveal the truth and enables participants to share and empathize about serious matters without the high levels of tension that often accompany such discussions. For example, in a women's codependent group, humor and laughter were regularly used. The group adopted this technique to talk about their "rescuing" and controlling behaviors. This group was composed of fragile individuals who grew up in abusive families. They worked hard at seeing, understanding, and changing their contribution to the destructive relationships they developed. The members brought examples of their "setting themselves up" to the group weekly and laughed as they were able to find humor in recognizing behavior that was similar to their own. The humor also allowed the members to give feedback in a less confrontive manner.

Groups with Co-Leaders

For a group, the presence of co-leaders may have advantages and disadvantages. When two clinicians share the leadership, the breadth of observation and the choice of interventions are greater than with one. For example, a male and female team may represent the family and offer the group members an opportunity to deal with issues related to parents or other significant male and female figures.

A male-female team also offers group members opportunities to observe a man and a woman working together with mutual respect and without exploitation, sexualizing, or putting each other down. A variety of transference reactions are available with experienced co-leaders to assist in learning and the resolution of problems. Exploration of the members' fantasies regarding the relationship between the leaders can give them a chance to see conflict and resolution. This can contribute significantly to the group's openness and power.

Disadvantages of the leadership team are often related to difficulties between the leaders. When there is competition, a major philosophical difference, or great variance in strategy or style, the group will not work effectively. Differences in levels of experience are handled if both are comfortable with their roles of apprentice and senior leader. Conflict between co-leaders could lead to the splitting of the group or the group developing an alliance with one of the leaders, which could be very damaging. Splitting needs to be openly interpreted in the group and dealt with by the group members and leaders.

NURSE-LED GROUPS

Nurses lead groups in a variety of health-care settings. Some types of groups that may be led by nurses are task groups, self-help groups, teaching groups, supportive/therapy groups, psychotherapy groups, and peer support groups. The type of group intervention provided by an individual nurse is determined by the needs and goals of the patients and by the education and experience of the nurse.

Task Groups

Task groups are designed to accomplish a particular task. Nursing care planning meetings and committees are examples of task groups. The emphasis of these groups is on decision making and problem solving. They often have specific goals to accomplish and a deadline for completion of the work.

Self-Help Groups

Groups organized around a common experience are labeled self-help groups. Some examples include smoking cessation groups, Overeaters Anonymous, Alcoholics Anonymous, Parents and Friends of Lesbians and Gays, Parents Without Partners, and numerous groups related to specific health problems. They may or may not receive consultation from a health-care provider, such as a professional nurse. Although some are established and organized by professionals, they are run by the members and often do not have a designated leader. Leadership evolves within the group depending on the need that arises. Nurses can support self-help groups by referring members and by offering advice and assistance if it is requested. They can also promote links between the self-help group and the health-care system. Kelly and associates[8] established a self-help group for people with serious mental illness. They found that the members who were coping well with their illnesses provided positive role models for the others.

Teaching Groups

The goal of teaching groups is to provide information. Examples are childbirth preparation and parent education groups. In-service education groups for staff are also included in this category. The nurse leader is able to educate more people more efficiently using a group format. The members themselves often become co-teachers as they share their information and experiences. Humphrey,[7] a school nurse, organized an Asthma Club to address the problems of asthmatic students who were doing poorly academically and felt stigmatized by their condition. Children discussed the disease and treatment. Positive outcomes included decreased absenteeism among the group members, use of inhalers in the classroom without embarrassment, and positive parent feedback. The group helped break the chain of illness, isolation, and self-perceived failure.

Mohr[11] developed a curriculum for a psychoeducation program for a heterogeneous group of inpatients. The only patients excluded from the group were those who were so narcissistic or psychotic that they would inhibit the work of the other group members. The groups were taught in six subject areas: stress management, medication management, life enrichment, social skills development, assertiveness skills, and games to help identify feelings and coping skills. Nurse leaders took the roles of teacher and facilitator. They thought the groups added concreteness and substance to the treatment program. Additional patient data were collected through participation in the sessions. Patients appreciated the increase in staff attention and an increase in the variety of activities.

Supportive Therapy Groups

The primary goal of supportive therapy groups is to help the members cope with life stress. The focus is on dysfunctional thoughts, feelings and behaviors. Nehls[12] identified successful interventions used with a group of community mental health center patients who had a psychiatric diagnosis of borderline personality disorder. Giving and receiving information was used to provide structure for the group. This enabled these patients, who had problems with appropriate limit-setting, to practice effective problem-solving techniques.

Koontz, Cox and Hastings[9] implemented a short-term support group to work with families of patients briefly hospitalized for evaluation and treatment on a general hospital psychiatric unit. During 10 months, over 120 persons attended these sessions an average of three times. The leaders discovered major gaps in information about illness and treatment. There was also a great need for family support. The short-term group provided emotional support and critical information to increase members' coping and problem-solving abilities, thereby strengthening patients' support systems.

Psychotherapy Groups

The goal of a psychotherapy group is the treatment of emotional, cognitive, or behavioral dysfunction. Group techniques and processes are used to help members learn about their behavior with other people and how it relates to core personality traits. The intent is for the members to change their behavior, not just understand or seek support for it. Members also learn that they have responsibilities to others and can help other members achieve their goals. An example of a psychotherapy group is a scheduled outpatient group that focuses on the behaviors that caused the member to seek help and the behavioral changes that will make life more satisfying. In a 2-year reality-based, ego supportive therapy group for mothers of incest victims, DelPo and Koontz[4] identified four strategies that they used to develop and maintain the group: noncritical acceptance and listening, appropriate nurturance and modeling of behaviors, restatement or reframing of paradoxical statements, and clarification. The effectiveness of the interventions was demonstrated by changes in the womens' perceptions and behaviors. Kreidler and Carlson[10] conducted a long-term group for women who were adult survivors of incest. Through the group these women were able to learn and experience positive self-esteem, give up the victim role, and feel empowered.

Peer Support Groups

Finally, peer support groups are an effective way for professionals to share the stresses and problems related to their work. An example of a peer support group is a group of advanced practice psychiatric nurse specialists who meet monthly. Group purposes may include case consultation, sharing information about educational opportunities, providing information about business management, and decreasing isolation for those who are in private practice. Another example is a group of nurses who work with people who are infected with the human immunodeficiency virus (HIV). They meet regularly for nursing consultation and support in coping with the continual loss associated with this disease.

As a head nurse, you decide to form a staff support group. How would this differ from a therapeutic group? Discuss in terms of the roles of the leader and the members. Would there be any similarities?

The types of groups led by nurses are limited only by the nurses' creative ability to assess the needs of the patients with whom they work. Group work is endlessly satisfying because the nurse leader nurtures and participates in the process of human growth and healing.

SUGGESTED CROSS-REFERENCES

SUMMARY

1. A group is a collection of individuals who are interrelated and interdependent and may share common purposes and norms.

2. Components of a small group including structure, size, length of sessions, communication, roles of members, norms, and cohesion were identified and described.

3. The phases of group development—pregroup, initial phase with orientation, conflict and cohesion stages, working phase, and termination were presented.

4. Small group evaluation is based on accomplishment of individual goals and expected group outcomes. Careful documentation of each group session is required.

5. The responsibilities and qualities of nurse group leaders include empathy, nurturance, genuineness, creativity, acceptance of confrontation, assertive communication skills, organization, and a sense of humor.

6. Types of nurse-led groups including task, self-help, teaching, supportive therapy, psychotherapy, and peer support groups were presented.

COMPETENT CARING
A CLINICAL EXEMPLAR OF A PSYCHIATRIC NURSE

Lynn Klair, MS, RN

While I was working as a clinical nurse specialist in a long-term inpatient psychiatric setting, I co-led a predischarge group. We were successful in preparing several patients for discharge. Five of the group members went to the same domiciliary care home. I was concerned about their adjustment to a community setting, so I arranged to continue providing group therapy in the community setting.

The group consisted of three women and two men. We met early in the morning, in part so I could stop on my way to work and in part so we could meet before the members became involved in their daily activities. All of the members attended the group on a fairly regular basis; two of them are particularly memorable to me because of the progress they made.

P was a former nurse who had depression and anorexia nervosa. One of her own goals was to get some new clothes, but her finances were very limited. I obtained some used clothing that I brought to her to replace her old clothes, which were several sizes too large for her. It took her a long time to try the new clothes because she believed that they were too tight on her. This was evidence of her distorted body image. P's greatest accomplishment was to reestablish contact with her family, who lived in another state. The group provided support to her as she struggled with the decision to write to them. They all felt a sense of accomplishment when she wrote and then later talked to family members on the telephone. By the time the group terminated, P was beginning to gain confidence and had stayed out of the hospital longer than she had after any previous hospital discharge.

R was a middle-aged man who had been hospitalized for 15 years following an arrest for a serious assault. He was college educated and had been employed in the past. He was a very large man, and I thought of him as a "gentle giant." He was very kind to the other group members and was liked by all of them, even the most paranoid member. R needed to learn to manage money; he carried his money in his sock. He also needed new clothing, but resisted the group's encouragement to go shopping. When I brought some catalogs to the group, I discovered that R had great difficulty making choices. He finally decided that he would give me money to use to buy clothing for him. Although I felt somewhat uncomfortable with this, I agreed because I knew that it was difficult for him to develop this much trust in another person. When he wore his new clothing to the group, the other members complimented him and I could see his self-esteem improving. R eventually moved into a smaller group home. The group mourned his loss,

but felt good about their role in helping him progress.

After several months of meeting at the house, we decided to have some of our meetings at a nearby fast-food restaurant. This was done to assist members to feel more comfortable out in the community, as well as to address their wish to have refreshments during the meetings. This change worked out well because we could work on socialization and community survival skills.

My experience leading this group was rewarding and resulted in professional growth for me. I gained a new understanding of the ability of some long-term patients to live successfully in the community and also developed an appreciation for the difficulties they face in doing this. I never stopped being impressed by their strength and courage as they met the challenges presented to them. ▼

REFERENCES

1. Bales R, Slater P: Role differentiation in small decision-making groups. In Parsons T, Bales RF, eds: *Family socialization and interactional process*, Glencoe, Ill, 1955, The Free Press.
2. Benne KD, Sheats P: Functional roles and group members, *J Soc Issues* 4:41, 1948.
3. Bennis W, Sheppard H: A theory of group development, *Hum Rel* 9:415, 1956.
4. DelPo EG, Koontz MA: Group therapy with mothers of incest victims: II. Therapeutic strategies, recurrent themes, interventions, and outcomes, *Arch Psychiatr Nurs* 5:70, 1991.
5. Guillory BA, Riggin OZ: Developing a nursing staff support group model, *Clin Nurse Spec* 5:170, 1991.
6. Hoge MA, McLoughlin KA: Group psychotherapy in acute treatment settings: theory and technique, *Hosp Community Psychiatr* 42:153, 1991.
7. Humphrey E: The politics of asthma: a lesson in confidence, *Nurs Times*, 88:31, 1992.
8. Kelly MK, Sauter F, Tugrul K, Weaver MD: Fostering self-help on an inpatient unit, *Arch Psychiatr Nurs* 4:161, 1990.
9. Koontz E, Cox D, Hastings S: Implementing a short-term family support group, *J Psychosoc Nurs Ment Health Serv* 29:5, 1991.
10. Kreidler MC, Carlson RE: Breaking the incest cycle: the group as a surrogate family, *J Psychosoc Nurs Ment Health Serv* 29:28, 1991.
11. Mohr WK: A nurse-led educational program in psychiatric settings: developing a curriculum, *J Psychosoc Nurs Ment Health Serv* 31:34, 1993.
12. Nehls N: Group therapy for people with borderline personality disorder: interventions associated with positive outcomes, *Issues Ment Health Nurs* 13:255, 1992.
13. Ripich S, Moore SM, Brennan PF: A new nursing medium: Computer networks for group intervention, *J Psychosoc Nurs Ment Health Serv* 30:15, 1992.
14. Schutz W: Interpersonal underworld, *Harvard Bus Rev* 36:123, 1958.
15. Tuckman B: Developmental sequence in small groups, *Psychol Bull*, 63:384, 1965.
16. vanServellen G et al: Methodological concerns in evaluating psychiatric nursing care modalities and a proposed standard group protocol format for nurse-led groups, *Arch Psychiatr Nurs* 4:117, 1992.
17. Yalom ID, Vinogradov S: *Group psychotherapy*, Washington, DC, 1989, American Psychiatric Press.

ANNOTATED SUGGESTED READINGS

*Abraham IL, Nerndoerfer MM, Currie LJ: Effects of group interventions on cognition and depression in nursing home residents, *Nurs Res* 41:196, 1992.

Describes a comparative study of three different types of group interventions for 76 depressed nursing home residents.

Corey G: Theory and practice of counseling and psychotherapy, Belmont, Calif, 1991, Brooks/Cole.

Clearly written, good basic text for the beginning nurse group leader.

*DiPasquale JA: The psychological effects of support groups on individuals infected by the AIDS virus, *Cancer Nurs* 13:278, 1990.

Report of a research study of the effects of support groups on the helplessness and anxiety experienced by people with AIDS.

*Evans M, Marad G: A triage model of psychotherapeutic group intervention, *Arch Psychiatr Nurs* 7:244, 1993.

Description of an interesting approach to group intervention with veterans suffering from posttraumatic stress disorder.

Hamilton JD et al: Quality assessment and improvement in group psychotherapy, *Am J Psychiatr* 150:316, 1993.

These authors developed a monitoring and evaluation program for the group therapies used on a large general hospital psychiatric unit.

*Heiney SP: Effects of group therapy on parents of children with cancer, *J Assoc Pediatr Oncol Nurses* 6:63, 1989.

Good example of an effective nurse-led group.

*Jenkins E: A strategy for managing change and stress: developing staff support groups, *Prof Nurse* 6:579, 1991.

Focuses on the benefit of group strategies for coping with stress and burnout prevention using a nurse peer support group.

*Kendall J: Promoting wellness in HIV-support groups, *J Assoc Nurses AIDS Care* 3:28, 1992.

Reports the results of research on a group formed of male homosexuals focusing on intimacy, group process, group structure, and the meaning of the group to the participants.

---

*Nursing reference.

*Kriedler MC, Hassan M: Use of an interactional model with survivors of incest, *Issues Ment Health Nurs* 13:149, 1992.

Through application of the interactional model, this article discusses dysfunctional communication patterns, boundary, and survival issues.

*Kurek-Ovshinsky C: Group psychotherapy in an acute inpatient setting, *Issues Ment health Nurs* 12:81, 1991.

Descriptive article on a conceptual model of group psychotherapy using reparative techniques.

Lentner E, Glazer G: Infertile couples' perceptions of infertility support group participation, *Health Care Women Int* 12:317, 1991.

Describes the use of a questionnaire to determine the benefits of participation in a support group.

*Pollack LE: Problem solving group therapy: two models based on level of functioning, *Issues Ment Health Nurs* 12:65, 1991.

Presents descriptions of two models of group interventions and discusses implications for practice and recommendations.

Rice CA, Rutan M: *Inpatient group psychotherapy: a psychodynamic perspective*, New York, 1987, Macmillan.

This book includes dealing with thought disordered, manic, borderline, and narcissistic patients.

*Shields JD, Lanza ML: The parallel process of resistance by clients and therapists to starting groups: a guide for nurses, *Arch Psychiatr Nurs* 7:300, 1993.

Delineates several ways in which group therapy trainees and patients who have been referred to groups resist initial group involvement.

---

*Nursing reference.

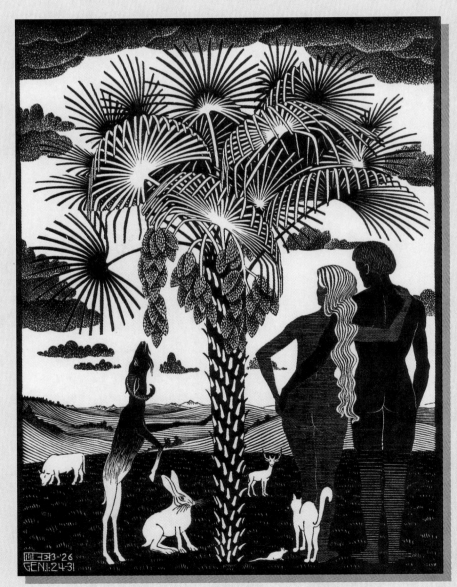

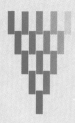

CHAPTER 30
Family Interventions

PATRICIA E. HELM

We are truly heirs of all the ages; but as honest men it behooves us to learn the extent of our inheritance. . . .

John Tyndall: *"Matter and Force" in vol. 2, Prayer as a Form of Physical Energy*

Psychiatric nurse generalists, without master's degrees, are exposed to families at all levels of functioning. Understanding principles of family interventions can allow nurses to make more acute observations, thus enhancing their assessment of families' needs and resources. It can also suggest new ways in which nurses can promote adaptive family functioning and enhance a family's use of positive coping skills. It can help nurses more readily identify problems within family systems and may assist the nurse generalist in initiating appropriate referrals.

Clinical training programs in family therapy are open to psychiatric nurses across the United States. They vary in duration, theoretical framework used, and the level of knowledge required. Usually they are limited to clinicians with graduate degrees in the mental health field. The psychiatric nurse doing family therapy should preferably have a master's degree with didactic content and clinical seminars focused on family work. The nurse also needs to obtain individual or group supervision to refine clinical skills and deepen theoretical understanding of family systems and interventions.

FAMILY FUNCTIONING

Contact with patients' families is a natural part of nursing care. For many years nurses have been making intuitive observations about functional and dysfunctional families. They have been intervening with families without formal training in family therapy. A well-functioning family can shift roles, levels of responsibility, and patterns of interaction as it experiences stressful life changes. A well-functioning family may, under acute or prolonged stress, produce a symptomatic member. This family rebalances in such a way that function of all members is restored and symptoms fade. A functional family has the following characteristics[28]:

1. It completes important life cycle tasks.
2. It has the capacity to tolerate conflict and to adapt to adverse circumstances without long-term dysfunction or disintegration of family cohesion.
3. Emotional contact is maintained across generations and between family members without blurring necessary levels of authority.
4. Overcloseness or fusion is avoided, and distance is not used to solve problems.
5. Each twosome is expected to resolve the problems between them. Bringing a third person in to settle disputes or to take sides is discouraged.
6. Differences between family members are encouraged to promote personal growth and creativity.
7. Children are expected to assume age-appropriate responsibility and to enjoy age-appropriate privileges negotiated with their parents.
8. The preservation of a positive emotional climate is more highly valued than doing what "should" be done or what is "right."
9. Within each spouse there is a balance of affective expression, careful rational thought, relationship focus, and care taking; each spouse can selectively function in the respective modes.

Dysfunctional families lack one or more of these characteristics. Some of the more common dysfunctional family patterns include the following:

1. The overprotective mother and distant father (distant through work, alcohol, or physical absence)
2. The overfunctioning "superwife" or "superhusband" and the underfunctioning passive, dependent, and compliant spouse
3. The spouse who maintains "peace at any price" and who denies difficulties in the marriage but who suddenly feels wronged and self-righteous when the mate is discovered to be in legal trouble or having an affair
4. The child who evidences poor peer relationships at school while attempting to parent younger siblings to compensate for ineffective or emotionally overwhelmed parents
5. The overclose three generations of grandparent, parent, and grandchild in which lines of authority and generational identity are poorly defined and the child is acting out because of a lack of effective limit setting by an agreed upon parental figure
6. The family with a substance abusing member
7. The family subject to physical, emotional, or sexual abuse perpetrated by one of its members

 Watch a popular television show that depicts a family situation and evaluate the family's level of functioning.

Competence Paradigm

The concepts of family functioning just discussed have most recently given way to a competence paradigm for professional practice.[17,18] This new approach was derived from the fact that older conceptual models tended to focus on pathologic states and dysfunction as opposed to family strengths, resources, and competencies. The competency paradigm values empowerment instead of a helper-helpee ideology and stresses the importance of treating people as collaborators who are the masters of their own fate (Table 30-1).

An empowerment model has been used increasingly as a framework for professional practice with families who are coping with a member who is mentally ill or mentally retarded. Its use is likely to increase the understanding of familial attributes that are relevant to coping with the mental illness of a relative, to facilitate the assessment of positive attributes among family members, to offer a blueprint for designing effective interventions for families, and to advance efforts to evaluate the outcome of family-oriented services. In addition, unlike pathology models that may stigmatize and alienate families, a competence paradigm attempts to foster positive alliances between families and health-care providers and enhance the delivery of services.

The competence paradigm emphasizes the following[6]:

1. Focus on growth-producing behaviors rather than on treatment of problems or prevention of negative outcomes
2. Promotion and strengthening of individual and family functioning by fostering the acquisition of prosocial, self-sustaining, self-efficacious, and other adaptive behaviors
3. Definition of the relationship between the help seeker and help giver as a cooperative partnership that assumes joint responsibility
4. Encouragement of assistance that is in line with

Table 30-1   Paradigms in Working with Families

Pathology paradigm	Competence paradigm
NATURE OF PARADIGM	
Disease-based medical model	Health-based developmental model
FAMILIES VIEWED AS	
Pathological, pathogenic, or dysfunctional	Basically or potentially competent
EMPHASIS ON	
Weaknesses, liabilities, and illness	Strengths, resources, and wellness
ROLE OF PROFESSIONALS	
Practitioners who provide psychotherapy	Enabling agents who assist families in achieving their goals
ROLE OF FAMILIES	
Clients or patients	Collaborators
ASSESSMENT BASED ON	
Clinical typologies	Competencies and competence deficits
GOAL OF INTERVENTION	
Treatment of family pathology or dysfunction	Empowerment of families in achieving mastery and control over their lives
MODUS OPERANDI	
Provision of psychotherapy	Strengthening of the relevant competencies
SYSTEMIC PERSPECTIVE	
Family systems framework	Ecological systems framework

From Marsh D: Working with families of people with serious mental illness. In VandeCreek L, Knapp S, Jackson T: *Innovations in clinical practice: a source book*, vol 2, Sarasota, Fla, 1992, Professional Resource Exchange.

the family's culture and congruent with the family's appraisal of problems and needs
5. Promotion of the family's use of natural support networks

In this framework it is expected that families will play a major role in deciding what is important to them, what options they will choose to achieve their goals, and whether or not they will accept help that is offered to them.[23,24]

NONCLINICAL INTERVENTIONS

An important development in the field of family intervention that is critically important to psychiatric nurses is the development of nonclinical interventions that are designed primarily to educate and support.[17] They are the result of the emergence of the family self-help movement in psychiatry.

In the 1970s some families began forming local self-help and consumer advocacy groups for families of the mentally ill. In 1979 about 100 such groups together formed the National Alliance for the Mentally Ill (NAMI). This strong and politically active group is organized with the following goals[13]:

1. Educating and informing families of services and treatment available for their ill member
2. Supporting families and friends of those with severe and disabling mental illness
3. Advocating for improved treatment and services for the chronically mentally ill
4. Promoting support for research into the neurophysiological, neurochemical, and genetic factors important in prolonged mental illness
5. Improving training for mental health professionals to foster a more enlightened understanding of the nature of prolonged mental illness
6. Working with the media to share accurate information and challenge stereotypes to overcome stigma about the mentally ill and their families

As enlightened consumers, NAMI members advocate for information about services needed for their ill family members and themselves during various phases of the illness. For participating families, local self-help and support groups offer mutual aid, intimacy with others, and involvement beyond the immediate family needs.[11,15]

Families of the mentally ill believe some family therapy theories stigmatize and blame families for their relatives' illness. Evaluate family systems, structural, and strategic therapies as presented in this chapter based on this criticism.

Psychoeducational Programs for Families

Due in large part to the efforts of NAMI and other family groups, a variety of psychoeducational programs have been developed for families of the mentally ill.[19] Although these programs vary, they share certain features. The program approach is mainly educational and pragmatic, and its aim is to improve the course of the family member's illness, reduce relapse rates, and improve the patient's and family's functioning. These goals are achieved through educating the family about the illness, teaching families techniques to cope with symptomatic behavior, and reinforcing family strengths.

Box 30-1

TEN-WEEK EDUCATIONAL PROGRAM FOR FAMILIES OF THE MENTALLY ILL

1. Nature and Purpose of Program
   a. Introductions of family members and staff
   b. Purpose and scope of program
   c. Description of treatment program, policies, and procedures
   d. Brief, written survey of specific family needs and requests

2. The Family Experience
   a. Family burden and needs
   b. The family system
   c. Family subsystems
   d. Life-span perspectives

3. Mental Illness I
   a. Diagnosis
   b. Etiology
   c. Prognosis
   d. Treatment

4. Mental Illness II
   a. Symptoms
   b. Medication
   c. Diathesis-stress model
   d. Recent research

5. Managing Symptoms and Problems
   a. Bizarre behavior
   b. Destructive and self-destructive behavior
   c. Hygiene and appearance
   d. Negative symptoms

6. Stress, Coping, and Adaptation
   a. The general model
   b. The stressor of mental illness
   c. The process of family adaptation
   d. Increasing coping effectiveness

7. Enhancing Personal and Family Effectiveness I
   a. Behavior management
   b. Conflict resolution
   c. Communication skills
   d. Problem solving

8. Enhancing Personal and Family Effectiveness II
   a. Stress management
   b. Assertiveness training
   c. Achieving a family balance
   d. Meeting personal needs

9. Relationships between Families and Professionals
   a. Historical context
   b. New modes of family-professional relationships
   c. Barriers to collaboration
   d. Breaking down barriers

10. Community Resources
   a. The consumer-advocacy movement
   b. Accessing the system
   c. Legal issues
   d. Appropriate referrals

While not all programs include the ill family member, they do promote regular contact of the family with other affected families.

In general, a comprehensive program of nonclinical family intervention should include the following components[17]:

1. A didactic component that provides information about mental illness and the mental health system
2. A skills component that offers training in communication, conflict resolution, problem solving, assertiveness, behavioral management, and stress management
3. An emotional component that provides opportunities for ventilation and sharing and mobilizing resources
4. A family process component that focuses on coping with mental illness and its sequelae for the family
5. A social component that increases use of informal and formal support networks

Although no single program will work equally well in all situations, it is possible to describe a general structure that can be modified to meet individual needs. The educational program outlined in Box 30-1 is time limited and didactic and is designed to primarily meet the cognitive and behavioral needs of families.[17] It is important that psychoeducational programs for families meet a range of family needs and that there be an opportunity for families to ask questions, express feelings, and socialize with each other and mental health professionals.

CLINICAL INTERVENTIONS

Deciding when family therapy is appropriate, or indicated over individual or group therapy, is not always easy. Resource availability is a factor; many settings do not have anyone trained in family therapy. When the resources are available, the therapist's bias may have an influence. Some family therapists conceptualize all emotional problems within the family framework. Others recommend certain guidelines in determining which problems should be treated in family therapy. They suggest that family therapy is indicated in the following situations:

1. The presenting problem appears in system terms, such as marital conflicts, severe sibling conflicts,

or cross-generational conflicts (parents versus off-spring; parents versus grandparents).

2. Various types of difficulty and conflict arise between the identified patient and other family members.

3. The family is experiencing a transitional stage of the family life cycle, such as beginning a family, marriage, birth of the first child, entrance of children into adolescence, the first child leaving home, retirement, or the death of one spouse.

4. Individual therapy with one family member results in symptoms developing in another family member.

5. No improvement occurs with adequate individual therapy. Enlarging the conceptual field to include the family in therapy may produce therapeutic movement.

6. The individual in treatment seems unable to use an intrapsychic or interpretive mode of individual therapy but primarily uses therapy sessions to talk about or complain about another member.

This chapter provides an overview of three theoretical approaches to clinical interventions with families: (1) family systems therapy, (2) structural therapy, and (3) strategic therapy. It describes some of the major techniques that are derived from each of these theories of family therapy. The principles and strategies proposed by these theories are distinct and sometimes conflicting, yet each defines a theoretical framework developed from clinical research with families, and each has some utility in clinical practice.

FAMILY SYSTEMS THERAPY

Family systems therapy was developed by Bowen[3] in the 1950s and continues to evolve.[32] A premise of this therapy is that a family is a homeostatic system. A change in functioning of one family member results in a change in the functioning of other family members. It resembles a centerless web in which, when one strand moves, the tensions in the entire web readjust.

Systems therapy explains emotional dysfunction in human relationships, specifically in the family system. Symptoms in any member of the family, whether social (e.g., child abuse, delinquency), physical (e.g., drug abuse, alcoholism, chronic illness), emotional (e.g., depression, schizophrenia), or conflictual (e.g., marital conflict), are viewed as evidence of dysfunction in the family relationship process. Although the family is only one emotional system in which an individual is involved, it is probably the most intense and influential one. Extrafamilial relationships rarely carry the intensity of the family emotional system. The family system does not totally determine behavior and function. Rather, the family system fosters or inhibits function. The

individual's responsibility for his or her actions is never lost.

The purpose of any theory is to understand, predict, and gain some control of the phenomena being studied. Understanding, as applied to family systems therapy, does not entail uncovering intrapsychic motivations. It identifies the functional facts of a relationship—what happened, when, where, how, and who was involved. These observable facts are more important than the reasons why the problematical behavior occurred. A systems therapist gathers from family members descriptions of behavior rather than feeling states. Conventional psychodynamic jargon is not present in family systems writing. Systems therapy uses simple, descriptive words.

Bowen[1-3] has described in detail the team research he conducted in the early 1950s on schizophrenic families in a live-in hospital setting. A new theory of family psychotherapy evolved from this live-in research. This theory, based on clinical observations of the research families' behavior, also applies to relationship patterns in more functional family systems. Bowen believed that "patterns originally thought to be typical of schizophrenia are present in all families some of the time and in some families most of the time."[2]

A cornerstone of systems therapy developed from a central pattern observed in research families. Some families failed to distinguish between the intellectual process of *thinking* and the more subjective process of *feeling*. It was as if the thinking processes were so flooded with feeling that members were unable to separate intellectual belief from subjective feelings. Routinely a person would say, "I feel that . . ." when "I think that . . ." would have been more accurate. The families focused on feelings in an attempt to foster togetherness and agreement. They avoided statements of opinion or belief that would make one member different or separate from the family "party line."

A key goal of systems therapy, therefore, is to clarify and distinguish thinking and feeling processes in family members. The observation of this fusion between thinking and feeling led to the concept of the "undifferentiated family ego mass." People with the greatest fusion between feeling and thinking function the most poorly. They inherit a high percentage of life's social, psychiatric, and medical problems.

Family systems theory consists of seven interlocking concepts. Three concepts apply to overall characteristics of family systems: differentiation of self, triangles, and the nuclear family emotional system. The remaining four concepts are related to the central family characteristics: the multigenerational transmission process, the family projection process, sibling position, and the emotional cutoff (Table 30-2).

All these concepts refer to family processes that inhibit or promote individual family members' rising out of the emotional "we-ness," or fusion. Bowen believes that a member's movement toward either increased emotional closeness or distance is reflexive and predictable. The higher the level of differentiation in a person, the higher the level of functioning. Differentiating the self from the "we-ness" is the ultimate goal of treatment.

Table 30-2 Central Concepts of Family Systems Therapy

Concept	Definition
Differentiation	Sufficient separation between intellect and emotions so that one is not dominated by the reactive anxiety of the family's emotional system
Triangle	A predictable emotional process that takes place in any significant relationship when difficulty exists in the relationship
Nuclear family emotional system	Patterns of interaction between family members and the degree to which these patterns promote emotional fusion
Multigenerational transmission process	The assumption that relationship patterns and symptoms in a family have their origin several generations earlier; a four- or five-generation genogram reveals such patterns
Family projection process	The projection of spouses' problems onto one or more children to avoid the intense emotional fusion between the spouses
Sibling position	Birth order and sex are seen as determining factors in a person's personality profile
Emotional cutoff	A dysfunctional way in which some family members deal with intense family conflict by using either emotional isolation or geographical distance

Differentiation of Self

The concept of differentiation of self is Bowen's attempt to measure all human functioning on a continuum. The continuum proceeds from the greatest emotional fusion of self boundaries, to the highest degree of differentiation or autonomy (Fig. 30-1). A concise description of the differentiated person is the person who is less anxious than the family system. This person is able to bring up emotion-laden issues in a nonassaulting way without anxiety. In his earlier work, Bowen refers to the "undifferentiated family ego mass" that exists in varying degrees of intensity in families. The intensity of emotional closeness in a family may allow members to know each other's thoughts, feelings, and fantasies.

There is a cyclical quality to this closeness. As the emotional intensity or fusion between two individuals increases and the self of one is incorporated into the other self, the relationship is perceived to be uncomfortably close. This is usually followed by distance-creating behavior characterized by hostile rejection of the overcloseness. The two individuals actively repel each other. Relationships can cycle through these phases, since anxiety in the relationship ebbs and flows. Relationships can also become fixed at an angry, repelling standoff. People who operate at the lower reactive end of the continuum are so fused that they are dominated by the automatic emotional system. These people are less adaptable, less flexible, and more emotionally dependent on those about them. They are easily stressed into dysfunction. People at the higher end of the continuum maintain a degree of separation between thought and emotion. In periods of stress they can retain a relative amount of intellectual functioning. They are more flexible, adaptable, and more independent of the reactive emotionality around them.

The concept of differentiation eliminates the notion

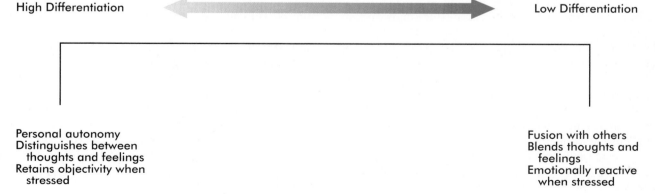

High Differentiation   Low Differentiation

Personal autonomy
Distinguishes between
   thoughts and feelings
Retains objectivity when
   stressed

Fusion with others
Blends thoughts and
   feelings
Emotionally reactive
   when stressed

Fig. 30-1   Continuum of differentiation of self.

of normalcy. It has no direct connection to presence or absence of symptoms, although Bowen believes people at the lower end of the scale tend to inherit more of life's problems. People at the higher end of the continuum recoup rapidly if they are stressed into dysfunction.

> How might a parent's level of self-differentiation affect their child's growth and development from infancy through adolescence?

Triangles

The concept of triangles is the key to understanding the systems approach to emotional function. Many techniques evolve from this concept. The idea of triangles is not a new one. Freud's theory of the oedipal complex describes a sexual triangle. Bowen has called the triangle the basic "building block of an emotional system." A triangle is a predictable emotional process that takes place in any significant relationship experiencing difficulty. The three corners of the triangle can be composed of three people; two people and a group, such as a religious affiliation or Al-Anon; two people and an issue, such as drinking or success; or two people and an object, such as the house or drugs. The possible list of groups, issues, or objects is endless; it must have an emotional significance equal to that of a person.

All people seek closeness in emotional systems. Emotional closeness but separateness is difficult for two people to maintain; the tendency is to fuse, to lose self, or parts of self, in the other. A natural urge exists to seek completeness of self by accumulating parts of the other. The old adage "opposites attract" reflects this assumption. It is difficult for two people to maintain sufficient emotional closeness without fusion. The inevitable result is emotional distancing. The system is then ripe for the formation of a triangle. For example, the husband wants more expression of affection from an emotionally constricted wife. The more he pursues her, the more she withdraws, most often into preoccupation with her child. The husband starts working longer hours. Husband and wife then start arguing circularly: "You care more about making a new account than you do about your wife and children!" "You expect to have nice things and then blame me for working extra hours!" Triangles stabilize by maintaining the status quo while avoiding tension, conflict, or talking about sensitive emotional areas. The two people can then focus on the new issue (or person or object) and avoid discussing the painful issues between them. Feelings are thus drained off, and the fo-

cus is removed from the self and one's own part in the problem. Change in self is avoided.

The reciprocal function of a triangle and the idea of equal responsibility can be difficult to convey to a couple. This is especially true when the distancing mechanism used by one spouse is as emotionally charged as an extramarital affair. Suppose the wife distances from the painful issues in the relationship. By "triangling" an affair, it is difficult for the husband to relinquish his self-righteous position of the "wronged husband." He does not see his behavior of working 14 to 16 hours a day as serving the same distancing function in the relationship. The nature of the distancing mechanism has meaningful content, whether it is overwork, extramarital affairs, homosexuality, psychotic symptoms, religious preoccupation, suicidal gestures, depression, or psychoanalysis. All serve the same function as a triangular relationship within the family.[20]

The concept of a family scapegoat originally broadened the individual pathological view to include the part the family played in the symptomatic behavior. The tendency, however, was to view the scapegoat as the helpless victim of a persecuting family. For example, a husband and wife who are unable to settle their differences and wish to avoid their marital discord may focus on the "victim child." This leads to blaming the parents. In contrast, the concept of triangles from the systems view holds each person in the triangle responsible, as evident in Fig. 30-2, a diagram of the family. Father and mother avoid conflict by focusing on the son. Mother and son avoid dealing with their overcloseness by having a common enemy in the father. Father and son avoid awareness of their emotional distance by relating through the mother as go-betweens. Thus the "victim" is eliminated. All members of a triangle participate equally in maintaining the triangle, and no triangle can persist without the active cooperation of all its members.

It is not a problem to be in a triangle; in fact, it is impossible to stay out of all triangles. Triangles form and re-form rapidly and are the daily way most people handle conflict or tension. Problems will arise if a tri-

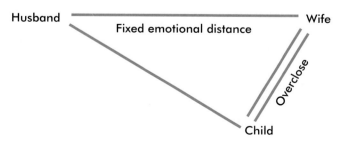

Fig. 30-2   Example of a family triangle.

angle becomes fixed and when it involves significant relationships of deep friendship, blood ties, or marriage. Triangles are not static but form and reform around emotion-laden issues, such as money, sex, child rearing, religion, alcohol, and education. A person's position in a triangle alters depending on the issue. A mother and father may be distant on the highly charged issue of how to spend their money. They may be close and in accord about their adolescent daughter's sexual activity. Judgments about these issues, however, are often based on emotion rather than careful thought.

 Many people marry thinking that they can change the parts of their spouse that they don't like after the honeymoon. What would a family systems therapist say about this?

Operating Principles. A person's operating principles are the laws that govern personal conduct. They must be inferred from what the person does in regard to an emotion-laden issue rather than what the person says. Operating principles vary from valuable ones based on conscious conviction to more immature, reactive, impulsive principles. Immature principles are other-focused rather than self-focused; they lead to a loss of freedom of self-determination. Any behavior that is predictable, as in behavior operated by a triangle, is not free. The loss of freedom impairs self-functioning, perpetuates problems, causes a deterioration in family functioning, and promotes symptom development.[14]

Other-focused, triangle-promoting operating principles are reflected in various ways. These include declaring feelings "right" or "wrong"; using plural pronouns "we" or "us" rather than "I"; accusing the other person of "you made me mad/do it"; stepping in to settle, side taking, or blaming in two other people's conflict; telling or holding secrets; telling the other person what to do; and assuming responsibility for the other person's feelings, for example, "I want to make her happy" or "I couldn't tell him because it would hurt him." These statements are typically interpreted as thoughtful or being very responsible. In fact, avoiding one's own feelings by focusing on the other person is irresponsible. Everyone falls into this pattern, especially in a marriage or parent-child relationship. When a person becomes anxious, it is more comfortable to project the problem onto the other person and then work to change the other. The implicit assumption here is, "I can't help my behavior, but he is behaving that way deliberately."[14]

In more dysfunctional, closed family systems, interaction between family members is determined by fixed interactional patterns. These fixed triangles are an effort to maintain a homeostatic balance and to avoid stress. When an additional stress occurs outside or within the family, such as a job change or the birth of a new member, symptoms may arise in a dysfunctional attempt to reduce stress and restore balance. This is evident in the following clinical example.

CLINICAL EXAMPLE

Mr. and Mrs. D, whose family consisted of six children, had a seventh unplanned child. The family was financially strained, and Mr. and Mrs. D had a conflictual and distant relationship. When the last child was born, a middle sibling, 13-year-old Andy, developed symptoms and became school phobic. The school insisted the child receive treatment. Late in the treatment the mother finally revealed that one of the reasons for the family's financial strain was the husband's work phobia and his occasional gambling sprees. The wife had covered for him for years, calling his boss to make excuses and taking part-time work herself. Until the birth of the last child, the family was able to maintain a precarious, minimally functional balance. The additional stress, however, produced symptoms that caused an outside agency, the school, to become involved.

Interventions. Treatment encourages key figures in key triangles to identify their emotional "triggers." The person identifies the verbal or behavioral cues of the other person, to which he reacts with a predictable behavior. When the person pinpoints these cues, he can take control of his part in the process. Once one person takes control and changes his part in a triangle, the whole system changes.

An example of this was a mother who was overclose to her 16-year-old daughter. The daughter had become school phobic and stayed home from school for a year before the family sought treatment. The father would come home from work, see the daughter had missed school another day, and angrily attack her with "shape-up speeches." The mother bitterly complained about the daughter being home all day doing nothing. However, when the father began his verbal attacks, she would then become protective of the daughter and launch an attack on the father: "How can you say those things to her; you know how upset she gets." When the mother was able to get a "handle" on her emotional trigger (the mother had always been terrified of her "drill sergeant" father), she was able to step back and permit the father to become more effective with his daughter.

Nurses must identify key triangles in a family and operating principles of its members. They must understand what sets off their emotional triggers and assume that the family will attempt to triangle them into its own emotional system to reestablish equilibrium. The nurse's job is to maintain sufficient emotional distance to watch the process unfolding between family members and at the same time to maintain emotional contact with each family member.

Therapist's reactions that indicate that the therapist is part of a triangle include feeling sorry for or pitying the other, feeling angry at the system or member, being overly positive about the system, wanting to correct behavior, and finding oneself without questions or responses in the session. The nurse must limit the action to the two family members and avoid becoming involved. Once the therapist steps in to take sides, progress stops and status quo is reestablished. Side taking should be a planned strategy in which the nurse maintains the freedom to realign with specific family members.[12]

Systems therapists do not believe they can change family members; change is possible only when it is generated within the self. Family members are encouraged to take responsibility for the self and not try to change the other. The therapist must avoid becoming part of a triangle in the system. To get out of an emotional process in the session, the nurse may elicit the members' responses. For example, if the nurse becomes irritated at a critical intrusive husband, the nurse can ask the wife, "What happens to your insides when your husband interrupts with criticism?" This feeds the process back into the system, keeping it between the spouses.

One of the areas of controversy in the field of family therapy is the importance of the therapist's working on his or her own family of origin. Systems therapists believe that it is a major aspect of training as a family therapist. "Working on" means the nurse differentiates herself in her own family of origin. She identifies the issues in her family that she is reactive to and with whom she is part of a triangle around these issues. She then works to get out of the triangle by gaining control of her reflexive distancing and fusing in her family. This way she has the freedom of emotional closeness and of some emotional distance with each family member (without using geographical distance to create emotional space). Unless a therapist is conscious of the triangles she is a part of in her own family, she will be vulnerable to the same roles and behaviors in the families she is treating.

Nuclear Family Emotional System

The nuclear family emotional system refers to patterns of interaction between family members and the degree to which these patterns promote emotional fusion (see Critical Thinking about Contemporary Issues). These patterns of interaction are the ways the person behaves

CRITICAL THINKING ABOUT CONTEMPORARY ISSUES

Does a Strong Mother-Daughter Attachment Imply Low Self-Differentiation?

Much attention has been given to the impact of the mother-daughter relationship on the development of women, particularly focusing on issues related to mental health and self-efficacy. Some theorists emphasize self-differentiation and devalue interpersonal attachment as a feminine behavior. Others analyze the concepts of caring, intimacy, closeness, and emotional reciprocity only when their absence is evident in intergenerational conflict, delinquency, broken homes, or family violence.

Recent research suggests, however, that a daughter's attachment to mother and her level of self-differentiation are not causally related, and that the concepts of self-differentiation and attachment appear to be separate variables in personality development.[5] Specifically, these researchers found that the daughters' levels of self-differentiation were positively related to positive energy, and women who were mentally healthy and functioning effectively also showed high levels of attachment. The findings from this research affirm the value of attachment behaviors and self-differentiation in adulthood, challenge the traditional bias against attachment behaviors of women, and provide psychiatric nurses with a focus for mental health promotion when working with women. ▼

in most significant relationships. All marriage relationships reflect a balance, or complementarity, of operating principles and reciprocal function.[9] For example, the reasonable, object-oriented, and emotionally distant spouse is married to the affectively expressive, relationship-oriented, emotional pursuer. These differences provide the attraction and the balancing stability to the marriage relationship. One spouse is the object-oriented overfunctioner, the other the emotion-oriented overfunctioner. Difficulty arises when dependence on attributes of the spouse reduces acquiring those attributes in the self. The self borrows on the functioning of the spouse, and self-boundaries are blurred. This is referred to as **ego fusion.** When they result in fixed positions of overfunction-underfunction, symptoms can occur, such as chronic depression or physical illness. In such a relationship, to view one spouse as strong and independent and the other as weak and dependent fails to recognize the overfunctioner's dependence on the underfunctioning of the other spouse. The underfunctioner must be one-down for the other to appear one-up.

Emotional fusion operates in all marriages to a lesser or greater extent. When the relationship is unstressed, the reciprocal function works smoothly. When stress occurs, each spouse becomes more as oneself. The distancer seeks space and objects (the job, art, alcohol); the pursuer seeks togetherness and expression of personal feelings. Both are efforts to avoid personal anxiety. The pursuer takes the distancer's withdrawal as personal rejection and reactively withdraws. No longer feeling crowded, the distancer then moves in emotionally, only to be met with, "Where were you when I needed you; get lost." The distancer then pulls back, baffled and angry at the rejection. A fixed emotional distance sets in.[9] These are the relationships seen just before the couple decides on a divorce. These relationships are ripe for triangulation with an affair or with an unsuspecting therapist.

People tend to pick spouses who have equivalent levels of differentiation of self.[3] The greater the undifferentiation, the greater is the tendency toward fusion and potential problems. If there is a high degree of ego fusion and intensity in the nuclear family, this intensity can be diffused and reduced through active contact with the family of origin. In periods of stress, contact with the extended family or family of origin can stabilize the nuclear family. Promoting such contact can be an effective therapeutic strategy.

Kerr and Bowen[14] have identified two patterns in the nuclear family emotional system, labeled the "explosive family" and the "cohesive family." Family units of a cohesive family are geographically close, in frequent contact and communication. The person who geographically separates from his family of origin because of the fusion or intensity of attachment there may marry a spouse from a cohesive family. The person's unresolved attachments to his own family of origin lie dormant until ritualized contact (at a wedding or funeral) stirs them up. In a nuclear family in which both spouses are detached from their families of origin, the spouses tend to be more dependent on each other. The process between them is more intense. These are the explosive families.

Bowen[3] proposes three mechanisms by which spouses maintain sufficient emotional distance from each other to handle the anxiety associated with fusion. All three mechanisms may be used by the couple, or tension may be focused in one area. If tension is great enough, it will spill over into other social systems, such as mental health centers or school counselors. The three mechanisms used are (1) marital conflict, (2) dysfunction in one spouse, and (3) projection of the problem onto one or more children.

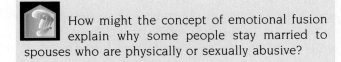

How might the concept of emotional fusion explain why some people stay married to spouses who are physically or sexually abusive?

Marital Conflict. Conflictual marriages are built on a constant struggle between spouses. They want "their fair share" of needs met, of freedom, of love, of attention, or of control. Neither spouse is willing to compromise. A high percentage of the self is wrapped up in the "happiness" of the other. Functioning of the self is enmeshed in the function of the other. These relationships tend to be stable, whether positive ("Anything to make her happy") or negative ("I sacrificed the best years of my life helping him be a success; I'll never let him go now"). They endure predictable cycles of intense closeness, distance-creating conflict, making up, then renewed closeness. It is commonly believed that this amount of conflict would harm the children of such marriages. Bowen believes, however, that the children are protected from overinvolvement because tension is focused between parents.

Intervention in conflictual marriages usually involves working with the most motivated spouse at first. If both spouses are seen together, frequently the uproar between them is too great to tolerate. They are very reactive to each other. Limit setting, such as prohibiting interruptions, and strategies such as a "listening chair" or turning one spouse's chair to the wall to listen are ineffective. In such situations spouses must be seen separately initially. The approach is to get the focus on the self and decrease efforts to change the other. The nurse focuses on what part the spouse plays in the situation. This spouse gains some self-control over reactive triggers. Once blaming is reduced, the spouse reevaluates beliefs and values without the need to attack the other. Such reevaluation entails contacting the family of origin by phone, letters, or planned visits. The goal is to understand better the source of the nuclear family conflict and to work to establish more personal relationships with the family of origin. Bowen calls this process "coaching." Usually, before this point is reached in the treatment, the absent, less-motivated spouse has sought to join the sessions because of the changes that have occurred.

Significant changes in the marriage system occur when one spouse reduces overinvestment in the other and focuses on self. The spouse making changes must be warned of predictable efforts by the other to reestablish status quo. This may occur in the other through an escalation of anger-provoking behavior, threats to leave, and so on. If the spouse making changes can maintain a self-focused position through the resistance, both partners may become active in the treatment. While temporarily working with one spouse, nurses must guard against becoming part of a triangle. They may emotionally side with the spouse initially in treatment or become the spouse's only support. This can be especially difficult for nurses when the unexpressed plan of the unmotivated spouse is to deposit the husband or wife in treatment and obtain a divorce. Nurses may then be expected to "take care of" the spouse.

Spouse Dysfunction. The second mechanism used by spouses to maintain emotional distance is the dysfunction of one spouse. As mentioned earlier, one spouse may be emotionally, socially, or physically disabled to varying degrees. The degree to which the one underfunctions is the degree to which the other overfunctions. This ensures that emotional equilibrium is maintained, since both partners are locked into a mutually dependent relationship. Interventions with such a relationship are similar to those used with the conflictual marriage. Herz Brown[12] suggests working with the overfunctioning spouse by first helping him to pull back. The underfunctioning spouse then moves in to take up the slack. This is evidenced in this clinical example.

 ## CLINICAL EXAMPLE

Mr. and Mrs. S are a couple who sought treatment because the husband was missing many days at work. The couple would have extensive arguments about the husband not wanting to work and the wife feeling outraged at the financial stress he was creating. It became apparent that Mrs. S treated Mr. S as one of their adolescent boys. She overfunctioned to the point of cleaning up after her husband's destructive temper tantrums. Over time, with considerable coaching, she was able to pull back in several areas, refusing to wake the husband or clean up after him, leaving it up to him to pay the bills, and generally holding back her critical nagging. The first sign of progress was at the husband's next temper tantrum (he did delicate electrical work and had a low frustration tolerance). He carefully selected which objects he would throw or smash in his workroom, for example, not throwing a box of small nuts and bolts. He cleaned up his own workroom and began going to work regularly. As the husband's functioning improved, the wife became significantly depressed and began addressing unresolved issues in her family of origin. This couple demonstrated the reciprocity in the mechanism of underfunctioning and overfunctioning in a marriage.

Projection on Child. The third distancing mechanism used by spouses to control the intensity of fusion between them is the projection of the problem to one or more of the children. Before the development of a family pathology theory, the parents of a symptomatic child would be excluded from therapy. This further reinforced the dysfunction in the family by focusing on the child as "the problem." Child-focused families either view the problem as exclusive to the symptomatic child or deny the existence of a problem entirely. When the school or probation officer recommends treatment, they passively comply but participate reluctantly. When a couple centers on their children, it is easier to avoid marital confrontations because there is always something to worry, criticize, or complain about with the children. These families strongly depend on the children's symptoms and resist exploring broader issues in therapy.

How one child becomes a parental concern is a complex process. It may have its roots in several previous generations. Key triangles tend to repeat themselves over generations; thus the parent's natural tendency is to put one child in the parent's past position in the triangle. Nodal events are the normative events that occur in every family life but generate anxiety because change ensues. These include such events as birth, death, sickness, marriage, job changes, school changes, divorce, and family relocation. The amount of stress generated around a nodal event depends on the amount of resultant change. If a significant developmental stage of the child (e.g., in utero, birth, entering school for the first time, adolescence) coincides with the occurrence of a nodal event, this child may be vulnerable to the focus of family stress and to impairment. The first-born and last-born children are also particularly vulnerable to family focus.

The primary goal of treatment is to remove the focus from the child and place the conflict between the parents where it belongs. The child's dysfunctions must be placed within the context of the family system by taking a family history and drawing a family genogram. A three-generation **family genogram** is a structured method of gathering information and graphically symbolizing much factual and emotional relationship data in the initial interview.[20] A sample genogram is presented in Fig. 30-3. Drawing a family genogram in full view of the family on large easel paper or a blackboard broadens the family's focus. The therapist's questions and comments are geared toward change of self rather than changing the child.

The therapist may identify problematic behavior in other family members to remove blame from the child. Another therapeutic strategy is to discuss how grandparents might handle the problem. With some families the nurse can coach the overinvolved parent, such as the mother, to pull back from the focused child and send a note to her own mother telling her one thing about herself that she does not want her to know. This reveals

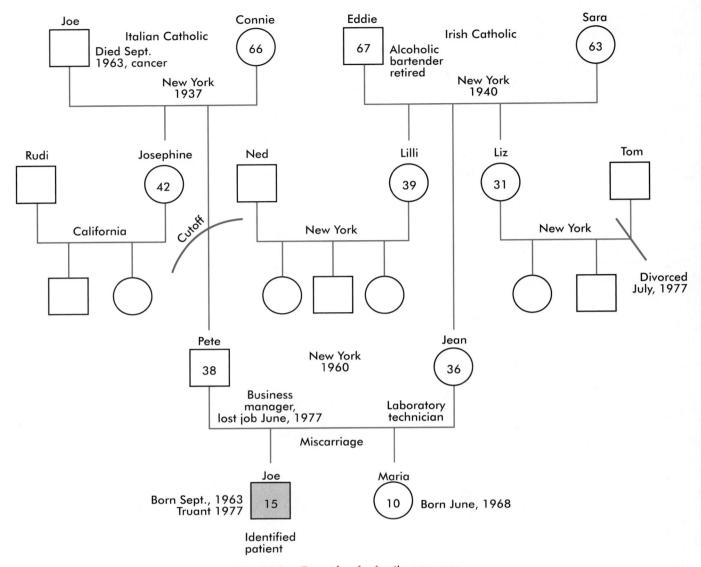

Fig. 30-3   Example of a family genogram.

the three-generational aspect of the presenting problem. It may also be helpful to work with the siblings at times, separately from the parents. This promotes a more positive support system among sibs. Frequently, sibs mimic their parents' negative behavior toward the focused child. They may also resent the excessive attention he receives from parents and act aggressively toward him.

Families with an acting-out child and two parents in the ineffective helpless position (or one parent set up as the "heavy" and the other as "the nice guy") need a direct approach initially. The parents may have given up their authority to the child. This may be determined by asking them the following extreme questions: "If your child had third-degree burns, could you get her to take the horribly painful treatments?" or "If your child had heart disease, could you limit her activities?" Following

are four guidelines for parents locked in a triangle with the acting-out "problem child":

1. The person who sets the rule must be present to enforce it.
2. With two parents in the home, divide the areas of responsibility (e.g., allowance, bedtime, nights out) so that when a dispute comes up, it is clear with whom the child must negotiate.
3. Yelling is ineffective and inhibits thinking. Parents need to control their reactions.
4. Decide the consequences of repeated disobedient behavior and inform the child of them. When the behavior occurs, without yelling, carry out the consequence even if the parent's personal plans must be changed to do so.

As soon as the child focus is sufficiently reduced, the child is removed from the sessions. The therapist then becomes the third corner of the triangle, actively relating to both spouses without taking sides and thereby keeping conflict between the spouses.

Multigenerational Transmission Process

The roots of the family emotional system extend back through generations. When emotional dysfunction occurs, it can be scattered throughout the family tree. Drawing a three-generation family genogram frequently reveals certain relationship patterns otherwise believed to be peculiar to one nuclear family. For example, suicide of younger brothers, divorce among female siblings, or alcoholism might be a pattern across a family system when four or five generations are mapped out on a genogram. In family therapy, a symptom in one family member in one generation has its origin several generations before.[7] This differentiates it from other forms of family therapy. Families seeking treatment, however, usually present symptoms as a nuclear family problem.

Family Projection Process

The family projection process refers to the way anxiety about specific issues is transmitted through the generations. These are emotionally powerful issues, such as money, sex, child rearing, religion, work or school achievement, alcohol, politics, illness and death, around which a rigid "party line" develops. Family members polarize around these issues, taking the family position or the direct opposite. Neither position allows freedom or flexibility of thought. Positions are reactive and fixed. Studying the family of origin helps identify a person's predictable position in family triangles involving specific issues. If individuals think about the issues they normally react to emotionally, they can plan strategies that will free them from triangled positions.

The family projection process also refers to the process that labels and assigns characteristics to certain family members. These labels may be overpositive ("Mary Sunshine," "The Genius") or overnegative ("The Crazy One," "Dummy"). They are equally unrealistic and confining. After years of family labeling, the labeled person will come to volunteer for the label and earn it.

Identify two emotionally powerful issues in your family of origin and think about your position related to them. Describe family labels you also heard while growing up.

Sibling Position

The concept of personality profiles based on sibling position is borrowed from Toman,[27] who believes that important personality characteristics are determined by the sex of one's siblings and one's birth order. For example, the younger brother of two older sisters will be quite different from the older brother of a brother. The personality profiles Toman developed can suggest marital discord or harmony on issues of rank or sex. For example, a younger brother of brothers may have more difficulty relating to his spouse than a younger brother of sisters. If this younger brother of brothers married a younger sister of sisters, they may both have discomfort with the opposite sex. In addition, they might struggle for juniority rights (who's going to take care of whom). The couple who recognizes sibling rank and sex as a possible source of their conflicts can help each other to cope with their differences.

Emotional Cutoff

The emotional cutoff is a way to deal with intense unresolved attachment between children and parents. The cutoff is emotional isolation, although members may still live geographically close. It also may be physical distance from the family of origin. The cutoff creates the illusion of separation from parents. The more intense the emotional cutoff, the more likely this problem will be reestablished in the next generation. Reconnecting emotionally with the cutoff family may prevent the same process from occurring with the parents and children of the next generation, since such patterns tend to be repeated.

Modes of Therapy

Several modes of therapy have been mentioned thus far, including therapy with both spouses. Another mode of family therapy involves only one family member. This is most frequently used with the young adult who is single and self-supporting. This method includes learning about the functioning of family systems and triangles. It also involves keeping an active emotional relationship with important family members by planned phone calls, letters, and visits. This therapy requires developing an ability to control emotional reactiveness to avoid becoming part of an emotional triangle during visits with the family.[25] The goal is to achieve more self-differentiation from the family of origin. The individual must also develop a person-to-person relationship with important family members. This therapy is referred to as coaching. Once the person is knowledgeable about triangles and methods of detriangling within the family, coaching sessions can be held as needed to supervise ongoing self-differentiation efforts.

The last mode of therapy is multiple family therapy (MFT), developed in its present form in the late 1960s. MFT is different from multiple family group therapy. The latter uses role playing and psychodrama and promotes interfamily group process to change family interaction and increase its sensitivity to the family environment.[26] MFT, from a family systems framework, is different. Sessions are structured to ensure against emotional exchange between families. Bowen believes this emotional exchange encourages a fusion of other families into a large, undifferentiated ego mass. The idea behind MFT is:

1. To conserve teaching time of families
2. To provide contact with a greater volume of families
3. To allow the opportunity for families to learn from the efforts and experiences of other families

While other families observe, the nurse therapist works with each family as if only one family was receiving therapy. While the family answers detailed questions about its problem, the nurse defocuses feelings and addresses one spouse while the other spouse listens. Then the silent spouse is asked to share thoughts or reactions to what the other spouse has said. The family members observing can talk to the therapist about another family but cannot directly talk to the other family.

STRUCTURAL FAMILY THERAPY

Structural family therapy is a body of theory and techniques based on the individual within a social context that is clearly described by Minuchin.[21,22] The assumption is that behavior is a consequence of the family's organization and the interactional patterns between members. Changing the family organization and the feedback processes between members changes the context in which a person functions. Thus the person's inner processes and behavior change.

The basic question of a structural family therapist is, "In what way is this family structure maintaining this maladaptive symptom?" Family structure is the invisible set of demands that determine the way in which family members interact. A family is a system that operates through transactional patterns. Repeated transactions establish patterns of how, when, and to whom to relate, and these patterns determine whether the system is functional or dysfunctional.

> What impact would sociocultural factors have on the effectiveness of a structural therapist's interventions with a family?

Components

Family in Transition. In this model the family is a social system in transformation. The family system must maintain its continuity so that family members can grow. At the same time it must adapt to both internal and external stresses to the system. Normal anxiety occurs during transitional stages. Traditional therapists call this anxiety pathological. This is described in the following clinical example by Minuchin.[21]

 CLINICAL EXAMPLE

An elderly widow decided to move from her apartment where she had lived for 25 years because she came home one day and found it had been robbed. Soon after moving, she sought treatment from a psychiatrist. She complained that the people who moved her were trying to control her and had purposely lost precious possessions. They were leaving sinister messages for each other on her furniture, and when she went outside, people followed her and signaled to each other. The psychiatrist diagnosed her as psychotic with paranoid delusions and prescribed tranquilizers. When this did not help, she sought a second psychiatrist, who recommended hospitalization. The third therapist she saw was a context-related therapist. He understood her symptoms as an ecological crisis. It was precipitated by feeling forced to move into an unfamiliar environment. He explained to her that she had lost her shell—the familiarity of objects in her apartment, the neighborhood, the neighbors. As any crustacean who has lost its shell, she felt vulnerable and was experiencing reality differently than before. He instructed her to go home, unpack, and place her familiar objects, books, and pictures in the new apartment. He told her to do her daily chores routinely, go the same shops and checkout counters, and for 2 weeks make no effort to meet neighbors. She was to visit old friends and family but not discuss her recent experiences. If anyone asked, she was to explain that those had just been the problems of an illogical, fearful old woman.

Structural family therapists change the relationship between a person and the familiar context in which the individual functions. This changes the subjective experience and enables new, more functional behavior to emerge. In the preceding clinical example, the therapist's interventions protected the woman from the unfamiliar and frightening environment until she could "grow a new shell." He blocked the environmental feedback that confirmed her paranoid fears as friends and family secretly discussed her frightening behavior. As her experience of her environment changed, her symptoms disappeared.

Stages of Family Development.

Every family undergoes predictable stages of development over time. These stages require adaptive restructuring. Each stage involves a process of transition and requires changes in family functioning for adaptive growth and development. The stages of the family life cycle are presented in Table 30-3.[4]

Family Structure.

A third component of Minuchin's model of a functioning family relates to the family structure. The major elements of structure are:

1. Power and influence within the family
2. Sets and family relationships including subsystems
3. Family boundaries that may be individual, sexual, or generational

Structure can become dysfunctional in any or all of these areas.[25]

First, as in any organization, the family system must have a power hierarchy with different levels of authority to function efficiently. Functions must be complementary, since the family needs to work together as a team. Over the years, mutual expectations of particular family members evolve. These expectations may be openly negotiated but are often implicit, with patterns of behavior developing around minor daily events. Critics of this aspect of structural therapy point out that too often, restoring the parent-child hierarchy means restoring a traditional male authority structure, which supports damaging gender inequalities existing in the family and society.[8] The nurse who focuses only on generational

Table 30-3 The Stages of the Family Life Cycle

Family life cycle stage	Emotional process of transition: key principles	Second-order changes in family status required to proceed developmentally
1. Leaving home: single young adults	Accepting emotional and financial responsibility for self	a. Differentiation of self in relation to family of origin b. Development of intimate peer relationships c. Establishment of self regarding work and financial independence
2. The joining of families through marriage: the new couple	Commitment to new system	a. Formation of marital system b. Realignment of relationships with extended families and friends to include spouse
3. Families with young children	Accepting new members into the system	a. Adjusting marital system to make space for child(ren) b. Joining in child rearing, financial, and household tasks c. Realignment of relationships with extended family to include parenting and grandparenting roles
4. Families with adolescents	Increasing flexibility of family boundaries to include children's independence and grandparents' frailties	a. Shifting of parent-child relationships to permit adolescent to move in and out of system b. Refocus on midlife marital and career issues c. Beginning shift toward joint caring for older generation
5. Launching children and moving on	Accepting a multitude of exits from and entries into the family system	a. Renegotiation of marital system as a dyad b. Development of adult-to-adult relationships between grown children and their parents c. Realignment of relationships to include in-laws and grandchildren d. Dealing with disabilities and death of parents (grandparents)
6. Families in later life	Accepting the shifting of generational roles	a. Maintaining own and/or couple functioning and interests in face of physiological decline; exploration of new familial and social role options b. Support for a more central role of middle generation c. Making room in the system for the wisdom and experience of the elderly, supporting the older generation without overfunctioning for them d. Dealing with loss of spouse, siblings, and other peers and preparation for own death; life review and integration

From Carter E, McGoldrick M: *The changing family life cycle: a framework for family therapy,* ed 2, Boston, 1989, Allyn & Bacon.

(parent-child) differences may ignore differences in power, resources, and needs among all family members. Thus the nurse could inadvertently promote gender-based power inequities that can result in destructive behavior. This dilemma highlights the need for family therapists to be particularly careful not to bring personal and sociocultural bias into their work with families.

> Describe how wife abuse and childhood incest can arise from a family structure that is based on male power and authority and female dependence and submission.

Second, the family system differentiates and functions through sets of relationships or subsystems. Subsystems can be made up of individuals or dyads. They are formed by generation, sex, interest, or function. Each person belongs to many subsystems. Each subsystem has different levels of power in which differentiated skills are learned.

Third, boundaries of a subsystem are the rules defining who participates in subsystem functions and how. Boundaries must be free of intrusion. Each subsystem has specific functions and interpersonal developmental tasks to be accomplished. Patterns of mutual accommodation as well as healthy competition cannot develop among siblings if parents or grandparents constantly interfere. Subsystem boundaries must be clear for proper family functioning but must also permit emotional contact among members.

Minuchin[21,22] describes families with extreme boundary problems as either enmeshed or disengaged. Enmeshed boundaries are weak and fluid; personal space and subsystem boundaries rapidly change and impact all subsystems. This diffuseness of boundaries prevents the development of autonomy and competence. Perceptions of self and others are poorly differentiated. A child in such a family might be so sensitized to conflict between parents that school performance may decline. The parents in such a family can become upset because the child refuses to eat vegetables at dinnertime. Such families flood with anxiety at times of stress and adapt poorly to change.

Disengaged families have rigid boundaries. Communication between subsystems is poor; supportive or protective contact is minimal. Members of such systems may function autonomously but have a skewed sense of independence. They lack feelings of loyalty and belonging and the capacity for interdependence. Some suggest that the product of a disengaged family is the sociopath. Because of the rigidity of subsystem boundaries, members may fail to respond adequately when one member is stressed. In such a family, a child's reading disorder might go unnoticed or a husband's suicidal behavior be disregarded.

In this model of family therapy the nurse often functions as a boundary maker and may clarify diffuse boundaries by discouraging interruptions and encouraging shutting bedroom doors. The nurse may also open overly rigid boundaries by recommending that a distant parent and child spend time together or by calling attention to a member's feeling that would otherwise go unnoticed by other members. The nurse's assessment of family subsystems and boundary functioning provides a rapid diagnosis of the family. It indicates the direction and goals of therapeutic interventions.

As mentioned earlier, each subsystem has specific functions and interpersonal developmental tasks to be accomplished. The spouse subsystem must develop patterns of mutual support. Couples must make decisions and settle arguments without domination or relinquishing of self by either spouse. Ideally, they will bring out the best in each other, with each promoting personal growth and creativity in their spouse.

Spouses typically engage in an "other-improvement program." They bring into the marriage certain expectations of their spouse and work hard to have the spouse meet them. Interpretations in this area should be directed to both spouses. The part each plays in the destructive process should be pointed out. A mutual interpretation would be to say to the wife, "In your efforts to make contact with your husband, you are driving him away," and to the husband, "Your strong silent style is alluring but elicits nagging." Balanced interpretations emphasize the complementarity of the system. Both positive and negative qualities are recognized in each spouse.

The parental subsystem socializes the children without sacrificing mutual support and accommodation between the spouses. Children must have access to each parent but be excluded from spouse functions. Minuchin advocates parental authority in an era that promotes "pure democracy" between parents and children. He recognizes the difficulty of parenting. Many parents are not satisfied with their own functioning. Parenting processes are different depending on the child's age. Part of promoting differentiation in the family is making the differentiation in ages clear. Adolescents have responsibilities and privileges that 12-year-old siblings do not. Children must learn to negotiate with their parents to live in a world of unequal power relationships.

Children first learn about peer relationships in the sibling subsystem. They learn to make friends, compete, negotiate, cooperate, and gain recognition of their skills. Knowledge of growth and development of children is valuable for the nurse who at times must translate age-appropriate skills, needs, and values to parents. The nurse should support the child's right to growing autonomy and the parents' responsible authority at the same time.

Interventions

A vital component to structural family therapy is the process of joining the family.[21,22] Nurse therapists temporarily become part of the family system. They adapt their behavior to the particular family's rules and manner. The aim is to accommodate to the family to gain experiential entrance into the family system. Unless this is accomplished at the outset, restructuring and change is impossible. Methods of joining the family are described in Table 30-4.

Another initial task of nurse therapists is to assume leadership in the session. They must join the family while still retaining the freedom to confront and challenge by presenting themselves as experts, gaining the family's confidence, and instilling hope. The nurse establishes the rules of the system by determining who attends the session, allowing no one to talk for another, and prohibiting interruptions. The nurse controls the flow and direction of communication.

At the beginning of the session, the nurse contacts each member. More than 15 to 20 minutes must not be spent with an individual or the nurse will become part of the system. Very soon the nurse asks two people to interact directly to enact a problem they have been describing. The nurse can now directly observe dysfunctional interactions. Rather than going from content issue to content issue, the nurse therapist can introduce the conflict inherent in small events and make conflictual events from nonevents.

Minuchin is a master of intensifying minute, simple nonevents for therapeutic intervention. For example, in a demonstration videotape, a father is "helping" the identified patient, the adolescent son, adjust his video microphone wire. Minuchin turns this into a therapeutic intervention focusing on the family's infantalization of the son. This occurs in the first 5 minutes of the tape. The amount of knowledge needed about the family to diagnose and begin restructuring dysfunctional interactions is available quickly. Structural family therapy does not explore or interpret the past—it is active and immediate.

Diagnosis in family therapy depends on the observation of how the family affects the nurse's behavior. It is also based on the nurse's impact on the family. The interactional diagnosis changes according to the family's acceptance or resistance of the therapist's restructuring interventions. It also varies depending on which family subsystem is active in the therapeutic situation at any one time. In this way, diagnosis and therapy are inseparable.

Intervention strategies transform the dysfunctional transactional patterns that maintain symptomatic behavior. The nurse is concerned about symptom removal and changes the family's organization to ensure that the symptom is not passed on. However, if an area of organization such as the parents' relationship does not contribute to the symptom, the therapist does not enter there. Therapy should be limited to the family's presenting symptom.

Minuchin identifies seven categories of restructuring operations: enacting family transactional patterns, marking boundaries, escalating stress, assigning tasks, using symptoms, manipulating mood, and supporting, educating, or guiding.[21]

Table 30-4   Methods of Joining the Family

Method	Description
Mirroring or mimicking	Matching the family's mood, pace, or communication patterns, such as by becoming jovial, somber, fidgety, or terse in conversing with them
Respecting family values	Supporting family hierarchies, such as by addressing all communication through the spouse that appears to be the "central switchboard"
Finding common elements	Keying in culturally or establishing areas of kinship, such as by offering "I have an adolescent boy, too"
Searching for strength	Observing for the smallest positive aspect of individual family members that the nurse can use to confirm that person's sense of self, such as by appreciating a clever phrase or a sense of humor
Supporting family subsystems	Confirming important family subsets, such as by giving small children toys to play with while talking with older ones, or by having parents sit together as they discuss their difficulty with the children
Tracking	Asking for elaboration with concrete details and examples of specific content in the family's discussion; this confirms individuals who are speaking and explores family structure, such as in tracking a mother's mentioning that she and her son are close by asking what time of the day and in which part of the house they are closest, thus learning that the mother and son sleep together while father sleeps in another room

Enacting Transactional Patterns. Enacting transactional patterns involves family members actively discussing an event that they might otherwise be describing to the nurse. Instead, the nurse instructs specific members to discuss the matter between themselves. The nurse disengages from the interaction to observe nonverbal confirmation or contradiction of the content, patterned sequences, interruptions, distractions, alliances, and coalitions.

It may be difficult to stay outside these transactions, and the family may drag the nurse back into direct discussion. Going behind a one-way mirror after giving the family directions is a way to avoid this temptation. Manipulating space by rearranging seating or position can be an effective way of encouraging or intensifying dialogue. The seating pattern a family assumes when it first walks into a session provides clues to alliances, coalitions, centrality, and isolation. The nurse's manipulation of seating and space can be a diagnostic probe to see how flexible the family is to such change. It is also a graphic indication to the family of a therapeutic goal. For instance, the nurse may seat the spatially isolated father next to his son where the mother was seated. The wife is placed next to the nurse. This encourages more direct involvement between father and son, with the mother outside that relationship.

Marking Boundaries. Boundaries must be marked in both individuals and subsystems. This promotes clarity in the enmeshed families and reduces rigidity in disengaged families. Simple rules promote individual autonomy. These include insisting family members to speak *to* each other and not *about* each other. No one speaks for another, no one may interrupt, and no one acts as another's memory bank. The nurse encourages subsystem boundaries by including or excluding various subsystems attending a session. She would ask children to leave or not attend a session in discussing spouses' sex life. The nurse may assign tasks to promote subsystem boundaries. She might instruct the father and daughter to go out for a pizza once a week without the mother or younger siblings. Having the sibling subsystem interact in a session, with the mother behind a one-way mirror, helps the children find alternative ways to resolve conflicts normally interrupted by mother's interventions. At the same time, this lets mother identify more positive interaction among the children. Previously, she could only reflexively react to their anger, rebelliousness, and selfishness by intruding on their boundaries. Rigid triads involving cross-generational interactions can be especially resistant to boundary marking.

Escalating Stress. Increasing stress in a family forces members to develop more functional ways of resolving stress. In families seeking treatment, dysfunctional patterns have developed around the symptomatic member. To escalate stress, the nurse may block usual transactional patterns and emphasize differences the family ignores. Asking for the silent spouse's opinion following the dominant spouse's statements highlights unspoken family disagreements. Developing implicit conflict involves making covert conflict overt.

Families develop methods for diffusing conflict rapidly. For example, siblings may tease and shove each other noisily just before their parents argue. This prevents the parents' conflict from surfacing. Blocking the sibling conflict forces the parents to contact directly. The nurse can polarize conflict to increase stress. If the mother and father appear equally concerned about their son's delinquent activities, the nurse may ask the husband if he had ever tried telling his wife she was "messing up" with the son. The positions of the overprotective mother and the "reasonable" distant father develop.

The nurse can also produce stress by temporarily joining one member or subsystem. This operation must be carefully planned and requires the nurse's ability to disengage, which can be done serially to help members take differentiated positions. Also, a coalition can be formed, usually with a spouse, when the system rigidly resists open conflict. Joining a husband's attack on the wife makes the conflict too intense for the wife to diffuse stress onto the son; she is forced to address the conflict between herself and the husband.

Assigning Tasks. The assigning of tasks structures the setting for alternative interactions and behavior. In designing tasks the nurse must have a clear idea of the family's structure and dysfunctional patterns. Specific interactional goals to accomplish through the task must be outlined. Tasks can be simple. The nurse may ask a husband and wife to sit next to each other as they discuss an issue. In a family in which the wife disciplines the children, the father is assigned the job. The mother handles only emergencies; otherwise, the father learns of infractions he does not directly observe. The wife may not interfere with her husband's disciplinary tactics. She takes notes. Both parents become active and effective.

In assigning tasks the nurse should give all critically involved members a portion of the task to complete. This reduces the likelihood of one member sabotaging another's new behavior if each member must remain self-focused. This also makes it easier to relinquish a fixed behavior if another behavior is assigned to replace it. Whether the task is completed or not, the family and nurse have new information about family patterns and progress.

Using Symptoms. Symptoms can be used in restructuring operations in various ways. Symptoms may be focused on, as in a family Minuchin describes in which the daughter was a fire setter. The focus remained on the daughter, but the mother was instructed to spend time daily teaching the daughter how to light matches safely. This promoted a closer mother-daughter relationship, which was previously obstructed. A helpful focus remained on the symptom. Symptoms can be exaggerated to increase their intensity and mobilize family resources. A symptom can be relabeled, as in the case of a mother who continually nagged the son. Redefining her nagging as concern encouraged caring interactions. A new symptom shifts the family's focus onto another family member temporarily. For example, the husband fails to go to work and the wife alternately protects and threatens to leave him. Identifying her behavior as seriously depressed reduces her intense focus on the husband. A symptom's affect can also be changed, thereby altering interactions around it. For example, the mother who interacts positively with her fire setter daughter evokes a new affect with the symptom.

Manipulating Mood.
Manipulating the family's mood is another restructuring operation. For example, by exaggerating the common family mood, the family reacts by showing a wide range of expressions. The nurse can also model a more appropriate affect for the family, for example, by reacting with strong indignation to a young boy's criticism of his mother. This promotes respect and clarifies the boundaries of a passive, enmeshed parental subsystem.

Supporting, Educating, Guiding.
Support, education, and guidance can be a restructuring operation. They can take the form of modeling, assigning tasks, or sharing concrete information. Minuchin shows families how they program each other in the circular process of a family system.

The goal of structural family therapy is not a change in behavior but a change in the whole family's organization. This allows individual members a new experience in the family. Using a model of an effectively functioning family, the therapist joins the family in a therapeutic system, hoping to restructure the family. The restructuring either helps to maintain functional subsystems or helps to form new subsystems that will promote healing and growth.

STRATEGIC FAMILY THERAPY

Strategic family therapy developed out of communication theory.[30] Communication theorists, such as Haley, contend that *all* behavior, not only verbal acts, is communication. They recognized that most communication consists of many levels between sender and receiver, and that the significance of any message depends on

how it is reinforced, contradicted, or framed by other messages. These, along with the setting and the relationship between sender and receiver, constitute the context that must be considered in interpreting any message.[31]

Another basic tenet of communication theory is that communication is an ongoing process. There is no beginning point or end point in the stimulus-response-reinforcement pattern of human interaction. In most relationships the behavior of each participant depends on the other's behavior. In families, complex, highly patterned, repetitive interactions become established. When a two-person (or more) system is dysfunctional in its communication, potential exists for problems. Three types of common communication problems are disqualification, disconfirmation, and incongruent communication.

Disqualification in communication includes self-contradictions, inconsistencies, subject switches, incomplete sentences, misunderstandings, obscure mannerisms of speech, and literal interpretation of metaphor.[30] An example of disqualification is a question an older brother used to baffle his younger sister: "Do you walk to school or carry your lunch?"

Disconfirmation in communication involves ignoring or invalidating essential elements of a significant other's self-image. It involves telling the person you do not feel the way you feel, need what you need, or experience what you experience.[30]

Incongruent communication is delivering two conflicting messages at the same time. If responding to either message, the receiver will be charged with "badness or madness." This is the basis of the double bind. An example is the command "be spontaneous!" or the direction to "be assertive, and don't make waves."

Components

Strategic therapists make a distinction between difficulties and problems. Difficulties are either (1) undesirable states of affairs that can be removed by a logical solution or (2) undesirable, common life problems that must be lived with. Problems arise from small difficulties that escalate. They are maintained by mishandling attempts to solve them. Mishandling frequently occurs around adaptation to ordinary life events and ranges from (1) ignoring or denying difficulties that require action to (2) attempting to resolve an ordinary life difficulty that is unnecessary (e.g., a husband who would not talk to his wife before breakfast) or impossible to resolve (e.g., the generation gap) to (3) difficulties where action is needed but the wrong kind is taken.[31]

Strategic family therapists are not concerned with the history of the problem or the motivation behind it. They are not interested in characteristics of people, and they place no importance on insight. Little distinction is made between acute and chronic problems. Chronic problems are ones that have been mishandled longer. The presenting problem behavior and the problem-maintaining behavior are the primary focus of treatment.

Communication theorists identified a positive feedback loop in human interaction. This is the vicious cycle that develops from efforts by family members, or the identified patient, to stop or "help" undesirable behavior. For example, the rebellious teenager, when faced with parental discipline, becomes increasingly rebellious. As discipline becomes harsher, the boy's behavior escalates further. Thus the action that is meant to alleviate the behavior of the other party aggravates it. From this view, the cause and the nature of a problem are essentially the same process. People try to change behavior in the most logical way possible. Common sense suggests prevention or avoidance of undesirable behavior by means of opposite behavior. If this does not work, they try harder with the same behavior. The resolution of problems therefore requires changing the problem-maintaining behaviors. This interrupts the vicious positive feedback cycles.[16]

Interventions

Intervention occurs with the patient, the unidentified patient, or both, depending on who is most concerned with the problem. This is the person most willing to change. Effective intervention can be made through any member of the system to break the positive feedback loop. This is illustrated in the following two clinical examples.

CLINICAL EXAMPLE

A colonel is being militarily strict with his son, and the boy is becoming increasingly defiant. The therapist tells the father his son is "going to the dogs." The therapist suggests that the father hold back on his discipline to get a baseline measurement of how bad the boy's behavior will become. As pressure on the boy is reduced, his behavior improves.

CLINICAL EXAMPLE

A woman had problems with urinary frequency. She was isolated at home, feeling unable to leave the house to socialize. She was also isolated at work because she had her machine set by the bathroom door where there were no co-workers. She worked from 12 to 8 PM. The therapist instructed her to urinate as many times as she felt

she had to each morning before going to work but to use the toilet only three times; after that she was to urinate sitting in the tub. She was to make no effort to change her pattern at work. The next week the woman reported she had been in agony the first morning but was unable to urinate sitting in the tub. She then figured that if she could limit herself at home, she could do so at work, and had no further problems with urinary frequency.

These examples demonstrate the use of reversal or symptom prescription. They carry the message "do not change" or "more of it," both of which stop the family or patient from trying to stop. Persuading people to change behavior that common sense tells them is correct often requires treatment strategies that appear weird, illogical, or paradoxical.

The nurse's first task is to obtain a statement from the patient of the presenting complaint in specific, concrete terms. After obtaining this statement, the nurse determines what about the behavior makes it a problem. The nurse asks what solutions the family has tried. This identifies which remedies to avoid and indicates the problem-maintaining behavior.

Next, the nurse asks what the family's or patient's minimum goal of treatment would be—what smallest identifiable change would signify progress or some success. General goals such as "improved communication" are not acceptable. Feeling changes such as "to feel happier" or negative goals such as "to stop certain behavior" are equally unacceptable. Rather, the nurse seeks positive, specific behavioral goals that reflect an attitude or feeling change. such as "the father will engage in one positive activity with his son each week." If a small but significant change can be made in what appeared to be a hopeless situation, a so-called ripple effect may occur. That is, once a patient is mobilized and regains confidence in the ability to solve a small problem, sometimes other difficulties can be surmounted.[16]

As soon as possible, the therapist attempts to grasp the patient's "language" and main ideas and values. "Tuning into" the family's view and then extending that view is a critical step known as **reframing.** It precedes the therapist's strategic intervention. To reframe means to change the conceptual or emotional setting or viewpoint in which a situation is experienced. Using language common to the family's worldview, the therapist places the experience in another frame that fits the "facts" of the same concrete situation equally well. The situation's entire meaning changes.[29]

An example of reframing includes using hostility when it is present in a woman's frigidity. The therapist may reframe the problem as one produced by her over-protecting the male. Assuming there is hostility and protecting the husband is the last thing the woman would want to do, the new frame to the problem uses hostility as an incentive to release her inhibited sexual feelings. Tom Sawyer reframed whitewashing the picket fence as an artistic, entertaining enterprise rather than a dreary chore. He used his friends' competitiveness to vie for the opportunity to whitewash. Reframing causes an attitudinal change and a change in emphasis of a situation's facts. This changes the situation's meaning to permit new behavior. The concrete facts remain unchanged.

Strategic therapists place no importance on the therapist having therapy as family systems therapists do. Nurses can be trained in this theoretical framework without understanding their involvement with their families. Structural therapists share this view.[14,21]

Strategic therapists are sometimes attacked for the "manipulative, insincere" nature of their approach. They acknowledge that this is the case. Communication research stresses that it is impossible not to communi-

cate. Likewise, it is impossible not to influence. A nondirective, dynamically oriented therapist influences the patient's communication in hundreds of subtle ways. These ways include body movement, intonation, and leading responses. The "insight" school and the nondirective school of therapy influence patients outside the patient's awareness. Strategic therapists do so openly. The patient's "awareness" of the manipulation itself is irrelevant as long as the strategy is given and followed. The difference between the "insight" school and the strategic school of psychotherapy is conceptual rather than ethical. The "insight" school believes that change in people occurs through the therapeutic relationship with a change in their understanding of themselves. The strategic school persuades a person to change "spontaneously." It arranges a situation so that the person initiates the change in behavior.[10,14]

The strategic therapist is an active and deliberate

Table 30-5   Models of Family Therapy

	Family systems (Bowen)	Structural (Minuchin)	Strategic (Haley)
View of normal family function	Differentiation of self in relation to others Balance between thinking and feeling	Generational hierarchy with strong parental authority Clear boundaries Flexibility of system for autonomy, interdependence, and adaptive change	Flexibility Large behavioral repertoire for problem solving and life cycle passage
View of symptoms/ dysfunction	Functioning impaired by relationship with family of origin Poor differentiation Emotional reactivity Triangulation Emotional cutoff	Symptoms result from current structural imbalance and malfunctioning generational hierarchy or boundaries Enmeshed or disengaged style Maladaptive reaction to internal or external demands	Symptom is embedded in interaction pattern Origin of problem not significant Symptoms maintained by unsuccessful problem solving Impasse at life cycle transition
Goals of therapy	Greater self differentiation Increased thinking Decreased emotional reactivity Detriangulate self	Reorganize family structure to achieve strengthened parental hierarchy, clear, flexible boundaries, and more adaptive patterns	Interrupt rigid feedback cycle Change symptom-maintaining sequence to attain new outcome
Role of the nurse in change	Stays detriangulated Change can occur only within the individual self Change in one member can bring about systemic change	Joining the family is prerequisite for restructuring Nurse is responsible for change while crediting the family for beneficial changes	If treatment fails, the fault lies with the nurse Success is credited to the family, thus enhancing its confidence in future problem-solving skills
Interventions	Teach how family systems work Coach individual to establish person-to-person relationship with key members of family of origin Use genogram to track triangles, myths, and themes, across the generations Ask factual who, what, when, where, and how questions to promote thinking and reduce emotionally reactive behavior	Joining Enacting Marking boundaries Escalating stress Assigning tasks Using symptom Manipulating mood Supporting Educating Advocacy	Detailed questions to track behaviors surrounding the problem Symptom prescription Reframing Strategies designed to interrupt self-reinforcing behavioral sequence maintaining the symptom

change agent. The therapist creates a strategy to bring about the change the patient is paying money to achieve. The responsibility for success or failure therefore rests on the nurse. The nurse never takes the credit for change in the patient's eyes. In this therapy the point at which termination takes place is clear. It occurs when the patient is satisfied with the improvement that has been made.

The theoretical views of family therapy presented in this chapter are summarized in Table 30-5. These models reflect current thinking in the field related to clinical interventions designed primarily to treat families.

 Compare and contrast strategic family therapy with cognitive behavioral therapy as described in Chapter 28.

SUGGESTED CROSS-REFERENCES

SUMMARY

1. Characteristics of the functional and dysfunctional family were described. The competence paradigm was also introduced with its emphasis on family strengths, resources, and competencies.
2. Nonclinical family interventions are designed primarily to educate and support. They are the result of the family self-help movement in psychiatry. Components of a comprehensive psychoeducational program were described.
3. Family systems theory conceptualizes all family systems on a continuum ranging from total dysfunction to high levels of functioning. Separating the thinking and feeling processes of family members is foundational to this therapy. The goal of systems therapy is for individual members to differentiate themselves from the family emotional "we-ness" system.
4. Structural family therapy assumes that behavior and the family's level of function are a consequence of the family's organization and the interactional patterns between members. The major elements of a family structure that enable viable family functioning are (1) a power hierarchy with different levels of authority, (2) differentiated subsystems with different functions and levels of power, and (3) subsystem boundaries sufficiently well defined to prevent intrusion but also able to allow emotional contact between members.
5. Strategic therapists are concerned with the removal of problematical behavioral patterns or symptoms. The goals of strategic therapy include obtaining a clear statement from the family of the presenting complaint in specific, concrete terms. The therapist reframes the problem, thereby changing the situation's meaning, permitting new behavior to occur.

 COMPETENT CARING
A CLINICAL EXEMPLAR OF A PSYCHIATRIC NURSE
Carole Bennett, MN, RN, CS

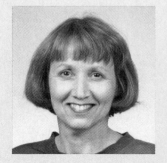 As a psychiatric nurse, it has always been difficult for me to describe the rewards I experienced for the years of hard work I have dedicated to my profession. Sometimes, the rewards elude even me. Then, quite unexpectedly, I have the opportunity to really help someone and I remember why I have been a psychiatric nurse for such a long time.

Recently, a nurse working on our youth unit was having difficulty with teaching parenting skills to a mother. It seemed that no matter how many times she demonstrated limit setting and reinforcement, this mother simply seemed unable to use these skills. The nurse asked me if I would see the mother and intervene using the family genogram and I agreed. The next day the family anxiously appeared—the mother, the father, and an aunt who flew down from New York. Well, I don't know about you, but when I hear the father's older sister from New York is waiting to be in family therapy, I think that this is going to be a rough one. So I drew a deep breath, offered coffee all around, poured myself a big cup, and began the meeting. Yes, they all knew why they were there. Yes, they all knew it might get uncomfortable. Yes, they all wanted to stay.

The father and his sister began with their family. They grew up in the projects, had different fathers, described years of struggle, related how the older sister was sent to New York to live with her natural father, and how their mother managed all the while to raise them from a wheelchair. But she had done it; she had shown them how to do it, too.

Then the mother began. She too was raised in the projects, but by her grandparents. Her mother never really visited often, and her grandmother was an alcoholic. Yes, she had a grandfather, but he was an alcoholic, too. She also lived with other family members at various times, but they were all heavy drinkers. In fact, every adult in her childhood was an alcoholic. But it was hard for her to recall facts. Had she been sexually abused? Well, she remembers being told something about that but she couldn't remember any details. She does remember being beaten regularly by various people, but that didn't seem unusual to her.

Everyone was quiet. It was hard for me to know quite what to say. By this time the husband was patting his wife lovingly. He had known only parts of the painful story he just heard his wife describe. And his sister from New York moved closer to her sister-in-law on the couch. They were very supportive while I suggested that perhaps no one had ever shown the wife how to be a mother. No one had ever shown her what to do, and so she really didn't know how to take care of the seven, yes seven, boys she was now raising.

As a group, we continued to talk until we came up with a plan. The sister was leaving for home soon, but there would be two other sisters who could help. The father said he could shorten his work day, and perhaps the mother could look for a job, which was something she wanted to do. The unit nurse said she could arrange for the mother to spend entire days on the unit so that she could begin to learn how to do this thing called "child rearing." And finally, we discussed the issue of therapy. Well, no thank you. The mother didn't think she was ready to talk to someone about what had happened to her so long ago, but maybe she would be sometime in the future.

We all stood up and shook hands smiling and sensing the partnership among us. The sister from New York gave my hand an especially firm squeeze and looked me right in the eye. I think she was saying she was glad I was there, and I was sending the same message back to her. At that moment I knew exactly why I have been a psychiatric nurse for such a long time. ▼

REFERENCES

1. Bowen M: Multigenerational process. In Haley J, ed: *Changing families*, New York, 1971, Grune & Stratton.
2. Bowen M: Theory in the practice of psychotherapy. In Guerin P, ed: *Family therapy theory and practice*, New York, 1976, Gardner Press.
3. Bowen M: Family therapy and family group therapy. In Kaplan H, Sadock B, eds: *Comprehensive group psychotherapy*, Baltimore, 1983, Williams & Wilkins.
4. Carter E, McGoldrick M: *The changing family life cycle, a framework for family therapy* ed 2, Boston, 1989, Allyn & Bacon.
5. Davis B, Jones L: Differentiation of self and attachment among adult daughters, *Issues Ment Health Nurs* 13:321, 1992.
6. Dunst C, Trivette C: *Enabling and empowering families: principles and guidelines for practice*, Cambridge, Mass, 1988, Brookline.
7. Giat-Roberto L: *Transgenerational family therapies*, New York, 1992, The Guilford Press.
8. Goodrich T, ed: *Women and power: perspectives for family therapy*, New York, 1991, WW Norton.
9. Guerin P: Theoretical aspects and clinical relevance of the multigenerational model of family therapy. In Guerin P, ed: *Family theory and practice*, New York, 1976, Gardner Press.
10. Haley J: *Problem solving therapy*, San Francisco, 1987, Jossey-Bass.
11. Hatfield A, Lefley H, eds: *Families of the mentally ill*, New York, 1987, The Guilford Press.
12. Herz Brown F: The therapeutic relationship. In Herz Brown F, ed: *Reweaving the family tapestry*, New York, 1991, WW Norton.
13. Howe C, Howe J: The National Alliance for the Mentally Ill: history and ideology, *New Directions for Mental Health Services*, no. 34, San Francisco, 1987, Jossey-Bass.
14. Kerr M, Bowen M: *Family evaluation: an approach based on Bowen theory*, New York, 1988, WW Norton.
15. Lamb R et al: Families of schizophrenics: a movement in jeopardy, *Hosp Community Psychiatry* 37:353, 1986.
16. Madanes C: Strategic family therapy. In Gurman A, Kniskern D, eds: *Handbook of family therapy*, vol II, New York, 1991, Brunner/Mazel.
17. Marsh D: *Families and mental illness: new directions in professional practice*, New York, 1992, Praeger.
18. Marsh D: Working with families of people with serious

mental illness. In VandeCreek L, Knapp S, Jackson T: *Innovations in clinical practice: a source book,* vol 11, Sarasota, Fla, 1992, Professional Resource Exchange.

19. McFarlane W: Family psychoeducational treatment. In Gurman A, Kniskern D: *Handbook of family therapy,* vol II, New York, 1991, Brunner/Mazel.
20. McGoldrick M, Gerson R: *Genograms and family assessment,* New York, 1986, WW Norton.
21. Minuchin S: *Families and family therapy,* Cambridge, Mass, 1974, Harvard University Press.
22. Minuchin S, Fishman H: *Family therapy techniques,* Cambridge, Mass, 1981, Harvard University Press.
23. Parker B: Living with mental illness: the family as caregiver, *J Psychosoc Nurs Ment Health Serv* 31:19, 1993.
24. Peternelj-Taylor C, Hartley V: Living with mental illness: professional/family collaboration, *J Psychosoc Nurs* 31:23, 1993.
25. Schwartzberg N: Single young adults. In Herz Brown F: *Reweaving the family therapy,* New York, 1991, WW Norton.
26. Strelnick A: Multiple family group therapy: a review of the literature, *Fam Process* 16:307, 1977.
27. Toman W: *Family constellation,* ed 4, New York, 1993, Springer Publishing.
28. Walsh F: Conceptualizations of normal family processes. In Walsh F, ed: *Normal family processes,* ed 2, New York, 1993, The Guilford Press.
29. Watzlawick P: Some basic issues in interaction research. In Framo J, ed: *Family interaction,* New York, 1972, Springer Publishing.
30. Watzlawick P, Beaven J, Jackson D: *Pragmatics of human communication,* New York, 1967, WW Norton.
31. Weakland J: Communication theory and clinical change. In Guerin P, ed: *Family therapy theory and practice,* New York, 1976, Gardner Press.
32. Wylie M: Family therapy's neglected prophet: Bowen's legacy, *Fam Ther Networker,* Mar/Apr:25, 1991.

ANNOTATED SUGGESTED READINGS

Boyd-Franklin N: *Black families in therapy: a multisystems approach,* New York, 1989, The Guilford Press.

Examines the social meaning race has acquired through stereotyping and differential power based on skin color. Helps the clinician deal with the issues of race, culture, class, and poverty.

*Bright M: Therapeutic ritual: helping families grow, *J Psychosoc Nurs Ment Health Serv* 28:24, 1990.

Describes the use of therapeutic rituals to help families resolve conflicts, negotiate new roles, and develop shared meanings about life together.

*Caroselli-Karinja M: Asthma and adaptation: exploring the family system, *J Psychosoc Nurs Ment Health Serv* 28:34, 1990.

Uses a family system approach to explore the physiology, case management, and treatment approaches for the child with asthma.

Carter E, McGoldrick M: *The changing family life cycle, a framework for family therapy,* ed 2, Boston, 1989, Allyn & Bacon.

Covers the developmental stages of the family life cycle and disruptive problems. Valuable for both beginning and advanced students.

*Clement J: Psychiatric nursing phenomena and the construct of family boundaries, *Arch Psychiatr Nurs* 5:236, 1991.

Presents theory, nursing interventions, and a case study based on family boundaries.

*Fawcett C: *Family psychiatric nursing,* St Louis, 1993, Mosby.

Presents information of mental health issues of families throughout the life span and the role of nurses in family mental health care.

Haley J: *Problem solving therapy,* San Francisco, 1987, Jossey-Bass.

Clearly presents the problem-focused, strategic approach to family therapy. Supports theory and technique with case examples.

Herz Brown F: *Reweaving the family tapestry,* New York, 1991, WW Norton.

Demonstrates the application of multigenerational theory to therapy with individuals, couples, and families. Issues of race, gender, and ethnicity are woven through chapters that examine life cycle changes and disruptions.

Kerr M, Bowen M: *Family evaluation: an approach based on Bowen theory,* New York, 1988, WW Norton.

Excellent reference for describing family work based on Bowen's theory of family therapy.

Marsh D: *Families and mental illness,* New York, 1992, Praeger.

Best text to describe the competence paradigm of family intervention. Includes practical intervention strategies and resources to enhance professional skills in working collaboratively with families.

McFarlane W: Family psychoeducational treatment. In Gurman A, Kniskern D: *Handbook of family therapy,* vol II, New York, 1991, Brunner/Mazel.

Describes the controversy surrounding the two basic approaches: the medical model approach, which includes a "psychoeducational" component, and the communication theory approach.

McGoldrick M, Anderson C, Walsh F eds: *Women in families for family therapy,* New York, 1989, WW Norton.

Addresses gender issues in family therapy theory, practice, and supervision and examines women's experience of family life from a variety of perspectives.

McGoldrick M, Gerson R: *Genograms and family assessment,* New York, 1986, WW Norton.

Presents a standard format for constructing genograms and clearly outlines the principles underlying their interpretation and application. Using genograms of famous people, introduces the beginner to this essential tool.

Minuchin S: *Families and family therapy,* Cambridge, Mass, 1974, Harvard University Press.

Provides definitive coverage of the techniques and skills used in structural family therapy. Describes techniques and includes excerpts of sessions.

*Peternelj-Taylor C, Hartley V: Living with mental illness: professional/family collaboration, *J Psychosoc Nurs Ment Health Serv* 31:23, 1993.

Describes objectives, agenda, and implementation issues of a family education program.

---

*Nursing reference.

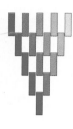

Treatment Settings

You may think that most people with emotional and psychiatric problems spend many days of their lives in an acute or long-term psychiatric hospital being cared for by specially trained staff. Years ago you would have been correct, but today, most people with such problems live in the community and receive their mental health care in outpatient settings. These are the people you pass on the street, see at the mall, and laugh with at the movies. Today, we no longer try to separate and isolate the mentally ill in large impersonal institutions. Rather, we ask our caregivers to reach out to these individuals and their families in the neighborhoods in which they live, love, and learn.

In this unit you will discover how contemporary psychiatric hospitals take care of patients. You will read how inpatient psychiatric care nurses protect and stabilize people in crisis and then turn their care over to a variety of community-based mental health care providers. As psychiatric treatment grows in the community, new and expanded roles are opening up for psychiatric nurses. These tap into nurses' spirit of innovation, creativity, and resourcefulness. And finally, you'll learn about how to ask for, receive, and provide consultation to others. In an era of health-care reform in which managing people and resources is an essential nursing skill, understanding the consultation process may very well be your ticket to personal satisfaction and professional success.

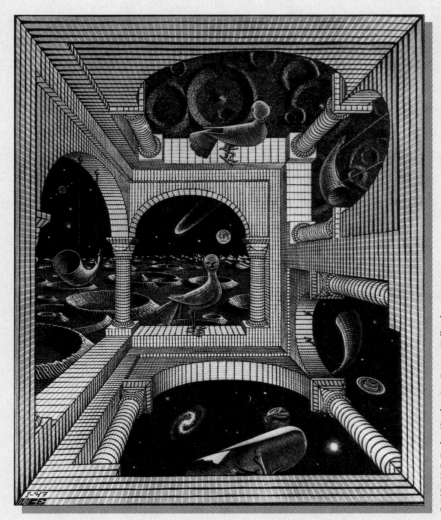

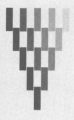

CHAPTER 31

Inpatient Psychiatric Nursing Care

VICTORIA A. QUEEN

"We're all mad here. I'm mad. You're mad."
"How do you know I'm mad?," said Alice.
"You must be," said the Cat, "or you wouldn't have come here."
Alice didn't think that proved it at all.

Lewis Carroll: *Alice's Adventures in Wonderland*

LEARNING OBJECTIVES

After studying this chapter the student should be able to:

▼ Describe recent changes in inpatient psychiatric care
▼ Identify the components of the therapeutic milieu and their implications for inpatient psychiatric nursing practice
▼ Discuss the caregiving activities of the inpatient psychiatric nurse
▼ Analyze the inpatient psychiatric nurse's role in integrating and coordinating patient care
▼ Evaluate outcomes related to inpatient psychiatric nursing practice

TOPICAL OUTLINE

The treatment of the mentally ill has always reflected the social values and public policy of the larger community. Before WW II effective medications were largely unavailable, and the mentally ill were separated from the community and housed in institutions for the protection of patients as well as society. Nursing care for these patients was primarily custodial. With changing social perspectives and the move toward more humane treatment, the psychiatric hospital came to be seen as a possibly powerful force that could influence patient behavior and help people recover from mental illness. More recently, scientific advances in biomedical practice have led to the use of effective medications and somatic therapies to treat symptoms of psychiatric illness. These, used in conjunction with therapeutic principles and management strategies of the inpatient milieu, offer psychiatric nurses valuable tools for the comprehensive care of the mentally ill.

Inpatient psychiatric nursing practice is rich in history and tradition. Psychiatric nurses are the only group of mental health professionals who are responsible for meeting the needs of inpatients 24 hours a day, 365 days a year. To deliver cost-effective, high-quality inpatient care, psychiatric nurses must manage the one-to-one nurse-patient relationship within a complex social and organizational environment. The full scope of contemporary inpatient psychiatric nursing practice therefore requires knowledge and expertise in four broad categories of functioning. These include:

1. Managing the therapeutic milieu
2. Implementing caregiving activities
3. Integrating and coordinating care delivery
4. Evaluating outcomes

It is through the integration of these four components that inpatient psychiatric nursing care positively influences a patient's overall treatment outcome.

All psychiatric nurses, regardless of education or experience, engage in these activities everyday. To do so requires that the nurse be aware of and value the breadth of professional psychiatric nursing functions and know about the changing mental health care delivery system. This chapter is organized around these four areas of functioning, since they represent both the structure and the process of inpatient psychiatric nursing care.

THE PSYCHIATRIC HOSPITAL IN TRANSITION

Health-care costs, changing reimbursement trends, and problems with accessibility of care among vast numbers of citizens have prompted major changes in how health care is delivered in the United States.[25] Specifically, in recent years the focus of psychiatric care has moved away from extended care in predominately inpatient settings toward shorter lengths of inpatient stays and a wider choice among continuum of care options.[24] For example, in 1987 the average length of stay for acute psychiatric inpatient treatment was about 25 days, as compared with 19 days in 1991 (Fig. 31-1). More recently, many inpatient psychiatric settings have an average length of stay of 7 to 10 days, and crisis stabilization inpatient programs may involve only a 2- or 3-day length of stay.

The treatment goals, process, and expected outcomes related to inpatient psychiatric care are also changing. Today there are considerably more treatment options being offered by inpatient facilities. Many psychiatric hospitals now provide day treatment, partial hospitalization, ambulatory, and even home care programs. These changes have required that mental health professionals reevaluate the care they provide based on the patient's treatment stage, setting, and resources. In previous years most patients with maladaptive coping responses entered the psychiatric hospital in the **acute** treatment stage and were able to stay in the hospital until the goal of symptom **remission** was attained (Fig. 31-2). Today, however, the majority of patients are admitted to hospitals in the **crisis** treatment stage with the treatment goal of **stabilization** rather than symptom remission.

The intensity of treatment has also drastically increased. Individuals who require hospitalization usually have high degrees of demoralization, hopelessness, and functional impairment. They are also likely to have experienced severe stress such as interpersonal loss, physical illness, unemployment, or collapse of support systems. This high level of symptomatology, combined with limited resources, calls for a vigorous and well-

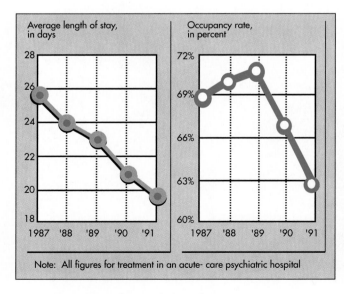

Note: All figures for treatment in an acute-care psychiatric hospital

Fig. 31-1 Hospital stays for psychiatric patients.

coordinated response from the inpatient treatment team.

Currently, approximately 72% of mental health insurance costs in the United States are spent on inpatient care, which is provided in general hospital psychiatric units, private psychiatric hospitals, and public psychiatric facilities that include long-term and forensic treatment.[16] The United States has about 300,000 psychiatric beds, or 130 beds per 100,000 people. The major psychiatric diagnoses of patients admitted to those beds are listed in Table 31-1.[4] The indications for inpatient hospital use have also become more focused in recent years. They now include the following:

▼ Prevention from harming self or others
▼ Need for a rapid, multidisciplinary diagnostic evaluation that requires frequent observation by specially trained personnel
▼ Stabilization to allow for treatment at a less-restrictive level of care

▼ Initiation of a treatment process with safety risks that need to be monitored by specially trained personnel
▼ Treatment of acute intoxicated states
▼ Management of agitation, overactivity, or acute psychosis resulting in significant confusion and disorganization

At this time the majority of psychiatric nurses continue to work in inpatient psychiatric settings.[17] Given the rapid changes in the mental health care environment, however, psychiatric nurses must continue to be progressive in designing models of care for patients. Nurses who staff inpatient units may no longer have their responsibilities limited to activities delivered exclusively in the hospital setting. Rather, inpatient psychiatric nurses must be ready and capable of providing their services throughout the continuum of care and in many traditional and untraditional mental health care settings (see Chapter 1). Psychiatric nurses must also

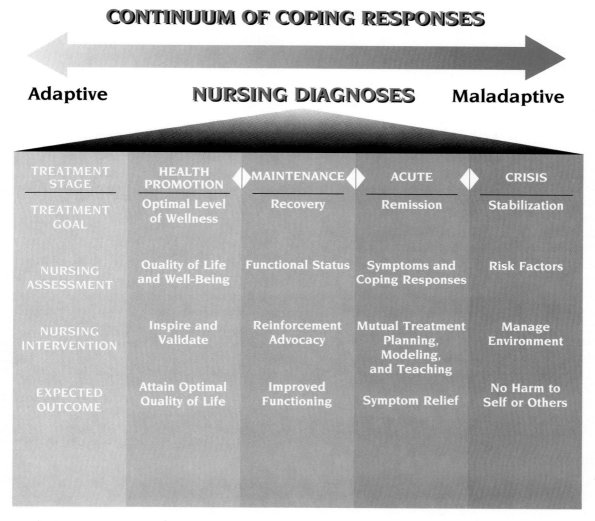

Fig. 31-2 Continuum of coping responses and treatment stages from the stress adaptation model.

Table 31-1 Major Diagnoses of Patients Admitted
to Inpatient Psychiatric Services

Diagnosis	Percentage
Affective disorders	32
Schizophrenia	23
Substance use disorders	21
Adjustment disorders	7
Organic mental disorders	3
Personality disorders	2

be flexible enough to move with patients from short-term inpatient units through a partial treatment program and ultimately to community-based settings (see Chapter 32). The challenge is for psychiatric nursing, as an essential mental health discipline, to be able to articulate what it can contribute in these various treatment settings and be ready to demonstrate outcomes of nursing interventions across the continuum of care.

How do you think the changes in inpatient psychiatric care affect the families and support systems of the mentally ill? How can nurses help them with the problems they now face?

MANAGING THE THERAPEUTIC MILIEU

The basic difference between inpatient and outpatient psychiatric care is the controlled environment, or milieu, in which it occurs. Inpatient treatment facilities generally provide a milieu that physically shelters patients from what they perceive to be painful and frightening stressors. This respite, although brief, provides patients with an opportunity to begin to stabilize while being protected from factors that would otherwise interfere with their treatment progress.

Understanding the concepts of the therapeutic milieu is an essential part of effective inpatient psychiatric nursing care. The aim of the therapeutic milieu is to provide patients with a stable and coherent social environment that facilitates the development and implementation of an individualized treatment plan. Many people have studied different aspects of the inpatient psychiatric environment and identified structures and principles that make it helpful in treating the mentally ill.

The Therapeutic Community

In 1953 Maxwell Jones[10] first described the inpatient environment as a **therapeutic community** with cultural norms for behaviors, values, and activity. He saw patients' social interactions among peers and health-care workers as treatment opportunities. For example, he believed that interpersonal difficulties between patients provided fertile material for psychodynamic intervention. He also believed that the clinical staff should share in the community governance with the patient group on an equal basis. He further emphasized the benefit of mutual participation of patients in each others' treatment, predominantly through sharing of intimate information and feedback in group settings like the community meeting.

Since its introduction, however, the concept of the therapeutic community has seemed to have lost some of its credibility and popularity. One reason for this is that its philosophy of democracy and egalitarianism among both patients and clinical staff is not compatible with the medical model. Others point out that the concept of the therapeutic community was developed when patients spent months and even years in the hospital. This is in sharp contrast to the short-term nature of most current inpatient psychiatric hospitalizations.

The therapeutic community is an example of the social model of psychiatric care described in Chapter 3. Discuss how it differs from the medical model in the roles of patient and therapist and the therapeutic process.

The Therapeutic Milieu

More than a decade later, Abroms[1] introduced the idea of the **therapeutic milieu**. He said that it served two main purposes:

1. It set limits on disturbing and maladaptive behavior
2. It teaches psychosocial skills

He described five categories of disturbing behaviors and related interventions that would help patients keep maladaptive behaviors under control and thus allow treatment to progress. These are listed in Table 31-2.

Once maladaptive behaviors were limited, Abroms stressed the use of the therapeutic milieu to foster the development of four important psychosocial skills in hospitalized mentally ill patients.

Orientation: All patients could achieve a greater level of orientation and reality awareness. Orientation refers to the patient's knowledge and understanding of time, place, person and purpose. Awareness of these elements can be reinforced through all patient interactions and activities. For example, introducing oneself, one's role, and rationale for an interaction helps disoriented patients better attend to their surroundings. Another intervention would be a "current events" group conducted with patients.

Table 31-2   Managing Disturbing Behaviors in the Milieu

Disturbing behavior	Intervention
Destructiveness—physically destructive behavior. It is a response to a variety of feelings, such as fear or anger.	In working with destructive behavior, the goal is to control or set limits on the maladaptive response but support the feeling underlying the behavior. Validation is essential to help the patient recognize the feeling and ultimately regain control of maladaptive behavior.
Disorganization—distorted or unusual behavior a psychotic patient may exhibit as symptomatic of the illness. It may be triggered by elevated anxiety, profound depression, or organic dysfunctions.	Reassure and assist the patient while reducing the degree to which these behaviors inhibit therapeutic processes.
Deviancy—behaviors often described as "acting out." They are the result of the patient expressing conflicts overtly in the environment. It is often difficult to determine precisely what "acting out" behavior is, as well as what is justifiable or even tolerable because much of it may be influenced by sociocultural factors.	The therapeutic goal in working with deviancy is to analyze how the behavior affects the inpatient milieu as a whole and how it inhibits the progress of the individual patient. Examining the behavior with the patient and identifying consequences and alternatives are useful approaches.
Dysphoria—patients with mood alterations may be dysphoric, which is evident in maladaptive responses such as withdrawal from the environment, obsessional behaviors, intrusiveness, or hyperreligiosity.	Establishing a therapeutic alliance is the first task of the nurse. From there, the nurse and patient can explore feelings and dysfunctional thoughts and begin to modify behavioral responses.
Dependence—evidenced by patients who do not identify and meet their own individual needs despite being able to do so. The avoidant nature of dependency interferes with therapeutic progress.	The initial therapeutic goal is to work with the patient to draw on any remaining areas of independence and strength. Once identified, situations can be identified in which the patient can apply these independent behaviors successfully.

Assertion: The ability to express one self appropriately can be modeled and exercised in a variety of ways in the hospital setting. Supporting patients in expressing themselves effectively and in a socially acceptable manner on a specific topic or issue is the overall goal. Some example interventions include assertiveness training groups, "focus" groups for lower functioning patients, or any facilitated, interactive patient group.

Occupation: Patients can feel a sense of confidence and accomplishment through industrious activity. Many therapeutic opportunities are provided through completion of individual or group "hands-on" activities. Spending time working with patients on something as simple as a jigsaw puzzle can provide purposeful activity, physical skill development, and the added benefit of practiced social interaction.

Recreation: The ability to engage in and enjoy constructive leisure activity is a beneficial outlet for pleasure and relaxation. Providing a variety of recreational opportunities helps patients apply many of the skills they have learned including orientation, assertion, social interaction, and physical dexterity. Some example interventions include informal games like cards, charades, bingo, or brief walks outdoors.

These are useful and practical ideas related to the inpatient environment that continue to have value today. They support the use of some of the different therapies patients receive in inpatient settings, such as recreational therapy, occupational therapy, and art therapy. However, their appropriateness in short-term inpatient settings is being reevaluated given the acute nature of contemporary inpatient psychiatric care in many settings.[23]

Perhaps the most important contribution to the concept of the therapeutic milieu came in 1978 when Gunderson[7] described five functional components of a therapeutic milieu: containment, support, structure, involvement, and validation. These components are commonly used to evaluate the therapeutic value of the inpatient treatment setting.

 How would you respond to a patient's wife who asks you why her husband is spending time in a fitness program and making crafts when he has only 7 days of insurance to pay for his hospitalization for severe depression?

Containment. The function of containment is to sustain the physical well-being of patients and to remove the patient's feelings of omnipotence. It refers to the provision of food, shelter, and medical attention, as well as the steps necessary to prevent the patient from harming self or others. As such it includes a continuum of interventions with the use of seclusion and restraints being the most extreme. It is intended to reinforce temporarily the internal controls of patients, thus allowing them to reality test their omnipotent beliefs concerning their own destructiveness.

Containment is necessary to provide safety and foster trust. Therapeutic use of containment communicates to patients that the nurse will impose external controls as necessary to keep them and the environment safe. Appropriate and consistent limit setting is essential to meeting this goal. Nursing examples of therapeutic containment include the use of time-outs, room programs, specified observation periods, and seclusion (see Chapter 27).

Support. Support has to do with the staff's conscious efforts to make patients feel better and enhance their self-esteem. It is the unconditional acceptance of the patient whatever their given circumstance. The function of support is to make patients feel comfortable and secure and to reduce their anxiety. It may take many forms on the inpatient unit, but it falls under the general heading of paying attention to the patient.

Support can be communicated through empathy, being available, appropriately offering encouragement and reassurance, giving helpful direction, taking the patient out of the hospital for various activities, offering food or beverages, and engaging patients in activities that they are reluctant to do. Other nursing examples include giving direction, advice and education, promoting reality testing, and modeling healthy relationships and interactions. To best accomplish this task, nursing staff activity must be coordinated, cohesive, and consistent with the patient's treatment goals. Supportive nurturance enhances self-esteem. Those milieus that offer support also provide nurturance and permit, encourage, and direct patients to become engaged in other therapeutic efforts on the unit.

Structure. Structure refers to all aspects of a milieu that provide a predictable organization of time, place and person. This dependability in activity, staff, and environment helps the patient feel safe. Having a predictable timetable of meeting, activities, and other unit activities is one feature of structure. Other nursing examples of it include the setting of limits within the unit and the use of contracts, token economies, and required meetings. The more these uses of structure are planned with the patient according to shared ideas of what is adaptive and maladaptive, the more the structure becomes therapeutic in itself.

The patient can then begin to accept responsibility for behavior and its consequences. Providing structure helps the patient control maladaptive behaviors. The nurse uses appropriate consequences if the patient is unable, for whatever reason, to either impose or honor effective limits. As natural consequences are consistently applied, the patient learns to delay impulsive and inappropriate responses through consistent expectations and behavioral responses.

Involvement. Involvement is a part of the unit structure that goes beyond compliance with rules and activities. It refers to those processes that cause patients to actively attend to their social environment and interact with it. The purpose of it is to strengthen a patient's ego and modify maladaptive interpersonal patterns. Interpersonal communication and shared activity provide patients with opportunities to interact with others in their immediate community.

Nursing examples of involvement include the use of open doors and open rounds and facilitating patient-led groups, community activities, and self-assertive experiences. Units that emphasize involvement encourage the use of cooperation, compromise, and confrontation. Through this involvement, patients learn appropriate interaction patterns and experience the consequences of unacceptable behaviors. For example, a patient who displays anger or offensive behavior that distances others can be encouraged to participate in activities that will assist in verbalizing feelings, working out differences, and receiving feedback. This supportive experience strengthens the patient's sense of self, behavioral control, and social interactive skills. Thus encouraging involvement provides corrective experiences for the patient.

Validation. Validation means that the individuality of each patient is recognized. It is the act of affirming a person's unique worldview. Validation can help patients develop a greater capacity for closeness and a more consolidated identity. The psychiatric nurse communicates this through individual attention, empathy, and nonjudgmental acceptance of the patient's thoughts, feelings, and perspective. Other nursing examples of validation include individualized treatment planning, showing respect for a patient's rights, and providing opportunities for the patient to fail as well as succeed. Therapeutic listening and acknowledging the feelings underlying the patient's personal experience reinforce individuality. Clarification of these feelings assists the patient in understanding and accepting one's unique experience. This strengthens the patient's sense of individuality and encourages the integration of pleasant and unpleasant aspects of one's personal experience.

Visit an inpatient psychiatric unit. Which of the five components of a therapeutic milieu did you observe? Which ones were missing? What barriers prevented the unit from fully implementing this concept?

Nursing Implications

One of the earliest advocates of the importance of the inpatient environment for the work of nursing was Florence Nightingale. She believed that the essential responsibilities of nursing included the provision of pure air and water, efficient drainage, cleanliness, and light. In addition, the "prudent" nurse prevented unnecessary noise and attended to the aesthetics and nutritional value of food and the comfort of bedding.[20] Since the time of this pioneer of nursing, the inpatient environment and the therapeutic management of the milieu have continued to be important aspects of the role of all nurses.

Managing the therapeutic milieu remains the domain of the inpatient psychiatric nurse. It is essential that psychiatric nurses working in inpatient settings realize the potential impact that the environment can have on the patient and consciously use it for the patient's benefit. The challenge is for psychiatric nurses to adapt to changes in the patient population and the mental health delivery system by evolving new approaches to managing the milieu as needed.[13,28,29] For example, milieus may need to be organized differently depending on the nature of the patient population. Box 31-1 compares descriptions of effective milieus for acutely psychotic and more long-term psychiatric patients.[19] Such approaches, however, need to be carefully documented and evaluated for their effectiveness.

Milieu management is a deliberate decision-making process. The psychiatric nurse should first identify what each patient needs from the therapeutic milieu while also taking into consideration the needs of the larger patient group. Weighing individual needs against group needs can be a difficult task, but it is essential for the successful implementation of a therapeutic milieu. The nurse can then engage aspects of the therapeutic milieu to meet the patient's individualized needs such as by providing specific:

▼ Limits and controls (containment)
▼ Education about the individual's illness and treatment plan (support)
▼ Therapeutic and predictable activity schedules (structure)
▼ Opportunities for social interaction (involvement)
▼ Acknowledgement of the patient's feelings (validation)

Activities related to each component of the therapeutic milieu can be incorporated in the nursing plan of care, thus maximizing the therapeutic effect of the environment on the patient.

The nature of inpatient psychiatry and the focus of treatment will continue to change with the influence of health-care reform and advances in the nursing and biomedical sciences. However, as long as some aspects of the treatment of the mentally ill is centralized in a con-

---

Box 31-1
EFFECTIVE MILIEUS BASED ON PATIENT CHARACTERISTICS

ACUTELY PSYCHOTIC PATIENTS

▼ Small (6-10 patients)
▼ High staff/patient ratio
▼ High interaction
▼ Real involvement of line staff and patients in decisions
▼ Emphasis on autonomy
▼ Focus on practical problems (for example, living arrangements, money)
▼ Positive expectations
▼ Minimal hierarchy

STABLE PERSISTENTLY ILL PATIENTS

▼ Clearly defined, specific behaviors requiring change
▼ Action (not explanation) oriented, structured program
▼ Reasonable, positive, progressive, practical expectations with increasing patient responsibility
▼ Continuation of treatment program into community settings
▼ Continuity of persons
▼ Extensive use of groups to facilitate socialization and network-building

---

trolled environment, the concept of the therapeutic milieu will remain viable.[8] The principles of patient participation in decision making, use of a multidisciplinary staff, and the belief that the environment can be a treatment agent continue to be a part of most inpatient settings. To be successful, however, the culture of the inpatient setting must have a value system that is congruent with the therapeutic milieu concept. The hospital's management team and interdisciplinary staff should have common goals, respect for the contribution of each other, and be able to communicate openly to truly enact the components of the therapeutic community.

 Compare the components of the therapeutic milieu with the responsive and action dimensions of the therapeutic nurse-patient relationship described in Chapter 2.

IMPLEMENTING CAREGIVING ACTIVITIES

Inpatient psychiatric nurses must possess clinical knowledge and skills and apply them for the benefit of their patients and families. The atmosphere created by the inpatient psychiatric nurse strives to provide patients with activities and interactions carefully designed to meet their needs. This includes both direct and indirect psychiatric nursing care functions, as well as dependent, independent and interdependent aspects of psychiatric nursing practice as evident in the following clinical example. A few of these caregiving activities in the inpatient setting merit special discussion.

 ## CLINICAL EXAMPLE

Ms. R was a 17-year-old, single, high school student who was admitted to an inpatient psychiatric unit with the diagnosis of bipolar disorder. She was admitted for uncontrollable behavior (i.e., sexual promiscuity, running away from home, hyperverbalization, extreme irritability).

The initial nursing assessment provided a data base that revealed a chaotic family system with a long history of mental illness on both sides of the family, a social and cultural environment in which drug and alcohol abuse were prevalent, and a community that, because of its low socioeconomic status, possessed limited mental health resources. However, the patient was very bright, cooperative, and motivated to benefit from her hospitalization.

The initial nursing actions were to carry out the functions of administering the prescribed medications, including lithium carbonate, and ensuring that blood levels were checked three times a week until a therapeutic level was reached. The nurse assessed that there was an immediate need to protect the patient from her impulsive uncontrollable behavior. The patient was placed under close nursing observation at all times until she was able to be in control of her own behavior.

Once the patient's mood had stabilized, she was presented in nursing rounds. During this time the patient was able to identify a great need for the nurse to teach her and her family about bipolar disorder and the importance of continued lithium treatment. The patient and staff agreed that a home visit would explore the pressures that the family placed on the patient to function as a surrogate mother to her eight siblings. The patient also believed that it was important that her illness not be viewed in exactly the same manner as that of her sister, who was diagnosed as schizophrenic. The patient viewed her intellectual ability and the "love" that existed in her family system as her best resources. She thought that, with the assistance of the nursing staff, she and her family could develop more understanding of her illness and decrease the chaos within the family system.

After discharge the patient was followed up in outpatient therapy by her primary nurse.

Discharge Planning

The most obvious goal for inpatient care is to discharge the patient to outpatient status. Thus discharge planning must begin on admission and be a focused nursing activity throughout the patient's hospital stay. The nurse must be knowledgeable about the patient's discharge environment. Potential needs and resources should be identified on admission (see Chapter 9). Once the nurse has decided what knowledge, skills, and behaviors will help the patient adapt to the discharge environment, creative and purposeful activities can be planned to provide the needed resources.

Throughout this process, the nurse should include family members, friends, significant others, and any other support system of the patient. Information regarding supportive resources and medications should be provided to patients and their families to encourage functional independence and decrease the chances of relapse once discharged from inpatient care. This can significantly influence patients' abilities to maintain adaptive coping responses when they return to their community environment. Nursing research suggests that family-centered discharge nursing interventions with a cognitive behavioral orientation can help patients adjust to the social, vocational, and psychological demands of their posthospital environment. Additional research on this important area of nursing intervention is needed.

Meeting Physical Needs

Studies have documented the prevalence of physical illness among psychiatric patients in both inpatient and outpatient treatment settings.[12] Yet too often, physical illness is undetected in this patient population. Physical illness, however, may:
1. Be the causative factor in a patient's presumed psychiatric illness
2. Exacerbate a psychiatric illness
3. Have no direct relationship to the psychiatric illness but still require medical and nursing intervention for the patient's well-being

The increase in medical and psychiatric comorbidity among psychiatric inpatients emphasizes the need for psychiatric nurses to stay current with their physical assessment and medical-surgical nursing skills. It is not uncommon for patients on psychiatric units to be receiving dialysis, hyperalimentation, intravenous therapy, or dressing changes. Thus completing a physical assessment on admission and monitoring the patient's physical and psychological status throughout the hospitalization are essential functions of the inpatient psychiatric nurse.

Activities, Groups, and Programs

Therapeutic nursing activities, groups, and programs provide a wide variety of opportunities for the nurse to influence the patient's progress toward treatment goals. In providing these corrective experiences, the psychiatric nurse must be clear on the purpose of these activities. They should be designed to accomplish specific nursing and patient goals in a constructive, efficient, and supportive way. The nurse's challenge is to plan these events to integrate the desired patient outcomes, the individual interests of the patient mix, and the ability of the patients to participate with feelings of pleasure and accomplishment.

Structured activities can accomplish several aspects of the nursing process at the same time. For example, encouraging a cognitively impaired patient to play a common table game, such as cards, allows the nurse to assess the patient's concentration, orientation, memory, and abstract thinking. Based on these observations, the nurse can better understand the patient's learning needs and incorporate them in the plan of care. This same activity can help the socially withdrawn patient try out newly learned interactive skills, experience the role-modeling of the nurse, and receive supportive feedback. In addition, the nurse can use these activities to evaluate the effect of nursing, somatic, and psychopharmacologic treatments. Thus planned nursing activities offer endless possibilities as supportive and corrective experiences for the psychiatric inpatient.

Therapeutic nursing groups and programs provide a cost-effective way to implement psychiatric nursing care. Nursing interventions applied in a group allow one or two nurses to work with many patients at the same time. Such interventions are productive not only in inpatient settings but across the continuum of care. For example, day treatment patients may join inpatients in the same groups or programs. This heterogeneity adds breadth of experience and perspective to the group. Each patient may accomplish a different goal within the same group or program, and such offerings can provide valuable structure to the inpatient milieu. Some examples of nursing inpatient groups are described in Box 31-2.

With the focus of psychiatric care shifting away from extended inpatient stays, opportunities for activity, group, and program development by psychiatric nurses are great. Nursing programs in the areas of social skills development, assertiveness, community-based support, crisis intervention, family preservation, and general health teaching are growing areas of inpatient psychiatric nursing responsibility.

Ask an inpatient psychiatric nurse if you can "shadow" her for a day. Group the nursing functions you see performed as direct or indirect and as dependent, independent, or interdependent. Did this experience change your perception of the inpatient psychiatric nursing role?

INTEGRATING CARE DELIVERY

The integrative function of the inpatient psychiatric nurse is a very important one, although it is often either overlooked or taken for granted. It includes all activities involved in the coordination of patient care such as those related to managing nursing resources, balancing costs and outcomes in patient care decision making, evaluating nursing care delivery modalities, ensuring compliance with professional and regulatory standards, and encouraging participative problem solving and conflict resolution among mental health team members. In addition, the clinical practice of the nurse involves ongoing implementation of new ideas and approaches for improving quality and decreasing costs.

Resource Allocation

Psychiatric nurses in the inpatient clinical setting must be able to articulate the value of nursing care and to justify the type and level of personnel needed to provide quality nursing care. This requires that all nurses become actively involved in examining patient needs, identifying realistic outcomes of care, and costing out the nursing services required. Determining the use of nursing resources by measuring the severity of the patient's illness is one way of accounting for the cost of nursing services. Nursing personnel costs are usually a major part of a hospital's operational expenses. As such, nursing personnel are often the first to be targeted in times of cost reduction. Thus attention to the most appropriate and efficient use of personnel and available resources is an important part of the psychiatric nurse's role in the prudent management of inpatient care. Assigning numbers and types of personnel based on patient care needs is an essential consideration for achieving quality outcomes.[9] The allocation of nursing resources must therefore be based on identified patient care needs, available resources, clinical competencies required to meet those needs, and the nursing care delivery modality employed to implement the care.

Box 31-2

EXAMPLES OF INPATIENT NURSING GROUPS OR PROGRAMS

MEDICATION EDUCATION GROUP

In this group basic concepts related to medications can be discussed. Providing general information about taking medications, such as the influence of slight dosage or schedule changes, serum levels, the therapeutic window, or how some medication potentiates the effect of other medications, can help the patient and family understand the specifics of the prescribed regimen. Common problems encountered by individuals taking psychotropic medication can be discussed, and strategies for dealing with these potential barriers can also be shared.

COMMUNITY RESOURCE GROUPS

These can be ongoing groups with rotating topics. Topics should be selected based on the learning needs of the group members and their ability to share individual knowledge about and experiences with varied community resources. For example, a pertinent topic might be the public transportation system of the city. Using maps and information from the local transit authority, exercises can be constructed where patients go from destination to destination practicing all that's involved in getting around the area independently. Another topic may be how to use the newspaper, library, or telephone book to learn about and contact nonprofit, social service, health-care, philanthropic, or other agencies, thus teaching the patient how to mobilize resources that may be beneficial after discharge.

NUTRITION GROUPS

Nutrition groups can be helpful in teaching patients the importance of balanced diets and how to recognize and prepare reasonable and appetizing meals for themselves. Food ingredients also provide excellent topics for discussion with psychiatric patients. For example, caffeine can be discussed, pointing out its subtle but pervasive effects on the body and its ability to interfere with the effectiveness of some medication. Other topics can include the basic food groups, shopping strategies, and the role of exercise in promoting balanced body weight.

SLEEP IMPROVEMENT PROGRAMS

Sleep improvement programs are often needed by psychiatric patients. Relaxation techniques such as simple yoga positioning, progressive muscle relaxation, and deep breathing may be helpful strategies for some patients. The importance of a healthy sleep-wake cycle can be discussed. Group members can be encouraged to share their individual sleep-inducing secrets. Commonly used ideas for encouraging sleep can be shared with the group, such as spending time in a soothing bath, sipping warm milk, or pleasure reading in bed with a soft light. Behaviors and influences that inhibit sleep may be discussed as well. Group members can be encouraged to try out the ideas and report back to the group on their effectiveness.

Because of the limited finances available for mental health care, the determination of acceptable levels of nurse staffing on inpatient units is a critical issue in inpatient psychiatric nursing care. Many methods have been developed to quantify nursing care delivered in an inpatient setting, and these have been used to make decisions regarding the allocation of nursing resources. Patient classification systems are the most popular of these methods.[26,27]

Patient Classification Systems. **Patient classification systems** were designed to determine the amount or intensity of nursing services needed by each patient based on patient acuity, or severity of illness. Within this system, patients' need for nursing care is typically grouped into four or sometimes five categories. Each higher level of grouping represents more intense needs for nursing services than the previous one (Table 31-3). A value (usually number of hours) is then assigned to each category representing the amount of nursing care required in a specific period of time (usually an 8-hour shift). This number is then multiplied by the number of patients on the unit who require each category of nurs-

ing care. These values are summed, and the final figure represents the number of nursing care hours required to care for all of the patients on that unit for the specified time period.

In the example shown in Table 31-3, 55 hours of nursing care are required to care for 18 patients during an 8-hour shift. To determine the number of staff needed to care for these patients, the number of required care hours is divided by the number of hours each staff member works in a shift. If nurses on the unit work 8-hour shifts, 55 would be divided by 8. This results in 6.875, or the determination that about 7 nursing staff will be needed to meet that unit's patient care requirements.

This example demonstrates how a patient classification system can be used as a framework for determining resources to meet patient care needs. It does not, however, offer insight into what kinds of nursing staff are required. Another disadvantage to this system is that the assignment of patients to a category is based on the judgment of the individual completing the report. Criteria or indicators related to each category can vary widely from person to person, unit to unit, and system to system. They can include frequently performed tasks,

Table 31-3   Example of a Patient Classification System

Category	Nursing services needed
Category I (1 nursing care hour per 8-hour shift)	The patient: ▼ Is able to perform activities of daily living with no or minimal supervision and assistance ▼ Actively participates in treatment regimen ▼ Independently attends scheduled activities and appointments on or off grounds ▼ Sleeps restfully during the night
Category II (3 nursing care hours per 8-hour shift)	The patient: ▼ Requires supervision or some assistance in performing activities of daily living ▼ Requires nursing supervision at all times while outside the inpatient unit ▼ Participates in treatment regimen with individual nursing intervention, redirection, or orientation required ▼ May or may not sleep restfully during the night requiring some nursing intervention
Category III (5 nursing care hours per 8-hour shift)	The patient: ▼ Requires intermittent, individual nursing intervention to complete activities of daily living ▼ Requires full visual observation by nursing at all times ▼ Is unable to understand or is resistant to treatment regimen ▼ Demonstrates disruptive perceptual, cognitive, or affective disturbance ▼ Is at risk of harm to self or others ▼ Requires redirection, orientation, or externally imposed limit setting ▼ Does not sleep restfully through the night requiring ongoing individual nursing intervention
Category IV (8 nursing care hours per 8-hour shift)	The patient: ▼ Is totally dependent in all activities of daily living ▼ Requires one-to-one nursing intervention throughout the shift ▼ Is unable to understand or is resistant to treatment regimen ▼ Demonstrates severe, persistent perceptual, cognitive, and/or affective disturbance ▼ Is at risk of harm to self or others ▼ Has a profound chronic sleep disturbance

Patient category	Nursing care hours required per shift		Patient census		
I	1	×	6	=	6
II	3	×	7	=	21
III	5	×	4	=	20
IV	8	×	1	=	8
		TOTAL	18	=	55 hours nursing care required
			55 ÷ 8	=	6.875 or 7 staff needed per 8-hour shift

nursing interventions, or behavioral indicators, such as the degree of containment, support, structure, involvement, or validation the patient may require. The more measurable the criteria, the less room for variation in judgment, and interrater reliability can be established to decrease this variability.

In developing criteria to identify the intensity of patients' needs, consideration must also be given to the range of resources that may be involved in providing patient care. The indirect nursing services that support the delivery of direct care, as well as direct caregiving activities, must also be considered. Indirect services include administrative support, management activities, staff development, infection control, and professional and regulatory standards compliance.

A major advantage of the patient classification sys-

tem is its flexibility. Not only can the criteria defining the categories be tailored to a specific clinical area, but also the method can be applied to individual patient care units, centers with greater costs, specialty programs and population-based DSM-IV or NANDA diagnostic groups. Other advantages are that the criteria may be weighted to reflect degrees of patient need and the system can be calculated on any specified time interval including by shift, day, or week. Thus it can be used in settings with different levels of care, such as units with inpatients and day treatment patients who share space and nursing resources.

The system allows nurses to track nursing care requirements over time, allocate resources appropriately, and justify the use of nursing resources. When applied to specific programs, it lets the nurse compare the nursing resource demands of the program with the costs recovered for the care provided. Thus program planning decisions can better reflect what can and should realistically be offered in a specific treatment setting.

> You report to work one evening and discover that you and one other staff member have been assigned to cover the 20-bed psychiatric unit. You realize that the hospital has been reducing costs, but you believe that this is unsafe staffing. How would you present your case for more staff to nursing and hospital administration?

Nursing Care Delivery Modalities

The nursing care delivery modality implemented in an inpatient setting reflects the professional values of the organization. It also influences the cost and quality of the nursing care provided and the outcomes achieved. Nurses prefer autonomous practice environments in which participation is elicited, professional competency is formally recognized, and administration is decentralized.[15,18] A professional practice environment encourages professional accountability and involves those who deliver the care in the decision making regarding care delivery.

Many nursing care delivery modalities have been described in the literature. Examples include primary nursing, team nursing, modular nursing, functional nursing, and case management.[14,22] Each one has distinct advantages and disadvantages, impacts differently on personnel costs, and varies in its application to the hospital setting (Table 31-4). Other factors to be considered in selecting a psychiatric nursing care delivery modality are the needs of the patient population served by the facility, goals and objectives of the nursing department, level of the nurses' education and experience, the organization's structure and governance, amount of staff turnover, nursing and nonnursing care priorities, professional expectations, and the presence or absence of union activity.[2,8,21] Finally, the selection of a delivery model is also influenced by the type of treatments and services given to patients and by how many continuum of care activities are provided in the particular setting.

> What nursing care delivery modality is used in your inpatient psychiatric facility? Do you think another modality would be better? Defend your position based on a cost-benefit approach.

Professional, Regulatory, and Accreditation Standards

Professional standards of the American Nurses' Association (ANA) for psychiatric–mental health clinical practice provide a basis for evaluating nursing care. In addition to the standards of care (see Chapter 9) and professional performance (see Chapter 10), other ANA standards are available to guide nursing activities in administrative and educational areas.

Regulatory and accreditation standards must be also considered by the inpatient psychiatric nurse. These include the state laws and regulations governing nursing scope and practice, the laws and regulations determining the payment of federal and state insurance monies (Medicaid and Medicare), and standards set forth by accrediting bodies. A health-care facility may be required to show how any of these standards are met, including those pertaining to the condition of the physical facility, credentialing of employees, or the documentation of the nursing process. Requirements vary depending on the type of facility, state government rules, and types of services offered.

The Joint Commission on Accreditation of Healthcare Organizations (JCAHO) has become a leading accrediting agency for many different types of health-care facilities. Their standards have served as a benchmark for many other regulatory agencies. JCAHO standards are a helpful and comprehensive guide for all aspects of health-care delivery in this country. In addition, the Health Care Financing Administration (HCFA) is the federal agency that oversees the spending of Medicare and Medicaid monies. Each state has an identified agency that implements HCFA policies locally. Often, for the care and treatment delivered by health-care agencies to be reimbursed by Medicare or Medicaid, HCFA consultants or the state agency will conduct surveys of the facility. They may review patient records, inspect the physical plant, and evaluate programs to ensure that their specific regulations are met. Once the facility has shown that all required standards are met, it is eligible to receive payment for treating patients insured by Medicaid and Medicare. These standards are often similar to those of other regulatory and credentialing bodies and focus mostly on the sanitation of the facility, competency of the providers, and the adequacy and pertinence of the care delivered.

Teamwork and Conflict Resolution

To integrate and coordinate patient care in the inpatient setting the psychiatric nurse must collaborate with professionals from other disciplines and manage a group of nursing care providers. Almost all inpatient units use a multidisciplinary team to deliver treatment. However, the degree of cooperation and cohesion among the dis-

Table 31-4 Comparison of Nursing Delivery Modalities

Delivery modality	Description	Advantages	Disadvantages
Primary nursing	The nurse assumes 24-hour accountability for an identified number of patients. The primary nurse is responsible for determining and evaluating all aspects of care for those primary patients. The nurse assumes accountability for the care of these same primary patients if later readmitted. The nurse assists in implementing the prescribed care for other nurses' primary patients. Other nurses and adjunct staff are utilized to implement the primary nurse's care plan. These providers are accountable for this care to the patient's primary nurse.	Opportunity for continuous care is greater. Patients and their primary nurse are able to establish a more profound nurse-patient relationship. Lines of accountability for clinical outcomes are clearer.	Motivation for assumption of this level of accountability varies among nurses. Higher personnel costs often result
Team nursing	A group of nursing personnel, called a team, work together to deliver comprehensive care to a larger number of patients. This team is led by a registered nurse who may supervise other nurses and adjunct staff. The whole team, and ultimately the registered nurse leading the team, is accountable for the care delivered to those patients for that shift.	Enables group cohesiveness to develop. Enables different types and skill levels of providers to share knowledge and expertise. Develops leadership abilities.	May fragment care delivery by dividing holistic care into tasks delegated to a number of providers.
Modular nursing	Similar to team nursing in that a group of patients receive care from a mixed group of providers. The patient group is designated by close geographic proximity, as on one hallway. Modules are often organized with access to all materials and documents needed for that team to care for those patients in that geographically distinct module.	Concentrates activity in a smaller area. Allows quicker, easier access to materials. Helpful with patients staying in their hospital rooms.	Not helpful in psychiatric settings where physical mobility and group activity are encouraged and access to materials is not a major concern.
Functional nursing	Functional nursing relegates nursing activity by task; one nurse may distribute medications, another may take vital signs and participate in somatic treatments.	Enables tasks to be done quickly and simultaneously.	Difficult to determine lines of accountability. Patient care is fragmented.
Case management	Similar to primary nursing, the case manager assumes responsibility for all aspects of care for a group, or caseload, of patients. With this modality, the care accountability extends before and beyond the inpatient phase(s) of treatment. Coordination of the patient's providers, medications, treatments, and resources are organized, evaluated and often determined by the case manager. All decisions are made with knowledge of all aspects of the patient's clinical and personal situation.	Greater opportunity for continuity of care. Accountability is clear. Greater emphasis on patient participation. Active, ongoing negotiation with the patient and significant others is integral to this modality.	Areas and agencies vary widely in application of this modality. Success of this method is closely linked with the amount of authority associated and autonomy assumed with this role.

ciplines varies widely. It is essential that the psychiatric nurse be an effective collaborator with peers, subordinates, superiors, and colleagues of other disciplines (see Chapters 1 and 10). Many interdisciplinary problems have been identified that could interfere with the quality of inpatient care (see Critical Thinking About Contemporary Issues). Problems between providers may involve poor communication, professional self-doubt, and role conflicts, all of which may be increased by work-related stress.[3]

Whenever there are multiple individuals each with a unique perspective working together there is the potential for conflict. Conflict is often an inherent part of the problem-solving process. Handling conflict productively is an ongoing challenge for the inpatient psychiatric nurse. When poorly handled or avoided, conflict can in-

terfere with the continuity of patient care and the management of a therapeutic milieu. However, effective management of conflict can facilitate stronger professional working relationships, model positive communication skills for patients, and contribute to the nurse's professional development. Through directly and effectively dealing with conflict, co-workers can express personal priorities and learn to appreciate the ideas and contributions of others.

 Observe a multidisciplinary treatment team in the inpatient psychiatric setting. Did you see any areas of team conflict, role blurring, or turf struggles? If so, how did the team handle these issues?

EVALUATING OUTCOMES

The last area of inpatient psychiatric nursing practice involves the evaluation of the care provided. Continuous evaluation of patient, process, and provider outcomes is mandatory for professional nursing practice (see Chapter 10). The evaluation process can focus on either quality, costs, or both as identified in Table 31-5.

Evaluation is an ongoing activity that ranges from simply raising questions to engaging in formal clinical research. All aspects of inpatient nursing care involve evaluation, from the staff assigned to work with a certain group of patients, to the value of a particular nursing group activity, to the piloting of a new nursing care delivery modality. From this perspective, evaluation is the validating activity of the inpatient psychiatric nurses' practice.

The psychiatric nurse is ultimately accountable for the outcomes of the inpatient nursing care provided. It is the responsibility of the psychiatric nurse to analyze pertinent data and, in negotiation with the patient and

CRITICAL THINKING ABOUT CONTEMPORARY ISSUES

Do Nurses and Psychiatrists View Patients in the Same Way?

It has been suggested that different members of the mental health care team perceive patients differently, and that this can create problems in developing cohesive treatment plans and maintaining a therapeutic inpatient milieu. One recent study compared characteristics attributed by nurses and residents to difficult-to-treat inpatients in a short-stay setting.[6] The researchers found that both groups identified self-harm behaviors, violence toward others, and treatment sabotage as characteristics of difficult patients, although these patient behaviors posed more problems for the nurses. Lack of response to medication and patient manipulation were the most important problems identified by the residents. Nurses, however, found difficulty with patients who were unable to form therapeutic alliances.

The researchers suggest that this may be because psychiatric nurses have seen their role as shaping the therapeutic milieu. Thus their interventions center on providing opportunities within the unit for improving interpersonal and coping skills and maximizing healthy aspects of the patient's ego functions. If the patient fails to engage or withdraws, these treatment goals are thwarted and the nurse's role as a therapeutic agent is blocked. Such findings suggest that differing perceptions of difficult patients may create communication problems for the treatment team. If the different disciplines do not share common concerns, they may not recognize the significance of their various observations and not respond to them. ▼

Table 31-5 Indicators for Evaluating Outcomes

	Direct	Indirect
C O S T S	Patient care charges	Staff productivity
	Use of resources	Staff satisfaction
	Length of stay	Staff turnover
	Complication rate	System inefficiencies
Q U A L I T Y	Patient adaptive-maladaptive responses	Caregiving process
	Discharge planning	Documentation
	Patient-family satisfaction	Communication
	Staff knowledge and skills	Organizational climate

other health-care providers, identify outcomes and a means of achieving them. Other staff work with the psychiatric nurse to accomplish this task. Given the varied education, skills, experience, and priorities of these other providers, success in achieving and evaluating patient care outcomes can often be a difficult and challenging task.

Costing Out Nursing Services

The current managed care environment is focusing much attention on accountability for outcomes and the costs involved in achieving those outcomes. Historically, inpatient settings have buried the costs of nursing care in with other services in a per diem or "bed" charge instead of separating out the cost of nursing care. There are good reasons, however, to support the separation of nursing care costs from per diem bed fees.

For one, many general hospital services are covered in the set bed charge, and it is difficult to factor out what each service actually costs when they are bundled all together. Yet consumers have the right to know how much they are paying for each service. Second, services such as environmental and physical plant, linen, and heating and air conditioning are usually fixed costs that are shared equally among inpatients. In contrast, nursing services vary greatly from patient to patient.[11] Thus it is not appropriate for all patients to be charged the same amount for nursing care when they receive different amounts of nursing care at different times during their inpatient stay. Finally, including nursing services in the per diem bed charge allows administrators to view nursing as a cost or expense to the hospital rather than as revenue generating. This has serious implications given the rising cost of health care and the increasing need to justify the use of resources. Thus it is clear that costing out nursing services needs to be a continued priority for inpatient psychiatric nurses.

> Inquire into the bed charge for 1 day of care in your psychiatric inpatient unit. How does that compare with the bed charge in a medical-surgical unit? How much of that charge do you think is related to nursing services?

Quality Monitoring Programs

Evaluating outcomes in inpatient settings is often referred to as **quality improvement** The emphasis on continuous quality improvement is reflected in the standards of JCAHO, which require that health-care agencies document that services provided have been reviewed based on standards of care.

Most quality monitoring programs in inpatient facilities are tiered. There is usually an overall interdisciplinary quality monitoring body. This group collects data from throughout the hospital and assesses the compliance and competence of all activities and providers within the organization. This group may also target specific activities or issues to evaluate based on health-care trends, feedback obtained from consumers, staff, or regulators, and concerns about costly or inefficient operations. Service groups, health-care disciplines, and individual professionals also engage in their own quality monitoring activities. They focus on issues pertaining to their interaction with others in the organization, as well as their own level of functioning.

Supervision, formal performance appraisals, self-evaluations, peer reviews, and clinical case reviews are additional methods for evaluating and maintaining the quality of care provided by inpatient psychiatric nurses (see Chapter 10). Through these evaluative activities, nurses in the hospital can share values, communicate expectations, and suggest professional development programs for the inpatient nursing staff. These evaluations should be reciprocal in that evaluative information should also be sought by administration from the direct care providers about job satisfaction, use of resources, and the availability and quality of general managerial support.

Risk Management

In an inpatient setting, evaluation also involves the assessment of **risk management** activities. These usually relate to situations that could result in legal action involving patients, families, the hospital, or the health-care provider. Issues related to involuntary admission, refusal of treatment, informed consent, confidentiality, duty to warn, least restrictive environment, and seclusion and restraint are confronted daily by the inpatient psychiatric nurse (see Chapter 8). It is recommended that all nurses become aware of the statutes governing the care of the mentally ill in their state and that systems be established within the inpatient setting to recognize any actual or potential breeches of the legal standard.

Utilization Review

Utilization review is a final but important aspect of evaluating outcomes in inpatient and outpatient psychiatric settings.[5,31] It is carried out by most hospitals and many health-care agencies, government-sponsored local agencies, third-party payors, managed care companies, and private insurers. The utilization review process is intended to ensure that health-care resources are appropriately used. Many believe, however, that it primarily involves saving money. If this is true, it is unfortunate, since utilization review has the potential of improving the quality and efficiency of health care.

Utilization review typically occurs in three stages. First, before admission, the patient or clinician requests approval to hospitalize the patient. This is called the *pre-authorization* or *preadmission screening*. This approval is usually good for a certain number of days. It is not done with court-ordered admissions. Next, *concurrent review* takes place after admission but before discharge. The reviewer may look at cases in which the patient has been hospitalized longer than the approved number of days or beyond some statistical norm, such as the average length of stay for that diagnosis in that hospital. The treatment team must justify any deviations from the norm. Finally, *retrospective review* occurs after discharge when the entire chart can be reviewed.

Psychiatric nurses need to be aware of this process because they may be asked to discuss the patient's status in any stage of the review process. In addition, nurses should be continually evaluating all patients' needs for care and the most appropriate use of limited mental health care resources to meet those needs.

SUGGESTED CROSS-REFERENCES

SUMMARY

1. The treatment goals, processes, expected outcomes, and length of stay related to inpatient psychiatric care are changing. The majority of psychiatric nurses currently work in inpatient settings, but they must be ready and able to provide their services throughout the continuum of care.
2. The aim of the therapeutic milieu is to provide patients with a stable and coherent social environment that facilitates the development and implementation of an individualized treatment plan. Components of the therapeutic milieu include containment, support, structure, involvement, and validation.
3. Inpatient psychiatric nursing includes both direct and indirect nursing functions, as well as dependent, independent, and interdependent aspects of practice. Discharge planning, meeting patients' physical needs, and implementing activities, groups, and programs are important caregiving activities.
4. The integrative function of the inpatient psychiatric nurse includes all activities involved in the coordination of patient care such as those related to managing nursing resources, balancing patient care costs and outcomes, evaluating nursing care delivery modalities, ensuring compliance with professional and regulatory standards, and encouraging participative problem solving and conflict resolution among mental health team members.
5. Continuous evaluation of patient, process, and provider outcomes is essential to inpatient psychiatric nursing practice. Relevant activities include costing out nursing services, quality monitoring programs, risk management, and utilization review.

COMPETENT CARING
A CLINICAL EXEMPLAR OF A PSYCHIATRIC NURSE

Therese Killeen, MSN, RN, CS

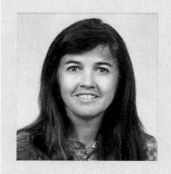

As I look back on my 16 years of experience in nursing, I find it's quite difficult to select one experience that stands out among the rest. I have had many fulfilling and rewarding memories. Probably if I had to choose an event that captures many of my emotions, I would travel back to a July 4th many years ago.

I was a young, energetic nurse just 2 years out of school and working as a staff nurse on an adolescent psychiatric unit. My youthfulness, as well as my excitement for nursing, enabled me to care for a large caseload of acutely ill patients and pull quite a few double shifts. On this particular day, I was just finishing up my 7:00-3:00 shift report to the 3:00-11:00 shift and ready to embark on my own 4th of July celebration. As I was collecting my purse to leave, I was annoyed by a fire alarm. "Now what idiot would order a fire drill on the 4th of July," I thought.

Mildly irritated by this delay, I made sure the unit fire doors shut as they should when this alarm sounds. As I happened to look out the window onto the next adjoining building, I was aghast at seeing black smoke emerging from the top of the building. Just as I realized that this was not a fire drill, a code 5 and 6 was announced on the intercom with all available personnel summoned to the emergency room.

Making sure that the 3:00-11:00 shift were settled in the unit, which was safe and under control, I reported to the ER. I received my first assignment, which was to assist with the evacuation of medical-surgical patients on the sixth floor of the burning building. It was my responsibility to make sure all patients were safely evacuated and accounted for. On the sixth floor, the air was thick with smoke and we protected ourselves by wearing dampened surgical masks. I finally got to actually use some of the patient transport techniques we all learn in fire safety classes. While I was on the sixth floor, the firemen arrived and together we safely got the patients to the psychiatric hospital across the street. Although quite fearful of being the only one left on the unit with the thickening smoke, I hastily checked the rooms, closed the doors, and made a quick exit.

My next assignment brought me to the intensive care unit located on the fourth floor. The smoke was quickly entering through the air conditioning vents and moving downward. The fire itself had completely engulfed the eighth and ninth floors and was considered out of control. We rolled ICU patients in their beds to an open, awaiting elevator in an adjoining building for transport to the ER. Most of these patients were discontinued off their respirators and ventilations were maintained manually with an Ambu bag during transport. The afternoon slowly turned into evening, then night, then early morning before I ever realized that I had been working nonstop for over 20 hours.

What struck me as so memorable about the situation was the spontaneous team effort put forth throughout this crisis. Housekeeping, security, lab technicians, couriers, and nursing all pulled together quite effectively. The light holiday schedule made the job even more difficult. Even the fire department, which arrived on the scene late, was in awe at the way the employees pulled together and put patient safety first. To me, this experience captured the special qualities of inpatient nursing care and the many different aspects of crisis intervention in a hospital setting. ▼

REFERENCES

1. Abroms G: Defining milieu therapy, *Arch Gen Psychiatry* 21:553, 1969.
2. Armstrong D, Stetler C: Strategic considerations in developing a delivery model, *Nurs Econ* 9:112, 1991.
3. Bair J, Greenspan B: Teams: teamwork training for interns, residents, and nurses. *Hosp Community Psychiatry* 37:633, 1986.
4. Center for Mental Health Services and National Institute of Mental Health: *Mental health, United States, 1992,* Washington, DC, 1992, US Government Printing Office.
5. Dorwart R, Epstein S: Issues in psychiatric hospital care, *Curr Opin Psychiatry* 4:789, 1991.
6. Gallop R, Lancee W, Shugar G: Residents' and nurses' perceptions of difficult-to-treat short-stay patients, *Hosp Community Psychiatry* 44:352, 1993.
7. Gunderson J: Defining the therapeutic process in therapeutic milieus, *Psychiatry* 41:327, 1978.
8. Gutheil T: The therapeutic milieu: changing themes and theories, *Hosp Community Psychiatry* 36:1279, 1985.
9. Harkness G, Miller J, Hill N: Differentiated practice: a three-dimensional model, *Nurs Manage* 23:26, 1992.
10. Jones M: *The therapeutic community,* New York, 1953, Basic Books.
11. Kicakulah M, Hanenow N, Cope F: The true costs of nursing care: a simple approach provides more accurate accounting of nursing services, *Health Prog* Dec 1990, p. 48.
12. Knutsen E, DuRand C: Previously unrecognized physical illnesses in psychiatric patients, *Hosp Community Psychiatry* 42:182, 1991.
13. LeCuyer E: Milieu therapy for short-stay units: a transformed practice theory, *Arch Psychiatr Nurs* 6:108, 1992.
14. McCausland M, Persing R, Kiley M: Primary nursing in a psychiatric setting, *Nurs Econ* 6:297, 1988.
15. McGinn N: Restructuring patient care delivery systems through empowerment, *J Nurs Adm* 22:21, 1992.
16. Mental Health Policy Resource Center: *Fact or fiction: interpretations of mental health expenditures data,* Washington, DC, 1992 The Center.
17. Merwin E, Fox J: Cost-effective integration of mental health professions, *Iss Ment Health Nurs* 13:139, 1992.
18. Moritz P: Innovative nursing practice models and patient outcomes, *Nurs Outlook* 39:111, 1991.
19. Mosher L, Burti L: *Community mental health: principles and practice,* New York, 1989, WW Norton.
20. Nightingale F: *Notes on nursing: what it is and what it is not,* New York, 1960, Dover Publications.
21. Rowland H, Rowland B: *Nursing administration handbook,* ed 2, Rockville, Md, 1985, Aspen.
22. Ryan J et al: A comparative study of primary and team

nursing models in the psychiatric care setting, *Arch Psychiatr Nurs* 2:3, 1988.

23. Santos A, McLeod-Bryant S: Strategies for operational efficiency in a general hospital inpatient unit, *Hosp Community Psychiatry* 42:66, 1991.

24. Schreter R: Ten trends in managed care and their impact on the biopsychosocial model, *Hosp Community Psychiatry* 44:325, 1993.

25. Sharfstein S, Stoline A, Goldman H: Psychiatric care and health insurance reform, *Am J Psychiatry* 150:7, 1993.

26. Sovie M: Variable costs of nursing care in hospitals, *Res Nurs Care Del* 6:131, 1988.

27. Treanor J, Cotch K: Staffing of adult inpatient facilities, *Hosp Community Psychiatry* 41:545, 1990.

28. Tuck I, Keels M: Milieu therapy: a review of development of this concept and its implications for psychiatric nursing, *Iss Ment Health Nurs* 13:51, 1992.

29. Watson J: Maintenance of therapeutic community principles in an age of biopharmacology and economic restraints, *Arch Psychiatr Nurs* 6:183, 1992.

30. Watson P, Lower M, Wells S, Farrah S, Jarrell C: Discovering what nurses do and what it costs, *Nurs Manage* 22:38, 1991.

31. Zusman J: Utilization review: theory, practice and issues, *Hosp Community Psychiatry* 41:531, 1990.

ANNOTATED SUGGESTED READINGS

*Armstrong D, Stetler C: Strategic considerations in developing a delivery model, *Nurs Econ* 9:112, 1991.

Excellent discussion of key components of a nursing care delivery model, evaluative criteria, and principles of strategic management success.

*Brown P et al: Linking psychiatric nursing care to patient classification codes, *Nurs Health Care* 8:157, 1987.

Links psychiatric nursing diagnoses to ICD9 codes and uses this system to describe nursing interventions and prepare discharge summaries.

*Emrich K: Helping or hurting? Interacting in the psychiatric milieu, *J Psychosoc Nurs Ment Health Serv* 27:26, 1989.

Describes the disturbing results of a study examining interactions between patients and psychiatric nurses. Nurse-patient interactions were more often parental with disconfirming messages, which raises interesting questions for psychiatric nurses.

Greenberg L et al: An interdisciplinary psychoeducation program for schizophrenic patients and their families in an acute care setting, *Hosp Community Psychiatry* 39:277, 1988.

Superb example of interdisciplinary teamwork in providing a quality psychoeducation program. This model should be adopted in many other inpatient settings.

---

*Nursing reference.

*Ingersoll G, Bazar M, Zentner J: Monitoring unit-based innovations: a process evaluation approach, Nurs Econ 11:137, 1993.

Excellent description of the process involved in implementing a professional practice model for nurses and evaluating it.

*LeCuyer E: Milieu therapy for short-stay units: a transformed practice theory, Arch Psychiatr Nurs 6:108, 1992.

Reviews historical milieu concepts and links them through theory with short inpatient stays, patient needs, outcomes, and nursing actions.

*Lewis L, Stuart G: Reconceptualizing the psychiatric head nurse role, Arch Psychiatr Nurs 7:125, 1993.

One of the few articles to describe the changing role of the head nurse in the psychiatric setting. Brings together issues of collaboration, delegation, and use of clinical nurse specialists in the inpatient setting.

*McDonald S: An ethical dilemma: risk versus responsibility, J Psychosoc Nurs Ment Health Serv 32:19, 1994.

Reports on the experience of nurses who spoke out when a hospital exploited certain psychiatric diagnoses by encouraging extended lengths of stay and restricting patients' rights. Should be read by all psychiatric nurses.

*Puskar K et al: Psychiatric nursing management of medication-free psychotic patients Arch Psychiatr Nurs 4:78, 1990.

Describes how a team of psychiatric nurses managed acutely psychotic patients on an inpatient unit without medications using interventions grounded in interpersonal psychiatric nursing practice and milieu therapy.

*Rittman M: Social organization of length of stay of psychiatric patients, J Psychosoc Nurs Ment Health Serv 31:21, 1993.

Examines a model used to explain the inpatient treatment process. Findings challenge traditional thinking and raise new questions.

*Ryan J et al: A comparative study of primary and team nursing models in the psychiatric care setting, Arch Psychiatr Nurs 2:3, 1988.

Reports on research comparing primary and team nursing in a psychiatric setting. Many variables were examined, and the results are quite thought provoking. More research like this is needed in the field.

*Smith T, Powers B: An integrative approach to quality assurance, Nurs Manage 21:28, 1990.

Describes how senior baccalaureate nursing students participated in planning and implementing quality assurance programs as part of their research course assignment.

*Tuck I, Keels M: Milieu therapy: a review of the development of this concept and its implications for psychiatric nursing, Iss Ment Health Nurs 13:51, 1992.

Reviews historical milieu concepts and the current role that psychiatric nurses have in its current effective implementation.

---

*Nursing reference.

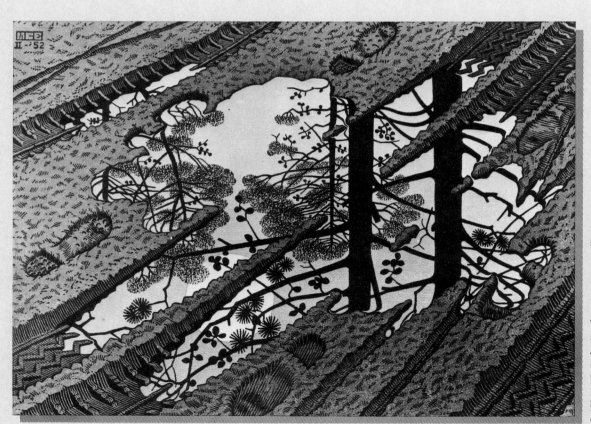

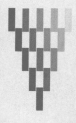

CHAPTER 32

Community Psychiatric Nursing Care

NANCY K. WORLEY

Every injury to the health of the individual is, so far as it goes, a public injury. It is an impediment to the general freedom; so much deduction from our power, as members of society, to make the best of ourselves.

Thomas Hill Green: *Works of Thomas Hill Green, vol. III, Miscellanies and Memoir*

LEARNING OBJECTIVES

After studying this chapter the student should be able to:

▼ Relate the goals of the community mental health movement

▼ Discuss the public health model of community mental health including interventions and the role of the nurse

▼ Discuss the biological-medical model of community mental health including interventions and the role of the nurse

▼ Discuss the systems model of community mental health including the interventions and the role of the nurse

▼ Discuss the patient-centered model of community mental health including interventions and the role of the nurse

▼ Analyze new psychiatric nursing roles in home health care, outreach services, collaborative practice, prevention, and family preservation

TOPICAL OUTLINE

Goals of Community Mental Health
Public Health Model
  Community Needs Assessment
  Identifying and Prioritizing Target Groups
  Intervention Strategies
  Role of Nurses
Biological-Medical Model
  Deinstitutionalization
  Role of Nurses
Systems Model
  Community Support Systems
  Case Management
  Role of Nurses
Patient-Centered Model
  Assertive Community Treatment
  Capitation and Managed Care
  Local Mental Health Authorities
  Role of Nurses
New Psychiatric Nursing Roles
  Home Health Care
  Outreach Clinical Services
  Collaborative Practice Arrangements
  Prevention and Wellness Programs
  Family Preservation

GOALS OF COMMUNITY MENTAL HEALTH

The Community Mental Health Centers Act of 1963 marked the beginning of a major federal effort to provide comprehensive community-based mental health services to all persons in need regardless of income. Each community mental health center was mandated by law to provide five essential mental health services. Four of these services—inpatient, emergency, partial hospitalization, and outpatient care—were to provide psychiatric care in the community to reduce the number of admissions to state hospitals. The goal of the fifth essential service, consultation and education, was to provide information about mental health principles to other community agencies, reduce the number of people at risk for mental illness, and increase community awareness of positive mental health practices through education. The dual nature of this mission, care of the diagnosed mentally ill and prevention of mental illness, has led to controversy in defining the purpose of community mental health.

Four models have dominated the community mental health movement since 1963. Each one has been influenced by the political, social, and economic climate of the time. Individually and together they have contributed much to the field, and the best parts of each model continue to be used today. They are summarized in Table 32-1.

PUBLIC HEALTH MODEL

Mental health professionals who believed in primary prevention through social change dominated the community mental health movement in its early years, using the public health model of service delivery. In this model the "patient" is the community rather than the individual, and the focus is on the amount of mental health or illness in the community as a whole, including factors that promote or inhibit mental health. The emphasis in this model is on reducing the risk of mental illness for an entire population by providing services to high-risk groups. Use of the public health model required that mental health professionals be familiar with a range of skills that were not a traditional part of their training. These included community needs assessment, identifying and prioritizing target or high-risk groups, and intervening with new treatment modalities such as consultation, education, and crisis intervention.

 Do you believe it is possible to prevent mental illness in an individual or a community?

Community Needs Assessment

In the public health model services are developed and delivered based on a culturally sensitive assessment of

Table 32-1 Models of Community Mental Health Services

Model	Conceptual framework	Intervention strategies	Nursing role
Public health (1960-1970)	Focuses on prevention Community as patient Services target high-risk groups	Community needs assessment Identifies high-risk groups Consultation Education Crisis intervention	Some group and family involvement Caring for the chronically mentally ill Limited preventive work
Biological-medical (1970-1980)	Focuses on the diagnosed mentally ill Stimulated by deinstitutionalization Views mental illness as brain disease	Medical management Psychotherapy Aftercare programs	Medication administration and monitoring Coordination of aftercare programs Psychotherapy
Systems (1980-1990)	Focuses on the role of the biological, psychological, and environmental in rehabilitation Developed comprehensive systems of care	Community support systems Service coordination Case management	Coordination of community services Case management activities
Patient centered (1990-present)	Focus on patients who overlap service systems Culturally relevant services Consumer participation	Assertive community treatment New reimbursement structures Formation of local mental health authorities	Medication management New initiatives such as home health, outreach, collaborative practice, prevention, and family preservation

community needs. Since it is not possible to interview each person in the community to determine mental health needs, four techniques are used to estimate service needs.

Social Indicators. Social indicators infer need for service from descriptive statistics found in public records and reports, especially those statistics that are highly correlated with poor mental health outcomes. Examples of statistics most commonly used as social indicators are income, race, marital status, population density, crime, and substance abuse.

Key Informant Surveys. Key informants are people knowledgeable about the community's needs. Typical key informants are public officials, clergy, social service personnel, nurses, and primary care physicians.

Community Forums. In a community forum, members of the community are invited to a series of public meetings where they can express their ideas and beliefs about mental health needs in their community.

Epidemiological Studies. Epidemiological studies examine the incidence and prevalence of mental disorders in a defined population. Because they are expensive to carry out, most community needs assessments use results from previously published studies and apply these findings to their situation. For example, several large epidemiological studies have estimated that the impairment rate (the number of persons with some form of emotional disorder) in the United States ranges between 15% and 30%.[5] These studies have shown that high impairment rates in a population are correlated with certain demographic and socioeconomic characteristics such as poverty, low educational status, and a high number of people who are divorced, separated, or widowed.[15] Applying this information to a particular community allows for an estimation of the impairment rate. It has been common to assign an impairment rate of 15% to a population that includes few high-risk individuals, 22.5% to populations with moderate risk factors, and 30% to populations with many high-risk individuals.

Identifying and Prioritizing Target Groups

When the data from the various community needs assessments are analyzed, specific high-risk groups begin to emerge. For example, socioeconomic data might show that a large number of elderly widows live in the community. Community forums and surveys of key informants may find there are few services and programs for the elderly, and epidemiological studies might suggest that elderly widows living alone are at

high risk for depression. Therefore elderly widows might become a target group for program development and intervention.

Demographic data might also show that a community has many preadolescent females, and socioeconomic indicators may suggest that many of these young women live in single-parent households and in poverty. Community forums and surveys of key informants may reveal few recreational and social services for children and adolescents. Finally, epidemiological studies may report high correlations among poverty, single-parent households, and adolescent pregnancy. Therefore community mental health administrators might consider adolescents in this community to be at risk for mental health problems and target them as a group for intervention.

Intervening with high-risk groups in the community can include primary, secondary, or tertiary prevention activities.

▼ **Primary prevention**—Targets people at risk for developing psychiatric illness and promotes their adaptive coping mechanisms
▼ **Secondary prevention**—Targets people who show early symptoms of an emotional disorder but regain pretreatment level of functioning through aggressive case finding and treatment
▼ **Tertiary prevention**—Targets those who are mentally ill and helps to reduce the severity, discomfort, and disability associated with their illness

Advocates of the public health model of community mental health are particularly interested in programs and interventions focused on primary prevention. These are described in Chapter 11.

Can you describe the characteristics of a group that was at high risk for developing mental illness in the community in which you grew up?

Intervention Strategies

The public health model of community mental health required the development of new interventions. Before the community mental health movement of the 1960s, most mental health outpatient services consisted of expensive, office-based, individual psychotherapy sessions. Although this may have been a good secondary prevention strategy, it did not promote mental health or prevent emotional problems on a communitywide basis. New treatment strategies that were developed to fulfill the goals of community mental health included mental health education (Chapter 11), crisis intervention (Chapter 12), and mental health consultation (Chapter 33).

Role of Nurses

The public health model had major consequences for the role of psychiatric nurses in community mental health. Social workers and psychologists who had years of experience in public sector roles dominated administrative and management positions in this model. Theoretically, nursing should have been readily accepted as one of the mental health disciplines because of public health nurses' long-standing presence in community care; however, public health nurses were seen as closely allied with secondary and tertiary prevention activities, the medical model, and care of the sick. Therefore while chronically mentally ill patients were referred to the public health nurse, few nurses were invited to join psychiatry, psychology, and social work as professional staff in most community mental health centers.[14] A 1962 national survey of nurses' role in outpatient psychiatric clinics found that fewer than 10% of these facilities included a nurse on the professional team.[17] The passage of the Community Mental Health Centers Act in 1963 did little to change that pattern. Specifically, the number of psychologists and social workers in community mental health centers increased between 1970 and 1980, while the number of psychiatrists and nurses declined.[46]

In addition, nursing education was slow to revise curricula and change clinical practice to reflect this shift in care from the hospital to the community. As a result, most nurses felt unprepared to function in the community and were unable to create a role for themselves. With few exceptions, the nurse's role in community mental health centers was limited to "traditional" nursing tasks, such as medication monitoring and caring for the chronically mentally ill.

BIOLOGICAL-MEDICAL MODEL

In the mid 1970s several events turned public attention to the second mission of the community mental health movement—the care of the diagnosed mentally ill. A new political administration, the waging of an expensive war in Vietnam, and a general economic downturn stimulated a national discussion regarding the best use of scarce health-care resources. At the same time, public disillusionment with the deinstitutionalization of the chronically mentally ill led to questions about the cost-effectiveness of community mental health centers with their focus on prevention rather than care of those who were already ill.[22]

Families of the mentally ill had also become a politi-

cal force in the late 1970s. Their agenda was at least two-fold: (1) to force as many resources as possible toward the care of those with severe and persistent mental illness and (2) to use their political strength to direct federal research dollars toward finding a biological basis for the major mental illnesses. Psychiatrists, with their new focus on the biological model of psychiatry, and family groups thus became allies and formed a coalition that put biological psychiatry in a strong leadership position in the mental health field.

Financial pressures also brought about a change in the focus of mental health centers. At the beginning of the community mental health movement the federal government had promised to pay 75% of the cost of each center. Regulations stated that federal support would decrease by 15% each year until by the eighth year of their existence the centers were expected to be self-supporting through a combination of state funds and third-party reimbursement. By the early 1970s many of the centers faced the end of federal funding, and state governments were unable or unwilling to take on the burden of funding these centers. The centers then had to rely heavily on third-party reimbursement through fee-for-service mechanisms, which were typically physician directed and illness oriented. Centers thus began to focus on the diagnosis and treatment of the deinstitutionalized severe and persistently mentally ill primarily through the reimbursable services of medication management and psychotherapy.

These factors led to major amendments of the Community Mental Health Centers Act in 1975, requiring centers to offer services for seriously mentally ill individuals who had been discharged from the state hospitals. These services included screening admissions to inpatient services, aftercare services, and transitional housing. Since centers were not allowed to reduce the five original essential services and were not given sufficient funds to add these new services, decisions about priorities had to be made. Because of political and social pressure to care for the mentally ill who were being discharged into the community in large numbers, the community mental health centers reluctantly decreased their preventive efforts and moved toward the increased use of the medical model and the care of the diagnosed mentally ill.

Deinstitutionalization

Between 1965 and 1975 nearly 500,000 patients were either discharged or diverted from state hospitals to care in the community. It was hoped that psychiatric treatment in community centers, combined with living arrangements provided by family or board and care homes, would allow these mentally ill persons to live more humane lives in their own communities. It rapidly became clear, however, that policymakers had seriously miscalculated both the service needs of this population and the ability of communities to accommodate the large numbers of mentally ill that had been discharged from the state hospitals. Frequently, these former patients had to be readmitted to the state hospital. In the early days of deinstitutionalization, as many as 70% of the patients discharged from the state hospital had to be readmitted within 1 year. Others who could not meet the increasingly strict admission criteria of the state hospitals drifted into the criminal justice system or into homelessness. Many who were elderly were admitted to nursing homes.[44]

In reviewing the failures of this early attempt to move mentally ill patients into community care, mental health experts agree that the following problems contributed to the lack of success[52]:

▼ Poor coordination between the state hospitals and the community mental health centers
▼ Underestimation of the support systems that were necessary to allow mentally ill persons to live in the community
▼ Lack of knowledge about psychiatric rehabilitation
▼ Underestimation of community resistance to deinstitutionalization
▼ Shortage of professionals trained to work with this population in the community
▼ Reimbursement systems that rewarded hospitalization

It was apparent by the 1980s that the biological-medical model of community mental health may not be able to provide the psychological and social supports that were needed to allow the severe and persistently mentally ill to live successfully in the community. Professionals began to search for a more comprehensive model of care that would take into account all aspects of a person's life.

Do you think that all psychiatric patients are better off living in the community rather than in public or private hospitals?

Role of Nurses

Nurses began to play a more important role in community mental health care during the 1970s and 1980s. This was partly because traditional nursing roles in the medical model were well known and readily accepted by physician team leaders and administrators of community mental health centers; also, the number of deinstitutionalized patients was growing. Initially, nurses worked in aftercare programs providing support, coordination of

care, and health teaching. Gradually, those responsibilities grew to those of nurse therapists in individual, group, and family therapies with a variety of community mental health center patients, not only the chronically mentally ill. Many psychiatric nurses with master's degrees opened private practices and initiated creative and innovative mental health services.

Nursing's expansion into less traditional roles in community mental health can be attributed to the influence of the National Institute of Mental Health (NIMH). In 1975 a NIMH task force examined the staffing needs in mental health and existing training programs. The result was a new NIMH policy mandating that to be eligible for NIMH training grants, educational programs had to address the needs of unserved and underserved populations including children, the chronically mentally ill, minorities, and women. By the fall of 1979 training grants were awarded only to educational programs that focused on one or more of these priorities, particularly those that focused on providing clinical training in community mental health centers.[11]

The outcome of this mandate was that nursing school faculty began to reach out to community mental health centers to develop clinical placements for nursing students. In this process, faculty were able to educate center administrators about the scope of nursing practice and the variety of skills, in addition to medication administration and monitoring, that nurses could bring to the community setting. At the same time, curricula in nursing schools were revised to reflect this new practice setting. Crisis intervention, brief therapy, counseling, assessment, and diagnosis skills were emphasized as nurses began to take their place as members of the interdisciplinary teams in community mental health centers while struggling to keep their unique identity.[16,25,31]

Why is the role of the psychiatric nurse on an interdisciplinary mental health care team more difficult to define in community settings?

SYSTEMS MODEL

The systems model of community mental health emerged in the 1980s and operated on the philosophy that all aspects of an individual's life needed to be cared for—basic human needs, as well as needs for psychiatric treatment and rehabilitation. The focus of this model was on developing a comprehensive system of care and coordinating needed services into an integrated package. This model of community mental health emerged as it became apparent that mental health treatment alone would not allow people with severe and disabling mental illnesses to live successfully in the community. A special federal initiative was launched in 1977 to assist states and communities to develop comprehensive services for this population. This initiative was led by NIMH, which began to fund demonstration programs for community support systems in all states.

Community Support Systems

Community mental health centers were given primary responsibility for the development and implementation of community support systems for individuals in their service areas. These systems were to be guided by the principles listed in Box 32-1.[42] In implementing these systems, case management became the primary means for ensuring that the components of the service system were available to every person with a chronic mental illness who needed them (Fig. 32-1). These components included client identification and outreach, mental health treatment, crisis response services, health and dental care, housing, support and entitlement, peer support, family and community support, rehabilitation services, and protection and advocacy.[3] These services are discussed in Chapter 13, Psychiatric Rehabilitation.

Case Management

Case management services are aimed at linking the service system to the individual and coordinating the service components so that the individual can achieve successful community living. It includes problem solving to provide continuity of services and overcome problems of rigid systems, fragmented services, poor utilization of resources, and problems of inaccessibility. The six activities that form the core of case management are the following:

- ▼ Identification and outreach
- ▼ Assessment
- ▼ Service planning
- ▼ Linkage with needed services
- ▼ Monitoring service delivery
- ▼ Advocacy

In addition, four components and thirteen interventions related to clinical case management have been identified by Kanter.[21] These are listed in Table 32-2.

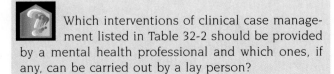

Which interventions of clinical case management listed in Table 32-2 should be provided by a mental health professional and which ones, if any, can be carried out by a lay person?

Box 32-1
PRINCIPLES OF COMMUNITY SUPPORT SYSTEMS

- ▼ Persons with long-term mental illness should have access to specialized mental health services and the supports needed by all individuals.
- ▼ The community is the best place to provide long-term care. Inpatient care is part of the needed community-based services and should be used for short-term evaluation, stabilization, and occasional long-term hospitalization.
- ▼ Services should be consumer centered and based on the needs of the individual rather than the needs of the system or provider.
- ▼ Services should empower people. Services should include consumer self-help approaches and allow people to retain the greatest possible control over their lives.
- ▼ Services should be racially and culturally appropriate.
- ▼ Services should be flexible. Services should be available whenever they are needed and for as long as they are needed.
- ▼ Services should focus on strengths.
- ▼ Services should be offered in the least restrictive and most natural settings possible.
- ▼ Services should meet special needs, including those of the severely mentally ill, homeless, elderly, mentally ill with substance abuse problems, and those mentally ill who have been inappropriately placed in the criminal justice system.
- ▼ Service systems should be accountable. Services should be monitored by the state to ensure quality of care and continued relevance. Consumers and families should be involved in planning, implementing, monitoring, and evaluating services.
- ▼ Services should be coordinated. Written agreements and linkages between participating agencies and various levels of government should be developed. Mechanisms should be in place to ensure continuity of care and coordination between hospitals and other community services.

Identification and Outreach. To encourage states to provide case management services, the federal government passed the State Comprehensive Mental Health Services Plan, which required that case management services be provided to every mentally ill individual in a state that receives a significant amount of public funds or services. A comprehensive mental health services plan must have strategies to locate potential individuals, inform them of available services, and ensure their access to these services. Establishing and maintaining close working relationships with potential referral sources such as public and community hospitals,

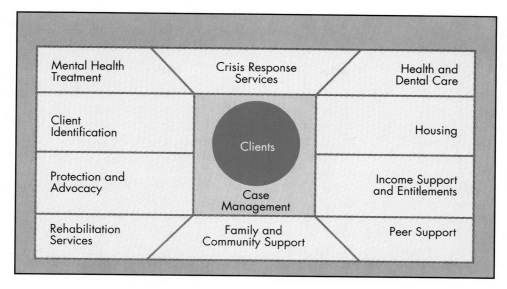

Fig. 32-1 Components of a community support system.
Department of Health and Human Services: *Toward a model plan for a comprehensive community-based mental health system*, October 1987.

community mental health centers, and social service agencies were essential to meeting this goal. Some case management agencies specialize in working with a particular target population, such as the homeless or those who carry the dual diagnosis of mental illness and substance abuse. These case managers establish contacts with potential individuals in homeless shelters, soup kitchens, drug treatment centers, and emergency facilities.

Assessment. A thorough assessment of an individual's strengths and deficits is required for an effective service plan. Assessments address all aspects of a person's life, including psychological, emotional, financial, medical, educational, vocational, social, and housing needs. Particular emphasis is placed on identifying patients' strengths that can be used to compensate for weaknesses and understanding patients' cultural and health-related values and beliefs. The knowledge and skills needed for a comprehensive assessment are generally beyond the ability of one case manager and often require a multidisciplinary approach. The expected outcome of the assessment is a detailed outline of the individual's present functioning, highest level of functioning, and needed services.

Service Planning. A comprehensive service plan guides all case management activities and must be carefully formulated with individual and family involvement. The goal of the service plan is to assist the person to live in the community successfully. Since many of these people have histories of numerous psychiatric hospital-

Table 32-2 Components and Interventions of Clinical Case Management

Component	Intervention
Initial phase	Engagement
	Assessment
	Planning
Environmental interventions	Linkages with community resources
	Consultation with families and caregivers
	Maintenance and expansion of social networks
	Collaboration with physicians and hospitals
	Advocacy
Patient interventions	Individual psychotherapy
	Training in independent living skills
	Patient psychoeducation
Patient-environment interventions	Crisis intervention
	Monitoring

izations, the service plan should include new approaches that might interrupt the chain of events that previously led to rehospitalization. Treatment objectives and specific actions that will be taken should also be clearly stated.

Linkage with Needed Services. A major component of case management is linking the mentally ill with the various social, medical, and rehabilitative services that they need to live successfully in the community. Once again, this activity often requires a team approach, since the services needed are often diverse and span a broad range of agencies.

MENTAL HEALTH TREATMENT. Clinical management of psychiatric disorders is an integral part of service delivery and may be provided on a long-term basis if needed. Clinical care should be directed at helping individuals manage symptoms, understand medications, recognize signs of relapse, and cope with daily living. Clinical care should also include diagnostic evaluation and ongoing monitoring of the patient's psychiatric condition. Supportive counseling and individual, family, or group intervention should be offered as appropriate.

An essential component of clinical management is medication management. Medication management services include prescribing medications, ensuring that needed medications are available, carefully monitoring medications to ensure maximal benefits and minimal side effects, and educating the patient and family about the medications.

CRISIS RESPONSE SERVICES. In spite of the provision of ongoing clinical care, individuals with serious and long-term mental illness tend to have crises. The primary goal of crisis services is to assist those in psychiatric crisis to maintain or quickly resume functioning within the community. Emergency services offered 24 hours a day must be provided by community mental health centers, and this can be accomplished in a variety of ways. It is common in large urban areas for this service to be provided by the emergency room of a local hospital. Other community mental health centers provide this service on site. In rural areas, where travel time and distance make a central crisis location unfeasible, mobile crisis outreach services visit the individual in the setting in which the crisis is occurring. Some community agencies provide 24-hour hot lines staffed by professionals or volunteers who offer crisis counseling or referral services over the telephone. However, when these services do not relieve the crisis situation, crisis residential services should be available in a residential nonhospital setting on a short-term basis.[43]

HEALTH AND DENTAL CARE. Severely mentally ill persons have been found to have higher rates of physical illness than the general population. One study found that more than 42% of such people were reported by their case managers as having at least one chronic medical problem that limited their functioning.[27] Another significant number of persons with long-term mental disorders have undetected physical disease that may contribute to their mental disorders.[7] Thus adequate health-care services for this population are important.

In spite of the fact that psychiatrically impaired persons also have serious medical problems, their use of general health-care services is often limited because of the barriers of access and availability.[35,51] Access is a problem because of active psychiatric symptoms, such as hallucinations regarding body functions and paranoid or delusional thinking. These symptoms may prevent individuals from seeking appropriate health care or from adhering to treatment. Another factor is that those psychiatrically ill people who do seek medical care are sometimes regarded with fear, hostility, and suspicion by health-care professionals who are inexperienced in working with this population. Finally, access and availability of general health care are also affected by current treatment and reimbursement mechanisms that are oriented toward specialization and episodic treatment of acute conditions.

HOUSING. An important goal of the community support system is to locate, secure, and maintain affordable housing for persons with long-term mental illness. Group homes where three to six mentally disabled persons live together with minimal supervision are becoming available, as well as apartment complexes that have several units rented to mentally ill persons scattered throughout the complex.[12] Training, supports, and services are provided to allow the mentally ill to live as independently as possible. Commonly offered services include social and recreational activities, on-site crisis intervention, and client advocacy. Most of the staff in these programs do not have professional training in a mental health field.[34] A variety of more structured residential settings are being used for more disabled individuals. Finally, foster care homes that provide accepting, normalized settings for persons with severe mental disabilities are also becoming more common.

Although great strides are being made to provide adequate and appropriate housing for the severely mentally ill, the greatest barrier continues to be community resistance to the placement of mentally ill persons in residential settings. In many places the outcome of this resistance has been "psychiatric ghettos" in which large numbers of psychiatrically impaired persons live in poorly supervised board and care homes in low-income areas or on the streets.[24]

 Would you and your family want a group home for the mentally ill to be built in your neighborhood?

Monitoring Service Delivery. Monitoring is an important part of case management and is often difficult to implement successfully. The monitoring function of case management serves two basic purposes: (1) it ensures that the objectives of the service plan are being met, and (2) it provides the information necessary for an ongoing reevaluation of the plan. The case manager assists the individual in obtaining the services identified in the service plan. Since the needs of the mentally ill are usually complex and require the services of multiple agencies, the case manager must develop coordinating and facilitating skills. Periodic review of the individual's progress with each of these service providers is part of the case manager's duties. Information gained from these contacts should also be used in regular reviews of the overall service plan.

Advocacy. Assisting people to receive the available services and influencing providers to improve existing services and develop new ones are also important roles of the case manager. Psychiatric patients and their families struggle with issues of discrimination, stigma, compromised rights, and inadequate resources on a daily basis. Advocacy activities are sensitive to these injustices and are proactive in nature. They include political negotiation, as well as consumer and professional collaboration. Finally, it is essential for advocacy efforts to be sensitive to the cultural background of the individual and the norms and values of the community.

Role of Nurses

The systems model of community mental health was based on a holistic approach that focused on the caring and the curative aspects of service delivery. Nursing, with a similar focus, thus had an opportunity to perform a variety of roles in this model. Case management, in particular, allowed nurses to assume direct care, supervisory, and consulting roles while working with patients and families by:

▼ Serving as their gatekeepers and facilitators in accessing the health-care system
▼ Assisting them in making informed decisions about their health-care needs
▼ Monitoring their health and human service plan of care
▼ Educating them to enhance their self-care ability

The American Nurses' Association states that[1]:

Psychiatric and mental health nurses are highly qualified to function as both case managers and providers within managed care systems. Psychiatric and mental health nurses are positioned to have a maximum impact on the managed care of psychiatric clients because:

1. They are committed to improving access, quality, and cost containment.
2. They understand prevention and wellness and know how to educate patients to improve health.
3. They know how to triage and assess the needs of patients.

4. They know how to accurately evaluate the necessity for inpatient admissions and continued hospital stays.

Others also believe that psychiatric nurses are well qualified to provide case management services.[26,50] The clinical example that follows illustrates the contributions a psychiatric nurse can make in providing case management services.

 ## Clinical Example

Jane M is single, 33 years of age, and has a history of multiple psychiatric admissions. She was referred to the community mental health center case management unit upon discharge from a 6-month stay at the state hospital. She had a diagnosis of undifferentiated schizophrenia in remission and was discharged to the care of her family on thioridazine 400 mg daily. Jane has occasional auditory hallucinations, is somewhat suspicious, and has a long history of disruptive family relationships and of noncompliance with medications.

The psychiatric nurse case manager volunteered to take the case and made an appointment with the family for a home visit. When she arrived, the family was visibly upset and related that in the week since Jane had been home, she slept much of the day and roamed around the house during the night, taking long showers, slamming kitchen cabinet doors, and playing loud rock music. When she was awake during the day, she would disappear for hours at a time causing great anxiety for the family. The mother was tearful and wringing her hands in an agitated manner while the father sat on the sofa with his head bowed. Jane sprawled in a chair and intermittently swore at her mother as the mother described these events.

In assessing the situation the nurse recognized that Jane's illness dominated the household, essentially putting her in control of the rest of the family. The nurse worked intensely with this family to restore generational boundaries by supporting the parents in making mutually agreed upon rules about behavior that would be tolerated in their household. She helped the family identify ways to support the patient, while also setting limits that would promote adaptive family functioning. The family found this exchange to be very helpful and they called on the nurse to validate their ideas and provide them with ongoing information on Jane's illness. The nurse also evaluated the impact of the medication on her patient's behavior. She arranged to have the time of Jane's medication changed so that the she received a dosage at bedtime.

Over the course of the next few weeks, Jane began to sleep at night. With continued support from the nurse, the parents became skilled and comfortable at presenting a united front. While Jane initially resisted, she adapted rather quickly to the new norms in the house, and a family crisis that might have resulted in Jane's readmission to the hospital was averted.

In reality, relatively few psychiatric nurses work in community mental health centers, and most case managers are social workers or paraprofessionals. During the 1980s the trend among psychiatric nurses with advanced training and education was to remain in inpatient settings, rather than to work with the serious mentally ill in the community. Thus many challenges remained for nursing as the community mental health movement moved to the next model of care.

 What factors encourage psychiatric nurses to work in inpatient settings and discourage them from working in community-based psychiatric programs?

PATIENT-CENTERED MODEL

Although the systems model of community mental health contributed to an improved and more coherent service delivery system for the mentally ill, new problems and populations began to emerge (see Critical Thinking about Contemporary Issues). Often, these were patients whose problems did not "fit" well in any service system, but instead required intervention by more than one of these systems simultaneously.

Dual-Diagnosis Patients

Individuals with a dual diagnosis have a substance abuse problem and a psychiatric disorder. Unfortunately, mental health and substance abuse services have traditionally been funded and staffed separately, and the substance abuse problems of patients treated in the mental health system have often received little attention. Mental health providers tend to treat the psychiatric condition and then refer the patient elsewhere for substance abuse treatment.

Young Seriously Mentally Ill

Young individuals with serious mental illness often do not fit into current programs and use the mental health system sporadically, primarily in times of crisis.

Homeless Mentally Ill

Mentally ill patients who are homeless reflect the tension between a mental health system that views hous-

ing as a social welfare problem and public housing agencies that believe that this population needs specialized residential programs provided by mental health agencies. This results in the needs of this population being underserved.

 Should individuals be allowed to "choose" to be homeless if they are not dangerous to themselves or others?

Individuals with AIDS/HIV

Those with AIDS/HIV require intensive services from the general health sector for their many life-threatening physical problems, but they also need psychiatric services to cope with the emotional impact of physical deterioration and impending death. In addition, 28% of men and 52% of women with AIDS are intravenous drug users[10]; thus they need to enter a third system of care, that of substance abuse treatment.

Mentally Ill in Jail

A nationwide survey reported that 1 of every 14 jail inmates in this country suffers from mental illness. This does not include mentally ill inmates in state or federal prisons. Twenty-nine percent of jails surveyed house seriously mentally ill individuals who have not committed any criminal actions. These people are often jailed because no other facilities are available to respond to their psychiatric emergencies.[48]

Have jails become today's substitute for yesterday's state hospitals for the mentally ill? If so, which alternative is better?

These system problems were frustrating to healthcare providers, consumers, families, and the public, and consumers of mental health services and their families became increasingly vocal about their lack of participation in the planning of mental health services. Thus in the 1990s a patient-centered model of community mental health emerged. In this model consumer participation in planning culturally relevant services is a guiding principle of service delivery.[9]

Patient-centered mental health services cannot be established merely by giving a greater voice to the mentally ill and their families. Rather, fundamental organizational and fiscal changes are also needed.[47] According to Mechanic,[29] a viable framework for organizing effective delivery of mental health services must include provision of assertive community treatment, use of capitation and managed care, and appointment of local health authorities.[29]

Assertive Community Treatment

In spite of the federal government's commitment, the use of case management to coordinate services for the mentally ill has not been universally implemented. When it is available, mental health workers often carry large caseloads, and the amount of time allocated to each client may be minimal. A study of the use of aftercare services by discharged patients revealed that, on average, patients received 2.5 hours of case management services in the year after discharge.[38]

However, studies have shown that intensive community intervention by case managers with small caseloads and 24-hour responsibility for their clients can serve as an alternative to hospitalization.[28] The best known intensive community treatment program is the Program for Assertive Community Treatment (PACT), which was developed by Stein and Test[41] in Wisconsin. In this program a multidisciplinary team works with patients in their homes, neighborhoods, and workplaces providing varying intensities of services depending on patient need. Teams also work with community members, act as gatekeepers to inpatient care, and help to coordinate all aspects of care (Table 32-3). The result of this intervention is that patients function better and report a higher quality of life than patients who receive traditional inpatient services and aftercare.

The PACT model has been duplicated in various settings around the country but still serves a small number of patients who could use this intensive community treatment. Implementation has been slowed by the changes needed in the training of mental health professionals, their assumption of new professional roles, and the restructuring of hierarchical status systems, all of which are necessary to implement this innovation.

Capitation and Managed Care

Reimbursement mechanisms that include fee-for-service payment for hospitalization and low reimbursement for community services favor the traditional system of repeated hospitalizations and low levels of aftercare. Any effort to change the patterns of services delivery requires a fundamental change in reimbursement structures. Capitation funding and managed care offer powerful incentives to move the service delivery system in new directions. According to Mechanic[29] capitation has three specific features:

1. All defined services for a specific period of time (usually 1 year) are provided for an agreed-upon payment.
2. Payment is tied to the care of a particular person or group of persons.
3. The provider agrees to be at risk for costs exceeding the agreed-upon amount.

This kind of reimbursement has incentives for the provider to manage the care of each patient cost effectively and to avoid expensive hospitalization if at all possible. Several capitation efforts are being tested in various parts of the country, and it promises to continue to be a part of future health-care reform initiatives.

Local Mental Health Authorities

Presently, reimbursement for mental health care comes from a variety of funding sources; federal and state governments and private insurance companies may pay for part or all of the costs. The result of these multiple payment sources is that there is no single authority responsible for providing the range of services needed by the

Table 32-3 Comparison Between the Program for Assertive Community Treatment (PACT) Model and Community Mental Health Center (CMHC) Services

	PACT	CMHC
Treatment base	*In the community*	*In a clinic*
Continuity of care	Team follows client through hospital, legal, health, and social services systems	Individual therapist or case manager less likely to follow client through health and social services systems
Staffing	10 to 1 ratio	30-50 to 1 ratio
Staff structure	Multidisciplinary team provides integrated clinical and case management services	Multiple providers who function fairly autonomously
Emergency treatment 24 hours a day	Team on-call	Hospital
Frequency of contact with client	Daily if needed	Weekly to monthly or less
Frequency of contact with families	Weekly	Occasionally
Responsibility for medication	Home delivery by team if required	Client or family
Responsibility for physical health	Actively monitored by team	Health care use encouraged
Responsibility for occupational rehabilitation	Direct client contact in work setting	Psychosocial programs
Responsibility for housing	Team	Usually client and family

From NAMI *Advocate* 14:5, 1993.

mentally ill. In an effort to overcome this systems problem, the Robert Wood Johnson Foundation funded demonstration programs in nine large cities throughout the United States for the development of central mental health authorities to consolidate administrative, fiscal, and clinical responsibility for care. One such program is described in the following clinical example.

 ## CLINICAL EXAMPLE

Before receiving the Robert Wood Johnson Foundation grant, Denver provided mental health services through four community mental health centers, each serving a different part of the city. Acute care was provided by a city-owned hospital and long-term care by a state hospital. Two specialty clinics served Denver's diverse ethnic groups. All of these agencies received funding from the state division of mental health and each operated independently of the others. In response to the Robert Wood Johnson initiative, Denver and the state of Colorado created the Mental Health Corporation of Denver. It was given responsibility for planning psychiatric services for the entire city, delivering clinical care, and developing housing for individuals who were mentally ill. All state and federal funds for services in Denver were channeled to this new corporation that provided services through contracts with providers. While evaluation of this project is ongoing, preliminary data suggest that significant change is possible in the organization and delivery of community mental health care.

It is clear that health-care financing reform will create changes in the current health-care delivery system.

Delivery sites will continue to shift from inpatient to community settings, increasing the amount of care that is delivered at traditional community agencies but also expanding to new delivery sites. School-based clinics that allow for health-care provision for all family members will increase, especially in rural areas. So too, home care will expand as efforts are made to decrease the use of hospitals.

 What benefits do you think should be included for psychiatric care in a reformed health-care system in the United States?

Role of Nurses

Current trends of shortened length of stays in psychiatric hospitals, use of alternatives for hospitalization whenever possible, increased focus on patients with complex treatment problems, and the growth of consumer and family movements have had major impacts on the ways in which mental health care is delivered in this country. A number of new approaches are being implemented to overcome the clinical and system problems that have interfered with providing patient-centered care for the mentally ill. These represent unique opportunities and challenges for nursing.

On one hand, psychiatric nurses continue to struggle with their involvement in community psychiatric care. Many community mental health centers are reluctant to hire psychiatric nurses because they are "too expensive" compared with other mental health care workers. Psychiatric nurses have also been slow to articulate the range and quality of services they can provide in community settings, thus demonstrating their cost effectiveness as health-care providers. In addition, community settings have difficulty differentiating among nurses based on education and experience, and they often underutilize psychiatric nurses by confining their activities to medication administration. Finally, psychiatric nurses have not been active enough in designing, organizing, and administering mental health delivery systems, so they are often viewed as implementors rather than decision makers.

NEW PSYCHIATRIC NURSING ROLES

Despite these problems, psychiatric nurses are beginning to play pivotal roles in emerging treatment modalities. They are fulfilling vital functions in day treatment facilities, psychotherapy clinics, vocational and rehabilitation centers, psychopharmacology clinics, psychiatric emergency rooms, and other community settings that provide care for the mentally ill. Other areas of role development will now be described.

Home Health Care

In recent years there has been an increased need for delivery of mental health services in the home, and the psychiatric nurse has become an important member of the interdisciplinary home health care team.[32] The psychiatric nurse engages in a variety of roles depending on the patient's needs, the home health agency, and the nurse's qualifications. These include direct caregiving, counseling, education, referral, health promotion, and consultation to family members or other direct care providers who lack knowledge of the principles of psychiatric care. Psychiatric nurses function as both generalists and specialists on home health care teams depending on the complexity of the problems. Figure 32-2 shows the many roles that the specialist in psychiatric nursing might assume.

Homebound status and the need for treatment are the major criteria for home visits by psychiatric nurses.[23] In general, patients are defined as homebound if their illnesses include refusal to leave their homes, inability to do so because of physical or mental impairment, or if it would be considered unsafe for them to leave home unattended. Soreff[39] found the program to be particularly effective in the following situations:

1. *People living alone, especially the elderly.* Because much has been written about the elderly in nursing homes, it is easy to forget the fact that 95% of those 65 to 74 years of age are living in the community. Many elderly exhibit a strong desire to be able to live independently for as long as possible. Since 18% to 25% of the elderly have significant mental health problems and persons over 65 years of age account for 20% of all suicides, home care that includes counseling and assessing for confusion, depression, dementia, and cognitive impairment by a psychiatric nurse may allow the individual extra years of independence.[19]

2. *Individuals with medical illnesses.* Patients with debilitating physical illnesses such as chronic obstructive pulmonary disease, cystic fibrosis, paraplegia, cancer, and AIDS/HIV often become isolated and depressed. The depression is often overlooked or too readily accepted by family and physicians as

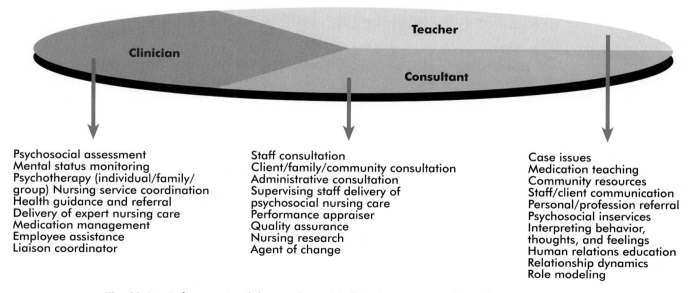

Fig. 32-2   Role aspects of the psychosocial clinical nurse specialist in home care.
From Klebanoff N, Casler C: *Home HealthC Nurse* 4:36, 1986.

an untreatable consequence of the medical illness. Psychiatric nurses, who are knowledgeable about both psychiatric and physical illness, can help treat the secondary psychiatric symptoms of the physical illness, thus improving the functioning and quality of life of these individuals.

3. *Persistently mentally ill individuals living at home.* Psychiatric nurses can provide valuable services to this vulnerable group. They can intervene directly with the patient in the home setting, assist the family in establishing appropriate structure, and provide psychoeducation and encouragement to relieve family burden.

4. *The housebound individual.* It is estimated that 2% of the general population suffer from panic disorder, many of whom experience the anticipatory anxiety and avoidance behavior associated with this disorder. A proportion of these individuals are housebound because of their fears. Because of the nature of the illness, the housebound patient is not often seen in physicians' offices or mental health clinics.

Outreach Clinical Services

Outreach implies that mental health workers literally "reach out" to patients wherever they are in the community, including family homes, board and care homes, group homes, fast food restaurants, homeless shelters, street corners, or prisons. This kind of assertive treatment is usually reserved for individuals with one of the following characteristics[40]:

1. *Unwillingness to seek out services.* Some patients are unwilling to go to community mental health centers for treatment. Others frequently miss appointments. This behavior is seen as part of the illness and requires more intensive outreach by the provider.

2. *Medication nonadherence.* Patients who are not willing, lack the money, or are too disorganized to take their medications require a treatment approach that can determine the problem, monitor the patient, and implement strategies to ensure needed medication is taken. Sometimes this can be accomplished by education, encouragement, titrating dosages, or switching medications. Depot injections of long-acting psychotropic medication may also be the recommended treatment. Packaging medications in daily doses with the date and time to take each pill can be an effective compliance tool. Sometimes legal procedures may be implemented by the treatment team, since many states have outpatient commitment laws in which patients are legally required to comply with outpatient treatment.

3. *Inability to self-monitor symptoms.* Patients sometimes respond to hallucinations and delusions by discontinuing their usual social and treatment contacts. They become isolated and withdrawn and must be visited frequently and encouraged to resume regular activities.

4. *Inability to structure daily activities.* While some patients have a social network and the ability to structure their daily activities, others have difficulty and need to be provided with structured daily activities by a professional team. Many are strongly encouraged to participate in day treatment programs or other community activities.

5. *Frequency of crises.* Patients who have frequent or severe crises need treatment from a program that provides intensive crisis intervention. The literature reflects the increasing participation of psychiatric nurses in assertive community treatment as members of mobile crisis teams,[45] assertive treatment teams in inner cities,[4,33] and similar outreach teams in rural areas.[6,36]

Collaborative Practice Arrangements

Many individuals are not receiving the mental health care they need. Some are undiagnosed in general medical settings. Others are correctly diagnosed but lack a consistent care provider. Still others have problems with their prescribed treatments and have relapses that could have been prevented. In response to these needs, psychiatric nurses are developing new collaborative models of care.

Psychiatric nurses are moving into the domain of primary care and working with other nurses and physicians in diagnosing and treating psychiatric illness in patients with somatic complaints.[13] Cardiovascular, gynecological, respiratory, gastrointestinal, and family practice settings are appropriate for assessing individuals for anxiety, depression, and substance abuse disorders. As health-care initiatives continue to move into schools and other community settings, psychiatric nurses can assume a leadership role in providing expertise through consultation and evaluation.

Another service that psychiatric nurses are providing is medical and medication management for selected groups of patients. For example, patients who are having difficulty being stabilized on their medications or those who have comorbid medical illnesses are seen in a psychiatric nursing clinic in which nurses and physicians collaborate to provide quality patient care.[30,49] As psychiatric nurses obtain prescriptive authority they will be able to further expand the services they provide and deliver cost-effective psychiatric care to communities that do not have access to a psychiatrist.

Prevention and Wellness Programs

Prevention and wellness programs are increasing as society moves away from a focus on illness to a focus on the maintenance of health and quality of life. Many of the serious, expensive, and chronic illnesses individuals have are "life-style" disorders, including obesity, smoking, lack of exercise, unhealthy diets, drug use, and unsafe sexual practices. Preventive programs that promote healthier life-styles have been found to be effective, and many corporations provide their employees with fitness and weight management centers and smoking cessation and stress management classes. These efforts have proven to be cost effective in the prevention of lost work days and expensive outpatient treatment and hospitalizations. Since they are partly educational and partly motivational, they are well within the expertise of psychiatric nurses.

In addition, certain groups who are at high risk and have been underserved in the past will be receiving more attention, and psychiatric nurses will be asked to expand the roles and services they provide to these targeted populations. The dramatic increase in child abuse and neglect in this country suggests one area needing new preventive interventions. An example of psychiatric nursing involvement in this area can be seen in South Carolina, where Medicaid is working with psychiatric nurses in planning a statewide initiative to reduce child abuse and neglect and the need for foster care. Once the program is in place, every infant will be screened for risk factors that have been associated with abuse and neglect, including poverty, being born into a single-parent family or to an adolescent mother, abuse in the mother's childhood, drug and alcohol abuse, and the presence of few social supports for the mother. Those mother-infant dyads with high-risk factors will receive intensive psychiatric nursing home intervention for the first year of life. Community mental health nurses will provide some of the direct care to the at-risk families and will supervise other providers.

> Describe an innovative psychiatric nursing service that you could provide the mentally ill in your community.

Family Preservation

Family preservation is an intensive home treatment modality for troubled youths and their families that has proven to be an effective community intervention. It focuses on the entire family system rather than the child, with the ultimate aim of preserving families whenever possible.[2,18] Services include crisis intervention, family

therapy, and coordination of other human service agencies.[20] Outcome research comparing the use of family preservation with more traditional treatment of serious juvenile offenders reveals significant decreases in conduct problems, immaturity, and associations with delinquent peers. In addition, parents and adolescents indicate more cohesive and adaptable family relationships and more positive mother-adolescent communications. Similar home-based crisis intervention programs have reported a great deal of success in reducing the need for psychiatric hospitalization or foster home placement for troubled youths.[8] These programs are ideal for the skills of psychiatric nurses.

These are a few of the activities of community-based psychiatric nurses. As the health-care system continues to change, more resources will be shifted to the community as an alternative to costly hospitalization. There will be exciting opportunities for psychiatric nurses to implement their skills and expertise across the continuum of health-care settings. Psychiatric nurses must be ready to articulate their knowledge base, demonstrate their skills, and advocate for high quality psychiatric care in this country. Given these events, community psychiatric nursing care promises to be the exciting frontier for psychiatric nurses well into the twenty-first century.

SUGGESTED CROSS-REFERENCES

Primary Mental Health Prevention	Chapter 11
Crisis Intervention	Chapter 12
Psychiatric Rehabilitation	Chapter 13
Consultation Liaison Psychiatric Nursing Care	Chapter 33

SUMMARY

1. The goals of community mental health are to care for the diagnosed mentally ill and prevent mental illness. There have been four models of community mental health.
2. The public health model (1960-1970) focused on the community and emphasized reducing the risk of mental illness for a population by providing services to high-risk groups. Intervention strategies included community needs assessment, identifying high-risk groups, consultation, education, and crisis intervention. The role of the nurse was minimal and often limited to caring for the chronically mentally ill.
3. The biological-medical model (1970-1980) focused on the diagnosed mentally ill and viewed mental illness as brain disease. Interventions included medication management and psychotherapy. Nurses became more involved in community roles ranging from medication administration to coordinating aftercare

programs and functioning as therapists for individuals, families, and groups.

4. The systems model (1980-1990) focused on developing a comprehensive system of care and coordinating needed services. Interventions included community support systems, service coordination, and case management. Nurses began to assume roles as coordinators of community services and case managers.

5. The patient-centered model (1990-present) focuses on patients who overlap service systems and emphasizes consumer participation and culturally relevant services. Interventions include assertive community treatment, creation of new reimbursement structures, and the formation of local mental health authorities. Nurses are struggling to demonstrate the range and quality of their services.

6. New psychiatric nursing roles include initiatives in home health, outreach, collaborative practice, prevention, and family preservation.

COMPETENT CARING
A CLINICAL EXEMPLAR OF A PSYCHIATRIC NURSE

Suzanne Smith, MSN, RN

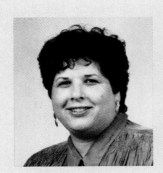

An experience I'll always remember involved a patient who was being discharged from the state psychiatric hospital and whom I interviewed for admission into an intensive case management program. R had been in and out of the state hospital for 3 years with the diagnosis of chronic schizophrenia. His frequent readmissions were related to the system's inability to place him in the community, which was due in part to his history of setting fires. Before this admission, he had burned down his residence during a psychotic episode. His psychosis, however, had resolved quickly after he was admitted to the hospital and started on a regimen of neuroleptics.

R was admitted into the intensive case management program, and his first 6 months had been very busy. He had been placed in an apartment with a roommate and became responsible for managing the apartment, cooking his own food, balancing his checkbook, and paying his bills. His adjustment to life in the community was progressing well. I was able to work with R on almost a daily basis, and all was going well.

On this specific day, I had called R to let him know that I would be coming to take him to the bank. We discussed in detail his checking account balance and financial obligations for that month. When I arrived at his home, R's roommate informed me that R had gone to the store to get a cup of coffee. While waiting, I walked into the hallway to check on a problem thermostat. As I glanced into R's room, I noticed that something was amiss. There were several cigarette burns in the carpet. On the bed there were a number of cigarette lighters. Propped on the pillows were cover photos from several women's magazines. The mouths on the models had been enlarged and a cigarette had been placed through the hole. In the bedside table, I found several more cigarette lighters. I noted all of these things, and added to my thinking the fact that R did not smoke.

On his return, we discussed some problems R was having with his roommate and banking affairs. His conversation was calm and rational. I then talked with him about what I had seen in his bedroom. Initially, he was silent and refused to discuss the matter. I realized that one of his greatest fears was returning to the state hospital to live for the remainder of his life, so I assured him that if something was wrong and he needed to go back to the hospital, it would be for a short-term hospitalization. At that point he began to explain that he had not taken his medication in a week and that recently he drank a six-pack of beer with several other patients in the program. Since then, he had been hearing messages from God in which she told him to smoke cigarettes because carbon monoxide was needed to clear all the pollution on the earth.

After a consultation phone call, I told R that I thought he was ill again and needed some time in the hospital. He agreed and we left in my car for an admission assessment at a local hospital. On the way, we stopped at the bank and R completed his banking business. When we arrived, several of my peers were astonished that I had let R ride in my car and go to the bank when he was obviously psychotic.

They exclaimed that they would have certainly called for backup from the office or the mobile crisis unit. I explained to them that I had assessed R and felt that this decision would not endanger either him or me. My decision was based on my skills as a psychiatric nurse, my experience in working with psychotic patients for a number of years, and my evaluation of R with whom I had worked closely for 6 months.

When I think back to this experience, I realize that it captured some of the critical essence of psychiatric nursing decision making. You see, I believe that it is calculated thinking woven into a fabric of clinical experience that guides psychiatric nursing practice. For R it was also a nursing act that expressed both "caring for" and "caring about." After 10 days in the hospital, R was stabilized once more and returned to the life he so wanted to live. ▼

REFERENCES

1. American Nurses' Association: *Position statement on psychiatric mental health nursing and managed care*, Washington, DC, 1993.
2. Amundson M: Family crisis care: a home-based intervention program for child abuse, *Issues Ment Health Nurs* 10:285, 1989.
3. Anthony W, Blanch A: Research on community support services: what we have learned, *Psychosoc Rehabil J* 12:55, 1989.
4. Arana J, Hastings B, Herron E: Continuous care teams in intensive outpatient treatment of chronic mentally ill patients, *Hosp Community Psychiatry* 42:503, 1991.
5. Ashbaugh J et al: Estimates of the size and selected characteristics of the adult chronically mentally ill population living in U.S. households. In Greenley J, Grenwich C, eds: *Research in community mental health*, vol 13, Greenwich, Conn, 1983, JAI Press.
6. Balacki M: Assessing mental health needs in a rural community: a critique of assessment approaches, *Issues Ment Health Nurs* 9:299, 1988.
7. Bartsch D et al: Screening CMHC outpatients for physical illness, *Hosp Community Psychiatry* 41:786, 1990.
8. Bishop E McNally G: An in-home crisis intervention program for children and their families, *Hosp Community Psychiatry* 44:182, 1993.
9. Campinha-Bacote J: Community mental health services for the underserved: a culturally specific model, *Arch Psychiatr Nurs* 5:229, 1991.
10. Centers for Disease Control: AIDS associated with IVDU—United States, 1988, *Morb Mortal Wkly Rep* 38:229, 1989.
11. Chamberlin J: The role of the government in development of psychiatric nursing, *J Psychosoc Nurs Ment Health Serv* 21:11, 1983.
12. Cutler D: Community residential options for the chronically mentally ill, *Community Ment Health J* 22:61, 1985.
13. Dashiff C, Greiner D, Cannon N: Physician and nurse collaboration in a medical clinic for indigent patients, *Fam Syst Med* 8:57, 1990.
14. De Young C, Tower M: *The nurse's role in community mental health centers: out of uniform and into trouble*, St Louis, 1971, Mosby.
15. Dohrenwend B, Dohrenwend B: Social and cultural influences on psychopathology. In Rosenzweig M, Porter L, eds: *Annu Rev Psychol* 25:417, 1974.
16. Fagin C: Psychiatric nursing at the crossroads: quo vadis, *Perspect Psychiatr Care* 19:99, 1981.
17. Glittenberg J: The role of the nurse in outpatient psychiatric clinics, *Am J Orthopsychiatry* 39:713, 1963.
18. Halvorson V: A home-based family intervention program, *Hosp Community Psychiatry* 43:395, 1992.
19. Harper M: Providing mental health services in the homes of the elderly, *Caring* 3:5, 1989.
20. Henggeler S, Melton G, Smith L: Family preservation using multisystemic therapy: an effective alternative to incarcerating serious juvenile offenders, *J Consult Clin Psychol* 60:953, 1992.
21. Kanter J: Clinical case management: definition, principles, components, *Hosp Community Psychiatry* 40:361, 1989.
22. Langsley D: The community mental health center: does it treat patients? *Hosp Community Psychiatry* 31:815, 1980.
23. Lesseig D: Home care for psych problems, *Am J Nursing* 87:1317, 1987.
24. Lieberman H: High needs and low priority of mentally ill residents of adult homes, *Hosp Commun Psychiatry* 43:486, 1992.
25. Marley M: Teaching and learning in a psychiatric–mental health clinical setting, *J Psychosoc Nurs Ment Health Serv* 18:16, 1980.
26. Maurin J: Case management: caring for psychiatric clients, *J Psychosoc Nurs Ment Health Serv* 28:7, 1990.
27. McCarrick A et al: Chronic medical problems in the chronically mentally ill, *Hosp Community Psychiatry* 37:289, 1986.

28. McGurrin M, Worley N: Evaluation of intensive case management for seriously and persistently mentally ill persons, J *Case Manage* 2:59, 1993.

29. Mechanic D: Strategies for integrating public mental health services, *Hosp Community Psychiatry* 42:797, 1991.

30. Nehls N et al: A collaborative nurse-physician practice model for helping persons with serious mental illness, *Hosp Community Psychiatry* 43:842, 1992.

31. Osborne O et al: The rise of public sector psychosocial nursing, *Arch Psychiatr Care* 7:133, 1993.

32. Pelletier L: Psychiatric home care, J *Psychosoc Nurs Ment Health Serv* 26:22, 1988.

33. Primm A, Houck J: COSTAR: Flexibility in urban community mental health. In Cohen N, ed: *Psychiatry takes to the streets,* New York, 1990, The Guilford Press.

34. Randolph F, Ridgway P, Carling P: Residential programs for persons with severe mental illness: a nationwide survey of state-affiliated agencies, *Hosp Community Psychiatry* 42:1111, 1991.

35. Roca R, Breakey W, Fisher P: Medical care of psychiatric outpatients, *Hosp Community Psychiatry* 38:741, 1987.

36. Santos A et al: Providing assertive community treatment for severely mentally ill patients in a rural area, *Hosp Community Psychiatry* 44:34, 1993.

37. Shore M, Cohen M: The Robert Wood Johnson Foundation Program on chronic mental illness: an overview, *Hosp Community Psychiatry* 41:1212, 1990.

38. Solomon P, Davis J, Gordon B: Discharged state hospital patients' characteristics and use of aftercare: effects on community tenure, *Am J Psychiatry* 141:1566, 1984.

39. Soreff S: Indications for home treatment, *Psychiatr Clin North Am* 8:563, 1985.

40. Stein L, Diamond R: A program for difficult-to-treat patients, *New Dir Ment Health Serv* 26:29, 1989.

41. Stein L, Test M: The training in community living model: A decade of experience, *New Dir Ment Health Serv* 26:7, 1985.

42. Stroul B: *Community support systems for persons with long-term mental illness: questions and answers,* Rockville, Md, 1988, National Institute of Mental Health.

43. Stroul B: Residential crisis services: a review, *Hosp Community Psychiatry* 39:1095, 1988.

44. Talbott J: Deinstitutionalization: avoiding the disasters of the past. In Talbott J, ed: *New Dir Ment Health Serv* 37:35, 1988.

45. Tamayo L et al: The systems impact of an urban mobile crisis team. In Cohen N, ed: *Psychiatry takes to the streets,* New York, 1990, The Guilford Press.

46. Thompson J, Bass R: Changing staffing patterns in community mental health centers, *Hosp Community Psychiatry* 35:1107, 1984.

47. Torrey E: Economic barriers to widespread implementation of model programs for the seriously mentally ill, *Hosp Commun Psychiatry* 41:526, 1990.

48. Torrey E, Wolfe S, Flynn L: Criminalizing the seriously mentally ill: the abuse of jails as hospitals, Arlington, Va, 1992, NAMI.

49. Wilkinson L: A collaborative model: ambulatory pharmacotherapy for chronic psychiatric patients, J *Psychosoc Nurs Ment Health Serv* 29:26, 1991.

50. Worley N: Advisor to the team, *Nurs Times* 87:38, 1991.

51. Worley N, Drago L, Hadley T: Improving the physical health–mental health interface for the chronically mentally ill: could nurse case managers make a difference? *Arch Psychiatr Nurs* 4:108, 1990.

52. Worley N, Lowery B: Deinstitutionalization: could the process have been better for patients? *Arch Psychiatr Nursing* 2:126, 1988.

ANNOTATED SUGGESTED READINGS

*Amundson M: Family crisis care: a home-based intervention program for child abuse, *Issues Ment Health Nurs* 10:285, 1989.
Reports on an intensive home-based crisis interaction and family education program developed by psychiatric clinical nurse specialists to reduce abuse and out-of-home placement of children, improve communication, and increase families' use of community resources.

*Campinha-Bacote J: Community mental health services for the underserved: a culturally specific model, *Arch Psychiatr Nurs* 5:229, 1991.
Addresses the need for culturally relevant services for African-American clients with the dual diagnosis of mental illness and substance abuse.

Chen A: Noncompliance in community psychiatry: a review of clinical interventions, *Hosp Community Psychiatry* 42:282, 1991.
One of the best articles written about the problem of noncompliance in the community with recommendations every nurse should know.

Cohen N, ed: *Psychiatry takes to the streets,* New York, 1990, The Guilford Press.
Excellent account of innovative community treatments such as outreach, case management, mobile crisis teams, and community residential care.

*Collins-Colon T: Do it yourself: medication management for community-based clients, J *Psychosoc Nurs Ment Health Serv* 28:25, 1990.
Describes the goals, content, format, and evaluation of a nurse-run medication education program for the chronically mentally ill living in the community.

*Dashiff C, Greiner D, Cannon N: Physician and nurse collaboration in a medical clinic for indigent patients, *Fam Systems Med* 8:57, 1990.
Describes an innovative collaboration between psychiatric clinical nurse specialists and a physician in an medical indigent clinic.

*Hicks L, Stallmeyer J, Coleman J: Nursing challenges in managed care, *Nurs Econ* 10:265, 1992.
Excellent article analyzing managed care and the opportunities, challenges, and threats it poses for nurses and nursing. Required reading for all nurses.

Hoge M et al: The promise of partial hospitalization: a reassessment, *Hosp Community Psychiatry* 43:345, 1992.
Reviews the trends in partial hospitalization since 1987 and includes timely recommendations for such community-based programs in the future.

*Journal of Psychosocial Nursing and Mental Health Services vol 27, 1989.
This entire volume is devoted to the homeless chronically mentally ill and is worth reading for the overview of issues it presents.

Mosher L, Burti L: *Community mental health: principles and practice,* New York, 1989, WW Norton.
The book to read for the clearest and most complete overview of contemporary community mental health. A welcome addition to one's library.

---

*Nursing reference.

*Nehls N et al: A collaborative nurse-physician practice model for helping persons with serious mental illness, Hosp Community Psychiatry 43:842, 1992.

Reports on nurse case managers working with consulting psychiatrists in a medical services unit for psychiatric patients who need medication services and supportive counseling.

*Pelletier L: Psychiatric home care, J Psychosoc Nurs Ment Health Serv 26:22, 1988.

Reviews opportunities and structures for nurses who work in psychiatric home care.

Robertson M, Greenblatt M: Homelessness: a national perspective, New York, 1992, Plenum.

Examines the many forces that contribute to homelessness in the United States and how to deal with the groups affected by it. Excellent overview.

*Wilkinson L: A collaborative model: ambulatory pharmacotherapy for chronic psychiatric patients, J Psychosoc Nurs Ment Health Serv 29:26, 1991.

Describes an outpatient medication clinic and group in which the patient, clinical nurse specialist, and psychiatrist share equal power and responsibility.

*Nursing reference.

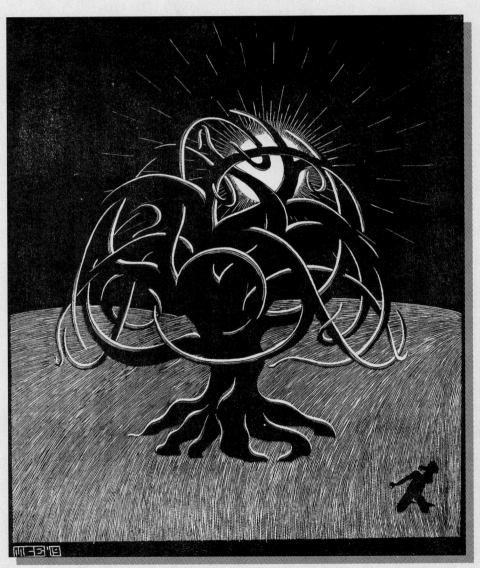

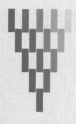

CHAPTER 33

Consultation Liaison Psychiatric Nursing Care

FRANCES G. LEHMANN

The greatest good we can do for others is not just share our riches with them but to reveal their riches to themselves.

Anonymous

All psychiatric nurses regardless of preparation engage in consultation activities at some time in their practice. Understanding the principles of consultation is necessary for the effective implementation of the psychiatric nursing role. In addition, psychiatric nurses often identify the need for a consultation and should be aware of what they can expect from the consultant and how they may best benefit from the consultation process. However, nurses need to remember that although the principles of consultation can be used by all psychiatric nurses, expertise increases with advanced education and experience.

Consultation liaison psychiatric nursing care is a model of nursing practice that has developed from the consultative process. It can be practiced in inpatient or community-based settings. This practice area originally grew out of the psychosocial needs of patients in the general hospital setting, and more recently, the need for nursing to provide care that is holistic and cost effective in a variety of practice environments. This nursing role is considered a psychiatric nursing specialty requiring a master's degree for practice, expertise in psychiatric nursing, and the ability to integrate this knowledge in general health-care settings to provide comprehensive nursing care.

ROLE CHARACTERISTICS

Problem solving is a function of all nurses, regardless of educational preparation or defined roles. Many essential qualities, however, contribute to the specialized problem-solving activity of consultation liaison nurses. It is important to differentiate commonly blurred activities, such as supervision and education, from consultation liaison nursing. Essential differences between this role and the supervisor role are the authority base and administrative responsibility for outcome. The consultation liaison nurse should have a coordinate professional relationship with the user with no administrative authority or coercive power over the user. The consultation liaison nurse is not responsible for implementing recommended changes, and the user is free to accept or reject any or all parts of the recommendation.

Organizationally, the consultation liaison nurse position should be a staff rather than a line position. This differs from a supervisory role, in which authority is based on hierarchical rank. By definition, the consultation liaison nurse is outside the user system, which means being outside the regular chain of command within the user organization. This aspect also provides the nurse with the necessary freedom to work with people at any level within any needed time frame rather than in a full-time line position that fills a slot within the organizational structure.

The power of the consultation liaison nurse rests in the authority of the nurse's ideas based on a specialized area of expertise. The user explicitly and voluntarily asks for help. The nurse respects the user as a professional partner in problem-solving activities. While dealing with the current problem, the nurse works to add to the user's knowledge, promoting more effective handling of similar situations in the future. Thus the nurse facilitates the user's potential by asking for and using the user's input. The nurse should project the attitude that the user is an active, interdependent partner who is ultimately responsible for implementing the proposed interventions.

Although the nurse may provide new information and knowledge to the user, the consultation process differs from an educational activity. The stated goal is not to teach a specific body of knowledge to the user. Rather, the nurse provides support and guidance while helping the user to gain understanding of the issues. The user can then develop more effective ways to handle the current problem and future similar situations.

 What problems could result if the consultant had direct authority over the consultee?

Settings and Functions

There are several ways of practicing consultation liaison nursing.[7-9,14] Some nurses are independent private practitioners who are employed for a specific assignment by the consultee organization on a fee-for-services basis. Other clinicians are staff members of an organization.

The consultation liaison nurse can provide either direct or indirect service. In both categories the nurse acts as an outside consultant, on a time-limited basis, facilitating and enhancing a person's, family's, group's, or organization's knowledge and skills. In direct service the nurse provides direct nursing care and intervenes so that the activity has a measurable effect on the health status of a person, group, or family. In indirect service the nurse functions as a resource, supporting key people directly responsible for the operation of the consultee system.

The setting in which a consultation liaison nurse may function is limited only by imagination and demand. The nurse's services may be used in acute or rehabilitative inpatient units of general hospitals, ambulatory health services, home health care organizations, community agencies, educational institutions, employee health components of industry or business, and special population settings such as extended care facilities, retirement communities, summer camp programs, and church-sponsored social support programs.

Types of Problems

The consultation liaison nurse intervenes in various types of problems. The identified problem can focus on:
▼ One client **(case problem)**
▼ A series of related problems **(program problem)**
▼ A particular administrative problem **(organization problem)**

In practice, these artificial categories generally overlap. However, the nurse's awareness of the identified problem and the target system with which one is interacting helps in working through the consultation liaison process. These categories are described in Box 33-1.

THE CONSULTATION LIAISON PROCESS
Theoretical Framework

There are many models of psychiatric consultation liaison nursing. A review of the literature reflects the diversity, complexity, and widespread use of the role.[3,4,6,12,15] The consultation liaison nurse should have a theoretical framework for practice. The model used in this chapter is based on a consultation process developed and used in community mental health by Caplan[2] in which the consultee asks the consultant who is an identified expert to assist in solving a work-related problem (Fig. 33-1). The term **consultation** refers to a specific professional process between two systems. One system (the user or consultee) has a problem and requests help from an outside system (the provider or consultant). In addition, the nurse is responsible for (1) using sound principles, (2) applying concepts to the information available, and (3) providing practical and useful interventions based on proven theories.[7]

The consultation liaison nurse uses knowledge and organizes theory from a variety of disciplines to formulate a unique model for nursing (see Critical Thinking

Box 33-1

PROBLEM CATEGORIES IN CONSULTATION LIAISON PSYCHIATRIC NURSING PRACTICE

CATEGORY: CASE PROBLEM

Definition: Focus is on a problem related to an individual client or patient

Role of nurse: Develop ways to increase the user's skills and knowledge

Clinical example: Mr. P was a 38-year-old man who was diagnosed with AIDS/HIV. He was admitted to the hospital in respiratory distress and was being treated aggressively with antibiotics. The nursing staff noted that he was despondent, withdrawn, and had little interest in eating or self-care activities. The staff were frustrated since their attempts to reach out to Mr. P had not been successful and he was responding poorly to treatment. The primary nurse requested a consultation from the consult liaison nurse employed by the hospital, who completed a nursing assessment and worked with the nursing staff to identify Mr. P's needs and formulate a mutual and realistic nursing care plan for him.

CATEGORY: PROGRAM PROBLEM

Definition: Focus is on a problem related to a program or unit of service delivery

Role of nurse: Help the user define and meet specific professional and programmatic goals

Clinical example: The teaching staff of a private preschool facility went to the director of the program and requested that she hire more teachers. The director of the program, who was a capable administrator, believed the present staffing pattern was adequate, but also recognized the staff were experiencing much frustration in providing high-quality care for children enrolled in the program. She requested that a clinical nurse specialist working in a community mental health center consult with the faculty regarding the problem.

CATEGORY: ORGANIZATION PROBLEM

Definition: Focus is on a problem related to an administrative or management issue

Role of nurse: Assist the user in bringing about organizational change to produce the desired outcomes

Clinical example: A small manufacturing plant was in the process of expanding its product line and corporate structure. With the expansion, the plant acquired a new board of directors and department managers. The growth and development of the organization had placed a tremendous strain on the newly appointed managers, and their work relationships had become strained and unproductive. The president of the plant had recently completed family therapy with a psychiatric clinical nurse specialist and decided that the company might profit from mental health intervention. He contacted the nurse who agreed to serve as a consultant to the management team during this time of administrative transition.

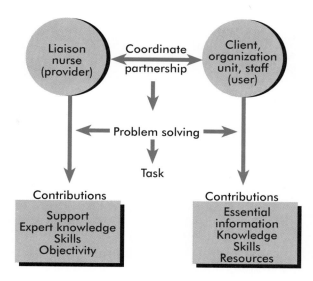

Fig. 33-1 Practice model used by the consultation liaison nurse.

About Contemporary Issues). The theory base should include knowledge of systems theory, change theory, staff management, organizational behavior, problem-solving theory, growth and development, cultural and ethnic norms, stress and stress reduction theory, and crisis theory, as well as environmental, interpersonal, and intrapersonal psychiatric dynamics. In one situation organizational theory may become the primary focus, at another time interpersonal relationships may be the frame of reference, and yet another situation will deal directly with an intrapersonal problem.

Phases of the Process

Although consultation liaison nursing is a specialty area, it can be compared to the traditional nursing process since both are:

1. Orderly, mutual, problem-solving activities
2. Relate to at least two people interacting to cause change
3. Hold the partners responsible for participation

The nursing process involves assessment, diagnosis, outcome identification, planning, implementation, and evaluation. These steps are incorporated within the orientation, working, and termination phases of the consultation liaison process.[1]

Orientation Phase. Initially, it is important that the nurse contact the appropriate authorities in the organization to make one's purpose and presence known. This contact also allows the nurse to gather data about the organizational structure and the communication networks. It is necessary that the nurse understand the ser-

CRITICAL THINKING ABOUT CONTEMPORARY ISSUES

Is There a Difference Between Consultation Liaison Nurses and Physicians?

Questions have been raised about the overlap between the consultation liaison roles of nurses and physicians in psychiatry. There have been challenges posed to the effectiveness and the costs of the services provided by each discipline. It is true that nurses and physicians who assume this role share a similar goal of improving patient care by addressing the psychosocial problems of patients, and that both assume the connectedness of the mind and body in promoting health. There are, however, significant differences between the two disciplines as well.[11]

Physicians are more often asked to make psychiatric differential diagnoses, distinguish between organicity and functional disorders, and prescribe medications to alter symptoms. Nurses are more frequently asked to assess behavioral problems, identify unmet psychosocial needs, and promote a patient's adaptive response to illness. When asked to provide direct patient care, physicians tend to do so from the medical model, which assumes pathology and is focused on cure. Nurse consultants strive to promote adaptation and optimize positive coping resources and behaviors. While it is obvious that consultation liaison nurses and physicians share common traditions, it is also apparent that the focus of their activities are distinct but complementary, and that both disciplines play an important role in the delivery of quality mental health care. ▼

vices provided by the organization, the philosophy, and any relevant operating policies or procedures.

The entire consultation liaison process is affected by the type of setting and professional background of the personnel involved in the relationship. Each setting will have its own unique philosophy, organizational structure, established protocols, and expectations of how the nurse will function in that particular setting. The effectiveness of the process is also influenced by the user's concept of the nurse's role. It is important for both sides to clarify this role to avoid two common causes of failure:

1. The staff has unrealistic expectations
2. The staff distorts the purpose for which the consultation was requested

The nurse should also evaluate the accuracy of the user's perception of the present consultation on the basis of past experience with other personnel in a similar role.

The nurse will have the opportunity to work with nurse colleagues, other disciplines, and nonprofessional personnel. Thus the nurse will have to maintain the strength of his or her identity as a nurse, as well as an awareness of the identities of others. The nurse should interact with other people under the assumption that they have a sense of accountability, responsibility, and competency in their own area of work regardless of their educational background or professional experiences.

EFFECTIVE COMMUNICATION. The nurse's ability to communicate effectively is a skill that makes the process much smoother (see Chapter 2). The communication process depends on the nurse, setting, and user of services. Developing communication channels involves identifying key formal and informal networks. It is important for the success of the consultation process that both sides have a working arrangement for giving and receiving information.

Basic conceptual differences will become apparent as people work together in the task of problem solving. Finding a common language in which both partners are comfortable and feel productive will minimize differences. It is helpful for the nurse to use words that are familiar to other people. This will prevent inappropriate discussions or skirting of the subject. Using abstract approaches or focusing on what seems to the users to be impractical or irrelevant will not promote their self-confidence. The nurse should not give advice or use declarative sentences when communicating with staff. It is preferable to use questions that guide the user to alternative ways of viewing the problem. Helping the user review and simplify relevant facts promotes clarity and mutual understanding of the situation.

It is important for the user to know that consultation discussions are confidential. This means that the nurse guards against being a "switchboard" or carrier for messages that should be delivered directly within the organization. Also the nurse should not take sides in differences of opinion among staff members. It is important to demonstrate that any information gathered will not be used to purposely harm any person or the reputation of the organization.

Finally, the focus of any interaction should be work difficulties and not the private personal needs of staff members. If personal issues are hindering a staff member's performance and interventions are needed, this recommendation is not transmitted within the official consultation process. The nurse restrains from gathering personal information that could turn the consultation into therapy. Instead, the nurse can tactfully encourage the troubled staff member to seek out an impartial skilled listener.

 A nurse colleague tells you that asking for a consultation about a patient or unit problem means that you're not doing your job and reflects badly on your nursing skills. How would you respond to this?

CONTRACT. Although consultation liaison nursing is an ongoing process, it is best guided and evaluated by a written agreement between the nurse and the user. This agreement is called a contract. It represents an exchange between the partners of the specific services to be provided and the nature of the complementary activity. If the request for services comes through informal channels (via telephone or face-to-face contact), the nurse needs to verify with the appropriate authority that permission is given for the liaison activity. The purpose behind requesting a letter of contract is to prevent misunderstandings between the parties.

To prevent possible misrepresentation or ambiguity, a letter or memorandum from a person in authority in the user organization should be directed to the consulting nurse. This document can describe the various aspects of the user's expectations and serve as a tool for outcome evaluation.

The contract is not so much a legal document as an agreement between professionals of two systems. It can be kept simple. It should be dated and signed by both user and consultant. The main points to cover in the contract are presented in Box 33-2.

The nurse can use the contract to better understand the informal relationship. By expanding and examining the statement of problem, the nurse can decide if it is a case, program, or organization problem. The nurse can gather more background information about what action has been taken so far to resolve the problem and what personnel have been involved in the activity to date. The stated goals may end up as part of the original problem. Viewing both the expected goals and stated problem will show how the user perceives the entire situation.

The contract also helps the nurse learn about the organization's perception of the time required and whether the organization sees the compensation as an hourly rate or a job rate. If the consultant is in-house, it should be clear to which department the time is to be charged. Finally, it is essential that the nurse become knowledgeable about the communication network to be used, the names of staff and their jobs, a list of people

---

Box 33-2

COMPONENTS OF THE CONSULTATION LIAISON CONTRACT

▼ Brief description of the problem
▼ Expected outcomes or goals
▼ Estimated time to be devoted to the project
▼ Amount of compensation for the consultant's time
▼ Key departments and personnel related to the consultation
▼ Name of contact person from the requesting agency

---

who are available for discussion, the scope of confidentiality expected, the kinds of information appropriate for discussion with whom, and who the authority source is for permission.

Compare and contrast the consultation liaison contract and the contract in the nurse-patient relationship.

Working Phase. After the orientation phase in which the initial contact and contract are completed, the actual consultation liaison process begins. This process can be used on case, program, and organization problems and can be applied to both direct and indirect care functions.

ASSESSMENT. This step begins when the contract is formulated. It continues with the two participants collecting data, clarifying the information available, and synthesizing and recording it in a standardized format. The nurse can ask questions to stimulate the staff's thinking and guide the discussion to a deeper level by asking questions about the complexities of the situation. By speculating aloud, the nurse promotes new understanding among the staff and demonstrates a willingness to risk and act as a role model for the problem-solving process. Beginning sentences with "I wonder if. . ." facilitates a feeling of mutuality. During this stage the nurse should:

1. Assess the strengths and weaknesses of the user
2. Identify the real and potential barriers to action
3. Determine what has prevented the user from resolving the problem
4. Assess the general problem-solving ability of the users

DIAGNOSIS. In this step the nurse identifies actual or potential problems, including sources of conflict, stress, or dysfunction within organizations or health-care delivery systems. These diagnoses are validated with the consultee or user and recorded to facilitate planning, evaluation, and research.

OUTCOME IDENTIFICATION. The nurse then proceeds to identify expected outcomes derived from the diagnoses. They should be realistic, attainable, and cost effective. Most important, they should be shared expectations of both the consultant and consultee. They serve as criteria to measure the success of the consultation process and thus are critical to effective role implementation.

PLANNING. This step starts with the nurse reframing the problem so that the user can view the situation objectively and without feeling threatened. The nurse uses theoretical concepts that promote learning and can be generalized to similar situations and listens to and values the staff's ideas. The nurse may also modify them by expanding the proposed interventions or by suggesting unusual but theoretically sound ways to implement them. All interventions should be feasible, practical, and in line with the skills and abilities of those responsible for implementation. This avoids upsetting the existing lines of communication and authority. The suggestions should also be sensitive to the rights and well-being of those affected by the potential change. The planning should reflect what currently exists and not what should be. It is unethical to propose interventions based on an ideal that cannot be reached.

This step ends when the nurse and the user arrive at a nursing care plan for the problem. Goals should be stated based on the expected outcome and prioritized. These goals provide a framework for interpreting, planning and evaluating ongoing activities.

IMPLEMENTATION. This step begins with the user selecting the interventions to be tried. It may take place after the nurse has left the physical environment and the actual consultation process is terminated. This stage includes testing alternative suggestions that came out of the planning step. It ends when the interventions have been in effect long enough to assess observable change.

EVALUATION. This step begins with asking to what extent the interventions met their stated goals. It may take place after the nurse has left, but it is still important that the nurse help the user find specific ways to measure the expected outcome and the interventions. The evaluation focuses on the effects of the planned interventions and not on the staff who implemented the plan. This is an important difference in that the total situation is examined, not how individual people are functioning. Another aspect of evaluation is identifying

that gaps of knowledge or lack of skill exist on the part of the staff. These needs may be met through an educational approach to the problem.

This step ends when the user determines whether the defined problem has been resolved, to what degree of success the solution worked, and what additional problems, if any, were uncovered during the process.

Some people believe that in the future nurses will be consultants to other caregivers who will actually provide the patient care. What would be the advantages and disadvantages of such an arrangement?

Termination Phase. Termination involves both physical and psychological closure. Tasks such as writing reports and leaving are included. Much of the work involved in this phase depends on the nurse's basic personality, the setting, and the formal contract. If the consulting nurse is a staff member of the user organization, his or her visibility will continue. If it is a one-time relationship, leaving will be more formal.

SUMMARY REPORT. Progress may have been verbally discussed throughout the liaison process, but at the end of the consultation activity a formal written report is required. This allows all members of the organization to have access to relevant information. The format of the report will vary with the type of consultation, the setting, the level of organization involved, and the issues addressed. Areas that should be included in the report are shown in Box 33-3. This formal report can be brief but explicit regarding what the nurse believed happened in the total process. The report should be consistent with the theoretical framework of the nurse's practice.

PROFESSIONAL DEVELOPMENT. The nurse uses the contract and summary report for self-evaluation of performance in the process and for making revisions in using

---

Box 33-3

COMPONENTS OF THE CONSULTATION LIAISON REPORT

▼ Purpose, dates, time, and activities of the consultation
▼ Statement of the identified problem
▼ Assessment of the problem and related diagnoses
▼ Proposed interventions for problem resolution
▼ Alternative problem-solving approaches
▼ Evaluation criteria and findings if available

the process on the next occasion. [7] Self-evaluation is a necessary part of the liaison process. Areas that need evaluation are goal setting, problem solving, communication skills, and theory application. Additional ways to evaluate performance are to survey consumers about their satisfaction with the consultation liaison service and to engage in peer review.[5,10,13]

DIRECT CARE ACTIVITIES

As a direct service provider, the consultation liaison nurse provides assessment, diagnosis, treatment, and evaluation services. The nurse may use individual, family, or group therapy, crisis intervention, health teaching, anticipatory guidance, or stress reduction counseling. The nurse intervenes on an interpersonal level to expand the mental health services available in nonpsychiatric settings.

In direct service the types of problems that arise are considered patient-centered case problems. Most of the nurse's time is spent with the patient, and the interaction is primarily supportive and goal directed. The identified case problem may be to:

1. Assess a patient's mental status
2. Assist a family through a crisis
3. Counsel and support the person who has impaired body functions; has loss of self-esteem; is grieving; has suffered family abuse, violence, or rape; demonstrates impaired mental or emotional functioning; or needs guidance in coping with a personal life situation that currently or in the future could interfere with optimal functioning

In direct service the patient and nurse are the primary participants. The nurse uses advanced nursing skills and knowledge to provide direct care that results in measurable changes in the patient's health. The nurse is directly responsible for implementing, evaluating, and documenting rendered services. The nurse must also collaborate with other team members and provide them with any information that may contribute to the patient's well-being.

The case study on p. 858 illustrates the role of the consultation liaison nurse as a direct care provider.

 How might a consultation liaison nurse be used in a large public high school as a direct and an indirect care provider?

INDIRECT CARE ACTIVITIES

When the consultation liaison nurse functions in an indirect manner, the consultee is responsible for resolving the identified problem. The nurse assists the consultees in improving their problem-solving skills in the specific presenting situation and in handling similar work problems that might arise in the future. The nurse is not expected to be an expert in the consultee-organization's specific operations. The nurse is acknowledged as an expert in maximizing human resources to resolve the current problem and to enhance the consultee's own abilities and efforts.

Psychiatric nursing indirect services of consultation, education, systems evaluation, and program development can be used by nurses in schools, industries, business corporations, civic and community organizations, or church-sponsored social groups. Problems can range from employee-assistance programs to interpersonal relationship enhancement among members of a corporate board of directors. The case study on p. 859 illustrates the role of the consult liaison nurse as an indirect care provider. Box 33-4 summarizes the direct and indirect care interventions of psychiatric consultation liaison nurses.[1]

BOX 33-4

INTERVENTIONS OF PSYCHIATRIC CONSULTATION LIAISON NURSES

DIRECT CARE INTERVENTIONS	INDIRECT CARE INTERVENTIONS
Psychotherapeutic	Consultation
Health teaching	Education
Anticipatory guidance	Maintenance of a therapeutic environment
Somatic therapies	Systems evaluation
Psychotherapies	Program development

SUGGESTED CROSS-REFERENCES

CASE STUDY—DIRECT CARE PROVIDER

Mrs. W, a 68-year-old widow, was admitted to a surgical unit of a general hospital for a colostomy after x-ray examination and biopsy revealed colorectal cancer. She had a history of three previous admissions for various somatic complaints over the last year since the death of her husband. During the presurgery workup, the attending physician asked for a consultation liaison nurse to establish a therapeutic relationship with Mrs. W in anticipation of the colostomy and to obtain an evaluation of Mrs. W's coping abilities.

▼ ASSESSMENT

The consultation liaison nurse, reviewed the patient's charts from the present and previous hospitalizations and talked with the family physician and the surgeon. She also talked with the ostomy service nurse and with Mrs. W's primary nurse. She then met with Mrs. W in her private room for an hour.

After a thorough assessment of Mrs. W's physical, social, mental, emotional, cultural, and spiritual health, the nurse explored with her the meaning Mrs. W gave to the situation she was experiencing. The nurse also talked with her about her family and social support network and received permission to talk with her adult daughter. Rapport was established, and they mutually decided subsequent visits would be helpful.

▼ DIAGNOSIS

The nurse made the following nursing diagnoses:
1. Severe level of anxiety related to medical diagnosis of cancer as evidenced by inability to focus on daily events
2. Disturbed body image related to the impending colostomy as evidenced by verbalized fears
3. Anticipatory grieving related to the loss of body functioning as evidenced by denial and sadness

▼ OUTCOME IDENTIFICATION

The nurse and Mrs. W agreed on the following expected outcomes:
1. Mrs. W will verbalize feelings related to the diagnosis of colorectal cancer and the colostomy.
2. Mrs. W will identify adaptive coping responses she may use to adjust to her colostomy.
3. Mrs. W will mobilize her social support network and other coping resources to help her at this time.

▼ PLANNING

The nurse conferred with the family physician and together they decided that Mrs. W, because of her high-risk stress factors, would benefit from six to eight sessions to be provided by the nurse. The scheduled surgery and Mrs. W's recuperation would be primary factors in the treatment plan. The nurse charted the assessment, diagnoses, treatment recommendations, and therapeutic goals in Mrs. W's chart. She also talked with Mrs. W's primary nurse and then stopped by Mrs. W's room to arrange another visit with her the next afternoon, the day before surgery.

▼ IMPLEMENTATION

Strategies were based on a continuous evaluation of Mrs. W's changing health status and surgical intervention. Theoretical considerations shaping the therapeutic relationship were life developmental stage, stress management, and the process of grieving for body changes. The nursing interventions included: (1) decreasing Mrs. W's level of anxiety, (2) providing therapeutic support for the grief and mourning process, and (3) reducing present and potential problems in the areas of self-esteem, body image, and personal control. The rationale for consultation liaison nursing participation was preventive intervention to reduce the negative effects of stress while improving Mrs. W's coping abilities at a time when she was dealing with a major health problem.

▼ EVALUATION

Evaluation of the patient's changing health status and how she was functioning was a shared responsibility of all health-care team members. The consultation liaison nurse functioned as a therapist and monitored the effectiveness of the interventions on Mrs. W's mental, emotional, and social health status.

Some of the therapeutic techniques used in this clinical example include:
1. Focus on time-limited interventions and well-defined goals
2. In promoting stress management, recognize the reality of the health-threatening situation and Mrs. W's compromised health status
3. Build on the strengths of the patient, her support network, and the team
4. Use the consultation liaison process as one component of the team's commitment to comprehensive care by participating in team conferences and collaborating with the team members in an ongoing manner

CASE STUDY—INDIRECT CARE PROVIDER

A psychiatric clinical nurse specialist received a telephone call from Ms. K, director of a retirement home. After discussing a problem she was having with one of the residents, Ms. K wrote a contract letter to the nurse: "Our home has a resident, Mr. C, whose lack of participation in planned activities keeps him isolated from other residents. We would appreciate your help in developing a treatment plan for him that would increase his involvement in group activities. As we mutually agreed, this project should require about 4 hours of consultation. Our standard rate for consultants is $75 per hour with no employee fringe benefits. Please feel free to talk with any staff or residents at their discretion.

▼ ASSESSMENT

The next day the clinical nurse specialist met with Ms. K and some of her staff, who described Mr. C's current status and the interventions that the staff had tried in the past. The nurse used nonthreatening questions to learn how the staff saw Mr. C in relation to his environment and his physical and psychosocial functioning. By speculating aloud to herself, the nurse brought out different aspects and broadened the focus of the problem. Ms. K then arranged for the nurse to talk with Mr. C, and she also spoke informally with other staff and residents. On returning to Ms. K's office and comparing information, they determined that Mr. C was having an anniversary reaction to his wife's death.

▼ DIAGNOSIS

They mutually agreed upon the following nursing diagnoses for Mr. C:
1. Delayed grief reaction related to his wife's death as evidenced by lack of interest and pleasure in usual activities
2. Social isolation related to the grieving process as evidenced by withdrawing from others

This identification of the problem made it easier for the staff to focus objectively on Mr. C and not be threatened by feelings of guilt or inadequacy in not meeting his socialization needs.

▼ OUTCOME IDENTIFICATION

The grief process was the theoretical concept the nurse used to help the staff reframe Mr. C's situation. The emphasis shifted away from engaging Mr. C in more activity to evaluating his behavior in relation to the stages of grief work. The expected nursing outcomes were:
1. Nursing staff would express satisfaction in the individualized care they were providing for Mr. C.
2. Mr. C. would begin to work through the grieving process.

3. Nursing staff would generalize information regarding grief and the grieving process to other retirement home residents.

▼ PLANNING

The treatment plan was written specific to the actions of the patient with the underlying assumption that present behaviors are meaningful in helping him work through the loss of his wife, his home, and his life-style. The nurse used a staff conference to help generate interventions that would facilitate his emotional release. The staff decided to reduce Mr. C's expected involvement in activities and provide him with a supportive environment. It was agreed that Mr. C should be included in the planning of his treatment program. Mr. C's participation in the assessment, planning, and implementation stages recognizes his strengths and allows him to remain self-reliant.

▼ INTERVENTION

The nurse used leading questions such as "Do you suppose Mr. C was in denial when he first came here? That might explain why he got involved in so many activities initially." The nurse also provided information on the various stages of grief and grieving and gave examples of behaviors and attitudes that would allow the staff to help Mr. C express his feelings and work through the grieving process.

In Mr. C's case "facilitating grief work" was one step toward helping him adjust to his life stressors. The interventions focused on specific, expected actions of Mr. C and were written in concise statements such as "Introduce Mr. C to Mr. O, who has successfully completed grieving for his wife." Expected measurable outcomes were established for staff interventions with Mr. C and a time frame was placed on each. The nurse also negotiated with the director to be available as a resource for 2 months as the planned interventions were tried and the results measured.

▼ EVALUATION

The nurse received a report from staff members regarding Mr. C's progress and a few revisions were made in the care plan. In addition to Mr. C's improvement, the nurse was told that the staff became more cohesive in problem solving and the knowledge they gained through the consultation benefited other residents as well. The nurse spent a total of 3 hours at the actual consultation site. The consultation ended when a summary report was sent to the director. The established relationship continued from time to time with other projects.

Some of the therapeutic techniques used in this clinical example include:

1. Focus on the patient's situation and not the staff's handling of it so that the users recognize that their work performance is not under investigation
2. Raise questions to discover additional details and enrich the staff's awareness
3. Use inquiry to show the staff the wealth of information they possess
4. Avoid asking for information that the staff would perceive as testing their knowledge base or questioning their competence
5. Allow the staff to know when you are confused. Being open to your own confusion allows the staff to recognize that clarifying is one of the steps in problem solving, and when the pieces are put together, the patterns and meaning become clear

SUMMARY

1. All psychiatric nurses request, receive, and provide consultation in their practices. The consultation liaison psychiatric nurse is considered a specialty area requiring a master's degree, expertise in psychiatric nursing, and the ability to integrate this knowledge in general health-care settings. Consultation liaison nurses practice in a variety of settings and intervene in case, program, and organization problems.

2. The consultation liaison process is based on a theoretical framework in which one system (the user or consultee) has a problem and requests help from an outside system (the provider or consultant). The phases of the process include orientation, working, and termination.

3. In direct service the consultation liaison nurse provides direct nursing care and intervenes so that the activity has a measurable effect on the health status of a person, group, or family.

4. In indirect service the nurse functions as a resource, supporting key people directly responsible for the operation of the consultee system.

COMPETENT CARING
A CLINICAL EXEMPLAR OF A PSYCHIATRIC NURSE

Paula E. Johnson, MSN, RN, CS

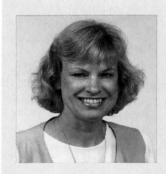

One of my most challenging experiences occurred while I was practicing as a consultation liaison nurse. I was called on by a colleague to deal with a situation that had become extremely difficult for nursing staff and administration alike. The intervention took place on a medical unit of a general hospital and involved a patient who had become essentially unmanageable for the nursing staff. This patient was a quadriplegic as the result of a motor vehicle accident incurred while driving intoxicated.

I first met with my nurse colleague, who thought she had begun to lose her objectivity in the situation and therefore her effectiveness with the staff. We discussed her assessment of the situation and what had been done up to this point in time. Many hours had been devoted to this patient, and all levels of staff had been involved at one time or another.

Next, I called and set up a meeting with the nurse manager. The patient was described by the nurse manager as a 65-year-old divorced black man who had served in the Army during World War II and had taught school for several years thereafter until his drinking apparently got out of control. He subsequently lost his job and was divorced, severing any relationship with his former wife. He had one daughter who seldom visited and appeared to be totally controlled by him, passively submitting to all his demands whenever she did visit. Since his motor vehicle accident, the patient had been ventilator dependent and required total nursing care. Several attempts to wean him from the ventilator had been unsuccessful. Placement had become a problem because of his dependence on the ventilator, lack of nursing home bed availability, and his limited financial resources.

In my initial introduction and meeting with the patient, he was pleasant and cooperative, but I noted that he focused on his past strengths and abilities in an almost grandiose fashion. I then met with the nursing staff. It was clear from the beginning that the staff's anger and frustration were interfering with their ability to cope with this stressful situation. They were angry not only with the patient but also with each other and on occasion would vehemently dispute the observations and interpretations of their fellow staff members. Sick calls on the unit had nearly doubled, and staff who rotated from other units felt uncomfortable and fearful of being caught in the middle between the patient and the unit nursing staff.

The staff reported that the patient had his call bell hooked up in such a way that he could use his mouth to press the button. They remarked that the patient made racial, seductive, and lewd sexual comments to them while they were providing nursing care. He had threatened to bring litigation, implied he had a method of punishing them, and verbally devalued their work. Clearly the intensity of the angry and helpless feelings the nurses held about this patient needed immediate attention. They asked for support in dealing with this problem and described feeling undermined by nursing administration and abandoned by the physicians.

With input from the nurse manager, I decided that my initial role was to defuse the anger. I would be supportive and provide education to the staff in an effort to help them give the best care they could to the patient. We arranged meetings twice a month on overlapping shifts. I also offered individual sessions for those nurses who felt uneasy discussing their feelings in a group or who were unable to make the meeting times. Several nurses took advantage of this individual time to share their feelings and discuss their interactions with the patient and other staff in a confidential and nonthreatening atmosphere.

The supportive group meetings were designed to let nurses talk about their feelings and thoughts, but because of the intensity of their responses, it was necessary to set limits and the group was led to focus more specifically on decreasing the stress associated with the situation. During this time the staff resisted trying new approaches to manage the patient, and every suggestion made was rebutted with "we've already tried that." Consequently, discussion about specific ways of managing the patient was placed on hold. Instead, group process was focused on staff strengths and resources. Specific strategies for combating their stress were identified, such as luncheons off the unit, and other planned activities that might encourage cohesiveness and teamwork were brainstormed. Since the nurses and I had established an alliance, I was able to identify various behaviors related to countertransference. As we talked, we emphasized the importance of honesty, and that what was said in the group stayed in the group. It took a while, but we eventually found some humor within ourselves and shared a few laughs.

My educational focus for the group was on taking care of the difficult patient. I remembered a favorite article I had saved from my med-surg nursing days entitled, "Taking Care of the Hateful Patient." I briefly summarized and outlined the article and shared it with the staff. They were able to recognize their patient and to begin to discuss his profound neediness. They acknowledged how the patient's attitude might be his shield from the awareness that they seemed to have power over his life and death. The article described a very specific and useful response to these patients that the nurses felt comfortable with and expressed a willingness to try. They posted the outline on the unit.

As I look back on this experience, I realize that not all problems were resolved. However, the benefits of me, as consultant, "meeting the nurses where they were" with this problem, and facilitating a support group interaction, proved useful to the nursing staff, as consultees. It also taught me once again that learning and growing in psychiatric nursing are reciprocal processes. ▼

REFERENCES

1. American Nurses' Association, Council on Psychiatric Mental Health Nursing: *Standards of psychiatric consultation-liaison nursing practice,* Kansas City, Mo, 1990, The Association.
2. Caplan G: *The theory and practice of mental health consultation,* New York, 1970, Basic Books.
3. Chiplin J, Geraghty M: Psychiatric liaison nursing: mental health needs in a burn unit, *Nurses Prax NZ* 5:15, 1990.
4. Griffin F: Advocating for seriously emotionally disturbed children and their families: an overview, *J Child Adolescent Psychiatr Ment Health Nurs* 6:33, 1993.
5. Harris J, Gallien E: Psychiatric mental health nursing specialist process evaluation criteria, *Nurs Manage* 23:54, 1992.
6. Kurlowicz L: Psychiatric consultation-liaison nursing interventions with nurses of hospitalized AIDS patients, *Clin Nurs Spec* 5:124, 1991.
7. Lewis A, Levy J: *Psychiatric liaison nursing: the theory and clinical practice,* Reston, Va, 1982, Reston Publishing.
8. Moschler L, Fincannon J: Subspecialization within psychiatric consultation-liaison nursing, *Arch Psychiatr Nurs* 6:234, 1992.
9. Nelson J, Schilke D: The evolution of psychiatric liaison nursing, *Perspect Psychiatr Care* 14:60, 1976.
10. Newton L, Wilson K: Consultee satisfaction with a psychiatric consultation-liaison nursing service, *Arch Psychiatr Nurs* 4:264, 1990.
11. Robinson L: Psychiatric consultation liaison nursing and psychiatric consultation liaison doctoring: similarities and differences, *Arch Psychiatr Nurs* 1:73, 1987.
12. Talley S, Davis D, Goicoechea N, Brown L, Barber L: Effect of psychiatric liaison nurse specialist consultation on the care of medical-surgical patients with sitters, *Arch Psychiatr Nurs* 4:114, 1990.
13. Titlebaum H, Hart C, Romano E: Interagency psychiatric consultation liaison nursing peer review and peer board: quality assurance and empowerment, *Arch Psychiatr Nurs* 6:125, 1992.
14. Tunmore R, Thomas B: Models of psychiatric consultation liaison nursing, *Br J Nurs* 1:447, 1992.
15. Yoest M: The clinical nurse specialist on the psychiatric team, *J Psychosoc Nurs Ment Health Serv* 27:27, 1989.

ANNOTATED SUGGESTED READINGS

*American Nurses' Association, Council on Psychiatric and Mental Health Nursing: *Standards of psychiatric consultation-liaison nursing practice,* Kansas City, Mo, 1990, The Association.
These practice and performance standards provide a framework for consult liaison nurses and should be essential reading for anyone in the specialty area.

*Campinha-Bacote J: Culturological assessment: an important factor in psychiatric consultation-liaison nursing, *Arch Psychiatr Nurs* 2:244, 1988.
Defines culture-bound illness and reviews the steps in a culturological assessment, including several known tools.

Caplan G: The theory and practice of mental health consultation, New York, 1970, Basic Books.
This is the classic text for consultation theory and practice. Excellent resource book for clinicians.

*Carnes B: Caring for the professional caregiver: the application of Caplan's model of consultation in the era a HIV, *Issues Ment Health Nurs* 13:357, 1992.
Excellent description of the development and implementation of a psychosocial support program based on Caplan's model using case, program, and organizational consultation.

*Fishel A: Psychiatric consultation: improving the work environment, *J Psychosoc Nurs Ment Health Serv* 29:31, 1991.
Presents an eight-stage process of consultation in reducing work stress for a group of nurses in a clinical setting.

*Hart C: The role of psychiatric consultation liaison nurses in ethical decisions to remove life-sustaining treatments, *Arch Psychiatr Nurs* 4:370, 1990.
Highlights the role of the psychiatric liaison nurse in facilitating the ethical decision-making process surrounding withdrawal of life-saving treatment from the terminally ill patient.

*Mallory G et al: Nursing care hours of patients receiving varying amounts and types of consultation/liaison services, *Arch Psychiatr Nurs* 7:353, 1993.
Describes the use computerized clinical databases to track the progress of consultation/liaison nursing interventions on patient outcomes and costs. Excellent example of research that is greatly needed in the field.

*Puskar K, Wargoe K: Difficulties with teens: can nursing consultation help? *J Child Adolescent Psychiatr Nurs* 5:34, 1992.
Reports on nursing consultation provided to a 15 bed adolescent unit to expand the knowledge base of direct care staff.

*Smith M, Buckwalter K, Albanese M: Psychiatric nursing consultation: a different choice for nursing homes, *J Psychosoc Nurs Ment Health Serv* 28:23, 1990.
Describes a consultation project focusing on the identification, assessment, treatment, and aftercare of the elderly in nursing homes who were in need of mental health treatment. Consultations were provided to the elderly, family members, and long-term and acute care providers.

*Titlebaum H, Hart C, Romano-Egen J: Interagency psychiatric consultation liaison nursing peer review and peer board: quality assurance and empowerment, *Arch Psychiatr Nurs* 6:125, 1992.
Reports on the advantages of a formal peer review process for psychiatric consultation liaison nurses and provides a model that represents a professionally accepted nursing quality assurance method.

Waldfogel S, Wolpe P: Using awareness of religious factors to enhance interventions in consultation-liaison psychiatry, *Hosp Community Psychiatry* 44:473, 1993.
Discusses approaches to incorporating religious factors in the psychiatric evaluation and treatment of hospitalized, medically ill patients.

*Nursing reference.

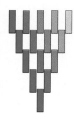

Special Populations in Psychiatry

*L*ife is unfair. It is unfair that people who are very young or very old should have to suffer in ways they may not even be responsible for. But that is a reality of life that nurses, more than many others, need to understand and incorporate in their practice. It has been said that a society can be judged by how it treats its most vulnerable groups. Given that criterion, how would you rank American society? What level of compassion, protection, and caring is needed to judge a society as humane? What resources are given to health-care providers to nourish, defend, and heal these most vulnerable groups? These are questions that you, as a nurse, may wrestle with the rest of your professional life.

In this unit you will enter the world of children, adolescents, and adults who are vulnerable to developing or being disabled by psychiatric illness. You will learn about their special needs and begin to search your heart and mind for ways to reach out and help them. In that sense, you have come to the end of your journey in this textbook. Your next passage as a professional nurse will be in other pages of your life. Good luck and godspeed.

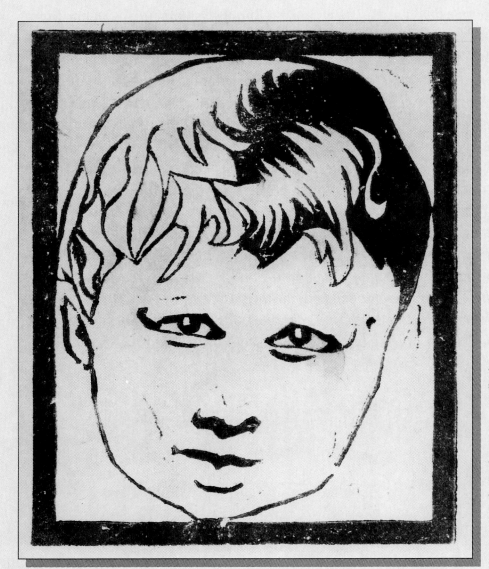

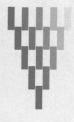

CHAPTER 34
Child Psychiatric Nursing

CAROLE F. BENNETT

Youth's love
Embracingly integrates
Successfully frustrates
And holds together,
Often unwittingly,
All that hate, fear, and selfishness
Attempt to disintegrate.

R. Buckminster Fuller: *And It Came to Pass—Not To Stay*

LEARNING OBJECTIVES

After studying this chapter the student should be able to:

▼ Discuss issues related to the psychiatric care of children including a framework for child psychiatric nursing practice

▼ Assess nine ego skills and adaptive responses that children need to become competent adults

▼ Identify nursing diagnoses and interventions related to ego competency skill deficits

▼ Implement therapeutic treatment modalities with children

TOPICAL OUTLINE

Recent studies suggest that about 7.5 million (12%) children in the United States have some type of psychiatric illness. These children have significant difficulty coping with the demands of school, family, and community life; however, less than one fifth, or 2 million, of the children who need mental health treatment actually receive it.[25] Psychiatric illnesses in children vary in the age at which they first appear, the types of symptoms or behaviors they produce, and the long-term effects they have on the child's development. Such disorders include states of depression and immobilizing anxiety, behavioral problems characterized by disruptive and antisocial acts, and developmental impairments that limit the child's ability to think, learn, form social relationships, and communicate with others.

Emotionally disturbed children need a variety of traditional and nontraditional services. In 1984 the National Institute of Mental Health[26] initiated the Child and Adolescent Service System Program (CASSP) in an effort to address the need for children's mental health services. Current research suggests that a range of services are needed by emotionally disturbed children, including the following[33]:

▼ Inpatient treatment
▼ Outpatient therapy
▼ Family support groups
▼ Intersystem case management
▼ School-based mental health services
▼ Training in independent living skills
▼ Intensive in-home therapy
▼ Psychological testing
▼ Supervised after-school activities

However, the majority of treatment resources continue to be focused on the relatively small number of children who receive care in hospitals, and most child psychiatric nurses currently care for emotionally ill children in inpatient treatment settings.[29]

For this reason, this chapter focuses on the nursing care of children in inpatient psychiatric units, although children who can benefit from these psychiatric nursing interventions receive care in a variety of settings. Children who are coping with trauma, abuse, and neglect are in pediatric hospitals, as well as residential facilities, homeless shelters, day-care centers, and schools. The nursing interventions described in this chapter can thus be easily adapted for general health-care settings, outpatient facilities, day-treatment programs, or in-home visitation.

PSYCHIATRIC CARE OF CHILDREN

Each year in the United States more than 130,000 children are hospitalized for psychiatric reasons. The decision to hospitalize a child is based on a complex set of factors, but a brief and appropriately timed hospitaliza-tion can enhance growth, reduce the suffering of the child and family, and shorten the duration of an illness.[8,10] In fact, many of the children who are currently hospitalized for psychiatric care could be managed in the community if their families and support systems had adequate resources.[16] Unfortunately, treatment resources for emotionally at-risk children are scarce, and inpatient care continues to be the dominant treatment setting. This promises to change in the future as psychiatric care makes the transition to new community-based programs and initiatives (see Chapter 32). The only question that remains is whether the money to implement these new community-based programs for children will follow them into the community.

Inpatient Treatment

Child psychiatric inpatient care has undergone dramatic changes in the last two decades. In the 1970s and 1980s inpatient child psychiatric units were typically structured around developmentally oriented milieu programs, and specialized treatment goals were identified for each child. These programs provided individual and group psychotherapy, special education, and collaborative work with families, and they were a vast improvement over the previous institutional model of care, which was basically custodial. Recommended lengths of stay ranged from 4 to 12 months. However, research showed that there were limited benefits of a prolonged, costly hospitalization over a more brief hospital stay, and so the need for change was identified.

Current developments in inpatient psychiatric care for children are the result of differences in the inpatient population, family and social structures, and the financing of health care.[17] For example, an increasing number of children referred for treatment are impulsive and aggressive. Many of these children have been neglected or physically or sexually abused.[4,27] The family structure has also changed to include more children in single-parent or foster care families. Finally, because of economic constraints, the length of stay for children has dramatically decreased from many months of hospitalization to a few inpatient days for brief stabilization. These changes in the delivery of psychiatric care to children have the following consequences[17]:

1. The current goals of hospitalization are focused on diagnosis and acute treatment strategies.
2. There has been a blurring of boundaries between hospital services and social system services.
3. The focus on understanding the psychodynamics of the child has decreased and been replaced by teaching coping skills and applying behavior management strategies.
4. Care has become more fragmented.

Do you think that the incidence of child abuse is increasing in this country or that it is the same as years before, only now it is being openly discussed?

A Framework for Nursing Practice

Because of these changes and the increased emphasis on the integrated biopsychosocial treatment of symptoms, child psychiatric nurses must have an organizing framework to conceptualize, implement, and research effective care of emotionally ill children. Nurses are challenged to derive realistic, well-defined goals, respond to the complex social needs of the child, understand and advocate for the child, and develop a comprehensive treatment plan that identifies and integrates the child's particular needs and resources. All of this needs to be done with the realization that the behavior of children is largely culturally based and must be viewed through a sociocultural perspective.[15,23]

Children who are hospitalized experience disabling symptoms that are responses to biological alterations, traumatizing situations, and maladaptive learning. During the course of hospitalization the children are medi-

cally evaluated and treatment is initiated.[13] The DSM-IV classifies disorders usually first evident in infancy, childhood, or adolescence by separating them into ten major groups.[2] These diagnostic categories and their essential features are listed in Table 34-1.

In addition to being knowledgeable about these psychiatric diagnoses, child psychiatric nurses must also be able to implement nursing care that has as its goal modifying a child's coping responses and strengthening a child's competency skills. Nursing care requires a comprehensive nursing assessment and the identification of treatment outcomes measured by a child's ability to adapt and function in life. Child psychiatric nurses should refer to the ANA *Standards of Child and Adolescent Psychiatric and Mental Health Nursing Practice* when implementing care.[1]

Regardless of the child's psychiatric diagnosis, nursing care must be focused on the child's response to illness and the nursing interventions designed to teach and model to the child and family more adaptive coping responses and improved methods of functioning. Thus nursing diagnosis and intervention proceed independently of and concurrently with psychiatric diagnosis and treatment. While nursing and medicine have collaborative roles, nursing has a critical and distinct contribution to make in the care of the emotionally ill child.

Table 34-1   DSM-IV Disorders of Infancy, Childhood, or Adolescence

Disorder	Essential feature(s)

Mental retardation	Significantly subaverage intellectual functioning with an IQ of approximately 70 or below.
	  Mild retardation = 55-70
	  Moderate retardation = 40-55
	  Severe retardation = 25-40
	  Profound retardation = below 25

Learning disorders	Functioning that is below that expected given the person's chronological age, measured intelligence, and age-appropriate education. May be evident in the areas of reading, mathematics, or written expression.
Motor skills disorder	Motor coordination is substantially below that expected given the person's chronological age and measured intelligence.
Pervasive developmental disorders	Impairment in a variety of indicators related to normal growth and developmental milestones including social interaction, communication, and the display of restricted, repetitive, and stereotyped patterns of behavior, interest, and activities (autistic disorder).
Disruptive behavior and attention-deficit disorders	Behaviors related to inattention that are maladaptive and inconsistent with the child's developmental level (attention-deficit or hyperactivity disorder); violation of the basic rights of others (conduct disorder); or negativism, hostility and, defiance (oppositional defiant disorder).
Feeding and eating disorders of infancy and early childhood	Behaviors related to eating of nonnutritive substances (pica); regurgitation and rechewing of food (rumination disorder); and failure to eat adequately (feeding disorder).
Tic disorders	An involuntary, sudden, rapid, recurrent, nonrhythmic, stereotyped movement or vocalization (Tourette's disorder).
Communication disorders	Difficulty with receptive or expressive language or the articulation of speech.
Elimination disorders	Repeated passage of feces in inappropriate places after 4 years of age (encopresis); or voiding of urine into bed or clothes after 5 years of age (enuresis).
Separation anxiety disorder	Inappropriate and excessive anxiety concerning separation from home or from those to whom the child is attached.

Organizing child psychiatric nursing care around ego competency skills is an effective and culturally sensitive way of planning and implementing nursing interventions for children regardless of psychiatric diagnosis or setting. Strayhorn[32] has identified the following nine skills that all children need to become competent adults:

1. Establishing closeness and trusting relationships
2. Handling separation and independent decision making
3. Negotiating joint decisions and interpersonal conflict
4. Dealing with frustration and unfavorable events
5. Celebrating good feelings and experiencing pleasure
6. Working for delayed gratification
7. Relaxing and playing
8. Cognitive processing through words, symbols, and images
9. Establishing an adaptive sense of direction and purpose

These skills give the child psychiatric nurse a framework with which to evaluate and intervene with emotionally ill children.[11]

Frequently a child's maladaptive responses are expressed differently from those of an adult. To develop the nursing plan, the nurse must learn to recognize and describe symptomatic behavior in children. It is helpful to use a specific assessment form, such as the one presented in Fig. 34-1, that identifies both competency skills and nursing diagnoses related to particular skill deficits to more fully describe the child's individual response or experience. Such a form would be used in addition to a standard nursing assessment tool that would also be completed by the nurse for each child (see Chapter 9).

The nurse should talk with the child about the child's strengths and then discuss the skills that need further development. Strategies used to teach these skills can then be explained to the child and the parents, which allows them to become active participants in the planning of nursing care. Children will be more motivated to cooperate if they are encouraged to sign a copy of their care plan after it has been explained to them. Even if they cannot write, a mark that represents their name is sufficient to signify their participation in the process. Nursing interventions can then be designed to improve the maladaptive responses and teach the accompanying skill.

Finally, child psychiatric nurses working in inpatient settings use individual, group, and milieu activities in working with children. Chapter 31 of this text discusses aspects of an inpatient therapeutic milieu,[9] which forms the context for many of the nursing interventions described in this chapter.

ASSESSING EGO COMPETENCY SKILLS

The child psychiatric nurse's assessment focuses on the specific skills all children need to become competent adults. Regardless of psychiatric diagnosis, a child should be assessed for mastery of each of the following skill areas.

Skill 1: Establishing Closeness and Trusting Relationships

A basic skill for positive growth and development is the child's ability to establish close and trusting relationships with others. The following questions are used to evaluate this skill:

▼ Does the child enjoy making friends?
▼ Does the child often feel picked on by other people?
▼ Does the child not know what to say when getting to know someone?

To reinforce this skill, a team of nursing staff should be assigned to each child during hospitalization. Members of this team can then engage the child in play and establish a therapeutic relationship. Nursing staff should encourage interaction and be attentive to the child without being intrusive. Talking with the child in a face-to-face position and offering nurturance are beginning nursing actions. Trust can then be demonstrated by the staff in their interactions with the child. If a child violates a trust, a discussion of the issue should take place, allowing trust to be reestablished. In this way, children learn about acknowledging mistakes and the importance of forgiveness in developing trusting relationships.

Skill 2: Handling Separation and Independent Decision Making

Individuation is an important mental health process. Being able to identify and express feelings and make independent decisions is critical to becoming a competent individual. The following questions are used to evaluate this skill:

▼ Does the child get upset or worry when away from his or her mother?
▼ Does the child get upset or worry if he or she thinks someone does not like him or her?
▼ When upset, is there something the child can do to feel better?

Nursing activities that focus on helping the child identify and clarify aspects of the self are critical exercises for promoting individuation. This may be done in many ways, such as by encouraging children to draw self-portraits, interview staff members to find out their opinions on an issue, or identify personality differences between themselves and others. Any experience that clari-

Questions used to evaluate competency skills are presented on the left. Nursing diagnoses related to these skills appear at the right. The screened response (N or Y) represents the appropriate competency skill. A patient score of 2 or 3 indicates a skill deficit, and the nurse should then select an appropriate nursing diagnosis based on the child's history and presenting problem.

SCORE 1._____	Establishing Closeness and Trusting Relationships	
N **Y**	1. I like making friends.	Fear
N Y	2. People pick on me a lot.	Anxiety
N Y	3. I don't know what to say when I am getting to know someone.	Post Trauma Response Family Processes Altered Growth & Development Altered

SCORE 2._____	Handling Separation and Independent Decision Making	
N **Y**	1. I'm upset when I am away from my mom and worry about her.	Self-Esteem, Chronic Low
N Y	2. If I think someone does not like me, I worry and get upset.	Anxiety Thought Processes Altered
N **Y**	3. When I am upset, there is something I can do to feel better.	Coping, Ineffective Individual

SCORE 3._____	Handling Joint Decision and Interpersonal Conflict	
N **Y**	1. When I have a problem, I can usually think of several solutions.	Social Interaction Impaired
N Y	2. If I do not get my way, it makes me mad.	Communication Impaired, Verbal
N Y	3. Other people get on my nerves a lot.	Violence, Potential for Decisional Conflict

SCORE 4._____	Dealing with Frustration and Unfavorable Events	
N **Y**	1. If I have hurt someone's feelings, I think about it and feel bad.	Trauma, Potential for
N Y	2. If someone disagrees with me, it makes me mad.	Social Interaction Impaired
N Y	3. I do not like playing a game if I lose.	

SCORE 5._____	Celebrating Good Feelings, Feeling Pleasure	
N **Y**	1. I worry about the future a lot.	Hopelessness
N **Y**	2. When people say good things to me, I don't like it for some reason.	Powerlessness Body Image Disturbance
N **Y**	3. There are things I do well, and it makes me feel good.	

SCORE 6._____	Working for Delayed Gratification	
N **Y**	1. Most rules are reasonable and I don't mind following them.	Growth & Development Altered
N Y	2. I find it hard to be honest; sometimes, lying is the only thing I do.	Sexuality Patterns Altered
N Y	3. I get mad if my mother dosen't get me what I want.	

Fig. 34-1 Competency skills assessment form.

SCORE 7. _____		Relaxing and Playing	
N	Y	1. There are some things I really enjoy doing.	Social Isolation Grieving-Anticipatory Sleep Pattern Disturbance
N	Y	2. I have lots of fun.	
N	Y	3. I enjoy sitting around and thinking about things.	

SCORE 8. _____		Cognitive Processing Through Words, Symbols, and Images	
N	Y	1. It is hard for me to describe how I feel to someone.	Growth & Development Altered Social Interaction Impaired Thought Process Altered Anxiety
N	Y	2. I never know how something is going to turn out for me.	
N	Y	3. I know what my strengths are.	

SCORE 9. _____		An Adaptive Sense of Direction and Purpose	
N	Y	1. I feel my life is going to get better.	Personal Idenity Disturbance Family Coping, Potential for Growth Hopelessness Powerlessness
N	Y	2. I am confused about growing up and don't know what to do about it.	
N	Y	3. I know school is important and going is my job in life right now.	

Fig. 34-1, cont'd   For legend see previous page.

fies differences between individuals assists the child to identify oneself as a unique individual within a social context. In the therapeutic milieu, opportunities also can be provided for the child to make choices and decisions, further supporting the child's growing sense of individuality and ego competency.

Skill 3: Handling Joint Decision Making and Interpersonal Conflict

Children who have not been allowed to participate in joint decision making or who have not been rewarded for cooperating may be deficient in this skill. This skill, however, is critical for success in interpersonal relationships. The following questions are used to evaluate this skill:

▼ When the child has a problem can he or she usually think of several solutions?
▼ Does the child get angry if he or she does not get one's way?
▼ Do other people get on the child's nerves alot?

The therapeutic milieu can provide an opportunity for the child to learn and practice these skills. For example, the nurse can set up opportunities for problem solving. Exercises may be developed for making group decisions in which cooperation and collaboration are heavily re-warded. The child should be helped to identify fears related to cooperating with others, and assertiveness can be modeled and taught. It is important that the nurse not resolve conflicts for the child. Rather, these situations should be used to teach negotiating skills and shape appropriate socialization through the use of reinforcement.

Games can be useful in teaching cooperation and compromise to children. What games can you identify that would be particularly helpful in teaching children this important skill?

Skill 4: Dealing with Frustration and Unfavorable Events

Tolerating frustration, although difficult, is critical to becoming a competent adult. The following questions are used to evaluate this skill:

▼ Does the child feel bad if he or she has hurt someone's feelings?
▼ If someone disagrees with the child does it make him or her mad?

▼ Does the child not like playing a game if he or she loses?

Children who have little frustration tolerance become angry easily and are often unable to complete tasks. Children typically learn this skill through cooperation and competition in playing childhood games. However, if a child has not had the opportunity to play games in this way and if tolerance has not been modeled for the child, he or she probably has not developed this skill. The child will experience numerous frustrations during the course of hospitalization. The nurse should use these opportunities to think through the process with the child and help increase the child's frustration tolerance.

> Do you think that a child's ability to handle frustration and stressful events is influenced by biological makeup? If so, does biology excuse individuals from being responsible for their actions?

Skill 5: Celebrating Good Feelings and Feeling Pleasure

Children who are raised in a healthy environment naturally experience good feelings and pleasure. However, in a maladaptive environment, shame is often used to control children's behavior with the result that they feel guilty for having angry or unacceptable thoughts. Consequently, they may lose the ability to celebrate life and feel pleasure. The following questions are used to evaluate this skill:

▼ Does the child worry about the future alot?
▼ Does the child not like it when people say good things about him or her?
▼ Does the child feel good about the things he or she does well?

A therapeutic milieu is one in which celebrating good feelings and feeling pleasure should be natural, spontaneous occurrences. Celebrating and having fun are important nursing interventions. These activities should not be confined to holidays alone but should be part of the weekly milieu activities. Children's families can be invited to participate in these celebrations where nursing staff model having fun with the children. In this way, children and their families learn the skill of celebrating good feelings and feeling pleasure.

> How often and in what ways did your family celebrate good feelings and experience pleasure when you were growing up? How do you incorporate this in your life today?

Skill 6: Working for Delayed Gratification

As children grow they are expected to delay needed gratification by following rules and waiting their turn. This skill is often difficult for anxious children to achieve. The following questions are used to evaluate this skill:

▼ Does the child believe that most rules are reasonable and does he or she not mind following them?
▼ Does the child find it difficult to be honest and think that lying is the only thing to do?
▼ Does the child get angry if his or her mother doesn't give them what they want?

Delayed gratification can be taught by the nurse through the earning of points for daily expectations, such as tidying one's room or completing homework assignments. Children's games, such as Red Light, in which they respond to "stop" and "wait" commands, are also useful in teaching this skill to younger age groups. As a child's behavior improves, the reward for the points earned can require the accumulation of many points or tokens. Thus the child is given the opportunity to delay the reinforcer for a reward of higher value to be received at a later time. As the child learns greater self-control, he or she will be better able to delay gratification for longer periods of time.

Skill 7: Relaxing and Playing

Given the stressful environment of current family life, many children may have little opportunity to learn the skill of relaxing and playing. For children and adults, learning to relax and play is an important skill. The following questions are used to evaluate this skill:

▼ Are there some things the child really enjoys doing?
▼ Can the child have lots of fun?
▼ Does the child enjoy sitting around and thinking about things?

In a therapeutic milieu, time should be devoted to learning this skill. Children should be given unstructured play time in which the staff participate with them in playing games. Having spontaneous talent shows or other forms of fun can contribute to a child's well-being. In this way relaxing and playing become part of the therapeutic milieu experience, and children learn to value and master this skill.

Skill 8: Cognitive Processing through Words, Symbols, and Images

Emotionally ill children may not have developed the important skill of cognitive processing. The following questions are used to evaluate this skill:

▼ Is it difficult for the child to describe how he or she feels to someone?

▼ Does the child feel as if he or she never knows how something is going to turn out?

▼ Can the child identify his or her strengths?

The therapeutic nursing milieu should be created to stimulate children's cognitive development. Furnishings and toys, communications and interactions, and community meetings and group experiences should all be designed to support the child's cognitive processing. The nurse can help the child learn this skill by encouraging abstract thinking whenever possible, such as by asking "What is the moral of the story?" or "What point do you think the movie was trying to communicate?" Children who are encouraged to express themselves in a responsive environment will gain greater competency in this important area of development.

Skill 9: Adaptive Sense of Direction and Purpose

Children, even as preschoolers, begin to think about their adult life. As they view adult life from watching those around them, they begin to draw conclusions about themselves in the world. The following questions are used to evaluate this skill:

▼ Does the child feel that his or her life is going to get better?

▼ Is the child confused about growing up and doesn't know what to do about it?

▼ Does the child believe that school is important and see it as his or her job in life at the present time?

Having role models for healthy, meaningful adult experiences is essential to healthy growth and development. Feeling value as an individual provides the child with an opportunity to learn to value others. This can be practiced in the therapeutic milieu by providing individualized nursing care. Nurses should actively listen to children in their interactions, and even young children should be encouraged to express their needs. The child's importance as a person can be shown through the approach the nurse uses in providing basic care. Older children can benefit from more in-depth discussions and the use of journals to gain perspective on the direction their life is taking. Above all, the nurse should actively assist all children in realistically assessing their abilities and potential to contribute to a better world.

> Many people believe that youth in contemporary society lack a sense of hope, direction, and purpose in life. Do you agree with this, and if so, what sociocultural factors might influence the learning of this skill?

NURSING DIAGNOSES AND RELATED INTERVENTIONS

Once the nurse has completed the ego competency skill assessment, the appropriate nursing diagnosis should be formulated. Nursing interventions can then be identified for each skill deficit, developmental stage, and related nursing diagnoses as summarized in Table 34-2.

Altered Family Processes

The family should be included in the child's treatment process as soon as possible. Psychiatric illness in any one family member affects all other family members as well. Thus the nurse can work with the individual needs of each family and either promote family competence through education and support or engage the family in focused clinical interventions, such as family therapy (see Chapter 30). In addition, some children with psychiatric problems may not have had consistent nurturing or may come from families that display maladaptive responses. Therefore activities that are less threatening should be used initially to teach the child about family relationships. Pictures of families cut out from magazines can provide opportunities for a child to interpret emotional content in the picture and describe what he or she thinks is happening in the picture. The nurse can then describe a healthy family scenario for the child to learn about adaptive family functioning.

> Many people believe that families are in crisis in this country. Describe the evidence for this conclusion and give specific ways to address each problem identified.

Altered Growth and Development

Normal growth and development in childhood requires a supportive, nurturing environment. A child who has a psychiatric illness often has delayed physical and emotional development (see Table 34-2). However, through carefully planned nursing interventions, a child can be taught the skills that have not yet been developed. For example, for the child to achieve independence in dressing, grooming, and room cleaning, a checklist can be made using pictures instead of words. Points can then be given for each accomplished task. Using similar behavioral interventions (see Chapter 28), the nurse can assist the child to make significant gains in the area of growth and development.

When considering altered growth and development, delays are often the presenting problem. However, many children who are unprotected by their parents and have

Table 34-2   Ego Competency Skills Summary

Competency skill	Developmental stage and tasks	Related nursing diagnosis	Nursing care for skill deficit
Trusting, closeness, relationship building	**Infancy** Trust Attachment Learning to walk, talk, and feed self	Fear Anxiety Posttrauma response Altered family processes Altered growth and development	Encourage interaction. Use face-to-face positioning. Use touch and nurturance. Offer food and transitional objects. Be attentive without being unnecessarily intrusive. Offer nurturance to the child's mother. Make attempts to connect family to child. Take time to develop relationship through play.
Handling separation and independence	**Toddlers** Autonomy Separation Toilet training Learning right from wrong	Chronic low self-esteem Anxiety Altered thought processes Coping, ineffective individual	Offer frequent exercise and motor activities. Allow child opportunities to make choices. Offer transitional object. Take control if child is out of control; otherwise let child have some control.
Handling joint decisions and interpersonal conflicts	**Preschoolers** Initiative Tolerance of others Sexual identity Socialization Developing a conscience	Impaired social interaction Impaired verbal communication Violence, potential for Decisional conflict	Set up opportunities for problem solving and cooperative thinking. Assist child to identify fears through books, art, play. Shape appropriate socialization using reinforcement. Become model for conflict resolution.
Dealing with frustration and unfavorable events Celebrating good things, feeling pleasure	**Middle childhood** Industry Physical skill development Peer relationships Learning to read, write, and calculate Development of morality and values	Trauma, potential for Social interaction impaired Hopelessness Powerlessness Body image disturbance	Assist the child to cope with frustration using stories and plays. Model cooperation and reinforce cooperative behavior. Do not use shame or humilation to gain control. Have fun with the child. Use community meetings for peer support and modeling. Use positive reinforcement for child's strengths and abilities.
Working for delayed gratification Relaxing and playing	**Early adolescence** Identity Role acceptance New relations with peers of both sexes	Altered growth and development Altered sexuality patterns Social isolation Anticipatory grieving Sleep pattern disturbance	Use daily expectations and games to teach delayed gratification. Encourage self-reinforcement. Encourage playfulness at appropriate times.
Cognitive processing Adaptive sense purpose and direction	**Later adolescence** Emotional and economic independence from parents Preparation for occupation Civic responsibility	Altered growth and development Social interaction impaired Altered thought process Anxiety Personal identity disturbance Family coping, potential for growth Hopelessness Powerlessness	Offer games that use cognitive processing. Discuss abstractions like the moral of stories or movies. Actively listen to and encourage the expression of needs and goals. In community meetings discuss relevant issues and life events. Assist the child in realistically assessing one's ability and potential.

early exposure to abuse or violence can develop a pseudomaturity. At times, they may have experienced a role reversal with their parents; the child may have become the more responsible person while the parent assumed the dependent role. These children will appear to be overcompliant with adults. Although this behavior may seem well-adapted, it is inappropriate developmentally and should not be reinforced. Rather, the child should be encouraged to choose developmentally appropriate play activities, and the parent encouraged to resume appropriate adult role responsibilities.

Altered Sexuality Patterns

Children who are exposed to sexual behavior prematurally may exhibit precocious sexuality. Appearing seductive, they may be particularly vulnerable to sexual abuse. Boys who have been sexually abused by a male may reenact the abuse experience by sexually acting out with other boys. If the other boy involved is considerably younger or coercion is used, this behavior is abusive and the other child then becomes the victim. These issues need to be discussed openly with children who have altered sexuality patterns by a supportive nurse who will provide them with needed insight about their behavior, information about prevention, and protection from repetition of the experience[5,14] (see Chapter 38).

Altered Thought Processes

Under stress, children often have difficulty thinking, identifying options, and making decisions. They become easily frustrated and may respond to their frustration with aggressive behavior. The most effective intervention for the school-aged child with this problem is to assist the child in thinking through options in a nonthreatening way. This thinking process can be practiced throughout the day by inventing a hypothetical situation that is potentially threatening and helping the child think through possible options. The created situations can gradually become more and more similar to the child's current life situation, and actual problems on the unit can be processed in a similar way. Through practicing identifying options and making decisions in nonstressful situations, the child can learn to respond more adaptively to stressful situations.

Although rare, children may have psychotic episodes. It is important that the child psychiatric nurse be able to discriminate between normal and abnormal thought processes in children. Healthy preschool and school-aged children typically have vivid imaginations, and their normal fears can become quite intense; however, these responses should not be confused with psychotic delusions or hallucinations. Children who are psychotic rarely discuss these experiences. Their symptoms are distinguished by their level of intensity, distress, and du-

ration. For example, a child may hallucinate seeing the devil or animals. These psychotic episodes are terrifying and should be treated as psychiatric emergencies. Antipsychotic medications are usually indicated to control these episodes.

Anticipatory Grieving

Children in chaotic families often experience many losses. With the chronic nature of life stressors, these children may experience the loss of stability, loss of security, and in many ways the loss of childhood. Children who have experienced repetitive losses begin to anticipate the future with grief. They may lose interest in playing and become withdrawn. Children who are withdrawn generally do not cause any disturbance in the milieu, so their needs can easily be overlooked. However, they need to be encouraged to actively express their grief by drawing or participating in play therapy, and then to join the other children in unstructured play. Rumination is discouraged, and participation is encouraged. Most importantly, the significance of their grief is never minimized.

Anxiety

Children who are anxious may become very active and appear to be uncooperative. Gentle touch and redirection is often effective in restoring a child's self-control. If this is insufficient, a child may need to be moved to a less stimulating environment, such as a small empty room to reduce anxiety and regain self-control. Also, children may have separation anxiety related to particular individuals, often their parents. While the child may have difficulty separating from a parent, the parent may similarly be ambivalent about leaving the child. Each may require a great deal of reassurance to tolerate the separation required for hospitalization. The nurse can help the child reduce anxiety by providing some attachment object, such as a small cuddly toy or something the parent brings from home. Often, drawing pictures of home, a family gathering, or the family's reaction to the hospitalization can be reassuring to a young child (Fig. 34-2). The nurse can also assist the parent by having frequent telephone contact to report the child's progress. Nursing interventions are then planned to help the child and parent anticipate the future, reduce anxiety related to each other, and focus on further development of the child's sense of self.

Body Image Disturbance

Some emotionally ill children may have distorted ideas about their body and experience gender identity confusion. This is usually identified in drawings in which a child may consistently delete important body parts or

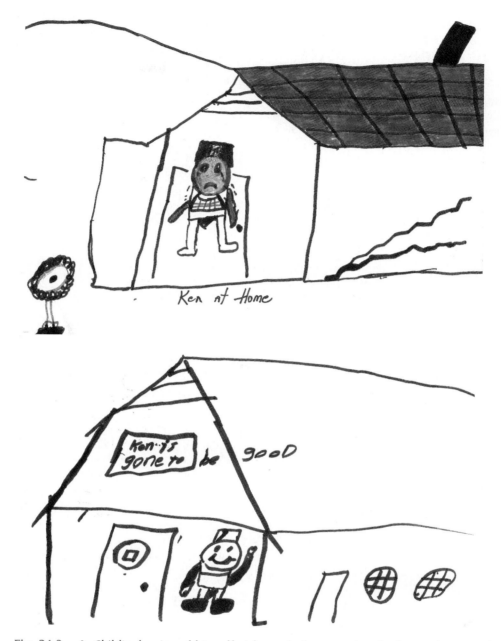

Fig. 34-2 **A,** Child's drawing of himself at home before entering the hospital: "I'm sad about the things I do and how people feel about me." **B,** Same child's drawing of himself entering the hospital.

draw gender-specific details that are confused, such as breasts on a boy or male genitalia on a girl. An effective nursing intervention is to have a child recline on a large piece of paper and draw a body outline. The child then draws in features, clothes, and other accessories. The children as a group may then have discussions about differences between boys and girls. At this time, open discussion can clarify any distortions or misperceptions. Also, children who have been sexually abused are often confused about body invasion for themselves and others. These children are frequently intrusive and

need to be taught about appropriate and inappropriate touching and respect for body boundaries. Nurses, male and female, can improve a child's body image disturbance through thoughtful, supportive care.

Chronic Low Self-Esteem

Children who have psychiatric illness often have low self-esteem. It may be expressed by infrequent eye contact, lack of motivation, or the use of negative behavior to seek attention. Specific therapeutic activities can be planned to improve a child's self-esteem.[28] Accomplishment of a goal, no matter how small, is very rewarding, and incremental goal setting can be an effective way to provide opportunities for success. For example, a child who is a chronic complainer could be rewarded for refraining from complaining for 15 minutes. The time can then be gradually increased. At the same time, new methods of communication, such as initiating a conversation, can be taught and rewarded. A bedtime review of accomplishments of the day in which the child lists personal strengths can also be positively reinforcing. Finally, the nurse can provide information and guidance to parents to help them enhance their child's self-esteem such as those listed in Table 34-3.[31]

Decisional Conflict

Children who have been abused or otherwise traumatized frequently respond to their experience by appearing defiant and oppositional. In evaluating a child's ability to handle interpersonal conflict, the child's developmental level should be considered. There are many tasks that are difficult for children to complete, particularly if they are developmentally delayed or anxious. Therefore expectations need to be carefully evaluated to determine if they exceed a child's capability. After a careful nursing assessment, an intervention should be planned to reward or positively reinforce a child's appropriate decision-making ability. For example, a point system in which a child earns points and then exchanges these for privileges may be very helpful. Parents may also be instructed in how to develop a similar program for the child at home.

Family Coping: Potential for Growth

Each family has an extensive history that has shaped and impacted the development of each family member. This collective family history and its adaptability for change has a powerful influence over a child's prognosis for learning, practicing, and applying new skills. Therefore the family's willingness to participate in the therapeutic process and interest in making change should guide the nursing intervention that is planned for the child. For example, if the child is returning home after discharge, the parents should be requested to participate in a parent training program early in the hospitalization process. During the parent training, a nurse models the effective use of reinforcement, communication, and behavior management techniques identified in Box 34-1, while another nurse watches the modeling of these skills with the parents and provides instruction about them (Fig. 34-3). The parents are then expected to practice these techniques with their child during the course of hospitalization. Throughout this time the par-

Table 34-3 Enhancing a Child's Self-Esteem

Targeted area	Strategy
Caregiver expectations	Describe expectations for the child
	Assess anticipated developmental milestones
	Review family patterns and influences
Personal value	Communicate confidence in the child
	Structure situations to promote success of the child
	Implement effective ways of praising the child
	Role model self-value
Communication	Listen attentively
	Encourage openness to feelings
	Avoid using judgmental statements
	Elicit different points of view
Discipline	Use effective methods of limit setting
	Discuss and implement appropriate consequences
	Review problem-solving techniques
	Discourage use of physical punishment
Guidance	Encourage open exchanges with the child
	Know the child's activities away from home
	Express interest in school events
	Become familiar with the child's friends
Autonomy	Demonstrate respect for the child
	Promote the child's responsible decision making
	Expect reciprocal respect

Adapted from Sieving R, Zirbel-Donisch S: J *Pediatr Health Care* 4:290, 1990.

ents are encouraged to function more and more independently in managing their child's behavior while being supported by the nursing staff. Before the child is discharged, specific plans are made for adapting these skills in the home.

 Do you think the strategies for behavior management of children described in Box 34-1 are "culture bound" or "culture free"? Defend your position.

Fear

Excessive or maladaptive fear in children may be displayed by aggressive or oppositional behavior. If children have been abused by someone they trusted, they will have fear associated with establishing close, trusting relationships. To minimize fears during hospitaliza-

Box 34-1

STRATEGIES FOR BEHAVIOR MANAGEMENT OF CHILDREN

1. Respond warmly to a child's positive behaviors.
2. Communicate approval by facial expression, tone of voice, and touch.
3. Express excitement around a child's accomplishments.
4. Ignore negative behavior whenever appropriate.
5. Refrain from giving unnecessary commands.
6. Respond calmly but effectively to negative behaviors. (Example: "No yelling," stated in a calm tone of voice.)
7. Use timeouts when necessary and appropriate. (30 to 60 seconds per year of a child's age.)
8. Avoid making unrealistic demands of a child.
9. Minimize negative remarks about the child.
10. Communicate frequently using the following techniques:
    a. The parent or staff member telling about personal experiences.
    b. The parent or staff member listening, paraphrasing, and asking "follow-up questions."
    c. Nightly review of positive behaviors noted during the day that the parent wants to be repeated. (Negative behaviors should not be mentioned at this time.)

Adapted from Strayhorn J, Weidman C: J *Am Acad Child Adolesc Psychiatry* 28:888, 1989.

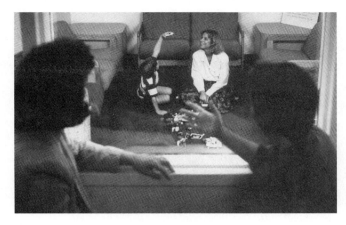

Fig. 34-3   A parent training program. The nurse with the child is modeling behavior management techniques, while a second nurse is providing instruction to the parent about them.

tion, consistent schedules should be maintained, and children should be prepared for changes in activities. For example, sometimes at change of shift children can suddenly become agitated as the oncoming staff is beginning to organize activities. The change of personnel is often difficult for young children to understand and tolerate. Therefore staggered scheduling and discussion about the changing of personnel may be helpful in reducing children's fears. If unexpected symptoms of fear or agitation appear, an assessment should be made to determine if this behavior is related to a change that has taken place in the nursing milieu.

Hopelessness

Many children live in chaotic and dangerous environments. Communities are often unsafe, and schools may be plagued with violence. Children in these situations may feel very hopeless. The hospitalization is an opportunity to teach these children and families about community helping agencies, to find advocates for the child, and to teach the child about self-protection. Trips to the police station, fire station, or community centers may help reduce the child's sense of hopelessness. Often a

child's relative, school teacher, guidance counselor, or church member can provide the child with a concerned adult in the community. Contact with some individual or agency that can provide safety for the child is an essential nursing intervention before the child is discharged.

Children who are frequently hospitalized or who live in foster care or in residential facilities often experience hopelessness. It can be helpful to make a scrapbook about the child's life. It should begin with the child's birth and biological family. By drawing pictures or using pictures from magazines, a book can be created. The current hospitalization should be included with a picture of the nursing staff. Accomplishments from the treatment program are featured as important life events. Autographs and words of encouragement may be written by staff members to the child. The child can then take this record to the next treatment facility or foster home. In this way the child begins to record life events so that hope for the future can be created.

> Imagine you are taking one of your school-age patients on a trip to the community. What helping agency would you visit, and what specifically would you like the child to learn from the experience?

Impaired Social Interaction

Children with emotional problems frequently have not learned basic social skills that help them relate to others. The therapeutic nurse-patient relationship can be used to learn these skills. Group therapy (see Chapter 29) and behavioral therapy strategies (see Chapter 28) such as social skills training and modeling socially appropriate responses that demonstrate respect for other individuals are also effective nursing interventions. Children can practice these skills by enacting plays or creating stories that demonstrate socially appropriate solutions to normal childhood dilemmas. Through guidance, demonstration, practice, and feedback, social interaction can be improved.

Some children who are hospitalized may not be able to control their behavior in a group setting. A child with this level of impairment requires intensive social training by a nurse with whom a positive relationship exists. This nurse models socially appropriate behavior and then asks the child to repeat the behavior. This "game" is played, gradually incorporating other staff members into it. Slowly, the child is incorporated into the milieu and becomes attached to other role models. Eventually the child begins to internalize these socialization behaviors and is able to become part of the group.

For children who are cognitively impaired, early social skills training is essential. These children are often small in stature. Consequently, they are often infantalized by their parents and the nursing staff. However, a cognitively impaired child needs to be encouraged to function as independently as possible. Therefore a plan of care should be developed and adhered to precisely. Because of the child's limited cognitive ability, exact repetition by all members of the nursing staff to the child's behavior is crucial. With repetition of responses from others, the cognitively impaired child who is poorly socialized will learn appropriate age-related behavior.

Impaired Verbal Communication

Being able to describe personal experience and express feelings is important to a child's mental health. The hospitalization experience provides the child with healthy role models and opportunities to practice clear communication. For example, the nurse can role model by initiating a conversation with a child about some recent life experience, such as something that happened on the way to work. The nurse can then prompt the child to tell about some personal life experience. As the child begins, the nurse reinforces communication with a smile, nod, and touch.

After the child has mastered the skill of talking about external experiences, the nurse can change the intervention to talking about an internal experience or feeling. Once again, the nurse may begin by describing a feeling that has become associated with an event, and then prompt the child, wait, and reinforce. A child who has never been encouraged to talk about feelings may require the use of therapeutic play involving animals or play figures to express feelings or may be better able to talk about feelings by drawing. This is evident in the artwork shown in Fig. 34-4 in which a 6-year-old boy was able to draw his different feelings.

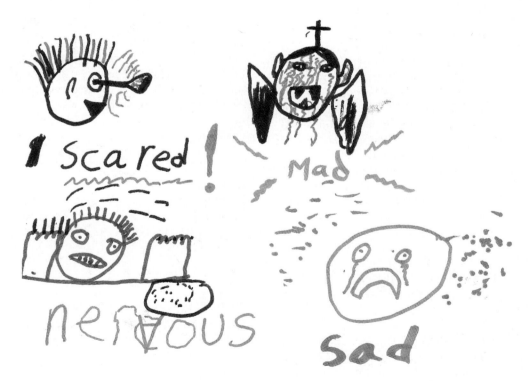

Fig. 34-4   Drawing by a hospitalized 6-year-old boy of his different feelings.

Have you ever tried to talk with a shy or unresponsive child? What techniques did you find to be effective in drawing the child out, and could these same strategies be applied to a child in a psychiatric setting?

Ineffective Individual Coping

Hospitalized children often have chronic overwhelming family stress with inadequate coping resources and support. The resulting dysfunctional behavior is often observed in a structured situation, such as school, where compliance is required. These children need to learn more effective methods of coping. School-age children may use a variety of coping strategies. Boys often report engaging in physical activities, such as riding bicycles, to cope with stress, while girls often find talking to friends to be helpful. Once a child learns to use more adaptive skills, the focus should shift to integrating them into the daily routines of home or school.

Personal Identity Disturbance

As children approach adolescence they begin to struggle with an individual identity. In adolescence, when they are able to use the skill of abstract thinking, they are able to conceive of the thoughts of others, and questions about their place in the world begin to emerge. Rapid changes occur in self-discovery, and this period is characterized by uncertainty and confusion. Even for healthy children, this period is emotionally difficult. Children who have not observed healthy adults negotiate successfully in life are unable to conceive of themselves as competent adults in the world.

Without role models for finding meaning in life, a child's personal identity formation becomes a crisis. If a child does not have successful adult models in life, fictional models can be used to help children imagine success in their own life. For example, nursing staff may select a movie, such as one of those listed in Box 34-2, that provides positive role models. After viewing the movie as a group, the nurse can lead a discussion about the hero's or heroine's life, talking about the obstacles the individual had to confront and overcome. It is useful to discuss the skills the characters applied in their efforts to overcome problems. The discussion will naturally flow into finding direction and purpose in life. It is within the context of important discussions such as this that a child with personal identity disturbance can develop a competent identity of self and meet the challenges of the adult world.

Posttrauma Response

Children who have been traumatized may have sudden and dramatic mood changes. Often, some unexpected event reminds them of a previous abuse episode, and they experience the anxiety associated with the earlier abuse. At that time their behavior may change without any identifiable cause. Nursing interventions such as art therapy and play therapy can be very useful in assisting a child to cope with a previous abuse incident and reduce a posttrauma response.[21,24] Through a guided process using play or drawings, a child may be able to identify those things that are associated with the trauma, for example, certain types of weather, body features such as mustaches, or experiences such as hearing loud voices. With this awareness, a child can learn to anticipate responses and may be able to gain some control over them.

Potential for Trauma

Safety from trauma in children is always a health concern. Children who have low frustration tolerance are particularly vulnerable to trauma, whether from accidents, self-injury, or assault from others. On the psychiatric unit these children may quickly provoke other children toward aggression. Therefore a nursing milieu plan to address this problem is essential. Teaching coping skills and using large motor exercises with an intermittent room program is effective until a child is able to achieve a higher level of tolerance and reduce the potential for trauma.

Potential for Violence

Being able to handle conflict without becoming aggressive toward oneself or others is very important for children to learn. In contemporary American culture, violence is widespread, and children may perceive it to be

---

Box 34-2
MOVIES WITH POSITIVE ROLE MODELS

The Black Stallion	D.A.R.Y.L.
Charlotte's Web	The Return of the Jedi
The Empire Strikes Back	School Ties
Fern Gully	The Secret Garden
Home Alone	Star Wars
Huckleberry Finn	Where the Red Fern Grows
The Last Starfighter	The Wizard of Oz
The Little Mermaid	Man Without a Face
The Neverending Story	My Girl
Old Yeller	Radio Flyer

an acceptable way of dealing with conflict. Therefore alternatives need to be taught so that a child will have a repertoire of solutions to use in conflict situations (see Chapter 27).

For a younger child, a brief timeout may be effective in interrupting behavior that is escalating or becoming out of control. Older school-age children may benefit from an intermittent room program in learning self-control. During these periods alone it may be helpful for a child to read a story about a similar conflict or for an older child to write thoughts and feelings in a journal.

Another useful strategy is to establish a contract with a child who is capable of understanding, writing, and adhering to it.[20] Such a contract would specify the level of precautions and restrictions that the child would face based on the specific behavior. Contracts allow the child to play an active role in the treatment process and provide immediate and constructive feedback about the child's actions.

As a last resort, seclusion may be needed. Seclusion is never used as punishment, for the convenience of staff, or as a substitute for individualized treatment[12] (see Critical Thinking about Contemporary Issues). During seclusion the child should be encouraged to express feelings so that the nurse can help the child gain insight into the interconnectedness of emotions, actions, relationships, and alternatives to aggressive behavior.

Powerlessness

Children who feel powerless have often been abused or may be trying to cope with a significant loss. They appear to be withdrawn and depressed and have difficulty eating or sleeping. Play therapy and bibliotherapy are effective in helping a child cope with these overwhelming experiences. In the milieu, small goals that a child accomplishes can reduce feelings of powerlessness. It must be remembered that children may, in fact, be powerless in protecting themselves from an abusive adult. Therefore a child's safety and risk for abuse or neglect should be carefully assessed. If necessary, referrals should be made to appropriate child protection agencies. The hospitalization itself, however, is an excellent opportunity to teach children about abuse prevention. Through an abuse prevention program, children can be taught how to better protect themselves and not feel as powerless.

Sleep Pattern Disturbance

Children who are experiencing anxiety may have sleep disturbances and nightmares. If a child is receiving psychostimulants, such as methylphenidate (Ritalin), and has disturbed sleep, the dosage or time of administration may need to be changed. Sleep disturbances can

 CRITICAL THINKING ABOUT CONTEMPORARY ISSUES

Is the Use of Seclusion and Restraints with Children Therapeutic?

The use of seclusion and restraints in the care and treatment of children with psychiatric problems has been the subject of considerable debate.[12] Advocates of these techniques cite the widespread problem of violent behavior among psychiatric patients, including children, and describe the clinical efficacy of these interventions.[3] In fact, seclusion and restraint appear to be widely used in inpatient settings by nurses who are the front-line professionals responsible for initiating emergency procedures and supervising the actions taken to prevent violent outbursts. On the other hand, these interventions have also been associated with punishment, custodial care, and institutional abuse and neglect. Some even view seclusion as a violation of a patient's civil liberties.

In examining the issue, Wong and colleagues[34] recommend a three-pronged approach to the reduction of dangerous, inappropriate behavior by children, including aggressive, destructive, and highly disruptive behavior. First, they recommend teaching and reinforcing acceptable ways for children to express themselves and satisfy their needs. Second, the authors advocate the use of procedures such as timeouts, room programs, or open-door seclusion to reduce inappropriate behavior. Third, they stress the need to evaluate the effect of these interventions on the individual child and to continuously monitor the efficacy of these interventions in research studies using objective measures and experimental controls. Thus like all other nursing interventions, the therapeutic value of seclusion and restraints for children is determined by the treatment goals, context of care, and respect shown by the nurse for the needs of the individual child and family. ▼

also be treated with various nursing interventions. Warm milk helps to induce sleep in some children. Back massage can also be helpful in encouraging relaxation in children. Many children's stories that deal with nightmares and fears related to bedtime can be read and talked about. In general, however, the most effective way to make a successful transition to bedtime and subsequently to sleep is to develop a consistent, predictable bedtime ritual, such as taking a bath followed by "quiet time" and a bedtime story. The consistent application of these activities usually reduces this maladaptive response in children.

Social Isolation

Dysfunctional families frequently isolate themselves from others. Young children may not have had normal socialization experiences with other children or adults. Therefore the opportunity for teaching positive social skills during hospitalization is critical. The simplest activity, such as looking out of a window with a child, can become an opportunity for learning. Cars and people provide an endless array of speculation and imagined scenarios about life. A trip for a diagnostic test can also be an adventure for a child. A sensitive nurse capitalizes on the opportunity to interest the child in people and the surroundings at all times. These experiences turn ordinary events into occasions for learning, relaxing, and playing.

THERAPEUTIC TREATMENT MODALITIES

Once a thorough assessment has been completed and nursing diagnoses have been formulated, the nurse can implement a variety of individualized interventions that are effective in treating maladaptive responses in children.[6,9,19] The following treatment modalities are particularly effective when caring for an emotionally ill child.

Therapeutic Play

Because play is normal and fun for children, it is a very effective tool for nurses to use in individual interventions.[30] Interventions that are enjoyable, arouse curiosity, and stimulate the imagination will capture the child's attention and interest. Many children with psychiatric problems may have lost interest in play or may have never experienced the joy of spontaneous play. Learning to play is critical not only to a child's development but also to mental health. Therapeutic aspects of play and their beneficial outcomes are listed in Table 34-4. The nurse should keep these elements in mind when incorporating play therapy into the plan of care.

The first step is for the nurse to develop a therapeutic alliance with the child so that life can be perceived from the child's perspective and the child's concerns can be anticipated. When a child feels understood, participation in therapeutic play with the nurse is common. If anxious, the child's developmental level may fluctuate rapidly, and this should be continuously assessed by the nurse. Care must be taken, however, to ensure that the child not fail at the activity, either because the develop-

Table 34-4   Therapeutic Aspects of Play

Therapeutic factor	Beneficial outcome
Overcoming resistance	Working alliance
Communication	Understanding
Competence	Self-esteem
Creative thinking	Problem solving
Catharsis	Emotional release
Abreaction	Perspective on traumatic event
Role-playing	Learning new behaviors
Fantasy	Compensation and sublimation
Teaching through metaphors	Insight
Relationship enhancement	Trust in others
Mastering developmental fears	Growth and development
Game play	Socialization

Adapted from Schaefer C: *The therapeutic powers of play*, Northvale, NJ, 1993, Jason Aronson.

mental level is too advanced or because of the severity of the child's symptoms. Children will become easily frustrated with play that is too difficult and thus feel a sense of failure at a time when their self-esteem is already compromised. Nursing interventions therefore need to be adapted to the child's presenting developmental level and gradually change as the child's anxiety is reduced.

Toys that are age appropriate and imaginative should be offered to a child. These may include blocks, a play house, family characters, soldiers, trucks, and rescue vehicles. The child is then encouraged to begin play without specific direction from the nurse. The nurse may ask the following clarifying questions:

▼ What is this person doing?
▼ How does this little boy feel?
▼ What is happening now?

The nurse can then follow up with some clarifying and validating statements such as, "This little girl looks afraid." The nurse, however, refrains from guiding the play, making unnecessary remarks, or making interpretations that may link the play to the child's life experience. The play should continue until the child is no longer engaged. The nurse can then evaluate the play intervention by considering the following questions:

▼ What did the play activity communicate about the child's development level?
▼ What emotions and behavioral responses were evidenced by the child while at play?
▼ What information can be added to the child's assessment or treatment plan based on observations during play therapy?

Art Therapy

Drawing is a valuable tool for children to use in describing an event or expressing a feeling.[18] Children often do not have the vocabulary to express themselves, and they feel pressured to answer questions they do not understand. Drawings provide the nurse with the child's perspective of an experience. Through drawings, a child can provide information about behavior and developmental maturity that the nurse can then use to assist the child in preparing for future change (Fig. 34-5).

Art is particularly useful in assessing a child's therapeutic needs. The nurse may begin by asking the child to draw a picture of something that happened before being admitted to the hospital. Children also can be asked to draw a picture of their family, a person or object they are afraid of, or where they are going after they leave the hospital. Children may find drawing stressful if they have been criticized about it in the past. However, with some encouragement, they will usually produce an interesting and often revealing picture. The nurse might ask the child what is happening in the picture or to name the people. The nurse should make notes about whatever the child reports the people are saying or thinking. This process can be continued until the child becomes disinterested in the activity or if the child's anxiety level becomes too great. In considering the effectiveness of this intervention, the nurse should consider the following:

▼ What was learned about the child's experience and perceptions from this intervention?

▼ What do the pictures reveal about the child's view of the world?

▼ Is there any gender confusion evident?

▼ Is there any distortion between the child's perception of personal experience and that which was reported?

Children's Games

Children with behavioral or emotional problems often have difficulty with motor control. These symptoms may be developmental or may be caused by anxiety. In either case, games that teach motor control can help the child. These games include Simon Says, Red Light, Musical Chairs, and many others. Games can also be used to increase a child's concentration and frustration tolerance. Games such as Candy Land, Hide and Seek, and Find the Button can be played with gradually increasing difficulty to teach these skills.

When initiating these activities the nurse should consider the child's motor development and level of anxiety and decide among games that engage large or small muscle groups. Thought should also be given to the child's tolerance for frustration and competition. Games may then be modified to meet the specific therapeutic needs of the child. Games can also be played with in-

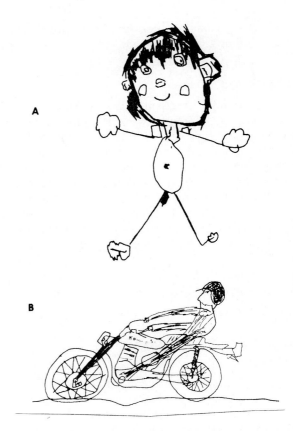

Fig. 34-5 Self-image drawings by two boys. **A,** Drawing by a 7-year-old boy. **B,** Drawing by a 13-year-old boy. Differences related to age, body perceptions, and interests are evident.

creasing demands placed on concentration and cognitive processing; however, it is important to stop playing a game that is too difficult or stressful for a child.

During the game it is important to keep in mind the therapeutic goal and for the nurse to be flexible about the rules. Although the goal is to challenge the child, it is also important to have fun and to use the game to shape and reinforce new adaptive behaviors for the child. The nurse should consider the following questions at the completion of the game:

▼ Was the game developmentally appropriate for the child?

▼ Was playing the game a pleasurable experience?

▼ If not, why not?

▼ Was the nurse's therapeutic goal met?

▼ How should the game be modified in the future to further the child's skill development and adaptive coping responses?

Bibliotherapy

Bibliotherapy is the use of literature to help children identify and express feelings within the structure and safety of the nurse-patient relationship[7] (Box 34-3). Because children actively engage in imaginary thinking, they can easily identify with the fictional characters in a story and gain insight into their own lives.

In implementing this activity, the nurse should carefully consider the child's age and attention span. To be effective, the story should have illustrations that capture the child's interest. The nurse should also think about the child's situation and try to select a book that describes a situation or issue relevant to the child's life situation. For example, hospitalized children who are separated from their families may be comforted by a story about a kitten who gets lost. It is often helpful to offer a choice of two books to the child. One book could be directly related to the child's experience and the other one less directly related, since the child may not be ready to confront life situations directly.

While reading the story the nurse should be sensitive to the child's response. If the text is wordy, the child may become bored or distracted. If this occurs, paraphrasing the story or asking what the child thinks is happening to the characters may be helpful. In this way the child's imagination becomes engaged and the experience will have value. It is also important to give the child an opportunity to reflect on the story and discuss any thoughts or feelings about the characters, since it is often easier to talk about the feelings of the characters than one's own.

After reading the story, the nurse should evaluate the usefulness of the intervention and assess the following:

▼ Was the story appropriate to the child's developmental age?
▼ Was the child engaged with the story?
▼ Did the child enjoy the experience?
▼ What was learned by the child and about the child as a result of this intervention?

 Traditional fairy tales are based on and convey many gender stereotypes. Do you think this is a problem, and how might you go about dealing with this issue in working with children?

Storytelling

The therapeutic use of storytelling for relieving distress and teaching new coping skills to children is a valuable intervention. Because children do not separate imaginary experiences from real experiences, stories that teach appropriate problem-solving skills can serve as models for real situations.

Initially the nurse needs to identify a social skill that the child needs to learn, such as assertiveness training. The nurse may then make up a story about a character who needs that particular skill, giving the hero or heroine similar characteristics to the child. It is important to select an ending to the story that will guide the child in learning the skill. Next, the nurse should plan a time and place for storytelling that is free from distractions and interruptions. Bedtime is often a natural time for individual storytelling. The story should be told using animated facial expressions and expressive voice inflections, and the child should be actively involved in the story as much as possible. At the end of the story the nurse should ask the child about the story and how it made the child feel. This may then lead to a broader discussion of other aspects of the child's life. In evaluating the outcome of the intervention, the nurse should consider the following questions:

▼ Could this story character be used to teach this child other skills through other stories?
▼ Could the child add to the story or make up one of his or her own?
▼ What was the moral of the story, and how did it apply to the child?
▼ Could the story be used in other creative ways such as by having the child enact the story or by including others?

Autogenic Storytelling

A similar version of storytelling is **autogenic storytelling**—a therapeutic activity in which the child participates in creating the story. Nurses may find this activity particularly valuable in helping children explore fears related to traumatic events. This intervention is particularly useful for a school-age child who has been traumatized or is having nightmares. A child will often reenact anxiety-related experiences in a story portrayed by animals or other fictional characters. Unlike real life, the child can have control over the experience if it is relived in play or storytelling.

Children often like audiotaping the story and then listening to their voice telling the story. The nurse should discuss the general structure of the story with the child, and together they can decide on the main characters and the beginning plot. The nurse should begin the story with the introduction and then stop, allowing the child to add the next event. The nurse picks up the storytelling when the child runs out of material or the child becomes particularly anxious or overstimulated. At the end of the story, if the child has chosen an unhealthy ending, the nurse begins the storytelling intervention again. In the retelling, however, the nurse takes on a more active role and adds adaptive responses at important moments in the story. This allows the child to explore a traumatic event while also learning healthy coping responses.

This intervention can be very useful for children who have had traumatic and abusive experiences. However,

it is critical that the nurse implementing this intervention be attentive to clues from the child indicating increased anxiety. The nurse should also avoid interpreting the story to the child, and this intervention should not be used to coerce the child to reveal information about an experience of abuse. Instead, the child should be given the freedom to explore the experience through storytelling with as much freedom as possible. At the conclusion the nurse should evaluate the following:

▼ What emotions and behaviors did the child portray in the story?
▼ What were the predominant themes?
▼ How did the child resolve the story, and what does it suggest about the child's ability to problem solve and resolve conflicts?

Enacting Plays

Enacting plays gives children the opportunity to practice new behaviors with peers in a structured activity. Using a story with a simple and familiar plot, the nurse can choose a play for social skill development. It can be performed by groups of children or by one child using a set of toy people characters.

In designing this activity, the nurse should consider a recurring social problem in the group or a symptom that has caused or is causing a child difficulty. The nurse can then find a book or write a story that depicts the problem and teaches an appropriate and adaptive response. The children should be allowed to select the characters, and dress-up props are particularly helpful to engage the children's imagination. The play may then be performed with the nurse prompting the children with the lines. Frequently, children will ask to repeat the performance and change characters. Each child needs to be given the opportunity to play each part so that all of the character options the story offers can be enacted. If a video camera is available, it can be therapeutic to videotape the performance and replay it for the children. At the conclusion the nurse should review the intervention considering how it affected each child:

▼ Was enacting the play fun for the children involved?
▼ Are there other social skills that the children need to practice in this format in the future?

Medication Management

Many emotionally ill children receive psychotropic medication as part of their treatment plan. Tables 34-5 and 34-6 list some of the drugs commonly used with children and adolescents along with their indications and dosages. Child psychiatric nurses need to be knowledgeable about these medications and develop interventions to monitor, educate, and evaluate medication

Table 34-5 Child Psychiatric Disorders and Drug Treatments

Disorder	Drug class	Comments/nursing considerations
Affective disorders: depression	Antidepressants	Careful diagnosis is necessary to differentiate depression from normal feeling states
Anxiety, impulse problems, transient insomnia, acute extrapyramidal symptoms	Antihistamines (Benadryl)	Tolerance to sedative effects may develop
Attention deficit–hyperactivity disorder (ADHD)	Stimulants	Used when primary symptoms are manifest in school Less reliable in preschooler and adolescent
	Antidepressants	Once-a-day dose and improved monitoring of compliance and toxicity using plasma levels Monitor cardiac status and signs of overdose
	Antipsychotics	Sometimes used in combination with stimulants for symptomatic relief
Conduct disorders	Antipsychotics, stimulants	May improve a child's capacity to benefit from social and educational interventions
Eating disorders	Antihistamines (cyproheptadine), antipsychotics	Anorexia nervosa
	Antidepressants (imipramine)	Bulimia
Functional enuresis	Antidepressants (imipramine)	Used when an immediate therapeutic effect is necessary because of severe emotional distress
Mental retardation with psychiatric symptoms and behavioral problems	Antipsychotics	Used to control behavioral and psychiatric complications
	Antidepressants	Treat affective symptoms
	Stimulants	Treat ADHD
	Lithium	Helps control aggression
	Carbamazepine	Anticonvulsant that can help control aggression
Obsessive-compulsive disorder (OCD)	Antidepressants (clomipramine)	Newly used to reduce OCD symptoms
Pervasive developmental disorders	Antipsychotics	Used to treat agitation, insomnia, sterotypic movements
Schizophrenia	Antipsychotics	As with adults, choice of drug depends on prior efficacy and the spectrum of pharmacological properties
Separation anxiety disorder	Antidepressants (imipramine)	Effective at high doses Speculative: panic disorder symptoms
Tic disorders: Tourette's disorder	Antipsychotics (haloperidol) Alpha-adrenergic agonist (clonidine)	Stimulants are avoided because they worsen symptoms

Table 34-6   Drugs Commonly Used in Childhood Psychiatric Disorders

Drug	Description	Daily dose (mg/kg of body weight)	Side effects
STIMULANTS: GENERIC (TRADE)			
Dextroamphetamine (Dexedrine)	Short-acting (2-4 hr)	0.3-1.5*; 1-3 doses daily	*Short term*: Decreased appetite, sleep disturbances
Methylphenidate (Ritalin)	Short-acting (2-4 hr)	0.3-1.5*;1-3 doses daily	*Long term*: Possible minor effects on growth; associated with onset of Tourette's syndrome in children with family history of tics
Pemoline (Cylert)	Long-acting (2-4 wk delay in therapeutic effect)	0.5-3.0*; 1 daily dose	*Abrupt discontinuation*: Behavioral deterioration
ANTIDEPRESSANTS			
Clomipramine (Anafranil)	20-40 hr half-life		
Imipramine (Tofranil)	10-17 hr half-life; immediate response with enuresis or ADHD; 2-4 week delay in response with depression	Usual daily dose should not exceed 5 mg/kg/day	*Short term*: Dry mouth, blurred vision, constipation, electrocardiogram changes, insomnia *Abrupt discontinuation*: Gastrointestinal (GI) symptoms, drowsiness, headaches
MOOD STABILIZERS			
Carbamazepine (Tegretol)	Peak effect in 7-10 days	10-30; maintain plasma level between 4-12 mm/L	*Short term*: GI symptoms, polyuria, polydipsia, tremors, sleepiness, impaired memory
Lithium	12 hr half-life	Maintain plasma level between 0.6 and 1.2 mm/L	*Long term*: Decreased calcium metabolism and thyroid function; possible kidney changes, blood dyscrasias, and hepatotoxicity
ANTIPSYCHOTICS			
Chlorpromazine (Thorazine)	Low potency	8-6	*Short term*: Drowsiness, weight gain, dry mouth, blurred vision, nasal congestion, acute dystonia, parkinsonism, postural hypotension, hyperpyrexia
Haloperidol (Haldol)	High potency	0.05-0.15	
Thioridazine (Mellaril)	Low potency	0.5-3.0	
Trifluoperazine (Stelazine)	High potency	0.1-0.5	*Abrupt discontinuation*: Withdrawal dyskinesias
ANTIANXIETY AGENTS			
Diphenhydramine (Benadryl)		37.5-50 mg/day, children ≤20 lb 37.5-100 mg/day, children >20 lb	*Short term*: Drowsiness; may cause excitation in young children *Contraindications*: Bronchial asthma; narrow-angle glaucoma; pyloroduodenal and bladder neck obstruction

*Doses are lower for younger children.

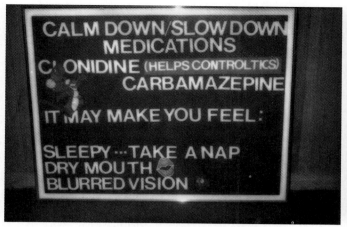
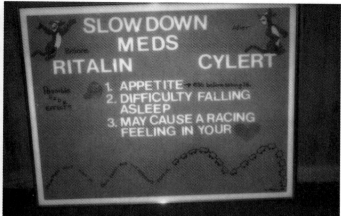

Fig. 34-6   Posters created by nurses to teach children about medications.

effects with children and their families. Nurses should also be aware that promoting a child's knowledge of medications can have a positive effect on self-esteem and feelings of control and self-worth. Thus numerous therapeutic outcomes can be achieved by effective medication teaching.

This is an area that allows for many creative nursing interventions.[22] A variety of puppet play, art, graphics, and audiovisual materials can be used to successfully teach and prepare children for managing their medications and their illness. Posters created by nurses to teach children about medications are presented in Fig. 34-6. Peer group participation is particularly effective in helping children describe common experiences, decrease their sense of isolation, and enhance the children's responses to the teaching materials. Through the use of imaginative but goal-directed nursing interventions, children can learn important information and experience greater control over the treatment of their illness and their future mental health.

SUGGESTED CROSS-REFERENCES

SUMMARY

1. Studies suggest that 12% of children in the United States have some type of psychiatric illness, and the majority of treatment resources are focused on those who receive care in hospital settings. Child psychiatric nurses need to be able to implement care that modifies a child's coping responses and strengthens a child's competency skills.

2. Strayhorn identified nine skills that all children need to become competent adults. Each of these skills and ways to assess a child's mastery of each skill were described.

3. Nursing diagnoses used by child psychiatric nurses were discussed and related nursing interventions were presented.

4. Child psychiatric nurses can also implement a variety of therapeutic treatment modalities when caring for children, including therapeutic play, art therapy, games, bibliotherapy, storytelling, autogenic storytelling, enacting plays, and medication management.

COMPETENT CARING
A CLINICAL EXEMPLAR OF A PSYCHIATRIC NURSE

Evelyn Middleton, BSN, RN, C
LeeAnn Welsh, RN

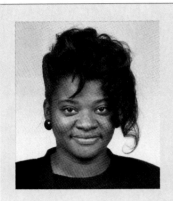

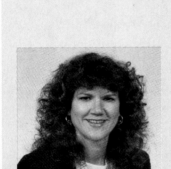

L, a 9-year-old black female, was admitted to our 25-bed combined child and adolescent psychiatric unit because of recent suicidal attempts and homicidal ideation. L was extremely depressed and had a difficult time talking about the situations that brought her to the hospital. Her family was dysfunctional. Her father was physically and sexually abusive to her mother in front of her.

Early in her hospitalization, L didn't trust anyone. She had suffered numerous traumatic events. She would lie in a fetal position, suck her thumb, and periodically talk about wanting to jump off a large bridge in the downtown section of our city. Working as a team on evening shift, we (with other members of the nursing staff) were able to assess the chronically low self-esteem and sadness this child was feeling. With a lot of one-to-one attention and therapeutic touch, we developed a bond with this child, who viewed us as caregivers, and we were able to establish a trusting relationship with her. She asked questions about our childhood and how we were brought up by our parents. She also asked about the way we treated our children. From this conversation, she understood she was not to blame for the beatings and the sexual abuse she endured. L continued talking to us with tears in her eyes and her hands clenched while hitting her pillow in an effort to control her anger. She would talk about a dream she often had, and we encouraged her to ventilate her feelings about this dream. The more this child spoke, the clearer it became to us that it was not only her father who repeatedly violated her, but also her grandfather. She constantly referred to these memories as a "dream" because she did not want to believe a grandfather could do this to his own "flesh and blood." We continued to sit with L at night consoling and reassuring her that she was not to blame and how great it was that she was finally able to release these ghosts.

During these conversations L had decided that she no longer wanted to be home with her father because she felt the beatings would continue. We prepared her for discharge by discussing different options for placement, her responsibility to keep herself safe, and other ways besides suicide to express her anger. At one point, the Department of Social Services failed to substantiate any sexual misconduct on the father's part toward L. It was their recommendation that she be returned to her father. This disappointment encouraged L to feel betrayed by the adults she had begun to trust. She cried, exclaiming that she told us everything and we had let her down. She stated she would kill her father if she went home. We again reassured her that we would help see that she not be returned home.

Because of the time factor and lack of support from the Department of Social Services, L had to be prepared to go to the state hospital. With a team effort, we were honest and positive about this placement at the state hospital. L was informed as to how she would be transported. We then called the state hospital and gathered some general information to share with her about the facility and different activities that went on there. On the day of discharge, L wanted to meet our children. LeeAnn brought her little boy in to have lunch with L. While interacting with us, L was able to see a healthy parent-child relationship. Once she was settled at the state hospital, she called the unit requesting to speak to Evelyn and LeeAnn. We encouraged her to trust the staff there and mentioned that she was welcome to call us anytime to let us know how she was doing.

Working as a team, we shared the hurt and love this child was feeling. As two experienced psychiatric nurses, we were able to assess, implement, and plan care for this suicidal patient. Together we established a trusting relationship and created a safe environment for her. Our expertise allowed this child to grow, develop self-esteem, and reclaim the will to live! For us, it truly reflected the essence of child psychiatric nursing practice. ▼

REFERENCES

1. American Nurses' Association: *Standards of child and adolescent psychiatric and mental health nursing practice*, Kansas City, Mo, 1985, The Association.
2. American Psychiatric Association: *Diagnostic and statistical manual*, ed 4, Washington, DC, 1994, The Association.
3. Barlow D: Therapeutic holding: effective intervention with the aggressive child, *J Psychosoc Nurs Ment Health Serv* 27:10, 1990.
4. Bennett C: Sexually abused boys: awareness, assessment, and intervention, *J Child Adolescent Psychiatr Nurs* 6:29, 1993.
5. Carrey N, Adams N: How to deal with sexual acting-out on the child psychiatric inpatient unit, *J Psychosoc Nurs Ment Health Serv* 30:19, 1992.
6. Clunn P: *Child psychiatric nursing*, St Louis, 1991, Mosby. Yearbook.
7. Cohen L: Bibilotherapy: using literature to help children deal with difficult problems, *J Psychosoc Nurs Ment Health Serv* 25:20, 1987.
8. Costello A: A checklist of hospitalization criteria for use with children, *Hosp Community Psychiatry* 42:823, 1991.
9. Delaney K: Nursing in child milieus, Part 1: What nurses do. Part 2: Mapping conceptual footholds, *J Child Adolesc Psychiatr Nurs* 5:10, 1992.
10. De Leon Siantz M: Children's rights and parental rights, *J Child Adolesc Psychiatr Nurs* 1:14, 1988.
11. Division of Psychiatric Nursing: *Competency in childhood: healthy development*, Charleston, SC, 1993, Medical University of South Carolina (videotape).
12. Fassler D, Cotton N: A national survey on the use of seclusion in the psychiatric treatment of children, *Hosp Community Psychiatry* 43:370, 1992.
13. Garfinkle B, Carlson G, Weller E: *Psychiatric disorders in children and adolescents*, Philadelphia, 1990, WB Saunders.
14. Gordon B, Schroeder C, Abrams J: Children's knowledge of sexuality: a comparison of sexually abused and non-abused children, *Am J Orthopsychiatry* 60:250, 1990.
15. Hendren R, Berlin I: *Psychiatric inpatient care of children and adolescents: a multicultural approach*, New York, 1991, John Wiley & Sons.
16. Hernandez J, Lineberger H, Baimbridge T: Development of an innovative child and youth mental health training and service delivery project, *Hosp Community Psychiatry* 43:375, 1992.
17. Jemerin J, Philips I: Changes in inpatient child psychiatry: consequences and recommendations, *J Am Acad Child Adolesc Psychiatry* 27:397, 1988.
18. Johnson B: Children's drawings as a projective technique, *Pediatr Nurs* 16:11, 1990.
19. Jones R, O'Brien P: Unique interventions for child inpatient psychiatry, *J Psychosoc Nurs Ment Health Serv* 28:29, 1990.
20. Jones R, O'Brien P, McMahon W: Contracting to lower precaution status for child psychiatric patients, *J Psychosoc Nurs Ment Health Serv* 31:6, 1993.
21. Kaufman B, Wohl A: *Casualties of childhood: a developmental perspective on sexual abuse using projective drawings*, New York, 1992, Brunner/Mazel.
22. Knight M et al: Medication education for children, *J Child Adolesc Psychiatr Nurs* 3:25, 1990.
23. Leininger M: Transcultural mental health nursing assessment of children and adolescents. In West P, Evans C: *Psychiatric and mental health nursing with children and adolescents*, Gaithersburg, Md, 1992, Aspen.
24. Malchiodi C: *Breaking the silence: art therapy with children from violent homes*, New York, 1990, Brunner/Mazel.
25. National Advisory Mental Health Council: *National plan for research on child and adolescent mental disorders*, Rockville, Md, 1990, US Department of Health and Human Services.
26. National Institute of Mental Health: *Program announcement: child and adolescent service system program*, Washington, DC, 1983, NIMH.
27. Polk-Walker G: What really happened? Incidence and factor assessment of abused children and adolescents, *J Psychosoc Nurs Ment Health Serv* 28:17, 1990.
28. Pope A, McHale S, Craighead W: *Self-esteem enhancement with children and adolescents*, New York, 1988, Pergamon Press.
29. Pothier P: Child mental health problems and policy, *Arch Psychiatr Nurs* 2:165, 1988.
30. Schaefer C: *The therapeutic powers of play*, Northvale, NJ, 1993, Jason Aronson.
31. Sieving R, Zirbel-Donisch S: Development and enhancement of self-esteem in children, *J Pediatr Health Care* 4:290, 1990.
32. Strayhorn J: *The competent child: an approach to psychotherapy and preventive mental health*, New York, 1989, The Guilford Press.
33. Trupin E, Forsyth-Stephens A, Benson P: Service needs of severely disturbed children, *Am J Public Health* 81:975, 1991.
34. Wong S, Martinez-Diaz J, Thorne-Henderson M: How therapeutic is therapeutic holding? *J Psychosoc Nurs Ment Health Serv* 28:24, 1990.

ANNOTATED SUGGESTED READINGS

Brett D: *More Annie stories: therapeutic storytelling techniques,* New York, 1992, Magination Press.

Teaches how to invent stories and tell them to children in ways that help distressed children deal with anxieties and solve problems.

*Carrey N, Adams L: How to deal with sexual acting-out on the child psychiatric inpatient ward, *J Psychosoc Nurs Ment Health Serv* 30:19, 1992.

Discusses practical interventions that nurses can implement for sexual acting-out behavior in children due to previous sexual abuse, delinquent acting-out, or age-appropriate exploration.

*Clunn P: *Child psychiatric nursing,* St Louis, 1991, Mosby.

Covers the field from foundations of practice, to developmental, behavioral, physical, and emotional disorders of children and psychotherapeutic interventions in a variety of settings.

*Delaney K: Nursing in child psychiatric milieus, Part 1: What nurses do. Part 2: Mapping conceptual footholds, *J Child Adolesc Psychiatr Nurs* 5:10, 1992.

Five therapeutic milieu processes that child psychiatric nurses can use—safety, structure, support, involvement, and validation are described in these two articles.

Garfinkle B, Carlson G, Weller E: *Psychiatric disorders in children and adolescents,* Philadelphia, 1990, WB Saunders.

Integrates the interpersonal and the biological-medical approach to develop an understanding of child and adolescent psychiatric disorders.

Green W: *Child and adolescent clinical psychopharmacology,* Baltimore, 1991, Williams & Wilkins.

Discusses current principles that guide the use of psychoactive medication with children.

Greenspan S, Greenspan N: *The clinical interview of the child,* Washington, DC, 1991, American Psychiatric Press.

Describes ways to conduct spontaneous, unstructured interviews with children. Includes age-appropriate behavior based on a developmental approach and is full of clinical illustrations.

Hendren R, Berlin I, eds: *Psychiatric inpatient care of children and adolescents: a multicultural approach,* New York, 1991, John Wiley & Sons.

Culturally responsive treatment of children and adolescents is discussed by psychiatrists, social workers, psychiatric nurses, and psychologists.

*Knight M et al: Medication education for children, *J Child Adolesc Psychiatr Nurs* 3:25, 1990.

One of the few articles in the field to describe various ways to teach children about their medication treatment.

Lewis M, Volkmar F: *Clinical aspects of child and adolescent development,* ed 3, Philadelphia, 1990, Lea & Febiger.

This text is divided into six sections making it particularly useful as a reference book for basic developmental issues, as well as for psychopathology and psychotherapeutic interventions.

Monahon C: *Children and trauma: a parent's guide to helping children heal,* New York, 1993, Lexington Books.

Provides parents with guidelines for seeking professional help for their traumatized children, as well as various psychotherapeutic approaches they can use to help the child's healing process.

Schaefer C, Cangelosi D: *Play therapy techniques,* Northvale, NJ, 1993, Jason Aronson.

Describes how structured play with familiar toys can be used with a variety of presenting problems in play therapy.

*Siantz M: The stigma of mental illness on children of color, *J Child Adolesc Psychiatr Nurs* 6:10, 1993.

Timely article that discusses the stigma that results from unreliable, invalid, unstandardized identification of psychiatric disorders, particularly among children from ethnic minority groups.

Strayhorn J: *The competent child,* New York, 1989, The Guilford Press.

Presents the complete theoretical framework of ego competencies developed by Strayhorn. A highly readable text.

*West P, Evans C, eds: *Psychiatric and mental health nursing with children and adolescents,* Maryland, 1992, Aspen Publishers.

Uses the nursing process and nursing diagnoses to organize a comprehensive text for child and adolescent psychiatric nursing.

---

*Nursing reference.

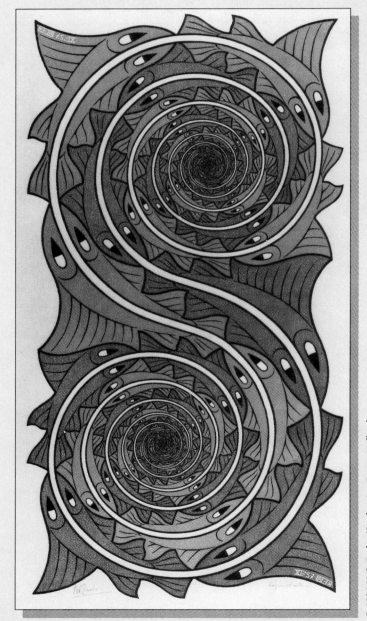

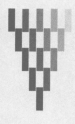

CHAPTER 35
Adolescent Psychiatric Nursing

AUDREY REDSTON-ISELIN

I'm so mixed up and lonely
Can't even make friends with my brain.
I'm too young to be where I'm going
But I'm too old to go back again.

John Prine: *"Rocky Mountain Time"*

LEARNING OBJECTIVES

After studying this chapter the student should be able to:
▼ List the developmental tasks of adolescence
▼ Compare and contrast the various theoretical views of adolescence
▼ Identify the major areas that should be included when assessing adolescents
▼ Describe maladaptive responses evident in adolescence
▼ Analyze nursing interventions useful in working with adolescents
▼ Evaluate nursing care provided for adolescents

TOPICAL OUTLINE

Developmental Stage
Theoretical Views of Adolescence
Assessing the Adolescent
   Body Image
   Identity
   Independence
   Social Role
   Sexual Behavior
Maladaptive Responses
   Inappropriate Sexual Activity
   Homosexuality Problems
   Unwed Motherhood
   Suicide
   Runaways
   Conduct Disorders
   Violence
   Drug Use
   Hypochondriasis
   Weight Problems
   Occult Involvement
   Parental Divorce
Working with Adolescents
   Health Education
   Family Therapy
   Group Therapy
   Individual Therapy
   Talking with Adolescents
   Parents of the Adolescent
Evaluating Nursing Care

Adolescence is a time of transition—an age when the individual is not yet an adult but is no longer a child. The intense feelings experienced at this time are meaningful, and the issues raised during adolescence are central to personal development. Adolescent psychiatric nurses focus on adolescents and their movement toward adulthood, considering social, emotional, and physical aspects of their adjustment in their family, school, and peer groups. These nurses concentrate on helping adolescents move successfully toward adulthood, and they have special expertise in identifying problems in the developmental process and working with support systems to enhance growth.

DEVELOPMENTAL STAGE

Adolescence is a unique stage of development that occurs between the ages of 11 and 20 when a shift in growth and learning occurs. The developmental tasks that emerge during adolescence threaten the individual's defenses. They can either stimulate new adaptive ways of coping or lead to regression and maladaptive coping responses. Old problems may interfere with the adolescent's coping abilities, and environmental factors may help or hinder the adolescent's attempts to deal with these issues. Previous coping skills, if used successfully, can assist healthy adaptation and integrated adult functioning.

An earlier, although still popular, view of adolescence described it as a time of conflict and upheaval that was necessary for later personality integration. More recent research suggests that this is not true; the complex changes in biological, social, and emotional development do not necessarily lead to psychological conflicts. Studies show that only 10% to 20% of adolescents have psychological disturbances, which is about the same percentage found in adults.[22]

During adolescence major events occur, and attempts are made to deal with them. This results in behavior uniquely "adolescent." Havighurst[11] identified the following tasks that should be accomplished during adolescence:

1. Achieving new and more mature relations with age mates of both sexes
2. Achieving masculine or feminine social roles
3. Accepting physical build and using the body effectively
4. Achieving emotional independence from parents and other adults
5. Preparing for marriage and family life
6. Preparing for an economic career
7. Acquiring a set of values and an ethical system as a guide to behavior and developing an ideology

Different theories describe these developmental tasks and how their positive resolution moves the adolescent toward adulthood. They will be briefly reviewed and are summarized in Table 35-1.

THEORETICAL VIEWS OF ADOLESCENCE
Biological Theory

Gesell, Ilg, and Ames[10] believe that biological influences are the major determinant of adolescent development and that growth patterns follow certain principles of maturation. Through maturation and environmental influences, a person learns how to adjust. They describe adolescent development as consisting of intense and dramatic physical growth changes that affect all aspects of the human being.

Psychoanalytical Theory

Freud also believed that human development was biological and was marked by stages. During puberty (ages 13 to 18), Freud's genital stage, a reawakening of sexual interest occurs. The adolescent with new sexual urges looks for gratification outside the home. This renewal comes from physiological maturing. The genitalia mature, and the release of sex hormones increases. Sexual exploration and maturation often occur. Freud stressed that the first years of life were important in establishing traits that become permanent in adolescence.[4]

More modern psychoanalytical theories define adolescence as the stage between childhood and adulthood correlated with the biological changes of puberty. Increased drives or impulses due to hormones cause a personality reorganization in adolescents as they attempt to adjust to their new physical status. These increased impulses confront a relatively weak ego. Adolescents therefore return to earlier coping skills in an effort to reestablish mastery over the environment.[2]

Psychosocial Theory

The classic psychoanalytical description of adolescence has been modified by Erikson, Sullivan, and others, who emphasize the effect of social factors on these developmental processes. Erikson[7] describes ego identity, or the relationship between a person's self-perception and how a person appears to others. To Erikson, adolescence represents an attempt to establish an identity within the social environment. This search is described as "normal adolescent identity crisis." He calls the stage of adolescence "identity versus identity diffusion," which is followed in young adulthood by the stage of "intimacy versus isolation." He stresses that identity must be established before intimacy can occur.

Table 35-1   Summary of Theoretical Views of Adolescence

Theory (contributor)	Definition	Description
Biological (Gesell, Ilg, and Ames)	Biological influences are the major determinant of adolescent development.	Emphasis is on physical growth, behavior, and the environment, which influence feelings, thoughts, and actions.
Psychoanalytical (Freud)	Adolescent development has its roots in resolution of earlier childhood developmental stages.	Puberty is called the genital stage in which sexual interest is reawakened. Biological changes upset the balance between the ego and id, and new solutions must be negotiated.
Psychosocial (Erikson, Sullivan)	Emphasizes social factors in the developmental process including how people view themselves and each other.	Adolescents attempt to establish an identity within the social environment. The task of development is "identity vs. identity diffusion."
Cognitive (Piaget)	Adolescence is accomplished by gradually internalizing actions, which evolves into a system of thought processes.	Adolescence is an advanced stage of cognition in which the ability to reason goes beyond the concrete to more abstract thinking described as "formal thought."
Cultural (Mead)	Adolescent behavior is a result of cultural determinants and reactions to social expectations.	Views adolescence as a time when a person believes that adult privileges are deserved but are withheld. This stage ends when society gives full power and status of an adult.
Multidimensional (Meeks)	Proposes no single concept of adolescence. Focuses on biological, sociological, psychological, and cultural integration.	Adolescence is seen as adaptation on a continuum of development. There is less emphasis on age and more on the developmental level and timing of biological, psychological, and environmental influences.

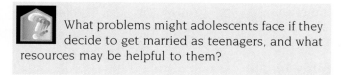

What problems might adolescents face if they decide to get married as teenagers, and what resources may be helpful to them?

Cognitive Theory

Cognitive theory views adolescence as an advanced stage of cognitive functioning in which the ability to reason goes beyond concrete objects to symbols or abstractions, or what Piaget calls "formal thought."[21] Piaget believes the adolescent has the ability to deal with logic, metaphors, and rational thought. This develops continuously from the concrete thinking of childhood to (at about age 12) when the concern with realities, tangible objects, and action is transferred to an ideational plane. This allows for conclusions to be made and for reflection to take place without the reality or object being present. Piaget calls this ability the "logic of operations."

Cultural Theory

Anthropologists report from studies of adolescents in different cultures that primitive cultures had less stressful periods than those experienced by American teen-

agers. Mead[17] concluded that adolescent rebellion was culturally determined and not biologically based. Anthropologists view adolescence as a period when the person believes that adult privileges are deserved but are being withheld. It ends when society gives the individual the social status of an adult. Anthropologists see growth as a continuous process and a cultural phenomenon, with individuals reacting to social expectations. The more clearly defined these expectations, the less stressful and ambiguous the adolescent period. The more culture changes, the greater the generation gap becomes.

Several issues in contemporary American society directly influence the support an adolescent can obtain from the environment. Blurring sexual roles is one such issue. Women have less traditional attitudes, expectations and behaviors. Men have become more involved in functions that were previously believed to be women's, and vice versa. Another social issue is the current concern about the economy. There are fewer jobs, particularly for adolescents. The cost of higher education has increased dramatically, which has resulted in prolonged economic dependency. These changes increase the complexity of society and add new pressures to adolescents, who are becoming adults and attempting to define their role in today's cultural milieu.

Multidimensional Theory

Multidimensional theory proposes that no singular view of adolescent development and mental health exists. Rather, these issues are related to the wide variation in adolescents' social relationships, behaviors, and attitudes and revolve around three main themes identified by Meeks:[18]

1. Profiles of ego and moral development are used to characterize adolescents for rates of progression, regression, and stability in age-related development.
2. Attention is given to biological, sociological, psychological, and cultural integration. These variables change rapidly during adolescence and affect the adolescent's behavior and view of self at any time.
3. The developmental issues of both psychological and biological maturation are viewed as affecting the adolescent's adaptation and functioning. For example, the timing of the adolescent's physical development in relation to a peer group has a direct influence on the teenager's self-esteem.

These issues may vary widely not only individually but also by culture and society.

The multidimensional view of adolescence sees adaptation on a continuum of development. Less emphasis is placed on specific age and more is put on developmental level and the timing of various biological, psychological, and environmental influences. This theory also proposes that severe family conflict need not necessarily occur. Rather, the degree and nature of conflicts change from childhood through the adolescent years and reflect both the diversity and the functional and dysfunctional aspects of family life.

ASSESSING THE ADOLESCENT

Nursing care of adolescents begins with a thorough assessment or evaluation of their health status. Data collection by the nurse is based on current and previous functioning in all aspects of an adolescent's life. A variety of approaches and tools may be used, but data collection should include the following information:

1. Growth and development (including developmental milestones)
2. Biophysical status (illnesses, accidents)
3. Emotional status (relatedness, affect, mental status, including evidence of thought disorder and suicidal or homicidal ideation)
4. Cultural, religious, and socioeconomic background
5. Performance of activities of daily living (home, attending school)
6. Patterns of coping (ego defenses such as denial, acting out, withdrawal)

7. Interaction patterns (family, peers)
8. Adolescent's perception of and satisfaction with health status
9. Adolescent's health goals
10. Environment (physical, emotional, ecological)
11. Available and accessible human and material resources (friends and school and community involvement)

These data are collected from adolescents and other significant persons through interviews, examinations, observations, and reports. In addition, the nurse may ask the following questions of the adolescent's family[1]:

1. What concerns you about your adolescent?
2. When did these problems start?
3. What changes have you noticed?
4. Have the problems been noticed in school as well as home?
5. What makes the behavior better or worse?
6. How have these problems affected your adolescent's relationship with you, siblings, peers, and teachers?
7. Has your adolescent's school performance changed?

An examination of typical adolescent behaviors reveals that adolescence is a time of change. The issues confronting adolescents are body image, identity, independence, social role, and sexual behavior. These issues can produce adaptive or maladaptive responses as the adolescent attempts to cope with the developmental tasks at hand.

Body Image

Chronological age is not a true guide for physical maturation, since growth often occurs in spurts and individual differences exist. Because the grouping of adolescents is usually done chronologically, the adolescent must face being with others who vary greatly in physical development and interests. This explains why adolescents often imitate behavior as an effort to keep within the expected range of conduct and be compatible with peers. The greater the divergence from the rest of the group, the greater the adolescent's anxiety. The lack of uniformity of growth often puts great demands on physical and mental adaptability. Growth being uneven and sudden, rather than smooth and gradual, causes a change in body image.

Adolescents reevaluate themselves in light of these physical changes, particularly the onset of primary and secondary sex characteristics, which are so pronounced. They tend to compare themselves and their physical development to that of their peers. They are very concerned about the normality of their physical status. The physical changes of puberty cause adolescents to be self-conscious of their changing bodies. Often they are reluctant to have medical examinations because they fear abnormalities will be found. Examinations may intensify masturbatory conflicts, sexual fantasies, and guilt feelings. The early and middle phases of puberty may also give rise to increased conflict, distance, and dissatisfaction in parental relationships.

Identity

In response to the physical changes of puberty, adolescents experience heightened periods of excitement and tension. They use defenses against these feelings that were helpful in childhood and experiment with new, more adultlike attempts at mastery. Thus, in their attempt to cope, adolescents sometimes act like adults and at other times behave like children. For example, adolescents show behavior marked with experimentation and test the self by going to extremes. This can be useful in establishing self-identity. The rebelliousness or negativism of the adolescent shows a movement toward individuation and autonomy that is more complex than but also similar to the 2-year-old's "no." Adolescents may also assert themselves by acting in a negative or contrary manner when relating to parents and other authority figures who they believe are not allowing them to be separate and unique. This is seen in the following clinical example.

 CLINICAL EXAMPLE

Scottie, although an avid football fan for several years, suddenly switched his interest to basketball. He quit his local football team despite his father's urgings to continue. His father, also a football fan, could not understand Scottie's sudden negative attitude toward football and newly found interest in basketball.

The individuation process of adolescence is accompanied by feelings of isolation, loneliness, and confusion, since it brings childhood dreams to an end and attributes them to fantasy. This realization of childhood's end can create intense fears or panic. Many adolescents therefore attempt to remain in this transitional stage. The awakening of emotional ties with the family also occurs in the establishment of new, more interdependent relationships. This fearful, yet exciting, entrance into adulthood is a profound personal experience that is not resolved in adolescence but is confronted throughout life. Adolescents mourn the loss of childhood, and the feelings of loneliness and isolation that accompany this loss establish an intense need for closeness, love, and understanding. If they are unable to obtain support during this struggle, depression may result.

Parenting styles that encourage individuality and relatedness to families are associated with support of adolescent identity exploration. Adolescents expressing high levels of identity exploration have parents who express mutuality and separateness, encourage member differences, and are aware of clear boundaries between themselves and their teenagers. These adolescents are also more likely to have competent approaches to peer and social relationships and more developed skills in initiating, diversifying, sustaining, and deepening peer friendships.[22]

Independence

Adolescents have an unconscious longing to give in to their dependency needs. It is also a time of movement toward independence. Adolescents show this ambivalence by responding to petty annoyances and irritations with intense outbursts. They see the process toward independence as being free of parental control. They do not see gaining independence as a gradual learning process but as an emancipation accomplished by acting "differently." If one acts adult, then one is adult. Therefore they expose themselves to situations beyond their capabilities and then become overwhelmed and frightened. They seek reassurance in an attempt to reduce their anxiety by returning to childlike ways and being dependent on those with whom they feel most secure, usually their parents. This accounts for the inconsistency of adolescent behavior.

Well-adjusted adults usually use a problem-solving approach and do not feel as threatened when inexperience requires dependency on others. Adolescents, however, already tempted to give in to dependency needs, feel as if they are regressing to childhood, which deflates their self-esteem. They must deny their need for their parents. Sometimes they will criticize their parents for treating them as a child and then remark that their parents are not helpful enough. When adolescents seem to be rebelling against their parents, they may be rebelling against their own childhood conscience or superego. They project their ambivalence onto their parents, since they were the original source of restrictions. This projection actually reveals a movement toward a more mature standard and also indicates their insecurity about giving up childhood standards. By blaming their parents for their childish actions, they can avoid blows to their fragile self-esteem and protest that their actions result from parental demands, not their own.

The interaction between adolescent changes in autonomy and family relationships is an important consideration. Three parenting styles have been described in relation to whether they help or hinder independent functioning in adolescence.[22]

1. Traditional parents tend to value a sense of continuity and order. They accept the patterns of understanding and value judgments that come from previous generations. Adolescents from these families tend to be more attached to their parents, more conforming, and achievement oriented. Often they avoid major conflicts in their teenage years.

2. Authoritarian parents are oriented toward shaping, controlling, and restricting the adolescent to fixed standards. Obedience is seen as a virtue. Power and responsibility are not shared with the adolescent. Harsh discipline is used to curb autonomous strivings that are viewed as willfulness. The approach here is often punitive and it can result in problems with the adolescent's development of autonomy.

3. Democratic parents do not believe that their standards are always right. They tend to be supportive and respond to the specific situation with solutions that promote the adolescent's autonomy. The environment fostered is one of stimulation and challenge. This parenting style combines limit setting with negotiation, thus encouraging the teenager's participation in the disciplinary process. It is shown to predict greater independent functioning in adolescents.

Did your parents have a traditional, authoritarian, or democratic parenting style, and what would you do different from them in raising children of your own?

Social Role

Adolescents respond intensely to persons and events. They may be totally invested in one interest and then suddenly change to something different. These intense and unstable feelings can account for their extreme sensitivity to the response of others. They are easily hurt, disappointed, and fearful of others. There is a tendency toward "hero worship" and "crushes," but with little evaluation of the persons to whom these feelings are directed.

Adolescent relationships serve many functions. Often adolescents relate to a friend as if neither person were a separate individual. They often mimic each other's dress, speech, language, and thoughts. These relationships help in the development of self-identity and establishment of a social role. The peer group is also very important, since within the security of the peer group, adolescents can attempt to resolve conflicts. With peers they can test out their thoughts and ideas. Their thoughts may differ, but through mutual sharing, they can try to find an answer. The peer group can also explore other ways of dealing with problems and offer its members companionship, protection, and security. In the peer group, adolescents can accept dependency, not as a child but as one of the gang, testing out ideas and trying new values. Within the safety of the peer group, they can observe, comment on, and evaluate the activities of others. Adolescents usually are very loyal to their group of friends. Sometimes group security is so important that it is necessary at all costs even if it involves destructive behavior.

Adolescents react to many stimuli and drain off the tension created by new drives and impulses by investment in many interests. They do this with great intensity, which is why adolescents are susceptible to fads. This is often seen in their dress, music, or hobbies. Close relationships with the opposite sex provide adolescents with security (often by "going steady") and a person with whom to discuss problems and evaluate solutions. Often the partner may take on similar characteristics. This reciprocal relationship enhances self-esteem by demonstrating sexual attractiveness to the self and to the world, and it indicates that one is lovable. It also allows for bisexual expression, since the girl expresses her partner's feminine parts and her boyfriend represents her masculine parts.

Think about a current television program that is a favorite among adolescents and describe why it is popular based on adolescent norms and developmental tasks.

Sexual Behavior

Adolescents use fantasy to discharge sexual tension. They may, however, feel guilt and shame about sexual feelings or fantasies. Fantasies usually are an attempt to find solutions and evaluate consequences. They may indicate a disturbance if they continually occupy the adolescent's thoughts, are not converted into constructive actions, or are not modified by reality. Then they may disrupt other activities important to adolescent functioning and indicate a withdrawal from reality.

Masturbation is another way in which adolescents discharge sexual tension. The value of masturbation may be lessened if shame and guilt accompany it. Male adolescents often fear discovery of evidence of ejaculation, and females often fear changes in their genitalia as a result of masturbation. Fears are not limited to discovery by others. They may also result from the loss of ego boundaries experienced during orgasm.

Mutual masturbation can also serve the purposes of tension release and fusing of identity. If mutual masturbation is the primary focus of the relationship, without the enrichment of other aspects of a relationship, it may be maladaptive. Mutual masturbation is often acceptable to adolescents as long as it does not lead to intercourse. It can help to dispel anxieties about sexuality by assuring adolescents that they are sexually adequate.

MALADAPTIVE RESPONSES

Behaviors that impede growth and development may require nursing intervention. The nurse should consider the nature of the adolescent's maladaptive responses and the harm resulting from them. If the difficulty is significant and ongoing, intervention may be needed. Table 35-2 lists some indicators of potential maladaptive responses evident in adolescence.

Inappropriate Sexual Activity

Sexual activity is often not as much an outlet for sexual passion as a desire to achieve closeness with another individual. Adolescents tend to use their sexuality to sublimate other needs such as those of love and security, and personal anxiety about sexual adequacy and peer group pressure may lead the adolescent to practice inappropriate sexual relations. For example, some adolescents engage in sexual relations as a means of punishing themselves. Their promiscuity elicits external control and criticism from others. This is especially true when there is an exhibitionistic quality, and subtle efforts to "get caught" are seen. This is evident in the following clinical example.

CLINICAL EXAMPLE

Isabel, a 14-year-old adolescent, had been sexually active since age 12. She was brought to the clinic by her parents when a neighbor told them Isabel had bragged of her sexual ventures. Two years before referral, her parents had placed her in a more controlled parochial school because they were concerned she was "acting wild." It became apparent that Isabel had wanted her parents to know about and put limits on her behavior. She admitted to not enjoying sexual intercourse very much. She seemed to be trying desperately to get approval from her distant mother. Her father, who was a

Table 35-2 Indicators of Potential Maladaptive Responses in Adolescence

Area affected	Indicator
School	Underachievement
	Recurrent truancy
	Disruptive behavior
Home	Continual disagreement plus acting out
	Increase in secretiveness and isolation
Peers	Inability to make friends
	Dropping of former friends
	Membership in a group involved in antisocial behaviors
Functional	Chronic sleep disturbances
	Major shifts in eating patterns
	Psychosomatic complaints
Appearance	Deterioration in dress
	Poor personal hygiene
Mood	Chronic depression or low self-esteem
	Chronic anxiety or nervousness
	Chronic anger or hostility
Substance abuse	Use of hallucinogens or narcotics
	Consumption of any drug or alcohol regularly or in large amounts
Antisocial behavior	Delinquency
	Trouble with the police
Sexual	Promiscuity
	Pregnancy
	Sexual abuse
	Gender identity or orientation problems
Medical	Chronic illness or handicap
	Any illness resulting in isolation from peer group

Modified from Hofmann A, Greydanus D: *Adolescent medicine*, Norwalk, Conn, 1989, Appleton & Lange.

policeman, was what she described as "a hopeless case," secretly wishing that he would be a better policeman for her.

It is also important to differentiate between inappropriate behavior and defects in socialization that may result from the absence of an adequate parental role model, physical disabilities, sexual abuse, and personality temperament.[18] The additional risk of sexually transmitted diseases, including AIDS/HIV, makes sexual experimentation more problematic because of its potential short-term and long-term effects. The nurse must therefore explore the meaning of the adolescent's sexual behavior by asking the following questions:

1. Does the adolescent desire sexual gratification for punishment?

2. Do the adolescent's goals match the situation, or is self-deception present?
3. Is the adolescent demanding adult privileges while acting irresponsible and dependent?
4. To what extent is the behavior a defense for depression, anger toward others, or experimentation?
5. Is the behavior a way to avoid anxiety-producing fantasies?
6. How close is the relationship to a mature one?

Homosexuality Problems

Sexual orientation develops during early childhood. Gender identity is usually established by age 2, and a sense of masculinity or femininity by age 5 or 6. Homosexual adults describe homosexual feelings during late childhood and early adolescence, years before engaging in sexual activity.[23]

Although between 5% and 10% of American youth acknowledge homosexual experiences and 5% feel that they could be gay, homosexual experimentation is common during late childhood and early adolescence.[6,27] Experimentation may include mutual masturbation and fondling of the genitals and does not by itself cause or lead to adult homosexuality. Theories about the cause of homosexuality include genetic, hormonal, environmental, and psychological models; however, there is no definitive explanation for causality (see Chapter 24). Thus nurses need to be aware of the following:

1. Not all homosexual adolescents are sexually active.
2. Many homosexual adolescents are heterosexually active.
3. Many heterosexual adolescents are homosexually active.
4. The relationship between sexual identity and sexual behavior is variable during adolescence.
5. Sexual issues produce stress and anxiety for adolescents of all sexual orientations.

The development of homosexual identity in youth commonly progresses through four stages.[28] The first is *sensitization*, which occurs before puberty and involves feeling "different" from same-sex peers. The second stage is *identity confusion*, which occurs when the adolescent feels inner turmoil related to the possibility of being gay. This confusion may be compounded by the absence of openly gay role models, the adolescent's inability to identify with negative stereotypes of homosexuals, and the lack of opportunity for open exploration of homosexual socialization and sexuality. The third stage is *identity assumption*, which usually occurs in late adolescence or early adulthood when sexual preference is accepted and sexuality and the gay subculture are explored. The fourth and final stage is *commitment*, in which a gay identity is integrated into the individual's life and personality. Because of society's bias and social stigma, this final phase may be difficult for the young person and the family, as seen in the following clinical example. However, many youth who identify themselves as gay or lesbian attain a positive sense of self-acceptance during the late teen years and begin the healthy task of forming stable and intimate relationships.[25]

 CLINICAL EXAMPLE

Stacy, an 18-year-old adolescent, was hospitalized for self-destructive behavior. She had talked of being distant from her peers through high school and felt self-conscious in spite of wishes for more closeness with others. She had attended an all-female high school and had approached some of her teachers for closeness without success. Upon graduation she began cutting her arms. She was hospitalized briefly, and 2 months after discharge she was able to reveal homosexual urges and fantasies. With therapy, she began to connect with others and explore her sexual feelings. Her self-destructive behavior diminished, and she engaged in relationships that helped her define her gender identity.

Unwed Motherhood

Pregnancy in adolescence is a complicated issue. Some adolescent girls have low self-esteem and fears of inadequacy. To ease these fears, they may become pregnant. Sometimes pregnancy is an effort to escape a difficult family situation or to force the parents to agree to a marriage that may be inappropriate, as shown in the clinical example that follows.

 CLINICAL EXAMPLE

Susie, a 15-year-old adolescent, had run away for the second time, only to return home to the same chaos. She had tried to run away with her boyfriend. Her alcoholic mother and angry 19-year-old brother were making life unbearable. Her mother was surprised to learn about 3 months after her return that Susie was pregnant. Susie was delighted because she had hopes that she could get out of the house, knowing her mother would now approve of her marriage to her boyfriend.

Occasionally, emotionally deprived adolescents hope to give their child what they believe they have never received (or, perhaps more accurately, receive from the child what they have not received). Sometimes pregnancy appears to be a way to allow parents to give up parental responsibility for the adolescent. In other cases the adolescent has lived out a scapegoat role as the bad one in the family, thereby justifying parental neglect and hostility. The pregnancy can then improve family relationships because, with the adulthood the pregnancy implies, parents may be freed of guilt and may then not need to encourage the adolescent to act in ways that make her unlovable.

Pregnancy in adolescence may have other origins. It can occur accidentally after sexual exploration. The adolescent may be unaware of contraceptive methods. Pregnancy for unmarried adolescents may also be associated with sexual promiscuity. If it is, the girl may be ostracized. Sometimes pregnancy occurs within a close, caring relationship. Peer groups can be supportive to a girl who becomes pregnant as a result of a meaningful relationship but intolerant of one whose pregnancy is the result of promiscuity. Both the circumstances and the adolescent's level of maturity need to be assessed. In some cultures, out-of-wedlock pregnancies are an accepted part of adolescence.

Decisions involving abortion, placement of the baby, and marriage are difficult. Attitudes and laws influencing these decisions are diverse. Many believe that to force the adolescent to have the baby and then give the infant up is more traumatic for her than abortion. Others believe that abortion can be more disturbing. Marriage is another alternative. Forcing a marriage to avoid societal stigma usually adds to the adolescent's problems, but a mature couple might do well in marriage. All the alternatives should be presented to the adolescent, with the consequences clearly stated. The adolescent makes her decision with the aid and support of her partner, her family, the nurse, and other involved health-care professionals.

Pregnancy among adolescents is increasing in the United States. Why is this, and what, if anything, should be done about it?

Suicide

Suicide is the second leading cause of death among adolescents.[3] One of the most common factors in adolescent suicide is lack or loss of a meaningful relationship. Many researchers think suicide is an attempt for attention and does not necessarily represent a true desire to die. Regardless, it is a bid for help that must be recognized. Subtle references, as well as attempts, should always be taken seriously and explored. Suicidal gestures are more often seen in girls, with boys expressing their depression by bravado that results in accidents, as in this clinical example. It is often difficult to distinguish between risk-taking behavior, accidents, and suicidal gestures, thus requiring a careful nursing assessment.

CLINICAL EXAMPLE

John, a 12-year-old depressed adolescent, had just gotten a small dirt bike. Six months earlier John's grandfather, his only friend, had died. John's father had died when he was 2 years old, and he had lived with his mother and grandparents ever since. John, feeling hopeless, had ridden his bike into a car. After medical treatment for his broken arm and rib and multiple bruises, John began to receive therapy. He described feeling helpless and lonely, especially without his grandfather.

Parent-adolescent relationships can influence suicidal behavior. For example, the adolescent may be prevented from acting on suicidal feelings by parental concern and the establishment of new relationships.[20] In contrast, feelings of helplessness and worthlessness can be caused by threatened abandonment, being asked to take the adult role, and lack of opportunities to be dependent. Sometimes these adolescents perceive themselves to be expendable because they believe that the family unconsciously wishes them dead.

The nurse must make it clear to the adolescent that suicidal behavior is something that is not confidential and that parents must be told. Family involvement is essential to avoid angry, hostile, and hopeless feelings of abandonment and to create support and caring.

In working with suicidal adolescents, the nurse should explore the following areas[13]:

1. The seriousness of the attempt
2. The mental status of the adolescent
3. The extent of environmental stress, especially family problems
4. The adolescent's wider social environment and the strength of support systems (social isolation, school performance, parental loss, disruption of friendship or romantic alliance)
5. The likelihood of repeated suicidal attempts, especially if conditions remain the same

Nursing interventions related to suicide are described in detail in Chapter 18. The next two clinical examples illustrate suicide attempts by adolescents.

CLINICAL EXAMPLE

Maria, a 15-year-old girl, was referred to her local community mental health center from the neighborhood emergency room after ingesting pills. Maria had taken five of her mother's "arthritis pills" after an argument with her father about her 17-year-old boyfriend, José. Her father, who came home only on weekends, told her to stay away from him. After he left, the other family members noticed Maria had become sleepy while playing cards in the living room. Maria admitted to taking the pills and was rushed by her mother to the emergency room.

She had performed poorly in school for the last year since her father had left the family. Maria had always been her father's favorite. When she reached puberty at age 13, that relationship changed. Maria's position as her father's favorite was delegated to a younger female sibling, causing Maria to feel angry and rejected. Her father left the family a year later and returned for weekend visits, during which he mainly disciplined the children. Maria's attempt to get close to José as a replacement for her father was sabotaged by her father as well. She thought her only recourse was to elicit her father's caring and concern through a suicide attempt.

 ## CLINICAL EXAMPLE

Donald, age 13, was brought to the emergency room after cutting his wrists one evening when he thought his family was asleep. His mother had awakened and found him bleeding. She rushed him to the local emergency room, where he received medical treatment. It was then revealed that this was Donald's second suicidal attempt. The first attempt occurred a year ago when he had ingested pills. Donald had received therapy for about a month. It was then discontinued because of the family moving to a new location, despite recommendations to continue with a new therapist. Donald was always an isolated child. He was never very close with anyone but had two friends. Since the move he had become more withdrawn. He had done well in school in the past but now had given up and was failing almost every subject. The youngest of nine children, Donald had little relationship with his siblings, who were all older than he and not at home much. Donald's parents, both approaching old age, seemed not to notice that he had become increasingly upset. Donald was hospitalized, since the risk of his attempting suicide again was high.

Runaways

Running away might be a cry for help or an attempt to escape from a unbearable living situation. It is sometimes a solution for an unmotivated youth who has little self-direction, drive, or ambition. Finally, it is a large phenomenon of inner cities, where an unknown number of older children and adolescents move among the homes of friends or relatives, the streets, and abandoned buildings. Usually victims of poverty and overburdened single-parent homes, these teenagers may have had little opportunity to gain any sense of security or loving discipline or to have a vision of a hopeful future.

Adolescent runaways often have been rejected by their parents since birth, and the parent may alternate between extreme punitive measures and a laissez-faire (do as you please) attitude toward the adolescent. Adolescent runaways are often conflicted, especially regarding dependency-independency, and feel embarrassed, helpless, and defeated by their dependency wishes. This can result in a panic that motivates running away to prove autonomy and escape painful circumstances. They usually run away from disappointment toward something viewed as favorable and supportive. Parents often feel guilty and ashamed and have difficulty acting on practical issues, although some, relieved of their responsibility, are secretly pleased. Often the adolescent becomes involved in dangerous activities after running away. Most runaway adolescents want to return home if they believe their parents really want them.[18] The clinical example that follows illustrates home conditions that may lead to an adolescent's running away.

 ## CLINICAL EXAMPLE

Karen, age 14, ran away from home to a friend's house. Her mother had often expressed a desire to leave; in fact, she had once left the family to the charge of Karen's father when Karen was 9 years' old. Karen's mother had suddenly told her she could not see her boyfriend for a month because she had come in late the night before. This caused a tremendous scene because Karen had been out late every night the week before without her mother even noticing. Karen's friend's mother was different. She spent a lot of money on her children, talked to them, and never limited their activity; thus the friend's home appeared attractive to Karen.

 How would you design a community-based program to prevent adolescents from running away from home?

Conduct Disorders

Adolescents with conduct disorders display behavior that violates the basic rights of others or societal norms and rules. Examples include fighting, cruelty, lying, truancy, and destroying property. Conduct-disordered adolescents often have poor relationships with their parents. Antisocial acts allow the adolescent to express anger toward parents, who are often punished for the adolescent's acts. Children are socialized mainly by their parents and, it is hoped, learn from their parents' acceptable behaviors that become part of the internalized self or conscience. A good relationship between parent and child facilitates this process.

However, adolescents learn not only from their parents but also from others. The school and peer groups are influencing factors, as are the social, economic, and cultural environments. The self-destructive behaviors seen in conduct-disordered adolescents may indicate the need for punishment, anger at the family, peer group pressure, depression, feelings of self-defeat, a search for opportunities to take what they feel emotionally deprived of, and testing omnipotence through exciting experiences. Alignment with delinquents gives a defeated adolescent a feeling of self-respect and companionship through a sense of belonging to a subculture.

Research supports the idea that when depression and conduct disorder occur together, the central problem is usually depression.[19] However, adolescents who report helplessness, with the expectation that someone should do something for them, and who report fewer sad moods and lethargy probably have conduct disorders. Finally, while both groups share problems with morals and superego, conduct-disordered adolescents tend to have more family problems than depressed adolescents.

CLINICAL EXAMPLE

Levar, 13 years of age, was referred by the juvenile court for therapy because he had been picked up for the second time after breaking into a store with another boy. Levar's parents were separated for the past 2 years after his father had served a sentence in jail for possession of drugs. Levar was extremely upset when his parents separated and rarely saw his father. His antisocial acts caused his father to become more involved with him, since his father claimed he did not want his son to go through what he had experienced in prison. Levar gained his father's attention during these times, even though his father was angry. His delinquent actions therefore enabled Levar to express his anger at his father's leaving, as well as to fantasize about having his father return.

The above clinical example of an adolescent who steals illustrates the many factors that may lead to adolescent delinquency. Adolescents may not differentiate between their stealing and their parent's business dealings. Stealing may also be an effective way to rebel against parents. Adolescents may perpetuate childhood by indulging in immediate gratification through stealing rather than maturely working for things. Sometimes adolescents steal in hopes of getting caught and obtaining help. Parents may consciously or unconsciously condone stealing. Adolescents may also act out their anger with the justification that they deserve the stolen items.

Finally, the conflict of dependence versus independence can be expressed in poor school adjustment. Some adolescents view teachers as parental surrogates who do not help or who merely apply rules of attendance and homework. Dependent feelings are sometimes elicited by these rules, and adolescents, in proving their independence, may become negative about learning. They may think that schoolwork is secondary to more important activities they are attempting to master. Daydreaming may interfere with schoolwork as adolescents concentrate on and fantasize about achieving independence.

Adolescents may drop out of school for financial reasons, or they may be rebelling against education laws. The adolescent may be part of a peer group that denounces school attendance and involvement. Parents may overtly or covertly discourage education. This is conveyed through lack of support and approval for education or by their making it difficult for the adolescent to follow through with school expectations, as illustrated by the clinical example that follows.

CLINICAL EXAMPLE

Debbie, a 15-year-old adolescent, dropped out of school after several years of poor school performance and truancy. She would occasionally go shopping with her mother on a school day. Her mother never knew the names of her teachers or guidance counselor, and no provisions for a place or time to study were made.

Violence

Most adolescents displaying aggression have experienced frustration and have had violent role models during their childhood. Aggression is a human impulse that must be channeled constructively by a learned process that occurs within a supportive, loving relationship. Under favorable conditions, a child learns the healthy expression of aggression by involvement in activities that result in pleasure and active problem-solving attempts. Under less ideal conditions, aggression can occur in destructive activities that are harmful to self and others. Violence can also be a maladaptive way of coping with adolescent anxiety and frustration, as evident in a "rage response."

However, not all violence in adolescence comes from violent impulses. Many teenagers are violent due to periods of overstimulation or because of strong desires for emotional contact. Empathic responses are most helpful with these teenagers. Some adolescents express hostility and violence to others who fail to live up to their idealized expectations. They try to rebuild a disintegrating self by turning the violent attack into a psychic victory.[14]

Much anxiety of adolescents is related to the fear that they may be unable to control their destructive aggression. Adolescents often have violent dreams and fantasies that they express in threats, even though in some the potential for violence is minimal. Pointing out the harmlessness of these thoughts is helpful to adolescents, since it shows them that these thoughts are not as powerful as they fear. Some adolescents, however, are genuinely fearful that they will be unable to stop their thoughts from becoming actions. They require the recognition of their fear and the reassurance of external limits. Pointing out to the adolescent the necessity of self-responsibility and control is very important. Their defenses against aggressive outbursts should be reinforced and supported. Focus should be on the behavior and feared loss of control, not on the roots of the anger. The following clinical example illustrates the management of a violent adolescent.

CLINICAL EXAMPLE

Ricky was a 14-year-old boy referred for treatment for violent outbursts at home. When frustrated, he would break and destroy objects in his path. Ricky was an only child, adopted shortly after birth by a couple in their forties who were unable to have children. Now Ricky's parents, who were about 55 years of age, were increasingly frightened by his aggressive outbursts. They had also felt powerless with his childhood temper tantrums and had consistently responded to outbursts by attempting to limit frustrating situations. They felt guilty and inadequate about his being an adopted child and continually made attempts to reassure Ricky of their love for him. They consequently reinforced his lack of control by assuming these outbursts were results of his fear of being unloved and would offer peace offerings of gifts and rewards. Ricky assumed he was omnipotent, successfully controlling his parents, but was fearful that he could not control his anger. Acknowledging Ricky's fear of loss of control, applying external controls, and pointing out areas of Ricky's ability for responsibility and control resulted in a gradual decrease in outbursts.

Adolescents who have committed extreme acts of violence or homicide are often from families in which

violence is the norm. These adolescents may have experienced physical or sexual abuse as described in Chapter 37. If not, they may have witnessed violence between their parents. Behavior toward them has often alternated between seductiveness and physical brutality, adding to the adolescent's confusion and arousing intense frustration. Often these adolescents are encouraged to be violent. Sometimes parents can predict the adolescent's ability to injure or kill. Often there is a history of dangerous assaults on family members and pets. In severely violent adolescents, violent acts can be followed by a calmness and lack of sorrow or guilt, or they may claim that outside forces provoked them. Many homicidal adolescents will freely discuss their violent plans or fears. These should be explored and homicidal intent evaluated. Does the adolescent have a victim, weapons, or plan? This information, along with the history, shows the level of success or failure in controlling feelings and delaying gratification.

What do you think society can do to decrease gang violence among adolescents in this country?

Drug Use

The onset of drug use before the age of 20 predicts more sustained use over time. Figure 35-1 shows the prevalence of drug use by high school seniors and reflects the extent of this problem among adolescents. From 70% to 90% of males and 50% to 60% of females who

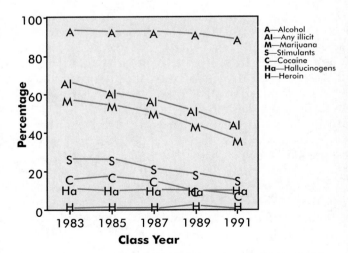

Fig. 35-1 Trends in lifetime prevalence of selected drugs of abuse by high school seniors.

National Institute on Drug Abuse: *Smoking, drinking, and illicit drug use among American secondary school students, college students, and young adults, 1975-1991,* vol I, Washington, DC, 1992, U.S. Government Printing Office.

abused drugs in adolescence continue to do so in adult life. Chemical dependency is the result of a gradual process. Table 35-3 presents the stages of adolescent substance abuse. It is important for the nurse to remember that not all adolescents progress through these stages, but the younger the user, the greater the risk for chemical dependency.

The meaning of drug use in adolescence is a complex question. The adolescent's motivation must be explored. The nurse must keep in mind that it may be an expression of rebelliousness with support of a peer group, as well as a way of obtaining gratification. It may also indicate an effort to come to grips with feelings of vulnerability and emptiness.

Adolescents often report a wish for closeness that is satisfied by sharing a drug experience with friends. Drug users can experience an illusion of closeness because drugs decrease anxiety and users can share anticipation of drug use. Some adolescents fill the void of isolated loneliness with drugs and would otherwise feel suicidally depressed. Drugs can be crippling and delay healthy maturity by promoting the avoidance of developing an adult identity in a real world, as illustrated in the next clinical example.

 ## CLINICAL EXAMPLE

Carlos was a 16-year-old adolescent who had been school phobic since age 10. He had been receiving home instruction since that age and was referred for a yearly assessment to obtain approval for a continuation of home instruction services. Carlos proudly spoke of his drug episodes. He and his small group of friends were close and had many exciting experiences induced by various hallucinogens and amphetamines. Carlos had little support in the real world, since he had been isolated at home and developed interpersonal relationships primarily through obtaining drugs and experiencing their effects.

One of the more frequently abused drugs is cocaine. This drug is snorted, free-based, injected, or smoked, producing euphoria, grandiosity, and increased feelings of confidence and esteem. In addition to emotional euphoria, it produces a sense of physical well-being that exceeds the normal body capacity.

The use of crack cocaine by adolescents has increased dramatically in the last few years. This is a combination of baking soda and cocaine, which is a powerful stimulant. When smoked, it directly reaches the brain from the lungs. An overdose can lead to a paranoid psychotic state that usually lasts a few hours. Overdose on crack cocaine can lead to excessive agitation followed by a "crash." This is a profound and prolonged depres-

sive state that may lead to suicidal behavior. Those adolescents who have smoked crack more than ten times are subject to grand mal seizures, stroke, and permanent brain damage.[12]

Alcoholism among adolescents is increasing. Some possible causes of alcoholism in adolescents include parental and social influence, peer pressure, and emotional disturbances. Many people believe that teenagers are currently switching from drugs to alcohol and that alcoholism is the greater social problem.

A final group of drugs often abused by adolescents are called "designer drugs." They are available in abundance and at low cost because they are easily produced by chemists. One designer drug of concern is steroids, which is often abused by athletes and adolescents who attempt to increase their physical strength, speed, and muscle mass. Steroids can give the adolescent a magical resolution to their lack of physical development, thereby enhancing their body image. Other designer drugs include opiate derivatives, or "knockoffs," which can produce aggressive or paranoid behavior, hallucinations, and euphoria. Substance abuse is discussed in detail in Chapter 22.

 You're concerned about your best friend's increasing use of drugs, but she denies it is a problem. How can you best help her?

Hypochondriasis

Adolescents are preoccupied with their bodies and body sensations. They are uncomfortable with their bodies because of the rapid changes in size, shape, and functioning. To establish their identity, adolescents try to become familiar with their changing bodies. They respond to sensations with increased intensity. When an adolescent appears overly concerned, it may indicate underlying difficulties in formation of self-image.

Hypochondriasis occurs when the adolescent has intense anxiety about personal health. This anxiety may be diffuse or directed toward one specific area. Adolescents' concern that their bodies are inadequate, that they will be rejected by others, or that they are unable to reach adulthood may predominate. Hypochondriasis may be a way of avoiding activities that expose these and other stressful fears. Fears such as inadequacy at school, either socially or in schoolwork, may be a projection of general fears of inadequacy. Lack of knowledge of normal body changes may be a simple precipitating factor. This can be tackled by reassurance that these changes are normal. If reassurance does not alleviate anxiety, other more intense fears may be involved.

Table 35-3 The Five Stages of Substance Abuse

Stage	Drugs	Sources	Frequency	Feelings	Behavior	Treatment
0: Curiosity	None	Available—but not used	—	Curiosity	Risk taking, desire for acceptance	Optimal time: anticipatory guidance to develop good coping skills and strong self-esteem; clear family guidelines on drug and alcohol use; drug education
1: Experimentation	Tobacco, alcohol, marijuana	House supply, friends, siblings	Weekend use for recreational purposes	Excitement, pleasure, few consequences; learning how easy it is to feel good	Lying, little change	Drug education; attention to societal messages; reduction of supply; strict, loving rules at home; establishment of drug-free alternative activities
2: Regular use	As above, plus hashish or hash oil, tranquilizers, sedatives, amphetamines	Buying	Progresses to midweek use; purpose is to get high	Excitement followed by guilt	Mood swings, faltering school performance, truancy, changing peer groups, changing style of dress	Drug-free self-help groups (Alcoholics or Narcotics Anonymous); family involvement; psychiatric counseling unhelpful unless family therapy and aftercare provided
3: Psychological or chemical dependency	As above, plus stimulants, hallucinogens	Selling to support their habit; possibly stealing or prostitution in exchange for drugs	Daily	Euphoric highs followed by depression, shame, guilt, and perhaps suicidal thoughts	Pathologic lying; school failure; family fights; involvement with the law over curfew, truancy, vandalism, shoplifting, driving under the influence, breaking and entering, violence	Inpatient or foster care programs that require family involvement and provide aftercare
4: Using drugs to feel "normal"	As above; any available drug, including opiates	Any way possible	All day	Euphoria rare and harder to achieve; chronic depression	Drifting, with repeated failures and psychological symptoms of paranoia and aggression; frequent overdosing, blackouts, amnesia; chronic cough, fatigue, malnutrition	Inpatient or foster care programs that require family involvement and provide aftercare

Adapted from MacDonald DI: *Pediatr Rev* 10:89, 1988.

It is important to communicate to adolescents that people are aware something is wrong and that their concerns will be taken seriously until the core problem is alleviated. Intense body concern is a signal that something is wrong and help is needed. Physical status must be assessed first before a psychological basis for concern is assumed. Sometimes body preoccupation is an effort to recreate infantile dependency by eliciting caregiving. This is particularly seen in adolescents who experienced early emotional deprivation. John, in the next clinical example, is an interesting example of this.

CLINICAL EXAMPLE

John, age 12, was referred for treatment from the local hospital after having been seen for chest pains. The physician found no medical problems. John was embarrassed and angry about the episode, insisting that the physician was wrong. The chest pains had disappeared, but he now had injured his arm. He also was often plagued by attacks of tonsillitis and middle ear infections. John had experienced early emotional deprivation because he was often moved around in his living arrangements. He was born out of wedlock and lived occasionally with his mother, often with his maternal grandmother, and infrequently with his father. He generally had the feeling that no one really cared for him. Further exploration revealed that John's body concerns were vocalized to initiate caregiving by those around him, who, he feared, really were not there for him. He performed well in school and had friends, but none of these compensated for his feelings of inadequacy.

Weight Problems

Eating disorders are another group of problems often seen in adolescence. They include anorexia nervosa, bulimia nervosa, and obesity. The sociocultural milieu for female adolescents in the United States has precipitated identity and body image confusion and anxiety in this age group. The emphasis on thinness, athletics, and physical attractiveness suggests that these are highly valued achievements for young women. These traits demonstrate self-control and social success and are culturally rewarded. The result is that fear of fat, restrained eating, binge eating, and body image distortion are common problems among teenage girls.

Recent understandings suggest that eating disorders represent a complex of issues related to many possible causes. Psychodynamics, family characteristics, physiology, and biochemical interactions all play a part in the development and treatment of these disorders.[17] They are discussed in detail in Chapter 23. The following clini-

cal example illustrates the development of anorexia nervosa in a young girl.

CLINICAL EXAMPLE

Janet, age 15, was admitted to the hospital because it was feared that her extreme loss of weight was endangering her life. Exploration revealed that Janet was afraid of her sexual feelings and the response of others to her budding sexuality. Her father, provocative and teasing toward Janet, was continually kidding her about her oncoming sexual attractiveness and implied that he really preferred her to her mother. This created panic, and Janet refused to eat. She liked her thinness, which was a protection from sexual desires. In the hospital, the area of concentration was not the behavior of not eating, but rather the underlying panic feelings about her sexuality and her relationship with her father. This provided freedom for normal sexual growth and development.

Occult Involvement

Adolescent risk-taking behavior has become evident more recently in the involvement of teenagers in the occult.[9,29] Individuals particularly prone to this involvement tend to be alienated from their family, be socially isolated, and have poor skills for interacting with others. They are cognitively curious and seek attention; they have their own belief system and are attracted to the bizarre. They are often negative, fatalistic, sensation seeking, poor judges of danger, and have low self-esteem. They rely on superstition to deal with their feelings of powerlessness and their fear of making decisions. In this way, their belief system establishes a sense of control for them. These adolescents depend on external rewards to make them feel good, and they conjure up spells to help them make decisions.

Satanism, the worship of Satan, is the dark side of the occult. Satanists do not necessarily believe in a personal devil, but rather that Satan symbolizes evil. Witchcraft includes a variety of magic with the goal of manipulating the spirits to do the will of humans. Astrology uses the earth-centered view of the solar system to interpret the influence of the heavenly bodies on human affairs.

Adolescent behaviors that are often associated with involvement in the occult include the following[29]:

▼ Sleep disturbances, including insomnia and nightmares
▼ Suicidal ideation with overwhelming feelings of guilt
▼ Chemical dependency and drug use

▼ Voyeurism, nudity, and sexual activity that includes thrill seeking
▼ Feelings of learned helplessness
▼ Fantasy role-play, including Dungeons and Dragons and various computer games
▼ Ritualistic use of objects such as knives and black clothing
▼ Preference for heavy metal music with hidden messages that ridicule society

Family systems that predispose adolescents to participate in occult practices may have unresolved conflicts and may use distancing to solve problems. A tolerance for deviance and a disengaged family structure may be present. Often the family structure has recently changed because of death or crisis. The adolescent's peer relations are often characterized by isolation and peer group rejection. Involvement in the occult therefore provides the teenager with an opportunity for acceptance. Environmental factors may include frequent exposure to the supernatural in movies, books, and games. These suggest magical solutions to life's problems. Finally, the adolescent may experience a disenchantment with formal religion and contempt for social norms and values.

Parental Divorce

Nearly one in four of all children and adolescents in the United States live in single-parent homes. Nearly half of all youngsters born in the past decade will experience a parental divorce. The effect of divorce on children varies with the child's age and developmental level. Adolescents are particularly vulnerable, and their initial reactions include depression, anger, and identification of one parent as the victim and rejection of the other. Over time, adolescents may become anxious or pessimistic about their own future involvement in intimate relationships. However, some adolescents become more mature and independent in perceiving that they have helped their parents in this time of crisis.

The most favorable outcome of divorce is seen when the divorced parents are able to put aside old conflicts and anger and return to meaningful caretaking relationships with their children. The adolescent's adaptation is also influenced by the amount of relief the divorce provides from predivorce marital strife and the young person's own emotional strengths, vulnerabilities, coping resources, and support systems. Major goals in the treatment of adolescents of divorced parents include helping the adolescent[26]:

1. Grieve the loss of the family unit
2. Maintain distance from parental conflicts
3. Express age-appropriate involvement in developmental tasks
4. Decrease anger, anxiety, depression, and acting out
5. Assess both parents realistically
6. Improve communication with both parents
7. Continue the separation-individuation process
8. Control overly aggressive and sexual drives

 How might growing up in a single-parent household positively and negatively affect an adolescent?

WORKING WITH ADOLESCENTS

Knowledge of normal adolescent development is necessary to differentiate between age-expected behavior and maladaptive responses. While there is some controversy over whether adolescent turmoil is normal (see Critical Thinking about Contemporary Issues), studies

 ### CRITICAL THINKING ABOUT CONTEMPORARY ISSUES

Is Adolescent Turmoil Normal?

Although it has been a commonly held belief that adolescence is a time of conflict and turmoil, recent research has disputed the notion that teenagers must experience a difficult adolescence.[22] Nonetheless, nurses should not underestimate the severity of adolescent problems. The National Adolescent Student Health Survey of more than 11,000 eighth and tenth graders in 20 states revealed many threats to the health and well-being of teenagers.[5] These included:

▼ 56% of students did not wear a seat belt the last time they rode in a car; 44% rode with a driver who had used alcohol or drugs before driving.
▼ 50% of the boys and 25% of the girls had been involved in at least one physical fight in the past year.
▼ 25% of the girls reported that someone had tried to force them to have sex in the past year.
▼ 23% of the boys carried a knife at least once in the past year; 7% carried one daily.
▼ 42% of the girls and 23% of the boys reported having seriously considered suicide at some time during their lives; 18% of the girls and 11% of the boys had attempted suicide.
▼ 60% of the girls had dieted during the past year; 16% had used diet pills; 12% had induced vomiting; and 8% had used laxatives. ▼

suggest that professionals view normal adolescents as being more disturbed than they really are, despite data refuting this view.

When dealing with the adolescent, it is advisable for the nurse to have an initial contact directly with the adolescent. Many adolescents are concerned that the nurse is aligned with the parents. Other adolescents take a passive role, letting the adults straighten things out for them. By initiating contact with the adolescent, an alignment is made with the individual's independent, mature aspects. Parents asking for advice on how to approach the adolescent about seeking treatment should be advised to be honest, stating the true nature of the visit and their reasons for requesting it. Many agencies and institutions use a child guidance approach, seeing the parents first to obtain a full developmental history. Family sessions have also been used in diagnostic evaluation, helping to reveal family interaction and later being helpful in establishing family support.

Health Education

The psychiatric nurse is in an excellent position to educate the adolescent, the parents, and the community. Basic health information can be given in such areas as drugs, sex and contraception, suicide prevention, and crime prevention. The nurse can also provide information on healthy emotional functioning. By educating parents and the community on normal adolescent behavior and by interpreting the underlying conflicts, parents, teachers, and other community members are better prepared to support adolescents and encourage healthy independent functioning. Often parents and others become frustrated, angry, and confused by the independent strivings of adolescents. Encouraging independence and lessening power struggles can produce a positive change in adolescents' relationships with adults and in their feelings about themselves.[24] However, adults should still set limits. Limit setting and providing structure can be done in a way to encourage the adolescent's independent functioning. Many parents are conflicted about their children becoming adults. This, together with the adolescent's own ambivalence and fears about independence, can create havoc.[8]

One of the best ways to educate parents on adolescent development is through a parents' group. In this way the nurse can inform parents on normal adolescent functioning, as well as provide them with much needed support from other parents in the same situation. Sharing mutual experiences and searching for solutions in a supportive environment can be extremely helpful to parents. It is important to remember that parents have nurtured children to reach this juncture of adolescence, moving toward adulthood. Many believe that "showing them how" is their primary parental responsibility. It is

a difficult change for them to suddenly switch from the "how to" of the child to the "try to" of the budding adult. Parents can learn the process of providing increased responsibilities based on a gradual progression of independent functioning. Despite their fears of their teenagers "getting into trouble," they can be educated to promote self-reliance in their adolescents. The next two clinical examples show the need to educate parents and community members.

 CLINICAL EXAMPLE

Mr. and Mrs. B came to the attention of the psychiatric nurse by their distressed calls to the community mental health center. Mrs. B tearfully explained that they had lost all control of their 14-year-old daughter. She had become arrogant and hostile, locking herself in her bedroom after an argument they had about her going to the movies with a 14-year-old boy she had met at school. Further exploration revealed that Emily was an honor student at school, maintaining a solid A average. She had many friends at school, was on the volleyball team, and babysat regularly on weekends for the neighbors' two children. She had always been pleasant, happy, and friendly. Suddenly this boy that the parents did not know called her at home. After many phone conversations he asked Emily to join him on a weekend evening at the movies. Mr. and Mrs. B felt Emily was much too young to date, that she could get involved with drugs, sexual promiscuity, and so on. They were sad and worried that they had lost their little girl who always did what she was told. Emily was hurt and furious. She thought her parents were being totally unreasonable and that they did not trust her. Further exploration revealed that Mrs. B had gotten into trouble sexually as a young girl. She did not want Emily to make the same mistake. Her parents had been very lenient. She blamed their lack of guidelines for her error. Mrs. B became aware of her overreaction. She was able to understand that dating was a normal part of adolescent development after discussion with a psychiatric nurse. A compromise was arranged when she recognized Emily's competent and responsible functioning. After Mr. and Mrs. B met the boy, Emily was able to go to the movies with him and two other friends on a Saturday afternoon.

 CLINICAL EXAMPLE

Lui Lee, an adolescent girl starting high school, had always functioned well. Beginning high school was a totally different experience. She became overwhelmed by the large building, increased academic responsibilities, and complex peer relationships. She began school in September with much anxiety. By October she began having numerous illnesses that prevented her from attending school. This came to the attention of the school guidance counselor, who noticed her increased absences. The guidance counselor saw her and, after no medical problems were found, offered to have Lui Lee come to her office whenever she felt sick at school. When this did not help, she suggested Lui Lee receive some home instruction until she felt less anxious. This suggestion validated Lui Lee's fears that she could not handle high school and its increased pressures. Her solution of retreat was supported. Fortunately, her parents sought the help of a psychiatric nurse, who encouraged immediate return to school with entry into a peer support group with individual sessions initially as needed. This enabled her to talk out her fears and receive support from her peers. This also strengthened her confidence and fostered healthy functioning. She found she could handle high school after all. The nurse educated the guidance counselor on ways to be supportive while encouraging independent functioning.

Another important part of health education is identifying teenagers at high risk for problems. The indicators identified in Table 35-2 interrelate to form a profile of the high-risk adolescent (Fig. 35-2). Nurses who work in schools and various community settings can engage in screening and early nursing intervention with these teenagers to promote their adaptive responses and prevent development of future problems.

 What teaching methods or aids would be particularly effective when implementing a health education program with adolescents?

Family Therapy

The nurse needs to assess the level of family functioning and determine how to best interact with and help the family of the adolescent. Family therapy is particularly useful to an adolescent when disturbed family in-

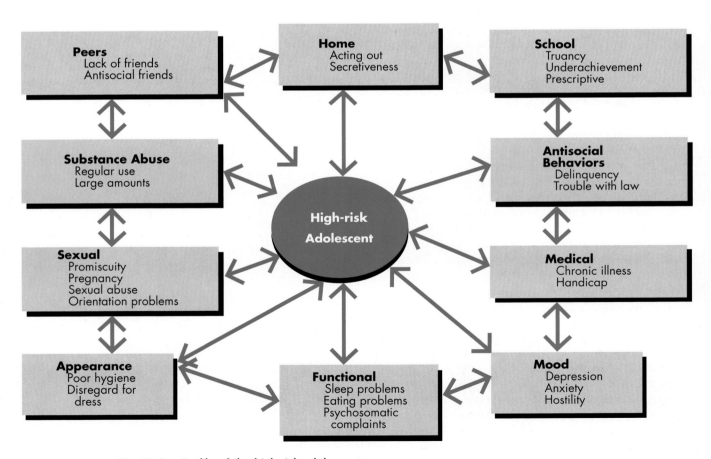

Fig. 35-2 Profile of the high-risk adolescent.

teraction is interfering with the adolescent's development.[16] Sometimes a series of family sessions may be enough, and the adolescent may benefit from either individual or group approaches to support the effort to separate emotionally from the family. Occasionally, after a few family sessions, it may become clear that the adolescent may not need the intervention directly. Engaging the parents may free the adolescent to progress on the developmental continuum.

The techniques used in family therapy are reviewed in detail in Chapter 30. Whichever modality is selected in working with the adolescent, a family orientation and the adolescent's attempt to separate from the family and become an independent adult should be considered.

Group Therapy

Group therapy addresses adolescents' need for peer support. The conflict of dependence-independence with adults becomes somewhat diluted by the presence of other adolescents. Conflicts, especially about authority, can be detected by peers rather than adults, making group therapy particularly helpful for adolescents. It is valuable in teaching skills in relating and dealing with others. Group therapy also helps fulfill the adolescent's need for a positive, meaningful peer group for ego identity formation.

Adolescent groups, in contrast to other groups, are difficult to manage because many adolescents react to peers defensively. Sibling rivalry often disrupts group cohesion. Many groups suffer from poor attendance, a high dropout rate, antisocial behavior, and a lack of group cohesion. However, group therapy with adolescents has proved to be successful in many community mental health centers, outpatient clinics, and hospital settings.

Often, beginning group sessions with some activity helps to provide a stabilizing factor for young adolescents. The number of members to include in the group depends on the type. For example, it may not be feasible to limit an outpatient "drop-in" group. Because of the age spread among adolescents, it is usually preferable to form at least two groups. A possibility is an early adolescence group consisting of 13- to 15-year-olds who have conflicts of separation from parents. An older adolescent group, ages 15 to 17, would probably consider issues such as the further establishment of identity, the beginning of dating, sex, experimentation with drugs, handling money, responsibilities of driving, and vocational plans.

Conflict between therapists, if there is an open and honest discussion, can provide a corrective experience because adolescents can see adults disagree without devastating consequences. If therapists are of the opposite sex, a parental similarity is often apparent; members often play on the therapist's feelings and try out tactics as they would with their own parents. Even if both therapists are of the same sex, one is usually more active, and a member may project a good or bad image onto each therapist that corresponds with how the parents are viewed. Group process with adolescents is often similar to that with adults, and specific aspects of working with groups are reviewed in Chapter 29.

Individual Therapy

Individual therapy done by the psychiatric clinical nurse specialist can consist of brief goal-directed therapy, behavioral therapy, or insight therapy. A description of insight therapy is presented here, since the principles are helpful in other types of individual therapy. Once the decision to engage in individual therapy is made, a pact or contract between the nurse and adolescent is established.

Therapeutic Alliance. This contract is described by Meeks[18] as a "therapeutic alliance" in which nurses align themselves with the healthy, reality-oriented aspect of the adolescent's ego and move toward an honest and critical understanding of the adolescent's inner experience. This alliance is created through the interpretation of the adolescent's feeling states and defensive behavior, especially toward the nurse.

Adolescents' alliances are focused toward links between their feelings and behavior in the present. The alliance is a central aspect of individual therapy. Once it is established, a feeling of working together is apparent. Meeks[18] mentions specific hints to establish and maintain this alliance:

1. Point out that behavior is motivated by feelings. Often, early in treatment, adolescents may express feelings of impatience, helplessness, and failure at having to seek treatment. Defenses are often seen in rebelliousness, passivity, shyness, negativism, and intellectualization. Adolescents generally have a tendency to act out and avoid examining their feelings.
2. Limit acting out by pointing out how it interferes with the therapeutic process and that it must be controlled to proceed. Maintain a neutral but interested attitude toward all behavior.
3. Point out the adolescent's tendencies to be judgmental and self-critical. This is supportive and helps to encourage the adolescent to look for sources of behaviors, attitudes, and feelings.
4. Establish that the adolescent's behavior is the end result of many inner feelings. Some of these un-

known feelings are interfering with the adolescent's happiness. This knowledge strengthens motivation for therapy and maintains an alignment with the adolescent's wishes for autonomy.

5. Point out the adolescent's tendency to see things in extremes; the desire to be complete master opposes the feelings of total helplessness. Reveal areas of strength and competence that are often unrecognized. Avoid focusing exclusively on problems and weaknesses. This shows neutrality and is supportive. Giving the adolescent as much information as possible to be prepared to make decisions helps the adolescent work toward self-direction.

6. Distinguish between thought and action, discouraging impulsiveness. Encourage open expression of strong feeling but not strong action. For example, anger does not mean killing; sexual feeling does not mean intercourse. Adolescents sometimes confuse discussion with permission to experiment with action, especially with sexual issues.

7. Encourage emotional catharsis in sessions by expressing interest in and acceptance of feelings involving the nurse and events outside the session. Point out the importance of feelings.

8. Be alert to the defenses of denial and reaction formation. Maintain neutrality and encourage objectivity without directly attacking needed defenses.

9. Adolescents often act provocatively to force punishment by adults. This puts the nurse in alignment with the self-hatred aspect of the adolescent's conscience and should be avoided. The nurse is supportive by continuing therapy even during these difficult periods.

The work of the nurse is to recognize the adolescent's anxiety and try to assist in finding ways to deal with emerging impulses. Accepting any healthy and adaptive responses of the adolescent strengthens the sense of ego mastery. Adolescents often have wishes that they regard as crazy and frightening. Open discussion of fears helps adolescents realize these feelings are uncomfortable but harmless thoughts.

Transference. Transference is an important aspect of adolescent treatment. The nurse must point out that these projections originate in the adolescent's mind and not in reality and that they usually represent a meaningful person such as a parent. It often helps to mention this is a common response. Several common transference patterns have been identified[18]:

1. **Erotic-sexual**—especially if the nurse is young and of the opposite sex. This transference typically is shown by awkward blushing and agitated confusion by the adolescent. It is usually best to emphasize the mutual work of emotional growth while establishing, tactfully, the nurse's unavailability as a sexual object. Focusing on origins or encouraging elaboration of these feelings is not helpful and is anxiety provoking.

2. **Omnipotent**—expecting the nurse will have answers to all questions. It is easy for the nurse to drift into this pattern, since often the adolescent appears to be helpless. The adolescent's secret desire for personal omnipotence is somewhat fulfilled by granting it to the nurse.

3. **Negative transference**—usually intense and pervasive. Negative feelings toward the nurse usually represent a negative attitude toward all adult authority figures. This transference is often defensive to cover feelings of shame, inadequacy, and anxiety, and it disappears as the adolescent respects the nurse's feelings. The adolescent tries to force the nurse's rejection. Open discussion to explore these feelings objectively and establish their origin is beneficial. Sometimes interpretations arouse anger toward the nurse because of the anxiety they create. These are reactions to the realities of therapy and are not to be confused with negative transference.

A true negative transference occurs when situations reactivate early experiences of negative feelings toward important others. The nurse unavoidably will frustrate the adolescent, who often has trouble delaying gratification to reach long-range goals. Negative transference, as with any other resistant behavior, is dealt with through objective exploration, which includes seeking causes of anger and pointing out irrationality. This is often followed by a period of regression and depression. Empathic understanding that the adolescent is mourning a loss is helpful, but it should be emphasized that what was lost was an illusion. Another common occurrence is for an adolescent to rebel against conscience and then respond to guilt through self-destructive behaviors. Pointing out this pattern helps the adolescent to eventually become aware of this.

Termination. Termination of therapy is an important part of the therapeutic process. Often, leaving therapy symbolizes the process of loosening bonds to parental images and giving up desires to be passive. One therefore expects defensive and regressive behaviors as the adolescent attempts to deal with the anxieties related to the termination process. This can mean the recurrence of emotional crises, symptoms, self-destructive fantasies, and even dependency behavior to provoke rescue.

Termination should be flexible and correctly timed. The decision should be made in line with adolescent norms, not adult ones. Often adolescents will verbalize appropriate interest in termination. When this occurs, it is often helpful to open it to discussion without commitment to a set time. This implies that further work needs to be done in a definite time span, and it maintains a focus on the adolescent's responsibility to finish. Gradually supporting and approving of the adolescent's independence and mature functioning prepares for a positive termination. Some adolescents leave therapy to return later. Some can never leave forever, seeing termination as a rejection rather than a vote of confidence. Gradual reduction of sessions without pressing for final termination may help as long as the overall situation is reviewed occasionally.

Sometimes terminations occur prematurely because either an alliance has not been established or some external event has occurred. Occasionally terminations are forced because of a nurse's change of location, death, or illness. The adolescent will express anger at the new therapist until the feelings about the lost therapist are accepted and resolved. In working out this attachment, a new therapeutic alliance can be established.

Talking with Adolescents

The following discussion focuses on some important considerations in communicating with adolescents.

Silence. Silence is often effective with adults but frightening to the adolescent, especially in the beginning stages of treatment or evaluation. This anxiety often reflects the adolescent's feelings of emptiness and lack of identity. Brief silences can be creative and productive when the adolescent is engaged in treatment; when the adolescent is able to tolerate them without anxiety, it indicates growth in self-confidence and acceptance of inner feelings. More often, however, silence is used defensively by adolescents to avoid discovery of hostile feelings or fantasies. Older adolescents may tolerate interpretive remarks, but with younger adolescents it is usually helpful to suggest an activity to help facilitate discussion and establish a relationship. For some adolescents, silence is a defense of inhibition and withdrawal, since they have never learned to communicate in a positive way. In these cases the therapist must be responsible for dialogue.

Confidentiality. Confidentiality is a concern to many, but especially to the adolescent who is fearful of the nurse reporting to parents. A blanket promise to tell nothing to the parents is not advised, since the nurse may need to contact the parents if the adolescent reveals suicidal or homicidal behavior or the use of illegal drugs. It is usually best to tell the adolescent that the nurse will not give out any information without informing the adolescent in advance. It is also helpful to explain that feelings are confidential but that actions considered dangerous to the adolescent or others may need to be shared.

Negativism. Negative feelings are often expressed by adolescents, especially initially, because they are frightened of the implications of coming for treatment. The young adolescent's lack of objectivity and upsurge of impulses, as well as the tendency to confuse fantasy and action, make the discussion of feelings threatening. Usually, gently noting in a supportive way defensive techniques the adolescent uses during the session helps to gain cooperation.

Resistance. Often adolescents begin by testing nurses to see if they will be authoritarian figures. The rebellious adolescent may deny the need for therapy or help. If the adolescent appears anxious, it is best to be supportive and sympathetic, expressing interest in getting to know the adolescent and then discussing a neutral area. A more angry, rebellious adolescent may require a direct approach, with the nurse saying openly that the adolescent is opposing the visit because of a false belief that no help is needed. This can lead to a further discussion of feelings about the visit (e.g., parental coercion to come to the session) or feelings about authority. Some adolescents are just baiting and testing to see if the nurse is an anxious, defensive adult. If so, it is best to ignore their comments about not wanting treatment and move on. Often adolescents with an angry facade depend on their omnipotent control of the environment and are often successful in manipulating their families. They are angry at attempts to disturb this power, and the anger is expressed in their lack of cooperation in the session.[15]

Arguing. Adolescents always argue and, although they do not admit it, learn from arguments. Often the adolescent goes against the viewpoint of the nurse and then in the next session adopts the nurse's opinion. It is best not to comment on this and accept it as a harmless defense. If the nurse admits having areas of ignorance, it is productive to the adolescent, who may fear the need to be perfect.

Testing. Adolescents often need and want limits. They are confused and cannot set their own limits. They experiment by trial and error to find a self-concept. Often, adolescents will test nurses to see how firm and consistent they will be. Controls frequently are effective if there is a basic positive relationship with the nurse. Limits should be set only when they are essential for current and future well-being, and the adolescent will value the security they provide. Adolescents will dare to be independent if it is conveyed that the nurse will serve as a control against carrying independence too far.

Dreams and Artistic Creations. Adolescents are often creative, and much can be learned from studying their works. As long as the discussion is relevant, it can be a productive source for exploring inner feelings. Along with dreams, these feelings can reveal valuable information about their real concerns, even when the adolescent attempts to avoid them.

Bringing Friends. The adolescent who brings a friend to a session may be attempting to avoid therapy. There is some benefit in sharing the experiences with the peer group, since this lowers anxiety. Telling the adolescent that bringing friends is not allowed may not be successful because the nurse cannot always enforce such a rule. The reason for bringing friends may vary, but it should be explored and understood. Sometimes adolescents want to refer friends. This may be positive but may also focus attention away from the original adolescent. The nurse should insist on exploring motives behind the referral before accepting the new patient, since the adolescent may think the nurse's acceptance of another is a betrayal of loyalty. If the friend clearly wants and needs therapy, referral to a colleague is usually best. If a friend is brought late in therapy, it may mean the adolescent is preparing to terminate.

Embarrassment about Being in Therapy. Embarrassment may occur in any age group, but it is prominent in adolescents, especially during the early stages of treatment. It also can become an issue as therapy progresses, since it often reveals the adolescent's embarrassment about a desire for dependency. Therefore adolescents may become uncomfortable in the therapeutic relationship. This is usually dealt with by indicating that these feelings are normal. Behind the fear of accepting help is the wish for care, and this can be dealt with by pointing out the adolescent's strengths and areas of independence.

Some adolescents, by expressing embarrassment about being in therapy, are actually revealing a fear or social stigma that they have heard from their parents. The adolescent who has feelings of inferiority often focuses these on the therapeutic process, blaming therapy for discomfort. It is best to encourage and support the adolescent, gently refusing to accept blame for this discomfort.

Requests for Special Attention. Some adolescents can develop intense dependency ties to the therapist. They reflect this in requests for additional appointments, extra time in appointments, frequent telephone calls, or social contact outside the therapeutic sessions. Focus should be on the exploration of feelings of inner emptiness, deprivation, and incompleteness that are responsible for these requests.

Parents of the Adolescent

If group or individual treatment is selected for the adolescent, the nurse must still consider the family. Parents cannot help the adolescent's treatment if they do not understand and accept it. The nurse can work with the parents without revealing confidential material.

Not all parents need treatment. It is helpful for parents to have treatment if the adolescent is asked to assume an inappropriate role at home, since this interferes with the adolescent's adaptive responses. If the parents are resistant, the nurse must usually begin with the adolescent until the parents are more receptive.

Telephone contact is a helpful way to ensure cooperation and support by having the parent call when necessary. Parents should tell the adolescent when they call. Parents should be told of normal adolescent behavior they can expect. The nurse should avoid advising the parents about specific actions and focus on attitudes and feelings, especially concerning discipline. Parents can be helped with understanding the purpose of limit setting. Some parents exclude themselves entirely from their adolescent's life. They have brought the adolescent to treatment to ease their guilt by doing all that is possible. They may want the nurse to take over parenting functions. This should not be permitted, especially during crises. If the adolescent is suicidal or homicidal, the parents are informed and helped to take responsibility for action.

Adolescents often need help in dealing with their parents. Parents should be discussed in an open exploratory manner, with emphasis on them having their own feelings and reasons for their actions. Adolescents should be helped to see their parents realistically and to work on their own strengths and weaknesses.

Sometimes adolescents want to leave home because they hope they will feel more adult away from their parents. It is usually best to explore the wish to leave, emphasizing that it must be done in an adult way. If leaving is an impulsive thought with no feasible plan, it will ensure failure, parental rescue, and continued dependency. This is often recapitulated in termination from therapy if the adolescent quits early to avoid the pain of separation that a planned termination would bring.

Do you think adolescents can benefit from treatment if their parents deny there is a problem, refuse to be involved, or are opposed to seeking help?

EVALUATING NURSING CARE

Problems presented by adolescents, more frequently than those of any other group, activate the nurse's own unresolved conflicts. Thus evaluating nursing care must begin with nurses monitoring their responses, including countertransference reactions. The nurse should watch for alignment with either the parents against the adolescent or the adolescent against the parents. Most adults are resistant to reexperiencing the feelings of adolescence and have repressed these experiences. As a result of anxiety, the nurse occasionally may have trouble listening or may encourage the adolescent (because of unrecognized wishes) to do what the nurse never dared do. The adolescent may be acting as the nurse did during adolescence. The nurse, in an effort to deny this, may see this adolescent behavior as nondeviant. Identification of the nurse with the adolescent can contribute to delays in exploring areas important for psychological growth. The nurse may relate well to the adolescent but because of unresolved, unrecognized conflicts or resentment toward the nurse's own parents, may be locked into adolescent rebellion. The nurse may overtly or covertly encourage adolescents to express rage toward their families. Both the adolescent and the nurse then avoid facing the reality of adult burdens.

Evaluation of psychiatric nursing care with adolescents also involves consideration of objective measurements of the adolescent's and the family's progress toward the goals of treatment. Specifically, the nurse may ask:

1. Were the concerns of the adolescent and family addressed?
2. Has the problematic behavior decreased and been replaced with more adaptive responses?
3. Have the adolescent's relationships with others improved?
4. Has school or work performance been enhanced?
5. Is the adolescent and family satisfied with the treatment outcome?

By reviewing areas of growth and progress, the adolescent is able to integrate the learning that has been accomplished and gain from the experience a greater sense of self-efficacy and mastery.

SUGGESTED CROSS-REFERENCES

SUMMARY

1. Adolescence is a unique stage of development that occurs between the ages of 11 and 20 and is accompanied by a shift in development and learning.
2. Various theories explain the adolescent's resolution of tasks, including biological, psychoanalytical, psychosocial, cognitive, cultural, and multidimensional.
3. Issues that are particularly problematic to adolescents include those of body image, identity, independence, social role, and sexual behavior.
4. Maladaptive responses impede growth and development and require nursing intervention. These are often related to inappropriate sexual activity, homosexuality problems, unwed motherhood, suicide, runaways, conduct disorders, violence, drug use, hypochondriasis, weight problems, occult involvement, and parental divorce.
5. Nursing interventions useful in working with adolescents include health education and family, group, and individual therapy. Special attention should be given to talking with adolescents and working with their parents.
6. Evaluation of nursing care requires special focus on countertransference issues and the need for objective measurements of the adolescent's and family's progress toward the treatment goals.

COMPETENT CARING
A CLINICAL EXEMPLAR OF A PSYCHIATRIC NURSE

Karen M. McHugh, BSN, RN, C

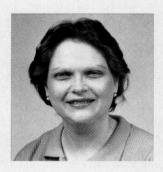

When I graduated with a bachelor of science degree in nursing, I never imagined I would be interested in psychiatric nursing. After 1½ years in medical-surgical nursing, I decided I wanted more interpersonal time with my patients rather than being so skill and task oriented. One of my first experiences as a psychiatric nurse was on a 32-bed adolescent unit in North Carolina. There I encountered a 14-year-old girl, S, who was admitted to our inpatient unit for depression. At that time patients typically stayed for about 3 months, which is much different from the current length of stay for adolescents in the hospital, which is most often 5 to 10 days.

S had several problems, most occurring within the previous year. She had a history of running away, crying spells, skipping school, failing grades, and suicidal threats. She lived at home with her father and 9-year-old brother. Her mother was no longer involved in her life because she had left the family and had given up custody of the children several years before.

S settled into the milieu but had a difficult time engaging with the staff. I began to spend time with her everyday to establish a trusting relationship. The first few days we would just sit in silence. Eventually we were able to talk about her history of oppositional behavior and low self-esteem. S trusted me more and more over time. Then, about 1 month after admission, she approached me and asked if we could talk again. S asked me if I could promise not to tell anyone (especially her father or doctors) if she confided in me about something. I knew then that something was troubling her, but I had to be honest with her. I told S that I couldn't make that promise because the treatment team works in the best interest of the patient and I would have to share pertinent information with them. She decided not to confide in me then, but the next day she approached me again.

S began to tell me that the past few months her father began to drink and had hit her several times, leaving marks on her legs and arms. She stated that one day she had to stay home from school because her legs were swollen and painful from the bruises. She said that her father always apologized once he was sober and promised that he would never hit her again. I gathered a few more details and was honest with her and informed her that I would have to collaborate with the treatment team and possibly seek help from the Department of Social Services. After meeting with the treatment team the next day, I told S that we had to report her father to Social Services. She began to yell and scream and blame me for telling everyone about her problems. Even though I had been honest with her, she couldn't understand that I was actually helping her.

At this point I had to examine my feelings, and I even questioned my judgment. I went home from work that evening quite upset. I began to ask myself such questions as, Did I do the right thing? Will S ever confide in me again or even talk with me? In spite of feeling a little guilty, I really knew that I had made the right decision, since protecting S and her future was of utmost importance. After a few days of cooling off S approached me and was able to express her feelings of relief and even apologized to me. We began to work on identifying and expressing her feelings of guilt, relief, sadness, and concern over the situation with her father. Social Services found no evidence of abuse to her 9-year-old brother, so he remained at home with the father.

At discharge, an aunt assumed foster care of S temporarily until her father could obtain the therapy he needed. S was referred to outpatient therapy as well. Several weeks after her discharge, I saw her at the mall, and she thanked me for helping and listening to her even though she didn't see it that way at first. She stated that she was happier now and was doing well in school and that she and her father were continuing therapy.

I had made the right decision. Being a child's advocate and maintaining a patient's safety during an inpatient stay and after discharge is always a nurse's first priority. As I reflected on this experience, I learned not to take things in my personal life so much for granted, such as a loving and supportive family. I also realized that psychiatric nurses do provide excellence in nursing and that we truly can make a difference. ▼

REFERENCES

1. Adams P, Fras I: *Beginning child psychiatry*, New York, 1988, Brunner/Mazel.
2. Blos P: The second individuation process of adolescence, *Psychoanal Study Child* 22:162, 1967.
3. Blumenthal S, Kupfer D: *Suicide over the life cycle: risk factors, assessment, and treatment of suicidal patients*, Washington, DC, 1990, American Psychiatric Press.
4. Brenner C: *An elementary textbook of psychoanalysis*, New York, 1974, Anchor Press.
5. Centers for Disease Control: Results from the national adolescent student health survey, MMWR 38:147, 1989.
6. Deisher R, Remafedi G: Adolescent sexuality. In Hofmann A, Greydanus D, eds: *Adolescent medicine*, Norwalk, Conn, 1989, Appleton & Lange.
7. Erikson E: *Childhood and society*, ed 2, New York, 1963, WW Norton & Sons.
8. Gabriel H, Hofmann A: Behavioral problems. In Hofmann A, Greydanus D, eds: *Adolescent medicine*, Norwalk, Conn, 1989, Appleton & Lange.
9. Galanter M: *Cults and new religious movements*, Washington, DC, 1989, American Psychiatric Press.
10. Gesell A, Ilg F, Ames L: *Youth: the years from ten to sixteen*, New York, 1956, Harper & Row.
11. Havighurst RL: *Developmental tasks and education*, ed 3, New York, 1972, David McKay.
12. Kalogerakis M: Emergency evaluation of adolescents, *Hosp Community Psychiatry* 43:617, 1992.
13. Klerman G: *Suicide and depression among adolescents and young adults*, Washington, DC, 1986, American Psychiatric Press.
14. Marohn R: Management of the assaultive adolescent, *Hosp Community Psychiatry* 43:622, 1992.
15. Marshall R: The treatment of resistances in psychotherapy of children and adolescents, *Psychother Theory Res Pract* 9:143, 1972.
16. Matorin S, Greenberg L: Family therapy in the treatment of adolescents, *Hosp Community Psychiatry* 43:625, 1992.
17. Mead M: *Culture and commitment: a study of the generation gap*, New York, 1970, Basic Books.
18. Meeks J: *The fragile alliance*, ed 4, Malabar, Fla, 1990, Robert Krieger.
19. Offer D, Ostrov E, Howard K, eds: *Patterns of the adolescent self-image*, San Francisco, 1984, Jossey-Bass.
20. Pfeffer C: *Suicide among youth: perspectives on risk and prevention*, Washington, DC, 1989, American Psychiatric Press.
21. Piaget J: *Six psychological studies*, New York, 1968, Vintage Books.
22. Powers S, Hauser S, Kilner L: Adolescent mental health, *Am Psychol* 44:200, 1989.
23. Remafedi G: Homosexual youth: a challenge to contemporary society, *JAMA* 258:222, 1987.
24. Riesch S, Forsyth D: Preparing to parent the adolescent, *J Child Adolesc Psychiatr Ment Health Nurs* 5:32, 1992.
25. Savin-Williams R: *Gay and lesbian youth: expressions of identity*, New York, 1990, Hemisphere Publishing.
26. Schwartzberg A: The impact of divorce on adolescents, *Hosp Community Psychiatry* 43:634, 1992.
27. Stein T: Overview of new developments in understanding homosexuality. In Oldham J, Riba M, Tasman A, eds: *Review of psychiatry*, volume 12, Washington, DC, 1993, American Psychiatric Press.
28. Troiden R: The formation of homosexual identities, *J Homosex* 17:43, 1989.
29. Wagner B, Stanley S: Occult involvement as a risk-taking behavior by adolescents. Paper presented at Advocates of Child Psychiatric Nursing Conference, New York, Sept 21, 1989.

ANNOTATED SUGGESTED READINGS

*Bender P: Multiple family therapy for adolescents: a case illustration, J *Child Adolesc Psychiatr Ment Health Nurs* 5:27, 1992.

Examines the mechanisms of change in multiple family therapy as used by nurses working with adolescents.

*Carbray J, Pitula C: Trends in adolescent psychiatric hospitalization, J *Child Adolesc Psychiatr Ment Health Nursing* 4:68, 1991.

Thought-provoking exploration of factors contributing to the increase in adolescent inpatient admissions and raises interesting questions about parental decision making.

Forgatch M, Patterson G: *Parents and adolescents living together: family problem solving,* Eugene, Ore, 1989, Castalia Publishing.

Teaches families with adolescents how to resolve conflicts concerning such problems as sexual behavior, drug and alcohol use, and school achievement.

Gibbs J, Huang L: *Children of color: psychological interventions with minority youth,* San Francisco, 1989, Jossey-Bass.

Explains cultural expectations, family structure, language, and discrimination concerns of Native Americans, Asian Americans, Hispanic Americans, and African Americans.

*Hogarth C: *Adolescent psychiatric nursing,* St Louis, 1991, Mosby.

This is a "must-own" book for all adolescent psychiatric nurses. It covers all aspects of the field in a thorough, practical, and highly readable way.

*Jones J: A proposed model of relapse prevention for adolescents who abuse alcohol, J *Child Adolesc Psychiatr Ment Health Nurs* 3:139, 1990.

Excellent article describing an effective relapse prevention program for adolescents who abuse alcohol.

Khan A: *Short-term psychiatric hospitalization of adolescents,* Chicago, 1990, Mosby.

Comprehensive but concise discussion of various aspects of inpatient care of adolescents from the medical point of view.

*McBride A: *The secret of a good life with your teenager,* New York, 1987, Times Books.

Explores the key developmental themes that characterize the experience of parents with teenagers. Full of insights, advice, warmth, and humor.

*Nixon M: Mental health care rights of adolescents: what mental health nurses need to know, J *Child Adolesc Psychiatr Ment Health Nurs* 5:14, 1992.

*Nursing reference.

Reviews issues of importance in the medical/legal rights of adolescents and their parents. Should be required reading for all nurses working with adolescents.

*Pushkar K, Lamb J, Martsolf D: The role of the psychiatric/ mental health nurse clinical specialist in an adolescent coping skills group, J *Child Adolesc Psychiatr Ment Health Nurs* 3:47, 1990.

Describes a nurse-led adolescent prevention program, including the specific adolescent coping skills group format used.

*Riesch S, Forsyth D: Preparing to parent the adolescent, J *Child Adolesc Psychiatr Ment health Nurs* 5:32, 1992.

Reviews the tasks of early adolescence and middle adulthood and analyzes family adaptability, cohesion, satisfaction, communication skills, and ability to resolve conflict.

*Sadler L: Depression in adolescents: context, manifestations, and clinical management, *Nurs Clin North Am* 26:559, 1991.

Overview article on the important problem of depression in adolescence.

*Scharer K, Challberg C, Rearick T: Young people and AIDS, J *Child Adolesc Psychiatr Ment Health Nurs* 3:41, 1990.

Reports the development and implementation of a health promotion and AIDS prevention program developed for junior high students, including learning strategies and the reactions of students, parents, and the educational system.

*Schepp K: A symptom management program for adolescents with psychotic illnesses: theoretical basis and preliminary clinical outcomes, J *Child Adoles Psychiatr Ment Health Nurs* 5:7, 1992.

These are two articles that describe the theoretical basis and outcomes of a nursing intervention program for adolescents who have experienced nondrug-related psychotic episodes. The program advocates self-management and family support.

Zera D: Coming of age in a heterosexist world: the development of gay and lesbian adolescents, *Adolescence* 27:849, 1992.

An excellent overview of the gay adolescent experience that should be required reading for all nurses to sensitize them to the needs of these adolescents and enable nurses to provide support and information.

*Nursing reference.

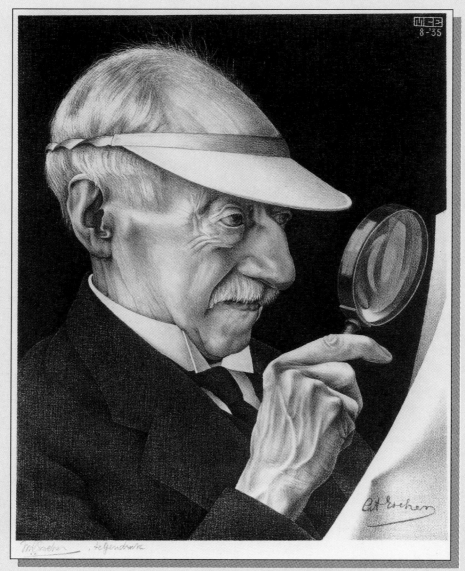

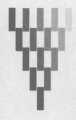

CHAPTER 36
Geriatric Psychiatric Nursing

BEVERLY A. BALDWIN
GEORGIA L. STEVENS
SUZANNE D. FRIEDMAN

Youth is like a fresh flower in May.
Age is like a rainbow that follows the storms of life.
Each has its own beauty.*

David Polis

LEARNING OBJECTIVES

After studying this chapter the student should be able to:

▼ Identify the role and functions of the geropsychiatric nurse
▼ Compare and contrast the major biopsychosocial theories of aging
▼ Identify and describe the elements of a comprehensive geropsychiatric nursing assessment
▼ Formulate nursing diagnoses for geropsychiatric patients
▼ Identify expected outcomes and short-term nursing goals for geropsychiatric patients
▼ Analyze nursing interventions for geropsychiatric patients
▼ Evaluate nursing care of geropsychiatric patients

TOPICAL OUTLINE

Role of the Geropsychiatric Nurse
Theories of Aging
   Biological Theories
   Psychological Theories
   Sociocultural Theories
Assessing the Geriatric Patient
   The Interview
   Cognitive Function
   Affective Status
   Behavioral Responses
   Functional Abilities
   Physiological Functioning
   Social Support
Diagnosis of the Geriatric Patient
   Altered Thought Processes
   Affective Responses
   Somatic Responses
   Stress Responses
   Behavioral Responses
Planning and Intervention
   Therapeutic Milieu
   Physical Restraints
   Somatic Therapies
   Interpersonal Interventions
Evaluating the Care of the Geriatric Patient

Persons 65 years of age and older make up the fastest growing age group in the United States. One in every nine Americans, or almost 13% of the population, is 65 or older; in the first half of the twenty-first century, this will increase to one in five. Women live an average of 7 years longer than men, and more older women live alone.[34] It is estimated that by 2030 there will be 60 million persons over 65—17% to 20% of the U.S. population.[39] By 2050 21% of those over 65 will be a member of an ethnic minority group, and 24% of these will be black.[2]

It has been estimated that over 4 million elderly Americans have moderate to severe psychiatric impairment resulting from dementia, psychosis, chronic alcoholism, or other conditions. The elderly account for over 25% of reported suicides, with the highest rate occurring in white men in their mid-eighties.[9] About 6 million older Americans require some type of community-based long-term care because of self-care deficits[34]; 28% of elders residing in the community have been found to have a mental disorder.[31] Prevalence of psychiatric disorders among institutionalized elders is significant. Recent studies have suggested that 51% to 94% of residents of long-term care facilities had some form of psychiatric disorder.[12,31,47] While the institutionalized population is only a small percentage of elders, this figure represents a challenge to nursing.

The extent of mental disorders in the elderly appears considerable; therefore nurses and other health-care professionals will be increasingly responsible for caring for older adults with mental and emotional health problems. Helping older adults to maximize their potential can be a challenging and rewarding experience for the nurse.

Stereotypes and myths often depict the elderly as a homogeneous group. On the contrary, the older adult represents a combination of multiple interpersonal, developmental, and situational experiences. The complexity and interaction of the needs and problems of old age are often underestimated and understated. Mental health in late life depends on a number of factors. These include physiological and psychological status, personality, social support system, economic resources, and usual life-style. This chapter addresses selected aspects of the psychiatric–mental health needs of geriatric patients and their families.

ROLE OF THE GEROPSYCHIATRIC NURSE

The nurse who works with mentally ill elders is challenged to integrate psychiatric nursing skills with knowledge of physiological disorders, the normal aging process, and sociocultural influences on the elderly and their families. Many nurses who work with these patients find that it is useful to combine nurse practitioner and psychiatric nursing skills. Mental health services are provided to this population in a variety of settings including general and psychiatric hospitals, nursing homes, outpatient mental health clinics, adult day-care programs, senior centers, and the person's own home.

As a primary care provider the geropsychiatric nurse must be proficient at assessing cognitive, affective, functional, physical, and behavioral status. Planning and nursing intervention may occur with the patient and family or other caregivers. Providing nursing care to these patients can be complex because they are often involved with a number of agencies.

As a consultant the geropsychiatric nurse assists other providers of services to the elderly to address the behavioral and cognitive aspects of the patient's care. Frequently this role is assumed by nurses in their own agency. For instance, a nurses may help nursing assistants understand how to respond to a patient who wanders or one who is aggressive. Advanced practice geropsychiatric nurses who have graduate education in this specialty may be employed by agencies to assist the entire staff to develop therapeutic programs for seniors with psychiatric or behavioral problems. Some nurses develop and market in-service education packages for nursing homes or other agencies that serve these patients.

Geropsychiatric nurses should become knowledgeable about the effects of psychotropic medication on elderly people. They often work closely with the physician to monitor complex medication regimens and assist the patient or caregiver with medication management. They may lead a variety of groups such as orientation, remotivation, bereavement, and socialization groups, whereas nurses with advanced degrees may provide psychotherapy.

THEORIES OF AGING

Ways of defining aging and explaining the causes and consequences of the aging process are based on two major approaches to aging:

1. The causes of the biological and psychological aging process
2. The psychosocial results of aging

Gerontologists disagree about the cause and adaptation to aging. No one theory can include all the variables that influence aging and the person's response to it. It is difficult to separate the effects of stress, disease processes, and specific age-related changes. Theories of aging may help, however, to clarify the physical and mental changes experienced by elderly patients.

Biological Theories

Biological Programming Theory.

The biological programming theory proposes that the life span of a cell is stored within the cell itself. Through laboratory studies, Hayflick et al.[29] demonstrated that normal human fibroblasts, when cultured, doubled a specific number of times and then died. The number of doublings is the same in male and female cells. This theory of a human biological clock views the decline of biological, cognitive, and psychomotor function as inevitable and irreversible, although diet changes or prolonged hypothermia may delay the process. The concept of programmed aging answers some questions about the human life span. It does not address hereditary and environmental influences on individual variations in aging.

> Give at least two examples that contradict the biological programming theory of aging. How do you feel about the idea of a biological clock determining life span?

Wear-and-Tear Theory.

The wear-and-tear theory suggests that structural and functional changes may be speeded by abuse and slowed by care. From a physiological standpoint, aging is viewed developmentally, beginning with conception and leading to decline and death. Problems associated with aging are the result of accumulated stress, trauma, injuries, infections, inadequate nutrition, metabolic and immunological disturbances, and prolonged abuse. This concept of aging is seen in widely accepted myths and stereotypes regarding the aged, as noted in such phrases as, "He's doing well for his age," or "What can you expect at that age?" Newer research on the value of exercise and cognitive stimulation in later years refutes the basic premise of this theory, since both body and mind seem to benefit from use and stimulation.

> Discuss how the wear-and-tear theory of aging compares with the present emphasis on nutrition and physical fitness in American culture.

Stress-Adaptation Theory.

The stress-adaptation theory emphasizes the positive and negative effects of stress on biopsychosocial development. As a positive influence, stress may stimulate a person to try new, more effective ways of adapting. A negative effect of stress would be inability to function because of feeling overwhelmed. The balance of positive and negative stress experiences must be examined. Although it is often assumed that stress accelerates the aging process, there is little evidence to support that conclusion. Stress may drain a person's reserve capacity—physiologically, psychologically, socially, and economically—increasing vulnerability to illness or injury.

Psychological Theories

Erikson's Stage of Ego Integrity.

Erikson's[19] theory of human development identifies tasks that must be accomplished at each of the eight stages of life. The last task, related to reflection about one's life and accomplishments, is identified as ego integrity. If this is not achieved, despair results. The end result of resolving the conflict between ego integrity and despair is acquired wisdom.

Life Review Theory.

The life review was identified in 1961 by Butler.[13] In elderly persons life review is a normal process brought about by the realization of approaching death. During the life review past experiences return to consciousness. There is also a resurgence of unresolved conflicts. The person examines and reintegrates these memories. Successful reintegration can give meaning to life and prepare the person for death by relieving anxiety and fear. According to the life review theory, this process occurs universally and is a functional preparation for the final stage of life. Although it occurs in all age groups to a certain degree, the emphasis and focused concentration are characteristic of the later stage of life. Aged persons have a vivid memory for past events and can recall early life experiences with clarity and imagination. They appear to be reviewing and sorting previous life events to better understand their present circumstances.

The life review may have positive or negative consequences. Anxiety, guilt, fear, and depression may surface if the person is unable to resolve or accept old, unsolved problems. On the other hand, the righting of the earlier wrongs can help establish a sense of serenity, pride in working through old conflicts, and acceptance of mortal life. Reflection is thus seen as a positive approach to aging. Further discussion of this process is found in the section on strategies for intervening in the mental health problems of the older adult.

Stability of Personality.

Some gerontologists contend that personality is established by early adulthood and remains fairly stable thereafter. Stability or continuity of personality has been observed in longitudinal studies of aging individuals at the National Institutes of Health Gerontology Research Center in Baltimore (the intramural research center for the National Institute on Aging). Usually no decline or change in personality, compared with other cognitive changes, was evident. Radical changes in personality in older persons may be indicative of brain disease. Researchers found that periods of psychological crisis in adulthood do not occur at regular intervals. This contradicts some theories such as Erikson's. Persons with a long history of emotional instability, however, were likely to encounter more crises. Finally, the researchers noted that changes in roles, attitudes, and situational demands created the need for new behavioral responses. The majority of elderly persons in these studies appeared to adapt effectively to those demands.

Can personality traits be altered in old age? If yes, how? If no, why are we interested in intervening in nonproductive behaviors of older adults?

Sociocultural Theories

Disengagement Theory. This controversial theory evolved from studies conducted by the University of Chicago Committee on Human Development.[16] It postulated that older adults and society mutually withdraw from active exchange with each other as part of the normal aging process. This was assumed to be a sign of psychological well-being and adjustment on the part of the elder. This theory did not consider the differences among the elderly and the personality variables important to coping with change. Stereotypes reinforced by this theory include the idea that older people only enjoy the company of people their own age and that retirement facilities should prohibit intergenerational living arrangements. Although many elders may desire such arrangements, others feel isolated and out of the mainstream of society.

Activity Theory. Disputes about the reliability of the disengagement theory led to the development of the current view that activity produces the most positive psychological climate for older adults. The activity theory developed as a reaction to the negative view of disengagement. Many gerontologists support the idea that aging is a phase in the developmental process; others contend that old age is only an extension of the middle years and can be modified or abolished by increased activity levels. The activity theory maintains that the aged should remain active as long as possible. Older adults who must stop working or participating in community activities should find substitutes. This theory emphasizes the positive influence of activity on the

older person's personality, mental health, and satisfaction with life.

The Family in Later Life. While theorists such as Erikson consider individual development throughout the life cycle, family theorists focus on the family as the basic unit of emotional development. This framework considers the interrelated tasks, problems, and relationships of the three-generational family system. Carter and McGoldrick[14] address multigenerational patterns, myths, developmental transitions, and external stressors. They theorize that the central process of the life cycle is changing the relationship system to support the functional entry, exit, and development of family members. Each transition requires a shift in emotional attitudes to support the relationship changes. In later life the emotional process involves accepting the shifting of generational roles, while the relationship changes include:

1. Maintaining functioning and interests during physiological decline
2. Exploring new role options
3. Supporting the middle generation in a more central role
4. Making room in the system for the wisdom and experience of the older generation
5. Supporting elderly family members without over-functioning
6. Dealing with the loss of significant others and preparing for death

Physical, emotional, and social symptoms are believed to reflect problems in negotiating the transitions of the family life cycle.

ASSESSING THE GERIATRIC PATIENT

Nursing assessment of the geropsychiatric patient is complex. The interplay of biological, psychological, and sociocultural factors related to aging sometimes makes it difficult to clearly identify nursing problems. For example, it can be quite difficult to sort out the behaviors related to the "4 D's" of geropsychiatric assessment—**depression, dementia, delirium,** and **delusions.** Aside from major psychotic disorders, delusions are also characteristic of depression in the elderly, and those with dementia may seem delusional because of the trouble they have in interpreting the environment.[40] Delirium may occur related to physical illness, medications, or sensory deprivation. Behaviors associated with delirium may include hallucinations, delusions, confusion, disorientation, and agitation. It may be mistaken for dementia, depriving the patient of treatment that could reverse the problem. Depressed elders often appear confused and cognitively impaired because of the lethargy and psychomotor retardation related to depression. Patients with dementia are sometimes also depressed, especially if they are aware of their declining mental functioning. A recent study found that depression is associated with multiinfarct dementia and mild to moderate Alzheimer's disease but not with severe Alzheimer's.[22] Gomez and Gomez[25] have identified some behaviors that help to differentiate between depression and dementia. Depressed patients are oriented and maintain socially appropriate behaviors. They are unlikely to undress in public or be incontinent. In response to questions, patients with dementia will try to answer but have trouble with logic and relevance. Depressed patients will be annoyed and reject the questioner with silence or short, unresponsive answers. Irritability and hostility are more characteristic of the depressed person.

Careful nursing assessment can be helpful in identifying the primary disorder. Nursing diagnoses are based on observation of patient behaviors and related to current needs. Cognitive responses including Alzheimer's disease and related disorders are discussed in Chapter 21 and emotional responses including depression in Chapter 17.

The Interview

Establishing a supportive and trusting relationship is essential to a positive interview with the geriatric patient. The elderly person may feel uneasy, vulnerable, and confused in a new place or with strangers. Patience and attentive listening promote a sense of security. Comfortable surroundings will help the patient relax and focus on the conversation.

Therapeutic Communication Skills. The nurse shows respect by addressing the patient by his last name: "Good morning, Mr. Smith." The nurse opens the interview by introducing herself and briefly orienting the patient to the purpose and length of the interview. Occasionally reinforcing the amount of time left may help direct a wandering discussion and give the patient the security of knowing the nurse is in control of the situation.

Older persons may respond to questions slowly, since ability to respond verbally slows with age. It is important to give the patient enough time to answer. Assuming the patient does not know the answer to a question, does not remember, or does not understand because of a slow response can lead the nurse to false conclusions about the patient.

The way the patient is interviewed is important. Baker[3] has suggested that using a life course interview format that is tied to significant historical events that have occurred during the person's lifetime may facilitate

interviews with black elders. Older people often are unfamiliar with new words, slang, or colloquialisms. Choice of words should also be based on knowledge of the person's sociocultural background. The nurse should avoid the use of medical abbreviations, terminology, or jargon. Questions should be short and to the point, particularly if the patient has difficulty with abstract thinking and conceptualization. Techniques such as clarification and summarization, described in Chapter 2, are important in validating information. The nurse should rephrase a question if the patient fails to answer appropriately or hesitates when answering.

Concentrated verbal interaction may be uncomfortable for the older person. The nurse can demonstrate interest and support by giving nonverbal cues and responses, such as direct eye contact, nodding, sitting close to the patient, and using touch appropriately. Touching the shoulder, arm, or hand of the patient in a firm, purposeful manner conveys support and interest (Fig. 36-1). Avoid stroking or patting the patient. Cul-

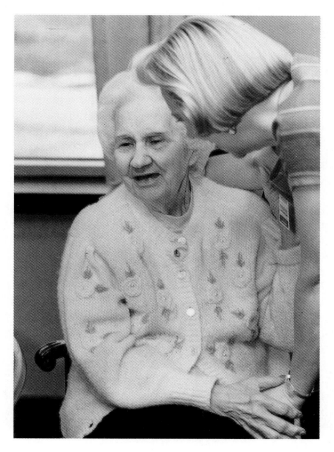

Fig. 36-1   Touching a patient's shoulder and hand is an appropriate nonverbal gesture that expresses interest and support.

tural background and altered tactile perception may result in misinterpretation.

The nurse's ability to collect useful data will depend greatly on how comfortable the nurse feels during the interview. Negative feelings toward the aged will surface in an interview. Older people are sensitive to others' lack of interest and impatience.

Although older people differ in their willingness to reveal life histories and personal experiences, most desire relationships with others and are anxious to share information with interested persons. Elderly patients have much to tell and may offer more information than the nurse needs at a particular time. Older patients often reminisce. The nurse should encourage this when possible. The patient is concerned with life review. The life review may serve as an excellent source of data about the patient's current health problems and support resources. Reminiscence and life review may make it difficult to keep the patient focused on the topic at hand; however, they allow the nurse to assess subtle changes in long-term memory, decision-making ability, judgment-making patterns, affect, and orientation to time, place, and person.

Many geriatric patients are aware of changes in their physical or psychological functioning. They may hesitate to have their fears confirmed. They may minimize or ignore symptoms, assuming they are age related and not related to current problems. Often these beliefs are reinforced by myths about aging and the false assumption of many health professionals that the problems of older persons are irreversible or untreatable.

Contrary to popular myths, most older people do not dwell unrealistically on their health and usually have a physical problem when they say they are not well. However, some older persons are preoccupied with the physical decline that occurs with age. The nurse must observe carefully for clues that help distinguish whether the patient's preoccupation reflects lifelong personality factors or current distress.

The geriatric patient may misunderstand the purpose of the nurse's questions. Questions regarding habits, previous life experience, or social supports may not seem to be related to current concerns. Careful and repeated explanations are necessary to gain the patient's cooperation. The nurse should never assume that the patient understands the purpose or protocol for the assessment interview. It is wiser to overstate than to increase the patient's anxiety and stress by omitting information. The nurse should take cues from the patient's responses by listening carefully and observing constantly.

The Interview Setting. The new and unfamiliar surroundings of the health-care agency may obstruct the initial interview by distracting the patient and increasing fear of the unknown. The physical environment should promote comfort. Many older persons are unable to sit for long periods because of arthritis or other joint disabilities. Chairs should be comfortable, The patient should be encouraged to move about as desired. Changing positions and range-of-motion exercises stimulate circulation and prevent stiffness.

Most older persons experience some form of sensory deficit, particularly diminished high-frequency hearing or changes in vision as a result of cataracts or glaucoma. The environment should be modified to decrease the impact of these deficits. The setting should be quiet and without distracting noises. A patient who is already under stress, may be annoyed by these distractions. The nurse should speak slowly and in a low-pitched voice. Shouting raises the pitch of the noise and makes hearing more difficult. Because fatigue may contribute to diminished mental functioning, morning may be the best time for the interview. Patients become tired as the day progresses and cognitive ability may diminish in the late afternoon or early evening.

The reliability of the data obtained from the assessment interview should be carefully evaluated. If there are questions about some of the patient's responses, the nurse should consult family members or other persons who know the patient well. The nurse should also consider the patient's physical condition at the time of the interview and other factors that may influence status, such as medications, nutrition, or anxiety level.

Cognitive Function

Mental status must be part of any geropsychiatric assessment for a number of reasons, including:
1. The increasing prevalence of dementia with age
2. The close association of clinical symptoms of confusion and depression
3. The frequency with which physical health problems present with symptoms of confusion
4. The need to identify specific areas of cognitive strength and limitation

An in-depth discussion of the assessment of mental status and other cognitive functioning scales used with the elderly is included in Chapter 6.

Affective Status

Affective status is an essential part of geropsychiatric assessment. The need to include a depression scale is based on:
1. The prevalence of depression in the elderly
2. The effectiveness of treatment for this disorder
3. The potential negative outcomes of depression (e.g., suicide, neglect)

4. Frequent misdiagnosis of depression as a physical problem
5. The tendency to dismiss elders as complainers or demanding

General estimates of the prevalence of depression among the elderly are 15% to 20%. However, the estimates are higher for special populations such as elders in long-term care facilities.[8]

In general, the prevalence of depression is lower in the elderly than in younger age groups.[33] There is also a higher incidence of depression among people of all ages who have disabilities. Since the number of physical disabilities tends to increase with age, this may account for some of the prevalence in the elderly.

Depression in the elderly differs in some ways from that in younger populations.[25] It may begin with decreased interest in usual activities and lack of energy. There may be increased dependence on others. Conversation may focus almost entirely on the past. There may be multiple somatic complaints with no diagnosable organic cause. The person may have pain, especially in the head, neck, back, or abdomen with no history or evidence of a physical cause. Other symptoms in the elderly include weight loss, paranoia,[7] fatigue, gastrointestinal distress,[38] and refusal to eat or drink with life-threatening consequences.

Physical illness can cause secondary depression (see Chapter 17). Some illnesses that tend to be associated with depression include thyroid disorders; cancer, especially lung, pancreas, and brain; Parkinson's disease; and stroke.[25] Some medications also increase the tendency for depression, including steroids, phenothiazines, benzodiazepines, and antihypertensives.[25]

Geriatric Depression Scale. The Geriatric Depression Scale (GDS)[23] is a reliable and valid measure of depression. It was designed specifically for screening elderly people for depression. The GDS consists of 30 yes-or-no questions. It may be administered orally or in writing. The versatility of the test makes it adaptable (i.e., oral format for an elder with visual problems). The simplicity of the answers (yes or no) and scoring is another advantage.

Behavioral Responses

A thorough behavioral assessment is especially important as a basis for planning nursing care for an elderly person. Behavioral changes may be the first sign of many physical and mental disorders. It is important to identify who is bothered by the behavior—the patient, the family, peers, or unrelated caregivers. It is also helpful to know why the behavior is bothersome. Elders and their families may be frightened by changes in behavior because they associate this with deterioration and the possible onset of dementia. The nurse can help them by explaining that behavior has many causes. Based on the assessment the cause of the problem may be treated and the person returned to normal. For instance, a woman who is agitated because of an undiagnosed urinary tract infection returns to her normal, calm self after the infection is treated. In other cases it may not be possible to remove the cause of the behavior, but nursing intervention can help the patient and family adapt to it. For example, a man is irritable because he is becoming forgetful. Early Alzheimer's disease is diagnosed. The patient becomes less irritable after the nurse teaches him and his family ways to maximize his memory. Behavioral changes that are related to declining cognitive functioning are often difficult to manage and require nursing creativity.

If possible, initial assessment should be completed in the home environment. This will capitalize on environmental factors that reduce the elder's anxiety. It will also give the nurse a chance to observe possible triggers of disruptive behavior. Family members or other caregivers can be asked about their usual responses to the patient's behavior, especially what is helpful and unhelpful. This may provide further clues about the source of the behavior.

Behavioral assessment involves defining the behavior, its frequency, duration, and precipitating factors or triggers. When a behavioral change occurs, it is important to analyze the underlying meaning. For instance, the person may be experiencing a threat to self-esteem or a change in sensory input. A complete physical examination is needed following any abrupt behavioral change. Caregiver response to behavior must also be assessed because it may reinforce or increase disturbed behavior. Frequently identified problem behaviors are listed in Box 36-1.

Box 36-1

PROBLEM BEHAVIORS FREQUENTLY OBSERVED IN GEROPSYCHIATRIC SETTINGS

Pacing	Scolding
Wandering	Hitting
Hand wringing	Kicking
Rapid speech	Threats of physical harm
Constant talking	Swearing
Repetitive movement	Isolating self
Biting	Refusal to eat or drink
Throwing things	Suspiciousness
Spitting	Delusions
	Hallucinations

Mr. Jones, an elderly gentleman, strikes out at the staff every morning when he is approached to take his bath. Describe the steps you would take to assess this behavior. What questions might you ask his family? What advice would you give to the staff who work with him?

Functional Abilities

Functional assessment of the geropsychiatric patient is not limited to indicators of mental health. Rather, the ability to function emotionally and cognitively depends greatly on the older person's overall functional ability. This discussion emphasizes the aspects of the functional assessment that have the greatest impact on mental and emotional status.

Mobility. Mobility and independence are important to the elder's perception of personal health. Three aspects of mobility should be assessed. These are the elder's ability to:

1. Move within the environment
2. Participate in necessary activities
3. Maintain contact with others

In assessing ambulation the nurse would address motor losses, adaptations made, use of assistive devices, and the amount and type of help that is needed. Restriction of joints due to degenerative diseases such as arthritis may affect ambulation. Orthostatic hypotension is possible when patients move rapidly from a lying to a standing position. The fit of footwear should be checked because gait may be unsteady. The motor ability of the arms can be tested by observing hair combing, shaving, dressing, and feeding.

In addition to altered functional ability caused by changes in physical or psychological status, many medications taken by geriatric patients alter perception, making ambulation and mobility difficult. This is particularly so with sedatives/hypnotics, tranquilizers, and cardiovascular and hypertensive drugs.[36] Patients should be cautioned about side effects of the medications and should be encouraged to take plenty of time when ambulating and moving from one position to another.

The incidence of falls and negative outcomes increases with age; 30% of people over 65 years of age fall every year, with women falling at twice the rate of men. Falls result in physical injuries such as hip fractures as well as psychological effects such as fearfulness. Risk factors must be assessed. A summary of these is presented in Table 36-1.

Activities of Daily Living. The assessment of self-care needs and activities of daily living (ADLs) is essen-

Table 36-1   Assessment of Risk for Falls

Risk factors	Assessment factors
Environmental hazards	Poor lighting
	Slippery or wet surfaces
	Stairs (no handrails, steep, poorly lit)
	Loose objects on the floor
	Throw rugs
	Small pets underfoot
Patient variables	History of falls
	Diurnal alertness level
	Familiarity with surroundings
	Emotional state (agitated, angry, etc.)
	Willingness to request help
	Confusion
	Usual activity level
	Type of activity
Assistive devices	Presence and adequacy of:
	Eyeglasses
	Hearing aid
	Ambulation aids (cane, tripod, walker)
	Prostheses
	Environmental aids (grab bars, hand rails, etc.)
Medications	Taking medications (prescribed or over-the-counter) that cause:
	Drowsiness
	Confusion
	Orthostatic hypotension
	Incoordination
	Decreased sensation
	Polypharmacy
Physical or mental disorders	Cardiovascular
	Orthopedic
	Neuromuscular
	Perceptual
	Cognitive
	Affective

tial for determining the patient's potential for independence. Activity may be limited because of physical dysfunction or psychosocial impairment. Although geriatric patients should be encouraged to become more independent in self-care, it is unrealistic to expect all patients to function independently. This is particularly so for people who are in a hospital or long-term care setting. Conforming to the routines and procedures of the institutional environment fosters dependence in the patient.

Activities of daily living (bathing, dressing, eating, grooming, and toileting) are concrete and task oriented. They provide an opportunity for purposeful nurse-patient interaction. It is important to encourage patients to be as independent as possible in performing their own ADLs. This helps elders meet their needs for safety/security, personal space, self-esteem, autonomy, and personal identity.

THE KATZ INDEX OF ACTIVITIES OF DAILY LIVING. The Katz Index[32] rates dependence versus independence for each of six ADL functions: bathing, dressing, toileting, transfer, continence, and feeding. One point is assigned for each observed item of dependency. The dependent-independent categories for each function are defined in observable terms ("gets clothes from closets and drawers"). One advantage of this tool is the ability to measure change in ADL function over time, allowing evaluation of rehabilitation activities.

Physiological Functioning

Assessment of physical health is especially important with elderly patients because of the interaction of multiple chronic conditions, the presence of sensory deficits, and the frequent behavioral presentation of physical health problems. Diagnostic procedures are described in detail in Chapter 5. These include the electroencephalogram (EEG), lumbar puncture, blood chemistry values, and brain visual imaging techniques such as the computed tomography (CT) scan and magnetic resonance imaging (MRI). In addition to these physiological factors, nutritional status and medication use must also be assessed.

Nutrition. Many elderly patients do not require help to eat or plan a nutritious diet. However, many geropsychiatric patients do have psychosocial problems that create a need for help with eating and monitoring dietary intake. These problems include the following:

- ▼ Depression or loneliness, resulting in decreased appetite
- ▼ Changes in cognition, such as confusion or disorientation
- ▼ Suicidal tendencies
- ▼ Removal from familiar ethnic and cultural eating patterns
- ▼ Fear of institutional routines or procedures

The range of physical problems varies greatly. The following areas should be assessed:

- ▼ Whether the patient has enough mobility and strength to open cartons of milk, cut meat, handle utensils
- ▼ The presence of neurological or joint conditions that interfere with hand and arm coordination
- ▼ The presence of vision problems
- ▼ Missing teeth and other losses of chewing ability
- ▼ Problems in swallowing or breathing
- ▼ The presence of ulcerations on the tongue or elsewhere in the mouth

- ▼ Periodontal disease
- ▼ Dry mouth because of medications

The nurse should routinely evaluate the patient's dietary needs. Nutritional needs are one of the most significant problems of the institutionalized elderly and can cause other problems, such as skin breakdown, inadequate absorption of medications, and impaired wound healing.

Nutritional assessment should also explore personal preferences, including prior routines (e.g., largest meal at lunchtime), time of day for meals, portion sizes, and food likes and dislikes. Serum cholesterol and albumin levels provide additional information about the person's nutritional status.

Medications. Special attention must be given to the older adult when assessing medication use. Four factors place the elder at risk for drug toxicity and should be included in any assessment: age, polypharmacy, decreased medication compliance, and comorbidity.[44]

As a person ages, physiological responses to medications change. Within the over-65 age group, drug dosages must be monitored carefully for continuing effectiveness. A medication dosage that is effective at age 65 may be toxic at age 75. Gastrointestinal absorption, hepatic blood flow and metabolism, and renal clearance may all decline. Also, the ratio of fat to lean muscle mass increases with age. Many of the psychoactive medications are lipophilic (attracted to fat), which increases the risk of drugs building up in fatty tissue and causing toxicity.[36] Drug testing is often done using a younger population. This does not allow evaluation of the differing effects of new drugs on older people.

Several surveys report that older adults take an average of eight to ten medications daily. It is also suggested that the use of over-the-counter medicines is underreported because they are not thought to be significant. Drugs such as alcohol and acetaminophen (Tylenol) are not always reported but can be toxic in combination with other drugs.[44]

Acute and chronic illnesses can alter the body's response to medications. Altered response to medications may result from such illnesses as chronic renal failure, congestive heart failure, and structural and functional changes in the central nervous system. Central nervous system changes may result in heightened sensitivity to drugs such as the benzodiazepines.[44]

Substance Abuse. Most studies of alcoholism have focused on a younger population, so the prevalence of alcohol abuse by elders has not been well documented. There is a risk for developing alcoholism in later life if there has been habitual drinking in the past. Significant loss and role changes or increased anxiety and concern over health add to the risk. Alcohol is the most commonly abused substance by the elderly because it is readily available and not usually perceived as a drug.[10] The abuse of prescription drugs, particularly antianxiety medications, is also frequent and may not be viewed as an addiction. Alcohol and substance abuse can lead to increased morbidity and mortality. Abuse of alcohol or any substance by any individual may be a means of attaining distance from painful issues such as loss and loneliness. Assessment tools for substance abuse are presented in Chapters 6 and 22.

Social Support

Positive support systems are essential for maintaining a sense of well-being throughout life. This is especially important for the geropsychiatric patient. With age, close family members and friends are lost. As a person's significant contacts decrease in number, it is important that the remaining support systems be consistent and meaningful.

Hutchison and Bahr[30] explored the caring behaviors that occur among elderly nursing home residents. They found that caring was "a major way in which residents maintained their personal identity, sense of value, and continuation of personhood." This demonstrates that support systems that develop among patients are beneficial to those who give and receive care.

The patient's ethnic background may be an important factor in identifying support systems. Strong family and ethnic ties promote feelings of security. Elderly people who live alone and are also without family ties generally have more serious problems than those who are not isolated. These problems may affect the patient's financial stability, as well as the desire to get well, be content with life, and perform self-care whenever possible. The nurse should assess the support systems available to the patient while at home, in the hospital, or in another health-care setting. Family and friends can help reduce the shock and stress of hospitalization and offer reassurance and comfort to the distressed elder.

Family-Patient Interaction. Family demographics are changing. Increased life expectancy, declining birth rate, and higher life expectancy for women all affect the availability of family to participate in caregiving and support of the elder. The majority of elders have a minimum of weekly contact with their children.[49]

Discuss the ways in which changing demographics in American society are affecting the social support systems of elderly people. What is the impact on their families?

Family expectations about caring for older members vary. The decision to care for an aging member at home or to include extended family members in the household is discussed over time within the family unit. The majority of caregiving in the United States is provided by family members. Lindgren[35] has identified three phases of caregiving (Table 36-2).

Significant issues that affect the family as it relates to the older adult are retirement, widowhood, grandparenthood, and illness. When assessing the older adult, the nurse should note previous success in dealing with life issues. The elder's adjustment to losses and changes associated with aging is affected by earlier life experiences.[49] Behavioral problems in the elderly may result from the family's inability to deal with the losses and increasing dependence of an older member.

Table 36-2 Stages of the Caregiving Career

Stage	Characteristics	Nursing activities
Encounter	Receiving and understanding the diagnosis Adjusting to the diagnosis Learning required caregiving skills Changing life-style	Provide information Teach caregiving skills Offer support and comfort Refer to support group of other new caregivers
Enduring	Heavy workloads Established routines of caregiving Little attention to personal well-being Feelings of hopelessness No planning for the future Social isolation Stress and burnout	Arrange respite care Refer to support group Encourage to pursue personal interests Focus on short-term and long-term goals Teach stress management and coping strategies Teach relaxation techniques
Exit	Decisions related to the end of caregiving Activities related to ending the role Adjustments to a changed role	Assist with nursing home placement Assist with grieving Discuss alternatives for activities, work, social relationships

Adapted from Lindgren CL: *Image* 25:214, 1993.

A comprehensive nursing assessment sets the stage for the rest of the nursing process. Table 36-3 summarizes the key components of a thorough geropsychiatric nursing assessment.

DIAGNOSIS OF THE GERIATRIC PATIENT

Although older adults may experience a wide range of psychiatric problems, the nursing diagnoses of greatest significance to the nurse and patient in promoting a therapeutic outcome will be discussed.

Altered Thought Processes

Memory Loss. The potential for memory loss is one of the most distressing and frustrating aspects of aging. Although memory loss may be caused by organic brain disease or depression, it is not necessarily related to a disease process. With age, loss of short-term memory (recall for recent events) is more likely to occur than loss of long-term memory (recall for events that occurred in the distant past). The network of past thoughts, images, ideas, and experiences that makes up memory develops and matures over a lifetime. Primary memory is the conscious control system for memory. It appears to be stable over the life span. There is little difference in primary memory among people of different ages. However, speed of access appears to slow with increasing age.[1] Long-term memory (secondary memory) is the storage system for what is commonly understood as memory.

Table 36-3 Key Components of Geropsychiatric Nursing Assessment

Component	Key elements
Interviewing	Therapeutic communication skills
	Comfortable, quiet setting
Cognitive function	Mini-Mental State Examination
	Mental Status Examination
Affective status	Mental Status Examination
	Geriatric Depression Scale
Behavioral responses	Description of behavior
	Assessment of behavioral change
	Frequently observed problem behaviors
Functional abilities	Mobility
	Activities of daily living
	Risk for falls
Physiological functioning	General health
	Nutrition
	Medication use
	Substance abuse
Social support	Social support systems
	Family-patient interaction
	Caregiver concerns

Failure in retrieval, original acquisition, or learning may cause loss in secondary memory.[1]

Many factors contribute to altered memory in older adults. Stress or crisis, depression, a sense of worthlessness, loss of interest in present events, cerebrovascular changes that affect cerebral function, loss of neural cells because of disease or trauma, and sensory deprivation or social isolation may all occur with advancing age.[19] Impaired memory for recent events may actually be a result of decreased vision or hearing. This may lead the older person to seek comfort in old memories and experiences, which replace the need to remain in touch with the present.

Institutionalized elderly persons appear to have more difficulty with memory than those who live at home or in other community settings. A stimulating environment and nursing intervention can counteract and often reverse withdrawal in the psychiatric patient. As the person becomes more involved in activities, memory may improve.

Confusion. Confusion is used by nurses "to describe a constellation of client behaviors, including inattention and memory deficits, inappropriate verbalizations, disruptive behavior, noncompliance, and failure to perform activities of daily living."[52] Frequently "confusion" is a nonspecific term used by staff to label apathetic, withdrawn, or uncooperative patients. Wolanin and Phillips[50] suggest that several categories of patients are particularly likely to be labeled as confused: the problem patient, the patient with communication problems (slurred speech, expressive dysphasia), the patient who challenges staff members' personal values, the physically unattractive patient, the depressed patient, and the "troublemaker" (one who does not improve despite nursing interventions.)

Institutionalized elders are at particular risk of confusion. From 40% to 80% suffer from some degree of organic brain disease, with disorientation to time, place, and person, remote and recent memory loss, and inability to do simple calculations. In many long-term care facilities, more than 30% of the patients have severe confusion.[18] The precipitating factors depend on both the physiological and psychological condition of the patient.

Early morning confusion, sometimes called **sunrise syndrome,** may result from the hangover effects of sedatives/hypnotics or other nighttime medications that interact with drugs for sleep. Sleep problems and insomnia are common in the elderly. Adverse reactions to drugs prescribed for sleep often occur. Increasing disorientation or confusion at night, resulting from loss of visual accommodation, is known as **sundown syndrome.** The nurse should take special precautions to prevent falls at these times.

A nurse's aide tells you that a patient is "wandering down the hall, staggering, pajama top unbuttoned." It is early morning, and the other patients are asleep. What would you do in this situation?

The nurse should never assume that confusion and disorientation are natural results of changes in cognitive or physiological status. Confusion is reversible in over half the patients who experience it. It is usually transient or short term. The nurse has primary responsibility for intervening in this problem. Well-planned nursing care can be a significant factor in preventing and intervening in this distressing condition.

Although the term *disorientation* is often used interchangeably with *confusion*, they are different. A disoriented patient is not necessarily confused, and a confused patient does not necessarily experience complete disorientation. Mental status tests differentiate disorientation to place, person, and time from components of confusion, such as alterations in memory, judgment, decision making, and problem solving. Cognitive responses are discussed in detail in Chapter 21.

Paranoia. Some older persons react to loss, isolation, and loneliness with paranoia and fear. Classic paranoia, involving a well-organized and elaborate delusional system, is rare in older persons. Delusions and disturbances in mood, behavior, and thinking may be temporary conditions caused by sensory deprivation or sensory loss, social isolation, or medications.[15]

Paranoid symptoms may be general or specific. The geriatric patient may feel threatened by certain persons (e.g., family, friends, neighbors) or at certain times (e.g., night). Relocation to a new home, new room, or strange environment causes fears, anxiety, and for some, paranoid ideation.

The personality of aging paranoid patients is characterized by withdrawal, aloofness, fearfulness, oversensitivity, and, often, secretiveness. As long as patients do not call attention to themselves or threaten themselves or others, their paranoia may remain hidden. Once they become a potential threat to themselves or others, institutionalization may be needed. Older persons who have transient or chronic paranoia are at high risk for victimization by others as well as self-neglect and abuse (e.g., refusal to eat, take prescribed medications, or attend to hygiene needs).

Affective Responses

Disturbances in mood, mood swings, or oversensitive emotional reactions are common to people of all ages.

An older person's reaction to physical limitations or disabilities, psychological loss (particularly of a spouse or other close person), or the possibility of institutionalization depends on past coping styles, support systems (especially family), and present psychological and physiological strength.

Extreme or sudden mood changes occur in response to stress or as inadequate coping mechanisms in people facing progressive loss or dependency. When this behavior is seen in elderly people who have been content and happy, physiological factors, including side effects of medications, should be considered. Reassurance and support are given to reduce the patient's anxiety and diminish the perceived threat.

Dysfunctional Grieving. Depression and sadness are sometimes viewed as a natural part of aging. In fact, depression, grief, and loss are common in later life. Prolonged grief and mourning over a real or imagined loss should be recognized and treated as depression. Common symptoms include weight loss, appetite loss, fatigue, apathy, loss of interest in friends, family, and usual activities, and psychomotor retardation. None of the symptoms are caused by increasing age; all are problems.[11]

The person's attitude toward aging, dying, and death influences whether the depression can be treated successfully. The loss of hope expressed by some older persons, particularly those with increasing disabilities, may cause or result from a depressive reaction.

Undiagnosed depression may have serious effects on the elderly, since depression always causes physical symptoms. Many of the medications routinely prescribed for older persons can increase depression. Examples include antianxiety drugs, neuroleptics, barbiturates, cardiotonics (digoxin), and steroids. A medication history is part of the evaluation and assessment.

It is important to understand the patient's and family's attitudes toward death and dying. The old differ from the young in their attitudes toward death in several ways: older people tend to integrate attitudes toward death with their religious beliefs, to have experienced the death of significant others, to be more accepting of death, and to approach problems primarily from an internal focus. The state of the older person's health, in addition to what he has learned from seeing people die, may signal that his life may be ending. Awareness of the older person's "stage of dying" is important to understanding his needs and concerns.

High Risk for Violence: Self-Directed. Intentional deaths among the elderly are not uncommon. Of all suicides committed in the United States each year, over 25% are persons over 65. White men who are over 85 are at the highest risk. Others at high risk include isolated elderly people who have lost family or friends through death; those with changes in body function and decreased independence because of pain, weakness, immobility, or shortness of breath; those with changes in body function because of surgery or stroke; or those who are terminally ill. Examples of intentional deaths include excessive risk taking, lack of caution in the management of ordinary affairs, refusal to eat, overuse or misuse of alcohol or drugs, and noncompliance with life-sustaining medical regimens, such as refusal to take insulin or digoxin.

Situational Low Self-Esteem.

Low self-esteem in the elderly is often expressed through preoccupation with physical and emotional health and expression of concern through body complaints. This may be labeled hypochondriasis but really represents the person's insecurity.

As a symbol of the geriatric patient's sense of defectiveness and deterioration, somaticism communicates the distress that accompanies decreased self-worth. The sick role is a legitimate and socially acceptable way to deal with stress and anxiety. The patient receives support, concern, and interest and experiences a sense of control.

One of the real problems encountered by elders with a history of somaticizing is health professionals' tendency to label them as a "crock" and dismiss their complaints, assuming there is no real illness. All symptoms should be taken seriously and investigated thoroughly. One must never assume the problem is "just a response to some emotional distress" and can therefore be dismissed. Whatever its cause, the problem and the patient's discomfort are real.

Somatic Responses

Sleep Pattern Disturbance.

Insomnia may be a symptom or a problem in itself for the geropsychiatric patient. Many older adults experience chronic or intermittent sleep problems. Complaints of interrupted sleep, loss of sleep, or "poor sleep," with frequent awakenings and morning exhaustion, are common. Daytime napping and drowsiness add to the problem.

Opinions vary regarding normal sleep patterns in older adults. Some researchers suggest that people need less sleep as they age. However, chronic fatigue, physical illness, pain, and decreased mobility may cause a need for more sleep. Geriatric patients often express distress over their inability to sleep or stay asleep. Perceived lack of sleep becomes a cyclical reaction. Worry about lack of sleep prevents falling asleep. Fatigue is the most common physical complaint of adults over the age of 75. It contributes to much of the insomnia of this age-group. Lack of exercise, limited mobility, and side effects

of drugs may also contribute to insomnia. It is also a symptom of depression.

Altered Nutrition: Less than Body Requirements.

Appetite loss is common in patients with depression. Inadequate dietary intake also occurs in confused or disoriented patients. Forgetting to eat or being unable to prepare meals may add to the problem of appetite loss. Side effects of some drugs (e.g., dry mouth, change in taste) contribute to lack of interest in food. The toothless patient or someone with gum disease avoids chewing when possible. The interaction of appetite loss and emotional dysfunction should always be considered in the nutritional evaluation. Poor nutrition contributes to fatigue, listlessness, and immobility.

Stress Responses

Relocation Stress Syndrome.

This condition involves physical and/or psychosocial disturbances related to transfer from one environment to another. Since 1950 the care of many elderly mentally ill has shifted from state psychiatric hospitals to nursing homes. In fact, the number of mentally ill elderly residing in nursing homes greatly exceeds that in state psychiatric hospitals. This shift in treatment site drew attention to the process and consequences of relocation. Although some data on mortality have been collected,[43] morbidity data are limited. Relocation will continue to be a fact of life, both to provide patients with less restrictive environments and to decrease the cost of long-term care of the mentally ill.

The stress of relocation should be anticipated for all geriatric patients. Intervention should be planned to reduce the impact. Allowing the patient to have personal belongings, liberal visiting hours for family or friends, and careful explanations of the purpose and routines of the institution are a few of the ways in which the stress of change can be minimized.

Establishing an effective support system within the new setting may prevent the negative behaviors often observed in isolated elders: apathy, depression, aggression, or hostility. In transfers between institutions, it may be helpful to arrange for the patient to visit the new location before the actual move. This allows the patient to meet other residents and staff, see the physical surroundings, and ask questions about the program. When possible, posttransfer visits by staff from the transferring agency also ease the transition, as well as offer staff from both agencies the opportunity to communicate about nursing approaches.

Risk factors[41] related to relocation stress syndrome include the following:

▼ Impaired psychosocial and/or physical health status

▼ Other recent losses
▼ Losses associated with the move
▼ Inadequate preparation for the move
▼ Feelings of powerlessness
▼ Moderate to great difference between the old and new environments
▼ Prior relocation experiences
▼ Inadequate support system

Behaviors associated with relocation stress syndrome are listed in Box 36-2.[41]

High Risk for Caregiver Role Strain. Disabled elderly people who live in the community rely on support and care from family members. As the percentage of elderly people in the population grows, family resources will be increasingly important to keep elders in the community and provide care that is less expensive than professional care. This role is stressful for those members who care for a frail elder. It has been well documented that providing elder care can result in emotional, physical, interpersonal, and occupational problems.[45,46] Research has also demonstrated that stress to the caregiver increases over time.[24]

A caregiver under stress is at risk for problems performing the family caregiver role. Risk factors have been identified for assessment by the North American Nursing Diagnosis Association.[41] They are listed in Table 36-4.

Behavioral Responses

Social Isolation. Multiple losses or fear of loss may lead to social isolation. Prolonged grief after the loss of a spouse, sibling, child, or close friend may make the elder hesitant to become involved in other close relationships. The person who has been close only to a few family members or friends will have even more difficulty with loss.

Elderly patients experiencing organic cognitive impairment (e.g., Alzheimer's disease and related disorders) frequently withdraw from social contacts, daily routines, and ADLs. They may deny having a problem or fear the consequences of memory changes. Social isolation can become a defense mechanism, reinforcing denial of perceived disability.

Self-care Deficit. Chronic illness is one aspect of aging that may result in the inability to care for oneself. With increasing years comes a greater chance of multiple chronic problems. Affective illnesses such as major depression or bipolar disorder may cause psychomotor retardation and lethargy preventing elders from meeting their basic needs. Medications may cause forgetfulness, lethargy, and physical impairment. Because of increasing frailty, cognitive impairment, or both many elders are unable to complete basic self-care activities such as bathing, toileting, grooming, and feeding. The underlying cause of the deficit must be determined and appropriate nursing interventions planned.

Box 36-2

BEHAVIORS ASSOCIATED WITH RELOCATION STRESS SYNDROME

▼ Anxiety, apprehension, restlessness, and verbalization of being concerned/upset about transfer
▼ Vigilance, dependency, increased verbalization of needs, insecurity, and lack of trust
▼ Increased confusion
▼ Depression, sad affect, withdrawal, and loneliness
▼ Sleep disturbance
▼ Change in eating habits, gastrointestinal disturbances, and weight changes
▼ Unfavorable comparison of posttransfer and pretransfer staff

From North American Nursing Diagnosis Association: NANDA *Nursing diagnoses: definitions and classifications* 1992-1993, Philadelphia, 1992, The Association.

Table 36-4   Risk Factors for Caregiver Role Strain

Category	Risk factors
Pathophysiological	Severe illness of elder
	Unpredictable illness course
	Addiction or codependency
	Elder discharged with serious home care needs
	Caregiver health impairment
	Caregiver is female
Psychosocial	Psychosocial/cognitive problems in care receiver
	Family problems before caregiving
	Marginal caregiver coping patterns
	Poor relationship between caregiver and receiver
	Caregiver is spouse
	Care receiver has deviant or bizarre behavior
Situational	Abuse or violence
	Other sources of stress on family
	Need for long-term caregiving
	Inadequate physical environment
	Family/caregiver isolation
	Lack of caregiver respite or recreation
	Inexperience
	Competing role commitments
	Complex/demanding caregiving tasks

From North American Nursing Diagnosis Association: NANDA *nursing diagnoses: definitions and classifications* 1992-1993, Philadelphia, 1992, The Association.

PLANNING AND INTERVENTION

Expected outcomes related to the nursing care of the geropsychiatric patient must be realistically based on the person's potential to change. If the person's behavioral problems result from a treatable disorder, expected outcomes and short-term goals may reflect a return to preillness functioning. For example, a goal for a patient with depression who is neglectful of personal hygiene might be:

The patient will bathe, dress, and brush his teeth independently.

If the condition is chronic and either no change or progressive deterioration is expected, then the outcomes of care focus on adaptation to this. For example, a goal for a patient with Alzheimer's disease who neglects personal hygiene might be:

The patient will assist with bathing, dressing, and brushing his teeth.

If the patient's condition is not expected to improve, the expected outcomes and goals may focus on the caregiver as well as the patient. For example, a goal for a caregiver of a person with Alzheimer's disease might be:

At least once a week the caregiver will participate in a recreational activity outside of the home while the home health aide is with the patient.

The plan of care needs to be developed with the active participation of the patient and the caregiver. It also needs to be reviewed frequently to be sure that it is relevant to the patient's current needs. Caregiver education is an important part of the plan.

Older adults respond well to both individual and group interventions. They need the opportunity to talk, be supported in their efforts to deal with day-to-day problems, and plan for a meaningful future. The type of nursing intervention selected depends on the nursing care problems identified, the interests and preferences of the elder, and the setting in which the care is to be provided. In the past most geropsychiatric care was provided in state psychiatric hospitals. Nurses will now find older patients with mental illness in these hospitals as well as in acute psychiatric units, nursing homes, and increasingly in community settings. The need for a comprehensive community-based system of care has been noted in the literature.[17]

Nursing care for cognitively impaired patients in inpatient settings is addressed in Chapter 21, including approaches to behaviors such as wandering, aggression, agitation, falls, and confusion.

Therapeutic Milieu

Whether in a hospital, nursing home, community program, or at home, the care environment should support effective intervention. There are several basic characteristics of a therapeutic milieu.

Cognitive Stimulation. Activities should be planned to maintain or improve the patients' cognitive functioning. Discussion groups help patients focus on topics of interest to them. Projects can reinforce skills and offer an opportunity for success. The nurse can collaborate with the rehabilitation therapist in planning interesting and appropriate activities.

Promote a Sense of Safety, Calm, and Quiet. Elders often do best in a setting that is designated for their care. In particular, inpatient units that admit all age groups may be too stimulating for confused patients. In general, the geropsychiatric setting should be decorated in soft colors. If music is played, it should be soothing and preferably familiar to the elderly. Bright lights that create glare should be avoided. Although the environmental background should be subdued, planned periods of increased activity help maintain interest and alertness.

Personal belongings can offer a sense of security. For people who are not in their own home, articles such as family pictures, religious objects, favorite books, afghans, or decorative objects are reassuring (Fig. 36-2).

Safety needs must be considered. The nurse should be alert for safety hazards and remove them. Because falls are a concern, floors should be free from slippery spots and obstacles. Hand rails and grab bars are helpful for frail elders. Fire is also a concern. Open flames

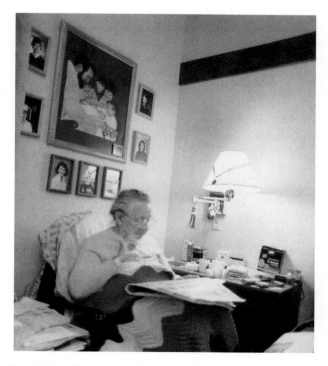

Fig. 36-2 This woman has many family pictures and other personal belongings that provide her with a sense of personal comfort and security.

should be avoided. If smoking is allowed, it may be necessary to provide supervision.

Consistent Physical Layout. In residential or inpatient settings, room changes should be avoided as much as possible. Furniture arrangements should be stable; this assists disoriented people to locate themselves and adds to their security.

Structured Routine. The daily schedule should be as predictable as possible. Bedtime, waking time, naptimes, and mealtimes should not vary. For elders who have recently moved to a new setting, it is helpful to give them and their families copies of the weekly schedule. Time should be allowed for reviewing the schedule with patients. Periodic reinforcement of the routines may be needed until patients adjust to the environment.

Focus on Strengths and Abilities. Most elders have strengths related to their past accomplishments. If the person is unable to communicate, family members can give information about the patient's life and suggest activities that are likely to be successful. Nursing creativity can find ways to capitalize on elders' strengths by planning opportunities for them to help staff or other patients or participate in activities based on their abilities.

Minimize Disruptive Behavior. Understanding the patient's behavioral patterns can help to reduce agitation and behavioral crises. Observation reveals situations that lead to disruptions. Adhering to the person's usual life-style as closely as possible reduces conflicts. For instance, a person who has always taken a bath in the evening before bed should not be forced to shower before breakfast. Patients who agitate each other should be kept apart as much as possible. Distraction can often interrupt a conflict before it gets out of control.

Minimal Demands for Compliant Behavior. Elders who are cognitively impaired often resist demands from others. They may not understand what is being asked of them or they may be frightened of an unexpected change in activity. Some older adults resent being under the control of others and need to assert themselves. It is best to avoid pressuring the patient to comply. Reapproaching the person after a few minutes is often successful. If the patient needs to be in control, it is helpful to negotiate a time of voluntary compliance.

 How would the therapeutic milieu differ if most patients were elderly and (a) depressed, (b) had dementia, or (c) delusional?

Physical Restraints

Physical restraints include a variety of devices such as mitts, posey vests, and geri chairs applied with a physician's order. Although such devices may assist staff to protect geropsychiatric patients, they limit freedom of choice and movement, as well as threaten dignity. Evans and Strumpf[20] have identified six myths related to physical restraint of elderly patients. These are summarized in Table 36-5.

Somatic Therapies

Electroconvulsive Therapy. Electroconvulsive therapy (ECT) has been found to be effective in the treatment of depression in the older adult. (See Chapter 26 for a detailed discussion of ECT.) Contraindications for this type of therapy are an intracranial space-occupying lesion with increased intracranial pressure, arrhythmias, and myocardial infarction within the last 3 months.

Psychotropic Medications. The addition of psychotropic medications to the drug regimen of elders must be approached carefully. Basic guidelines for medication administration for elders include the slow initiation of medications using lower dosages. Special consideration needs to be given to psychotropic medications and elders because drugs that affect behavior also affect the central nervous system. It has been documented that elderly patients are especially vulnerable to developing tardive dyskinesia.[51] Many of the drugs take up to 6 weeks to exert a change in affective disorders. In the interim elders may see no benefit to continued compliance and may abandon their medication regimen. Education regarding the purpose, therapeutic value, and side effects of medications should be provided to elders to enhance medication compliance and awareness. Table 36-6 describes recommended dosages of psychotropic medications for the elderly. (See Chapter 25 for a thorough discussion of psychopharmacology.)

Interpersonal Interventions

Psychotherapy. Elderly patients participate in both individual and group psychotherapy sessions. Nurses who have advanced degrees in geropsychiatric nursing are qualified to provide this service. The issue of the appropriateness of psychotherapy for this population is addressed in Critical Thinking about Contemporary Issues.

Turner[48] has identified themes that emerge during psychotherapy with this age group. They include "maintenance of self-esteem, fear of pain and suffering, helplessness and hopelessness, isolation and loneliness, physical and mental impairment, loss of competency, need to rely on those who may abandon them, and an

Table 36-5   Myths and Realities about Physical Restraint

Myths	Realities
Restraints reduce the risk of injury related to falls.	Restraints do not reduce the risk of injury from falls and may increase it. Falls do increase the likelihood of future restraint.
Restraining meets the nurse's moral duty to protect the patient from harm.	Restraints may increase the risk of injury as well as leading to problems related to immobility, confusion, aggression, depression, and incontinence.
Failure to restrain results in legal liability.	Federal and state laws and regulations prohibit the unnecessary use of restraint.
Older people do not mind being restrained.	Older people do not wish to be restrained. They feel angry, hurt and embarrassed by the experience.
Inadequate staffing justifies restraining patients.	Federal and state laws and regulations forbid restraining patients for staff convenience. Providing adequate nursing care to a restrained patient takes at least as much time as caring for an unrestrained one.
There are no adequate alternatives to physical restraint.	Nursing care alternatives have been identified in several categories: ▼ Physical care: comfort, relief of pain, positioning ▼ Psychosocial care: remotivation, communication, attention ▼ Activities ▼ Environmental manipulation: improved lighting, removal of restraint devices, redesigned furniture ▼ Administrative support and staff training

Adapted from Evans LK, Strumpf NE: *Image* 22:124, 1990.

TABLE 36-6
PSYCHOACTIVE MEDICATIONS

Category		Recommended dosage range for older adults
Selective serotonin reuptake inhibitors (SSRIs)	Fluoxetene/Prozac	20-80 mg/day
	Sertraline/Zoloft	50 mg/day
	Paroxetene/Paxil	20 mg/day
	Effexor	175-225 mg/day
Neuroleptics	Haloperidol/Haldol	0.25-6.0 mg/day
	Fluphenazine/Prolixin	0.25-6.0 mg/day
	Trifluoperazine/Stelazine	4-20 mg/day
	Thioridazine/Mellaril	10-300 mg/day
	Chlorpromazine/Thorazine	10-300 mg/day
Tricyclic antidepressants (TCAs)	Amitriptyline/Elavil	10-75 mg/day
	Imipramine/Tofranil	10-75 mg/day
	Desipramine/Norpramin	10-75 mg/day
	Nortriptyline/Aventyl	10-50 mg/day
	Trazodone/Desyrel	25-400 mg/day
Monoamine oxidase inhibitor antidepressants (MAO inhibitors)	Isocarboxazid/Marplan	10-30 mg/day
	Phenelzine/Nardil	15-45 mg/day
	Tranylcypromine/Parnate	10-30 mg/day
Lithium	Lithium	300 mg tid/qid
Anxiolytic benzodiazepines	Clonazepam/Klonopin	0.5 mg q8h
	Oxazepam/Serax	10-45 mg (divided in 3-4 doses)
	Lorazepam/Ativan	0.5-1.0 mg bid to tid
Sedative/hypnotic benzodiazepines	Flurazepam/Dalmane	15-30 mg qhs
	Temazepam/Restoril	7.5-15 mg qhs

Adapted from Salzman C: *Clinical geriatric psychopharmacology*, ed 2, Baltimore, 1992, Williams & Wilkins.

existential perspective on death." She believes that these are important concerns that can be addressed in therapy. She also notes that transference and countertransference issues are related to the ages of the patient and therapist. Child/parent or grandchild/grandparent themes are common. Therapists often have particular difficulty responding to sexual transference with elders. This may be related to the therapist's beliefs and feelings about sexuality and aging.

Group psychotherapy is another intervention for el-

CRITICAL THINKING ABOUT CONTEMPORARY ISSUES

Is Psychotherapy an Appropriate Intervention for Geropsychiatric Patients?

Some believe that psychotherapy for elderly patients is inappropriate and not helpful. Psychotherapy requires confronting and working through basic personality traits. It is argued that the elderly do not have the capacity, stamina, or interest to take on such a challenging task. Is this based on an accurate estimate of the elder's cognitive ability and interpersonal potential? Psychotherapy may be a long-term process. Is it reasonable to ask a person who is nearing the end of life to make a commitment to an effort that might not be completed? People in therapy often change their relationships with others. Should the elderly be put in the position of possibly jeopardizing their support systems by changing their expectations of themselves and others?

Geropsychiatric nurse specialists have begun to document their experiences in providing psychotherapy to elders.[29,42,48] These nurses believe that elderly patients benefit from this intervention. They describe the elder's ability to change and grow. Psychotherapists have noted that older patients are more focused on therapeutic work, perhaps because they know they do not have unlimited time to achieve their goals. Elders have a wealth of life experiences to bring to therapy and a need to find meaning in their lives that is often aided by therapeutic intervention. In groups, they also benefit from the mutuality and cohesion that they find. Based on this, is it worth the investment to improve the life experience of one who may or may not have enough time left to experience long-term rewards of the psychotherapy experience? ▼

derly patients. Pearlman[42] has described several benefits of group therapy for this population, including giving and receiving help, decreasing social isolation, receiving support by sharing common experiences, and improving self-esteem.

Life Review Therapy. Life review therapy was first described by Butler.[13] It has a positive psychotherapeutic function, providing an opportunity for the person to reflect on life and resolve, reorganize, and reintegrate troubling or disturbing areas. The life review works well with groups or individuals. In a group, members may positively reinforce each other and stimulate mutual learning. Developing individual autobiographies to share with the group is one way to introduce common experiences and interests among the members and put them at ease. The group cohesion and sharing can build self-esteem and a feeling of belonging, in addition to the positive effect of the review itself.

Haight and Burnside[26] have differentiated between life review and reminiscence. Both are planned interventions that are led by a mental health professional. Reminiscence is usually a pleasant experience in which the patient reviews life events without any particular structure and talks about meanings and feelings. The nurse listens and responds but does not try to interpret or probe for deeper meanings. The life review is structured, with the emphasis on analyzing life events. The nurse assists the patient to look for the meaning of experiences and to resolve conflicts and lingering feelings. Life review assists the elder to achieve the ego integrity and wisdom identified by Erikson as the goal of the last stage of life.

Reality Orientation. Reality orientation was developed as a specific therapeutic program for institutionalized geriatric patients. Both 24-hour and classroom (structured) reality orientation can prevent confusion and keep patients oriented to time, place, person, and situation. The environment reinforces contact with reality, the here and now, when it is kept simple and focused. Helpful physical props include clocks, directional signs, calendars, and orientation boards (season of the year, weather, etc.). Classroom reality orientation is an intensive small-group experience that is especially effective for the moderately to severely impaired elderly. It provides an opportunity to reinforce time, place, and person orientation with patients who have short attention spans and need extra verbal and visual stimulation. Reality orientation, along with a discussion of current events, stimulates patients to maintain contact with the real world and their place in it. Current events discussions, used alone, may be structured in various ways, such as sharing of newspaper articles or group viewing of television news programs. The scope of the group depends on the patients' abilities and the other therapeutic modalities at hand.

Validation Therapy. Although reality orientation is effective for many institutionalized and community-based elderly with confusion and/or disorientation, some evidence indicates that for some older adults, especially those with minimal organic impairment, disorientation may be a form of denial of unpleasant realities. These elders may become more anxious or agitated if constantly reminded of environmental realities. An alternate approach to confused and disoriented older adults was developed by Feil[21] and discussed in relation to working with the patient who does not respond to reality orientation. This approach involves searching for the emotion and meaning in the patient's disoriented or confused words and behavior (such as wandering) and validating them verbally with the patient. A series of verbal cues or steps are involved that allow the patient to simply focus on key words or phrases in the confused interaction and the nurse validates by asking for description, more detail, or clarification. What is sometimes identified as meaningless or incoherent conversation may often have significant meaning for the patient and can be related to current or past events. Validation is being used successfully with both mild and moderately impaired elderly and shows promise for providing an effective avenue for reaching older adults who are experiencing cognitive dysfunction. Little documentation is available on the use of this strategy in group settings or with severely impaired elders.

Cognitive Training and Therapy.

Much research is under way using cognitive training and stimulation (see Chapter 28). Problem-solving situations, formal or didactic memory training, and selected memory exercises have been effective in increasing attention span, efficiency of recall, and the ability to learn new skills (e.g., mathematical calculations and vocabulary). Intelligence does not decline with progressive age but may be dulled by depression, drugs, or lack of use. Cognitive training can keep older adults active mentally, which in turn will enhance emotional well-being. The "use it or lose it" adage holds as true for maintenance of intelligence as it does for physical functioning.

Clinical studies and experience to date indicate that cognitive training and therapy may be especially effective for cognitively intact, motivated elderly persons with minor or major depressions. Cognitive therapy supports higher-level defense mechanisms, such as rationalization and intellectualization, and encourages active participation of patients in a highly structured treatment. One positive aspect of this approach is its time-limited nature, reinforcing the goal of a positive change within a specific time period. Research has demonstrated that cognitive therapy is effective with depressed elderly patients.[53]

Stimulating cognitive skills can challenge the nurse's creativity in relating to geropsychiatric patients. To be able to capitalize on the patient's interests and skills, the nurse must be familiar with the patient's past occupation, hobbies, and leisure activities. The nursing interview should focus on gathering as much of that information as possible on admission and adding to the database as the nurse builds a trusting relationship with the patient and family.

Relaxation Therapy.

Besides promoting a sense of physical well-being, relaxation can release tension and reduce stress, reducing barriers to communication. Additional information about relaxation therapy is presented in Chapters 14 and 28. Relaxation, combined with mild isometric exercises, increases cardiovascular output, energy, and mobility and reduces stress. Relaxation and exercise strategies, used in group or individual contexts, do not require advanced skills of the nurse or the patient. They may begin with simple tension-releasing muscle exercises, coupled with verbal instructions about breathing and concentration.

Supportive and Counseling Groups.

Gerontological psychiatric patients respond well to both supportive and counseling groups. These interventions may use either a nondirective or unstructured format or a more structured, didactic approach. Group members can ventilate feelings, try out problem-solving approaches, and resolve conflict in a rational, systematic manner. These groups may incorporate some aspects of cognitive training or reminiscence, described earlier in this chapter. Older adults respond well to a supportive group structure, which increases self-esteem, self-confidence, risk-taking and empathy. Humor may be an effective way to reach the nonverbal or withdrawn elder. The ability to laugh at oneself and see the irony in everyday events provides an effective outlet for frustration, anger, stress, and anxiety. Promoting humor by telling jokes and stories and watching cartoons or situation-comedies can be therapeutic in a group or with individual patients. Expressions of humor and active laughter allow older adults an opportunity to step out of their situation, releasing some of the tension related to coping with changes accompanying aging.

Patient Education.

Older adults often question the physiological and cognitive (memory) changes that occur naturally in aging. Slowed response time, benign memory loss, altered gait, and interrupted sleep patterns are a few of the normal changes of aging that elders may interpret as pathological. The nurse has an opportunity to teach patients about their own developmental changes during the assessment phase of the nurse-patient relationship. Dispelling myths and stereotypes related to aging is a primary goal for patient education.

Depressed older adults are particularly receptive to the educative process, since it is in the depressive state that they are most vulnerable and open to suggestion. Exercises for promoting positive thoughts and images, visualization, and repetitive cognitive games can be used as a basis for teaching new patterns of behavior. Cognitive training, relaxation, and life review approaches are well suited to patient education formats.

Family Education and Support. Because 80% of the elders living at home are cared for by a spouse, sibling, or adult child, family caregiver education and support groups are becoming essential to maintain this living situation as long as possible.[4] Many community agencies, clinics, and senior citizen centers are responding to the needs of this group with special activities, classes, and support groups.

Family members often view nurses as the most approachable health-care professional for understanding family relationships, conflicts, needs, and resources. Family education related to the normal aging process, family dynamics and family systems, and stress inherent in the caregiver role can be integrated into counseling sessions with family members, referral conferences, or part of the family history on admission of the patient.[5]

A more formal approach to family education can be developed using the numerous books now available commercially that address the caregiving role with older adults. These materials provide practical, step-by-step guides to handling common problems of the frail elderly, including agitation, wandering, withdrawal, resistance, anxiety, insomnia, incontinence, anorexia, and restlessness. These books, which have been written specifically for the consumer, supply the text for nurse-family teaching sessions as well as excellent resource materials for use in the home.[37]

EVALUATING THE CARE OF THE GERIATRIC PATIENT

Specific nursing interventions designed to promote optimum cognitive function and emotional well-being have been considered as the role of the geropsychiatric nurse. Increasingly, research is being initiated to determine the most appropriate approach to meet the needs of the patient and the most effective intervention to use.

Hall[27] suggests that evaluation of patient care should be based on a model that explains the progression of dysfunctional behavior from normative to anxious to stress behaviors. The type of care and the evaluation of outcome would be directly related to the level of behavior targeted for intervention.

Beck and Heacock[6] note that the goal of nursing intervention is to promote maximum independence of the older adult, based on capacity and functional abilities. Evaluation of outcomes of nursing care would not be based on reversal of behaviors or elimination of patient needs but on the change the patient demonstrates based on individual abilities. This approach reinforces the emphasis on the individual as a unit for evaluation and allows for patient differences and for the process of change over time.

Harris, Marriott, and Robertson[28] have identified the issues to be addressed in the evaluation of community geropsychiatric programs. They include the outcome of treatment; the satisfaction of the patient, significant others, referring professionals, the community, the agency, and the staff; the expectations of those who fund the program; the compliance with accreditation and quality assurance standards; and cost effectiveness. The nurse plays an important part in ensuring that these goals are met.

In the final analysis, the most important evaluation criterion is the feedback from the patient and caregivers that nursing care was helpful and growth producing. The challenge to the nurse is to be creative in producing a positive experience for each elder for whom care is provided.

SUMMARY

1. The role of the geropsychiatric nurse includes providing primary mental health nursing care, including intervening with caregivers and consulting with other care providers. Advanced practice nurses provide individual and group psychotherapy and take leadership in program development.

2. Biopsychosocial theories of aging were identified. Biological theories include biological programming, wear-and-tear and stress adaptation. Psychological theories include Erikson's stage of ego integrity, life review, and stability of personality. Sociocultural theories include disengagement, activity, and the family in later life.

3. A comprehensive geropsychiatric nursing assessment includes application of interviewing skills. The areas to be assessed include cognitive, affective, behavioral, functional abilities, physiological, and social support.

4. NANDA nursing diagnoses related to geropsychiatric patients include altered thought processes, dysfunctional grieving, high risk for violence: self-directed, situational low self-esteem, sleep pattern disturbance, altered nutrition: less than body requirements, relocation stress syndrome, high risk for caregiver role strain, social isolation, and self-care deficit.

5. Expected outcomes and short-term goals for nursing care are related to the patient's identified problems and prognosis. If recovery from the problem cannot reasonably be expected, the goals should focus on adaptation to life changes. Caregivers must be involved in planning.

6. Nursing interventions with geropsychiatric patients include creation of a therapeutic milieu, use of physical restraints, involvement in somatic therapies, and interpersonal interventions.

7. Evaluation of geropsychiatric nursing care focuses on the patient's ability to reach maximum independence.

COMPETENT CARING
A CLINICAL EXEMPLAR OF A PSYCHIATRIC NURSE

Beth Greco, MSN, RN

A frail ghost of a man sat silently in his easy chair. He did not raise his head nor speak as I entered the room with his wife. He made no eye contact as I introduced myself as his new home health nurse. He simply remained quiet, barely moving even as he breathed. I was struck by his appearance. He was not the person I had expected to meet that day.

Mr. R had been reported to be "very difficult," "demanding," "noncompliant," "an impossible patient." Emergency visits by nurses were frequently necessary to fix a leaky catheter, assess a drastic decrease in urinary output, unclog a clogged feeding tube, and assess reported changes in cardiac and respiratory status. His wife and primary caretaker made numerous calls to the home health office and continually asked questions about Mr. R's medicines, diet, heart problems, breathing difficulties, and general overall health status. After meeting Mr. R, it occurred to me that caring for this patient would involve not only extensive medical management but also intensive psychiatric nursing care for him and his family. I was very glad that I had a few years of psychiatric nursing experience under my belt before I met this family.

My immediate response in assessing Mr. R's needs was to increase the frequency of home visits to three times per week. During these visits I carefully reviewed Mr. R's medications, diet, and treatments with him and his wife at the same time. I was very careful to include Mr. R in these discussions by asking him questions and providing him opportunities to make decisions about his care. At first he was very reluctant to participate in these teaching sessions, but gradually he began to show some interest. As he became more engaged in conversations with me I began showing him how to take care of his feeding tube and catheter. I encouraged his wife to let Mr. R do his care when he felt up to it. I thought it would be very important for Mr. R to have some control over what was happening to him. I also thought it would be necessary for Mrs. R to let go of the total responsibility for her husband's care. Her anxiety level had reached almost unmanageable proportions several weeks before I had received the case.

I encouraged Mrs. R to arrange some time for herself away from the home on a regular basis. She agreed that she would have her daughter come in once a week so that she could spend time with her church friends. Mr. R stated that it would be good for his wife to get out more often and he would be all right in her absence. After a few weeks of concentrating on the "tasks" to be learned, Mr. R became more open to discussion of his illness's impact on his life and his family. He talked about his past work and leisure activities and his disbelief over his current situation. He felt that his retirement years were supposed to be full of travel and leisure pursuits, and instead he was confined by his failing health to his home. He was angry, very angry, as he talked to me about these things, and as I glanced at a picture on his dresser of a broad-shouldered, confident military man, I better understood his anger and his pain. He had been that man in the picture, and his losses were great.

Grief work became an important focus of my nursing care in the remainder of the time that I worked with Mr. R and his family. We talked about the changes in their lives, their disappointments over missed opportunities, their anger, and their fears. We explored ways to cope with Mr. R's limitations, and I was happy to hear one day that Mr. and Mrs. R had ventured out to dinner at a restaurant. A wheelchair and some courage were the necessary ingredients for an enjoyable evening for the couple.

As time went on, Mr. R's condition stabilized, and weekly maintenance visits were all that was needed.

His condition remained acute, but he and his wife were managing his care very well at home. Emergency visits were no longer needed, and this once-"difficult" patient was rarely heard from between home visits.

My last visit to Mr. R's home was prompted by an early morning telephone call from my office. There, indeed, was an emergency at his home on that day. When I arrived at the house I found Mr. R in bed clutching his chest. His wife explained that he had awakened with chest pain. My quick physical assessment indicated that his pulse was rapid and thready and his blood pressure was lower than his normal baseline. He was alert but looked pale and was diaphoretic. I instructed Mrs. R to call EMS, and as she did so I sat with Mr. R. I held his hand and asked him if he was afraid. He nodded and met my eyes with his. In them I saw only his courage. He remained conscious until EMS arrived, and they promptly started an IV line and provided oxygen and whisked him off to the nearest hospital. He died later that same day, but I will always remember him for the bravery of his struggle for life. ▼

REFERENCES

1. Albert MS: Cognition and aging. In Hazzard WR et al, eds: *Principles of geriatric medicine and gerontology*, ed 2, New York, 1990, McGraw-Hill.
2. Angel IL, Hogan DP: The demography of minority aging populations. In Harootyan LK, ed: *Minority elders: longevity, economics, and health: building a public policy base*, Washington, DC, 1991, Gerontological Society of America.
3. Baker FM: Psychiatric treatment of older African-Americans, *Hosp Community Psychiatry* 45:32, 1994.
4. Baldwin BA: Community management of Alzheimer's disese, *Nurs Clin North Am* 23:47, 1988.
5. Baldwin BA et al: Family caregiver stress: clinical assessment and management, *Inter Psychoger* 1:185, 1989.
6. Beck C, Heacock P: Nursing interventions with patients with Alzheimer's disease, *Nurs Clin North Am* 23:95, 1988.
7. Blazer D: Current concepts: depression in the elderly, *N Engl J Med* 320:164, 1989.
8. Blazer DG: *Emotional problems in later life: intervention strategies for professional caregivers*, New York, 1990, Springer.
9. Blazer DG: The epidemiology of psychiatric disorders in late life. In Busse EW, Blazer DG, eds: *Geriatric psychiatry*, Washington, DC, 1989, American Psychiatric Press.
10. Blazer DG: Alcohol and drug problems in the elderly. In Busse EW, Blazer DG, eds: *Geriatric psychiatry*, Washington, DC, 1989, American Psychiatric Press.
11. Blazer DG: Affective disorders in late life. In Busse EW, Blazer DG, eds: *Geriatric psychiatry*, Washington, DC, 1989, American Psychiatric Press.
12. Burns BJ et al: Mental health service use by the elderly in nursing homes, *Am J Public Health* 83:331, 1993.
13. Butler RN: Re-awakening interest, *Nurs Homes* 10:8, 1961.
14. Carter EA, McGoldrick M: *The family life cycle: a framework for family therapy*, ed 2, New York, 1989, Gardner Press.
15. Christison C, Christison G, Blazer DG: Late-life schizophrenia and paranoid disorders. In Busse EW, Blazer DG, eds: *Geriatric psychiatry*, Washington, DC, 1989, American Psychiatric Press.
16. Cumming E, Henry WE: *Growing old: the process of disengagement*, New York, 1961, Basic Books.
17. Draper B: The effectiveness of services and treatment in psychogeriatrics, *Aust NZ J Psychiatry* 24:238, 1990.
18. Ebersole P: *Caring for the psychogeriatric patient*, New York, 1989, Springer.
19. Erikson EH: *Childhood and society*, New York, 1963, WW Norton.
20. Evans LK, Strumpf NE: Myths about elder restraint, *Image* 22:124, 1990.
21. Feil N: Communicating with the confused elderly patient, *Geriatrics* 39:131, 1993.
22. Fischer P, Simanyi M, Danielczyk W: Depression in dementia of the Alzheimer type and in multiinfarct dementia, *Am J Psychiatry* 147:1484, 1990.
23. Gallo JJ, Reichel W, Andersen L: *Handbook of geriatric assessment*, Rockville, Md, 1988, Aspen.
24. Gaynor SE: The long haul: the effects of home care on caregivers, *Image* 22:208, 1990.
25. Gomez GE, Gomez EF: Depression in the elderly, *J Psychosoc Nurs Ment Health Serv* 31:28, 1993.

26. Haight BK, Burnside I: Reminiscing and life review: explaining the difference, *Arch Psychiatr Nurs* 7:91, 1993.

27. Hall GR: Care of the patient with Alzheimer's disease living at home, *Nurs Clin North Am* 23:31, 1988.

28. Harris AG, Marriott JAS, Robertson J: Issues in the evaluation of a community psychogeriatric service, *Can J Psychiatry* 35:215, 1990.

29. Hayflick L et al: The serial cultivation of human diploid cells, *Exp Cell Res* 25:585, 1961.

30. Hutchison CP, Bahr RT Sr: Types and meanings of caring behaviors among elderly nursing home residents, *Image* 23:85, 1991.

31. Junginger J, Phelan E, Cherry K, Levy J: Prevalence of psychopathology in elderly persons in nursing homes and in the community, *Hosp Community Psychiatr* 44:381, 1993.

32. Katz S et al: Studies of illness in the aged: the index of ADL; a standardized measure of biological and psychosocial function, *JAMA* 185:914, 1963.

33. Kurlowicz LH: Social factors and depression in late life, *Arch Psychiatr Nurs* 7:30, 1993.

34. Lebowitz BD, Cohen GD: Introduction: older Americans and their illnesses. In Salzman C, ed: *Clinical geriatric psychopharmacology*, ed 2, Baltimore, 1992, Williams & Wilkins.

35. Lindgren CL: The caregiver career, *Image* 25:214, 1993.

36. Luke EA Jr: Psychotropic drugs. In Hogstel MO, ed: *Geropsychiatric nursing*, St Louis, 1990, Mosby.

37. Mace NL, Rabins PV: *The 36-hour day*, New York, 1991, Warner Books.

38. McCullough PK: Geriatric depression: atypical presentations, hidden meanings, *Geriatrics* 46:72, 1991.

39. Moritz DF, Ostfeld AD: The epidemiology and demography of aging. In Hazzard WR et al, eds: *Principles of geriatric medicine and gerontology*, ed 2, New York, 1990, McGraw-Hill.

40. Morriss RK, Rovner BW, Folstein MF, German PS: Delusions in newly admitted residents of nursing homes, *Am J Psychiatry* 147:299, 1990.

41. North American Nursing Diagnosis Association: NANDA *nursing diagnosis: definitions and classifications* 1993-1994, Philadelphia, 1994, NANDA.

42. Pearlman IR: Group psychotherapy with the elderly, *J Psychosoc Nurs Ment Health Serv* 31:7, 1993.

43. Saathoff GB, Cortina JA, Jacobson R, Aldrich CK: Mortality among elderly patients discharged from a state hospital, *Hosp Community Psychiatry* 43:280, 1992.

44. Salzman C: *Clinical geriatric psychopharmacology*, ed 2, Baltimore, 1992, Williams & Wilkins.

45. Sayles-Cross S: Perceptions of family caregivers of elder adults, *Image* 25:88, 1993.

46. Stevens GL, Walsh RA, Baldwin BA: Family caregivers of institutionalized and noninstitutionalized elderly individuals, *Nurs Clin North Am* 28:349, 1993.

47. Tariot PN, Podgorski CA, Blazina L, Leibovici A: Mental disorders in the nursing home: another perspective, *Am J Psychiatry* 150:1063, 1993.

48. Turner MS: Individual psychodynamic psychotherapy with older adults: perspectives from a nurse psychotherapist, *Arch Psychiatr Nurs* 6:266, 1992.

49. Walsh F: The family in later life. In Carter E, McGoldrick M, eds: *The family life cycle: a framework for family therapy*, ed 2, New York, 1989, Gardner Press.

50. Wolanin MO, Phillips LRF: *Confusion: prevention and care*, St Louis, 1981, Mosby.

51. Yassa R, Nastase C, Dupont D, Thibeau M: Tardive dyskinesia in elderly psychiatric patients: a 5-year study, *Am J Psychiatry* 149:1206, 1992.

52. Yesavage JA et al: Senile dementia: combined pharmacologic and psychologic treatment, *J Am Geriatr Soc* 29:164, 1981.

53. Zerhusen JD, Boyle K, Wilson W: Out of the darkness: group cognitive therapy for depressed elderly, *J Psychosoc Nurs Ment Health Serv* 29:16, 1991.

ANNOTATED SUGGESTED READINGS

*Baldwin BA, Stevens GL: Family caregiving: education and support. In Eliopoulos C, ed: *Caring for the elderly in diverse care settings*, Philadelphia, 1990, JB Lippincott.

This chapter describes the recent trends in family caregiving, identifies causes and manifestations of caregiver stress, and discusses ways in which nurses can assist family caregivers through education and support groups.

*Baldwin BA, Beck CM, Stevens GL: *Resident care planning system*, Crofton, Md, 1992, PAL Associates.

Contains instruction manual and 18 ready-to-use Resident Care Planning Guides. Developed to meet the OBRA '87 regulatory mandates, as well as maximize teamwork, individualized quality care, and effective problem solving.

Busse EW, Blazer DG, eds: *Geriatric psychiatry*, Washington, DC, 1989, American Psychiatric Press.

Provides scientific facts and applied skills and knowledge needed in dealing with the mental disorders of late life.

*Ebersole P: *Caring for the psychogeriatric client*, New York, 1989, Springer Publishers.

Designed for those who deal directly with the mental health needs and emotional disorders of the aged. Emphasis is on management strategies.

*Farran CJ, Popovich JM: Hope: a relevant concept for geriatric psychiatry, *Arch Psychiatr Nurs* 4:124, 1990.

The authors identify the importance of developing nursing interventions to assist older adults who are in the community to maintain hope.

Glickstein JK: *Therapeutic interventions in Alzheimer's disease*, Rockville, Md, 1988, Aspen.

Provides health-care professionals with therapy material that can be used in the development of individualized programs. Contains overview of Alzheimer's disease, workbook with specific lesson plans, and how-to suggestions for working with dementia clients.

*King S, Collins C, Given B, Vredevoogd J: Institutionalization of an elderly family member: reactions of spouse and nonspouse caregivers, *Arch Psychiatr Nurs* 5:323, 1991.

The authors report on their research, which challenges the notion that caregivers always feel a sense of relief after an elderly family member is institutionalized. This is a good example of longitudinal nursing research.

---

*Nursing reference.

*Kjervik DK: Empowerment of the elderly, J Prof Nurs 6:74, 1990.

The author, who is a nurse-attorney, discusses the consequences of empowerment and the need for effective advocacy for elderly patients.

Maclay E: *Green winter,* New York, 1977, McGraw-Hill.

A book of poems whose pages surprise with wit and the grit and tenderness of human spirit. A celebration of old age.

Suess Dr, Geisel AS: *You're only old once!* New York, 1986, Random House.

Theodor Seuss Geisel, better known as Dr. Seuss, celebrated his eighty-second birthday on March 2, 1986, the publication date of this book. With the humor typical of Dr. Seuss's books, we follow our hapless hero through his checkup with the experts at the Golden Years Clinic.

*Stevens GL, Baldwin BA: Optimizing mental health in the nursing home setting, J Psychosoc Nurs Ment Health Serv 26:27, 1988.

Suggests that the physical and social environment of the nursing home setting can be manipulated by staff to support functional behavior, rather than behavioral decline.

*Stevens GL, Baldwin BA, Friedman SD, Eigelsbach LM: *Stress and behavioral management: a motivational training manual,* Baltimore, 1991, National Health Publishing.

Provides an in-depth motivational training manual in stress management for caregivers and behavior management for elders including 18 mental health content modules, each of which includes module outline, content, handout materials, references and resources, and teaching tips.

*Vaughn K, Young BC, Rice F, Stoner MH: A retrospective study of patient falls in a psychiatric hospital, J Psychosoc Nurs Ment Health Serv 31:37, 1993.

The authors describe the profile of patients who fell while in a psychiatric hospital. The largest percentage of were over 65.

*Walter K: That was then: elderly survivors of incest, J Psychosoc Nurs Ment Health Serv 30:14, 1992.

Incest is not usually considered when elderly patients are being assessed. The author presents evidence that past incest experiences continue to be an issue for patients into old age.

*Wright L: Alzheimer's disease and marriage: an intimate account, Newbury Park, Calif, 1993, Sage Publications.

Excellent discussion from nursing research about how Alzheimer's disease affects married couples. Important findings sensitively written.

*Nursing reference.

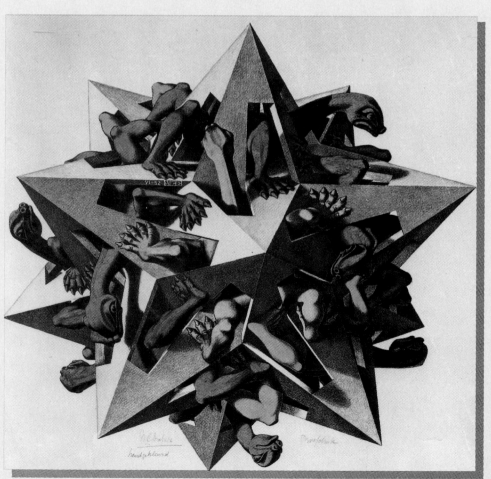

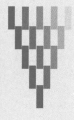

CHAPTER 37

Care of Survivors of Abuse and Violence

BARBARA PARKER
JACQUELINE C. CAMPBELL

When I was a laddie I lived with my granny
And many a hiding my granny di'ed me.
Now I am a man and I live with my granny
And do to my granny what she did to me.

Traditional rhyme, anonymous

LEARNING OBJECTIVES

After studying this chapter the student should be able to:

▼ Define and describe family violence
▼ Identify factors influencing family violence
▼ Identify characteristics frequently observed with violent families
▼ Compare and contrast theories of family violence
▼ Identify behaviors and values of nurses related to family violence
▼ Describe physiological, behavioral, and psychological responses of survivors of family violence
▼ Describe nursing actions related to the prevention of family violence
▼ Analyze characteristics of abuse and violence related to specific populations
▼ Describe common reactions of survivors of rape or sexual assault

TOPICAL OUTLINE

Definition of Family Violence
    Societal Influence on Family Violence
    Characteristics of Violent Families
    Nursing Attitudes Toward Survivors of Violence
    Responses to Family Violence
    Preventive Nursing Interventions
Special Populations
    Child Abuse
    Wife Abuse
    Elder Abuse
Rape and Sexual Assault
    Definition of Sexual Assault
    Marital Rape
    Nursing Care of the Sexual Assault Survivor

Nurses encounter victims of abuse and violence in many settings. However, since experiencing violence is generally devastating, survivors of abuse and violence are frequently seen in psychiatric settings. At times the violence is openly discussed and recognized as a precipitating factor for the current hospitalization, such as a victim of sexual assault treated in an emergency room.

Frequently, however, violence is disclosed only following the establishment of a trusting nurse-patient relationship. Although there are various forms of violence, such as gang behavior and drug-related violence, the types most frequently described by psychiatric patients are family violence and nonfamily rape and sexual assault. Since the dynamics of these two forms of violence are different, they are covered in two separate sections of this chapter. Rape and sexual assault also can be forms of family violence. In addition, attention is given to populations that are particularly at risk for abuse. These include children, spouses, and the elderly.

The words used to describe people who have experienced violence are important. Traditionally the term *victim* has been used, along with discussions of *syndromes*. These labels distance nurses from the person who has been abused as they search for differences between themselves and the survivors to decrease their feelings of vulnerability. In this chapter the term *survivor* is used to emphasize that the person who has experienced abuse has many strengths and coping strategies that can be incorporated into the plan of care.

 Do you agree with the use of the term *survivor* instead of *victim* in this chapter? What do you think of when you hear the words *victim* and *survivor*?

DEFINITION OF FAMILY VIOLENCE

Family violence refers to a range of behaviors occurring between family members. It includes physical and emotional abuse of children, child neglect, spouse battering, marital rape, and elder abuse. There are several different issues related to abuse within families. Although each family is unique, there appear to be characteristics common to most violent families. Furthermore, regardless of the type of abuse occurring within a family, all members, including the extended family, are affected. Family violence, although often unnoted, is at the core of many family disturbances. Violence may be the "family secret" and often continues through generations.[41]

Although numerous research studies and theories have been directed toward the causes, treatment, and prevention of family violence, there are more questions unanswered than answered. Hotaling and Straus[26] note that "the family is the training ground for violence" and ask why the social group designated to provide love and support is also the most violent group to which most people belong. They point out that behaviors that would be unacceptable between strangers, co-workers, or friends are frequently tolerated within families.

Feminist authors note that most victims of family violence are the most vulnerable and powerless family members: women, children, and the elderly.[11,17] They propose that the root cause of violence is the abuser's need for power and control, which is acted out by violent behavior. Social norms that support or at least allow male dominance and violence is also considered crucial in the feminist analysis.[54]

Violence and abuse are generally believed to be caused by an interaction of personality, demographic, situational, and societal factors that impact on a family. Many of the unique characteristics of the family as a social group—time spent together, emotional involvement, privacy, and in-depth knowledge of each other—can facilitate both intimacy and violence. Thus a given family can be both loving and supportive as well as violent.

Societal Influence on Family Violence

To understand violence in American families the influence of the society on the family must be examined. The United States has a high level of violence compared with other Western nations. Many believe that society's willingness to tolerate violence sets the stage for family violence. Social norms are sometimes used to justify violence to maintain the family system. For example, a husband's use of violence may be considered legitimate if the wife is having an extramarital affair. Historical attitudes toward women, children, and the elderly, economic discrimination, the nonresponsiveness of the criminal justice system, and the belief that women and children are property have been cited as factors maintaining norms allowing violence (Fig. 37-1).[11,17] Changing norms related to definitions of family privacy and when government should be allowed to intervene in family matters have also influenced the definitions and recognition of family violence.

Why do you think more violence occurs in American society as compared with other Western nations? What societal factors influence the use of violence?

Characteristics of Violent Families

There are several factors common to violent families. These include the multigenerational family process, social isolation, the use and abuse of power, and the effect of alcohol and drug abuse.

Multigenerational Transmission. Multigenerational transmission means that family violence is often perpetuated through generations by a cycle of violence. Fig. 37-2 illustrates multigenerational transmission of family violence. Several theories have been proposed regarding this phenomenon. The most enduring is social learning theory, in which violence is viewed as a learned behavior.

Social learning theory related to violence states that

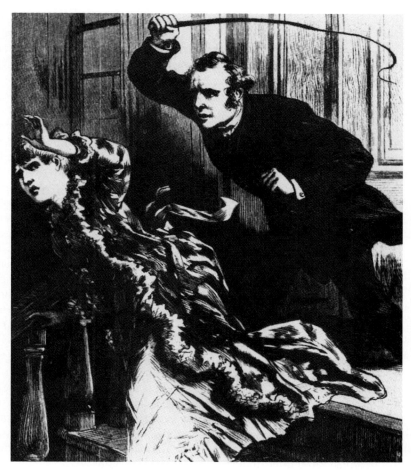

Fig. 37-1   Spouse abuse is a recent psychological concern but an age-old reality. This 1887 woodcut depicts wife-beating in a "proper" family.
From the Bettmann Archive.

a child learns this behavior pattern in a family setting by taking a violent parent as a role model. In this case, violence and victimization are behaviors learned through childhood experience. The child learns both the means and the approval of violence. Children who witness violence not only learn specific aggressive behaviors but also acquire the belief that violence is a legitimate way to solve problems within a family. When frustrated or angry as an adult, the individual relies on this learned behavior and responds with violence.

Social learning theory was first applied to child abuse when it was noted that many child abusers were abused as children. Many studies have suggested the intergenerational transmission of child abuse within families.[51] However, other studies examining parental punishment history and current child abuse found no differences between abusive and nonabusive parents. Experiencing abuse as a child does not totally determine an adult's later behaviors. Many people who were abused as children are able to avoid violence with their own children. Straus and Gelles[51] suggest that the key factor may be

the age at which the child was abused or which parent was abusive. Experiencing abuse from a father at age 4 years may be totally different from experiencing abuse from a mother as an adolescent.

The incidence of violence in the families of both the survivors of wife abuse and their abusers supports multigenerational transmission in this case as well. A literature review conducted by Hotaling and Sugerman[27] identified witnessing parental violence during childhood or adolescence as one of the strongest risk factors for the abuse of wives in adulthood. It is less clear that women learn to be victims of wife abuse from childhood experiences with violence.

To date, there is limited evidence of multigenerational transmission of violence in elder abuse. Pillemer and Suitor,[44] however, suggest that elder abuse could be the result of formerly abused children displaying both retaliatory and imitative behavior or behavior role modeled by their parents with their grandparents.

Many treatment modalities, especially cognitive approaches, are based on the social learning model that

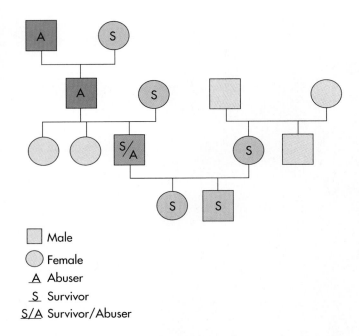

☐ Male
◯ Female
A̲ Abuser
S̲ Survivor
S̲/A̲ Survivor/Abuser

Fig. 37-2 Genogram demonstrates the multigenerational transmission of family violence.

violent reactions can be unlearned and replaced with constructive responses to conflict.

Social Isolation. It has been observed that violent families are also socially isolated. One reason may be that some types of violence are considered abnormal or illegitimate and become a "family secret." Exposure of family violence can result in both formal and informal sanctions from other family members, neighbors, the police, or the judicial system; therefore the abuser often purposely keeps the family isolated. Social isolation has been found to be a factor in elder abuse,[43] wife abuse,[33] and child abuse.[11]

Use and Abuse of Power. Another common factor within the various forms of family violence is the use and abuse of power. In almost all forms of family violence the abuser has some form of power or control over the victim. For example, with the sexual abuse of children, the abuser is usually a male in an authority position victimizing a child in a subordinate position.[53] A study of sexual abuse of children by caregivers[40] also noted the unequal power between the violator and the child victim.

Power issues appear to be a central factor with wife abuse. Although wife abusers will justify the use of violence for trivial events such as not having a meal ready or not keeping the house tidy, violence often is related to the husband's need for total domination of his wife. Wife abuse often begins or escalates when the woman behaves more independently by working or attending

school. Finkelhor and Pillemer[21] found that the largest category (60%) of physical abuse of the elderly was actually spouse abuse, thereby incorporating the issues of power and control central in that form of family violence.

Alcohol and Drug Abuse. The relationship between alcohol and drug abuse and family violence has been studied extensively. Survivors of violence frequently report concurrent substance abuse by the abuser. Most researchers, however, deny that substance abuse is a direct cause of violence because one behavior is not necessary for the other to occur. That is, people who abuse alcohol are not consistently violent, and people who are violent are not always intoxicated. Instead, it has been suggested that the person uses alcohol as a more socially acceptable explanation for the behavior. Family and friends may also attribute the conduct to the effects of alcohol, which to some extent decreases the degree of blame. The use of alcohol or drugs may also increase violent behavior by reducing fear or inhibitions and decreasing sensitivity to the impact of the behavior.

Cross-cultural studies suggest that behavior while drinking varies from culture to culture. In societies where it is believed that alcohol removes inhibitions, people become less inhibited. If they believe it is a depressant, they become depressed when drinking. If people in America believe that normal rules of behavior are suspended when one is drinking, people will behave antisocially.

Leonard and Jacob[36] conducted an extensive literature review of the relationship between alcohol abuse and family violence. They concluded that there was some evidence relating alcohol use and alcoholism to marital violence, but the evidence related to child abuse was much weaker. In addition, with marital violence, other factors such as the stress of alcoholism on the family system or familial expectations that drinking will increase aggressive behavior have not been adequately studied.

Connections between drug abuse and family violence have been less well researched. Early research on aggressiveness and illicit drugs has established that marijuana and heroin use are not related to violence. In contrast, drugs such as "crack" cocaine, amphetamines, mescaline, "angel dust" (PCP), and steroids used illegally have been associated with increased violence, but the specific relationships with various forms of family violence are not yet established.[4]

Nursing Attitudes Toward Survivors of Violence

It can be extremely difficult and frustrating to provide nursing care for survivors of violence. The attitudes nurses bring to these situations help shape their responses. Studies of health-care professionals' attitudes indicate that myths about battered women are accepted even though there is sympathy toward the survivor.[54] Nurses have been found *not* to blame rape victims in general. However, the tendency to blame the victim increases when a vignette describes the woman as having gone out late at night, not locked her car doors, or gone shopping for beer rather than milk for the baby.[15]

Although most nurses do not actually blame survivors for what has happened to them, they do dislike certain behaviors. They are not happy with sexual assault survivors within and outside the family who do not resist "enough." They have difficulty understanding abused children who want to return to abusive parents. They especially dislike battered women who do not leave their abusers. Kurz[32] published a classic study describing the subtle blaming and distancing of battered women by emergency department personnel, including nurses. Stark and Flitcraft[50] used emergency room chart reviews to document the lack of recognition, negative labeling, and inappropriate treatment that all too often happens to battered women. Other studies describe how survivors find the health-care system to be unhelpful and even traumatizing when they have gone for assistance.[2] King and Ryan[31] note that nurses most often use a paternalistic and individualistic model of helping battered women. The paternalistic model may be contrasted with the empowerment model. Table 37-1 compares the characteristics of these models. When the paternalistic model is used, the nurse is more likely to be frustrated because the survivor does not follow the nurse's advice. Therefore the empowerment model is not only more helpful to the survivor but also more professionally satisfying for the nurse.

Origins of Negative Attitudes. There are several theories that can help in understanding nurses' attitudes. The "just world" hypothesis was first advanced by Lerner and Simmons.[37] Basically this proposes that people believe that others generally get what they deserve. Therefore good things happen to good people, and bad things happen to bad people. This belief helps one feel safe because oneself is seen as basically good and therefore protected. When a person is victimized by violence, there is a need to make sense of this horrible idea. The easiest way is not to see it at all, which explains some of the lack of recognition. However, when family violence is unmistakable, one needs to understand why that particular person is the victim. If bad things happen to bad people, the victimized person must have done something wrong or at least something stupid, something different from what oneself would have done.

The whole process of victim blaming is easier if the victim is of "a type" who is already the focus of bias. It is easier to blame and distance oneself from women or minority groups if there is already bias against them. Conversely, the more the person resembles oneself, the harder it is to recognize the violence at all. Thus it is not reported as often; the abuse is just not "seen" when the people are middle class and especially professionals. Consequently, child abuse is more likely to be reported if the family is poor and of a racial minority.

Ryan[47] discusses similar dynamics in the book *Blaming the Victim*. Ryan describes how blaming the victim helps the person avoid blaming the system in which violence is perpetuated. If the battered woman is to blame for at least not ending the violence, society is less at fault for perpetuating the notions that power, aggression, and dominance are the marks of a successful man and a successful country. Consequently the issue can be avoided. If the family who abuses elders is dysfunctional, others need not worry about a society that fails to provide help to the caregivers of the elderly. As another example, consider the family member who has always been the most despised in cases of incest, the "collusive" mother. Despite the lack of research evidence to support this,[19] professionals are still eager to find out the mother's role in sexual abuse of her daughter. Since it is difficult to blame the child, they have shifted the blame to another female family member. Professionals should try to understand the mother's normal responses to a horrible dilemma. Even though some of the societal forces that lead to incest have been exposed, they are generally not addressed in recommendations for clinical interventions. The focus is on the "dysfunctional family unit" rather than the real issue: a criminal who has violated the safety and health of a child in a society uncomfortable with the attitudes that may encourage such behavior.

Another perspective—theories of deviance as explained by Schur[48] is especially relevant for nursing. Deviance theory proposes that making the survivors and perpetrators of violence into objects to be studied or

Table 37-1 A Comparison of the Paternalistic and Empowerment Models of Intervention with Battered Women

Paternalistic model	Empowerment model
Nurse is perceived to be more knowledgeable than the survivor	There is mutual sharing of knowledge and information
Responsibility for ending the violence is placed on the survivor	The nurse strategizes with the survivor
	Survivors are assisted to recognize societal influences
Advice and sympathy are given rather than respect	The survivor's competence and experience are respected

diagnostic categories creates further distance between them and the nurse. This is the problem with the proposed medical diagnosis of "battered woman syndrome" or a psychiatric diagnosis specific to victims of violence.[3,14] If adults receive diagnoses only because they were abused sometime in their past, the assumption of pathology becomes concrete. The survivor of family violence is officially sick and has the responsibility to become well. There is no chance that the person's responses will be seen as survival strategies or normal reactions; they become symptoms. Survivors become a "deviant group" to be studied and "fixed."

It has been suggested that more nurses have been victimized by violence than other groups, which might explain their negative attitudes toward other survivors. Research has not established whether there are more battered women among nurses than among other populations of women. However, Rew[46] found the percentage of nursing students who had experienced childhood sexual exploitation (62%) to be similar to that in another survey of female college students. Regardless of the specific violence experience of nurses, there are certainly power, control, and exploitation issues that have shaped the history of the nursing profession and continue to influence nurses' daily reality. Therefore, according to "oppressed group" behavior literature,[25] nurses would tend to have negative attitudes toward another oppressed group, the predominantly female victims of family violence.

Overcoming Negative Attitudes. The first step in providing effective nursing care is exploring one's own attitudes toward survivors of family violence. Understanding the mechanisms that help create such attitudes is also helpful. It has been suggested that nurses who have had clinical experience with survivors and gotten to know them as persons may be less blaming than nurses who have not.[15] Therefore it is important to gain this experience either through educational programs or as a volunteer in programs such as rape crisis centers, battered women's shelters, or child protection programs. Formal continuing and in-service education on family violence should be directed toward recognizing and changing feelings, as well as learning facts about violence. Nurses can also increase their own understanding and appreciation of the experience of survivors by reading novels and watching media programs about these issues.[10]

Responses to Family Violence

There is a growing body of knowledge that describes how people are likely to respond to violence from other family members. Since the definition of nursing is the diagnosis and treatment of human responses to health problems, these biopsychosocial responses to violence

as a major health problem are the primary focus of nursing.

Physical Responses to Battering. One area of study has been the types and patterns of physical injuries received. A characteristic pattern of injuries, especially to the head, neck/face/throat, trunk, and sexual organs has been seen in all forms of family violence. For all groups experiencing family violence, sexual abuse frequently accompanies physical abuse. This has been best documented in battered women; several studies have found that approximately 40% were also sexually assaulted by their partners. All survivors of family violence tend to have injuries at multiple sites in various stages of healing.

Survivors of family violence frequently experience a range of physical symptoms not obviously related to their injuries, such as headaches, menstrual problems, chronic pain, and digestive and sleeping disturbances.[3,8,14] Frequently, communicable diseases are a problem in shelters for battered women and their children.

Many characterize these types of symptoms as evidence of psychopathology, but similar symptoms occur after rape and other forms of violence, as well as in widows and divorcees. They have failed to consider that past injuries could cause such symptoms as headaches and other forms of chronic pain. Stress is known to affect the immune system. Thus, rather than labeling such symptoms "hysterical," "psychosomatic," or "evidence of somaticizing," they can be identified as part of a physical stress reaction. Such responses to stress are common to those who have experienced many types of emotional trauma.

Behavioral Responses to Battering. There have been many attempts to understand the behavior of survivors of family violence, especially their continued involvement with an abuser. This has been especially damaging in literature addressing the question of why battered women remain in the relationship. It is assumed that she *should* leave rather than stay. In actuality, when a battered woman leaves, she is in the most danger of being killed by a partner obsessed with power and control.[7,24] At the other end of the continuum, some battered women are able to end the violence but maintain their relationships using a variety of strategies.

However, family violence usually escalates in severity and frequency. In cases where the violence does not end, it is normal and healthy for a battered woman to consider her entire existence and that of her significant others for a long time before ending her most important attachment relationship.[9,34] Constraints that make it difficult to leave include cultural sanctions, an intense attachment to the man, and lack of resources. Gilligan[22] has observed that women usually make moral decisions by weighing the consequences to others more heavily than consequences to themselves. Thus concern for her children is a major issue in the woman's decision making.

Most battered women eventually leave a relationship that is continuously violent, but there is often a pattern of leaving and returning many times before making a final break. Rather than a sign of weakness, this can be viewed as a normal behavioral pattern. It is influenced by the quality of social support and assistance to the woman and the batterer's behavior rather than the woman's psychological factors. Leaving and returning are purposeful and meant to achieve one or more of the following: (1) pressure the abuser into meaningful change, (2) test external and internal resources, and (3) evaluate how the children are reacting without their father.

Similar long processes of ending attachment relationships are seen with wives of alcoholics, divorced and separated women, and persons experiencing anticipatory grief. Grief can explain the denial that is frequently described in battered women.[11] This coping mechanism has been renamed as "forgetting and minimizing" by Kelly[30] in her exploration of responses to sexual violence (rape, incest, battering). The women in Kelly's sample saw this response as generally very useful rather than a problem, as is often implied.

 Discuss the issue of women remaining in abusive relationships. What factors keep them in these relationships? How do health professionals usually respond to a woman who has remained in an abusive relationship? What approach would be helpful to her?

Clinical reports also describe the reluctance of abused children and elderly family members to leave their families as pathological rather than normal. These responses seem more understandable and healthy if they are related to normal grief and fear of foster homes or nursing homes. An important nursing research study by Humphreys[28] documented that the children of battered women take significant action to try to protect their mothers. Although these actions are sometimes viewed as unhealthy, Humphreys described them as an instance of Orem's concept of dependent care. This way of viewing responses to family violence is congruent with nursing's emphasis on physical and mental health.

Psychological Responses to Battering.
More work has been done to explore psychological responses to abuse in battered women than in either child abuse or elder abuse. Most of our knowledge about the emotional responses to incest describes delayed reactions rather than immediate ones. Psychological responses studied most frequently include the cognitive responses of attribution and problem solving and the emotional responses of depression and lowered self-esteem.

ATTRIBUTIONS. Attributions can be defined as the reasoning processes people use to explain events. A relationship to future mental health has been found in a variety of situations, including serious violence. A discussion of the impact of attributions on the survivor of violence is presented in Critical Thinking about Contemporary Issues.

PROBLEM-SOLVING TECHNIQUES. Several studies have found that battered women have trouble with problem solving.[35] School problems have also been reported in abused children.[14] In contrast, another researcher[9] describes a variety of approaches used and factors considered by battered women that suggest appropriate decision making. Undoubtedly, some battered women, children, and elders are so frequently and severely beaten and controlled that their ability to problem solve is severely and chronically affected.

? CRITICAL THINKING ABOUT CONTEMPORARY ISSUES

Do Most Victims of Violence Believe That They Are To Blame for What Happened to Them?

Attributions affect how people feel about their behavior and how they interpret life events. It is often said that victims of violence tend to blame themselves. Research shows that only about 20% of battered women do so.[9] Battered women tend to blame themselves less over time. In contrast, one report showed that the majority of adult survivors of repeated childhood sexual abuse by a person they knew blamed themselves. However, these women were in a clinical setting rather than the community.[29]

It has been argued that internal self-blaming attributions may be adaptive for survivors of violence as a way of maintaining control over their lives. Others think that self-blame may contribute to long-term depression. To date, research has not resolved this issue for battered women or for other survivors of family violence. There is insufficient evidence to assume that self-blame is either widespread among survivors or always pathological. Nurses who work with these patients using the empowerment model will assist them to identify their attributions and explore the effect on their feelings and relationships. ▼

Extreme difficulty in problem solving could be explained by "posttraumatic stress disorder," described in the DSM-IV[1] as including symptoms of memory impairment or difficulty concentrating. Problem-solving difficulties noted in widows and divorcees have been explained as normal responses to loss. Such problems could also be explained as one of the cognitive aspects of depression.

DEPRESSION. Depression has been noted in many research studies of battered women, adult survivors of incest, and abused children.[3,38,52] Depression has also been described in survivors of other forms of violence, as well as in divorcees and widows. Depression is a complex process. Detailed information about predisposing factors and precipitating stressors related to depression is discussed in Chapter 17.

Walker[52] hypothesized that learned helplessness was the best explanation of depression in battered women. Although her research generally supported the model, she found that women who had left the abusive relationship had higher scores on the depression measure than those still with the batterer. This finding may indicate a problem in her assumption that learned helplessness is an explanation for some battered women staying in the relationship. It could also mean that depression experienced by the women who left was a result of grief rather than learned helplessness. Campbell[9] found support for both grief and learned helplessness using theory comparison research. However, both models left almost half the variation in depression unexplained. This may reflect the emphasis in both models on the individual situation. The wider influences that contribute to both healthy and unhealthy responses to violence are not included in either model. Furthermore, only a small minority of the battered women in the Campbell sample exhibited all aspects of the syndrome of learned helplessness: depression, low self-esteem, apathy, and difficulty with problem solving.

Mackey and associates[38] studied depression in female survivors of sexual assault. They found that 60% were at least somewhat depressed. Factors associated with more severe depression included lack of disclosure of the assault to significant others related to stigma, having children at home, and involvement in a civil lawsuit. Women who reported being sexually active were less depressed.

SELF-ESTEEM. Although most research has found low self-esteem in battered women and incest survivors, there have been some exceptions.[3,9,52] For instance, Kelly[30] reported that a greater proportion of the incest and battering survivors in her study felt more "independent and stronger" than more "insecure in self" as a result of the abuse.

One way to resolve these differences is to compare groups who are experiencing the same situational dynamics, except for the violence. Using this approach, Campbell[9] found no significant difference in self-esteem between battered women and other women considering leaving an intimate relationship, even though both groups were below norms. Similarly, DiPietro[16] found no significant difference in the self-esteem of incest survivors compared to young women in treatment for other family problems. Both groups were again lower than norms. However, sexual abuse had a direct detrimental effect on battered women's self-esteem independent of severity and frequency of physical beatings.[9]

In summary, responses to family violence can be interpreted as symptoms of pathology of a certain group of people. The same responses can be interpreted as how normal people respond to incredible physical and emotional trauma and yet survive. Research regarding this latter approach is beginning to document survivor mechanisms and a recovery process from abuse.[33]

Preventive Nursing Interventions

Preventing family violence requires the use of a variety of approaches. These include the primary prevention strategies of changing norms and values, preventive education with a variety of populations, and secondary prevention strategies of effective treatment.

Primary Prevention. Primary prevention refers to an activity that stops a problem before it occurs. Changing society's acceptance of violence and abuse is an important first step in prevention. Consider, for example, the changing view of cigarette smoking that has occurred in America in the past 15 years. In less than 2 decades perceptions of cigarette smoking have changed from an attractive, sophisticated behavior to a health hazard that is prohibited in most public places.

Effective primary prevention includes eliminating cultural norms and values that accept and glamorize violence. This would begin by severely limiting the amount of violence permitted on television and in other media. The prevalence of violence on television plays a role in creating a social climate that says violence is exciting and appropriate. The average child watches television for 20 hours a week. It has been estimated that American children observe 18,000 killings before they graduate from high school. A report summarizing studies on the effect of media violence noted, "Of the 85 major studies into the effects of television violence, only one concluded that television violence did not cause increased aggressiveness in children. It was paid for by NBC."[13] Video games are becoming increasingly popular with children also, and there is a great deal of concern about the violence in these games. Some video game manufacturers have agreed to place ratings on video games according to age appropriateness and level of violence (Fig. 37-3).

A related area of primary prevention would be the elimination of pornography, especially violent pornography. Violent pornography has been particularly associated with sexual violence.[49] However, the rate of subscription to even a mild form of pornography as *Playboy* magazine has been positively correlated with state rape rates.

Primary prevention of abuse also includes strengthening individuals and families so they can cope more effectively with stress. Nurses can conduct programs in the schools, workplace, or community. Strategies such as nurse-developed educational programs in high-school parenting classes or childbirth education classes can be used to prepare families for the stress of child rearing. Topics could include normal child development and expectations, basic skills of infant care, and means of disciplining children that do not involve physical punishment. Additional educational strategies are teaching family members that conflict resolution does not always mean one party wins while the other loses and that they should respect individual differences among family members.

Nurses can be involved in teaching family life and sex education courses in elementary and middle schools. Child sexual abuse can be prevented or detected when children are taught about inappropriate sexual contact and what they should do if it occurs. Middle-school students need information about how to have relationships in which jealousy is not viewed as a sign of love and domination of one partner over the other is not expected. Peer discussions can help change the definition

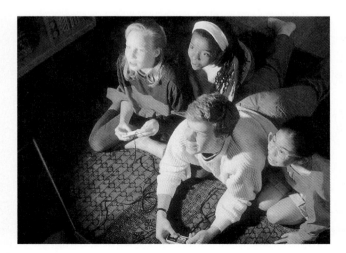

Fig. 37-3 Some video games contain a great deal of violence. This has led to concern about how the games are influencing the behavior of the children who play them.
From Superstock, Inc.

of manliness based on confrontation and control.

Family violence prevention also includes anticipatory guidance while working with families. For example, respite care is needed for families with chronically ill or incapacitated members, including the elderly and children. Planning in advance for relief from responsibility will prevent strained relationships and potential violence or abuse. Families also need to anticipate the difficult developmental stages of children. Parents need to know that infants are not intentionally frustrating to parents, that toddlers' obstinance is necessary for independence in later childhood, and that bed-wetting is a signal for increased positive attention and not punishment.

As a society we must develop programs and policies that support families and reduce stresses and inequities. This includes adequate and appropriate day care for children and incapacitated elders, equity in salary and wages to make women less financially dependent, public education that ensures an adequate foundation for full employment of all, and sufficient financing of prevention and treatment programs.

Secondary Prevention. Secondary prevention of family violence is aimed at its cyclic nature. Although there is not a perfect relationship, we do know that children raised in violent, noncaring homes are more likely to become spouse and child abusers. Therefore one of the most effective methods of preventing violence and abuse in future generations is to stop current abuse.

Even when the violence has ended, those affected will need help. The children of battered women and siblings of abused children are groups who have witnessed violence and need assistance to counteract that learning. Frequently it is believed that abused children are "out of the woods" when they have been removed from the home or the family is no longer violent. Even if there are no identifiable long-term effects, there may have been "trauma encapsulation." This may not be evident until many years afterward.[6] In addition, the child will believe that family members are violent to each other. Conscious resolve alone may not overcome this.[46]

Secondary prevention also involves identification of families at risk or those who are beginning to use violence. Table 37-2 lists characteristics common to violent families. These can be used for nursing assessment. Additional early indicators of families at risk include violence in the family of origin of either partner, communication problems, and excessive family stress such as an unplanned pregnancy, unemployment, or inadequate family resources. Pregnancy is an ideal time to identify women at risk to become battered or in the early stages of an abusive relationship. This is also the best time to identify the infant's risk for abuse. Pregnancy is when healthy women are most often seen in the health care system. A comprehensive assessment should include in-

Table 37-2 Indicators of Actual or Potential Abuse

Nursing history	Physical examination	Nursing observations
PRIMARY REASON FOR CONTACT Vague information about cause of problem Discrepancy between physical findings and description of cause Minimizing injuries Inappropriate delay between time of injury and treatment Inappropriate family reactions (e.g., lack of concern, overconcern, threatening demeanor) **INFORMATION FROM FAMILY GENOGRAM** Family violence in history (child, spouse, elder) History of violence outside of home Incarcerations Violent deaths in extended family Alcoholism/drug abuse in family history **HEALTH HISTORY** History of traumatic injuries Spontaneous abortions Psychiatric hospitalizations History of depression Substance abuse **SEXUAL HISTORY** Prior sexual abuse Use of force in sexual activities Venereal disease Child with sexual knowledge beyond that appropriate for age Promiscuity **PERSONAL/SOCIAL HISTORY** Unwanted or unplanned pregnancy Adolescent pregnancy Social isolation (difficulty naming persons available for help in a crisis) Lack of contact with extended family Unrealistic expectations of relationships or age-appropriate behavior Extreme jealousy by spouse Rigid traditional sex-role beliefs Verbal aggression Belief in use of physical punishment Difficulties in school Truancy, running away **PSYCHOLOGICAL HISTORY** Feelings of helplessness/hopelessness Feeling trapped Difficulty making plans for future Tearfulness Chronic fatigue, apathy Suicide attempts	**GENERAL APPEARANCE** Fearful, anxious, hyperactive or hypoactive Poor hygiene, careless grooming Inappropriate dress Increased anxiety in presence of abuser Looking to abuser for answers to questions Inappropriate or anxious nonverbal behavior (e.g., giggling at serious questions or questions related to abuse) Flinching when touched **VITAL STATISTICS** Overweight or underweight Hypertension **SKIN** Bruises, welts, edema Presence of scars and indications of injuries in various stages of healing Cigarette burns **HEAD** Bald patches on scalp from pulling hair Subdural hematoma **EYES** Subconjunctival hemorrhage Swelling Black eyes **EARS** Hearing loss from prior injury or untreated infections **MOUTH** Bruising Lacerations Untreated dental caries Venereal infection **ABDOMEN** Intraabdominal injuries Abdominal injuries during pregnancy **EXTREMITIES** Bruising to forearms from attempts to protect self from blows Broken arms Radiological indications of previous fractures	**GENERAL OBSERVATIONS** Observations differ significantly from history Family members inadequately clothed or groomed **HOME ENVIRONMENT** Inadequate heating Inappropriate sleeping arrangements Total household disorganization Inadequate food Spoiled food not discarded **FAMILY COMMUNICATION PATTERN** One parent answers all questions Looking for approval of other family members before answering questions Members continually interrupt each other Negative nonverbal behavior in other members when one member speaking Members do not listen to each other Taboo topics (family secrets) **EMOTIONAL CLIMATE** Tense, secretive atmosphere Unhappiness Lack of affection Apparent fear of other family members Verbal arguing

Table 37-2   Indicators of Actual or Potential Abuse—cont'd

Nursing history	Physical examination	Nursing observations

FINANCIAL HISTORY

Poverty

Finances rigidly controlled by one family member

Unwillingness to spend money on health care or adequate nutrition

Complaints about spending money on family members

Unemployment

Use of elders' finances for other family members

FAMILY BELIEFS/VALUES

Belief in importance of physical discipline

Autocratic decision making

Intolerance of differing views among members

Mistrust of outsiders

FAMILY RELATIONS

Lack of visible affection or nurturing between family members

Extreme dependency between family members

Autonomy discouraged

Numerous arguments

Temporary separations

Dissatisfaction with family members

Lack of enjoyable family activities

Extramarital affairs

Role rigidity (inability of members to assume nontraditional roles)

NEUROLOGICAL

Developmental delays

Difficulty with speech or swallowing

Hyperactive reflex response

GENITAL/URINARY

Genital lacerations or bruising

Urinary tract infections

Sexually transmitted disease

RECTAL

Rectal bruising

Bleeding

Edema

Tenderness

Poor sphincter tone

---

formation about relationships and child-rearing beliefs and practices. It may also be possible to identify abuse early in a relationship before abusive patterns become entrenched.[42] When the nurse hears an indication of risk, immediate nursing intervention is required. Taking the time to explore the risk factors, to discuss perceptions and attitudes, and to brainstorm with the patient about possible alternatives is time well spent.

SPECIAL POPULATIONS
Child Abuse

The earliest form of family violence recognized in the health professional literature was physical abuse to children. Although violence to children was identified as a social problem in the nineteenth century, it was not until the 1940s that it became a medical problem, even a unique "syndrome." In 1962 the classic article by C. Henry Kempe and his associates, "The Battered Child

Syndrome," created interest in the problem of physical abuse to children. By the end of the 1960s every state had enacted legislation mandating the report of suspected child abuse and neglect. Under current laws, nurses and any other professionals providing services to children are required to report suspected incidents of child abuse and neglect.

There are many forms of abuse to children. These include physical abuse or battering, emotional abuse, sexual abuse, and neglect. There is still much that is unknown about the causes, treatment, or prevention of child abuse. In addition, research has failed to identify any factors that are present in all abusing and absent in all nonabusing parents.

Sexual Abuse of Children and Adolescents. Sexual abuse is defined as the involvement of children and adolescents in sexual activities they do not fully comprehend and to which they do not freely consent.[20] Sexual abuse results in both long-term and short-term problems. Physical problems include:

▼ Venereal disease or infection
▼ Vaginal or rectal bleeding, itching, or soreness
▼ Recurrent urinary tract infections
▼ Pregnancy

Emotional changes as identified by Morris and Bihan[39] include:

▼ Sexual acting-out
▼ Physical aggression
▼ Excessive masturbation
▼ Withdrawal
▼ Low self-esteem
▼ Drop in school performance
▼ Disturbed sleep

Morris and Bihan found that physical and sexual abuse often were not considered as possible causes of these behaviors in a review of the records of 100 former child psychiatric hospital patients.

The long-term effects of sexual abuse as a child include:

▼ Sexual problems
▼ Difficulty trusting others
▼ Anxiety and panic attacks
▼ Depression
▼ Substance abuse

A study by Feinauer[20] of adult women who had been sexually abused as children found that they experienced more emotional distress and long-term effects when the perpetrator was a person who was known and trusted by them. Feinauer found that the kinship relationship between the victim and the abuser was less important in creating distress than the emotional bond the victim felt toward the perpetrator. Thus a critical factor seems to be the violation of the child's trust, as well as the physical trauma.

Nursing Assessment. Nursing assessment of actual or potential child abuse begins with a thorough history and physical examination. Gathering a history of child abuse can be a stressful experience for both the nurse and the family. It is therefore essential for the nurse to examine personal values and past experiences to maintain a therapeutic and nonjudgmental clinical approach.

It is important to use an honest, open approach that is not intended to punish or shame either the child or the parent.[11] Most abusive parents are genuinely embarrassed about their behavior and would like assistance in developing alternative approaches to discipline. Knowledge of this can be used by the nurse to establish an environment that will facilitate honesty and sharing. The setting for the interview needs to be quiet, private, and uninterrupted.

In general, the child and the adult(s) should be separated for the initial interview. This decision, however, depends on the child's age and other extenuating circumstances. The nurse should honestly state the purpose of the interview, type of questions being asked, and describe the subsequent physical examination. The approach needs to be calm and supportive because both the child and the family will be uneasy.

The interview with the parent(s) can begin with a discussion of the problem that first brought the child to a health-care facility. During this discussion the nurse should pay particular attention to the parent's understanding of the problem, discrepancies in the stories, and the parent's emotional responses. The interview can then be expanded to discussions of how the parent "disciplines" the child or spanks the child. The initial interview is not the time to confront a suspected abuser directly, since measures must be taken to document and report the abuse in a way that will ensure the child's safety.

Nursing Interventions. When child abuse is suspected, the nurse must report this to protective services. An investigation by the state protective service agency is legally mandated and also reinforces to the family the seriousness of the problem. When protective services are involved, the nurse should explain to the family precisely what will happen in an investigation and the amount of time involved. The nurse should maintain frequent contact with the assigned worker to ensure a comprehensive, consistent approach. Nurses who work with violent families need to know exactly how protective services in their community operate. Ongoing professional relationships with colleagues at the agency will enable the nurse to remain informed about policies and reporting protocols and ensure successful coordination and continuity.

Wife Abuse

The term *wife abuse* includes all forms of physical violence toward a female partner in an ongoing intimate relationship. It also refers to emotional degradation and intimidation, which almost always accompany physical abuse, of female partners, and to sexual abuse (or marital rape), which is part of the violence in about half of the cases.[9] The violence is part of a system of coercive control that may also include financial coercion, threats against children and other family members, and destruction of property. Wife abuse is the most widespread form of family violence. At least one in every six wives is hit by a husband sometime during their relationship. At least 1.6 million women each year are severely and repeatedly beaten by their spouses.[51] Although wives do hit husbands, female violence is much more likely to be in self-defense. It seldom takes the intentional repeated, serious, and controlling form characteristic of wife abuse. Therefore using the terms *spouse abuse* and *domestic violence* obscures the gender specificity of the violence. However, the nurse must be aware that both husband abuse and homosexual partner abuse are possibilities, although apparently rare.

One of the most frightening realities of wife abuse is the potential for murder. The majority of female homicide victims in the United States are killed by a husband, lover, or ex-husband or -lover. The majority of these murders are preceded by abuse.[7] There is evidence that a battered woman is in most danger of homicide when she leaves her abusive partner or makes it clear to him that she is ending the relationship.[24] Battered women also kill their spouses. Many of the risk factors are similar. They include having a handgun in the house, a history of suicide threats or attempts in either partner, battering during pregnancy, sexual abuse, severe substance abuse, and extreme jealousy and controlling behavior.[4,8] A frequent statement heard by potentially murderous abusers is, "If I can't have you, no one can."

Stark and Flitcraft[50] assert that battering may be the most important precipitating stressor for female suicide attempts and that 10% of battered women have considered suicide. Therefore, when an abused woman is depressed, suicide potential must be carefully assessed.

 Discuss social reaction to wife abuse in relation to the Loreena Bobbitt and O.J. Simpson trials.

Nursing Assessment. It has been documented that the most prevalent cause of trauma in women treated in emergency rooms is wife abuse. It is also a frequent cause of female visits to psychiatric emergency departments and other mental health treatment centers. We now recognize that nursing assessment for all forms of violence is critical. Assessment for wife abuse should be mandatory in mental health settings, as well as in emergency rooms, prenatal settings, and primary care facilities.[12,42]

When there are no obvious injuries, assessment for abuse is best included with the history about the patient's (both genders) primary intimate attachment relationship. Answers to general questions on the quality of that relationship should be assessed for feelings of being controlled or needing to control. A relationship characterized by excessive jealousy (of possessions, children, jobs, friends, and other family members, as well as potential sexual partners) is more likely to be violent. The patient can be asked about how the couple solves conflicts; one partner needing to have the final say or frequent and forceful verbal aggression also can

be considered risk factors. Finally, the patient should be asked if arguments ever involve "pushing or shoving." Questions about minor violence within a couple relationship help to establish the unfortunate normalcy of wife abuse and to lessen the stigma of disclosure. If the patient hesitates, looks away, displays other uncomfortable nonverbal behavior or reveals risk factors for abuse, she or he can be asked again later in the interview about physical violence.

If abuse is revealed, the nurse's first response is critical. It is important that an abused woman realize that she is not alone; important affirmation can be given with a statement about the frequency of wife abuse. The extent and types of the abuse need to be identified and described in the record. Careful documentation using a body map (Fig. 37-4) is necessary for potential legal actions, which are frequently child custody suits as well as criminal actions related to the violence.[42]

The woman's responses to the violence are also a critical area for mental health assessment. It is important to interpret these responses to the woman as normal within the circumstances. Signs of posttraumatic stress disorder, depression, and low self-esteem need to be assessed and recorded. Attribution regarding the abuse is also important. One nursing study[9] revealed that women who blamed abuse on an unchanging personality characteristic within themselves had lower levels of self-esteem and increased depression. The nurse must carefully assess the woman's beliefs regarding the abuse and responsibility for the abuse. Since many wife abusers find an excuse for the violence, the woman may be unnecessarily accepting the blame for his actions.

If the patient is an abuser, mental state is also important, with the potential for further violence carefully assessed. The safety of the abused partner is a concern, as is treatment for the abuser. Consultation with legal advisors about the nurse's "duty to warn" would be warranted (see Chapter 8).[24]

Nursing Interventions. Most communities have treatment programs for abusive men. They have been found to be most effective when the court has ordered treatment with punishment for noncompliance.[18] Severely abusive men seldom admit they have a problem and frequently need to be mandated to enter and remain in treatment. The nurse needs to confront the violence and clarify that the responsibility lies with the abuser. A combination of strategies may be needed to get the abuser into treatment if he is not involved with the court.

The type of referral chosen is extremely important. Long-lasting change is more likely if the treatment combines behavioral therapy around anger control with a program designed to change attitudes toward women.[23] (Managing anger is discussed in Chapter 27 and cogni-

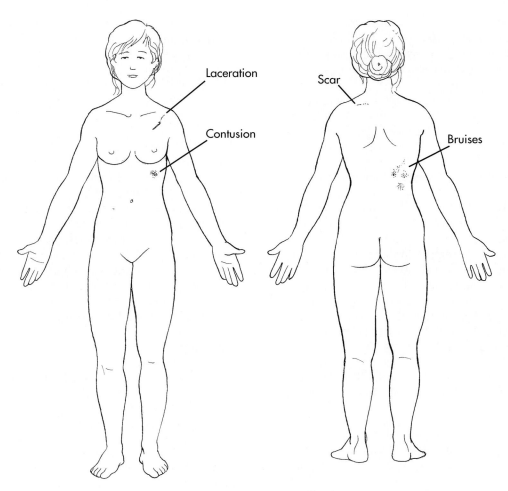

Fig. 37-4 Body map demonstrating evidence of physical abuse.

tive behavioral theory in Chapter 28.) Traditional marriage therapy or couple counseling as the only treatment is potentially dangerous to the woman because of the unequal power in the relationship and the possibility of retaliatory violence.

To empower an abused woman, one must first make sure she has the information she needs. This includes illegality of wife assault and the related state and local laws and ordinances. She also needs to be aware of the local battered woman's shelter(s) available for advice, support, and group participation, even if she does not intend to enter the shelter at this time.

Mutual goal setting is particularly important when working with abused women. Nurses can be frustrated if they impose their goals on the women, who may not be ready for drastic action. Ideally they will have a long-term relationship during which the nurse and patient can work through the normal denial and minimization that takes place when the primary attachment relationship is threatened. The nurse and patient can then consider all the options the woman has thought about and devise others. Dealing with an abusive situation is a re-

covering process that takes time and ongoing support.[34] The nurse, whether in a short- or long-term relationship, can help the patient mobilize both natural and system support so that her economic as well as emotional needs are addressed.

Evaluation of nursing interventions is based on mutual goals not on a preconceived notion of what a battered woman should do. Since most abused women eventually leave a seriously violent situation or end the violence in some other way and seek help when the violence becomes severe,[23] the nurse can be optimistic about the eventual outcome. Interventions may not result in an immediately happy ending, but they can plant the needs of empowerment that facilitate the woman's recovery process.

Elder Abuse

Estimates of the numbers of elderly persons abused vary widely. Finkelhor and Pillemer[21] found 32 victims of physical abuse, physical neglect, or chronic verbal aggression per 1000 elderly in Boston. However, the majority of the abuse was committed by spouses (60% of the physical abuse and 58% of the overall maltreatment). Thus spouse abuse and elder abuse are often overlapping categories.

This also contradicts the notion that elder abuse is most likely a case of children abusing an elderly parent for whom they are providing physical care. Although caregiver stress is an important nursing concern, it may not play the central role in elder abuse that was previously assumed. In fact, Finkelhor and Pillemer[21] found that an important risk factor for elder abuse was the abuser's financial dependence on the abused. Research has not found abused elders to be more functionally impaired than control groups. Rather than the condition of the elder, characteristics of the abuser, such as mental and emotional problems including substance abuse, create a family situation at risk for elder abuse.

Nursing Assessment. Based on this information, it would be important to assess for elder abuse in families where a mentally ill person is financially dependent on aging parents. Consequently, family interviews would not focus exclusively on the patient but would also assess the interactions among family members for indications of verbal and physical aggression.

It is difficult for abused elders to admit being physically hurt by a child or spouse. Again, gentle inquiry about the family's usual approach to resolving interpersonal difficulties is useful. At least part of this assessment needs to take place with the elder alone. An elder may be reluctant to disclose abuse because of fear of being abandoned to a nursing home or a life of total isolation. Only by establishing a trusting relationship over time or utilizing an already established relationship with someone else will the nurse be able to explore the abusive situation completely (Fig. 37-5).

Assessment is even more difficult when the elder is severely mentally or emotionally impaired. In those cases physical assessment plus careful attention to nonverbal behavior is critical. Bruises to the upper arms from shaking are especially common in elder abuse. Although bruises from abuse are difficult to differentiate from those normal in aging, bilateral upper outer arm bruises are relatively definitive. Lacerations, especially to the face, are not usually caused by falls and should be regarded with suspicion. Vaginal lacerations and/or bruises and twisting bone fractures are particularly indicative of abuse. Signs of neglect are more frequent than those of physical abuse. Determining whether or not the neglect is intentional is the key to planning a nursing course of action.

Whenever a dependent elderly person is being cared for by another, their interaction will give important clues about the relationship. Flinching or shrinking away by the elder or rough physical treatment accompanied by

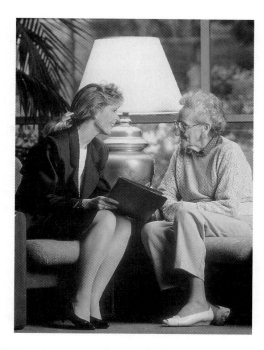

Fig. 37-5   A nurse and an elderly person establishing a trusting relationship.
From Index Stock Photography and Lonnie Duke.

verbal denigration by the caretaker are possible indicators of abuse. As with all types of family violence, the nurse needs to analyze the data from the history, physical examination, and direct observations to make an assessment of abuse. The decision to report is difficult, especially if it appears likely that the outcome will be a nursing home placement unwanted by the elder. However, most states have laws that mandate nurses to report suspected elder abuse.

You are providing home care services to an elderly person who shows evidence of physical abuse. The patient's caregiver handles her roughly and is impatient with her. The patient denies that she is unhappy or abused. Describe your response to this situation. What is your obligation to report your suspicions?

Nursing Interventions. When the nurse must report elder abuse, it is usually less damaging to the therapeutic relationship to inform the family first. Deciding whether to discuss reporting beforehand will be influenced by the likelihood of the abusing family member disappearing and the severity of the abuse. If the abuse is less severe or mainly a neglectful or caretaker stress situation, discussing the intent to report first will make the action seem less a condemnation, allow protective services to be perceived as a helping agency rather than a punitive one, and enhance the possibilities that the nurse will be seen as a continuing source of help. Respite care or other stress relievers may be the key interventions for an overburdened caretaker situation.

In other cases the primary intervention may be therapeutic assistance for the abusers. This may include counseling, therapy for mental disorders, or substance abuse treatment. The success of various interventions for elder abuse is not yet known, since research into this issue is scant. However, one should assume that the treatment will need to involve specific components aimed at the violence as well as at whatever other problems are involved.

RAPE AND SEXUAL ASSAULT

Rape and sexual assault are concerns for individuals, families, and the community. Sexual assaults against women and children (the most prevalent survivors) result in physical trauma, psychic and spiritual disruptions, and deterioration of social relationships. In addition, fear of rape and sexual assault has major effects on women as they restrict their activities in attempts to ensure their safety. Survivors of sexual assaults include women and men of all ages, social classes, races, and occupations. Sexual assault disrupts every aspect of the survivor's life, including social activities, interpersonal relationships, employment, and career. Although males may be sexually assaulted and women sexual offenders,

in this section the survivor is referred to as "she" and the offender as "he." It must be recognized, however, that men and young boys are also victimized and that assessment must not be limited to women.

> How would you respond to a roommate who returned from a date tearful and saying that her boyfriend forced her to have sex even though she refused? Would it make any difference if she had been sexually active with him in the past? Why or why not?

Definition of Sexual Assault

Sexual assault is generally defined as forced perpetration of an act of sexual contact with another person without consent. Lack of consent could be related to the victim's cognitive or personality development, feelings of fear or coercion, or the offender's physical or verbal threats. Most authors agree that sexual assault is not a sexual act but is instead motivated by a desire to humiliate, defile, and dominate the victim. Sexual assault has occurred for centuries but is now recognized as a social and public health problem.

Consent can be conceptualized as a continuum, as seen in Box 37-1. This continuum demonstrates degrees of coercion, including bribery, taking advantage of one's position of power or trust in a relationship, or the victim's inability to consent freely.

Box 37-1

SEXUAL BEHAVIOR: THE FORCE CONTINUUM

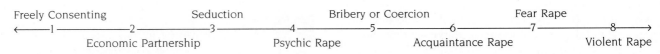

Freely Consenting   Seduction   Bribery or Coercion   Fear Rape

←——1——————2——————3——————4——————5——————6——————7——————8——→

Economic Partnership   Psychic Rape   Acquaintance Rape   Violent Rape

1. **Freely consenting.** Partners with equal power mutually choosing sexual activity. Equal power means each partner has equal status, knowledge, and ability to consent. This includes one partner agreeing to engage in sexual activity, even if not interested, as an expression of love and caring for the other person.
2. **Economic partnership.** One person agrees to sexual activity as part of an economic agreement. The types of sexual behavior permitted are mutually determined as part of the economic agreement.
3. **Seduction.** One party attempts to persuade the other to engage in sexual activities.
4. **Psychic rape.** Assault to another person's dignity and self-respect, such as verbal abuse, street harassment, or the portrayal of violence or pornography in the media.

5. **Bribery or coercion.** The use of emotional or psychological force to persuade the other to take part in sexual activities. This includes situations of unequal power between the individuals, especially when one person is in a position of authority.
6. **Acquaintance rape.** Sexual assault occurring when one party abuses the trust of a relationship and forces the other into sexual activities.
7. **Fear rape.** When one party engages in sexual activities out of fear of potential violence if she resists.
8. **Violent rape.** When violence is threatened or occurs. This includes forced sexual activity between spouses, acquaintances, or strangers.

Marital Rape

It is important to recognize that most cases of sexual assault do not occur between strangers. Marital rape has recently been recognized in most states. Child sexual abuse by family members, family friends, and caretakers is being reported in record numbers.

Marital rape is frequently reported concurrently with physical abuse. Campbell[9] found that the husbands of most of the abused women in her study believed it was their right to have sex whenever they wanted. This included when the women were ill, had recently given birth, or were discharged from a hospital. These women described forced vaginal intercourse, anal intercourse, being hit, burned, or kicked during sex, having objects inserted into their vagina and anus, or being forced to perform sexual acts with animals or while their children were observing. Many women were threatened with weapons or beaten when they refused to take part in these activities. Marital rape may be especially devastating for the survivor. She often must continue to interact with the rapist because of her dependence on him. In addition, many survivors do not seek health care or the support of family members or friends because of embarrassment or humiliation.

Rape and sexual assault are important issues for nursing because nurses treat people in the hospital and the community. Several aspects of nursing practice place nurses at an increased risk for sexual assault by strangers: hours of employment, home visiting in the community, and for some a reluctance to create a scene or defend themselves aggressively. Recently, nurses who were sexually assaulted in hospital parking lots or on hospital property have successfully sued the hospital for negligence in not providing adequate security.[45]

Nursing Care of the Sexual Assault Survivor

Nursing Assessment. The initial assessment is an important phase of the treatment of rape and sexual assault victims. Although most nurses would quickly recognize the woman brought to the emergency department by the police following an attack by a stranger, many survivors of sexual assault are not so easily identified. Therefore all nursing assessments need to include questions to determine current or past sexual abuse. Since people have different definitions of rape, the assessment question needs to be broadly stated, such as that suggested by Russell[11]: "Has anyone ever forced you into sex that you did not wish to participate in?" This question may uncover other types of sexual trauma, such as incest, date rape, or sexual abuse as a child. When the answer is affirmative, it can be gently followed with broad questions, such as "Can you tell me more about it?" or "How often has it happened?" Often the response may be hesitant, questioning, or an embarrassed laugh. When this occurs, the nurse can increase the patient's comfort by explaining that the question is routine because sexual assault is not uncommon. The nurse can offer assistance in obtaining legal or social services.

Nursing Interventions. When it is assessed that abuse has occurred, it cannot be ignored. Disclosing sexual abuse is an indication of trust. If nurses immediately refer the patient elsewhere, they communicate that the problem is too distasteful or delicate to handle or that there are serious psychological implications. Therefore assessment requires an immediate response of nonjudgmental listening and psychological support. In addition, if a recent attack is disclosed, physical evidence will be needed. Evidence collection is an appropriate nursing responsibility. Later interventions may include referrals to survivors' groups, shelters for battered women (in instances of marital rape), or legal services.

People respond to sexual assault differently depending on their past experiences, personal characteristics, and the amount and type of support received from significant others, health-care providers, and the criminal justice system. Burgess[5] describes a two-phase reaction to sexual assault. The acute stage, immediately following the attack, is characterized by extreme confusion, fear, disorganization, and restlessness. Some survivors, however, may mask these feelings and appear to be outwardly calm or subdued.

The second phase involves the long-term process of reorganization. It generally begins several weeks following the attack. This phase may include intrusive memories of the traumatic event during the day and while asleep; fears; or phobias such as extreme fears of being alone, in a crowd, or traveling. The survivor frequently has a sense of living in a dangerous, unpredictable world and may become preoccupied with feelings of victimization and vulnerability. She may encounter difficulties in sexual relationships or her ability to relate comfortably to men. Some survivors develop secondary phobic reactions to people or situations that remind them of the attack.

> How do you think the woman's movement and feminist thinking have influenced society's views on family violence? On rape and sexual assault?

Coping strategies may include changing one's phone number or residence, talking with friends or family, or taking classes in self-defense. Nursing actions to assist the survivor of sexual assault include active listening, empathetic responses, active concern and caring, assistance in problem solving, and referral to sexual assault crisis centers. A sample Nursing Care Plan for the victim of sexual assault is presented below.

SUGGESTED CROSS-REFERENCES

SUMMARY

1. Family violence refers to a range of behaviors occurring between family members and includes physical and emotional abuse of children, child neglect, spouse battering, marital rape, and elder abuse.

2. Violence and abuse are believed to be caused by an interaction of personality, demographic, situational, and societal factors.

3. Characteristics of violent families include multigenerational transmission, social isolation, abuse of power, and substance abuse.

4. Many nurses have a negative response to survivors of violence. It is important to identify and overcome these attitudes.

NURSING CARE PLAN SUMMARY
Survivors of Abuse and Violence

Nursing Diagnosis: Rape Trauma Syndrome

Expected Outcome: The patient will resume one's usual life-style and social relationships.

Short-term Goals	Nursing Interventions	Rationale
The patient will express feelings related to the assault, including guilt, fear, and vulnerability.	Allow patient to discuss feelings regarding assault Communicate knowledge and understanding of emotional responses to sexual assault to assist in identification of feelings Provide anticipatory guidance regarding common physical, psychological, and social responses	Women often experience various feelings including guilt, shame, anger, and embarrassment. It is necessary to identify and express these feelings to develop coping skills. Knowing what to expect reassures the patient that her reactions are normal and can be managed.
The patient will identify supportive people to assist in dealing with this crisis.	Explore relationships with significant others Encourage the patient to discuss the situation with trusted and supportive people.	According to the principles of crisis intervention, it is important for the person in crisis to identify and use a social support system.
The patient will seek medical care for physical problems related to the assault.	Advise patient of the potential for sexually transmitted diseases or pregnancy Assist in identifying a medical care provider Offer to accompany to the medical examination	Early identification of physical problems provides the patient with the maximum number of treatment choices. Many women relive the assault during a gynecological examination. Support from a trusted person can be helpful
The patient will be actively involved in mobilizing support systems.	Support decision making and active problem solving Provide written information about community services and encourage use of them Plan for a follow-up phone contact within a few days	Active involvement in seeking resources gives the patient a sense of control over life, counteracting the helplessness related to the assault.

5. Physical responses to battering are described including a characteristic pattern of injuries and the occurrence of a variety of stress-related symptoms.
6. Behavioral responses to battering are explained including reluctance to leave the violent situation.
7. Psychological responses to violence are described including attributions, problem-solving techniques, and depression.

8. Nursing actions related to violence prevention are discussed.
9. Nursing interventions related to abuse of specific populations including children, wives, and the elderly are presented.
10. Common reactions and the nursing care of survivors of sexual assault are discussed.

COMPETENT CARING
A CLINICAL EXEMPLAR OF A PSYCHIATRIC NURSE

Pat Engdahl, RN, C

When thinking about how I made a difference in a patient's life, I remembered an experience I had with a young woman just over 30 years of age who was admitted in a state of extreme panic, hardly able to process a simple request such as "I need you to please move away from the door." She told me this later, saying her first memories of being on our floor included a voice saying the above words "in the kindest, firmest, most caring tones" she had ever heard—and she felt safe. She said she didn't want to move away from the locked door, but she did it anyway and she said, "I think it was your voice."

We worked very hard together, this patient and myself. She was a victim of childhood sexual and physical abuse and, as often happens, married to a man who also abused her. She talked; I listened. She said she had shed enough tears and wasn't going to cry anymore. I replied she needed to "cry a river" for the therapeutic process to begin. We role-played. We practiced handling verbal abuse and daring to express anger—the latter frightened her more than the former. But she was not able to deal with issues related to her abusive husband and her angry feelings of victimization in the marriage.

The night before her discharge she began to discuss these feelings, as they had suddenly risen to the surface during a group meeting. In this meeting a male patient had boasted that he never struck his wife except when he was drunk, and then he "only slapped her around a few times, not enough to send her to the hospital or such—nothing like that." When my patient heard this, she got up in a rage and ran out of the group. It was several hours later during our one-on-one when she was finally able to discuss the episode. She berated herself for being "gutless" and not being able to say something right then. She paced and questioned whether she "really was ready to go home" and maybe she "wasn't as strong as she thought."

We continued exploring her feelings of childhood helplessness. She talked until her rage was spent, but did not seem to reach closure in her thoughts or feelings. She was discharged the next morning before I came to work for my evening shift. However, in my mailbox, I found a powerful note in which, among other things, she simply wrote, "I was able to confront that male patient in group today. . . . I guess I was ready for discharge after all. Thanks." It was now my turn to become a little emotional as my eyes filled with tears and I whispered, "you're welcome, you'll never know how welcome." ▼

REFERENCES

1. American Psychiatric Association: *Diagnostic and statistical manual for mental disorders*, ed 4, Washington, DC, 1994, The Association.
2. Brendtro M, Bowker HL: Battered women: how can nurses help, *Issues Ment Health Nurs* 10:169, 1989.
3. Briere J, Runtz M: The trauma symptom checklist (TSC-33) early data on a new scale, *J Interpersonal Violence* 4:151, 1989.
4. Browne A: *When battered women kill*, New York, 1987, The Free Press.
5. Burgess A: Rape trauma syndrome: a nursing diagnosis, *Occup Health Nurs* 33:405, 1985.
6. Burgess AW et al: Child molestation: assessing impact in multiple victims, *Arch Psychiatr Nurs* 1:33, 1987.
7. Campbell JC: Misogyny and homicide of women, *Adv Nurs Sci* 3:67, 1981.
8. Campbell JC: Nursing assessment for risk of homicide with battered women, *Adv Nurs Sci* 8:36, 1986.
9. Campbell JC: A test of two explanatory models of women's responses to battering, *Nurs Res* 38:18, 1989.
10. Campbell JC: Ways of teaching, learning, and knowing about violence against women, *Nurs Health Care* 13:464, 1992.
11. Campbell JC, Humphreys JC: *Nursing care of survivors of family violence*, St Louis, 1993, Mosby.
12. Campbell JC, Sheridan D: Emergency nursing interventions and battered women, *J Emerg Nurs* 15:12, 1989.
13. Cannon C: Violent verdict: connecting TV and real-life aggression, *The Washington Post*, p D5, 1989.
14. Conte JR, Scheurman JR: The effects of sexual abuse on children, *J Interpersonal Violence* 2:380, 1988.
15. Damrosch S et al: Nurses' attributions about rape victims, *Res Nurs Health* 10:245, 1987.
16. DiPietro SB: The effects of intrafamilial child sexual abuse on the adjustment and attitudes of adolescents, *Violence Vict* 2:59, 1987.
17. Dobash RE, Dobash RP: Research as social action: the struggle for battered women. In Yllo K, Bograd M, eds: *Feminist perspectives on wife abuse*, Newbury Park, Calif, 1988, Sage.
18. Dutton DG: *The domestic assault of women*, Newton, Mass, 1988, Allyn & Bacon.
19. Faller KC: The myth of the "collusive mother," *J Interpersonal Violence* 3:190, 1988.
20. Feinauer L: Comparison of long-term effects on child abuse by type of abuse and by relationship of the offender to the victim, *Am J Fam Ther* 17:48, 1989.
21. Finkelhor D, Pillemer K: The prevalence of elder abuse: a random sample survey, *Gerontol Soc Am* 28:51, 1988.
22. Gilligan C: *In a different voice*, Cambridge, Mass, 1982, Harvard University Press.
23. Gondolf EW: The effect of batterer counseling on shelter outcome, *J Interpersonal Violence* 3:275, 1988.
24. Hart B: Beyond the "duty to warn": a therapist's "duty to protect" battered women and children. In Yllo K, Bograd M, eds: *Feminist perspectives on wife abuse*, Newbury Park, Calif, 1988, Sage.
25. Hedin BA: A case study of oppressed group behavior in nurses, *Image* 18:53, 1986.

26. Hotaling GT, Straus M: *The social causes of husband-wife violence*, Minneapolis, 1980, University of Minnesota Press.
27. Hotaling GT, Sugerman D: An analysis of risk markers in husband to wife violence: the current state of knowledge, *Violence Vict* 1:101, 1986.
28. Humphreys JC: Children of battered women: worries about their mothers, *Pediatr Nurs* 17:342, 1991.
29. Jehu D: Mood disturbances among women clients sexually abused in childhood, *J Interpersonal Violence* 4:164, 1989.
30. Kelly L: How women define their experiences of violence. In Yllo K, Bograd M, eds: *Feminist perspectives on wife abuse*, Newbury Park, Calif, 1988, Sage.
31. King MC, Ryan J: Abused women: dispelling myths and encouraging interventions, *Nurse Pract* 14:47, 1989.
32. Kurz D: Emergency department responses to battered women: resistance to medicalization, *Soc Problems* 34:501, 1987.
33. Landenburger K: Conflicting realities of women in abusive relationships, *Commun Nurs Res* 21:15, 1988.
34. Landenburger K: A process of entrapment in and recovery from an abusive relationship, *Issues Ment Health Nurs* 10:209, 1989.
35. Launius MH, Jensen BL: Interpersonal problem-solving skills in battered counseling and control women, *J Fam Violence* 2:151, 1987.
36. Leonard K, Jacob T: Alcohol, alcoholism, and family violence. In Van Hasselt VB et al, eds: *Handbook of family violence*, New York, 1988, Plenum.
37. Lerner JM, Simmons CH: Observer's reaction to the "innocent victim," *J Pers Soc Psychol* 4:203, 1966.
38. Mackey T et al: Factors associated with long-term depressive symptoms of sexual assault victims, *Arch Psychiatr Nurs* 6:10, 1992.
39. Morris PA, Bihan SM: The prevalence of children with a history of sexual abuse hospitalized in the psychiatric setting, *J Child Psychiatr Nurs* 4:49, 1991.
40. Newbern V: Sexual victimization of children and adolescent patients, *Image* 21:10, 1989.
41. Parker B, Schumacher D: The battered wife syndrome and violence in the nuclear family of origin: a controlled pilot study, *Am J Public Health* 67:760, 1977.
42. Parker B et al: Physical and emotional abuse in pregnancy: a comparison of adult and teenaged women, *Nurs Res* 42:173, 1993.
43. Pillemer K: Social isolation and elder abuse, *Response Victimization Women Children* 8:1, 1985.
44. Pillemer K, Suitor J: Elder abuse. In Van Hasselt VB et al, eds: *Handbook of family violence*, New York, 1988, Plenum.
45. Regan W: Rape on hospital property: now you can sue, *RN* 69:70, 1983.
46. Rew L: Long-term effects of childhood sexual exploitation, *Issues Ment Health Nurs* 10:229, 244, 1989.
47. Ryan W: *Blaming the victim*, New York, 1976, Vintage.
48. Schur EM: *The politics of deviance: stigma contests and the uses of power*, Englewood Cliffs, NJ, 1986, Prentice Hall.
49. Sommers EK, Check JVP: An empirical investigation of the role of pornography in the verbal and physical abuse of women, *Violence Vict* 2:189, 1987.
50. Stark E, Flitcraft A: Violence among intimates: An epidemiological review. In Van Hasselt VB et al, eds: *Handbook of family violence*, New York, 1988, Plenum.

51. Straus MA, Gelles RJ: Societal change and change in family violence from 1975 to 1985 as revealed by two national surveys, J Marriage Fam 45:465, 1986.

52. Walker LE: The battered women syndrome, New York, 1984, Springer.

53. Walsh D, Liddy R: Surviving sexual abuse, Dublin, 1989, Attic Press.

54. Yllo K, Bograd M, eds: Feminist perspectives on wife abuse, Newbury Park, Calif, 1988, Sage.

ANNOTATED SUGGESTED READINGS

*Campbell JC: A survivor group for battered women, Adv Nurs Sci 8:13, 1987.

Describes nurse-facilitated group intervention focusing on the importance of control, body image, alternatives to end the violence, and decision making about ending the relationship.

*Campbell JC, Alford P: The dark side of marital rape, Am J Nurs 89:946-949, 1989.

Documents the serious physical effects of marital rape.

*Campbell JC, Humphreys J: Nursing care of survivors of family violence, St Louis, 1993, Mosby.

The only nursing text totally concerned with family violence, this book presents theory, research, and nursing care for child abuse, wife abuse, sexual assault, and elder abuse.

*Corman BJ: Group treatment for female adolescent sexual abuse victims, Issues Mental Health Nurs 10:261, 1989.

Describes the dynamics of traumatic sexualization, betrayal, powerlessness, and stigmatization and group intervention strategies for each.

Counts D, Brown J, Campbell J: Sanctions and sanctuary: cultural perspectives on the beating of wives, Boulder, Colo, 1992, Westview Press.

An ethnographic description of the range and diversity of wife beating around the world. Describes societies with frequent, infrequent, and no battering of women and places wife battering in the economic, political, and social context in which it occurs.

*Damrosch S et al: Nurses' attributions about rape victims, Res Nurs Health 10:245, 1987.

Discusses the feelings of registered nurses who were given one of four written accounts of a woman's rape while she was driving to a drugstore.

Draucker C: Counselling survivors of childhood sexual abuse, Newbury Park, Calif, 1992, Sage.

Describes counselling techniques for adults in therapy who disclose sexual abuse as children. A detailed case study is included.

*Glod C: Long-term consequences of childhood physical and sexual abuse, Arch Psychiatr Nurs 7:163, 1993.

Superb review of state-of-the-art knowledge of the long-term sequelae of childhood physical and sexual abuse. Critically reviews the initial uncontrolled investigations and mounting evidence from controlled studies.

Gondolf E, Fisher E: Battered women as survivors, Lexington, Mass, 1988, Heath & Co.

Based on research with over 6000 survivors of abuse in Texas. Challenges current assumptions regarding abused women as helpless and passive. Describes help-seeking strategies employed by the survivors, a typology of abusers, and policy implications.

*Houck GM, King MC: Child maltreatment: family characteristics and developmental consequences, Issues Ment Health Nurs 10:193, 1989.

Presents a comprehensive research review of the cognitive, social, and emotional outcomes for children who have been abused and neglected.

NiCarthy G, Davidson S: You can be free, Seattle, 1989, Seal Press.

This book is written in an easy to read format, designed for women with limited reading skills. The chapters offer advice on identifying abuse, making decisions, and finding helpful assistance from the legal, medical, and judicial systems.

*Parker B et al: Physical and emotional abuse in pregnancy: a comparison of adult and teenage women, Nurs Res 42:173, 1993.

A sample of 691 African-American, Hispanic, and white pregnant teen and adult women were interviewed in the prenatal setting. Women were assessed on their first prenatal visit, and 26% reported physical or sexual abuse within the past year.

*Phillips L: Abuse and neglect of the frail elderly at home: an exploration of theoretical relationships, J Adv Nurs 8:379, 1983.

Explores the correlates of elder abuse, such as economic strains, social isolation, and environmental problems.

Walsh D, Liddy R: Surviving sexual abuse, Dublin, 1989, Attic Press.

For survivors of childhood sexual abuse. Includes a summary of the types of assaults, common responses of survivors, strategies for long-term healing and recovery and case studies and vignettes.

White E: Chain, chain, change: for black women dealing with physical and emotional abuse, Seattle, 1985, Seal Press.

Covers topics such as the psychology of abuse, effects of violence on the children, and dealing with the legal, police, and medical systems from the perspective of black women.

---

*Nursing reference.

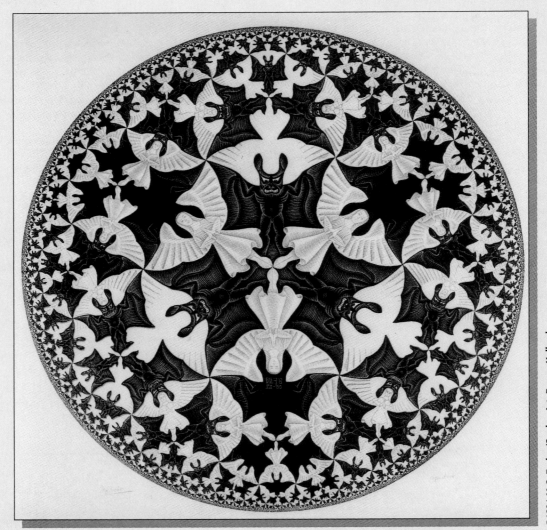

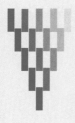

CHAPTER 38
Psychological Care of the Patient with HIV/AIDS

PAULA C. LASALLE
ARTHUR J. LASALLE

While we were fearing it, it came,
But came with less of fear
Because that fearing it so long
Had almost made it fair.
There is a fitting—dismay;
A fitting—a despair.
'Tis harder knowing it is due
Than knowing it is here.
The trying on the utmost,
The morning it is new,
Is terribler than wearing it
A whole existence through.

Emily Dickinson: *While we were fearing it, it came*

LEARNING OBJECTIVES

After studying this chapter the student should be able to:
▼ Describe the characteristics of HIV disease
▼ Discuss ways to decrease the risk of contracting HIV infection
▼ Identify behaviors associated with HIV disease
▼ Formulate nursing diagnoses for patients related to HIV disease
▼ Discuss multidisciplinary planning related to the needs of the patient who has HIV disease
▼ Analyze nursing interventions for patients related to HIV disease
▼ Evaluate nursing care for patients related to HIV disease

TOPICAL OUTLINE

Characteristics of HIV
Assessing the Patient with HIV Disease
   Psychological Behaviors
   Behaviors Related to Depression
   Behaviors Related to Dementia
   Social Behaviors
Planning and Implementing Care
   Case Management
   Interventions Related to Risk Reduction
   Interventions Related to Changing Levels of Functioning
   Interventions Related to Changes in Body Image
   Interventions Related to AIDS Dementia Complex
   Interventions Related to Preparation for Death
   Interventions Related to Significant Others
   Response of the Nurse to the Person with HIV Disease
Psychiatric Consultation Liaison Nursing
Evaluating Care of the Patient with HIV Disease

HIV *Disease* is the term used to describe all of the disorders resulting from infection with the human immunodeficiency virus. It includes acquired immunodeficiency syndrome (AIDS) and its associated opportunistic infections. It involves the physical, psychological, emotional, and social aspects of the patient. The psychosocial aspects of this disease are varied and complex and relate directly to the patient's health care. Knowledgeable and compassionate nurses have an opportunity to contribute greatly to the HIV patient's quality of life.

HIV disease has become a leading killer of young adults in the United States. What started as a disease predominantly affecting homosexual men has now spread to other populations including heterosexual men and women, intravenous drug users, children, and hemophiliacs. The HIV virus is transmitted through direct exposure to infected blood, blood derivatives, and other body fluids. It is transmitted through various sexual behaviors with infected persons, use of HIV-contaminated intravenous needles, transfusion of infected blood or blood derivatives, and from infected mother to fetus.

CHARACTERISTICS OF HIV

The Centers for Disease Control and Prevention (CDC)[3] defines HIV as a retrovirus that has as its primary target the CD4+T-lymphocyte because of the affinity of the virus for the CD4 surface marker.

The CD4+T-lymphocyte coordinates a number of important immunologic functions and a loss of these functions results in progressive impairment of the immune response. Studies have documented a wide spectrum of disease manifestations, ranging from asymptomatic infection to life-threatening conditions characterized by severe immunodeficiency, serious opportunistic infections, and cancers.[4]

Opportunistic infections, such as toxoplasmosis and *Pneumocystis carinii* pneumonia are common. Infections can develop in the central nervous system and cause dementia. In other cases, depression related to the diagnosis of HIV may erode immunological functioning and decrease the patient's motivation to engage in health-promoting behaviors.

In the spring of 1993 the World Health Organization's (WHO) Global Programme on AIDS[3] estimated that approximately 2.5 million people now have AIDS, and an additional 14 million people are infected with HIV disease. WHO estimates that during this decade mothers or both parents of more than 10 million children will have died of HIV infection. As of September 1993 the CDC reported a cumulative total of 339,250 Americans diagnosed with AIDS. AIDS cases in women increased 17% between 1990 and 1991, and 4% in men during the

same period. One out of every four AIDS cases now being diagnosed is a young person who became infected with HIV as a teenager. Additional 1993 figures on the incidence of AIDS are presented in Box 38-1.

> Have you known someone with HIV disease? What were your feelings about that person? Did you worry about becoming infected? Have your feelings changed since entering your nursing program?

ASSESSING THE PATIENT WITH HIV DISEASE

Table 38-1 lists the major domains of patient needs that are related to the health care of people who have HIV disease.[1] Because their lives are affected in so many ways, assessment of each of these areas is an important aspect of nursing care planning. For example, a person's financial, transportation, and housing needs may directly relate to one's ability to participate in treatment.

Psychological Behaviors

HIV disease presents the patient and loved ones with a series of stressors, sometimes occurring simultaneously, sometimes sequentially. Nurses need to pay special attention to the psychosocial needs of HIV patients because these stressors may directly affect the patient's health and the patient's willingness and ability to fully utilize the health-care system. Flaskerud[9] has identified factors to be addressed in the psychosocial nursing assessment of patients with HIV (Table 38-2).

Box 38-1

INCIDENCE OF AIDS IN THE UNITED STATES (AS OF SEPTEMBER 1993)

Number of AIDS cases reported to CDC	339,250
Number of AIDS cases in males	293,642
Number of AIDS cases in females	40,702
Number of AIDS cases in children (under 13)	4906
Number of cases in men who have had sex with men	183,344
Number of cases in intravenous drug users	80,713
Number of cases in hemophiliacs	2963

From United States Centers for Disease Control and Prevention, 1993, Atlanta, US Department of Health and Human Services.

Table 38-1 Major Domains of Health-Care Needs of People Who Have HIV Disease

Domain	Subdomain
Environmental	Finances
	Housing
Psychosocial	Community networking
	Family system
	Emotional response
	Individual growth and development
Physiological	Sensory function
	Respiratory and circulatory function
	Neuromusculoskeletal function
	Reproductive function
	Digestion/elimination
	Structural integrity
Health behaviors	Nutrition
	Personal habits
	Health management

Modified from Berk RA, Poe SS, Baigis-Smith JA: *J Assoc Nurse* AIDS *Care* 3:10, 1992.

Table 38-2 Psychosocial Assessment Factors Related to HIV Disease

Assessment factors	Characteristics
Psychosocial history	Identifies vulnerabilities and strengths; important to note past psychiatric disorders and substance abuse
Current distress and crisis	Includes assessment of depression, fear, anxiety, anger, and behavioral disorganization
Past and current coping	Identifies usual coping mechanisms and coping resources
Social support needed and available	Compares current social support systems with anticipated needs related to illness
Life cycle phase	Considers developmental stage, goals, social roles, personal resources, and skills
Illness phase	Includes pretesting and posttesting, postdiagnosis, infection without symptoms, symptomatic related to specific concurrent disorders, and terminal
Individual identity	Includes self-esteem, role definition, and life plans
Experience with loss and grief	Particular emphasis on past experience with terminal illness and involvement with others who have died of HIV disease

From Flaskerud JH: AIDS/HIV *infection: a reference guide for nursing professionals*, Philadelphia, 1989, WB Saunders.

Stigma. Some of the psychosocial problems associated with HIV disease are a result of stigma. HIV stigma is closely connected to the risk behaviors that lead to infection. The illness was first identified in homosexual men, a stigmatized group. Later, it became prevalent in intravenous drug users, another stigmatized population. Because of these risk behaviors, assumptions are often made about the life-styles of people with HIV disease. Some believe they are immoral and that the illness is a punishment for their behavior. Stigma may inhibit individuals from seeking HIV testing. It also fosters reluctance to inform others of their diagnosis and to adopt risk-reduction behaviors. It is reflected in the difficulty people with HIV disease face in keeping their jobs, getting insurance, finding housing, and acquiring health care. Stigma is very difficult to overcome, but the best way to confront it is through health education. Nurses can also model nonstigmatizing attitudes by providing sensitive and competent care to people with HIV disease.

Field[7] believes that stigma contributes to the development of "AIDS phobia," a condition in which people who are not infected fear acquiring HIV and worry about it constantly. Some even become convinced they have AIDS to the extent of developing a somatoform disorder or a somatic delusion.

Identify a situation in which you noticed stigmatizing behavior toward people with HIV disease. What did you do (or could you have done) to change this behavior?

Crisis Points and Emotional Response. Several potential crisis points occur during the course of HIV disease.[9] The diagnosis of HIV seropositivity may be the first crisis. However, the patient may already have had a crisis based on anticipation of the potential diagnosis. With the initial diagnosis the person frequently feels intense anxiety, fear, anger, guilt and may have impulsive behavior. High levels of anxiety and depression may continue for 2 to 3 months and may be exhibited in agitation, risky sexual behavior, crying, and suicidal ideation and attempts. The patient should not be left alone nor expected to make decisions immediately after learning the diagnosis. Safety precautions and taking the necessary time to allow the person to process the initial reaction are critical. The nurse should share information regarding HIV disease when the patient requests it. Assisting the patient to recognize and verbalize beliefs regarding HIV may be helpful.

McCain and Gramling[17] refer to this phase of coping with HIV disease as "living with dying." The person is learning to live with the knowledge of having a terminal illness. It is essential that structure be provided during this time by implementing crisis intervention techniques (see Chapter 12). Medications may be indicated, but safety must be considered. Medications are not a means of suppressing the natural reactions to crisis but enable the person to function, to sleep, and to cope during the crisis. The following clinical example highlights some of the issues around notification of the HIV diagnosis.

CLINICAL EXAMPLE

Mr. and Ms. G are a prominent couple in the community. Mr. G was hospitalized for a severe case of herpes zoster (shingles). With his informed consent he was tested for HIV and was found to be positive. Mr. G is fearful of his wife's reaction to his diagnosis. They have been married for 24 years. He had one incident of homosexual marital infidelity 3 years ago while on a business trip. He is angry over the "unfairness" of how one experience will alter not only his health but also the state of his relationship with his wife. He is also worried that his children will reject him and his employer will fire him. Another concern is that his high public profile will lead to unwanted negative publicity for him, his family, and the community organizations in which he has been active.

Selected Nursing Diagnoses:

▼ Anxiety related to diagnosis of AIDS as evidenced by verbalized concerns about impact of the diagnosis on relationships

▼ Altered family processes related to changed role of husband and father as evidenced by concern over reactions of wife and children

▼ Altered role performance related to change in health status as evidenced by concern that job and community activities will be affected

There may be a quiet phase between the initial diagnosis and the first opportunistic infection. During this transition period the patient moves into the phase of coping identified by McCain and Gramling[17] as "fighting the sickness." There is a focus on learning about HIV disease and often the adoption of a healthier life-style including attention to diet, exercise, and adequate rest. Attempts to cope may include denial of the illness. However, when the first infection occurs, a crisis that is more intense than the first may be precipitated. Denial is no longer effective. The treatment phase may be char-

acterized by alienation, depression, and discouragement. Patients may fear or experience disfigurement, pain, and loss of health. The process of treatment with medical side effects, testing, and awaiting results may cause self-absorption, frustration, and irritability. HIV patients may experience a loss of control especially in dealing with the medical system. They may become fearful, demanding, and dependent on health-care providers. As treatment continues, they may be frightened to be away from the close supervision of the hospital staff or health-care provider. They may become hypervigilant and seek reassurance that they will know when to ask for help.

Finally the person enters the phase of coping called "getting worn-out."[17] During this phase of preparation for death, there is a gradual decline and deterioration of the person's functional ability. Recurrence and relapse are accompanied by feelings of depression, dependency, isolation, suicidal ideation, and fear of abandonment. There is usually ambivalence, dependence, and withdrawal from the world combined with increased self-absorption. Patients often review their lives. They may finalize their wishes related to their death and postmortem arrangements. Support and physical assistance must be given because important decisions regarding the last phases of life are being made and important goodbyes are shared.

The person who is living with HIV disease often experiences conflict about the implications of the illness. These have been identified by Flaskerud[8] and are summarized in Table 38-3. Concerns related to the person's life-style are illustrated in the next clinical example.

Table 38-3 Internal Conflicts and Emotional Responses Related to HIV Disease

Internal Conflicts	Emotional Responses
Concerns about transmission	Sadness, anxiety, fear, anger, suspicion, guilt
▼ Blaming self or others for own infection	
▼ Concern for those one has placed at risk	
Protection from opportunistic infections	Anger, suspicion, guilt, loneliness, withdrawal
▼ Fear of others who may carry infections	
Life-style issues	Internalization of cultural disapproval resulting in self-hate or blame
▼ Sexual behavior	
▼ Intravenous drug use	
Concerns about intimate relationships	Fear of abandonment and isolation

Adapted from Flaskerud JH: *AIDS/HIV infection: a reference guide for nursing professionals*, Philadelphia, 1989, WB Saunders.

CLINICAL EXAMPLE

Mr. J was diagnosed as HIV positive 4 years ago and has been asymptomatic. On his forty-fifth birthday, he noticed a Kaposi's sarcoma spot on his cheek and is now in a state of panic. He has not told anyone about his discovery. His parents are scheduled to arrive on the next day to celebrate his birthday. They are not aware that he is HIV positive nor that he is homosexual. He knows his mother will question him about the spot. His father is vehemently antihomosexual, consistent with his religious beliefs. Mr. J is uncertain and anxious about how his father would accept this information. Mr. J's lover, however, is pressuring him to tell his parents so that their relationship can be open.

Selected Nursing Diagnoses:
▼ Anxiety related to parental response to sexual preference as evidenced by secrecy about his homosexuality
▼ Body image disturbance related to discovery of facial lesion as evidenced by not telling anyone
▼ Situational low self-esteem related to guilt about sexual preference as evidenced by hiding relationship with lover

Behaviors Related to Depression

Depression related to HIV disease is a psychological response to the diagnosis and prognosis. Marzuk et al.[16] reported that the suicide rate for men with HIV disease is 66 times that of the general male population. Depression may be a reaction to the multiple losses experienced during the course of the disease. Also, it is often related to feelings of isolation, changes in body image, guilt over sexual or drug-related behavior, and fear of death.[10] Depression is discussed in detail in Chapter 17 and suicide in Chapter 18.

Behaviors Related to Dementia

A major complication of HIV disease is AIDS dementia complex (ADC), which is a subcortical encephalopathy characterized by progressive dementia. Boccellari and Dilley[2] note that it is difficult to identify the incidence of ADC because of a lack of clear guidelines. They cite estimates ranging from 12.8% to 67% of AIDS patients.

Although some opportunistic infections may involve the brain, ADC is believed to result primarily from direct infection with HIV.[20] The virus is believed to be transported to brain tissue by infected monocytes that cross the blood-brain barrier or by infected endothelial cells in the brain capillaries. Once the virus is in brain cells, several disruptions are believed to occur (Table 38-4).

Table 38-4 Possible Brain Disruptions in AIDS Dementia Complex

Disruption	Characteristics
Increased calcium in neurons	HIV envelope protein (gp 120) increases intraneuronal calcium; this is toxic to neurons
Loss of myelin sheath	HIV triggers an autoimmune response either related to shared surface proteins or to infection of oligodendrocytes, which are the cells that produce myelin
Increased tumor necrosis factor-alpha	HIV-infected monocytes in the brain release tumor necrosis factor-alpha as a response to the virus; it causes inflammation and damage to brain tissue

Adapted from Swanson B et al: *Arch Psychiatr Nurs* 7:74, 1993.

The progression of behaviors related to ADC is described in the abbreviated neuropsychiatric AIDS rating scale developed by Boccellari and Dilley (Table 38-5).[2] The equivocal stage is the time during which it is uncertain whether the patient is developing ADC. Mild, moderate, severe, and end stage are all levels of ADC.

Because ADC and depression may both present with apathy and psychomotor retardation, the nurse needs to be able to distinguish between them. Swanson and colleagues[19] state that, unlike demented persons, depressed persons typically appear sadder and express feeling hopeless and worthless. Demented persons have difficulty drawing, whereas the drawing ability of depressed persons is relatively unaffected. Nurses can ask patients to draw simple figures such as squares or triangles to assess whether their behavioral changes are caused by depression or dementia. Depressed persons can also generate a list of words, for example, a list starting with the same letter, without much difficulty. Demented persons are unable to produce more than a few words. Cognitive responses are described in more detail in Chapter 21.

Social Behaviors

A number of social conflicts such as fear of exposure of diagnosis and being a member of a stigmatized group are also commonly experienced by individuals who have HIV disease.[9] Patients often need the nurse's support and assistance in dealing with whom to tell about their status, as well as when and how. Physical changes such as Kaposi's sarcoma, wasting, or rashes may force the

Table 38-5   Abbreviated Neuropsychiatric AIDS Rating Scale

Impairment stage	Orientation	Memory	Motor	Behavioral	Problem solving	Activities of daily living
Normal	Fully oriented	Normal	Normal	Normal	Can solve everyday problems	Fully capable of self-care
Equivocal	Fully oriented	Complains of memory problems	Fully ambulatory; slightly slowed movements	Normal	Slight mental slowing	Slight impairment in business dealings
Mild	Fully oriented but may have brief periods of "spaciness"	Mild memory problems	Balance, coordination, and handwriting difficulties	More irritable, labile; or apathetic and withdrawn	Difficulty planning and completing work	Can do simple daily activities; may need prompting
Moderate	Some disorientation	Memory moderately impaired (new learning)	Ambulatory but may require a cane	Some impulsivity or agitated behavior	Severe impairment; poor social judgment; gets lost easily	Needs assistance
Severe	Frequent disorientation	Severe memory loss; only fragments remain	Ambulatory with assistance	May have an organic psychosis	Judgment very poor	Cannot live independently
End stage	Confused and disoriented	Virtually no memory	Bedridden	Mute and unresponsive	No problem-solving ability	Nearly vegetative

From Boccellari AA, Dilley JW: *Hosp Community Psychiatry* 43:32, 1992.

patient to reveal the illness before feeling prepared to do so.

Conflict regarding sexual activity may leave the person socially isolated and alone if sexual activity is discontinued. This is especially true for persons who used sex to establish interpersonal contacts. Even people in stable relationships may find their sexual relationship dramatically changed, affecting feelings of closeness and the ability to give and receive love, comfort, and affection.

Employment and insurance issues are sources of stress because patients are in the position of being rejected and stigmatized. Although employers are not legally able to fire someone because of HIV, now considered a legally protected disability, subtle means may be used to encourage the person with AIDS to leave the work setting. Allocation of work, reassignment, evaluation, or redefinition of a job may result in a person with AIDS being terminated by an employer. Others have lost positions because of being physically unable to work. Loss of a job there is frequently associated with loss of health insurance.

Social support limitations are common especially in a mobile society in which friends and family are scattered around the world. Persons who have chosen to keep their life-style secret frequently move away from

their family of origin and may or may not have a group in whom they confide. For many people, work colleagues make up a major portion of their social support system. When the job is lost the isolation increases. Resources that can be used to provide social support include community agencies that offer services such as shopping, Meals on Wheels, and housekeeping. Some clergy and churches have become involved in transportation or other services for persons with AIDS. The homosexual community has also organized support services in many areas.

Nurses can assist patients with psychosocial issues if a trusting, confidential relationship is established. At times the boundaries of confidentiality are not clear. See Critical Thinking about Contemporary Issues for a discussion of this issue.

HIV disease and related opportunistic infections involving pathogens such as *Pneumocystis carinii* and *Cryptococcus*, as well as Kaposi's sarcoma, affect multiple body systems. A complete nursing assessment will result in nursing diagnoses related to all of the identified behaviors. Nursing diagnoses related to physiological disruptions are discussed in medical-surgical nursing textbooks. Box 38-2 lists NANDA nursing diagnoses that are particularly associated with the psychosocial aspects of HIV disease.

CRITICAL THINKING ABOUT CONTEMPORARY ISSUES

Should a Person Be Obligated To Reveal HIV Positive Status?

Harding and colleagues[12] cite conflicting opinions in the literature regarding the conditions under which confidentiality about HIV positive status may be breached. The conflict focuses mainly on the duty to warn others who may be in danger of being infected by the patient. For example, a man who is HIV positive informs the nurse that he will not share the information with his wife and he intends to continue having sexual relations with her. The patient claims that he will protect his wife from infection but will not be specific about the method that he plans to use. The nurse is caught between maintaining a confidential relationship with the patient and protecting a third party, while being unsure of the degree of "clear and present" danger to the wife.

A similar conflict exists regarding the responsibility of health-care workers who know that they are HIV positive to inform their patients, supervisors, and co-workers. Since several patients were believed to have been infected by a Florida dentist there has been political pressure to require reporting. Health-care workers fear that revealing HIV disease will result in job loss. They cite evidence that HIV is not transmitted in health-care situations as long as universal precautions are observed.

Since serious consequences exist for the individual related to personal relationships and continued employment, there are no easy answers to this question. The nurse must consider the facts related to each situation and assist the patient to consider all of the alternatives, including the likely consequences. ▼

Do you believe that a person who is HIV positive should engage in sexual activity? What types of sexual expression would you recommend? Do you feel comfortable discussing this with your patients?

PLANNING AND IMPLEMENTING CARE

The complexity of the biopsychosocial needs of the person with HIV disease demands a team approach to

---

> **Box 38-2**
> ## NANDA DIAGNOSES RELATED TO PSYCHOSOCIAL ASPECTS OF HIV DISEASE
>
> Adjustment, impaired
> Anxiety
> Body image disturbance
> Caregiver role strain, high risk for
> Communication, impaired verbal
> Defensive coping
> Denial, ineffective
> Family processes, altered
> Fear
> Grieving, anticipatory
> Grieving, dysfunctional
> Health maintenance, altered
> Hopelessness
> Individual coping, ineffective
> Management of therapeutic regimen (individual), ineffective
> Parental role conflict
> Parenting, high risk for altered
> Powerlessness
> Role performance, altered
> Self-esteem, situational low
> Sexual dysfunction
> Sexuality patterns, altered
> Social interaction, impaired
> Social isolation
> Spiritual distress
> Thought processes, altered

From North American Nursing Diagnosis Association: NANDA *nursing diagnoses: definitions and classifications* 1992-1993, Philadelphia, 1992, The Association.

health-care planning and implementation. The physician prescribes the course of medical treatment, frequently involving prophylactic medication or pharmacotherapy for identified physiological disorders. Occupational or physical therapy may be needed to assist the patient to adjust to changing neuromuscular and cognitive functioning. Social workers assist the patient and significant others to find and contact community resources. Nursing care centers around providing support and counseling while assisting the patient to conserve energy and set priorities for activities. Nurses are also responsible for being sure that the patient is informed about the disease and options related to intervention.

Nurses in AIDS care have opportunities to develop close relationships with patients and their significant others. The reaction to the HIV disease process is unique to each individual. A frequently encountered counseling issue is concern about the course of disease and the length of survival. This is reflected by a commonly asked question when people with HIV disease meet: "How long have you known your diagnosis?" This is a way of determining how far along the other person is in dealing with HIV. Also, there is the underlying hope that the question will identify a long-term survivor, serving as reassurance that a person with HIV disease can live a long and fruitful life.

Case Management

Although many communities are involved in attempts to organize the necessary services for people with HIV disease, services and funds are not coordinated and are often difficult to find. The person who is struggling with the HIV diagnosis has the additional burden of locating needed help. Case management by the nurse, social worker, or other professional is a system that can help to locate available services. The case manager can assist in identifying medical providers, dentists, therapists, housing, and other resources.

Interventions Related to Risk Reduction

Currently the only effective way of combating HIV disease is by preventing it through risk reduction. Because of their credibility with the general public, nurses are in a good position to provide health education related to prevention. Nurses should familiarize themselves with the routes of transmission of HIV and the currently recommended ways of preventing infection. Patients can be encouraged to inform sexual partners of their illness and to practice safe sex. Intravenous drug users can be referred to treatment programs, discouraged from needle-sharing, and taught how to disinfect used needles. Pregnant women who are HIV positive should be assisted to find obstetrical care from a provider who understands the implications of the disease for the mother and infant.

People who have serious and persistent mental illnesses are often vulnerable to infection with HIV. In one study of this population[13] many patients traded sex for money, drugs, or a place to stay; were coerced to engage in unwanted sex; had casual sexual encounters; and engaged in sexual activity after using drugs or intoxicants. These are high-risk activities related to acquiring HIV. Another study[5] of high-risk activities among the seriously mentally ill found the following:

▼ There was no relationship between diagnosis and high-risk activity
▼ Heterosexual behavior was the most common high-risk activity
▼ Younger patients did not have more sexual activity, although they did have more partners

Nurses need to be aware of these findings so that they can provide relevant health education to patients.

Interventions may include self-esteem enhancement, assertiveness training, education about sexuality and HIV prevention, and role playing of potentially risky social situations. Condoms should be readily available to patients in all treatment settings. Graham and Cates[11] describe an educational program to inform group home residents about HIV prevention. They conducted a series of three sessions using a videotape in each, followed by a discussion period. Patients in this study responded best to a same-sex presenter. Patients with psychotic episodes sometimes incorporated the educational material into their delusional thinking. Others who tended to somaticize began to report symptoms of HIV. It was important for group home staff to be well-informed about HIV disease before the training and be prepared to respond to questions and concerns afterwards.

People infected with HIV are often asymptomatic up to 10 years. Testing for the presence of HIV antibodies is is the only way of determining whether a person is infected with the virus. Inferences based on sex, race, socioeconomic status, habits of cleanliness, nutrition, and sexual and drug behavior are not valid. Nurses should treat all patients as potential sources of HIV infection and protect themselves by using universal precautions.

 Describe patient behaviors related to the medical diagnoses of bipolar disorder and schizophrenia that might contribute to increased risk for HIV.

Interventions Related to Changing Levels of Functioning

The unpredictability of the course of HIV disease is itself a stressor because persons with the infection cannot prepare for disease events and frequently feel surprised by the onset of new symptoms. They cannot determine if a common cold is the serious *Pneumocystis carinii* pneumonia that they have heard about or if a new mole is actually Kaposi's sarcoma. With each opportunistic infection they need to redefine what they can reasonably expect from themselves regarding energy output and physical and mental abilities.

People with HIV disease have been living longer because of medical breakthroughs and greater knowledge of the disease. This means that a person may have multiple opportunistic infections over years of time. People may question, "Is all this worth it?" during periods of fatigue and discouragement. They may consider suicide as a solution. At this time it is helpful for nurses to listen receptively to patients' feelings and not discourage them from talking because of nurses' own discomfort or fear. Information about suicide assessment and intervention is presented in Chapter 18. Nurses can remind patients that there is no need to go through this alone because others will be there to help. The respectful and careful use of physical touch may be a powerful intervention. Persons with HIV disease frequently express the feeling of being "lepers" and may isolate themselves at times. A touch on the hand or a hug may convey the sense of being there for the patient.

 The partner of a person who is terminally ill with AIDS asks for your opinion about assisted suicide. How would you respond?

Support Groups. Nurse-led support groups may supply the person with a safe place to express feelings regarding HIV and the physical threats that are being experienced. The patient can give and receive information and learn more effective coping strategies. The group also serves as a social network for people who are gradually losing their sociocultural roles of worker and provider. Subjects such as living wills, new medications, suicide, responses of friends and family, and the future can be discussed. Group members grieve for themselves as well as their fellow members. Life-style and medical questions may be asked at this time. Education about exposing others to HIV and the dangers of reexposure to themselves is important. Safer sex techniques and the responsibility to inform past sexual or needle-sharing partners need to be addressed.

Some people with HIV disease strive to learn to live for today, not allowing unnecessary worry about the future to rob them of a high quality of life. One woman, who was called "Amazing Grace" by other support group members, was repeatedly hospitalized for opportunistic infections. Between hospitalizations, however, she sought ways to be with her children to the limits of her physical abilities. Two months before she died she drove her children on a six-state touring vacation. One week before her death, with the help of her family, she took her children to the zoo.

Encouraging Productive Activity. The course of HIV disease is characterized by periods of relative wellness, but inconsistent health may result in unstable employment. It is important for the nurse to help patients maintain themselves as contributing members of society by offering outlets for their energy and skills. Such activities could include acting as a "buddy" for another with HIV disease, joining political movements to pro-

mote legislation in which they believe, volunteering at a museum or library, and expanding talents in music, poetry, and other arts.

Interventions Related to Changes in Body Image

Persons with HIV disease often face the impairment of disfigurement. Some examples are:

▼ Kaposi's sarcoma, which may cause large, purple, bruiselike blotches on the face, hands, and legs

▼ "AIDS hair," which resembles the thinning, fine hair of people who have received chemotherapy

▼ Wasting, during which a person continuously loses weight and becomes skeletal in appearance

The nurse should offer opportunities for the patient and significant others to talk about feelings related to body changes. Encouraging the patient to consider oneself as a whole person with both strong, attractive components as well as less pleasing ones may be helpful in establishing perspective. Often, the visible changes caused by HIV disease are viewed as evidence of approaching death. This needs to be discussed openly and accurate information about the cause and meaning of physical symptoms should be given.

Interventions Related to AIDS Dementia Complex

Nursing interventions for the person with HIV disease must address the limitations related to ADC if the patient has behaviors related to a cognitive disorder. The nursing care of patients with cognitive problems is addressed in Chapter 21. Memory problems may be especially troubling to young patients who want to remain actively involved in life, including work. The nurse may suggest ways to improve memory such as writing notes and establishing set routines for activities. Many patients are well informed about HIV disease and may worry about cognitive changes. The nurse needs to provide an opportunity for expression of fears about this and give accurate feedback about cognitive functioning. Some may interpret normal forgetfulness as a sign of pathological deterioration. Significant others should also be provided with information about this aspect of the disease.

What is your reaction to the following statement: Patients should not be informed about potential cognitive changes related to HIV disease; since these changes cannot be prevented, they would only worry unnecessarily.

Interventions Related to Preparation for Death

Spiritual Concerns. Awareness of impending death often leads HIV patients to think about the meaning of life and their spiritual belief system. For some, this means seeking comfort from a religion with which they are already connected. Others may wish to establish a connection with a member of the clergy or a lay representative of a religion. Some patients may choose not to become involved with a particular religion but may want to discuss spiritual and philosophical beliefs. The nurse should assess the patient's spiritual needs and preferences, facilitating access to the selected manner of expression. Some patients appreciate the nurse sitting quietly while they think, providing relevant reading materials or reading, and discussing religious or philosophical writings. If the nurse is comfortable with praying with the patient, this may also be helpful. If the nurse is not comfortable, it is best to be candid and perhaps suggest a few moments of silent meditation.

Advance Directives. Taking charge of the practical aspects of their lives helps people with HIV disease feel in control. For example, making decisions about medical power of attorney, living will, and a last will assists patients in taking control during the later stages of their lives. For single parents, one of the most difficult decisions is selecting a custodian for their surviving children, as illustrated in the following clinical example.

 CLINICAL EXAMPLE

Ms. B is a 30-year-old divorced woman who is the mother of a 7-year-old child. She was diagnosed as HIV positive 2 years ago but has had a rapid progression of opportunistic infections and is now in the acute phase of her illness. As part of trying to write her durable power of attorney, living will, and will, she is trying to decide who she will ask to care for her son. The child's father has had no contact with them, and Ms. B believes he is unfit and probably unwilling to assume responsibility for his child. Ms. B's parents are elderly and in frail health. Her older sister is married with four children. Her older brother is unmarried and travels a great deal for business. Ms. B's best friend, who is divorced and childless, has expressed a willingness to care for her son. Ms. B is depressed about leaving her son and highly anxious regarding the best situation for him.

Selected Nursing Diagnoses:

▼ Anxiety related to conflict over arranging for son's care as evidenced by indecision over completing will

▼ Anticipatory grieving related to expected loss of the relationship with her son as evidenced by depressed mood

Many people wish to make decisions regarding their funeral. Some write their own obituaries; others design or even make their own quilt panel for the National AIDS Quilt. Some people prepare videotapes and letters for their family members to be presented after their death. It is important that the nurse support these efforts to maintain control, allowing the person to live and die in one's own style. Even though these decisions and activities may be very difficult and emotional, the patient frequently feels a sense of relief and completion when these tasks are accomplished.

Interventions Related to Significant Others

Families, partners, and friends of people who have HIV disease need a great deal of support to enable them to meet the needs of the patient. One nursing study of people living with HIV disease and their families revealed higher levels of psychological distress than in a nonpatient normative sample but lower than in psychiatric patients.[18] The investigators recommended the following interventions to assist patients and their families:

▼ Anxiety reduction
▼ Assistance with control and appropriate expression of anger
▼ Teaching calming techniques to be used during acute distress
▼ Sleep enhancement
▼ Cognitive restructuring to develop a more realistic world view

Another nursing study[6] focused on family members, partners, and friends of young men who had HIV disease and identified their needs. At the time that they became aware of the diagnosis, they reported feeling shocked but also needing information. The other concern at this time was related to the patient's reluctance to inform others of the diagnosis, sometimes limiting the access of significant others to their own support systems. The nurse can be helpful by discussing the anticipated response of others to the diagnosis and supporting the patient and significant others during and following disclosure.

Significant others described the emotional stress of feeling hopeful when the patient was asymptomatic and then hopeless when an opportunistic infection occurred. Nurses need to provide support and relevant information about the patient's changing condition. Interpersonal relationships often changed as a result of the HIV disease. Positive changes were related to expressions of concern and offers of help from others. Some felt increased closeness in their relationship. Negative changes were more frequent. Some resulted from a family member's rejection of the patient upon learning of the diagnosis. Others were related to significant others' reluctance to tell others about the diagnosis, increasing their own stress. Nurses can be very helpful by inquiring about the status of relationships with family members and others and by exploring negative responses. Family meetings may facilitate the sharing of feelings and clarification of misconceptions.

Response of the Nurse to the Person with HIV Disease

As a progressive disease is discouraging to patients, so too it may be discouraging to nurses. It is essential that nurses monitor their reactions and investment in patients. Professional nurses must allow themselves the necessary time and opportunities to grieve the multiple losses their patients experience and the death of patients they know well. Nurses may confront many challenges when working with patients with HIV.

Fear of Contagion. The nurse needs to know, understand, and use universal precautions. Careful planning during procedures and taking the time for necessary steps such as gloving will eliminate most opportunities for infection from contact with a patient. Since 1978 there has been documented job-related transmission of HIV to nurses in 13 cases.[3] They were exposed to the virus via percutaneous (e.g., needlesticks) or mucotaneous routes. There are 15 additional instances of possible occupational transmission where HIV seroconversion specifically resulting from an occupational exposure was not documented.

Cultural and Behavioral Differences. Nurses work with patients whose backgrounds and past behaviors may vary markedly from their own and challenge the nurse's beliefs and values. Although a nurse is entitled to have private views, there is an obligation to provide the best nursing care available to each patient. Disapproval of the patient's past behavior is the nurse's prerogative. The challenge is to keep that view from interfering with care while accepting the patient as a person.

Identification. As HIV disease spreads throughout society, it will become increasingly common for the nurse to have many similarities with the patient. Patients will have more characteristics in common with the nurse, including age, life-style, and socioeconomic status. In some cases it is difficult for the nurse to manage the

feelings aroused by patients with HIV disease and maintain an objective approach. For example, a pregnant nurse may care for a young woman who has recently delivered an HIV-infected baby. Anger, fear, confusion, disgust, and pity toward the patient are some of the reactions with which a nurse may have to cope to provide quality care. The clinical example that follows illustrates this problem.

CLINICAL EXAMPLE

TJ, a 2-year-old girl, entered the hospital with a broken wrist suffered during a fall from her porch. Upon admission the treatment team was notified by her parents that she was HIV positive. She has had no opportunistic infections, has a T-cell count of 950, and is of normal weight and height for her age group. She shows no symptoms of HIV disease. Ms. K, her primary nurse, has approached her senior clinical nurse with a dilemma. She believes that the only way TJ could have become infected was in utero. Ms. K is experiencing great anger toward TJ's parents, whom she believes should have taken precautions against the birth of children once they knew TJ's mother was HIV positive. Ms. K wants to be removed as TJ's primary nurse not only because of her anger against her parents, but also because Ms. K has a 2-year-old daughter and finds that she is too distressed to work with TJ.

When a nurse identifies that a patient is arousing strong feelings or if colleagues question one's objectivity, it is essential to seek out supervision or consultation from an experienced nurse.

Fear of Death and Dying. For many nurses, dealing with death is an occasional stressor. But for the nurse caring for patients with HIV disease, death and the preparation for it are common issues. Nurses may get to know patients during the course of repeated hospitalizations or work with patients who are young and energetic but are showing signs of decreasing vitality. Unresolved grief on the nurse's part, lack of acceptance of death as an outcome, and the nurse's own religious and cultural values related to death are factors that may inhibit the nurse's ability to cope with the losses experienced while caring for HIV patients.

Would you apply for a nursing position in a setting that specialized in the treatment of people with HIV disease? What considerations would influence your decision?

Psychiatric Consultation Liaison Nursing

Of special note is the role of the psychiatric consultation liaison nurse in the general hospital setting. This nurse provides consultation to, collaborates with, and educates nurses in addressing the interactive effects of the biopsychosocial aspects of AIDS care. Among the services the nurse consultant can provide or coordinate are educational and informational programs on all aspects of HIV disease; consistent policies and procedures for infection control practices for all staff; postexposure education and support; institutional resources and support for patients and staff; attention to work and personal stress-reduction techniques; encouragement of acknowledgment and appreciation by supervisors and peers of work well done; regular and as-needed group meetings to provide emotional support for staff caring for patients and their families; and group forums for nurses to verbalize their feelings, attitudes, values, and concerns.[14] More information about the role of the consultation liaison nurse is provided in Chapter 33.

It has been observed that nurses are accustomed to trying to cure, to fix, and to solve.[15] HIV disease requires nurses to recognize no cure for the disease to date, and no solution to the many family and personal issues the patient confronts. Nurses may be burdened with their own feelings of helplessness and frustration. They do not have all the answers and may feel they have failed the patient they have come to know well. Nurses may find it helpful to remember a note received by one of the authors from a patient: *"I see evidence of God's loving hand in the concern and support coming from so many people. I've had so much help in getting through a difficult period, frequently from people I hadn't met before all this began. And even in that honored company, you stand out. Thanks for your efforts to help me and for being a good friend."*

EVALUATING CARE OF THE PATIENT WITH HIV DISEASE

In working with the psychosocial aspects of HIV disease, evaluation of nursing interventions focuses on the patient's reduction of maladaptive responses to the stressors associated with the disease. The primary issue for the patient is adjustment to loss. Self-esteem, social acceptance, employment and financial independence, family relationships, and future goals are all threatened by HIV disease. The nurse's assessment and counseling skills, the teaching of coping skills, and referrals to support services are appropriate areas for evaluation. Nurses also need to conduct periodic self-evaluation to prevent becoming overwhelmed by the stresses of working with patients who have HIV disease.

SUMMARY

1. HIV disease includes all of the disorders resulting from infection with the retrovirus, human immunodeficiency virus. It has multiple effects on all aspects of biopsychosocial functioning.
2. Behaviors related to HIV disease may be related to stigma, crisis, depression, AIDS dementia complex, or social relationships.
3. Nursing diagnoses related to the psychosocial aspects of HIV disease are particularly related to body image, sexuality, and grieving.
4. Planning health care for the person who has HIV disease must involve the multidisciplinary team.
5. Interventions include case management, risk reduction, support groups, crisis intervention, encouragement of productive activity, enhancement of self-esteem, grief counseling, support during terminal stages, and support of significant others.
6. Evaluation focuses on the patient's adjustment to the multiple losses associated with HIV disease.

COMPETENT CARING
A CLINICAL EXEMPLAR OF A PSYCHIATRIC NURSE

Donna Green, RN

A special moment for me, as a psychiatric nurse who influenced a patient's treatment, happened several years ago at the beginning of the AIDS epidemic. It involved a relationship I formed with a patient who was diagnosed with AIDS. I spent time with him when others stayed away and allowed him to share his thoughts and feelings. I encouraged him to talk about his feelings concerning problems in his relationships in an atmosphere of unconditional acceptance of his sexuality. I promoted this by showing no fear of contracting the disease from him and no judgment of his life situation.

Slowly, he began to interact more on the unit by initiating conversations with the staff, although not with other patients. When he consented to a case conference, he requested that I accompany him because he felt more at ease when I was with him.

It was at this point that I realized the time that I spent with him and the efforts I made to reach out to him had made a difference in this man's hospital stay. My efforts were also recognized by my supervisor and were a large factor in my receiving a performance award for the excellent care I delivered as a psychiatric nurse. Such are the difficult challenges and special rewards of our profession and the specialty area in which we practice the art and science of psychiatric nursing. ▼

REFERENCES

1. Berk RA, Poe SS, Baigis-Smith JA: Healthcare needs scale for patients with HIV/AIDS: content validation, J Assoc Nurse AIDS Care 3:10, 1992.
2. Boccellari AA, Dilley JW: Management and residual placement problems of patients with HIV-related cognitive impairment, Hosp Community Psychiatry, 43:32, 1992.
3. Centers for Disease Control and Prevention: HIV/AIDS surveillance report, Georgia, 1993, US Department of Health and Human Services.
4. Centers for Disease Control and Prevention: 1993 revised classification system for HIV infection and expanded surveillance case definition for AIDS among adolescents and adults, Georgia, 1992, US Department of Health and Human Services.
5. Cournos F et al: HIV risk activity among persons with severe mental illness: preliminary findings, Hosp Community Psychiatry 44:1104, 1993.
6. Cowles KV, Rodgers BL: When a loved one has AIDS: care for the significant other, J Psychosoc Nurs Ment Health Serv 29:6, 1991.
7. Field HL: Biopsychosocial aspects of AIDS, New Dir Ment Health Serv 57:51, 1993.
8. Flaskerud JH: AIDS: psychosocial aspects, J Psychosoc Nurs Ment Health Serv 25:8, 1987.
9. Flaskerud JH: AIDS/HIV infection: a reference guide for nursing professionals, Philadelphia, 1989, WB Saunders.
10. Frierson RL, Lippman SB: Psychologic implications of AIDS, Am Fam Practitioner 35:109, 1987.
11. Graham LL, Cates JA: How to reduce the risk of HIV infec-

tion for the seriously mentally ill, J Psychosoc Nurs Ment Health Serv 30:9, 1992.
12. Harding AK, Gray LA, Neal M: Confidentiality limits with clients who have HIV: a review of ethical and legal guidelines and professional policies, J Couns Dev 71:297, 1993.
13. Kelly JA et al: AIDS/HIV risk behavior among the chronically mentally ill, Am J Psychiatry 149:886, 1992.
14. Kurlowicz LH: Psychiatric consultation-liaison nursing interventions with nurses of hospitalized AIDS patients, Clin Nurse Spec 5:124, 1991.
15. LaSalle AJ, LaSalle PM: Care of people living with HIV disease: counseling issues for the nurse practitioner, Nurse Pract Forum 2:137, 1991.
16. Marzuk PM et al: Increased risk of suicide in persons with AIDS, JAMA 259:1333, 1988.
17. McCain NL, Gramling LF: Living with dying: coping with HIV disease, Issues Ment Health Nurs 13:271, 1992.
18. McShane RE, Bumbalo JA, Patsdaughter CA: Psychological distress in family members living with human immunodeficiency virus/acquired immune deficiency syndrome, Arch Psychiatr Nurs 8:53, 1994.
19. Swanson B, Cronin-Stubbs D, Colletti MA: Dementia and depression in persons with AIDS: causes and care, J Psychosoc Nurs Ment Health Serv 28:33, 1990.
20. Swanson B et al: Characterizing the neuropsychological functioning of persons with human immunodeficiency virus infection; Part 1. Acquired immunodeficiency syndrome dementia complex: a review, Arch Psychiatr Nurs 7:74, 1993.

ANNOTATED SUGGESTED READINGS

*Andrews S, Williams AB, Neil K: The mother-child relationship in the HIV-1 positive family, *Image J Nurs Sch* 25:193, 1993.

Describes the relationship between an HIV positive mother and her child as both a source of support and a stressor.

*Carmack BJ: Balancing engagement/detachment in AIDS-related multiple losses, *Image J Nurs Sch* 24:9. 1992.

Nursing study of gay men who had experienced many losses as result of AIDS identifying four categories of response.

*Corless IB, Halloran EJ, Belyea MJ: Nursing dependency needs of HIV-infected patients: Part 1. Methods and clinical findings, *Nurs Admin Q* 18:1, 1994.

Demonstrates application of the nursing process to the care of individuals with HIV disease, including impact of nursing diagnoses on hospital stay. Particularly relevant for nurse managers.

Kalichman SC, Kelly JA, Johnson JR, Bulto M: Factors associated with risk for HIV infection among chronic mentally ill adults, *Am J Psychiatry* 151:221, 1994.

Study found high risk for exposure to HIV related to both unsafe sexual behavior and drug use. Findings are helpful for preventive interventions.

Kelly JA: Changing the behavior of an HIV-seropositive man who practices unsafe sex, *Hosp Community Psychiatry* 42:239, 1991.

Addresses treatment planning for a patient who demonstrates behavior that is often a source of concern for nurses. Provides practical suggestions for intervention.

*Korniewicz DM, O'Brien ME, Larson E: Coping with AIDS and HIV: psychosocial adaptation, *J Psychosoc Nurs Ment Health Serv* 28:14, 1990.

Report of a nursing study that identifies the psychosocial support needs of people who have HIV infection but do not yet have AIDS. Emphasizes that newly diagnosed individuals should receive particular attention from the nurse.

Leserman J, Perkins DO, Evans DL: Coping with the threat of AIDS: The role of social support, *Am J Psychiatry* 149:1514, 1992.

Focuses on the need for social support experienced by asymptomatic HIV-positive men. Discusses therapeutic approaches, with particular attention to the needs of black patients.

Markowitz JC, Klerman GL, Perry SW: Interpersonal psychotherapy of depressed HIV-positive outpatients, *Hosp Community Psychiatry* 43:885, 1992.

Describes the effectiveness of interpersonal psychotherapy with HIV-positive people who are depressed. Identifies six therapeutic factors.

*Regan-Kubinski MJ, Sharts-Engel N: The HIV-infected woman: illness cognition assessment, *J Psychosoc Nurs Ment Health Serv* 30:11, 1992.

Identifies the special concerns of women who have HIV disease. Nursing assessment of the woman's perception of her illness is especially important for effective care planning.

Sewell DD et al: HIV-associated psychosis: a study of 20 cases, *Am J Psychiatry* 151:237, 1994.

Study suggests that psychosis related to HIV disease may be a result of encephalopathy.

*Sowell RL et al: The lived experience of survival and bereavement following the death of a lover from AIDS, *Image J Nurs Sch* 23:89, 1991.

Describes the grief experience of individuals who have lost lovers to AIDS. Identifies experiential categories of isolation/disconnectedness, emotional confusion, and acceptance/denial.

*Swanson B et al: Characterizing the neuropsychological functioning of persons with human immunodeficiency virus (HIV) infection: Part II. Neuropsychological functioning of persons at different stages of HIV infection, *Arch Psychiatr Nurs* 7:82, 1993.

Relates levels of impairment to stage of illness and functional ability. Suggests related nursing interventions.

---

*Nursing reference.

Glossary

abreaction The release of feelings that takes place as a patient talks about emotionally charged areas.

accountability To be answerable to someone for something, focusing responsibility on the individual for personal actions or lack of actions.

action cues A category of nonverbal communication that consists of body movements and is sometimes referred to as kinetics.

addiction The psychosocial behaviors related to substance dependence.

adolescence The period from the beginning of puberty to the attainment of maturity. The transitional stage during which the youth is becoming an adult man or woman. This period is described in terms of development in many different functions that may be reached at different times. Only conventional limits may be stated: 12 to 21 years for girls, 13 to 23 years for boys.

advanced directives Documents, written while a person is competent, that specify how decisions about treatment would be made if the person were to become incompetent.

adventitious crisis An accidental, uncommon, and unexpected event that results in multiple losses and major environmental changes.

advocacy Assisting people to receive the available services and influencing providers to improve existing services and develop new ones.

affect Feeling, mood, or emotional tone.

affective Relating to an individual's affect.

agnosia Difficulty recognizing well-known objects.

agonist In pharmacology, a substance that acts with, enhances, or potentiates a specific activity.

agoraphobia Fear of open spaces and the marketplace.

AIDS dementia complex Subcortical encephalopathy characterized by progressive dementia; believed to result primarily from direct infection with HIV.

akathisia A motor restlessness ranging from a feeling of inner disquiet, often localized in the muscles, to an inability to sit still or lie quietly; a side effect of some antipsychotic drugs.

alcohol hallucinosis A medical diagnosis referring to an alcohol withdrawal syndrome that is characterized by auditory hallucinations in the absence of any other psychotic symptoms.

alcohol withdrawal delirium A medical diagnosis for a serious alcohol withdrawal syndrome that is characterized by delirium and autonomic hyperactivity occurring within 1 week of reduction of alcohol intake.

alexithymia Difficulty naming and describing emotions.

altruism A sense of concern for the welfare of others that can be expressed at the level of the individual or the larger social system.

amotivational syndrome A cluster of symptoms apparently related to prolonged marijuana use which includes apathy, lack of energy, loss of desire to work or be productive, diminished concentration, poor personal hygiene, and preoccupation with marijuana.

anaclitic depression A deprivational reaction in infants separated from their mothers in the second half of the first year of life. The reaction is characterized by apprehension, crying, withdrawal, psychomotor slowing, dejection, stupor, insomnia, anorexia, and gross retardation in growth and development.

anhedonia Inability or decreased ability to experience pleasure, joy, intimacy, and closeness.

anorexia nervosa An eating disorder in which the person experiences hunger but refuses to eat because of a distorted body image leading to a self-perception of fatness. Starvation ensues.

antecedent The stimulus or cue that occurs before behavior that leads to its occurrence.

antisocial personality disorder A disorder occurring in adult patients with a history of conduct disorder; behavior is often characterized by poor work record, disregard for social norms, aggressiveness, financial irresponsibility, impulsiveness, lying, recklessness, inability to maintain close relationships or to meet responsibilities for significant others, and a lack of remorse for harmful behavior.

anxiety A diffuse apprehension vague in nature and associated with feelings of uncertainty and helplessness. It is an emotion without a specific object, is subjectively experienced by the individual, and is communicated interpersonally. It occurs as a result of a threat to the person's being, self-esteem, or identity.

apathy Lack of feelings, emotions, interests, or concern.

aphasia Difficulty finding the right word.

appraisal of stressor An evaluation of the significance of an event for one's well-being that takes place on the cognitive, affective, physiological, behavioral, and social levels.

apraxia Inability or difficulty in performing a purposeful organized task or similar skilled activities.

assertive community treatment An intensive community intervention program, undertaken by case managers with small caseloads and 24-hour responsibility for their clients, in which a multidisciplinary team works with patients in their homes, neighborhoods, and workplaces, providing varying intensities of services depending on patient need.

assertiveness The midpoint of a continuum that runs from passive to aggressive behavior. Assertive behavior conveys a sense of self-assurance but also communicates respect for the other person.

attention The ability to focus on one activity in a sustained, concentrated manner.

attributions Reasoning processes used to explain events.

autogenic storytelling A therapeutic version of storytelling in which the child participates in creating the story.

autonomy Self-determination that fosters independence and self-regulation; the condition that allows for definition of and control over a domain.

aversion therapy Reduces unwanted but persistent maladaptive behaviors by applying an aversive or noxious stimulus when that maladaptive behavior occurs.

axon The presynaptic cell membrane of a neuron.

behavior Any observable, recordable, and measurable act, movement, or response of the individual.

behavioral Relating to an individual's behavior.

bibliotherapy Use of literature to help children identify and express feelings within the structure and safety of the nurse-patient relationship.

binge eating The rapid consumption of large quantities of food in a discrete period of time.

biofeedback The use of a machine to communicate physical changes; used to train an individual to reduce anxiety and modify behavioral responses.

biological psychiatry A school of psychiatric thought that emphasizes physical, chemical, and neurological causes and treatment approaches.

bipolar affective disorder A subgroup of the affective disorders characterized by at least one episode of manic behavior, with or without a history of episodes of depression.

bisexuality A sexual attraction to persons of both sexes and the engagement in both homosexual and heterosexual activity.

blood levels The concentration of a drug in the plasma, serum, or blood. In psychiatry the term is most often applied to levels of lithium or some tricyclic antidepressants. Maximum clinical responses to these agents have been correlated with specific ranges of blood levels.

body dysmorphic disorder A somatoform disorder characterized by a normal-appearing person's belief that he or she has a physical defect.

body image Sum of the conscious and unconscious attitudes the individual has toward his or her body. It includes present and past perceptions as well as feelings about size, function, appearance, and potential.

borderline personality disorder A specific personality disorder having the essential features of unstable mood, interpersonal relationships and self-image; characteristic behaviors may include unstable relationships, exploitation of others, impulsive behavior, labile affect, problems expressing anger appropriately, self-destructive behavior, and identity disturbances.

brain electrical activity mapping (BEAM) Images brain activity and function by using CT techniques to display data derived from EEG recordings of brain electrical activity that has been sensory evoked by specific stimuli or cognitive evoked by specific mental tasks.

bulimia nervosa An eating disorder that is characterized by uncontrollable binge eating, alternating with vomiting or dieting.

capitation A funding mechanism in which (1) all defined services for a specific period of time are provided for an agreed-upon payment, (2) payment is tied to the care of a particular person or group, and (3) the provider agrees to be at risk for costs exceeding the agreed-upon amount.

case management Services aimed at linking the service system to the individual and coordinating the service components so that the individual can achieve successful community living.

catatonia A stuporous state.

catharsis Release that occurs when the patient is encouraged to talk about things that bother him or her most. Fears, feelings, and experiences are brought out into the open and discussed.

certification A formal review process of clinical practice.

certified generalist A psychiatric nurse who demonstrates expertise in practice, knowledge of theories concerning personality development and behavior patterns in treating mental illness, and the relationship of such treatments to nursing care.

certified specialist A nurse showing a high degree of proficiency in interpersonal skills, in the use of the nursing process, and in psychological and milieu therapies.

circadian rhythms The correlation between human activities and behaviors and external environmental stimuli.

classical conditioning A theory describing the process by which involuntary behavior is learned, in which an event occurs when one stimulus, by being paired with another stimulus, comes to produce the same response as that other stimulus.

clinical pathway A shortened version of the plan of care for a particular individual that lists key nursing and medical processes and corresponding time lines to which the patient must adhere to achieve standard outcomes within a specified period.

cognition The mental process characterized by knowing, thinking, learning, and judging.

cognitive Relating to an individual's cognition.

cognitive distortions Positive or negative distortions of reality that might include errors of logic, mistakes in reasoning, or individualized views of the world that do not reflect reality.

collaboration The shared planning, decision making, problem solving, goal setting, and assumption of responsibilities by individuals who work together cooperatively and with open communication.

collaborative practice The diagnosis and treatment of psychiatric illness in patients with somatic complaints.

collegiality An essential aspect of professional practice that requires that nurses view their nurse peers as collaborators in the caregiving process who are valued and respected for their unique contributions.

commitment Involuntary admission in which the request for hospitalization did not originate with the patient. When committed, the patient loses the right to leave the hospital when he or she wishes. It is usually justified on the ground that the patient is dangerous to self or others and needs treatment.

communication Process of influencing the behavior of others by sending, receiving, and interpreting messages; feedback and consideration of the context complete the cycle.

community support systems Systems developed by community mental health centers to provide patients with necessary specialized mental health service. Includes such community-based components as crisis response services, health and dental care, rehabilitation services, and protection and advocacy.

compensation Process by which a person makes up for a deficiency in self-image by strongly emphasizing some other feature that the person regards as an asset.

competence building The health education strategy of primary prevention that involves the strengthening of individuals and groups and is based on the assumption that many maladaptive responses result from a lack of competence.

compulsion A recurring irresistible impulse to perform some act.

computed tomography (CT) Depicts brain structure with a series of x-rays that is computer-constructed into "slices" of the brain that can be stacked by the computer, giving a three-dimensional view.

concreteness Use of specific terminology rather than abstractions in the discussion of the patient's feelings, experiences, and behavior.

conduct disorder Disorder with the essential feature of behavior that violates the basic rights of others or societal norms and rules.

confidentiality Disclosure of certain information to another specifically authorized person.

conflict Clashing of two opposing interests. The person experiences two competing drives and must choose between them.

confrontation An expression by the nurse of perceived discrepancies in the patient's behavior. It is an attempt by the nurse to bring to the patient's awareness the incongruence in feelings, attitudes, beliefs, and behaviors.

confusion A nonspecific term used to describe a constellation of behaviors related to cognitive impairment, usually including disorientation, memory loss, loss of social skills, disruptive behavior, and difficulties with self-care.

congruent communication A communication pattern in which the sender is communicating the same message on both the verbal and the nonverbal levels.

consequence What kind of effect (positive, negative, or neutral) the person thinks a behavior has.

consultation A specific professional process between two systems in which the consultee has a problem and requests help from an outside system, the consultant.

consultation liaison nursing care Expert psychiatric consultation provided by a psychiatric mental health nurse in various other health-care settings.

context Setting in which an event takes place.

contingency contracting A formal contract between the patient and the therapist defining what behaviors are to be changed and what consequences follow the performance of these behaviors.

conversion disorder A somatoform disorder characterized by a loss or alteration of physical functioning without evidence of organic impairment.

coping resources Characteristics of the person, group, or environment that are helpful in assisting individuals in adapting to stress.

countertransference An emotional response of the nurse that is generated by the patient's qualities and is inappropriate to the content and context of the therapeutic relationship or inappropriate in the degree of emotional intensity.

crisis A disturbance caused by a stressful event or a perceived threat to self.

crisis intervention Short-term therapy focused on solving the immediate problem and allowing the individual to return to a precrisis level of function.

cultural sensitivity Having an understanding of and respect for the importance of social and cultural forces on the individual.

decatastrophizing Helping patients to evaluate if they are overestimating the catastrophic nature of a situation.

decision making Arriving at a solution or making a choice.

defense mechanisms Coping mechanisms of the ego that attempt to protect the person from feelings of inadequacy and worthlessness and prevent awareness of anxiety. They are primarily unconscious and involve a degree of self-deception and reality distortion.

deinstitutionalization At the patient level, the transfer to a community setting of a patient hospitalized for an extended time, generally many years; at the mental health care system level, a shift in the focus of care from the large, long-term institution to the community, accomplished by discharging long-term patients and avoiding unnecessary admissions.

delinquency A relatively minor violation of legal or moral codes, especially by children or adolescents. Juvenile delinquency is such behavior by a young person (usually younger than 16 or 18 years of age) as to bring him or her to the attention of a court.

delirium The medical diagnostic term that describes an organic mental disorder characterized by a cluster of cognitive impairments with an acute onset and the identification of a specific precipitating stressor.

delirium tremens A medical diagnostic term that has been replaced with the diagnosis of alcohol withdrawal delirium.

delusion A false belief that is firmly maintained even though it is not shared by others and is contradicted by social reality.

dementia The medical diagnostic term that describes an organic mental disorder characterized by a cluster of cognitive impairments that are generally of gradual onset and irreversible. The predisposing and precipitating stressors may or may not be identifiable.

dendrite The postsynaptic membrane of a neuron.

denial Avoidance of disagreeable realities by ignoring or refusing to recognize them.

depersonalization A feeling of unreality and alienation from oneself. One has difficulty distinguishing self from others, and one's body has an unreal or strange quality about it. The subjective experience of the partial or total disruption of one's ego and the disintegration and disorganization of one's self-concept.

depression An abnormal extension of overelaboration of sadness and grief. The term *depression* can denote a variety of phenomena, a sign, symptom, syndrome, emotional state, reaction, disease, or clinical entity.

detoxification The removal of a toxic substance from the body, either naturally through physiological process, such as hepatic or renal functions, or medically by the introduction of alternative substances and gradual withdrawal.

differentiated practice Distinguishing among professionals with role descriptions and functional assignments based on education, experience, and competency; responsibilities reflect each individual's unique knowledge base.

differentiation Sufficient separation between intellect and emotions so that one is not dominated by the reactive anxiety of the family's emotional system.

direct self-destructive behavior (DSDB) Suicidal behavior.

disadvantagement The lack of socioeconomic resources that are basic to biopsychosocial adaptation.

discrimination Differential treatment of individuals or groups not based on actual merit.

disengaged A transactional style in a family reflecting inappropriately rigid boundaries requiring a high level of individual stress to activate family response.

displacement Shift of an emotion from the person or object toward which it was originally directed to another usually neutral or less dangerous person or object.

dissociation The separation of any group of mental or behavioral processes from the rest of the person's consciousness or identity.

diurnal mood variation Changes in mood that are related to the time of day.

double bind Simultaneous communication of conflicting messages in the context of a situation that does not allow escape. (See *incongruent communication*.)

drug interaction The effects of two or more drugs being taken simultaneously, producing an alteration in the usual effects of either drug taken alone. The interacting drugs may have a potentiating or additive effect, and serious side effects may result.

drug tolerance Repeated use of some substance or drug (e.g., narcotics) so that larger and larger doses are required to produce the same physiological and/or psychological effect obtained previously by a smaller dose.

drug trial The time it takes to administer a drug at adequate therapeutic doses for a long enough period to determine its efficacy for a particular patient. The trial culminates with (1) acceptable clinical results, (2) intolerable adverse effects, or (3) poor response after an appropriate blood level is reached or after the drug is administered for a time specific for the illness.

DSM-IV Commonly used abbreviation for the *Diagnostic and Statistical Manual of Mental Disorders*, which contains standard nomenclature of emotional illness used by all health-care practitioners. DSM-IV is a revised version published in 1994; it updates and classifies mental illnesses and presents guidelines and diagnostic criteria for various mental disorders.

dual diagnosis Simultaneous occurrence of a mental illness and a substance abuse disorder.

dyspareunia Recurrent or persistent genital pain occurring before, during, or after intercourse (male or female).

dystonia Acute tonic muscle spasms, often of the tongue, jaw, eyes, and neck but sometimes of the whole body. Sometimes occurs during the first few days of antipsychotic drug administration.

echopraxia Purposeless imitation of other's movements.

ego defense mechanisms See *defense mechanisms*.

elder abuse A variety of behaviors that threaten the health, comfort, and possibly the lives of elderly people, including physical and emotional neglect, emotional abuse, violation of personal rights, financial abuse, and direct physical abuse.

electroconvulsive therapy (ECT) Artificial induction of a grand mal seizure by passing a controlled electrical current through electrodes applied to one or both temples. The patient is anesthetized and the seizure attenuated by administration of a muscle relaxant medication.

empathetic understanding Ability to view the patient's world from his or her internal frame of reference. It involves the nurses's sensitivity to the patient's current feelings and the verbal ability to communicate this understanding in a language attuned to the patient.

enabler The role that is frequently assumed by the significant others of substance abusers, characterized by covert support of the substance-abusing behavior.

encounter group therapy An application of the existential model of psychiatric care in a group setting. The focus is on here-and-now experience and the expression of real feelings verbally and nonverbally as members react to events in the group.

endogenous Developing or originating within the organism or arising from causes within the organism.

enmeshed A transactional style in a family reflecting diffuse subsystem boundaries resulting in stress in one family member that emotionally reverberates quickly and intensely throughout the family system.

ethic A standard of behavior or a belief valued by an individual or group.

ethical dilemma Exists when moral claims conflict with one another, resulting in a difficult problem that seems to have no satisfactory solution because of the existence of a choice between equally unsatisfactory alternatives.

ethnicity An individual's racial, national, tribal, linguistic, or cultural origin or background.

exhibitionism Intense sexual arousal or desire and acts, fantasies, or other stimuli involving exposing one's genitals to an unsuspecting stranger.

existential (therapy) A school of philosophical thought that focuses on the importance of experience in the present and the belief that humans find meaning in life through their experiences.

exogenous Developing or originating outside the organism.

extinction The process of eliminating the occurrence of a behavior by ignoring or not rewarding that behavior.

extrapyramidal syndrome A variety of signs and symptoms, including muscular rigidity, tremors, drooling, shuffling gait (parkinsonism); restlessness (akathisia); peculiar involuntary postures (dystonia); motor inertia (akinesia); and many other neurological disturbances. Results from dysfunction of the extrapyramidal system. May occur as a reversible side effect of certain psychotropic drugs, particularly antipsychotics.

family A group of people living in a household who are attached emotionally, interact regularly, and share concerns for the growth and development of individuals and the family.

family burden The impact of a family member's mental illness on the entire family.

family preservation Intensive home treatment modality for troubled youths and their families.

family projection process Transmission of anxiety of one or both parents onto a target child, establishing an overly protective or conflictual relationship with the child and resulting ultimately in impairment of the child.

family violence Refers to a range of behaviors occurring between family members, including physical and emotional abuse of children, child neglect, spouse battering, marital rape, and elder abuse.

fetishism Intense sexual arousal or desire and acts, fantasies, or other stimuli involving nonliving objects by themselves.

flight of ideas Overproductive speech characterized by rapid shifting from one topic to another and fragmented ideas.

flooding Exposure therapy in which the patient is immediately exposed to the most anxiety-provoking stimuli.

Food and Drug Administration (FDA) One of a number of health administrations under the assistant secretary of health of the U.S. Department of Health, Education and Welfare (in April 1980 Department of Health and Human Services) to set standards for, to license the sale of, and in general to safeguard the public from the use of dangerous drugs and food substances.

frotteurism Intense sexual arousal or desire and acts, fantasies, or other stimuli involving rubbing against a nonconsenting person.

fusion A blurring of self-boundaries in a highly reactive emotional relationship with another.

genogram A structured method of gathering information and graphically symbolizing factual and emotional relationship data.

genuineness A quality of the nurse characterized by openness, honesty, and sincerity. The nurse is self-congruent and authentic and relates to the patient without a defensive facade.

Gestalt therapy A therapeutic approach based on the existential model of psychiatric care. It was developed by Perls and focuses on the development of enhanced self-awareness.

glial cells Support cells that form myelin sheaths; thought to remove excess transmitters and ions from the extracellular spaces in the brain, provide glucose to some nerve cells, and direct the flow of blood and oxygen to various parts of the brain.

grief An individual's subjective response to the loss of a person, object, or concept that is highly valued. Uncomplicated grief is a healthy, adaptive, reparative response.

habeas corpus A right retained by all psychiatric patients that provides for the release of an individual who claims being deprived of liberty and being detained illegally. The hearing for this determination takes place in a court of law, and the patient's sanity is at issue.

half-life The amount of time it takes the body to excrete approximately half of an ingested drug; after this time the effects of the drug usually begin to deteriorate.

hallucination Perceptual distortion arising from any of the five senses.

hallucinogens A class of abused drugs that cause a psychotic-like experience.

hardiness A measurement of an individual's psychological capability to resist illness when faced with a stressful life event.

health education A teaching strategy related to health issues that involves the strengthening of individuals and groups through competence building.

HIV disease Describes all of the disorders resulting from infection with the human immunodeficiency virus.

home health care Delivery of health services in the home, including mental health services.

homosexuality Sexual attraction to members of the same sex.

hypersomnia Disorders of excessive somnolence.

hypochondriasis A somatoform disorder characterized by the belief that one is ill without evidence of organic impairment, involving somatic overconcern with and morbid attention to details of body functioning.

hypomania A clinical syndrome that is similar to, but less severe than, that described by the term *mania* or *manic episode*.

hypoxia Inadequate oxygen at the cellular level, characterized by cyanosis, tachycardia, hypertension, peripheral vasoconstriction, dizziness and mental confusion.

ideas of reference Incorrect interpretation of casual incidents and external events as having direct personal references.

identification Process by which a person tries to become like someone else whom he or she admires by taking on the thoughts, mannerisms, or tastes of that individual.

identity Organizing principle of the personality system that accounts for the unity, continuity, uniqueness, and consistency of the personality. It is the awareness of the process of "being oneself" that is derived from self-observation and judgment. It is the synthesis of all self-representations into an organized whole.

identity confusion Lack of clarity and consistency in one's perception of the self, resulting in a high degree of anxiety.

identity diffusion An individual's failure to integrate various childhood identifications into a harmonious adult psychosocial identity.

identity foreclosure Premature adoption of an identity that is desired by significant others without coming to terms with one's own desires, aspirations, or potential.

illusions False perceptions of or false responses to a sensory stimulus.

immediacy State that occurs when the current interaction of the nurse and the patient is focused on.

impulsivity A maladaptive social behavior characterized by unpredictability, unreliability, inability to plan or learn from experience, and overall poor judgment.

incompetency A legal status that must be proved in a special court hearing. As a result of the hearing, the person can be deprived of many civil rights. Incompetency can be reversed only in another court hearing that declares the person competent.

incongruent communication A communication pattern in which the sender is communicating a different message on the verbal and nonverbal levels and the listener does not know to which level he or she should respond. (See *double bind*.)

indirect self-destructive behavior (ISDB) Any activity that is detrimental to the person's well-being and could cause death, accompanied by lack of conscious awareness of the self-destructive nature of the behavior.

informed consent Disclosure of a certain amount of information to the patient about the proposed treatment and the attainment of the patient's consent, which must be competent, understanding, and voluntary.

insanity defense Legal defense proposing that a person who has committed an act that in a usual situation would be criminal should be held not guilty by reason of "insanity."

insight The patient's understanding of the nature of the problem or illness.

insomnia Disorders of initiating or maintaining sleep.

intellectualization Excessive reasoning or logic used to avoid experiencing disturbing feelings.

interdisciplinary team A team with members of different disciplines involved in a formal arrangement to provide patient services while maximizing educational interchange.

introjection An intense type of identification in which one incorporates qualities or values of another person or group into one's own ego structure.

isolation Splitting off the emotional component of a thought. It may be temporary or long term.

Kaposi's sarcoma A malignant, multifocal neoplasm or reticuloendothelial cells that begins as soft, brownish or purple papules on the feet and slowly spreads in the skin; associated with AIDS.

learned helplessness A behavioral state and personality trait of persons who believe they are ineffectual, their responses are futile, and they have lost control over the reinforcers in the environment.

lethality An estimation of the probability that a person who is threatening suicide will succeed on the basis of the method described, the specificity of the plan, and the availability of the means.

libido Freud's term for psychic energy.

life review Progressive return to consciousness of past experiences.

limbic system An area in the brain associated with the control of emotion, eating, drinking, and sexual activity.

limit setting Nonpunitive, nonmanipulative act in which the patient is told what behavior is acceptable, what is not acceptable, and the consequences of behaving unacceptably.

living will Determining in advance one's participation in heroic measures during the dying process.

logotherapy An approach to psychotherapy based on the existential model and developed by Frankl. The focus is on the search for meaning in present experiences.

loose associations Lack of a logical relationship between thoughts and ideas that renders speech and thought inexact, vague, diffuse, and unfocused.

magical thinking Belief that thinking equates with doing; characterized by lack of realistic relationship between cause and effect.

magnetic resonance imaging (MRI) Depicts brain structure and activity using a magnetic field that surrounds the head and induces brain tissues to emit radio waves that are then computerized for clear and detailed construction of sections of the brain.

malingering Deliberate feigning of an illness.

malpractice Failure of a professional person to give the type of proper and competent care provided by members of his or her profession in the community. This failure causes harm to the patient.

mania A condition characterized by a mood that is elevated, expansive, or irritable.

manipulation A maladaptive social response in which individuals treat others as objects, enter relationships that are centered around control issues, and are self- or goal oriented rather than other oriented.

masochism Intense sexual arousal or desire and acts, fantasies, or other stimuli involving being humiliated, beaten, bound, or otherwise made to suffer (real or simulated).

maturational crisis A developmental event requiring a role change.

medical diagnosis A physician's independent judgment of the patient's health problems or disease states.

memory The retention or storage of knowledge learned about the world.

mental status examination Represents a cross-section of the patient's psychological life and the sum total of the nurse's observations and impressions at the moment, serving as a basis for future comparison to track the progress of the patient.

message A unit of communication.

methadone maintenance A treatment program in which methadone is given to a patient recovering from heroin abuse to prevent the characteristic withdrawal symptoms, as methadone will substitute for the heroin without causing withdrawal symptoms or impaired functioning.

modeling Strategy used to form new behavior patterns, increase existing skills, or reduce avoidance behavior in which the patient observes an individual modeling anxiety provoking behavior, and is then encouraged to imitate it.

mood The patient's self-report of prevailing emotional state and a reflection of the patient's life situation.

mourning Includes all the psychological processes set in motion within the individual by a loss. The process of mourning is resolved only when the lost object is internalized, bonds of attachment are loosened, and new object relationships are established.

multidisciplinary team A team with members of different disciplines, each providing specific services to the patient.

multigenerational transmission process The repetition of relationship patterns and anxiety associated with toxic issues passed through generations in a family.

multiple personality The existence within an individual of two or more distinct personalities or personality states, with each having its own pattern of perceiving, feeling, and thinking.

myelin sheath Provides insulation to the nervous system (see *glial cells*.)

narcissism A maladaptive social response characterized by egocentric attitude, fragile self-esteem, constant seeking of praise and admiration, and envy.

narcissistic personality disorder A specific personality disorder having the essential features of a pattern of grandiosity, lack of empathy, and hypersensitivity to the evaluation of others, beginning in early adulthood; characteristic behaviors may include rageful reactions to criticism, exploitation of others, inability to recognize how others feel, sense of entitlement, envy, belief that one's problems are unique, preoccupation with grandiose fantasies, and search for constant attention and admiration.

narcolepsy A condition characterized by brief attacks of deep sleep.

National Institutes of Mental Health (NIMH) Responsible for programs dealing with mental health, NIMH is an institute within the Alcohol, Drug Abuse, and Mental Health Administration (ADAMHA). ADAMHA is an agency in the U.S. Department of Health and Human Services that provides leadership, policies, and goals for the federal effort to ensure the treatment and rehabilitation of persons with alcohol, drug abuse, and mental health problems; this agency is also responsible for administering grants to advance and support research, training, and service programs.

negative identity Assumption of an identity that is at odds with the accepted values and expectations of society.

negative reinforcement Increases the frequency of a behavior by reinforcing the behavior's power to control an aversive stimuli.

neologisms New word or words created by the patient; often a blend of other words.

neurosis A mental disorder characterized by maladaptive anxiety responses associated with moderate and severe levels of anxiety.

neurotransmission The process whereby neurons communicate with each other through chemical messengers called *neurotransmitters*.

neurotransmitters Chemical messengers of the nervous system, manufactured in one neuron and released from the axon into the synapse and received by the dendrite of the next neuron.

nihilistic ideas Thoughts of nonexistence and hopelessness.

noncompliance The failure of an individual to carry out the self-care activities prescribed in a health-care plan.

nonverbal communication Transmission of a message without the use of words. It involves all five senses.

nuclear family emotional system Patterns of interaction between family members and the degree to which these patterns promote fusion.

nursing diagnosis A nurse's independent judgment of the patient's behavioral response to stress. It is a statement of the patient's nursing problems, which may be overt, covert, existing, or potential, and includes the behavioral disruption or threatened disruption, the contributing stressors, and the adaptive or maladaptive health responses.

nursing process An interactive, problem-solving process; a systematic and individualized way to achieve the outcomes of nursing care. The phases of the nursing process as de-scribed by the *Standards of Psychiatric–Mental Health Clinical Nursing Practice* are assessment, diagnosis, outcome identification, planning, implementation, and evaluation.

object cues A category of nonverbal communication that includes the speaker's intentional and unintentional use of all objects, such as dress, furnishings, and possessions.

obsession An idea, emotion, or impulse that repetitively and insistently forces itself into consciousness; unwanted, but cannot be voluntarily excluded from consciousness.

operant conditioning A theory concerned with the relationship between voluntary behavior and the environment that states that behaviors are influenced by their consequences and that operant behaviors are cued by environmental stimuli.

outreach clinical services Delivery of health services where health workers literally reach out to patients wherever they are in the community.

pain disorder A preoccupation with pain in the absence of physical disease to account for its intensity.

panic An attack of extreme anxiety that involves the disorganization of the personality. Distorted perceptions, loss of rational thought, and inability to communicate and function are evident.

paraphilia Characterized by sexual arousal in response to objects or situations that are not normally arousing for affectionate sexual activities with human partners (e.g. pedophilia, exhibitionism, zoophilia).

parasomnia Disorders associated with sleep stages, such as sleepwalking, night terrors, nightmares, and enuresis.

patient classification system Designed to determine the amount or intensity of nursing services needed by each patient based on patient acuity or severity of illness.

pedophilia Intense sexual arousal or desire and acts, fantasies, or other stimuli involving one or more children, 13 years of age or younger.

perception Identification and initial interpretation of a stimulus based on information received through the five senses of sight, hearing, taste, touch, and smell.

perseveration Involuntary, excessive continuation or repetition of a single response, idea, or activity; may apply to speech or movement, but most often verbal.

personality fusion An individual's attempt to establish a sense of self by fusing or belonging to someone else.

pharmacokinetics The study of the process and rates of drug distribution, metabolism, and disposition in the organism.

phobia A morbid fear associated with extreme anxiety.

phototherapy Light therapy that consists of exposing patients to artificial therapeutic lights about 5 to 20 times brighter than indoor lighting.

physical abuse Harm or threatened harm to an individual's health or welfare that occurs through nonaccidental physical or mental injury, sexual abuse, or maltreatment.

physical dependence A characteristic of drug addiction that is present when withdrawal of the drug results in physiological disruptions.

polypharmacy Use of combinations of psychoactive drugs in a patient at the same time; more than one drug may not be more effective than a single agent, can cause drug interactions, and may increase the incidence of adverse reactions.

positive reinforcement Increases the frequency of a behavior by reinforcing the behavior's power to achieve a rewarding stimuli.

positron emission tomography (PET) Depicts brain activity and function using an injected radioactive substance that travels to the brain and shows up as a bright spot on the scan; different substances are taken up by the brain in different amounts depending on the type of tissue and activity level.

postpartum blues Brief episodes lasting 1 to 4 days of labile mood and tearfulness that occur in about 50% to 80% of women within 1 to 5 days of delivery.

postvention Therapeutic intervention with the significant others of an individual who has committed suicide.

precipitating stressors Stimuli that the individual perceives as challenging, threatening, or harmful. They require the use of excess energy and produce a state of tension and stress within the individual.

predisposing factors Conditioning factors that influence both the type and the amount of resources that the individual can elicit to cope with stress. They may be biological, psychological, or sociocultural.

prejudice A preconceived, unfavorable belief about individuals or groups that disregards knowledge, thought, or reason.

premature ejaculation Ejaculation that occurs with minimal sexual stimulation or before, on, or shortly after penetration and before the individual wishes it.

primary prevention Biological, social, or psychological intervention that promotes health and well-being or reduces the incidence of illness in a community by altering the causative factors before they have an opportunity to do harm.

projection Attributing one's own thoughts or impulses to another person. Through this process the individual can attribute intolerable wishes, emotional feelings, or motivations to another person.

pseudodementia A depressive condition of the elderly characterized by impaired cognitive function.

psychiatric nursing An interpersonal process that strives to promote and maintain behavior that contributes to integrated functioning. It employs the theories of human behavior as its science and the purposeful use of self as its art. Psychiatric nursing is directed toward both preventive and corrective impacts on mental disorders and their sequelae and is concerned with the promotion of optimum mental health for society, the community, and those individuals who live within it.

psychoanalysis A therapeutic approach based on the belief that behavioral disorders are related to unresolved, anxiety-provoking childhood experiences that are repressed into the unconscious. The goal of psychoanalysis is to bring repressed experiences into conscious awareness and to learn healthier means of coping with the related anxiety.

psychobiological resilience A concept that proposes that there is a recurrent human need to weather periods of stress and change throughout life. The ability to weather successfully each period of disruption and reintegration leaves the person better able to deal with the next change.

psychoeducation Education or training of a person with a psychiatric disorder in subject areas that serve the goals of treatment and rehabilitation.

psychoimmunology Field that explores the psychological influences on the nervous system's control of immune responsiveness.

psychological autopsy A retrospective review of the individual's behavior for the time preceding death by suicide.

psychological dependence A characteristic of drug addiction that is manifested in a craving for the abused substance and a fear that it will not be available in the future.

psychological factors affecting physical condition A category of psychophysiological disruptions in which organic impairment is evident. Examples include migraine headache, asthma, hypertension, colitis, and duodenal ulcer.

psychoneuroimmunology The scientific field exploring the relationship between psychological states and the immune response.

psychopharmacology Drugs that treat the symptoms of mental illness and whose actions in the brain provide us with models to better understand the mechanisms of mental disorders.

psychosis A mental disorder characterized by maladaptive anxiety responses associated with panic levels of anxiety.

psychotic disorders A category of health problems that are distinguished by the following characteristics: severe mood disorder, regressive behavior, personality disintegration, reduced level of awareness, great difficulty in functioning adequately, and gross impairment in reality testing.

punishment Decreases the frequency of a behavior by causing an aversive stimuli to occur after that behavior.

purging A variety of maladaptive behaviors intended to prevent weight gain, including vomiting, excessive exercise, and use of diuretics, diet pills, laxatives, and steroids.

quality improvement The process of evaluating treatment outcomes in inpatient settings, usually monitored by an interdisciplinary body.

racism The belief that inherent differences between races determine individual achievement and that one race is superior.

rational-emotive therapy (RET) A therapeutic approach based on the existential model of psychiatric care and developed by Ellis. The emphasis is on risk taking and the assumption of responsibility for one's behavior.

rationalization Offering a socially acceptable or apparently logical explanation to justify or make acceptable otherwise unacceptable impulses, feelings, behaviors, and motives.

reaction formation Development of conscious attitudes and behavior patterns that are opposite to what one really feels one would like to do.

reality orientation Formal process of keeping an individual alert to events in the here and now.

reality therapy A therapeutic approach based on the existential model of psychiatric care and developed by Glasser. The focus is on recognition and accomplishment of life goals with emphasis on development of the capacity for caring.

receptor A specialized area on a nerve membrane, a blood vessel, or a muscle that receives the chemical stimulation that activates or inhibits the nerve, blood vessel, or muscle.

recurrence Return of a new episode of illness.

reframing To change the conceptual and/or emotional viewpoint in how a situation is experienced and to place it in a different frame that fits the "facts" of the concrete situation equally well; this changes the situation's entire meaning. Attributing positive motivations behind undesirable behavior often constitutes reframing.

regression A retreat in the face of stress to behavior that is characteristic of an earlier level of development.

rehabilitation The process of enabling a mentally ill individual to return to the highest possible level of functioning.

relapse Return of symptoms.

relaxation response A protective mechanism against stress that brings about decreased heart rate, lower metabolism, and decreased respiratory rate. It is the physiological opposite of the fight-or-flight, or anxiety, response.

relaxation training Training an individual to relax and thus reduce anxiety. Procedures include rhythmic breathing, reduced muscle tension, and an altered state of consciousness.

reminiscence Recounting early life experiences and events.

remission Occurs when a patient is symptom-free at the end of a phase of preillness functioning, which generally lasts 6 to 12 weeks.

repression Involuntary exclusion of a painful or conflictual thought, impulse, or memory from awareness. It is the primary ego defense, and other mechanisms tend to reinforce it.

residual Remaining, or left behind; those symptoms that remain after treatment has reached its maximum effect.

resistance Attempt of the patient to remain unaware of anxiety-producing aspects within the self. Ambivalent attitudes toward self-exploration in which the patient both appreciates and avoids anxiety-producing experiences that are a normal part of the therapeutic process.

respect An attitude of the nurse that conveys caring for, liking, and valuing the patient. The nurse regards the patient as a person of worth and accepts the patient without qualification.

response Improvement with treatment.

response cost Decreases the frequency of a behavior through the experience of a loss or penalty following the behavior.

response prevention Patient is encouraged to face a particular fear or situation without engaging in the accompanying behavior.

restraint The use of mechanical or manual devices to limit the physical mobility of the patient.

reuptake The process of neurotransmitters returning to the presynaptic cell after communication with receptor cells.

risk management Assessment of activities related to those situations that could result in legal action involving patients, families, the hospital, or the health-care provider.

role ambiguity A type of role strain that occurs when shared specifications set for an expected role are incomplete or insufficient to tell the involved individual what is desired or how to do it.

role conflict Frustration experienced by the individual because of role demands that are incompatible or confusing regarding appropriate role behavior.

role overload A type of role strain that occurs when a person is faced with a role set that is too complex or overwhelms available resources.

role playing Acting out of a particular situation. It functions to increase the person's insight into human relations and can deepen one's ability to see a situation from another point of view.

role strain Stress associated with expected roles or positions and experienced as frustration.

roles Set of socially expected behavior patterns associated with one individual's function in various social groups. Roles provide a means for social participation and a way to test out identities for consensual validation by significant others.

room program A titration of the amount of time patients are allowed in the unit milieu, with patients asked to stay in their rooms for certain lengths of time, and conversely allowed out of their rooms for a specific amount of time.

sadism Intense sexual arousal or desire and acts, fantasies, or other stimuli involving the infliction of real or simulated psychological or physical suffering (including humiliation).

schizoaffective disorder Diagnosis given to a patient who meets the diagnostic criteria for schizophrenia as well as one or both of the major mood disorders of bipolar disorder and major depression.

seasonal affective disorder (SAD) Depression that comes with shortened daylight in winter and fall and that disappears during spring and summer.

seclusion Separating the patient from others in a safe, contained environment.

secondary prevention A type of prevention that seeks to reduce the prevalence of illness by interventions that provide for early detection and treatment of problems.

self-actualization Process of fulfilling one's potential.

self-concept All the notions, beliefs, and convictions that constitute an individual's knowledge of self and influence relationships with others.

self-disclosure Revelation that occurs when a person reveals information about self, ideas, values, feelings, and attitudes.

self-esteem The individual's judgment of personal worth obtained by analyzing how well his or her behavior conforms to self-ideal.

self-help groups Groups composed of members who organize to solve their own problems; the members share a common experience, work together toward a common goal, and use their strengths to gain control over their lives.

self-ideal The individual's perception of how he or she should behave on the basis of certain personal standards. The standard may be either a carefully constructed image of the type of person one would like to be or merely various aspirations, goals, or values that one would like to achieve.

self-injury The act of deliberate harm to one's own body.

sensory integration A category of perceptual behaviors including pain recognition, stereogenesis, graphesthesia, right/left recognition, and recognition and perception of faces.

sexual abuse The involvement of children and adolescents in sexual activities they do not fully comprehend and to which they do not freely consent.

sexual assault Forced perpetration of an act of sexual contact with another person without consent.

shaping Introduces new behaviors by reinforcing behaviors that approximate the desired behavior.

situational crisis Occurs when a life event upsets an individual's or a group's psychological equilibrium.

sleep deprivation therapy A possible therapy for depressed and bipolar patients based on reports that as many as 60% of depressed patients improve immediately after a night of sleep deprivation.

social skills training Teaching smooth social functioning to those who do not manifest social skills, utilizing the principles of guidance, demonstration, practice, and feedback, resulting in the acquisition of behaviors that will support community living.

somatization disorder A somatoform disorder characterized by multiple physical complaints with no evidence of organic impairment.

somatoform disorder A category of psychophysiological disruptions with no evidence of organic impairment.

splitting Viewing people and situations as either all good or all bad. Failure to integrate the positive and negative qualities of oneself and of objects.

steady state Exists when the body has reached a state of drug level equilibrium: a drug has been taken long enough that the amount of drug excreted equals the amount ingested. This occurs in approximately four to six half-lives.

stereotype A depersonalized conception of individuals within a group.

stigma An attribute or trait deemed by the individual's social environment as different and diminishing.

sublimation Acceptance of a socially approved substitute goal for a drive whose normal channel of expression is blocked.

substance abuse The use of any mind-altering agent to such an extent that it interferes with the individual's biological, psychological, or sociocultural integrity.

substance dependence A severe condition of addictive behaviors often resulting in physical problems as well as serious disruptions of work, family life, and social life; usually considered a disease.

subsystems Smaller components of the larger system composed of individuals or dyads, formed by generation, gender, interest, or function.

suicide Self-inflicted death.

suicide attempt An action deliberately undertaken by the individual that, if carried to completion, will result in death.

suicide gesture A suicide attempt that is planned to be discovered in an attempt to influence the behavior of others.

suicide threat A warning, direct or indirect, verbal or nonverbal, that the individual plans to attempt suicide.

sundown syndrome Cognitive ability diminishing in the late afternoon or early evening.

sunrise syndrome Unstable cognitive ability upon rising in the morning.

supervision Guidance provided through a mentoring relationship between one nurse and a more experienced, skilled, and educated nurse.

suppression A process that is the conscious analogy of repression. It is the intentional exclusion of material from consciousness.

synapse The gap between the membrane of one neuron and the membrane of another. The synapse is the point at which the transmission of nerve impulses occurs.

systematic desensitization Designed to decrease avoidance behavior linked to a specific stimulus by helping the patient change the response to a threatening stimuli.

tardive dyskinesia Literally, "late-appearing abnormal movements," a variable complex of choreiform or athetoid movements developing in patients exposed to antipsychotic drugs. Typical movements include tongue writhing or protrusion, chewing, lip puckering, choreiform finger movements, toe and ankle movements, leg jiggling, and movements of neck, trunk, and pelvis.

target symptoms Symptoms of an illness that are most likely to respond to a specific treatment, such as a particular psychopharmacological drug.

tertiary prevention Rehabilitative measures designed to reduce the severity, disability, or residual impairment resulting from illness.

testamentary capacity Competency to make a will, which requires that persons know they are making a will, the nature and extent of their property, and who their friends and relatives are.

testimonial privilege A term used in court-related proceedings to refer to the communication between two parties. The right to reveal information belongs to the person who spoke, and the listener cannot disclose the information unless the speaker gives permission. This includes communication between husband and wife, attorney and client, and clergy and church member.

themes Underlying issues or problems experienced by the patient that emerge repeatedly during the course of the nurse-patient relationship.

therapeutic community The inpatient environment described as a community with cultural norms for behaviors, values, and activity.

therapeutic impasses Roadblocks in the progress of the nurse-patient relationship. They arise for a variety of reasons and may take different forms, but they all create stalls in the therapeutic relationship.

therapeutic milieu The controlled environment of treatment facilities that shelters patients from what they perceive to be painful and frightening stressors, thus providing patients with a stable and coherent social environment that facilitates the development and implementation of treatment.

therapeutic nurse-patient relationship A mutual learning experience and a corrective emotional experience for the patient, in which the nurse uses self and specified clinical techniques in working with the patient to bring about behavioral change.

therapeutic touch The nurse's laying of hands on or close to the body of an ill person for the purpose of helping or healing.

thought blocking Sudden stopping in the train of thought or in the midst of a sentence.

thought stopping Teaching a patient to interrupt dysfunctional thoughts.

time-out Short-term removal of the patient from overstimulating and sometimes reinforcing situations.

token economy A form of positive reinforcement in which patients are rewarded with tokens for performing desired target behaviors.

tolerance A characteristic of drug addiction that refers to the progressive need for more of the abused substance to achieve the desired effect.

transactional analysis A model of communication developed by Eric Berne that consists of the study of the communication or transactions between people and the sometimes unconscious and destructive ways ("games") that people relate to each other.

transference An unconscious response of patients in which they experience feelings and attitudes toward the nurse that were originally associated with significant figures in their early life.

transsexual A person who is anatomically a male or female but who expresses, with strong conviction, that he or she (1) has the mind of the opposite sex, (2) lives as a member of the opposite sex part-time or full-time, and (3) seeks to change his or her original sex legally and through hormonal and surgical sex reassignment.

transvestism Condition in which a male (less often a female) has a sexual obsession for or addiction to women's (men's) clothes.

triangle A predictable emotional process that takes place when there is difficulty in a relationship. Triangles represent dysfunctional efforts to reduce fusion or conflict in a relationship. The three corners of a triangle can be composed of three people, two people and an object or group, or an issue.

undoing An act or communication that partially negates a previous one.

unidisciplinary team A team with members of the same discipline.

utilization review A three-part process intended to ensure that resources are appropriately used. It includes a review of the initial request to hospitalize the patient, the length of the patient's stay, and a retrospective review after discharge.

vaginismus Recurrent or persistent involuntary spasm of the musculature of the outer third of the vagina that interferes with coitus.

value clarification A method whereby a person can assess, explore, and determine personal values and what priority they hold in personal decision making.

values The concepts that a person holds worthy in personal life. They are formed as a result of one's life experiences with family, friends, culture, education, work, and relaxation.

visualization The conscious programming of desired change with positive images.

vocal communication Written or spoken transmission of a message.

vocal cues A category of nonverbal communication that includes all the noises and sounds that are sounds outside speech. They are sometimes referred to as paralinguistic cues.

voyeurism Intense sexual arousal or desire and acts, fantasies, or other stimuli involving the observation of unsuspecting people who are either naked, in the act of disrobing, or engaging in sexual activity.

wear-and-tear theory Structural and functional changes of humans may be accelerated by abuse and decelerated by care.

wife abuse Includes all forms of physical violence toward a female partner in an ongoing intimate relationship, as well as emotional degradation and intimidation.

word salad Series of words that seem totally unrelated.

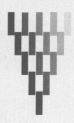

Index

A

Abnormal Involuntary Movement Scale, 688, 694
Abortion during adolescence, 901
Abreaction
  in crisis intervention, 288
  definition and example of, 289
Abstraction, selective, definition and
    example of, 751
Accountability, 236-237
  defined, 236
Acetylcholine
  location, effect, and function of, 107t
  loss of, in Alzheimer's disease, 695
Acquired immunodeficiency syndrome
  dementia in, 552
  incidence of, 970
  mentally ill patient with, 840-841
  neuropsychiatric rating scale in, 974t
  psychological care of patient with, 969-982
  therapeutic groups for, with computer
    networks, 777
Acting out in borderline personality
    disorder, 526
Activities of daily living
  for elderly, 928-929, 935
  Katz Index of, 929
  in serious mental illness, 306, 307t
Activity therapist, training and role of, 250t
Acute stress disorder, characteristics of, 342
Adapin; see Doxepin
Addiction; see Alcoholism; Chemically
    mediated responses; Drug abuse;
    Substance abuse
Adenosine in panic disorder, 119
Adolescence
  conduct disorders in, 902-903
  maladaptive responses in, 899-915
    indicators of, 899t
  parental divorce during, 908
  pregnancy during, 900-901
  tasks of, 894
  theoretical views of, 894-896
    cognitive, 895
    cultural, 895
    multidimensional, 896
    psychoanalytical, 894
    psychosocial, 894
    summary of, 895t

Page numers in *italic* indicate illustrations;
page numbers followed by *t* indicate tables.

Adolescent(s)
  assessment of, 896-899
  body image of, 896-897
  developmental stage of, 894
  drug use by, 572, 904, 904-905
  DSM-IV disorders of, 867t
  family therapy for, 910-911
  group therapy for, 911
  health education for, 909-910
  high-risk, 910
  homosexuality of, 900
  hypochondriasis of, 905, 907
  identity of, 897
  identity problems in, 390
  independence of, 897-898
  individual therapy for, 911-913
  occult involvement of, 907-908
  parents of, 914
  rate of psychological disturbance in,
    versus adult rate, 894
  runaway, 902
  sexual abuse of, 957-958
  sexual behavior of, 898-899
  social responses of, 519-520
  social role of, 898
  suicide of, 901-902
  talking with, 913-914
  violent, 903-904
  weight problems of, 907
  working with, 908-915
Adolescent psychiatric nursing, 893-918
  clinical exemplar of, 916-917
  evaluation of, 915
Adoption studies, 108
Advance directives
  for HIV-infected patients, 978
  legislation pertaining to, 189
Advocacy, 188-189
  for mentally ill, 839
Affect; *see also* Emotion; Feelings
  disorders of, 484
  in elderly, 926-927, 932-933
  mental status examination evaluation of,
    145
  negative, disease proneness associated
    with, 360
  terms related to, 484
  withdrawal of, in borderline personality
    disorder, 526
Affective disorders; *see also* Mood disorders;
    specific disorders
  behavioral rating scales for, 153t
  bipolar-unipolar, 432-433

Affective disorders—cont'd
  in children, drug therapy for, 885t
  DSM-IV classification of, 416, 417t
  primary versus secondary, 432
  supportive therapy in, 72
Affective states, psychotic versus neurotic,
    432
Age; *see also* Aging
  questions related to, 165
  as risk factor in mental illness, 160
Ageism, 269
Aggressive behavior, 719-744; *see also*
    Violence
  assessment form for, 728
  background associated with, 724
  behaviors associated with, 727
  biological etiology of, 727-728
  characteristics of, 721
  clinical example of, 722
  compared with passive and assertive, 722
  dimensions of problem of, 720
  emergencies involving, management of,
    736
  environmental factors in, 726
  hierarchy of, 727
  interventions in, 729-740
    assertiveness training in, 730
    behavioral, 732-734
    behavioral contracts, 733-734
    clinical exemplar of, 742-743
    communication strategies in, 730-731
    crisis management, 735-737
    limit setting in, 732
    nurse's self-awareness in, 729-730
    patient education in, 730
    restraints, 737-739
    room program in, 732, 733
    seclusion, 737, 738
    staff development for, 740-741
    terminating, 739-740
    time-outs, 734
    token economy, 734
  media and, 724
  mental illnesses characterized by, 726
  nursing assessment of, 727-729
  predicting, 725-726
  provocation of, 726
  against staff, interventions in, 740-741
  theories of, 722-725
    behavioral, 723-724
    neurobiological, 724-725
    psychoanalytical, 723
    psychological, 723